Textbook of
Pulmonary Diseases

Textbook of Pulmonary Diseases

Fifth Edition

VOLUME II

Edited by

Gerald L. Baum, M.D.

Professor of Medicine, Sackler Faculty of Medicine, Tel Aviv University;
Medical Director, Israel Lung Association, Tel Aviv, Israel

Emanuel Wolinsky, M.D.

Professor Emeritus of Medicine and Pathology, Case Western
Reserve University School of Medicine; Attending Physician,
Infectious Diseases, MetroHealth Medical Center, Cleveland

Little, Brown and Company
Boston/New York/Toronto/London

Library of Congress Cataloging-in-Publication Data

Textbook of pulmonary diseases / edited by Gerald L. Baum, Emanuel Wolinsky.—5th ed.
    p.   cm.
   Includes bibliographical references and index.
   ISBN 0-316-08410-7 (set)
   1. Lungs—Diseases.   2. Pleura—Diseases.   I. Baum, Gerald L.
II. Wolinsky, Emanuel, 1917–
   [DNLM: 1. Lung Diseases.   WF 600 T355 1993]
   RC756.T48   1993
   616.2′4—dc20
   DNLM/DLC
   for Library of Congress   93-19164
                                                   CIP

Printed in the United States of America

MV-NY

Second Printing

Sponsoring Editor: Elizabeth Thompson
Development Editor: Laurie Anello
Production Editor: Karen Feeney
Copyeditors: Mary Babcock, Libby Dabrowski, and Lois Hall
Indexer: Nancy Weaver
Production Supervisor/Designer: Louis C. Bruno, Jr.
Cover Designer: Linda Dana Willis

Contents

VOLUME I

VOLUME II

VI. Respiratory Insufficiency

VII. Pulmonary Vascular Diseases

VI

Respiratory Insufficiency

37

The Morphologic Basis for Diseases of Airways Obstruction

Richard E. Sobonya

Several general principles of pulmonary pathology apply to the pathologic appearances of various types of chronic airflow obstruction. First of all, for this group of diseases, structure is largely useless in determining pathogenesis. Unlike the pulmonary infectious diseases, in which histologic examination of the affected lung may even disclose the offending agent, the pathologic alterations in chronic airflow obstruction are nonspecific. Similarly, morphologic forms of response to injury that characterize chronic airflow obstruction are relatively stereotyped, and histologic variation is meager. This may be contrasted with the variety and histologic richness of primary pulmonary neoplasms. A third important consideration, which is probably most crucial in the study of chronic airflow obstruction, is the realization that the lung is an organ of extremely variable volume. Most of our understanding of diseases of chronic airflow obstruction comes from the examination of autopsy specimens. However, uninflated specimens are usually not representative of the degree of pulmonary inflation present during life, and it is unrealistic to imagine that the pulmonary parenchyma, vascular tree, and distal airways can be examined satisfactorily in irregularly or poorly inflated specimens.

It is not surprising that our modern understanding of emphysema, which began in the late 1950s, was simultaneous with the development of techniques of inflation fixation. Inflation fixation is usually accomplished by the instillation of formalin into the bronchial tree under a constant physiologic pressure, usually 25 to 30 cmH$_2$O. Both hot and cold formalin steam also have been used, with similar results. The parenchyma is uniformly expanded to a degree suggestive of total lung capacity during life. Comparison among lungs is facilitated, since all specimens have been handled identically. Finally, when liquid formalin is used, fixation for histologic examination is greatly improved.

The easiest inflation fixation technique, and the one recommended for general use, is that described by Heard [23]. Liquid 10% formalin is instilled into the main bronchus from a reservoir 25 to 30 cm above the level of a formalin bath in which the specimen floats. A small recirculating pump keeps the level of formalin in the reservoir constant. The specimen is so perfused for a minimum of 1 day. Lacking the above perfusion apparatus, for general diagnostic pathology it is adequate to inflate the lung endobronchially with 10% formalin until the normal shape of the lung is restored and the pleura is not wrinkled. The main bronchus can then be clamped and the specimen floated in formalin until completely fixed. Inflation-fixed lungs are usually sectioned parasagittally in 1- to 2-cm intervals; they also may be sectioned in the coronal plane to be compared to posteroanterior chest roentgenograms.

Disadvantages of perfusion fixation are the loss of areas of atelectasis and the displacement of edema fluid from the alveoli. However, atelectasis is best recognized with the lungs in situ or immediately after removal from the body and should be noted before inflation fixation is performed. Edema similarly can be recognized by frothy pink fluid exuding from the incised lung or bronchial tree and can be quantitated by lung weight (in the absence of other pathologic processes). One lung from the autopsy can be sectioned fresh to preserve the edema, while the other is perfusion-fixed. It should be noted that thromboemboli and pneumonic infiltrates are not significantly disturbed by perfusion fixation.

Even mucous plugs tend to stay in place and rarely interfere with fixation.

The development of inflation fixation of lungs and standardization in the handling of pulmonary tissue enabled quantitative techniques to be developed to complement qualitative observations. It will become evident that most of the pathologic changes in chronic airflow obstruction are important not because they are there but because they are there to an extent that correlates with limited function. The quantitation of morphologic changes is known as morphometry. A detailed discussion of common morphometric techniques is available [1,62]. An example of an application of one of the simplest techniques, that of point counting, can be seen in the gross examination of the lung. The underlying principle is that the percentage of various components of a surface of known dimensions reflects the volume percentage of these components, assuming that they are randomly distributed. To estimate the percentage area of each component, a uniform grid of points is superimposed on the total area and the number of points falling on each type of component is counted. A midparasagittal section of lung typically contains 90 percent alveolar parenchyma and 10 percent nonparenchyma (e.g., bronchi, vessels). This number can then be regarded as a fairly accurate percentage of the volumetric distribution of these components in the lung. Similarly, for microscopic sections of bronchi, the percentage of glands, muscle, cartilage, and interstitium can be computed and regarded as proportionate volumes. Additional morphometric techniques are discussed when various types of chronic airflow obstruction are treated in detail.

Structure and function are probably more closely correlated in the lung than in any other single organ. Because of this, comprehension of the lung in terms of either discipline alone leads to a skewed and ultimately erroneous understanding of the diseased and the normal lung. The following discussion should provide the structural basis for specific correlations of structure and function dealt with in later chapters. For more detailed information about the pathology of various forms of chronic airflow obstruction, the monograph by Thurlbeck [57] is recommended.

Chronic Airflow Obstruction

Several terms historically have been used to designate the group of conditions we recognize by obstruction to airflow. *Chronic obstructive lung disease* (COLD) (or *chronic obstructive pulmonary disease*, COPD) is a clinical term denoting a group of diseases "characterized by persistent slowing of airflow during expiration" [49]. Thus, the term is a clinical rather than a pathologic diagnosis, and it embraces entities such as chronic bronchitis, emphysema, and sometimes asthma and bronchiectasis. Thurlbeck [58] and others have questioned the appropriateness of the term *disease* for these entities and prefers the term *chronic airflow obstruction* (CAO), a phrase which emphasizes that airflow is obstructed but not necessarily by intrinsic airway lesions. In either case, the idea is the same. More recently the term *chronic airflow limitation* has been proposed, with the thought that *limitation* describes more precisely the physiologic impairment than does *obstruction*. In general, a patient who dies of symptomatic CAO will at autopsy show a mixture of emphysema, chronic bronchitis, and probably another more recently described entity that fits under COLD (i.e., small airways disease).

The use of such designations as COPD or CAO derives from the fact that for many years the pathologic components of these diseases were inseparable clinically. With recent sophistication in physiologic evaluation of patients with CAO, the various contributions of emphysema, small airways disease, and chronic bronchitis to CAO now may be better appreciated during life. However, as a general designation, the term *CAO* is still appropriate; if known, the form or type of CAO should then be indicated.

Emphysema

Emphysema is best defined as "a condition of the lung characterized by abnormal, permanent enlargement of airspaces distal to the terminal bronchiole, accompanied by the destruction of their walls, and without obvious fibrosis" [45]. This definition, published in 1985, refines and updates the American Thoracic Society definition of 1962 [2]. Let us now examine the components of this definition.

First of all, emphysema is now a *condition*, while previously it was an *anatomic alteration*, but the definition is still in anatomic terms. However, the advent of thin-section computed tomography has allowed visualization of the actual airspace enlargement seen in emphysema, a sort of gross pathology [26]. The term *airspaces* as used here refers to those pulmonary structures grossly seen to contain air but having no discernible wall. These include alveolar ducts, second- and third-order respiratory bronchioles, and emphysema lesions. In the preceding definition, the enlarged airspaces of emphysema are given a specific location. They lie entirely within the gas-exchanging portion of the lung, that is, distal to all purely conducting airways. Thus, respiratory bronchioles, alveolar ducts, and alveolar sacs may be involved. Stated another way, emphysema is intraacinar and thus involves only alveolated structures.

The requirement of destructive changes in alveolar walls implies two points: (1) Since alveolar tissue is destroyed and is largely incapable of regeneration, the changes of emphysema are essentially irreversible; and (2) such conditions as hyperinflation and overdistension are not true emphysema, since there is no destruction of alveolar tissue. Another way of looking at the distinction between emphysema and hyperinflation is that emphysema is a disease in itself, whereas hyperinflation is a change secondary to another process. The British classification of emphysema as discussed by Spencer [56] prefaces the term *emphysema* with either *destructive* or *nondestructive*, the former corresponding to what is here simply called emphysema and the latter including the various types of hyperinflation.

Two other uses of the term *emphysema* that do not conform to the preceding definitions exist but are accepted because of widespread use and the lack of alternative terms. These are *infantile lobar emphysema* and *interstitial emphysema*. The former is a heterogeneous collection of pulmonary parenchymal alterations, from simple hyperinflation to developmental anomalies in alveolar number and size. The latter is the presence of air dissecting into the connective-tissue framework of the lung and thus is akin to subcutaneous and mediastinal emphysema. In the latter case, the term *emphysema* could just as well be replaced by the word *air*. Again, as in hyperinflation, interstitial emphysema usually is secondary to some other disease.

The revised definition [45] uses the term *respiratory airspace enlargement*, which would include simple enlargement, either congenital or acquired, emphysema, and airspace enlargement with fibrosis. Infantile lobar emphysema and the airspace enlargement in Down's syndrome are examples of congenital simple airspace enlargement; hyperinflation or airspace enlargement in the aging lung illustrates acquired simple airspace enlargement.

Emphysema lesions should not be confused with those of honeycombing fibrosis, since the suggested causes, pathogenesis, and physiologic abnormalities of the two are quite distinct. However, since both appear as enlarged airspaces involving the pulmonary parenchyma and grossly may be somewhat similar, the possibility for confusion arises. A crucial difference is the presence of fibrous tissue in the wall of the lesion of honeycombing fibrosis. In general, fibrosis is not a noticeable component of typical emphysema lesions [33]. However, fibrosis may be seen in relation to emphysema lesions associated with parenchymal scarring. Thus, it is entirely possible to see, in one area of the lung, parenchymal scarring, honeycombing fibrosis, and emphysema in various mixtures. In fact, experimental emphysema and pulmonary fibrosis may result from the same lung injury [46]. The proposed category of *airspace enlargement with fibrosis* reflects the separation of this entity from emphysema. Nonetheless, the lack of appreciable fibrosis in most emphysema lesions is important and makes emphysema unique among chronic destructive diseases that involve various organs of the human body.

In general, the morphologic types of emphysema are centrilobular (centriacinar), panlobular (panacinar), paraseptal (distal acinar, including subpleural), perifocal (including paracicatricial), and other. Bullae are usually considered a form of emphysema as well, and these lesions (and blebs) also are considered under this heading.

CENTRIACINAR AND PANACINAR EMPHYSEMA
Centrilobular emphysema is characterized grossly by enlarged airspaces, generally measuring from 1 to 10 mm in diameter, surrounded by normal lung tissue. A typical centrilobular lesion involves respiratory bronchioles, which gives the lesion a centriacinar location. The definition of *acinus* used here is that of the airways and parenchyma arising distal to a terminal bronchiole. The term *lobule* is used to designate the secondary lobule of Miller, that is, a group of terminal bronchioles and their tissues (acini) originating from the same lobular bronchus, sometimes surrounded by sheets of delicate fibrous tissue, the interlobular septa. Obviously, centriacinar lesions (Fig. 37-1) are also more or less centrilobular, and either term can be used. Centriacinar emphysema lesions smaller than 1 mm in diameter are

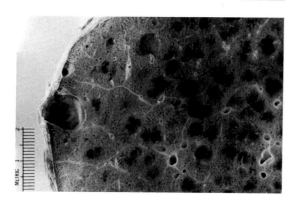

Fig. 37-1. Portion of lung showing centriacinar emphysema lesions. Lobular outlines occasionally are discernible as thin white lines. Note that virtually all lesions have a surrounding rim of normal parenchyma. A subpleural bulla and a subpleural emphysema lesion are also present (barium sulfate impregnation).

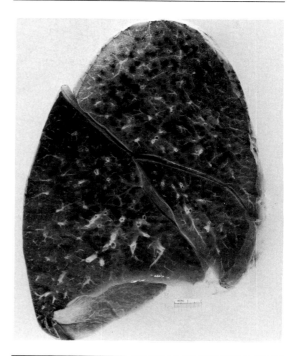

Fig. 37-2. Parasagittal slice of right lung showing the characteristic distribution of centriacinar emphysema lesions in the upper half (barium sulfate impregnation).

difficult to detect grossly, since alveolar ducts may be as large as 0.7 mm. Centriacinar lesions larger than 10 mm will have occupied so much of the acinus that their centriacinar character will be lost. An alternate and more anatomically precise term for centriacinar emphysema is *proximal acinar emphysema*, as described by Thurlbeck [57]. It is indeed the proximal part of the acinus (the respiratory bronchioles) that is primarily involved, whether or not in the gross lung the emphysematous lesion appears centriacinar, centrilobular, or otherwise.

Centriacinar lesions favor the superior half of the lung (Fig. 37-2). The lesions will be sharply circumscribed but will not have an obvious wall. A single spherical lesion may be present, or several smaller lesions may form a more or less spherical lesion. If consisting of several smaller holes, thin incomplete bits of delicate parenchyma subdivide the lesion. These have been referred to by some as "baffles." Very frequently, black pigment will be trapped in the area of the lesion. If a specimen of lung with centriacinar emphysema is examined floating in water and is then lifted out of the water, the emphysema lesions will tend to collapse below the cut surface of normal parenchyma and will be readily apparent.

Microscopically, the centriacinar lesion is undramatic. It appears again as a punched-out hole. The wall resembles normal alveolar septa in com-

position and is of normal thickness or only mildly thickened. In a typical lesion, few alveolar septa protrude from the wall of the lesion into the airspace. Alveolar ducts communicate with the lesion freely and are morphologically normal. At the edge of the lesion, the remains of a respiratory bronchiole or the proximal terminal bronchiole are often seen with an accompanying small muscular artery. Again, black pigment is frequently seen in the interstitium in this area. While such changes as fibrous narrowing, chronic inflammation, and mucous plugging may be seen in the terminal bronchiole adjacent to an emphysema lesion, in most sections it appears normal (Figs. 37-3 and 37-4). A feature not appreciated in the usual microscopic sections of centriacinar lesions is the abnormality of the wall of the emphysema lesion itself. The wall frequently contains holes of 20 to 280 μm called *fenestrae* [5], which are considerably larger than the pores of Kohn (these are approximately 2 to 12 μm in diameter). These holes are generally regarded as evidence of the destructive nature of the centri-

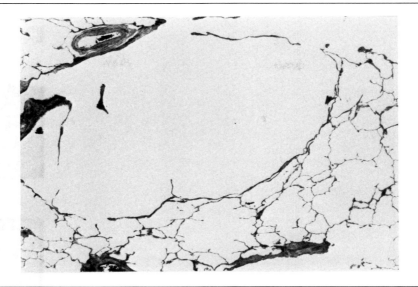

Fig. 37-3. Centriacinar emphysema lesion. Note
the tortuous bronchiole entering the lesion in the
upper left; the thin, sharply defined wall of the
lesion with few protruding alveolar septa; and
surrounding normal parenchyma (H&E, ×45).

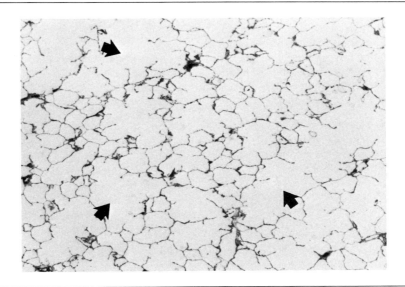

Fig. 37-4. Normal alveolar parenchyma. Alveolar
ducts (*arrows*) are often mistaken for emphysema
lesions but are smaller (H&E, ×45).

acinar lesion. Similarly, en face views of the capillary vascular bed show marked decrease in the usual extremely dense capillary network.

Panacinar emphysema appears grossly as enlarged airspaces like those in centriacinar emphysema, but involving the entire acinus or more commonly entire lobules (Fig. 37-5). The size range is the same, from 1 to 10 mm. With aging, the alveolar ducts in the acinus dilate, reaching a diameter approaching 1 mm [61], and elastic tissue is decreased [20]. This change may mimic mild panacinar emphysema; however, in the senile lung, portions of normal alveolar parenchyma will be found in the same acinus. This change of aging corresponds to what was once called *senile emphysema*. It is now generally agreed that there is no such clinicopathologic entity. In general, panacinar emphysema is found in the basilar segments of the lung (Fig. 37-6) or is diffuse. Microscopically, again, the panacinar lesions resemble the centriacinar lesions except that the centriacinar location is not seen. One has the impression of a large number of abnormal airspaces and a general diminution of small airways and small arteries (Fig. 37-7).

From the foregoing discussion, it would seem easy to separate the two most common forms of emphysema. However, such is certainly not the case. Since most of the destructive characteristics of emphysema are appreciated grossly, whole-lung sections (Gough sections) were circulated among several noted lung pathologists [59]. The lack of agreement among observers was obvious; one person's mild centriacinar emphysema was another's moderate panacinar emphysema. Intraobserver differences were far less, implying that criteria rather than ability to apply them accounted for much of the variation.

Several other good reasons can be found for the differences in classifying emphysema. First, since large centriacinar lesions will essentially fill an entire acinus, several such lesions in one lobule will reproduce the gross pattern of panacinar emphysema. Similarly, a portion of an acinus or lobule may be injured in some fashion that results in emphysema lesions conforming to neither the panacinar nor the centriacinar pattern. At autopsy, the most common form of significant pulmonary emphysema will appear as large areas of emphysema lesions in the apical portions of the upper lobe as well as the apical portion of the superior segment of the lower lobe, with somewhat less emphysema in the more basilar areas of the lung. While much of the emphysema will look centriacinar, the most severe apical foci will look decidedly panacinar. An example of both centriacinar and panacinar emphysema in the same slice of lung is shown in Figure 37-8. Be-

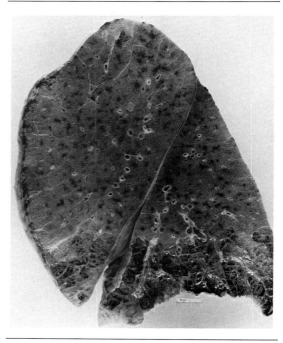

Fig. 37-6. Panacinar emphysema confined to the lower quarter of the lung. The majority of the dark centriacinar areas represent black pigment deposition without emphysema (barium sulfate impregnation).

Fig. 37-5. Panacinar emphysema. Entire acini and usually lobules show emphysema lesions. A diffusely emphysematous lobule is indicated by arrows (barium sulfate impregnation).

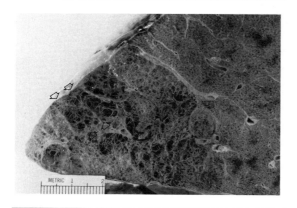

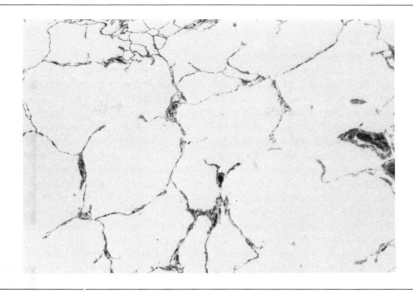

Fig. 37-7. Panacinar emphysema. A pattern of enlarged, thin-walled airspaces is seen without centriacinar circumscription. Note the few normal-size alveoli in the upper center (H&E, ×100). Compare with Figure 37-4.

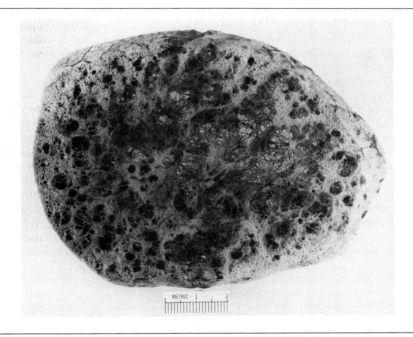

Fig. 37-8. Coexisting apical centriacinar and panacinar emphysema. The lesions toward the periphery of this slice, particularly on the right, are clearly centriacinar by virtue of the surrounding rim of normal parenchyma. The central lesions fill whole lobules and are clearly panacinar and panlobular (dried lung, horizontal section).

cause of the most severe involvement of the upper portion of the lung, one observer may regard this as centriacinar emphysema throughout; another would call it centriacinar emphysema with panacinar confluence in the upper lobe; a third would call it panacinar emphysema in the superior portion of the lung and centriacinar emphysema elsewhere. There is merit in all these approaches, but unfortunately, without additional understanding of emphysema, there can be no recommended best terminology. At this stage it is most important to be sure that those with whom you are communicating understand what you mean.

The recognition of types of emphysema and lesions of varying severity (size) raises two questions: (1) Do centriacinar emphysema lesions grow into panacinar lesions? (2) Do individual emphysema lesions grow (increase in size)? A third question that arises from these first two is, Are centriacinar emphysema and panacinar emphysema two different diseases? I have previously noted that centriacinar lesions can become so large that they are not clearly distinguishable from panacinar lesions. However, it is not known whether individual emphysema lesions increase in size; thus, a 2-mm centriacinar lesion is not necessarily an early lesion, nor is an 8-mm centriacinar lesion one of necessarily longer duration. Several authors have argued as to whether panacinar and centriacinar emphysema should be regarded as two different diseases [3,32,40]. The major differences in the two forms lie in the tendency for centriacinar emphysema to be more severe in the superior half of the lung, while pure panacinar emphysema is usually basilar or diffuse. Finally, the association of the latter form with alpha$_1$-antitrypsin deficiency is well known. However, it is entirely possible for persons with abnormalities in alpha$_1$-antitrypsin (such as Pi$_{MZ}$ heterozygotes; see below) to have only centriacinar emphysema at autopsy. Patients with centriacinar emphysema are not statistically different from those with panacinar emphysema in regard to clinical symptoms, pulmonary function abnormalities, and a myriad of other measurements. Thus, it is convenient to regard the two as separate but closely related diseases, although there is no compelling reason for doing so. No one has ever seen an emphysema lesion grow; thus, whether centriacinar lesions enlarge with time and whether they turn into panacinar lesions can only be speculated on.

CAUSE

Two discoveries in the 1960s shed considerable light on the cause of emphysema. It was found that certain individuals were markedly deficient in the serum antiprotease alpha$_1$-antitrypsin and that these individuals were particularly prone to develop pulmonary emphysema [19]. Also, it was found that a pulmonary lesion closely resembling human emphysema could be produced by the instillation of papain into the lungs of laboratory animals [22]. From these observations and the numerous studies that followed, a coherent hypothesis of the development of human emphysema has been realized. Several articles [11,15, 27,29] summarized the bulk of the clinical and experimental observations considering the morphogenesis of emphysema. Alpha$_1$-antitrypsin and its deficiency were reviewed by Kueppers and Black [34], Pierce [48], and Morse [41].

Alpha$_1$-antitrypsin, now often called alpha$_1$-proteinase inhibitor, comprises approximately 90 percent of serum alpha$_1$ globulin and is the most important antiprotease in humans. However, there are over 20 phenotypes of alpha$_1$-antitrypsin, designated by letters, that can be separated by electrophoresis and represent alleles of the same genetic locus. Although intraspecies differences exist, over 90 percent of persons are homozygous for the M type of alpha$_1$-antitrypsin. In the nomenclature of the protease inhibitor (Pi) system, this would be designated as Pi$_{MM}$. The second most common phenotype is Pi$_{MZ}$. These individuals sometimes have decreased levels of circulating alpha$_1$-antitrypsin. Less than 1 percent of populations studied are Pi$_{ZZ}$ and are severely deficient in circulating alpha$_1$-antitrypsin; their serum has a markedly reduced ability to inhibit proteases. Most present data indicate that the MZ heterozygotes are not at a greater risk for developing emphysema, but approximately 80 percent of ZZ homozygotes will develop clinically significant emphysema in their lifetime [34,41]. Other phenotypes of alpha$_1$-antitrypsin are uncommon and may or may not be associated with the development of emphysema [15].

The pathogenesis of emphysema currently is explained by an imbalance between protease release and destruction of alveolar parenchyma on the one hand and the neutralization of tissue proteases by antiproteases such as alpha$_1$-antitrypsin on the other. Pulmonary neutrophils are rich in elastase, and elastase is the active ingredient in the papain used to produce experimental emphysema. This has been substantiated by the production of experimental emphysema with purified elastase. With the dissolution of the alveolar parenchymal elastic skeleton by elastase, remodeling of the lung takes place in such a way that the enlarged airspaces of emphysema result. Elastic tissue regenerates, but its geometry is much different from that of the preexisting parenchyma [35] and it differs ultrastructurally [20]. There is probably also similar and more subtle remodeling in portions of the alveolar parenchyma that show no apparent emphysema by light microscopy.

The development of emphysema lesions probably extends over many years. There are increased numbers of neutrophils in the lungs of chronic cigarette smokers as detected by bronchoalveolar lavage. This observation may help to explain the close link between the development of emphysema and smoking, for neutrophil elastase is presently thought to be responsible for tissue destruction in human and experimental emphysema [11,30]. The excess of elastase in pulmonary secretions can be presently explained both by excess secretion from inflammatory cells and by inactivation of antiproteases by cigarette smoke [29]. Thus, because of increased subclinical pulmonary injury with the release of proteolytic agents, especially elastase, and incomplete neutralization of these proteases by the antiprotease system, there is a continuous slow remodeling of the alveolar parenchyma that eventually culminates in grossly apparent emphysema lesions and clinical symptoms. This proposed pathogenesis also would explain why emphysema is different from other chronic forms of injury to visceral organs, such as hepatic cirrhosis or regional enteritis, in which fibrosis is a prominent histopathologic feature. It is most likely that the injury-producing emphysema is relatively low grade compared with other forms of chronic tissue injury, and the duration of injury is much more protracted. Thus, an inflammatory response sufficient to induce fibrogenesis does not occur.

OTHER FORMS OF EMPHYSEMA
Several other anatomic forms of emphysema are recognized, including paraseptal, subpleural, and paracicatricial. Paraseptal and subpleural emphysema are similar, being emphysema lesions adjacent to interstitium, whether interlobular septa, peribronchial or perivascular interstitium, or visceral pleura. Paraseptal emphysema is also known as *distal acinar emphysema*, since the lesion primarily involves alveolar ducts and sacs. A subpleural emphysema lesion is shown in Figure

37-1. This form of emphysema is generally a curiosity and is not regarded as giving rise to clinical symptoms in itself [18]. Paracicatricial emphysema consists of more or less typical emphysema lesions forming adjacent to cicatrix (i.e., a scar). Often the scar is stellate and the lesions are a single row of emphysematous airspaces nestled within the arms of the scar.

The terms *bulla* and *bleb* are used in many ways and are frequently used synonymously. Some use *bleb* as a diminutive for *bulla*. The elaboration of Miller's definitions in the publication of Edge and colleagues [18] is recommended. A *bulla* is an emphysema lesion with a diameter greater than 1 cm. While the subpleural location is most common, bullae also may be entirely intraparenchymal. Bullae often extend prominently into the pleural space, but also extend into lung parenchyma (see Figs. 37-1 and 37-9). The apical location is most common, and the medial surface of the lung, especially at sharp margins, is prone to develop bullae. A *bleb* is an intrapleural lesion consisting of a collection of air between the two layers of pleura, analogous to an intraepidermal vesicle in the skin. Blebs are usually the result of barotrauma, with a dissection of air into the interstitium and eventually into an intrapleural location. Those lesions seen on chest x-ray films are virtually always bullae. Bullae may be associated with a bit of fibrosis, unlike the vast majority of emphysema lesions. This may be because of their close association with the pleura,

Fig. 37-9. An apical bulla. Note the thinness of the wall of the bulla, the delicate residual strands of fibrous tissue traversing the bulla, and the extension of the lesion into the parenchyma of the lung.

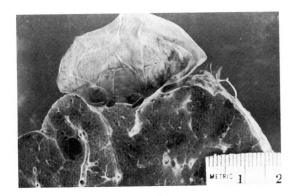

which by and large contains more interstitium with fibroblasts than does the alveolar parenchyma. Bullae may coexist with other forms of emphysema or may occur by themselves. Generally it is only in the latter case that surgical removal of bullae is of significant benefit.

Chronic Bronchitis

The clinical definition of chronic bronchitis (also known as *simple* chronic bronchitis) is well known and is repeated only to avoid the misconception of regarding chronic bronchitis as a pathologic entity. A committee of the American Thoracic Society [2] defines *chronic bronchitis* as a "clinical disorder characterized by excessive mucous secretion in the bronchial tree . . . manifested by chronic or recurring productive cough." The definition also states time limits for the duration of symptoms and points out that other known causes of productive cough should be absent, such as abscess or tumors. The pathologic equivalent to chronic bronchitis is a nonspecific series of changes in the bronchial wall, generally characterized by an increase in seromucous glands. The word *increase* is used because it is apparent that there are both hyperplasia and hypertrophy of glands (Figs. 37-10 and 37-11). Histologically, it appears that mucous glands are more numerous than usual, but this is not always the case. Goblet cells in the epithelium are usually increased as well, but since the vast majority

of mucus comes from the glands themselves, the glandular changes are more important. Additional findings in many cases consist of some degree of muscular prominence, increased numbers of chronic inflammatory cells in the lamina propria, dilatation of bronchial gland ducts (making the histologic alterations in chronic bronchitis apparent on a bronchogram), vascular engorgement, and nonspecific epithelial changes, including shedding and squamous metaplasia. Edema of the wall may be seen in some cases as well. The bronchial basement membrane is slightly thickened, but usually this does not approach the degree of thickening seen in asthma.

In severe cases, the bronchial gland enlargement may be seen grossly. The best way to visualize these changes is with low magnification, noting the thickness of the bronchial wall between the epithelium and the cartilage plate. If this reaches or exceeds 1 mm, bronchial gland enlargement is quite probable.

The degree of glandular enlargement in individuals, however, does not allow one to distinguish completely between groups with clinical chronic

Fig. 37-10. Bronchial gland enlargement in chronic bronchitis. A cartilage plaque can be seen on the left. Adjacent to it are masses of mucous (*lighter*) and serous (*darker*) glandular acini, which occupy most of the wall between cartilage and epithelium. The lamina propria contains bundles of smooth muscle and dilated blood vessels. Some mucus is present in the bronchial lumen (*far right*) (H&E, ×100).

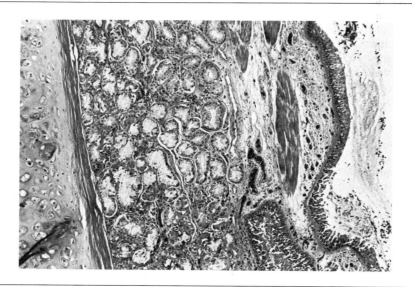

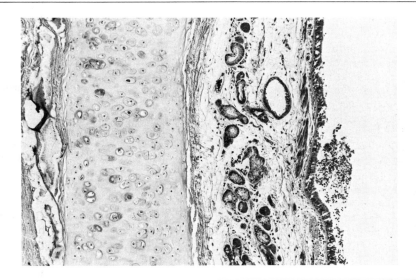

Fig. 37-11. Normal large bronchus. The cartilage plate is present on the left, and scattered glands are located in the bronchial lamina propria. Compare the bronchial wall thickness from cartilage to epithelium with that in Figure 37-10 (H&E, ×100).

bronchitis and those without. Similarly, bronchial gland enlargement does not correlate extremely well with past years of cigarette smoking or amount of sputum production. Thus, a population of subjects with clinical chronic bronchitis and the population of normal persons would show considerable overlap in bronchial morphology [60].

Several morphometric techniques have been devised for assessing chronic bronchitis [4]. One of the first and easiest is the Reid index [51]. In a transverse microscopic section of bronchus, a series of perpendicular lines is dropped from the epithelial basement membrane to the perichondrium of the cartilage. The ratio of the portion of the line that passes through bronchial glands to that of the whole line, averaged over many places in the bronchial wall, is the Reid index. A normal Reid index is usually less than 0.40, while that in chronic bronchitis is frequently in the range of 0.55. Other more laborious techniques involve determining the percentage of glands in the whole bronchial wall, such as by tracing out the various components of the bronchial wall on cardboard and weighing the portions of cardboard, by superimposing a grid of points over the histologic

section and determining the portion of points falling on bronchial glands, or by using a quantitative digital image analysis system.

With the shift in interest to the smaller airways of the lung, chronic bronchitis is still recognized as a reflection of chronic bronchial irritation, probably due to environmental factors such as cigarette smoking, airborne pollutants, and infection, but it is not now regarded as a major cause of morbidity and mortality in CAO.

Small Airways Disease

In 1968, Hogg and associates [25] partitioned pulmonary resistance in human lungs into that of airways 2 mm or less in internal diameter and airways larger than 2 mm. They realized that a major portion of pulmonary expiratory resistance was present in airways 2 mm or less and finally gave physiologic respectability to some very old ideas about bronchiolitis and emphysema. The term *small airways* refers to small bronchi and bronchioles that contain no cartilage, glands, or alveoli in their walls and measure 2 mm or less in internal diameter. There are approximately 30,000 in a 5-liter lung [36]. While in some cases abnormalities of these small airways had been seen histologically in patients with emphysema, the lesions were frequently scattered, and a vast majority of small airways looked reasonably normal. With the rising interest in airflow obstruction at the level of the small airways, the "silent zone" of the lung, morphometric studies determining the diameter of small airways were done. These showed that in many patients with CAO, the diameter of small airways was significantly less than that in normal individuals [6,36,38]. The histologic lesions were probably so infrequent and spotty because areas of bronchiolar stenosis in emphysema are probably quite localized, and the average histologic section would frequently transect a normal area rather than the functionally stenotic lesion.

The term *small airways disease* has come to be used for a group of nonspecific histologic changes of peripheral airways found in patients with CAO, including such reversible features as mucous plugging, chronic inflammation, and muscular enlargement of small airway walls (Figs. 37-10 through 37-14). Epithelium may show goblet cell or squamous metaplasia [13,14]. It also includes progressive fibrosis with stenosis of small airways (Fig. 37-15), an irreversible change [50]. The nonspecificity of these lesions should be obvious. Small airways disease is present in some patients with the clinical picture of chronic bronchitis as well as in some, though not all, patients with significant emphysema [42,43]. The term *chronic obstructive bronchitis* refers to patients with chronic bronchitis and airflow obstruction (CAO); the obstruction in these bronchitic patients is due to small airways disease, and the term is thus misleading. Severe small airway lesions typically are seen in patients with bronchiectasis. Typical of these changes is the small airways disease in cystic fibrosis (see Fig. 37-15).

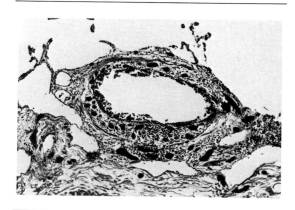

Fig. 37-13. Chronically inflamed small airway. The darker collections are engorged blood vessels in the airway wall. The wall is thickened by edema and infiltrates of lymphocytes (H&E, × 100).

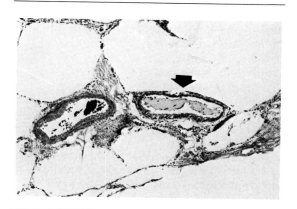

Fig. 37-14. Atrophy and mucous plugging in small airway. Muscle is not appreciated in the wall of the small airway (*arrow*). A mucous plug, which has probably shrunken during fixation, fills most of the lumen (H&E, × 100).

Fig. 37-12. A normal small airway. Note the intimate relationship with alveolar septa, which radiate from the airway (H&E, × 100).

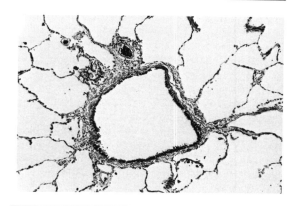

It should also be recognized that small airways can be narrowed functionally, although they have no intrinsic anatomic abnormality. This can be due to lack of supporting alveolar septa (see Chap. 38, Fig. 38-5), which is a structural alteration that is part of emphysema [44] and leads to collapse with forced expiration. One might term this sort of functional obstruction *extrinsic small airways disease.*

Emphysema is relatively easy to recognize grossly and histologically in inflated lungs, and

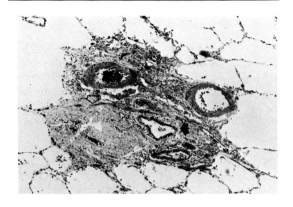

Fig. 37-15. Fibrosis and stenosis in small airways disease. A remnant of the small airways lumen is seen (*solid arrow*). Dense fibrous tissue is present to the left of this lumen and surrounds the bronchial wall. Smooth muscle (*hollow arrow*) outlines the extent of the previous small airways wall (H&E, ×100).

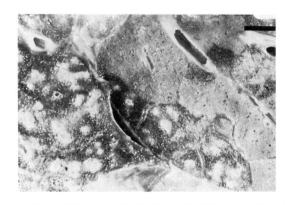

Fig. 37-16. Inflammatory small airways disease. The left side and lower portion of this picture show discrete inflammatory infiltrates around small airways, separated by normal parenchyma. The remainder shows lobular pneumonic consolidation (bar = 5 mm).

the glandular enlargement of chronic bronchitis is obvious. However, the average pathologist still has much difficulty in appreciating small airways disease unless it is quite severe. Inflammatory disease of small airways can be seen grossly in properly inflated lungs; it appears as tiny infiltrates in a centriacinar location (Fig. 37-16). Calculation of evidence of small airways disease, such as mean bronchiolar diameter, number of bronchioles per square centimeter of lung tissue, and histographic distribution of percentage of small airways by diameter, is beyond the range of all but larger research labs. The grading system first suggested by Cosio and coworkers [13] may provide a solution to this problem. Small airways in a specimen are examined for the presence of such changes as mucous plugging, inflammation, and fibrosis, and the lesions are graded on a semiquantitative 0 to 3 scale. A numerical score (the pathology score) is derived from this scale and seems to correlate fairly well with functional disability. A similar set of standards with semiquantitative grades (0 to 3+) for small airways disease, including both membranous bronchioles (small airways) and respiratory bronchioles, has been published [64]. One can also measure the wall thickness of specific small airways. A study by Boskin and coworkers [6], which quantitated small airways wall thickness, as well as mural muscle, connective tissue, and epithelium by

point counting, found that patients with physiologically documented CAO had thicker small airways walls with more epithelium, muscle, and connective tissue.

Asthma

Asthma is included here, although it is not considered part of CAO by many, but rather a more treatable disease to be separated clinically from CAO. Asthma frequently is divided clinically into extrinsic and intrinsic asthma, separating asthma triggered by environmental allergens from that in which atopy does not appear to play a major role. However, if those patients who have asthma-like symptoms due to other diseases are excluded, intrinsic asthma and extrinsic asthma are identical histologically.

The term *chronic asthmatic bronchitis* has no clearly defined pathologic equivalent. These patients, who have the chronic productive cough of those with chronic bronchitis, also have episodes of bronchospasm and never seem to be completely free from airflow obstruction [39]. The term *chronic asthma* and the older term *eosinophilic bronchitis* describe the same sort of CAO. Clinically these patients appear to have a combination of chronic bronchitis with small airways disease (chronic obstructive bronchitis), and asthma, and the pathology presumably would be that of those conditions. A study of autopsy lungs from patients with chronic asthma [55] included such patients, though prolonged corticosteroid treatment probably had altered the basic pathology.

Our knowledge of the pathology of asthma was derived initially from the lungs of those who died during an acute asthma attack, or status asthmaticus. The three cardinal changes of asthma [10], which are best seen in bronchi from 3 to 5 mm in diameter (i.e., subsegmental bronchi larger than small airways), are (1) tenacious mucous plugging, (2) thickening of the basement membrane, and (3) infiltration of the bronchial wall with eosinophils (Fig. 37-17; see Fig. 37-11). Other changes frequently noted include muscular hypertrophy of bronchial walls, excessive lymphoplasmacytic infiltrates in bronchial walls, glandular enlargement, shedding of the bronchial epithelium, and goblet cell metaplasia. The thickening of the bronchial basement membrane in asthma may be in part due to deposition of immunoglobulins, particularly IgE and IgG [9], but it is mostly due to subepithelial collagen deposition by myofibroblasts [8].

In patients with asthma who have died of other diseases, a thickened basement membrane may be the only evidence suggesting a history of asthma. Similarly, even in some patients dying with active asthma, eosinophilic infiltration may be absent due to corticosteroid therapy. Glandular enlargement and muscular thickening in the bronchial walls of chronic allergic asthmatics

may be absent or only mild in degree [55]. Airway narrowing in asthmatics may be due to chronic mural inflammation as well as smooth muscle contraction [28]. With metachromatic stains, mast cells in the bronchial wall can be detected. In some cases of asthma these are quite numerous, but in other cases they are difficult to see, presumably because they have been degranulated and are no longer easily detectable [12,54]. It is generally thought that mast cell populations of the bronchial wall are quite increased in asthma, however. Small airways disease sometimes complicates asthma and may explain the long-standing lack of complete reversion to normal expiratory airflow between asthmatic attacks [53,55].

Grossly, in fatal asthma the lung is hyperinflated, and on sectioning, tenacious mucous plugs are evident diffusely. Despite a history of repeated attacks of asthma, emphysema is extremely uncommon unless its usual risk factors, such as cigarette smoking, are also present.

With the advent of fiberoptic bronchoscopy and the need to investigate the pathology of mild asthma, most recent studies of the pathology of

Fig. 37-17. Bronchial changes in asthma. The cartilage plate lies along the lower border. Smooth muscle bundles in the lamina propria are prominent, and the basement membrane is thickened. The epithelium shows an abundance of goblet cells, and the lumen is filled with mucus (H&E, × 100). Compare with normal bronchus in Figure 37-11.

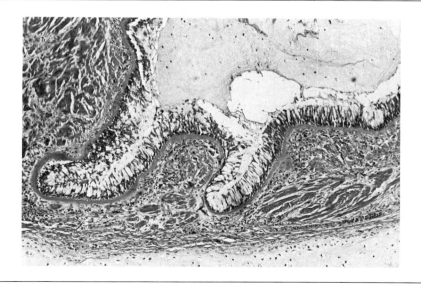

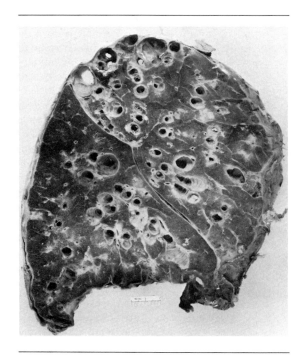

Fig. 37-18. Bronchiectasis. Cylindrical dilatation is seen, and bronchi do not taper as they approach the pleura. The subpleural cysts are actually dilated bronchi.

Fig. 37-19. Bronchiectasis. The epithelium is preserved but the bronchial lumen is filled with purulent secretions. Chronic inflammatory cells lie under the epithelium, and dense fibrous tissue is external to this infiltrate. Smooth muscle, cartilage, and glands are absent (H&E, ×100).

asthma have been based on examinations of bronchial biopsy specimens and bronchoalveolar lavage fluid. Mucosal inflammation with epithelial injury and denudation are constant findings in active asthma [17,31], and the severity of asthma is correlated with the degree of eosinophilic inflammation [7]. Release of major basic protein by eosinophil granules may be responsible for epithelial injury in asthma [21]. Bronchoalveolar lavage studies suggest that the onset of the late asthmatic response is due to an influx of eosinophils and neutrophils in airways [47].

Bronchiectasis

In the past, *bronchiectasis* (i.e., fixed dilatation of bronchi) was a much more common disease. With the advent of appropriate antibiotic therapy for pulmonary infections, bronchiectasis is now seen mostly in those infections not appropriately treated, in patients with cystic fibrosis, in occasional asthmatics, or in immune deficiency states characterized by repeated episodes of bronchitis and pneumonia. The localized bronchiectasis seen distal to occluding airway lesions (tumors, foreign bodies) is pathologically similar to other forms of bronchiectasis and is not considered further (see Chap. 26).

Grossly, bronchiectasis can be classified as saccular, cylindrical, or varicose [63]. Frequently it is a mixture of all these. Peribronchial fibrosis is sometimes seen but frequently is absent, and

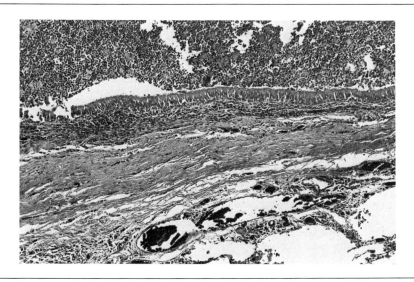

typically the bronchial wall appears quite thin. Prominent transverse ridges on the mucosal surface of the bronchial wall may be easily seen and are due to muscular hypertrophy. Bronchiectasis in cystic fibrosis is illustrated in Figure 37-18. Within bronchi is a mixture of mucinous and purulent secretions. Histologically, the bronchial wall is characterized by fibrosis and chronic inflammatory cells with a relative or absolute loss of normal bronchial wall components, such as cartilage, glands, and smooth muscle (Fig. 37-19). The epithelium may be completely normal or may show goblet cell or squamous cell metaplasia. In acute inflammation superimposed on chronic bronchiectasis, the epithelial surface may be ulcerated, and neutrophils are abundant. An interesting histologic form called *follicular bronchiectasis* is characterized by lymphoid follicles in the bronchial walls [63]. This type of bronchiectasis has been linked to adenoviral infection, but a recent study using in situ hybridization techniques failed to identify adenoviral genomes in such cases [24].

A notable feature of bronchiectasis is the absolute loss of bronchial subdivisions, especially after the first several subsegmental bronchial generations [52]. Thus, it seems that the most severe injury to the bronchial tree in bronchiectasis is at the level of the small and slightly larger airways. At these sites the changes of small airways disease, particularly chronic inflammation, stenosis, and fibrosis, are quite evident.

Acknowledgments

The author thanks Jean Aspen for the gross photography. This work was supported in part by Specialized Center of Research grant HL-14136 from the National Heart, Lung, and Blood Institute.

References

1. Aherne WA, Dunnill MS. *Morphometry.* London: Edward Arnold, 1982.
2. American Thoracic Society. Chronic bronchitis, asthma, and pulmonary emphysema: A statement by the committee on diagnostic standards for non-tuberculosis respiratory diseases. *Am Rev Respir Dis* 85:762, 1962.
3. Anderson AE Jr, Foraker AG. Centrilobular emphysema: Two different diseases. *Thorax* 28:547, 1973.
4. Bedrossian CWM, Greenberg SD, Duran ES. Bronchial gland measurements: A continuing search for a "yardstick." *Exp Mol Pathol* 18:219, 1973.
5. Boren HG. Alveolar fenestrae: Relationship to the pathology and pathogenesis of pulmonary emphysema. *Am Rev Respir Dis* 85:328, 1962.
6. Bosken CH, et al. Small airway dimensions in smokers with obstruction to airflow. *Am Rev Respir Dis* 142:563, 1990.
7. Bousquet J, et al. Eosinophilic inflammation in asthma. *N Engl J Med* 323:15, 1990.
8. Brewster CEP, et al. Myofibroblasts and subepithelial fibrosis in bronchial asthma. *Am J Respir Cell Mol Biol* 3:507, 1990.
9. Callerame ML, et al. Immunologic reactions of bronchial tissues in asthma. *N Engl J Med* 284:459, 1971.
10. Cardell BS, Pearson RSB. Death in asthmatics. *Thorax* 14:341, 1959.
11. Cohen AB (Ed). Proteases and antiproteases in the lung. *Am Rev Respir Dis* 127(Suppl, Part 2):S2, 1983.
12. Connell JT. Asthmatic deaths: Role of the mast cells. *JAMA* 215:769, 1971.
13. Cosio MG, Ghezzo H, Hogg JC. The relations between structural changes in small airways and pulmonary-function tests. *N Engl J Med* 298:1277, 1978.
14. Cosio MG, Hale KA, Niewoehner DE. Morphologic and morphometric effects of prolonged cigarette smoking on the small airways. *Am Rev Respir Dis* 122:265, 1980.
15. Crystal RG, et al. The alpha₁-antitrypsin gene and its mutations. *Chest* 95:1, 1989.
16. D'Errico A, et al. Changes in the alveolar connective tissue of the ageing lung. *Virchows Arch A Pathol Anat Histopathol* 415:137, 1989.
17. Djukanovic R, et al. Mucosal inflammation in asthma. *Am Rev Respir Dis* 142:434, 1990.
18. Edge J, Simon G, Reid L. Periacinar (paraseptal) emphysema: Its clinical, radiological, and physiological features. *Br J Dis Chest* 60:10, 1966.
19. Eriksson S. Alpha₁-antitrypsin deficiency: Lessons learned from the bedside to the gene and back again. *Chest* 95:1, 1989.
20. Fukuda Y, et al. Morphogenesis of abnormal elastic fibers in lungs of patients with panacinar and centriacinar emphysema. *Hum Pathol* 20:652, 1989.
21. Gleich GJ, et al. The eosinophilic leukocyte and the pathology of fatal bronchial asthma: Evidence for pathologic heterogeneity. *J Allergy Clin Immunol* 80:413, 1987.
22. Gross P, et al. Enzymatically produced pulmonary emphysema. A preliminary report. *J Occup Med* 6:481, 1964.
23. Heard BE. Pathology of pulmonary emphysema: Methods of study. *Am Rev Respir Dis* 82:792, 1960.
24. Hogg JC, et al. In situ hybridization studies of adenoviral infections of the lung and their rela-

tionship to follicular bronchiectasis. *Am Rev Respir Dis* 139:1531, 1989.

25. Hogg JC, Macklem PT, Thurlbeck WM. Site and nature of airway obstruction in chronic obstructive lung disease. *N Engl J Med* 278:1355, 1968.

26. Hruban RH, et al. High resolution computed tomography of inflation-fixed lungs. *Am Rev Respir Dis* 136:935, 1987.

27. Hugh-Jones P, Whimster W. The etiology and management of disabling emphysema. *Am Rev Respir Dis* 117:343, 1978.

28. James AL, Pare PD, Hogg JC. The mechanics of airway narrowing in asthma. *Am Rev Respir Dis* 139:242, 1989.

29. Janoff A. Elastases and emphysema: Current assessment of the protease-antiprotease hypothesis. *Am Rev Respir Dis* 132:417, 1985.

30. Karlinsky JB, Snider GL. Animal models of emphysema. *Am Rev Respir Dis* 117:1109, 1978.

31. Kay AB. Asthma and inflammation. *J Allergy Clin Immunol* 87:893, 1991.

32. Kim WD, et al. Centrilobular and panlobular emphysema in smokers. *Am Rev Respir Dis* 144:1385, 1991.

33. Kleinerman J, Boren HG. Morphologic Basis in Chronic Obstructive Lung Disease: Anatomy of the Tracheal Bronchial Tree and Lung. In GL Baum (Ed), *Textbook of Pulmonary Diseases* (2nd ed). Boston: Little, Brown, 1974. P 507.

34. Kueppers F, Black LF. Alpha₁-antitrypsin and its deficiency. *Am Rev Respir Dis* 110:176, 1974.

35. Kuhn C, et al. The induction of emphysema with elastase: II. Changes in connective tissue. *Lab Invest* 34:372, 1976.

36. Matsuba K, Thurlbeck WM. The number and dimensions of small airways in nonemphysematous lungs. *Am Rev Respir Dis* 104:516, 1971.

37. Matsuba K, Thurlbeck WM. The number and dimensions of small airways in emphysematous lungs. *Am J Pathol* 67:265, 1972.

38. Matsuba K, Thurlbeck WM. Disease of the small airways in chronic bronchitis. *Am Rev Respir Dis* 107:552, 1973.

39. Matthay RB. Chronic Airways Diseases. In JB Wyngaarden, LH Smith Jr (Eds), *Cecil Textbook of Medicine* (18th ed). Philadelphia: Saunders, 1988. Pp 410–418.

40. Mitchell RS, et al. Are centrilobular emphysema and panlobular emphysema two different diseases? *Hum Pathol* 1:443, 1970.

41. Morse JO. Alpha₁-antitrypsin deficiency. *N Engl J Med* 299:1045 (Part 1), 1099, (Part 2), 1978.

42. Nagai A, et al. The National Institutes of Health intermittent positive-pressure breathing trial: Pathology studies: I. Interrelationship between morphologic lesions. *Am Rev Respir Dis* 132:937, 1985.

43. Nagai A, West WW, Thurlbeck WM. The National Institutes of Health intermittent positive-pressure breathing trial: Pathology studies: II. Correlation between morphologic findings, clinical findings, and evidence of expiratory airflow obstruction. *Am Rev Respir Dis* 132:946, 1985.

44. Nagai A, et al. Alveolar attachments in emphysema of human lungs. *Am Rev Respir Dis* 144:888, 1991.

45. National Heart, Lung, and Blood Institute, Division of Lung Diseases Workshop. The definition of emphysema. *Am Rev Respir Dis* 132:182, 1985.

46. Niewoehner DE, Hoidal JR. Lung fibrosis and emphysema: Divergent responses to a common injury? *Science* 217:23, 1982.

47. O'Byrne PM, Dolovich J, Hargreave FE. Late asthmatic responses. *Am Rev Respir Dis* 136:740, 1987.

48. Pierce JA. Antitrypsin and emphysema. *JAMA* 259:19, 1988.

49. Pulmonary terms and symbols: A report of the ACCP-ATS Joint Committee on Pulmonary Nomenclature. *Chest* 67:583, 1975.

50. Ranga V, Kleinerman J. Structure and function of small airways in health and disease. *Arch Pathol Lab Med* 102:609, 1978.

51. Reid L. Measurement of the bronchial mucous gland layer: A diagnostic yardstick in chronic bronchitis. *Thorax* 15:132, 1960.

52. Reid LM. Reduction in bronchial subdivisions in bronchiectasis. *Thorax* 5:233, 1950.

53. Saetta M, et al. Quantitative structural analysis of peripheral airways and arteries in sudden fatal asthma. *Am Rev Respir Dis* 143:138, 1991.

54. Salvato G. Some histological changes in chronic bronchitis and asthma. *Thorax* 23:168, 1968.

55. Sobonya RE. Quantitative structural alterations in long-standing allergic asthma. *Am Rev Respir Dis* 130:289, 1984.

56. Spencer H. *Pathology of the Lung* (3rd ed), Vol 1. Philadelphia: Saunders, 1977. P 506.

57. Thurlbeck WM. Chronic Airflow Obstruction in Lung Disease. In JL Bennington (Ed), *Major Problems in Pathology*, Vol 5. Philadelphia: Saunders, 1976. P 98.

58. Thurlbeck WM. Aspects of chronic airflow obstruction. *Chest* 72:341, 1977.

59. Thurlbeck WM, et al. A comparative study of certain measurements of emphysema. *Am Rev Respir Dis* 98:217, 1968.

60. Thurlbeck WM, Angus GE. The distribution curve for chronic bronchitis. *Thorax* 19:436, 1964.

61. Vincent TN, et al. Duct ectasia. An asymptomatic pulmonary change related to age. *Lancet* 84:331, 1964.

62. Weibel ER, Kistler GS, Scherle WF. Practical stereological methods for morphometric cytology. *J Cell Biol* 30:23, 1966.

63. Whitwell F. A study of the pathology and pathogenesis of bronchiectasis. *Thorax* 7:213, 1952.

64. Wright JL, et al. Morphologic grading scheme for membranous and respiratory bronchioles. *Arch Pathol Lab Med* 109:183, 1985.

38

Structure-Function Correlations in Chronic Obstructive Pulmonary Disease

Dennis E. Niewoehner   Richard E. Sobonya

Chronic obstructive pulmonary disease (COPD) is characterized functionally by a decrease in maximal expiratory flow rates. In addition, patients with COPD have uneven ventilation, which results in arterial hypoxemia and hypercapnia. These functional abnormalities can be detected and quantitated by relatively simple pulmonary function tests. Similarly, pathologic lesions in lungs of patients with COPD have been described in exhaustive detail, and efforts have been made to quantitate the severity of the lesions.

Structure-function relationships in COPD are imperfectly understood. Optimally, it should be possible for the pathologist to predict accurately the nature and severity of dysfunction from gross and microscopic examination of lung tissue. Unfortunately, this ideal has not been realized, since there may be striking discrepancies between the extent of disease as determined by the pathologist and the severity of dysfunction as measured by physiologic tests. These disparities can partly be attributed to the formidable methodologic problems that the pathologist faces in studying a structurally complex organ such as the lung. However, the lack of better structure-function correlation in COPD also may indicate that certain pathophysiologic mechanisms occurring in COPD have not been explained.

In this chapter we attempt to summarize the state of knowledge concerning pathologic-physiologic correlations in this disorder. The mechanisms that are thought to determine maximal expiratory flow rates and ventilatory distribution are reviewed. The effects of emphysema and intrinsic airways disease on pulmonary function are examined. Finally, the question of whether or not different pathologic lesions give rise to recognizable clinical or physiologic types of COPD is addressed.

Determinants of Maximal Expiratory Airflow

The interaction of air molecules with each other and with the internal surface of a cylinder impedes their movement, so that energy in the form of a pressure difference is necessary to cause flow through the cylinder. *Flow resistance* is defined as the ratio of the longitudinal pressure difference to the flow rate which that pressure differential produces ($R = \Delta P/\dot{V}$). The magnitude of flow resistance depends on the physical properties of the gas and on the length and diameter of the cylinder.

Individual bronchi and bronchioles are imperfect cylinders, so that flow resistance is dependent on their internal geometry. Because the bronchial tree branches through many generations, each airway can be viewed as a resistive element existing in series and in parallel with literally tens of thousands of other resistive elements. The energy necessary to move air through this resistive network is provided by the bellows action of the thoracic cage.

For a constant resistance, flow through the conducting airways is proportional to applied pressure. In Figure 38-1, transairway (alveolar–airway opening) pressure is plotted against flow rate at a fixed lung volume in a normal subject. On inspiration, the relationship of flow to pressure is approximately linear, which means that resistance is relatively constant over a wide range of applied pressures. Maximal inspiratory flow is limited by the magnitude of the applied pressure, which is largely dependent on muscle strength. With expiration, the relationship is quite different. At low values for flow and pressure, the relationship is nearly linear, but beyond a certain critical point, flow remains constant despite fur-

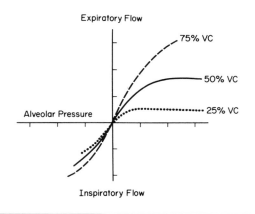

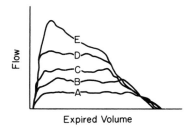

Fig. 38-1. Inspiratory and expiratory airflow as a function of alveolar pressure at various lung volumes. With inspiration, flow increases as the driving pressure between airway opening and alveolus increases. With expiration, flow increases with pressure only to a point, beyond which flow remains constant despite further increases in pressure. This is called flow limitation, and the effect is most marked at small lung volumes. *VC* = vital capacity.

Fig. 38-2. Flow-volume relationships in a normal subject who expired from total lung capacity to residual volume with progressively greater effort (*A* through *E*). The latter portion of the maximal effort is superimposed on the tracings from lesser efforts, demonstrating flow limitations at smaller lung volumes.

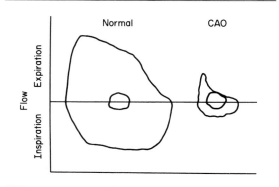

Fig. 38-3. Expiratory and inspiratory flow rates as a function of lung volume in a normal subject and in a patient with severe COPD. The outer envelopes represent maximal efforts; the inner tracings are from tidal breathing. The patient with COPD has very limited ability to increase ventilation with exercise.

ther increases in pressure. This phenomenon is described as *flow limitation*, which indicates that expiratory airflow resistance increases in a dynamic fashion with greater effort.

Flow limitation can be demonstrated by a simple experiment utilizing flow-volume curves. Figure 38-2 shows a series of flow-volume tracings in a normal subject who was instructed to expire repeatedly from total lung capacity (TLC) to residual volume (RV) with progressively greater effort. With minimal effort (*A*), flow rates are low and relatively constant over much of the vital capacity. With increasing effort (*B* through *D*), flow rates at large lung volumes increase correspondingly. However, the tracing from each submaximal effort contains an inflection, and below that volume the flow tracing is superimposed on those from previous, lesser efforts. At each lung volume, flow rates over the lower two-thirds of the vital capacity have a maximum which is relatively independent of effort, but which, as will be described, is dependent on intrinsic mechanical properties of the lung.

The clinical significance of flow limitation can be appreciated by examining flow-volume curves in normal subjects and in patients with COPD. In Figure 38-3 flow-volume relationships with maximal inspiratory and expiratory efforts are com-

pared with those during tidal ventilation in a normal person. Since a large reserve normally exists, ventilatory capacity is not a limiting factor, even with vigorous exercise. In the patient with COPD, both inspiratory and expiratory flow rates are diminished, with expiration being relatively more affected than inspiration. Tidal expiration may actually be superimposed on the tracing from a maximal forced effort. Such an individual has little reserve and can increase total ventilation only marginally in response to exercise demands. The decrease in ventilatory capacity results not from decreased expiratory effort but from abnormalities intrinsic to the lung.

Models of varying complexity have been used to analyze the physical behavior of the lung during forced expiratory maneuvers [58,72,76]. A simple model, shown in Figure 38-4, consists of a distensible balloon, representing the gas-exchanging regions of the lung, contained within a box, representing the thoracic cage. The balloon is connected to the environment by a compliant tube (conducting airways) and is surrounded by a space between the balloon and box (intrapleural space). The action of respiratory muscles, which actively alter intrapleural pressures, is represented by a bellows situated at the bottom of the box.

If the lung is inflated above its resting volume, it will deflate to its original volume, unless this tendency to recoil is opposed by an outward-acting transpleural pressure difference. The transpleural pressure required to keep the lung statically inflated at a particular volume is referred to as elastic recoil pressure (Pel). Alveolar pressure (Palv) is at all times greater than intrapleural pressure (Ppl) by the amount of Pel; Palv = Pel + Ppl. For air to flow through the conducting airway, there must be a pressure gradient between the alveolus and the airway opening (Pao). With no flow, Palv is equal to Pao and Ppl is negative, equal in magnitude but opposite in sign to Pel, in order to keep the lung distended. At functional residual capacity in normal subjects, Ppl is typically 4 to 3 cmH$_2$O less than ambient pressure.

Inspiration creates a more negative Ppl. Since Palv is the algebraic sum of Ppl and Pel, Palv becomes negative with respect to Pao and air is drawn into the lung. Expiration reverses this process; Ppl becomes less negative, Palv becomes positive with respect to Pao, and air flows out of the lung. During the normal breathing cycle, pressure fluctuations in the pleural space are only a few centimeters of water, and during expiration, Ppl ordinarily remains negative with respect to ambient pressure. During expiration, pressure at all points within the conducting airways is positive with respect to ambient pressure. Hence, during tidal expiration, there is a net pressure gradient acting outward on those conducting airways that are exposed to pleural pressure. However, with forced expiration, this transmural pressure gradient may be reversed; it is these compressive pressures acting on compliant bronchi that narrow the airway lumen and limit maximal expiratory flow rates.

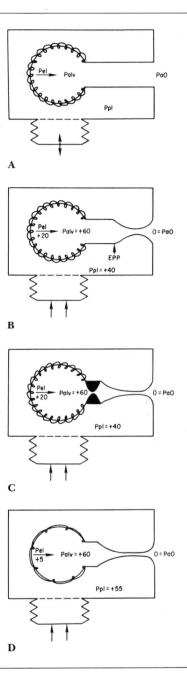

Fig. 38-4. Model of forced expiratory airflow. See text for explanation. *A* and *B* represent the normal relationships. *C* illustrates the effects of intrinsic airways obstruction on forced expired airflow. *D* demonstrates the effects of decreased lung elastic recoil, as might occur with emphysema. *Pel* = elastic recoil pressure; *Palv* = alveolar pressure; *PaO* = airway-opening pressure; *Ppl* = intrapleural pressure; *EPP* = equal-pressure point.

Representative pressure relationships during a forced expiration are shown in Figure 38-4B. Assume that Pel is $+20$ cmH$_2$O, Ppl is $+40$ cmH$_2$O, and Palv is $+60$ cmH$_2$O. The alveolar driving pressure is dissipated by flow resistance along the length of the airway so that intraairway pressure progressively decreases to that of ambient pressure at the airway opening. Since Ppl is $+40$ cmH$_2$O, and intraairway pressure varies from $+60$ to 0 cmH$_2$O, there is a point where intraairway pressure is equal to Ppl and the transmural pressure gradient is zero. Distal (meaning in the direction of the alveolus) to this "equal-pressure point" (EPP), pressures within the airway are positive with respect to Ppl, and this outward-acting force distends the airway lumen. Proximal to the equal-pressure point, intraluminal pressures are negative with respect to Ppl, creating a compressive force. Because bronchi are not rigid tubes, inward-acting transmural pressure gradients tend to compress the airway lumen, which in turn increases flow resistance.

As Ppl increases, Palv $-$ Pao increases by the same amount and would for a constant resistance cause an increase in expiratory flow. However, increases in Ppl subject the proximal bronchi to greater compressive pressures, which narrow their lumina even more. The increase in driving pressure between alveolus and airway opening is balanced by the increase in flow resistance so that flow rates remain relatively constant. Thus, it is the flow-limiting segment of the conducting airways, usually located in the proximal bronchi, that sets an upper limit to expiratory flow rates.

From this simple model several factors can be recognized which may affect the mechanical behavior of the flow-limiting segment and determine the magnitude of expiratory flow rates. One factor relates to the intrinsic elastic behavior of the flow-limiting segment itself. It is evident that the same compressive pressure might cause greater flow resistance in a highly compliant airway than in an airway with relatively rigid walls. Experimental studies suggest that pathologic conditions that create overly compliant bronchi may cause a decrease in maximal expiratory flow rates [39,70]. Degenerative changes have been observed in the bronchi of patients with severe COPD; however, it has not been determined whether such lesions play a significant role in causing airflow obstruction [49].

The mechanical behavior of the flow-limiting segment is also influenced by flow resistance in more distal portions of the conducting airways. This is illustrated in Figure 38-4C, which shows airway stenosis immediately proximal to the alveolar unit. Under these conditions, a relatively greater portion of the alveolar driving pressure, Palv $-$ Pao, is dissipated over the obstructed segment of airway. Compared with the pressures in Figure 38-4B, intraairway pressures at each point between the obstruction and the airway opening are necessarily less positive and the compressive pressures are correspondingly greater. Since a longer segment of normal airway is exposed to larger compressive forces, it is reasonable to expect that airflow resistance would be greater and maximal expiratory flow rates less.

Intrinsic airway narrowing may occur from pathologic conditions such as inflammation and fibrosis in airway walls and from excessive luminal mucus. These lesions and others are frequently observed in lungs from patients with COPD. If such lesions are sufficiently severe and widespread, they may cause significant expiratory airflow obstruction.

The possible functional significance of pathologic conditions that directly alter airway dimensions is apparent. However, the pathologic state that may be most important in causing airflow obstruction, emphysema, does not directly affect the conducting airways, but rather involves the lung parenchyma. How does a condition affecting lung parenchyma give rise to expiratory airflow obstruction?

Emphysema is characterized by destruction of alveolar walls and disruption of the normal parenchymal architecture. These morphologic changes are associated with a loss of lung elastic recoil, which may be regarded as the primary functional defect in emphysema. The loss of elastic recoil affects both the dimension of intrapulmonary airways and the behavior of the flow-limiting segment.

Intrapulmonary airways are surrounded by lung parenchyma and are intimately connected to the elastic and collagen fibers in the alveolar walls (Fig. 38-5). In the inflated lung, alveolar walls are stressed, and a tethering effect on airways is created at their points of attachment. As lung volume increases, the radial distending force increases airway length and diameter [37]. This mechanism accounts for the volume dependence of airflow resistance in the lung, resistance being greater at small volumes and less at large volumes. With loss of lung elastic recoil, distending forces acting on the airway at any particular volume would be less, and increased airflow resistance would occur.

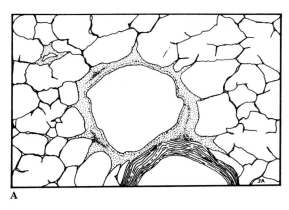

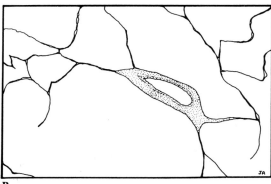

Fig. 38-5. Camera lucida drawings (approximately ×50) from lungs inflation-fixed at 25 cmH$_2$O. (*A*) Normal small airway and surrounding alveolar parenchyma, showing tethering effect of alveolar septa. (*B*) Small airway adjacent to emphysema lesions is narrowed due to loss of tethering alveolar walls.

Lung elastic recoil also influences maximal expiratory flow rates through an indirect effect on the elastic behavior of the flow-limiting segment. This mechanism can be appreciated by again considering the model. In Figure 38-4D, the effect of emphysema has been simulated by a decrease in Pel from +20 cmH$_2$O to +5 cmH$_2$O. For the sake of the argument, let Ppl increase from +40 cmH$_2$O to +55 cmH$_2$O, a change that could be realized simply by more forceful chest constriction. The sum of Pel and Ppl in this example provides the same driving pressure between alveolus and airway opening, +60 cmH$_2$O, as in Figure 38-4B. While the driving pressure is the same, pressure relationships across the airway wall are quite different. Since Ppl has been increased by

15 cmH$_2$O, external pressures at each point on the airway in Figure 38-4D are necessarily increased by a like amount. The larger compressive forces on the flow-limiting airways would, in comparison with Figure 38-4B, cause greater luminal narrowing, resulting in decreased maximal expiratory flow rates. Thus, Pel effectively opposes compressive forces of Ppl on intrathoracic airways. In experimental models of emphysema it has been demonstrated that the decrease in maximal expiratory flow rates is nearly proportional to the decrease in Pel [66].

Mechanisms of Impaired Gas Exchange

In patients with COPD, ventilatory capacity may be a limiting factor in determining oxygen uptake and carbon dioxide excretion during exercise. However, even at rest most COPD patients have evidence of impaired gas exchange. With mild COPD, impaired gas exchange may be manifest only as mild arterial hypoxemia. However, with severe disease, hypoxemia may be profound, and it, along with hypercapnia, contributes to the clinical signs and symptoms of this disorder.

The mechanisms by which certain pathologic conditions may impair gas exchange are well understood. For example, widespread emphysema is associated with a substantial loss of alveolar-capillary surface area. With extensive destruction of parenchyma, the lung cannot function effectively in exchanging oxygen and carbon dioxide. However, current thinking suggests that mechanisms other than a simple loss of surface area are more important as a cause of hypoxemia and hypercapnia. These other mechanisms relate to the distribution of ventilation and perfusion within the lung.

Gas exchange is most efficient when the ratio of ventilation to perfusion ($\dot{V}/\dot{Q}$) is uniform. To the extent that regional $\dot{V}/\dot{Q}$ deviates from unity, gas exchange is impaired.

If an alveolar region is ventilated but not perfused ($\dot{V}/\dot{Q} = \alpha$), no gas exchange can occur. Alveolar regions receiving some blood flow but still relatively overventilated behave functionally as though a portion of that region were normally perfused and the remainder received no blood flow. The excess ventilation in both situations is wasted, a condition that is described as a *high $\dot{V}/\dot{Q}$ abnormality*. High $\dot{V}/\dot{Q}$ abnormalities can be detected as an increase in the dead space to tidal volume ratio (V$_D$/V$_T$). In normal subjects, V$_D$/V$_T$

is 0.3 to 0.4, but in patients with severe COPD, it may be as high as 0.7 to 0.8. In these patients, a major portion of each inspired breath contributes nothing to gas exchange.

Alveolar regions that are perfused but not ventilated ($\dot{V}/\dot{Q} = 0$) also do not participate in gas exchange. The proportion of the cardiac output that passes through unventilated lung zones is termed the *shunt fraction*, and the admixture of shunted blood into pulmonary venous blood results in arterial hypoxemia. If an alveolar region receives some ventilation but relative to its blood supply is underventilated, there also will be arterial oxygen desaturation. Underventilated alveolar regions, called *low $\dot{V}/\dot{Q}$ abnormalities*, are thought to be the principal cause of hypoxemia in COPD.

Theoretically, pathologic states affecting the pattern of either ventilation or perfusion may cause the regional $\dot{V}/\dot{Q}$ to deviate from unity. Abnormal ventilation and perfusion patterns have been demonstrated by radioactive scanning methods in patients with COPD [2]. With diffuse emphysema, hypoperfusion can be attributed partly to loss of the capillary bed. However, abnormal perfusion patterns in COPD also may represent normal homeostasis in the pulmonary vasculature. According to this concept, pathologic changes in COPD create regions of hyperventilation and hypoventilation. Hypoxic vasoconstriction occurs in regions that are underventilated; this reduction in blood flow tends to restore the $\dot{V}/\dot{Q}$ ratio toward unity. Over long periods of time, hypoxic vasoconstriction may induce permanent histopathologic changes in the pulmonary arteries. However, since these changes may be regarded as secondary, attention in this discussion is directed at those pathologic mechanisms that alter the distribution of ventilation.

Ventilation is the process by which ambient air is transported to the alveolar-capillary interface and alveolar air is removed to the environment. *Regional ventilation* may be defined as the volume of ambient air that reaches a given lung region relative to the volume of gas that resided in that same region at the beginning of the breath. Regional ventilation is determined by the relative volume expansion of that region and by the manner in which inspired air mixes with resident gas.

Expansion of alveolated zones depends on both the elastic behavior of that region and external forces acting on it. Distending forces are closely equated to intrapleural pressure. For the same change in intrapleural pressure, compliant regions expand more than noncompliant regions

do and, other things being equal, receive more ventilation. Therefore, any pathologic state resulting in nonhomogeneous elastic behavior in lung parenchyma can be expected to cause uneven ventilation.

Emphysema is the prototype of diseases that alter lung elastic properties. In most instances, lung parenchyma is not uniformly involved by emphysema; severely diseased regions lie adjacent to histologically normal lung tissue. Therefore, one would anticipate abnormal ventilation patterns in emphysematous lungs, and this is observed. However, emphysematous regions may be either overventilated or underventilated. This may seem surprising in view of the fact that emphysematous lungs are generally said to be overly compliant and that compliant lungs should theoretically receive more ventilation. This seeming paradox can be understood by comparing pressure-volume curves in normal and emphysematous lungs (Fig. 38-6). With emphysema, there is a loss of lung elastic recoil and a leftward shift of the pressure-volume curve. At low volumes, the emphysematous lung undergoes greater volume change than does the normal lung. However, at large volumes the emphysematous lung is less compliant than the normal lung and undergoes less volume change for the same change in pressure. Thus, the distribution of ventilation between normal and emphysematous zones would be determined by relative differences in the pressure-volume relationships and by the magnitude

Fig. 38-6. Pressure-volume relationships in normal and emphysematous lungs. At small lung volumes the emphysematous lung is more compliant than the normal lung but the reverse is true at large lung volumes. ΔP = change in pressure; ΔV = change in volume.

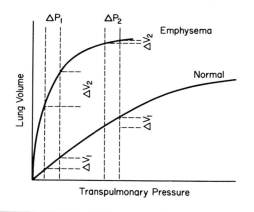

of external forces acting on each region. Existing evidence suggests that emphysematous areas are underventilated compared with normal lung parenchyma [3,36]. However, if perfusion were even more severely impaired than ventilation, emphysematous regions might still represent high $\dot{V}/\dot{Q}$ zones.

Not all the volume change that a lung region undergoes with each breath cycle is effective ventilation. At the end of expiration, all gas-transport pathways are filled with alveolar gas. With the next inspiration, this "dead-space" gas precedes ambient air into the gas-exchanging zones. If the volume expansion of a given lung region consisted solely of dead-space gas, net transfer of gas molecules could not occur. Dead-space gas represents a significant portion of each tidal breath so that its distribution and mixing with ambient air affect the efficiency of gas exchange.

Gas is transported from the airway opening to the alveolar-capillary interface by two mechanisms: convection and diffusion. Gas moves through the proximal airways principally by convection, but in the distal alveolated zones diffusion predominates.

At the beginning of inspiration one can imagine a front forming at the airway opening with ambient air on the proximal side and resident gas on the distal side. If no mixing occurs across the interface, the front would migrate distally as inspiration proceeds. The location of this front at the end of inspiration marks the limit of convective flow, and beyond this point gas transport is solely dependent on diffusion. (In reality, of course, mixing between ambient air and residual gas begins at the airway opening, but the notion of a convective front is conceptually useful.)

Calculations based on known dimensions of the respiratory tract suggest that with tidal breathing, this imaginary convective front penetrates to the level of the alveolar ducts. From there gas diffuses radially into the alveoli and axially into more distal alveolar ducts and alveoli. Because distances are short, radial mixing between the alveolar duct and alveoli probably is complete within a fraction of a second. However, axial pathways are much longer. Theoretical studies suggest that because distal pathways are of uneven length, mixing between proximal and distal alveolar ducts may not be complete within the span of a single breathing cycle [63]. If so, certain proximal alveolated regions would behave as high $\dot{V}/\dot{Q}$ zones, while other more distal regions would represent low $\dot{V}/\dot{Q}$ abnormalities. The length of the transport pathways within the

alveolated zones of the lung may be a critical factor in the efficiency of gas mixing.

Gas mixing within alveolated regions may be impaired by any pathologic state that alters the dimensions of transport pathways. While precise mechanisms are not known, two examples serve to illustrate how this may occur.

Centriacinar emphysema primarily involves the respiratory bronchiole, leaving more distal portions of the acinus intact (Fig. 38-7). To reach normal alveoli, gas molecules must pass through the increased dead-space volume of the pathologically enlarged respiratory bronchiole. With inspiration, ambient gas preferentially fills the proximal emphysema lesion, while distal regions tend to be filled by resident dead-space gas. This creates a region of relative alveolar hypoxia in the distal acinus but a high $\dot{V}/\dot{Q}$ zone within the emphysema lesion itself.

Another mechanism by which a specific structural abnormality may impair gas exchange is depicted in Figure 38-7C. Adjacent acini are shown, one with a normal supplying bronchiole, the

Fig. 38-7. Postulated mechanisms of uneven ventilation in COPD. (*Shading* represents resident dead-space gas.) (*A*) Normally inspired air is mixed evenly with resident gas throughout the acinus. (*B*) A disproportionate amount of inspired air remains within a proximally located centriacinar emphysema lesion, while the distal acinus contains relatively more dead-space gas. (*C*) Alveolated regions distal to an obstructed bronchiole are ventilated through a collateral channel. Because the pathway for gas transport is longer, mixing between inspired air and resident gas is incomplete.

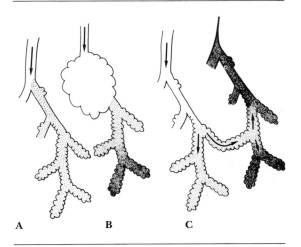

A   B   C

other in which the bronchiole is occluded by a mucous plug. If the latter bronchiole remained closed throughout the respiratory cycle and if no other bronchial connections existed, gas in the distal acinus would be absorbed. Atelectasis probably does not occur in such instances because of ventilation to the obstructed acinus through collateral channels. However, collateral pathways are likely to be longer with a corresponding increase in the dead-space volume. In the example shown, alveolated regions behind the obstructed bronchiole might function as a low $\dot{V}/\dot{Q}$ abnormality, whereas portions of the unobstructed acinus might represent regions with a high $\dot{V}/\dot{Q}$ ratio.

These examples illustrate how abnormal ventilation distribution may occur as a result of specific anatomic lesions. The relative importance of various types of pathologic changes as a cause of $\dot{V}/\dot{Q}$ disturbances in COPD has not been determined. Gas exchange is similarly dependent on factors relating to the distribution of blood flow. The final common expression of gas-exchange function in the lung, arterial blood gases, represents a summation of events at literally millions of different sites. Because of this complexity, it perhaps is not surprising that efforts to relate lung pathology with abnormal gas exchange have met with limited success.

Correlations between Anatomic Emphysema and COPD

Emphysema is defined as "a condition characterized by abnormal enlargement of the airspaces distal to the terminal bronchiole, accompanied by destruction of their walls, and without obvious fibrosis" [65]. Airspace enlargement may be due to actual departitioning of alveolar walls or to destructive changes that result in simple rearrangement of acinar shapes without fenestration. Airspace enlargement is also observed in conditions other than emphysema, and distinctions may at times be very difficult. For example, the aging lung is characterized by progressive enlargement of the alveolar ducts with effacement of adjacent alveoli. The enlarged alveolar ducts in aged lungs can be readily appreciated when viewing whole-lung sections, and this condition has been termed *senile emphysema*. Whether it is appropriate to regard this condition as emphysema or whether it represents a normal, nondestructive process is an unsettled question.

Emphysema is strictly an anatomic entity, and its presence and severity can best be determined in specimens obtained at surgery or autopsy. The accurate diagnosis of emphysema severity requires that lungs be fixed in an inflated state, which is usually accomplished by instilling a fixative into the mainstem bronchus at a constant pressure. Assessments of emphysema severity are then made either from whole-lung slices or from histologic sections.

Although a variety of techniques have been used, a method introduced by Thurlbeck and associates probably represents the "gold standard" for measuring emphysema severity at the present time [92]. Paper-mounted whole-lung slices are scored by comparing them to a standard picture panel depicting progressively more severe grades of emphysema. This method has been shown to be highly reproducible, and it is also quite sensitive in detecting mild grades of emphysema. Other investigators have assessed emphysema by comparing water-submerged and barium-impregnated lung slices against the same picture panel, and the results appear comparable [32]. There also have been efforts to quantitate the extent of emphysematous involvement on whole-lung slices by point-counting methods [17]; but these methods involve more difficult subjective judgments on the part of the observer and probably are less reproducible.

Emphysema severity also can be assessed by more direct measurements of airspace size from histologic sections [24]. A test line of known length, contained within the eyepiece reticule, is superimposed over lung parenchyma at multiple sites. The number of intersections of the test line with alveolar walls is counted, and from this is calculated the average distance between alveolar walls (mean linear intercept). Provided that adequate attention is given to sampling, the mean linear intercept can be quickly determined with an error of only a few percent. The correlation between estimates of severity from the panel-scoring method and from the mean linear intercept is generally good in lungs involved by moderate to severe grades of emphysema [88]. The mean linear intercept method has the advantage of being truly quantitative, but it suffers the disadvantage of lacking sensitivity. There is considerable variability in the mean linear intercept of normal lungs [88]. Milder forms of emphysema are usually focal in their distribution, and these abnormalities can be recognized from visualization of whole-lung slices or histologic sections. However, focal disease may have little effect on the mean linear intercept when this is determined as the average for the whole lung. Hence considerable overlap exists between mean linear intercept values determined in normal lungs and in those with mild emphysema.

Another recently described histologic method for evaluating emphysema, the *destructive index*, has been compared to the grading of whole-lung slices and the measurement of the mean linear intercept [78]. The destructive index was not of increased value in relating the severity of emphysema to pulmonary function test results, and the method was found to be quite time-consuming.

The problem of assessing emphysema presence and severity is further compounded by the fact that this condition has been categorized into morphologic subtypes, the most important of which are centriacinar and panacinar. The panacinar form predominates in the severe $alpha_1$-antiprotease deficiency state, whereas centriacinar emphysema is more closely linked to cigarette smoking by etiology [1,25]. In their earlier stages, these two forms of emphysema can usually be distinguished, but mixed forms are the rule in most cases of advanced COPD, and the relative proportion of each cannot be reliably distinguished. In most studies, assessment of emphysema has been made without reference to morphologic type, but there is some evidence that the panacinar and centriacinar forms of emphysema may have distinguishing functional features [43].

Patients with physical impairment due to COPD nearly always have emphysema, but severity varies widely. Occasionally, emphysema may be absent or present in only trace amounts. Advanced grades of emphysema can be strongly suspected from certain characteristic pulmonary function abnormalities, but it bears emphasizing that none of the available pulmonary function tests is capable of predicting emphysema severity with a high degree of precision.

The enlargement of the airspaces in emphysema is due to loss of alveolar walls. The loss of surface area available for gas exchange, as well as in homogeneities in ventilation and perfusion, impair oxygen and carbon dioxide exchange between ambient air and capillary blood. However, the extent of anatomic emphysema correlates poorly with abnormalities in arterial blood gas measurements, but it does correlate somewhat better with reductions in the diffusing capacity for carbon dioxide (DLCO) [9,74,86]. A study by

Berends and colleagues is representative [4]. They assessed emphysema by the picture panel method in surgically resected lobes and compared this to the DLCO obtained prior to surgery. In 22 patients, emphysema severity ranged from 0 to 50 units, and the correlation coefficient with the DLCO was -0.72. This correlation exceeded that with any other test. However, a correlation coefficient of -0.72 means that only about half the variance in the DLCO is attributable to emphysema, and in individual patients, discrepancies between the two measurements were large.

Severe emphysema is also associated with characteristic abnormalities in the lung pressure-volume relationships, these include an increase in maximal lung capacity and a decrease in lung elastic recoil pressure at each lung volume. Efforts have been made to use the pressure-volume relationship and parameters derived from it as tests for emphysema severity. When pressure-volume relationships have been measured in excised human lungs, correlations with emphysema grade and/or the mean linear intercept have been quite good in some studies [31,81]. Similarly high-order relationships have been shown in an animal model of emphysema [66]. Unfortunately, these relationships have been less consistent when the pressure-volume relationships have been measured in live humans and compared to emphysema severity in excised lungs [9,73,74]. Correlations were found to be variable and not always statistically significant.

These disappointing results may partly result from large errors inherent in the measurements of pressure-volume relationships in live subjects in comparison to those in excised lungs. Additionally, in human disease there are usually mixed elements of panacinar and centriacinar emphysema, and these two subtypes of emphysema may have different effects on lung elasticity [43]. Thurlbeck raised another possibility [90]. He suggested that loss of lung elastic recoil may relate only indirectly to airspace enlargement, but more directly to other, more subtle abnormalities in the lung's connective-tissue skeleton. He showed that the maximal distended lung volumes may be considerably increased over normal when only traces of emphysema are present.

In a preceding section it was pointed out that emphysema would be expected to cause a reduction in maximal expiratory flow rates both because of a loss of lung elastic recoil and because of the loss of tethering on intraparenchymal airways. Several correlative studies have shown that with increasing emphysema severity, maximal expiratory flow rates, as measured by spirometry, decrease [8,20,73,82]. Spirometric variables distinguish those patients with severe emphysema from those with no or trivial airspace enlargement, but in general the correlation coefficients are relatively poor, so that spirometry is not a good predictor of emphysema severity.

Another finding in emphysema that also can be attributed to the loss of elastic recoil is the tendency for lung overinflation. TLC on average is increased in patients with severe emphysema, as are the vital capacity, functional residual capacity, and RV [9,13,85,89]. However, none of these correlations is sufficiently good to permit their use as indices of emphysema in individual subjects.

Thus, the principal conclusion to be drawn is that currently there is no physiologic test that allows an accurate assessment of the severity of anatomic emphysema in the living patient. In most studies, emphysema severity has been shown to correlate most closely with the D$_{LCO}$ and less well with spirometric variables, lung volumes, and parameters of the pressure-volume relationships.

Conventional roentgenographic techniques are also of limited value. However, computed tomography (CT) appears quite promising as a method for estimating the severity of emphysema in the live patient. This application of the CT scan permits accurate quantitation of regional variations in lung tissue density, with the areas of lowest density representing the greatest involvement by emphysema. Estimates of the extent and severity of airspace enlargement by CT correlate quite closely with quantitative estimates of emphysema in surgically resected lung tissue [5,30].

Correlation between Intrinsic Airways Disease and COPD

The diverse pathologic conditions that affect the conducting airways in COPD are frequently lumped together as chronic bronchitis. Since not all these lesions can be described as bronchial inflammation, and since *chronic bronchitis* has another clinical definition, the practice of using this term to describe a variety of histopathologic changes in the conducting airways is not recommended. In this discussion we describe the entire complex of lesions affecting the conducting airways in COPD as *airways disease* or, to clearly distinguish this category of disease from emphysema, as *intrinsic airways disease*.

As discussed in the previous section, the importance of emphysema as a cause of airflow obstruction is firmly established from theoretical, experimental, and correlative studies. However, it bears emphasizing that the extent of anatomic emphysema does not always explain the patient's clinical status. Occasionally, patients with well-documented, severe COPD are found to have little emphysema when the lungs are examined at autopsy. Though unusual, cases have been reported in which fatal COPD was associated with no emphysema whatever [28,82]. Widespread emphysema is occasionally an incidental finding at autopsy in persons without known respiratory symptoms. One might suspect that had careful pulmonary function testing been carried out in these individuals, some degree of airflow obstruction would have been found. Yet it is clear that the same amount of emphysema may be associated with severe disability and death in one person and cause few, if any, symptoms in the next. This indicates that other factors act in concert with emphysema to determine the severity of airflow obstruction. It has long been suspected that the most important of these other factors is the presence and severity of intrinsic airways disease.

Reid [77] provided a comprehensive description of airway pathology in lungs from persons with productive cough and airflow obstruction. She emphasized hypertrophy and hyperplasia of the mucus-secreting elements (i.e., bronchial mucous glands and epithelial goblet cells) as being the essential feature of COPD. It was suggested that excessive mucus predisposed to recurrent infection and that other pathologic changes—purulent bronchiolitis, microabscess formation, and tortuosity of the peripheral airways—were secondary phenomena. Because mucus hypersecretion was considered of paramount importance in the pathogenesis of COPD, *chronic bronchitis* was defined clinically as the presence of a productive cough, and to the pathologist it became virtually synonymous with bronchial mucous gland enlargement.

Other investigators emphasized the importance of abnormalities in the peripheral airways of patients with COPD. Laennec, in his treatise on the emphysematous lung published in 1834 [45], commented on abnormalities in the smaller airways and suggested that these lesions might be responsible for air trapping and obstruction. Spain and Kaufman [84] observed mural thickening and inflammation in many noncartilaginous bronchioles of severely emphysematous lungs. McLean [57] noted similar abnormalities and suggested that extension of the inflammatory process from the airway to adjacent lung parenchyma might be a factor in the pathogenesis of emphysema. Leopold and Gough [46] observed widespread inflammation and fibrosis in the membranous and respiratory bronchioles in cases of centriacinar emphysema, whereas these lesions were usually absent with panacinar emphysema. In the latter type of emphysema, chronic inflammatory reactions were more common in the large, cartilaginous airways.

Morphometric methods also have been employed to study disease in the peripheral airways. Bignon and associates [7,8] measured internal bronchiole diameters on histologic sections of lungs from patients with severe COPD. They observed that the proportion of bronchioles with internal diameters less than 350 μm was consistently greater in diseased lungs than in normal lungs. In similar studies, Matsuba and Thurlbeck [52–54] observed that diameters of membranous bronchioles were on the average slightly less than normal in emphysematous lungs and in lungs from patients with COPD.

While various pathologic lesions are commonly observed throughout the bronchial tree of patients with COPD, their mere presence gives no clue as to their functional significance. Efforts to correlate the extent of intrinsic airways disease with the severity of COPD as assessed clinically and physiologically have until recently been largely unsuccessful.

The relationship between ventilatory dysfunction and mucous gland enlargement has been most thoroughly investigated [10,47,51,56,91]. In most studies cited, the extent of mucous gland enlargement was assessed at autopsy by the Reid index or by other quantitative methods and was compared to pulmonary function measured within 1 or 2 years before death. With one exception, each of these studies showed a relationship between ventilatory function and gland hypertrophy that either was not statistically significant or, if significant, was so only with a very low correlation coefficient. The one exception is a study of Australian coal miners performed by McKenzie and associates [56]. They found that the percent predicted forced expiratory volume (FEV_1) and the Reid index were correlated with a coefficient of -0.74. This divergent result remains unexplained and cannot be attributed to coal mining per se, since Lyons and coworkers [47] found no significant relationship between the Reid index and various measures of lung function among Welsh coal miners. This one study excepted, physiologic and pathologic correlative studies indicate that at most, mucous gland enlargement plays a very minor role in the genesis of airflow obstruction. This conclusion is further substantiated by studies of lung mechanics and morphology in postmortem lungs; no relationship has been found between the volume of bronchial gland mass and any of the flow-resistive properties of the conducting airways [67,69]. Also, no significant relationship exists between the volume of sputum production and long-term changes in spirometric function [75].

A number of earlier studies were unsuccessful in showing that other disease features, including inflammation, fibrosis, and goblet cell metaplasia, involving either the large or small airways correlated to any appreciable extent with antemortem spirometric abnormalities [42,51,62]. While these studies with largely negative findings suggest that airways disease plays only a small role in the causation of airflow obstruction, it is important to keep in mind that pathologic features such as inflammation and fibrosis do not lend themselves readily to quantitative assessment. Sampling is another potential problem, since a single lung may contain as many as 30,000 separate airways. Hence, the results of the studies cited can only be regarded as inconclusive.

With tidal breathing, most patients with COPD have an elevated pulmonary resistance. The increase in airflow resistance, particularly when measured on inspiration, correlates with clinical status but not with the extent of anatomic emphysema. This measurement is thought to reflect more directly intrinsic airways disease than does spirometry, which, for reasons previously outlined, is also closely dependent on lung elastic recoil.

Hogg and associates [35] provided an important clue as to the site of increased airflow resistance in COPD. They positioned a retrograde catheter in the bronchial tree of postmortem lungs so as to partition flow resistance between central airways and those peripheral airways of less than 2-mm internal diameter. Their measurements suggested that in normal lungs, peripheral resistance was negligible in comparison with the central component. In lungs from patients known to have COPD, central airways resistance was on average increased only slightly, but the peripheral component was increased between 10- and 20-fold.

These observations have had an enormous impact on subsequent research. Contrary to the opinion prevailing at that time, their studies indicated that it was disease in the distal airways and not the large bronchi that was principally responsible for increased flow resistance in COPD. In addition, these investigators introduced novel ideas concerning the natural history and pathophysiology of COPD. They reasoned that if peripheral resistance was negligible in the normal lung but predominated in clinically overt COPD, clinically quiescent disease might exist in the distal airways for many years before clinical symptoms of airflow obstruction became manifest.

It was further suggested that routine spirometric tests may not be sufficiently sensitive to detect early disease in the distal airways [48]. This premise provided an impetus to develop and evaluate so-called tests of small airways disease, such as the closing volume. Whether or not any of these newer tests offer any advantages over spirometry for either clinical or investigational purposes remains conjectural. Current evidence from epidemiologic and correlative studies indicates that both early COPD and small airways disease are reflected by spirometric abnormalities and that, at best, newer tests offer only marginal advantages [18,44,69,71].

However, the suggestion that disease in the peripheral airways may antedate the clinical manifestations of COPD has been largely substantiated by physiologic and pathologic studies. Most of these studies have been directed at young smokers, a logical choice, since cigarette smoking causes COPD but only after at least 20 years of heavy consumption.

Evidence of subtle ventilatory dysfunction in young smokers has been provided by several studies utilizing a variety of pulmonary function tests [12,15,23,38,80]. The pathologic lesions thought to be responsible for these minimal physiologic abnormalities have been identified in studies of lungs from youthful victims of sudden death [68]. The characteristic lesion in cigarette smokers (Fig. 38-8) is located in the respiratory bronchiole and consists of clumps of brown-pigmented macrophages lying within the airspaces with edema, epithelial hyperplasia, and minimal fibrosis involving adjacent alveolar and bronchiolar walls. Frequently, a sparse mononuclear inflammatory infiltrate is seen within the walls of the terminal membranous bronchioles. These lesions were noted in each of the lungs from cigarette smokers, but only occasionally in nonsmokers. In complementary studies, detailed

Fig. 38-8. Terminal airway in a lung from a youthful cigarette smoker. Clusters of pigmented macrophages can be seen in the respiratory bronchiole. There is also a mild inflammatory reaction in the walls of the bronchiole and adjacent alveoli.

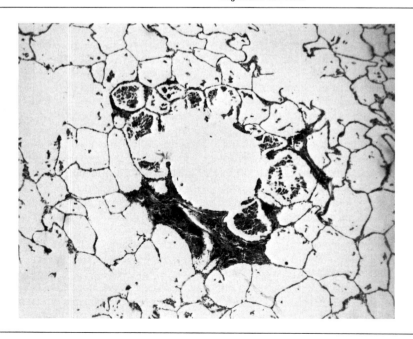

morphometric analyses of central cartilaginous bronchi revealed no differences between young smokers and age-matched controls [83]. Hence, the suggestion from physiologic studies that the earliest morphologic abnormalities in smokers might be found in the distal airways has been largely substantiated.

Functional and morphologic correlative studies in postmortem human lungs lend further support to the concept that peripheral airways are the site of increased resistance in COPD [67,69]. In a population of largely normal lungs, it was found that pulmonary resistance and maximal expiratory flow rates correlated closely with the diameter of the membranous bronchioles and not with any other morphologic variable. For example, pulmonary resistance was correlated to average bronchiole diameter with a coefficient of -0.85, whereas the correlations between pulmonary resistance and both bronchial gland mass ($r = -0.10$) and large airways diameter ($r = -0.21$) were not statistically significant.

These results suggest that the peripheral component of resistance in most normal lungs may

be considerably greater than suggested by the studies of Hogg and associates [35]. Indeed, a subsequent study utilizing a similar retrograde catheter technique indicated that the peripheral component of airways resistance in normal lungs was seriously underestimated in that original study [93]. This finding has important implications concerning the pathophysiology of COPD. If the peripheral airways are an important determinant of ventilatory function in the normal lung, it logically follows that lung function may be critically vulnerable to minor degrees of pathologic narrowing in those same airways.

The sensitivity of ventilatory function to minor degrees of bronchiolar narrowing can be appreciated in Figure 38-9, which shows the frequency distribution of internal bronchiole diameters in two normal adult lungs from persons of the same age. The average diameter in one lung is nearly twice that in the other. Because airflow resistance through cylinders varies with higher powers of diameter, the seemingly modest difference in average bronchiole diameter is associated with pronounced functional differences. Pulmonary resistance in the second lung is more than five times greater than that in the first lung, and maximal expiratory flow rates are correspondingly less. Subtle pathologic changes that diffusely affect the distal air passages may have profound functional consequences.

Cosio and associates [18] provided the first convincing evidence that disease in the small air-

Fig. 38-9. Ventilatory function is sensitive to minor degrees of narrowing in the membranous bronchioles. Postmortem flow-volume loops and pulmonary resistance (R_{pulm}) were measured in two normal lungs (A, B) from men 40 years old. The lower panel shows the distribution of internal bronchiole diameters in the same two lungs. TLC = total lung capacity; MEF = maximum expiratory flow.

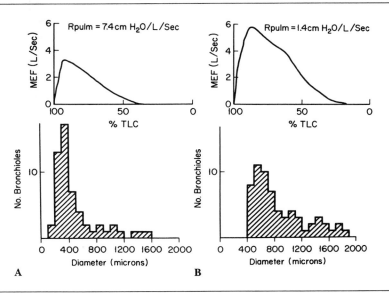

A   B

ways is a major determinant of functional impairment in patients with COPD. They obtained lung tissue from patients undergoing thoracotomy in whom extensive pulmonary function tests had been performed immediately before surgery. They studied 36 patients ranging in age from 24 to 73 years. A few subjects had normal pulmonary function, but most had evidence of COPD varying in severity from minimal to moderately severe. Emphysema was quantitated from thick lung slices, while the extent of small airways disease was assessed on multiple histologic sections from each lung. Each bronchiole was individually evaluated and assigned a score appropriate to the severity of each morphologic abnormality, including luminal mucus, squamous and goblet cell metaplasia of the epithelium, and inflammation, fibrosis, pigment, and smooth muscle hypertrophy in the airway wall. The reproducibility of this semiquantitative scoring method was assessed carefully and found to be excellent.

These investigators observed a close relationship ($r = +0.85$) between composite scores for small airways disease and the severity of airflow obstruction as assessed by various physiologic tests. Functional disturbances were closely related to fibrosis and inflammation within the wall of the bronchioles but correlated less well with epithelial abnormalities and with the amount of intraluminal mucus. In 12 patients, mild to moderate emphysema also was present. While lungs with emphysema were associated with impaired ventilatory function, the severity of airflow obstruction, overall, correlated better with small airways disease than it did with the presence or severity of emphysema.

The contribution of peripheral airway narrowing and disease to impaired ventilatory function was confirmed in subsequent studies [32,55,96], and it is reasonable to presume that small airways disease is a significant factor in the causation of airflow obstruction in most patients with COPD. Minimal pulmonary dysfunction in young cigarette smokers is associated with scattered inflammatory lesions located principally in the respiratory bronchioles. In patients with established COPD, the degree of dysfunction correlates with inflammation and fibrosis in both the respiratory and the noncartilaginous membranous bronchioles.

Relative Contribution of Emphysema and Intrinsic Airways Disease to COPD

Peripheral airways disease is clearly a more important factor than chronic bronchitis in the causation of airflow obstruction, but several studies suggest it to be somewhat less important than emphysema in patients with advanced COPD. Mitchell and colleagues [62] compared a clinical assessment of physical impairment from COPD with pathology studied in autopsied lungs. Emphysema severity was most closely correlated with clinical status, whereas peripheral airways disease and other abnormalities in the conducting airways were of secondary importance. Hale and coworkers [32] studied lungs obtained at autopsy from patients with known COPD, and they found that the percent predicted FEV_1, measured premortem, correlated substantially better with

Table 38-1. **Pathologic features of COPD and their relationship to clinical and ventilatory abnormalities**

	Pathologic features	Clinical and physiologic correlates
Chronic bronchitis	Inflammation, mucous gland enlargement in central cartilaginous airways	Cough and sputum expectoration; no exercise intolerance; little or no effect on spirometry
Emphysema	Airspace enlargement with destruction of alveolar walls	Exercise intolerance; abnormal pressure-volume curve and spirometry when severe; variable effects on arterial blood gases; DLCO single best correlate
Small airways disease	Inflammation, fibrosis, goblet cell metaplasia, and smooth-muscle hypertrophy in terminal bronchioles; inflammation in respiratory bronchioles	Mild spirometric abnormalities in young smokers; secondary cause of airflow obstruction and exercise intolerance in advanced COPD

emphysema severity than with peripheral airways disease. Nagai and associates [64] performed a similar study and came to substantially the same conclusion. A summary of the principal pathologic changes found in COPD and their relationship to clinical and physiologic abnormalities is provided in Table 38-1.

Clinical and Pathologic Subtypes

Patients having in common irreversible airflow obstruction may exhibit otherwise diverse clinical and physiologic features. The variability in the clinical expression of COPD was commented on by Dornhurst [22], and based on clinical, roentgenographic, and physiologic criteria, subsequent investigators described two contrasting categories of disease, the so-called emphysematous and bronchial subtypes of COPD [11,16,29,41,61]. As implied by the descriptive terms applied to each subgroup, it was presumed that extensive anatomic emphysema provided the principal morphologic basis for dysfunction in the first group, whereas enlargement of the mucus-secreting elements was the major pathologic lesion in patients with bronchial disease. There is general agreement as to the basic clinical and physiologic features of each syndrome; whether there are distinguishable patterns of lung pathology associated with each subtype is open to conjecture.

The patient thought to have predominant emphysema (type A disease) has been described in vivid terms as a "pink puffer." He is said to be a cachectic, elderly man who relates a long history of progressive and unrelenting breathlessness. Sputum production and recurrent chest infections are notable by their absence and, except in the preterminal stages of the disease, heart failure (cor pulmonale) is not clinically evident. The chest roentgenogram reveals a small cardiac silhouette along with the roentgenographic signs of advanced emphysema: lung hyperinflation, attenuated peripheral lung markings, and frequently the thin ring shadows pathognomonic of bullae. At rest, arterial blood gas values reveal mild hypoxemia with little or no elevation in the arterial carbon dioxide tension. The hematocrit is seldom greater than 45 to 50 percent, reflecting the relative absence of arterial oxygen desaturation. In addition to the decrease in expiratory flow rates, pulmonary function studies show large lung volumes, with TLC being 130 percent or more of predicted. Because of the loss of alveolar tissue, lung elastic recoil is decreased and the D_LCO is severely impaired. In the absence of intrinsic airways disease, pulmonary resistance measured either during tidal breathing or during the panting maneuver is normal or only slightly elevated.

The patient considered to have predominant bronchial disease (type B patient) is known as the "blue bloater." In contrast to the asthenic appearance of the pink puffer, this patient is described as a stocky and sometimes overweight individual with a plethoric facies and pronounced cyanosis. Because enlargement of the mucus-secreting elements has been thought the principal cause of airflow obstruction in these individuals, the presence of chronic cough and sputum production has been considered an essential feature of type B disease by most authors. The other essential feature is cor pulmonale, which appears early and remains a prominent feature throughout the course of the disease. Cor pulmonale is manifest clinically as peripheral edema, cardiac enlargement, and classic electrocardiographic signs of right ventricular enlargement. Arterial blood gas values show evidence of severe arterial oxygen desaturation and a strong tendency to retention of carbon dioxide. Secondary polycythemia with a hematocrit in excess of 55 percent develops as a consequence of severe, chronic hypoxemia. As with the type A patient, spirometry shows severe airflow obstruction, but there is less hyperinflation of the lung. Because alveolar tissue is thought to be preserved, lung elastic recoil is normal, as is the D_LCO.

Filley and associates [27] provided detailed information concerning the physiologic features of emphysematous and bronchial patients. They classified patients principally on the basis of associated heart disease; emphysematous patients had normal cardiac silhouettes on chest roentgenogram, no history of heart failure, and hematocrits of less than 55 percent; bronchial patients had enlarged hearts, recurrent congestive heart failure, and marked polycythemia.

Emphysematous patients were found to have larger lung volumes, more nearly normal arterial blood gases, and a larger volume of total ventilation per unit of oxygen uptake. Consistent differences were noted between the two groups with regard to pulmonary vascular hemodynamics and systemic oxygen transport. In the pink puffers, cardiac output was subnormal both at rest and with exercise, whereas this physiologic variable was normal under both conditions in the blue bloaters. Calculated pulmonary vascular resistance was not significantly different in the two groups, but because cardiac output was higher in the bronchial group, mean pulmonary artery pressures also were greater. Despite a greater degree of arterial oxygen desaturation, systemic oxygen transport was better preserved among the blue bloaters because of their secondary polycythemia and because of their higher cardiac output.

Burrows and coworkers [14] came to many of the same conclusions regarding hemodynamic differences between emphysematous and bronchial patients. Patients who conformed to earlier established criteria of type A disease had relatively well-preserved blood gases, low cardiac outputs both at rest and with exercise, and pulmonary artery pressures that became elevated only with exercise. Patients conforming to type B criteria had more severe hypoxemia, relatively normal cardiac outputs, and elevated mean pulmonary artery pressures even at rest. The latter group frequently had classic and electrocardiographic manifestations of cor pulmonale.

Other investigators have studied exercise performance in patients with COPD [40,50]. Minute ventilation in relation to oxygen consumption and to carbon dioxide excretion was higher in the type A patient than in the type B patient. Maximum work load and the exercise level associated with the threshold of anaerobic metabolism tended to be less in the emphysematous patient.

Wagner and associates [94] used a sophisticated multiple inert-gas elimination technique to study ventilation-perfusion relationships in patients with COPD and to compare patients with type A and type B disease. Much overlap was observed between the two groups, but in general patients with type A disease had patterns of high $\dot{V}/\dot{Q}$ abnormalities with relatively few areas of low $\dot{V}/\dot{Q}$ abnormality. They postulated that high $\dot{V}/\dot{Q}$ disturbances in such patients reflected loss of blood flow to emphysematous zones. There was a greater tendency for low $\dot{V}/\dot{Q}$ patterns to be found in type B disease, but most patients with this clinical syndrome had mixed patterns of both high and low $\dot{V}/\dot{Q}$ disturbances.

While clinical and physiologic features that distinguish COPD subtypes can be recognized in some patients, it is also generally acknowledged that most patients with COPD appear to have features of both groups and cannot be categorized. It has been proposed that the population of COPD patients represents a spectrum, with the emphysematous patients at one end and the bronchial patients at the other [28]. Because of extensive overlap between the two groups, only

those few patients at the extreme ends of the spectrum can be recognized as distinct subtypes.

Although the existence of the emphysematous and bronchial patient is widely accepted, it is to be emphasized that these distinctions in most instances have been clinical or physiologic and not pathologic. There have been relatively few efforts to correlate lung pathology with the clinical type of COPD, and when these efforts have been made, findings frequently have been contradictory and inconclusive.

A clinicopathologic study by Burrows and associates [13] provided the strongest evidence that the type A and type B subtypes are associated with distinctive lung pathology. Clinical diagnosis of type A disease was based principally on roentgenographic evidence of advanced emphysema, whereas type B patients were diagnosed on the basis of having chronic expectoration, disproportionate hypercapnia, a well-preserved $D_{L}CO$, a relatively small TLC, and right-sided heart failure.

At autopsy those patients with type B disease had only mild emphysema, whereas type A patients without exception had widespread emphysema. The two clinical types were almost perfectly separated, based on the extent of anatomic emphysema. Whether type B patients had a greater incidence of intrinsic airways disease is uncertain because the authors did not comment on the presence and severity of bronchial and bronchiolar disease in the lungs studied.

This study seemed to provide a sound basis for believing that emphysematous patients do in fact have severe anatomic emphysema. However, it is evident that these authors weighted roentgenographic criteria very heavily in distinguishing the type A from the type B patient. Other investigators also showed that the extent of anatomic emphysema can be predicted with reasonable accuracy from chest roentgenograms. Also, in the Burrows group study [13], four patients with severe bronchiectasis were included as having type B disease, and many authorities would regard bronchiectasis as being an entity apart from what is ordinarily regarded as COPD.

Mitchell and associates [59] proposed a relationship between bronchial mucous gland enlargement and the blue bloater syndrome based on their clinical and pathologic correlative studies. Of 46 patients considered to have mucous gland enlargement on the basis of the Reid index, 21 had clinical features of the blue bloater type, whereas only 3 resembled the pink puffer. It was also reported from this same series that patients with the pink puffer syndrome had more severe emphysema. However, these morphologic distinctions became blurred as additional patients were studied. In a subsequent report, autopsy findings in 22 patients classified as pink puffers were compared with findings in 15 patients who by clinical criteria were considered to be blue bloaters [62]. The severity of anatomic emphysema was found to be nearly identical in the two groups. Mitchell and coworkers did find a small though statistically significant increase in the degree of mucous gland enlargement and in the extent of bronchiolar inflammation among the blue bloaters. However, such minor differences scarcely constitute a clear-cut pathologic basis for distinguishing pink puffers from blue bloaters. Cullen and associates [20] also failed to find a consistent relationship between bronchial disease and the type B clinical syndrome.

Many of the criteria used to categorize clinical subtypes are descriptive and not quantitative. It is evident that selection criteria are nonuniform in the various studies cited even for the same group of investigators at different periods. These factors may explain partly the relative lack of success in correlating clinical COPD subtypes with pathology.

It may be more rational to consider whether cor pulmonale alone is more closely associated with intrinsic airways disease or emphysema. It is generally agreed that right-sided heart failure is an essential feature of the type B patient but not the type A patient. Clinical right-sided heart failure relates closely to right ventricular enlargement, and this morphologic feature can be accurately assessed at autopsy.

It is fair to conclude from available evidence that the presence of emphysema alone is not the predominant factor in the pathogenesis of cor pulmonale. Numerous autopsy studies have been performed in which right ventricular size was compared to the severity of emphysema. It has been variously reported that this correlation is positive, negative, or not statistically significant [7-9,19,33,60,87,95]. However, even when a positive correlation has been observed, the correlation coefficients have generally been low. In no study has more than approximately 25 percent of the total variance in right ventricular weight been explained on the basis of the amount of emphysema, and in most studies the figure is much lower. Since the methods for assessing emphysema and right ventricular size are reasonably accurate, these low levels of correlation cannot be attributed to measurement error. It also has been suggested that right ventricular enlargement might be more closely related to certain types of emphysema. However, even here the evidence is conflicting; some investigators reported that right ventricular size is more closely related to the presence of centriacinar emphysema, while others found larger right ventricles in lungs with predominantly panacinar emphysema [34,85].

The dissociation between the severity of emphysema and right ventricular size is in accordance with the notion that type A or emphysematous patients have little tendency to develop right-sided heart failure. However, it has not been shown that bronchial mucous gland enlargement, thought to be an essential pathologic feature in type B patients, relates to right ventricular size either. Carefully performed pathologic studies by several groups of investigators failed to demonstrate a statistically significant relationship between right ventricular weight and bronchial gland enlargement in patients known to have had COPD [7-9,60,91]. This provides no support for the hypothesis that excessive mucus production in the large airways initiates a chain of events leading to pulmonary arterial hypertension and cor pulmonale. Perhaps these negative conclusions should not be surprising in light of the previously cited evidence that bronchial mucous gland enlargement is also unrelated to airflow obstruction.

There is suggestive evidence that cor pulmonale may be associated with disease in the distal airways. Bignon and associates [7,8,21] performed detailed morphometric studies on inflated lungs from patients with fatal COPD. Emphysema was quantitated both from gross lung slices and from histologic sections. Areas of bronchial mucous glands were measured. As an index of small airways disease, the internal diameters of approximately 100 bronchioles were measured in each lung. In accord with other studies, these investigators found only weak correlations between right ventricular weight and either the severity of emphysema or the extent of mucous gland enlargement. However, right ventricular weight did bear an impressively close relationship to bronchiolar diameter; those cases with the largest right ventricles also had the highest percentage of bronchioles less than 350 μm in internal diameter.

These same investigators studied selected lungs with bronchial casts and with serial histologic sections [21]. In those cases with most severe cor pulmonale, multiple stenoses were identified in membranous bronchioles. Fibrosis and inflammation were commonly observed in airway walls at the site of luminal narrowing. Esterly and Heard [26] described similar abnormalities in two patients with documented COPD and cor pulmonale but with no anatomic emphysema.

Scott and Steiner [79] insufflated tantalum into the bronchial tree of postmortem lungs to evaluate the size, shape, and patency of the distal airways. Many fewer patent airways were observed in lungs from patients who died of COPD and cor pulmonale than in normal lungs or in lungs matched for comparable degrees of emphysema. Alternating regions of dilatation and stenosis were noted even in those airways that did fill. By histologic examination, nonfilling airways were fibrotic and contained a purulent exudate within their lumen.

These elegant morphologic studies suggest an association between small airways disease and the development of cor pulmonale. However, Mitchell and associates [60] found no relationship between right ventricular weight and histologic assessment of peripheral airways disease in a larger population of patients with COPD. Similarly, Hale and coworkers [32] found that hypertensive changes in the small muscular arteries related equally well to the amount of emphysema as to the severity of small airways disease.

Recently, Biernacki and associates [6] measured gas-exchange and pulmonary hemodynamics in a group of patients with COPD who had a wide range of arterial carbon dioxide and oxygen pressures. The severity of emphysema was assessed by CT in the same subjects. They found no significant correlations between the extent of emphysema and either arterial blood gases, cardiac output, mean pulmonary artery pressure, or pulmonary vascular resistance.

Certain patients with COPD do have a greater predisposition toward developing hypoxemia, hypercapnia, and pulmonary hypertension, so that the terms *pink puffer* and *blue bloater* may have some validity as clinical and physiologic descriptive terms. However, it is not known why these differences exist. Since they have no clearly defined anatomic basis, there is no justification for describing such patients as having emphysematous or bronchitic types of COPD.

References

1. Anderson AE Jr, et al. Pulmonary emphysema: Prevalence, severity, and anatomical patterns in macrosections, with respect to smoking patterns. *Arch Environ Health* 12:569, 1966.
2. Anthonisen NR, et al. Regional lung function in patients with chronic bronchitis. *Clin Sci* 35:455, 1968.
3. Barter CE, et al. Radiology compared with xenon-133 scanning and bronchoscopic lobar sampling for assessing regional lung function in patients with emphysema. *Thorax* 28:29, 1973.
4. Berend N, Woolcock AJ, Marlin GE. Correlation between the function and the structure of the lung in smokers. *Am Rev Respir Dis* 119:695, 1979.
5. Bergin C, et al. The diagnosis of emphysema: A computed tomographic-pathologic correlation. *Am Rev Respir Dis* 133:541, 1986.
6. Biernacki W, et al. Pulmonary hemodynamics, gas exchange, and the severity of emphysema as assessed by quantitative CT scan in chronic bronchitis and emphysema. *Am Rev Respir Dis* 139:1509, 1989.
7. Bignon J, Andre-Bougaran J, Brouet G. Parenchymal, bronchiolar, and bronchial measurements in centrilobular emphysema. Relation to weight of right ventricle. *Thorax* 25:556, 1970.
8. Bignon J, et al. Morphometric study in chronic obstructive bronchopulmonary disease: Pathologic, clinical, and physiologic correlations. *Am Rev Respir Dis* 99:669, 1969.
9. Boushy SF, et al. Lung recoil pressure, airway resistance, and forced flows related to morphologic emphysema. *Am Rev Respir Dis* 104:551, 1971.
10. Boushy SF, et al. Clinical, physiologic, and morphologic examination of the lung in patients with bronchogenic carcinoma and the relation of the findings to death. *Am Rev Respir Dis* 101:685, 1970.
11. Briscoe WA, Nash ES. The slow space in chronic obstructive pulmonary disease. *Ann NY Acad Sci* 121:706, 1965.
12. Buist AS, van Fleet DL, Ross BB. A comparison of conventional spirometric tests and the test of closing volume in an emphysema screening center. *Am Rev Respir Dis* 107:735, 1973.
13. Burrows B, et al. The emphysematous and bronchial types of chronic airways obstruction: A clinicopathological study of patients in London and Chicago. *Lancet* 1:830, 1966.
14. Burrows B, et al. Patterns of cardiovascular dysfunction in chronic obstructive lung disease. *N Engl J Med* 286:912, 1972.
15. Burrows B, et al. Quantitative relationships between cigarette smoking and ventilatory function. *Am Rev Respir Dis* 115:195, 1977.
16. Burrows B, et al. Clinical types of chronic obstructive lung disease in London and Chicago: A study of one hundred patients. *Am Rev Respir Dis* 90:14, 1964.
17. Butler C. Lung surface area in various morpho-

logic forms of emphysema. *Am Rev Respir Dis* 114:237, 1976.

18. Cosio MG, et al. The relation between structural changes in small airways and pulmonary function tests. *N Engl J Med* 298:1277, 1978.

19. Cromie JB. Correlation of anatomic pulmonary emphysema and right ventricular hypertrophy. *Am Rev Respir Dis* 84:657, 1961.

20. Cullen JH, et al. A prospective clinical-pathologic study of the lungs and heart in chronic obstructive lung disease. *Am Rev Respir Dis* 102:190, 1970.

21. Depierre A, et al. Quantitative study of parenchyma and small conductive airways in chronic nonspecific lung disease. *Chest* 62:699, 1972.

22. Dornhorst AC. Respiratory insufficiency. *Lancet* 1:1185, 1955.

23. Dosman J, et al. The use of helium-oxygen mixture during maximum expiratory flow to demonstrate obstruction in small airways in smokers. *J Clin Invest* 55:1090, 1975.

24. Dunnill MS. Quantitative methods in the study of pulmonary pathology. *Thorax* 17:320, 1962.

25. Eriksson S. Studies in alpha₁-antitrypsin deficiency. *Acta Med Scand Suppl* 432:1, 1965.

26. Esterly JR, Heard BE. Multiple bronchiolar stenoses in a patient with generalized airways obstruction. *Thorax* 20:309, 1965.

27. Filley GF, et al. Chronic obstructive bronchopulmonary disease: II. Oxygen transport in two clinical types. *Am J Med* 44:26, 1968.

28. Fishman AP. The roads to respiratory insufficiency. *Ann NY Acad Sci* 121:657, 1965.

29. Fletcher CM, et al. The diagnosis of pulmonary emphysema in the presence of chronic bronchitis. *Q J Med* 323:33, 1963.

30. Gould GA, et al. Measurements of lung density in life can quantitate distal air space enlargement—An essential defining feature of human emphysema. *Am Rev Respir Dis* 137:380, 1988.

31. Greaves IA, Colebatch HJH. Elastic behavior and structure of normal and emphysematous lungs postmortem. *Am Rev Respir Dis* 121:127, 1980.

32. Hale KA, et al. Lung disease in long-term smokers with and without chronic airflow obstruction. *Am Rev Respir Dis* 130:716, 1984.

33. Hasleton PS. Right ventricular hypertrophy in emphysema. *J Pathol* 110:27, 1973.

34. Hicken P, Heath D, Brewer D. The relation between the weight of the right ventricle and the percentage of abnormal air space in the lung in emphysema. *J Pathol Bacteriol* 9:519, 1966.

35. Hogg JC, Macklem PT, Thurlbeck WM. Site and nature of airway obstruction in chronic obstructive lung disease. *N Engl J Med* 278:1355, 1968.

36. Hogg JC, et al. Elastic properties of the centrilobular emphysematous space. *J Clin Invest* 48:1306, 1969.

37. Hyatt RE, Plath RE. Influence of lung parenchyma on pressure-diameter behavior of dog bronchi. *J Appl Physiol* 21:1448, 1966.

38. Ingram RH Jr, O'Cain CF. Frequency dependence of compliance in apparently healthy smokers versus nonsmokers. *Bull Physiopathol Respir* 7:195, 1971.

39. Jones JG, Fraser RB, Nadel JA. Effect of changing airway mechanics on maximum expiratory flow. *J Appl Physiol* 38:1012, 1975.

40. Jones NL. Pulmonary gas exchange during exercise in patients with chronic airway obstruction. *Clin Sci* 31:39, 1966.

41. Kahana LM, Aronovitch M, Place R. A comparative study of the clinical and functional pattern in emphysematous patients with and without chronic respiratory failure. *Am Rev Respir Dis* 87:699, 1963.

42. Karpick RJ, et al. Pathological findings in respiratory failure: Goblet cell metaplasia, alveolar damage, and myocardial infarction. *Ann Intern Med* 72:189, 1970.

43. Kim WD, et al. Centrilobular and panlobular emphysema in smokers. Two distinct morphologic and functional entities. *Am Rev Respir Dis* 144:1385, 1991.

44. Knudson RJ, Lebowitz MD. Comparison of flow-volume and closing volume variables in a random population. *Am Rev Respir Dis* 116:1039, 1977.

45. Laennec RTH. *A Treatise on the Diseases of the Chest and on Mediate Auscultation* (4th ed). Translated by Sir John Forbes. London: Longmans, 1834.

46. Leopold JG, Gough J. The centrilobular form of hypertrophic emphysema and its relation to chronic bronchitis. *Thorax* 12:219, 1957.

47. Lyons JP, et al. Pulmonary disability in coal workers' pneumoconiosis. *Br Med J* 1:713, 1972.

48. Macklem PT. Obstruction in small airways: A challenge to medicine (editorial). *Am J Med* 52:721, 1972.

49. Maisel JL, et al. The significance of bronchial atrophy. *Am J Pathol* 67:371, 1972.

50. Marcus JH, et al. Exercise performance in relation to the pathophysiologic type of chronic obstructive pulmonary disease. *Ann Intern Med* 49:14, 1970.

51. Martin CJ, Katsura S, Cochran TH. The relationship of chronic bronchitis to the diffuse obstructive pulmonary syndrome. *Am Rev Respir Dis* 102:362, 1970.

52. Matsuba K, Thurlbeck WM. The number and dimensions of small airways in nonemphysematous lungs. *Am Rev Respir Dis* 104:516, 1971.

53. Matsuba K, Thurlbeck WM. The number and dimensions of small airways in emphysematous lungs. *Am J Pathol* 67:265, 1972.

54. Matsuba K, Thurlbeck WM. Disease of the small airways in chronic bronchitis. *Am Rev Respir Dis* 107:552, 1973.

55. Matsuba K, et al. The changes in airways structure associated with reduced expiratory volume in one second. *Eur Respir J* 2:834, 1989.

56. McKenzie HI, Glick M, Outhred KG. Chronic bronchitis in coal miners: Antemortem-postmortem comparisons. *Thorax* 24:527, 1969.

57. McLean KH. The pathogenesis of pulmonary emphysema. *Am J Med* 25:62, 1958.

58. Mead J, et al. Significance of the relationship between lung recoil and maximum expiratory flow. *J Appl Physiol* 22:95, 1967.

59. Mitchell RS, et al. The significance of morphologic chronic hyperplastic bronchitis. *Am Rev Respir Dis* 93:720, 1966.

60. Mitchell RS, et al. The right ventricle in chronic airway obstruction: A clinicopathologic study. *Am Rev Respir Dis* 114:147, 1976.

61. Mitchell RS, et al. Chronic obstructive bronchopulmonary disease: IV. The clinical and physiological differentiation of chronic bronchitis and emphysema. *Am J Med Sci* 247:513, 1964.

62. Mitchell RS, et al. The morphologic features of the bronchi, bronchioles, and alveoli in chronic airway obstruction: A clinicopathologic study. *Am Rev Respir Dis* 114:137, 1976.

63. Mon E, Ultman JS. Monte Carlo simulation of simultaneous gas flow and diffusion in an asymmetric distal pulmonary airway model. *Bull Math Biol* 38:61, 1976.

64. Nagai A, West WW, Thurlbeck WM. The National Institutes of Health Positive-Pressure Breathing Trial: Pathology studies: II. Correlation between morphologic findings, clinical findings, and evidence of air-flow obstruction. *Am Rev Respir Dis* 132:946, 1985.

65. National Heart, Lung, and Blood Institute, Division of Lung Diseases. Workshop report: The definition of emphysema. *Am Rev Respir Dis* 132:182, 1985.

66. Niewoehner DE, Kleinerman J. Effects of experimental emphysema and bronchiolitis on lung mechanics and morphometry. *J Appl Physiol* 35:25, 1973.

67. Niewoehner DE, Kleinerman J. Morphologic basis of pulmonary resistance in the human lung and effects of aging. *J Appl Physiol* 36:412, 1974.

68. Niewoehner DE, Kleinerman J, Rice DB. Pathologic changes in the peripheral airways of young cigarette smokers. *N Engl J Med* 291:755, 1974.

69. Niewoehner DE, Knoke J, Kleinerman J. Peripheral airways as a determinant of ventilatory function in the human lung. *J Clin Invest* 60:139, 1977.

70. Olsen CR, Stevens AE, McIlroy MB. Rigidity of trachea and bronchi during muscular contraction. *J Appl Physiol* 23:27, 1967.

71. Oxhoj H, Bake B, Wilhelmensen L. Ability of spirometry, flow-volume curves, and the nitrogen closing volume test to detect smokers: A population study. *Scand J Respir Dis* 58:80, 1977.

72. Pardaens J, van de Woestijne KP, Clement J. A physical model of expiration. *J Appl Physiol* 33:479, 1972.

73. Pare PD, et al. Exponential analysis of the pressure-volume curve as a predictor of emphysema. *Am Rev Respir Dis* 126:54, 1982.

74. Park SS, et al. Relationship of bronchitis and emphysema to altered pulmonary function. *Am Rev Respir Dis* 102:927, 1970.

75. Peto R, et al. The relevance in adults of air-flow obstruction, but not mucus hypersecretion, to mortality from chronic lung disease. *Am Rev Respir Dis* 128:491, 1983.

76. Pride NB, et al. Determinants of maximal expiratory flow from the lungs. *J Appl Physiol* 23:646, 1967.

77. Reid LM. Pathology of chronic bronchitis. *Lancet* 1:275, 1954.

78. Saito K, et al. The "destructive index" in nonemphysematous and emphysematous lungs. Morphologic observations and correlation with function. *Am Rev Respir Dis* 139:308, 1989.

79. Scott KW, Steiner GM. Postmortem assessment of chronic airways obstruction by tantalum. *Thorax* 30:405, 1975.

80. Seely JE, Zuskin E, Bouhuys A. Cigarette smoking: Objective evidence for lung damage in teenagers. *Science* 172:741, 1971.

81. Silvers GW, Petty TL, Stanford RE. Elastic recoil changes in early emphysema. *Thorax* 35:490, 1980.

82. Simonson T, Heard B, Laws JW. Severe irreversible airways obstruction without emphysema. *Thorax* 18:361, 1963.

83. Sobonya RE, Kleinerman J. Morphometric studies of bronchi in young smokers. *Am Rev Respir Dis* 105:768, 1972.

84. Spain DM, Kaufman G. The basic lesion in chronic emphysema. *Am Rev Tuberc* 68:24, 1952.

85. Sweet HC, et al. Panlobular and centrilobular emphysema: Correlation of clinical findings with pathologic patterns. *Ann Intern Med* 55:565, 1961.

86. Symonds G, Rensetti AD Jr, Mitchell MM. The diffusing capacity in pulmonary emphysema. *Am Rev Respir Dis* 109:391, 1974.

87. Thurlbeck WM. A clinicopathologic study of emphysema in an American hospital. *Thorax* 18:59, 1963.

88. Thurlbeck WM. Internal surface area and other measurements in emphysema. *Thorax* 22:483, 1967.

89. Thurlbeck WM. *Chronic Airflow Obstruction in Lung Disease.* Philadelphia: Saunders, 1976. Pp 370–378.

90. Thurlbeck WM. Postmortem lung volumes. *Thorax* 34:735, 1979.

91. Thurlbeck WM, et al. Chronic obstructive lung disease. A comparison between clinical, roentgenologic, functional, and morphologic criteria

in chronic bronchitis, emphysema, asthma, and bronchiectasis. *Medicine,* 49:81, 1970.

92. Thurlbeck WM, et al. A comparison of three methods for measuring emphysema. *Hum Pathol* 1:215, 1970.

93. van Brabrandt H, et al. Partitioning of pulmonary impedance in excised human and canine lungs. *J Appl Physiol* 55:1733, 1983.

94. Wagner PD, et al. Ventilation-perfusion inequality in chronic obstructive pulmonary disease. *J Clin Invest* 59:203, 1977.

95. Watanabe S, Mitchell M, Renzetti AD Jr. Correlation of structure and function in chronic pulmonary disease. *Am Rev Respir Dis* 92:221, 1965.

96. Wright JL, et al. The detection of small airways disease. *Am Rev Respir Dis* 129:989, 1984.

39

Clinical Aspects of Chronic Obstructive Pulmonary Disease

Dennis E. Niewoehner

Definition

Despite the efforts of several expert committees, some disagreement still surrounds the nomenclature of the obstructive lung disorders. In particular, there has been disagreement as to the best term to describe the clinical condition characterized by "persistent slowing of airflow during expiration" [2,3,46] in patients who are not thought to have more specific entities such as asthma, bronchiectasis, or cystic fibrosis. Popular usage currently favors *chronic obstructive pulmonary disease* (COPD), and this term is used throughout.

COPD is sometimes diagnosed as chronic bronchitis or emphysema, or both. This practice has caused no great harm, but both emphysema and chronic bronchitis have other meanings agreed on by expert committees, and these official definitions relate only indirectly and imperfectly to the functional disturbance of airflow obstruction.

Emphysema is a pathologic entity "characterized by abnormal, permanent enlargement of airspaces distal to the terminal bronchiole, accompanied by the destruction of their walls, and without obvious fibrosis" [3,178]. Emphysema is an important cause of airflow obstruction in COPD, but the relationship between the extent of emphysema and the severity of airflow obstruction is imperfect. An occasional patient with fatal COPD may have no emphysema at all, whereas other patients with extensive emphysema may have only modest functional impairment. Thus, it seems prudent to restrict the use of emphysema to that condition which is recognized from pathologic examination or which may be diagnosed from specialized roentgenographic imaging procedures.

The greatest confusion arises with regards to the use of the term *chronic bronchitis*. Chronic bronchitis is properly a pathologic term meaning chronic inflammation of the large bronchi. However, chronic bronchitis also came to be defined as excess mucus secretion in the bronchial tree. Since this can be recognized in patients only as an increase in sputum expectoration, chronic bronchitis was further defined as a clinical condition characterized by "chronic cough and sputum production occurring on most days for at least 3 months in the year for at least 2 successive years" [3,46]. This definition was agreed on at a time when excess mucus secretion was thought to be an important cause of airflow obstruction, and many physicians used "chronic bronchitis" interchangeably with "COPD." Since it is now known that excess sputum expectoration is largely unrelated to airflow obstruction in COPD, this practice is clearly unacceptable. In this discussion, the use of "chronic bronchitis" is avoided wherever possible, and when mentioned, its definition conforms to that agreed on by expert committees.

There have also been efforts to delineate subsets of patients with COPD who were thought to have predominant "emphysema" or predominant "bronchitis." It is my opinion that a basis for making these distinctions has not been firmly established, and this subject is not addressed subsequently.

Symptoms and Signs

The typical patient with COPD is a middle-aged person with a long history of cigarette consumption who seeks medical care because of increasing breathlessness; less often, previously undiagnosed COPD is recognized during medical evaluation for another problem. Even in these cases, careful questioning usually elicits the history that the patient has voluntarily limited his or her activities because of breathlessness.

Symptoms commonly associated with COPD include dyspnea, wheezing, cough, and sputum expectoration. Of these, only dyspnea bears a consistent relationship to the presence and severity of airflow obstruction [177]. Dyspnea is less well understood than many other aspects of COPD, and because it is subjective and so difficult to quantitate, the central importance of the symptom to the patient may be forgotten.

The severity of dyspnea as judged by patient questionnaire tends to parallel the severity of airflow obstruction as determined by spirometry. Clinical studies indicate that in men the threshold for discernible exercise limitation occurs with 1-second forced expiratory volume (FEV_1) values of between 1.50 and 2.00 liters (representing approximately 50 to 60 percent of the predicted mean for middle-aged men of medium height) [177]. Below these values there is a reasonably consistent relationship between worsening ventilatory function and increasing dyspnea. Most patients with an FEV_1 of less than 1.50 liters admit that even though they can walk long distances on the level, they cannot maintain a normal pace. With a FEV_1 of less than 0.50 liter, few patients can walk more than 100 yards without resting, and many have dyspnea at rest.

While the FEV_1 parallels clinical disability, the relationship is not a perfect one. Certain patients with grossly impaired ventilatory function admit to little or no breathlessness, while others complain of disability that seems out of proportion to the degree of airflow obstruction. Because the sensation of breathlessness is subjective, much of the discrepancy can be explained by individual variation in the perception of the reaction to the same stimuli. However, the mechanism by which airflow obstruction causes dyspnea is not well understood, and other physiologic factors may be equally important [42,201].

The breathlessness associated with COPD cannot be reliably distinguished from dyspnea due to other cardiorespiratory disorders. Dyspnea is usually gradual in onset and frequently has been present for several years by the time the patient is first seen by a physician. Occasionally, patients date the onset of the symptoms to a severe, persistent "chest cold" in the recent past, but the significance of this is uncertain in view of evidence that episodic chest infections do not usually cause permanent loss in ventilatory function. The presence of episodic dyspnea, particularly in conjunction with increased cough and wheezing, suggests the existence of reversible airflow obstruction (asthma). Patients with severe COPD may report that their dyspnea varies with body position and it worsens at night; these symptoms do not distinguish COPD from congestive heart failure. The presence of COPD may be strongly suspected on the basis of the medical history, but laboratory evaluation is required to establish the diagnosis.

Dyspnea is usually the only symptom that can be directly attributed to COPD. Chronic productive cough is frequently present with COPD but is not essential to the diagnosis and does not correlate closely with physiologic abnormalities [57]. In terminal stages of COPD, patients may experience lassitude, anorexia, sleep disturbances, depression, and weight loss. Whether these signs and symptoms are a direct result of COPD, such as might be caused by derangements in systemic oxygen and carbon dioxide transport, or whether they are nonspecific effects of chronic invalidism is uncertain.

The physical signs of COPD are familiar to most physicians. Hyperexpansion of the chest wall imparts to it a barrel shape. The increase in thoracic gas volume is also responsible for the hyperresonance of the chest to percussion, the diminished vocal fremitus, the widened subcostal margin, and the low, relatively immobile diaphragm. Displacement of other organs by the overinflated lung explains the diminished area of cardiac dullness and the absent apical heart impulse. Distant or absent inspiratory breath sounds result both from the increased thoracic air volume and from decreased flow rates. Wheezing and rhonchi suggest local airways obstruction, either from mucous plugs or from airway stenosis. Increased resistance to airflow and the disadvantageous mechanical position of the overexpanded thoracic cage increase the work of breathing so that the patients frequently use their accessory muscles of respiration. The greater-than-normal forces required to move air in and out of the lungs result in wide intrathoracic pressure swings during the respiratory cycle. These pressure fluctuations are large enough to influence hemodynamic function. This is manifest as venous distension in the neck during expiration and as a paradoxical pulse. Systolic blood pressure may decrease by as much as 15 to 20 mmHg during inspiration in patients with severe COPD. Cyanosis of the lips and nail beds occurs with severe hypoxemia, particularly when associated with secondary polycythemia. COPD is not usually associated with clubbing of the fingers and the presence of this sign should alert the physician to the possibility of concurrent disease such as bronchiectasis or lung carcinoma. Cachexia, weight loss, and signs of neurologic dysfunction may be prominent features of near-terminal COPD. Cor pulmonale is a frequent complication of severe COPD, and it may be manifest as increasing dyspnea along with signs of fluid retention and increased systemic venous pressures.

A careful examination with an effort to identify the classic physical signs of COPD is an important part of patient evaluation. However, the physical examination should not be relied on to establish the diagnosis of COPD or to determine its severity. For example, the barrel-shaped chest was shown to be a normal finding in many older people [169]. The poor correlation between a physical examination diagnosis of COPD and spirometric values has been nicely documented [182]. In addition, interobserver agreement in identifying specific physical signs is surprisingly poor [74]. The agreement among different physicians as to the presence of certain common physical signs in patients with COPD fell midway between perfect concordance and that expected by chance alone, a finding confirmed in several studies [78,182,193]. It is unlikely that these disparities can be reduced appreciably because they persist even after careful physician training [78]. However, physical examination during initial evaluation remains valuable for excluding other causes of dyspnea and for guiding subsequent diagnostic efforts. Repeated physical examination during follow-up in patients with COPD is an important part of total patient care and provides information about the patient's state of well-being that is not otherwise available.

Roentgenographic Signs

A chest roentgenogram is an essential part of the initial medical evaluation of all patients with an undiagnosed complaint of dyspnea. However, its chief diagnostic value may lie in what it does not reveal, namely, roentgenographic signs that suggest some cause for dyspnea other than COPD. The chest roentgenogram is a relatively insensitive test for COPD, and it may appear normal or near-normal in the face of severe airflow obstruction. The criteria for the roentgenographic diagnosis of COPD have been established in several studies and these criteria fall into two main categories: lung hyperinflation and irregular radiolucencies of the lung fields [150,191,203].

LUNG HYPERINFLATION

The standard chest roentgenogram in a patient with severe COPD reveals a diaphragm that is depressed with an altered contour (Fig. 39-1). The diaphragm is abnormally low if the dome is at the level of the anterior aspect of the seventh rib or below, and it is considered flattened if the maximum curvature is less than 1.5 cm [191]. It has also been suggested that the sternodiaphragmatic angle on the lateral chest film may be a useful sign [203]. In normal subjects this angle is acute, but in patients with COPD it is frequently greater than 90 degrees. Lung hyperinflation is also indicated by an increase in the retrosternal clear space. This distance is measured horizontally between the posterior edge of the sternum and the most anterior portion of the ascending aorta. Some experts have considered a distance of 2.5 cm or more as being abnormal, but others believe a value of 4.5 cm to be a more specific criterion for COPD [150,191,203].

IRREGULAR RADIOLUCENCY OF THE LUNG FIELDS

Emphysema results in a loss of alveolar tissue and a diminution in the number of blood vessels. As a consequence, affected areas are less dense, and these abnormalities can be appreciated roentgenographically as areas of radiolucencies in the peripheral lung fields. On the standard chest roentgenogram these changes may be quite subtle, and the presence of radiolucencies can be appreciated only by comparison against more normal-appearing regions. The edges of bullae can frequently be identified by the presence of thin, curved lines on the plain chest roentgenogram, and these changes can be regarded as pathognomonic for bullous emphysema.

The irregular radiolucencies associated with emphysema can be much better appreciated with tomography, particularly with the superior resolution provided by computed tomography (CT). When regional variations in lung tissue density are quantitated by CT scans, remarkably good correlations with the extent of anatomic emphysema can be demonstrated [20,79]. At present, this type of study remains an investigational tool, as precise knowledge concerning the anatomic distribution and severity of emphysema only rarely has practical implications in clinical management.

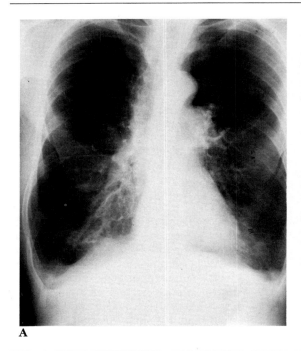

A

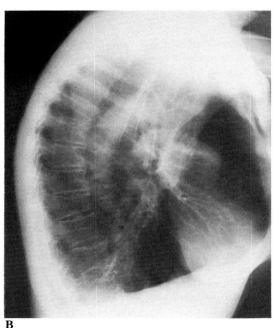

B

Laboratory Diagnosis

Pulmonary function testing is essential for establishing the diagnosis of COPD. It is evident from the foregoing discussion that clinical and roentgenographic evaluations are not reliable even in patients with more advanced disease, yet many patients are misdiagnosed as having COPD on the basis of vague clinical criteria or because a chest roentgenogram has been overinterpreted. Whenever there is a suspicion of COPD, pulmonary function testing is indicated. Several categories of testing may be helpful.

Measures of Airflow Obstruction

The most practical and useful physiologic test of airflow obstruction is spirometry. The conventional instrument is the water-sealed spirometer from which the expired volume-time relationship is obtained. With newer types of instruments, the same data can be replotted as a flow-volume relationship. Identical information is obtained by both methods (Fig. 39-2). Various indices of maximal expiratory flow rates, including the FEV_1, the forced expiratory flow between 200 and 1200 ml of forced vital capacity ($FEF_{200-1200}$), the mid–expiratory phase forced expiratory flow

Fig. 39-1. Chest roentgenogram from a patient with severe chronic airflow obstruction. In the posteroanterior projection (*left*), the lungs appear hyperinflated with attenuation of the peripheral lung markings. The lateral projection (*right*) shows loss of the normal contour of the hemidiaphragms and an increase in the retrosternal clear space.

($FEF_{25-75\%}$), and other less frequently used values, are calculated from the spirogram. There is a high degree of concordance among these different indices, but because of individual variations in the slope of the expired volume-time relationship, the correlation is not perfect.

The maximal breathing capacity (MBC), or maximal voluntary ventilation (MVV), is an older test for demonstrating airflow obstruction. In this test, the patient is instructed to inhale and exhale maximally for a short time, usually 15 to 20 seconds, and the volume of expired air is measured. When this test is properly performed, abnormalities closely parallel spirometric abnormalities [112,177]. However, it is unclear that it provides independent information that is diagnostically useful, and for this reason it has fallen out of favor.

Airflow obstruction also may be evaluated by measurement of total pulmonary resistance and airway resistance [58,136]. These measurements

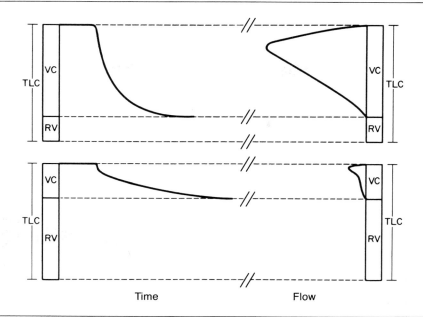

Time   Flow

Fig. 39-2. Characteristic spirometric and lung volume abnormalities in a patient with severe COPD (*lower panel*). Spirometry is shown on the left as a volume-time relationship and on the right as a flow-volume relationship. In comparison with the normal subject (*upper panel*), the patient with COPD has a reduction in mid–maximal flow rates, a decrease in the forced expiratory vital capacity (*VC*), and a corresponding increase in the residual volume (*RV*). TLC = total lung capacity.

require more sophisticated instrumentation than does spirometry, and while they may be useful for investigation, they provide little practical information in the clinical management of patients with COPD. Some patients with advanced COPD as assessed by spirometry may have normal or near-normal pulmonary resistance. An increase in pulmonary resistance is generally regarded as evidence that the patient has relatively more airway disease than emphysema, even though this interpretation has not been rigorously proved from physiologic and pathologic correlative studies.

Lung Volume

The characteristic lung volume abnormalities in COPD are (1) a decrease in the vital capacity (VC), (2) an increase in the residual volume (RV) and the residual volume–total lung capacity (RV/TLC) ratio, (3) an increase in the functional residual capacity (FRC), and (4) a variable increase in TLC. The interpretation of abnormalities in lung volumes is limited by the large normal variation in lung size. For this reason, a scaled volume, such as the RV/TLC ratio, is probably more useful than any absolute lung volume. It is unclear whether the measurement of lung volumes adds independent and useful information about the patient with COPD. Increases in the RV/TLC ratio are observed relatively early in the natural history of COPD, and the magnitude of these changes continues to parallel spirometric abnormalities in more advanced stages of the disease [14,177]. The measurement of lung volumes may in certain circumstances be useful in differentiating interstitial fibrosis and other forms of restrictive lung disease from COPD. However, these distinctions are usually evident from other clinical and roentgenographic findings.

Lung volumes can be measured either by the washin or the washout of tracer gases such as helium or by plethysmography [59,139]. Because of the long equilibration times for tracer-gas methods in the presence of severe COPD, plethysmography is probably the preferred method. Surprisingly accurate estimates of TLC can also be made from the standard chest roentgenogram [151].

Ventilation Distribution and Gas-Exchange Abnormalities

An early and characteristic physiologic abnormality in COPD is arterial hypoxemia. Mild hypoxemia has been observed in the very early stages of COPD when spirometry values are normal or nearly normal [119]. As COPD worsens, hypoxemia also tends to worsen, although the relationship between the severity of COPD and the severity of hypoxemia is imperfect for unknown reasons. Elevation of the $PaCO_2$ is usually a manifestation of advanced disease, but it may at times be much greater or much less than expected from the FEV_1. With severe COPD, the $PaCO_2$ increases at an average rate of about 1 mmHg each year [104].

It is now generally believed that the major mechanism underlying the arterial blood gas derangements in COPD is the mismatching of ventilation and perfusion in different lung units. This results principally from the uneven distribution of inspired ventilation and to a lesser extent from pathologic alterations in the distribution of blood flow to the lung. Tests using various tracer gases have been devised to assess the distribution of ventilation.

The single-breath oxygen test was introduced as a means for assessing the evenness of ventilation [76] (Fig. 39-3). The subject inspires a single breath of pure oxygen and then slowly exhales while expired volume and nitrogen concentration at the mouth are measured and plotted against each other. A positive slope in phase III, the "alveolar plateau," indicates that different portions of the lung with different concentrations of residual nitrogen are emptying asynchronously. In normal subjects, this slope is usually not more than a 2 percent rise in nitrogen concentration per liter of expired volume, but this value may rise to as much as 10 or 15 percent/liter in patients with COPD.

The evenness of ventilation also can be assessed by the multibreath washin or washout of tracer gases. One such method is the multiple-breath washout of nitrogen, in which the patient inspires pure oxygen and the nitrogen concentration of expired air is measured on a breath-by-breath basis [180] (Fig. 39-4). In normal subjects, the decrease in nitrogen concentration with each succeeding breath can be fitted by a single exponential function, which is interpreted to mean that all regions of the lung are emptying at very nearly the same rate. In patients with COPD, the washout time is prolonged and the curve cannot

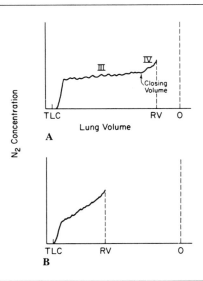

Fig. 39-3. Representative tracings from the single-breath oxygen test in a normal subject (A) and a patient with COPD (B). In normal subjects, the slope of phase III (the "alveolar plateau") is no more than a 2 percent change in nitrogen fraction for each liter of expired air. Phase III is delineated from phase IV by an inflection point, the closing volume. In the patient with COPD, the slope of phase III is much steeper, suggesting less even ventilation, and frequently the closing volume cannot be identified. TLC = total lung capacity; RV = residual volume.

be fitted by a single exponential function, which indicates the presence of slowly ventilated functional compartments. Similar information is gained by measuring equilibration times for tracer gases in closed systems, such as the helium-mixing efficiency index [15].

The uneven distribution of ventilation and perfusion results in some lung regions having a relative excess of ventilation over perfusion (high $\dot{V}/\dot{Q}$ zone) and other regions with less ventilation relative to perfusion (low $\dot{V}/\dot{Q}$ zone). High $\dot{V}/\dot{Q}$ abnormalities can be detected by a relatively simple laboratory test, the measurement of the physiologic dead space. Direct quantitative assessment of low $\dot{V}/\dot{Q}$ abnormalities requires specialized techniques that are beyond the capabilities of all but the most sophisticated laboratories [217]. Combined ventilation and perfusion scanning with radioactive xenon allows a rather crude assessment of $\dot{V}/\dot{Q}$ disturbances, which have been found even in early COPD [5].

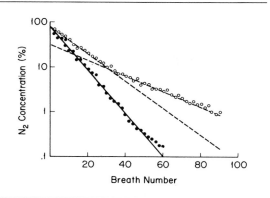

Fig. 39-4. Multiple-breath nitrogen washout in a normal subject (*solid circles*) and in a patient with COPD (*open circles*). The logarithm of end-expired nitrogen concentration measured at the mouth is plotted as a function of breath number. In the normal subject, this relationship is accurately described by a straight line, which suggests that various regions in the lung are emptying synchronously. In the patient with COPD, this relationship cannot be accurately described by a single linear function, which suggests that some regions of the lung are emptying more rapidly than others.

Various laboratory methods are available to measure the diffusing capacity for carbon monoxide (DLCO), and most patients with advanced COPD have a reduced DLCO. The impairment in the DLCO in patients with COPD correlates to some degree with the extent of anatomic emphysema, presumably because the destruction of alveolar walls reduces the surface area available for gas exchange [28,159]. The DLCO, particularly as measured by the single-breath methods, may also be affected by $\dot{V}/\dot{Q}$ abnormalities [120].

Blood gas measurements are important in the initial evaluation of patients with COPD, as a means for evaluating the severity of the disease and for assessing the need for and response to chronic oxygen therapy. Repeated blood gas measurements are also invaluable during the treatment of acute respiratory failure caused by COPD.

Interpretation of Pulmonary Function Tests in the Diagnosis of COPD

COPD has been defined as a functional disorder so that its presence and severity are logically determined from pulmonary function tests. Questions arise both about the interpretation of individual tests and about diagnosis when the many available tests are used in combination.

Ideally, COPD in an individual patient would be defined as a reduction in ventilatory capacity below that which would have existed in the absence of disease. Since there is usually no way of knowing accurately what disease-free ventilatory function should be in a given individual, test values can only be compared against values for normal subjects who are matched for age, sex, and height. Unfortunately, the ranges of normal values for all tests are sufficiently large to severely limit diagnostic sensitivity.

The test most commonly used to assess ventilatory function, the FEV_1, serves as an example. The FEV_1 in normal subjects correlates with height, sex, and age, but even after adjusting for these variables, the residual variance remains large [109,112,144]. For example, in a study of several hundred apparently healthy men, the predicted FEV_1 for 50-year-old men 70 in. tall is 3.59 liters [112]. One standard deviation of the regression mean is 0.52 liter, so that assuming normally distributed values, the FEV_1 for approximately 63 percent of the men in the group would fall into the range of 3.07 to 4.11 liters and that for approximately 95 percent it would fall into the range of 2.55 to 4.63 liters.

Patients with dyspnea or exercise intolerance attributable to COPD generally have an FEV_1 of 1.50 to 2.00 liters or less. Since a normal 50-year-old man should not have an FEV_1 of less than 2.00 liters, little problem exists in distinguishing most patients with symptomatic COPD on the basis of the FEV_1. However, the distinction between normal and abnormal may be less clear in those patients with milder disease. In the case of the 50-year-old man mentioned above, an FEV_1 of 2.50 liters would fall within the lower limits of what could be considered normal values. However, if this man's FEV_1 had been 4.50 liters in the absence of disease, the measured value would represent a substantial loss in function, and he might well have symptoms attributable to ventilatory limitation. This example is extreme but it illustrates the problem of distinguishing milder forms of disease using parameters that have an inherently high variability in the normal population.

Some clinicians consider any spirometric value that is less than 80 percent of the predicted mean to be abnormal. This practice has little scientific justification, as the various parameters derived from the spirometric tracing do not have the same variability in the normal population [194]. It seems appropriate to set limits of normal for each test parameter on the basis of the predicted means and the standard deviations about the mean. If a test value is considered abnormal when it falls more than two standard deviations below the mean, only a small percentage of the "normal" population will be diagnosed as having COPD, and few individuals with COPD so severe as to cause symptoms will be excluded. For most purposes, this criterion appears reasonable.

Which test(s) should be utilized in the diagnosis of COPD? Most tests of airflow show a high degree of intercorrelation, but this concordance is imperfect, so that a patient may be judged normal by some tests and abnormal by others. Whether the patient has COPD cannot be answered definitely. However, no spirometric indices have been shown to relate more closely to clinical disability or to prognosis in COPD than has the FEV_1 [36,177]. Since reductions in the FEV_1 are also observed in lung diseases that are not obstructive, it is useful to normalize the FEV_1 with respect to the forced vital capacity (FVC) (FEV_1/FVC). Obstructive lung diseases are associated with a reduction in the FEV_1/FVC ratio, whereas it is preserved in restrictive lung disorders. The FEV_1 and the FVC are the most reproducible of the commonly calculated spirometric variables, and this is one factor in their diagnostic superiority [121]. It has been suggested that the FEV_1 is relatively insensitive in the diagnosis of milder forms of COPD; however, careful studies have not indicated that any single test or combination of tests is appreciably more sensitive than the FEV_1 alone [108,156]. For most purposes, COPD is best defined from the FEV_1 and its ratio to the FVC.

Prevalence and Mortality

COPD is an important public health problem, but accurate estimates of prevalence and mortality are difficult to obtain. Mortality figures and hospital admission rates for patients with a primary diagnosis of COPD provide some measure of the magnitude of the problem, even though both are subject to well-recognized classification errors.

The enormous impact of cigarette smoking and COPD on mortality was first shown by Doll and Hill [55]. In their classic study of British physicians, they attributed a standardized annual death rate of 34 per 100,000 directly to chronic bronchitis (which is presumed to mean COPD principally) over the 10-year period from 1951 to 1961. Among cigarette smokers, this rate increased to 51 per 100,000 and was about 10 times greater than among nonsmokers. Subsequently, a significant number of physicians stopped smoking, and overall mortality rates have fallen accordingly [75]. Currently in the United States, COPD is thought to account for approximately 100,000 deaths per year, or 3.6 percent of deaths from all causes, making it the fifth leading cause of death [91]. As might be expected, death rates from COPD are much higher among older-aged groups, but they are appreciably higher in men than in women. The influence of gender undoubtedly reflects historical patterns in cigarette use, and this can be expected to narrow as sexual differences in cigarette consumption have narrowed.

Mortality rates do not reflect the fact that COPD also may contribute to death from other causes and that COPD causes much morbidity and disability in those patients in whom COPD is not the primary cause of death. Governmental reports indicate that COPD is the primary diagnosis in more than 2 percent of all disabled persons in the United States and that in persons less than 65 years old, this figure is substantially higher [149]. COPD is the principal reason for about 13 percent of all general hospital admissions in the United States. The costs of hospitalization do not include the additional expenses of outpatient care for this condition or the cost of lost working days, expenses that probably total in the tens of billions of dollars.

Cross-sectional community surveys provide the most reliable data concerning the prevalence of COPD, though these data are heavily dependent on the screening tests employed and the criteria chosen to indicate the presence of disease. Using spirometric data and clinical evaluations, Ferris and associates [69] determined that 8.5 percent of adult men and 8.1 percent of adult women in Berlin, New Hampshire, had COPD. This figure rose to 13.4 percent in men between the ages of 55 and 64 years. In a study of white subjects in Tucson, Arizona, Knudson and associates [107] concluded from spirometric data that as many as 20 to 25 percent of the total population had some evidence for COPD. In a similar cross-sectional study of Swedish men, Oxhoj and associates [156] found functional abnormalities in about one-half of middle-aged smokers. In a 15-year prospective study in Tecumseh, Michigan, Higgins and coworkers [92] determined that the prevalence of COPD (defined as an FEV_1 of less than 65 percent of the predicted value) was 16.3 percent in men 45 to 54 years old and was 5.0 percent in women of the same age.

Causes

COPD will not develop unless age-related losses in pulmonary function exceed the normal expected losses by a considerable margin. Causes of COPD should be recognizable from their association with an excessively rapid fall in ventilatory function over time. Current knowledge about the causes of COPD has been provided primarily by population studies in which the effects of specific factors have been isolated through sophisticated sampling and analytic techniques.

It is clear that COPD does not have a single cause, and that multiple factors must act in concert for the disorder to become clinically evident. Cigarette smoking is the principal identified risk factor in the causation of COPD, yet only a minority of persons who smoke develop COPD while an occasional lifelong nonsmoker may develop severe disease. Other factors are clearly operative, but their identity remains largely unknown.

Aging and Ventilatory Function

Severe COPD is uncommon in persons less than 40 years old, but it becomes increasingly prevalent in patients beyond that age. This is apparent from survey studies of the general population and is also evident from observations in general medical clinics [107,108,156]. Most patients with COPD seek medical attention because of symptoms when they are between 55 and 65 years old [36,177]. It is believed that the loss of ventilatory function that characterizes COPD occurs at a relatively slow rate, so that the cumulative effects of lung damage become clinically manifest only in older people. However, the relationship between aging and COPD can also be attributed to the deleterious effects of the normal aging process on lung function.

Advancing age in the adult is associated with a decrease in maximal expiratory flow rates [109,112,144], an increase in pulmonary resistance measured during tidal breathing [77], and a loss of lung elastic recoil [213]. Other tests of ventilatory function, including the closing volume and the frequency dependence of dynamic compliance, are also strongly age-dependent [18,33]. Except for TLC, the subdivisions of lung volumes

also change with advancing age; the FRC and the RV increase as the FVC decreases [25]. The directions of age-related changes are the same as those seen in COPD; differences are only quantitative. Therefore, it is necessary to define the normal aging effects so as to assess their contribution to the development of COPD.

The effects of normal aging have been best characterized in the case of spirometry. Earlier studies suggested that the FEV_1 declined throughout adult life, but more recent data indicate that the maximal FEV_1 occurs between 25 and 30 years old and that it declines only thereafter [109]. Most studies indicate that the loss in function is linear, but others have suggested that the rate of decline may accelerate slightly with advancing age [72].

Values for the average decline in FEV_1 from representative studies are given in Table 39-1. The FEV_1 in the average man declines at an average rate of approximately 30 ml/year. When expressed as a percent of the original FEV_1, the rate of decline is the same for men of different heights [47]. That is, tall men with large lungs and a large FEV_1 experience a more rapid decline with age when the FEV_1 is expressed in absolute units, but with normalization, tall men and short men lose function at the same rate. Available data suggest that with appropriate scaling factors, sex and race are also unimportant factors in determining the age-related rate of decline in the FEV_1 [221].

Averaged losses in the FEV_1 with advancing age might conceal interesting information about individual variations, as accelerated rates of "normal" aging in some people might make them more susceptible to the development of COPD. Reliable data on this subject are unavailable, as the data are difficult to obtain and the estimates of individual FEV_1 losses are associated with large errors, even when measurements are performed over an extended period [72].

Although the average annual losses in ventilatory capacity are small, the cumulative effects over an adult's lifetime are substantial (Fig. 39-5). The nomograms developed by Knudson and associates [109] predict an FEV_1 of 4.22 liters for a 25-year-old man 175 cm tall. With an annual loss of 27 ml, the FEV_1 of this same person will have fallen to 3.14 liters at age 65 years. Symptoms from COPD are not usually manifest until the FEV_1 has fallen to less than 2.0 liters. It is evident that aging alone will not cause COPD in the average person. However, aging does cause an appreciable loss of functional reserve, and this is an

Table 39-1. Age-related losses in FEV_1

Study	Subject population	Age range (yr)	No. of subjects	Annual FEV_1 loss (ml/s)	Comments
Kory et al. [112]	Hospital personnel and patients	18–66	389	28	Asymptomatic smokers included
Berglund et al. [21]	Swedish population	20–70	296	33	Smoking history not given
Ferris et al. [71]	Community cross section	25–74	157	28	Healthy nonsmokers
Cotes et al. [50]	Community cross section	20–64	275	33	Includes smokers
Morris et al. [144]	Members of church group	20–84	517	32	Healthy nonsmokers
Knudson et al. [109]	Community cross section	25–79	128	27	Healthy nonsmokers without respiratory symptoms

important factor, when coupled with the cumulative effects of lung damage from cigarette smoking and other insults, in allowing clinical expression of the disease.

Cigarette Smoking

Expert and unbiased observers no longer question the causal relationship between cigarette smoking and COPD. This relationship was long suspected by physicians, and these suspicions were definitively supported by the report of the Advisory Committee to the Surgeon General in 1964 [214]. This opinion has subsequently been updated [215] and even more strongly affirmed. Cigarette smoking is so important as a cause that COPD would disappear as an important public health problem if cigarette smoking were to cease.

Several independent lines of evidence link cigarette smoking to COPD. Most general physicians have long been aware that patients with COPD almost invariably describe a long history of heavy cigarette consumption. Allowing for a lag time of 20 to 30 years while the disease develops, the apparent increases in mortality from COPD in western nations closely parallels increases in per capita consumption of tobacco [214]. Longitudinal observations in British physicians indicated that mortality from COPD was increased by approximately a factor of 10 in smokers are compared to nonsmokers [55]. Several necropsy studies revealed a marked increase in the prevalence and severity of emphysema in lungs from cigarette smokers [4,9,195].

Functional abnormalities have consistently been demonstrated in survey studies in male and female smokers of all ages [8,38,184,211,222]. The extent of these abnormalities worsens with advancing age and increased tobacco consumption. However, subtle spirometric abnormalities have been demonstrated both in teenage and in college-age smokers [162,183]. Functional abnormalities in young smokers have also been demonstrated with tests of the closing volume, the frequency dependence of dynamic compliance, and helium-oxygen flow-volume curves [35,56,97]. The studies in younger smokers suggest that mild lung damage occurs within a short time after the onset of cigarette smoking, an interpretation that has been confirmed by pathologic studies [152].

The magnitude of the average cigarette smoke–induced losses in ventilatory function is known from population studies. A representative and excellent study of this type was performed by Fletcher and colleagues [72]. They prospectively followed several hundred London postal and transport workers for 8 years. They measured ventilatory function at regular interviews while collecting information relating to several suspected factors in the development of COPD. Their results and conclusions concerning cigarette smoking are of particular interest. Nonsmokers in their study experienced an annual decline in the FEV_1 that averaged 36 ml/year.

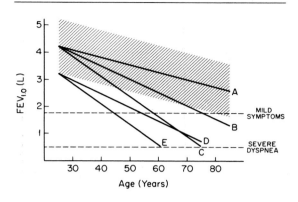

Fig. 39-5. Age-related and smoking-related changes in the FEV_1. *A* represents average prediced FEV_1 losses (27 ml/s/year) in a nonsmoking white man who is 175 cm tall [102]. (*Shaded area* represents range of normal values.) If that individual smokes cigarettes regularly, the predicted annual loss in the FEV_1 is approximately 50 ml/s (*B*) but may be as much as 100 ml/s (*C*). *D* and *E* represent average and accelerated smoking effects in an individual whose FEV_1 at age 25 years is already at the lower limits of normal.

Depending on consumption (heavy or light, regular or irregular), smokers suffered a loss in FEV_1 that on average was 10 to 20 ml/year greater than that for nonsmokers. This had the characteristics of a causal relationship in that heavier smokers experienced the more rapid decline in function.

Burrows and associates [38] obtained similar results from their cross-sectional and longitudinal population studies in Tucson, Arizona. The data are presented in a manner that does not allow direct comparison with the London workers, but the magnitude of the average losses in lung function due to smoking appears closely comparable in the two studies. The relationship between heavier cigarette consumption and more rapid decline in function is more clearly evident in the Tucson study.

These and similar investigations have shown conclusively that cigarette smoking does cause an excessively rapid decline in lung function. However, they also show that the usual added effect of smoking on annual FEV_1 decline (between 10 and 25 ml/year) is relatively modest and somewhat less than that which can be attributed to normal aging alone. This average effect is sufficiently small so that most people who smoke will not develop severe COPD. Consider again the example of the average 25-year-old man with an FEV_1 of approximately 4.0 liters (see Fig. 39-5). Normal aging will reduce his FEV_1 at an annual rate of 27 ml to about 3.0 liters at age 65 years. Even if these losses are doubled by heavy cigarette consumption, his FEV_1 would still be at about 2.0 liters at age 65 years. At this level of function he might experience mild exercise intolerance, but not incapacitating COPD.

Cigarette smoking appears to cause COPD in some smokers because they experience smoking-related losses in lung function that far exceed the mean. Fletcher and associates [72] showed that the variability in annual FEV_1 losses was considerably larger in smokers as compared to nonsmokers. Some heavy smokers experience declines in lung function that differ little from those in nonsmokers, whereas in other susceptible smokers, the losses are more precipitous. Among the London workers in Fletcher's study, the overall decline in smokers' FEV_1 was about 50 ml/year, but 7 percent of the light smokers and 11 percent of the heavy smokers suffered FEV_1 decreases of greater than 90 ml/year. As shown in Figure 39-5, an FEV_1 loss of 100 ml/year beginning at age 25 will result in symptoms by age 55 years and severe disability by age 70 years. Although there is presently little insight as to what distinguishes "susceptible" and "nonsusceptible" smokers, the concept may be a useful one in identifying those persons at greatest risk for developing COPD.

Inspection of Figure 39-5 suggests another factor that might place certain smokers at greater risk for developing COPD. In the example cited, 25-year-old men who are 170 cm tall have a predicted FEV_1 of 4.22. However, due to apparently normal biologic variability, a small proportion of this group will have an FEV_1 of 3.50 liters or less. If these individuals sustain the expected losses from cigarette smoking, it is evident that they are much more likely to develop COPD. For a man with an FEV_1 of 3.25 liters at age 25 years, sustained losses of 50 ml/year will result in symptomatic COPD at about 55 years old. With more rapid losses, the onset of symptoms will occur at a correspondingly younger age. The importance of baseline pulmonary function as a predictor of future COPD risk has been clearly ascertained in longitudinal population studies [92,164].

Air Pollution

The potentially harmful effect of air pollution on lung function is understandably a subject of great concern, because of the large numbers of persons at risk in urban settings. Despite intense investigative efforts over the past several decades, there remains a very incomplete understanding of the overall impact that air pollution has on human health and more specifically on the development of lung disease. The chemistry of air pollutants is extraordinarily complex, and it varies appreciably from region to region. Most attention has focused on the potentially deleterious effects from particulates, sulfur oxides, ozone, the oxides of nitrogen, and carbon monoxide.

Extreme levels of air pollution, particularly those associated with high concentrations of particulate matter and sulfur dioxide, are clearly a cause of illness and death. The most notable example is the London smog of December 1952, which caused an estimated 4000 deaths [31]. The persons who died tended to be older and many had preexisting cardiorespiratory disorders. Subsequent studies demonstrated a consistent relationship between indices of air pollution in London and daily morbidity and mortality [130]. The very high levels of air pollution encountered in London during the 1950s were rapidly controlled by legislative measures. Such extreme cases are rarely encountered. The more important question is whether the lower levels of air pollution as they currently exist have a significant impact on lung function.

Ambient levels of certain pollutants are clearly capable of inducing short-term, detrimental effects on lung function. It has been shown that concentrations of ozone that sometimes occur in urban areas cause modest decrements of lung function both in children attending summer camp and in exercising, normal adults [197,198]. Abnormalities in lung function are associated with cough and chest discomfort, and all may be related to an acute inflammatory response involving the airways [111]. Somewhat surprisingly, subjects with preexisting COPD appear to tolerate ozone exposures nearly as well as normal subjects [125]. Ambient levels of nitrogen dioxide or particulate matter also cause mild changes in lung function but the evidence is less convincing than is the case for ozone.

Whether chronic exposure to ozone and other air pollutants is a factor in the development of COPD is less certain, but there is some supportive evidence from epidemiologic studies in which lung function and respiratory symptoms have been compared in population cohorts from regions with greater and lesser degrees of air pollution. Differences in the study groups, particularly as they relate to ethnic and socioeconomic composition, are only some of the problems encountered in performing these difficult investigations.

Postal workers residing in London were found to have more respiratory symptoms and lower levels of pulmonary function as compared to their rural counterparts [93]. It was also reported that children living in heavily polluted areas of Japan had lower levels of ventilatory function than did their counterparts in less polluted regions [212]. Ferris and his colleagues [70] detected a slight increase in the prevalence of COPD in a heavily polluted city (Berlin, New Hampshire) compared with a lightly polluted city (Chilliwack, British Columbia). In a study comparing cohorts of office workers from two cities with different levels of photochemical smog (Los Angeles and San Francisco), workers residing in the more heavily polluted city (Los Angeles) had more cough and phlegm but no detectable impairment in pulmonary function [124]. Over a 5-year period nonsmokers from a heavily polluted southern California community sustained slightly greater losses in spirometric function than did residents of a nearby city with much lower average levels of photochemical smog [53].

Although the issue is not settled, available evidence suggests that urban air pollution might be a factor in the development of COPD. However, if the effect does exist, it is much less important than cigarette smoking.

Mucus Hypersecretion and Bronchial Infection

A major role for mucus hypersecretion and bronchial infection in the pathogenesis of COPD was proposed on the basis of pathologic studies of patients who died from this disorder and from clinical studies in which an association of sputum production and bronchial infection with impaired ventilatory function was noted [73,176]. It was postulated that irritants such as cigarette smoke and air pollutants and other unknown factors caused hypersecretion of mucus into the bronchial lumen, which created favorable conditions for recurrent infection. Widespread inflammation and fibrosis of the conducting airways caused by repeated infections and blockage of the airway lumen from mucus itself were thought to be the major mechanisms responsible for airflow obstruction. Mucus hypersecretion was deemed to be of such central importance that chronic bronchitis was defined clinically as persistent cough and sputum production [3,46]. This hypothesis heavily influenced the research on COPD for many years.

It is now evident that the relationship of mucus secretion and bronchial infections to COPD is less direct than was previously thought. Population studies repeatedly confirmed a weak association between mucus hypersecretion and airflow obstruction, but several lines of evidence suggest this is not a causal relationship.

Mucus in the bronchial lumen is secreted both by bronchial mucous glands and by epithelial goblet cells. The bronchial mucous glands are thought to be the principal source of sputum that is expectorated, and a correlation between gland size and the amount of expectorated sputum has been demonstrated [99]. Enlargement of the bronchial mucous glands is regarded as the major criterion for the pathologic diagnosis of chronic bronchitis [174]. If excessive mucus production were essential to the development of COPD, then a relationship between the extent of gland enlargement and the severity of airflow obstruction would be anticipated. However, numerous physiologic and pathologic correlative studies have failed to demonstrate a strong and consistent relationship between gland size and the degree of ventilatory impairment [131,141,209].

Clinical observations also fail to show a consistent relationship between either mucus secretion or infection and the evolution of COPD. Some patients with severe COPD give no history of sputum expectoration or purulent sputum, while other patients with those symptoms have no demonstrable impairment of ventilatory function [140]. The best studies demonstrating the variable relationship of mucus hypersecretion and infection to airflow obstruction are those performed by Fletcher and colleagues [72] on London transport workers. They found that cigarette smoking, sputum production, and an excessively rapid decline in the FEV_1 were all strongly intercorrelated. However, cigarette smoking correlated more closely with loss of ventilatory function than did sputum production. Moreover, stepwise regression analysis indicated that for a given level of cigarette consumption, mucus hypersecretion is not associated with a more rapid fall in the FEV_1.

Fletcher and associates [72] also found that in a given individual, variations in sputum volume with time bore no relationship to changes in the FEV_1. Sharp and colleagues [186] also observed an inconstant relationship between sputum production and the development of COPD in a cohort of industrial workers. In another British epidemiologic study extending over a 20- to 25-year period, mortality from COPD was closely related to the initial level of ventilatory function, but was entirely independent of sputum production [164].

Based on the studies described above, it has been proposed that mucus hypersecretion and airflow obstruction should be regarded as largely separate entities but ones that share a common cause, cigarette smoking. Mucus hypersecretion causes morbidity because it is associated with chronic cough and it may predispose to recurrent bronchial infections. However, airflow obstruction is the more important consequence of cigarette smoking because it is responsible for disability and death.

Fletcher and associates [72] did show that those subjects with the greater sputum volume also suffered more bouts of purulent bronchitis. However, recurrent infection, like mucus hypersecretion, does not independently relate to FEV_1 loss once cigarette smoking has been taken into account. Individual episodes of acute bronchitis may occasionally be associated with a decrease in the FEV_1, but as the infection subsides, the FEV_1 usually returns to its premorbid level. Other longitudinal studies also indicate that individual episodes of bronchial infection seldom cause a decrease in ventilatory function and that the frequency of infections does not relate to long-term changes in spirometric abnormalities [81,94].

The lower respiratory tract in patients with advanced COPD is frequently contaminated by a variety of bacterial species, particularly *Streptococcus pneumoniae* and *Hemophilus influenzae* [132]. Patients with COPD frequently have agglutinating antibodies against *H. influenzae* and these antibodies disappear when *H. influenzae* is eradicated from the respiratory tract with antibiotic therapy [101,133]. However, once adjustment has been made for smoking habits, there is no significant association between the presence of *H. influenzae* antibodies and either the level of ventilatory function or its rate of decline [134]. Further evidence against a role for bacterial infection in the development of COPD is provided by clinical studies showing that prolonged antibiotic use in patients with mild airflow obstruction does not appreciably affect the rate of decline in the FEV_1 [30,65,103].

Most available evidence suggests that bronchial infections are not an important factor in the development of COPD, but it is also important to appreciate the limitations of such studies. It remains possible that one or more discrete infections with a specific pathogen might contribute to the development of COPD, but subtle long-lasting changes in ventilatory function cannot be detected against background noise. For example, uncomplicated viral upper respiratory tract infections have been shown to compromise lower airway function for extended periods in young healthy adults [167]. There are also suggestions that respiratory infections during the formative period of lung growth in childhood might predispose to COPD in later life. Recurrent respiratory infections in children have been correlated with a lower level of ventilatory function [40]. Although recall bias might have influenced the findings, a childhood history of respiratory symptoms has been shown to be associated with lower levels of ventilatory function in adults. However, a prospective study in children demonstrated an association between viral upper respiratory tract infections in children and the persistence of subtle spirometric abnormalities [48]. The precise role of infection in the development of COPD remains to be defined through additional clinical and epidemiologic studies.

Sex and Race

Mortality rates from COPD are presently higher in men than in women, and this gender-related predisposition probably reflects differing historical patterns of tobacco use [214]. This difference can be expected to narrow as gender patterns of cigarette consumption have largely disappeared. For equivalent cigarette consumption, symptoms of cough and phlegm may be more common in men [206], but losses in ventilatory function are nearly identical [8,38,184,222].

COPD occurs in all major ethnic groups, but studies of relative risk are hampered by the inability to control other environmental variables. Some data suggest that white males may be somewhat more susceptible to developing COPD than black males. In a study of New York transit and postal workers, the percentage decline in white smokers was considerably greater than for black smokers, but no racial differences were seen in nonsmokers [199]. In a survey of 65,000 people who attended health screening clinics in San Francisco, a deleterious effect of cigarette smoking on lung function was readily discernible in whites of all ages, but these differences were less evident in blacks and Orientals [184].

Allergic and Bronchial Hyperreactivity

Because asthma and COPD appear to coexist in some patients and because most patients with COPD exhibit some degree of airflow reversibility after the use of bronchodilators, it has been suggested that allergic factors and/or bronchial hyperreactivity might play some role in the development of COPD. Among London transport workers, neither the FEV_1 nor the slope of the FEV_1 against age correlated with a personal or family history of allergic disorders, but there was a weak relationship of lung function to sputum eosinophilia [72]. In the Tucson population study, ventilatory impairment was found to be significantly correlated with skin test reactivity, blood eosinophilia, and serum levels of IgE [41]. However, when these data were reanalyzed to exclude subjects with a known diagnosis of asthma, the relationships of allergy variables to lung function were no longer apparent [39].

Bronchial hyperreactivity is defined as an abnormal degree of bronchial constriction in response to a standard stimulus. Nonspecific bronchial hyperreactivity appears to play a central role in the pathogenesis of asthma, and it has been suggested that a similar mechanism might represent a risk factor for the development of COPD. Apparent bronchial hyperreactivity, of considerably smaller magnitude than is usually observed in asthma, has been detected in many patients with COPD [155]. However, it has also been observed that the magnitude of the spirometric response in response to a methacholine challenge is closely related to the level of lung function existing prior to challenge; patients with the worst baseline spirometric values exhibit the greatest sensitivity to the stimulus [196]. What is termed *bronchial hyperreactivity* in patients with COPD may be largely a consequence of the disease, involving factors such as abnormal airway geometry and the altered disposition of inhaled aerosols. At the moment it is difficult to judge whether bronchial hyperreactivity plays any significant role in the development of COPD.

Hereditary Factors

Laurell and Eriksson [66,116] first noted that a deficiency in the alpha$_1$-globulin component of serum proteins is associated with diffuse emphysema and severe disability at a relatively young age. Subsequent work by these investigators and others determined that the specific deficiency involves a glycoprotein, alpha$_1$-protease inhibitor; that the deficiency is hereditary; and that it follows the pattern of mendelian inheritance [113]. The data are consistent with a single autosomal locus, designated Pi, with multiple codominant alleles, designated Pi$_M$, Pi$_Z$, and so on. Pi$_M$ is the common form with an allele frequency of greater than 95 percent, but approximately 75 percent Pi alleles have been identified with Pi$_S$ and Pi$_Z$ being the most frequent variant subtypes. Phenotypes are recognized from specialized electrophoretic studies of the alpha$_1$-protease inhibitor fraction; homozygous phenotypes are designated as MM, ZZ, and so on, and heterozygous phenotypes are designated as MS, MZ, and so on. MM subjects have serum alpha$_1$-protease inhibitor levels of between 150 and 250 mg/ml. Certain phenotypes, particularly ZZ, are associated with severely depressed serum levels of alpha$_1$-protease inhibitor (usually 25 percent or less of normal), whereas intermediate levels are observed in other homozygous and heterozygous states, including SS, MZ, and MS.

Severe depression of serum alpha$_1$-protease inhibitor levels, most commonly occurring with the ZZ phenotype, is clearly a major risk factor for the development of COPD. Most affected individuals have widespread panacinar emphysema, which frequently develops into large bullae, and the onset of symptoms may occur at a relatively young age. Early studies suggested that as many as 80 percent of persons with severe alpha$_1$-protease inhibitor deficiency states might develop symptomatic airflow obstruction [113]. However, more recent population studies provide a truer picture of the natural history of the disorder [100,190]. As is the case with persons having the normal amount of alpha$_1$-protease inhibitor, cigarette smoking markedly increases the risk for developing disabling airflow obstruction in those persons who have severe deficiency states. Among nonsmokers with severe deficiency states, many will develop a mild impairment of lung function as they age, but only a few will develop clinically apparent COPD.

It is also evident that genetic deficiencies in the serum levels of alpha$_1$-protease inhibitor do not explain the widespread prevalence of COPD. The frequency of the ZZ phenotype among patients with COPD is low [88]. The frequency of phenotypes associated with very low levels of alpha$_1$-protease inhibitor is no more than one in several thousand among Caucasians, whereas approximately 10 percent of smokers in the same

populations may develop COPD [67,69]. Phenotypes associated with intermediate levels of alpha$_1$-protease inhibitor, particularly MZ, are considerably more prevalent, and they might be suspected as constituting a smaller but significant risk factor. A few small studies suggested a modest increase in the prevalence of COPD in MZ subjects who smoke [49,51,106]. However, the best available information on this subject indicates that any increased risk of developing COPD among smokers with intermediate levels of alpha$_1$-protease inhibitor is at most extremely small [32].

Genetic influences other than those related to alpha$_1$-protease inhibitor may also influence the risk for developing COPD, but these factors have not been well characterized. Familial clusterings of COPD have been noted from clinical observations [115]. Significant familial aggregations for respiratory symptoms and impaired ventilatory function have also been detected in epidemiologic studies [89,205]. Some of these studies suggest that the risk may be associated with genetic markers, such as the ABO blood type. These associations are generally weak and they have added little to our understanding as to why COPD develops only in certain individuals.

Socioeconomic Level

An increased mortality rate from COPD among lower socioeconomic groups is observed consistently. This increased risk can be attributed in part to smoking habits, and perhaps to other factors such as occupation and residence in more polluted regions. However, even when these factors are taken into account, people in lower socioeconomic groups, particularly blue-collar workers, appear to have slightly lower levels of ventilatory function and correspondingly increased risks for developing COPD than do their wealthier counterparts [90]. The reasons for this effect are not known.

Occupational Risks

There is widespread concern that noxious fumes, dust, and smoke encountered in the workplace may permanently impair ventilatory function and contribute to the development of COPD. This concern has prompted numerous longitudinal and cross-sectional surveys of workers in various occupations and occupational exposures to determine the presence and magnitude of this risk.

A number of occupational exposures appear to be associated with some added risk for developing COPD; some of these are listed below. Some types of occupational lung disease cannot be clearly categorized as "obstructive," and the list is restricted to those occupations in which the functional abnormality observed is principally irreversible airflow obstruction.

OCCUPATIONS:
Coal miners [143]
Fire fighters [189]
Grain handlers [54]
Copper smelters [192]

OCCUPATIONAL EXPOSURES:
Poison gas (mustard gas and lewisite) [153]
Granite dust [147]
Carbon black [216]
Cotton (byssinosis) [27]
Hemp [26]
Toluene diisocyanate [161]

For most occupation exposures, the risk of developing COPD appears to be more pronounced in those workers who also smoke cigarettes. In general, the magnitude of the occupational effect is substantially less important than is the smoking effect, and occupation alone would rarely lead to the development of clinically apparent COPD. Coal miners have been studied as extensively as a single occupational group. Critical review of the literature suggests that time spent underground in coal mines has only a minor effect on ventilatory capacity, and that cigarette smoking is by far the more important factor in the development of COPD among coal miners [143].

Natural History

The natural history of COPD can be divided into two parts; the earlier subclinical stage, which is associated with modest impairment in ventilatory function and no symptoms that can be attributed to airflow obstruction, and the later stage, which causes clinical disability and eventually death. The earlier stage is longer and less well understood.

As noted previously, the importance of other identified risk factors pales in comparison with cigarette smoking, so that the natural history of COPD is largely defined by the combined effects of tobacco exposure and advancing age. Cigarette smoking causes some loss of ventilatory function in nearly all exposed subjects, but only

the susceptible minority with greater-than-average loss rates will develop disabling COPD. Even in this susceptible group, at least 20 to 30 years of exposure are required for the emergence of clinical symptoms. Available data suggest that loss in function from smoking occurs at a relatively constant rate from the time the individual begins to smoke. Large functional decrements over relatively short time periods have been observed [95], but longitudinal studies involving large numbers of subjects indicate that precipitous spirometric losses are unusual [14,72]. Different studies suggest that rates of ventilatory decline may either accelerate or decelerate as the disease progresses [64,72]. The disease may follow a very unpredictable course in the individual patient.

More is known about natural history and prognostic factors in established COPD than in its earlier stages. Tests of ventilatory function, particularly spirometry, as well as certain other clinical findings, have been shown to have prognostic significance in COPD.

A number of long-term clinical studies of patients with COPD have been reported; those by Renzetti and associates [177], by Burrows and Earle [36], and by Boushy and colleagues [29] are representative. The typical patient, when admitted to these studies, was a 60-year-old man with an FEV_1 of about 1.0 liter. Overall mortality was between 40 and 50 percent after 5 years, and in each study, life expectancy was most closely related to the FEV_1 at the time of entry into the study. For patients with an FEV_1 of less than 0.75 liter, only 20 to 25 percent will survive 5 years, whereas an FEV_1 of about 1.50 liters is associated with a survival rate of about 70 to 80 percent at 5 years. In the studies cited, the average annual decrease in the FEV_1 was between 50 and 60 ml/year, figures that are somewhat less than what has been reported for other groups of patients with COPD [30,94].

Renzetti and associates [177] observed that for a given FEV_1, abnormalities in blood gases and particularly the presence of cor pulmonale worsened prognosis. The D_LCO, elastic recoil pressure, roentgenographic presence of emphysema, $PaCO_2$, and single-breath nitrogen washout test had some prognostic significance beyond that seen in the study by Boushy and associates [29]. Burrows and Earle [36] identified resting heart rate, a physician's assessment as to the severity of disease, a history of edema, the serum albumin-globulin ratio, and the response to bronchodilators as significant, though weak determinants of prognosis. It has been suggested by some investigators that pulmonary hypertension worsens prognosis independently of the FEV_1 [37], but this has been disputed by others [29].

Available short-term studies indicate that the functional abnormalities observed in COPD are largely irreversible. The damaged lung will likely continue to exhibit usual aging losses in function even though no further injury is sustained. Thus, the best that one might hope to achieve through treatment is that the patient with COPD lose no more than 25 to 30 ml in his or her FEV_1 each year. The difference between normal aging losses and the losses observed as part of the usual progression of COPD, 50 to 100 ml/year, may represent the only therapeutic leeway in altering the natural history of the disease. Because short-term changes in ventilatory function are small, and because individual variations are large, beneficial effects of therapy may be difficult to detect. Although a reduction in annual loss of 50 or 100 ml to between 25 and 30 ml may appear to be of marginal clinical significance, the cumulative effects may have a large impact on prognosis when viewed against the long natural history of the disease.

These effects are illustrated graphically in Figure 39-6. For a 50-year-old man with mild disability from an FEV_1 of 1.50 liters, continued losses of 100 ml/year will in less than 10 years reduce the FEV_1 to about 0.50 liter, a level that is associated with severe disability and imminent death. If, on the other hand, annual losses are reduced to a normal 27 ml/year, this same level of impairment would not occur for another 35 years. The benefits of an altered slope obviously diminish as COPD worsens. Yet, even with advanced disease, successful intervention might delay severe disability and death by several years.

Treatment

The structural damage to the lung that is responsible for airflow obstruction is largely irreversible, so most patients will experience little improvement in function despite what is considered optimal therapy. Therefore, the goals of therapy in COPD are (1) to prevent further deterioration in lung function, (2) to provide relief of symptoms, and (3) to deal with complications as they arise.

Presently, there is firm scientific evidence that only two treatment modalities significantly alter the natural history of COPD. Cessation of smoking clearly slows the rate of ventilatory deterioration, at least in patients with mild disease, and chronic oxygen therapy prolongs life in patients with severe COPD who are also hypoxemic. Whether other treatment modalities also alter the natural history of COPD is not known, as adequately designed studies for assessing their impact have not been completed.

Even if they do not prolong life, some of the therapies employed in COPD clearly provide some symptomatic benefit and improvement in the overall quality of life. The physicians caring for patients with COPD should be flexible in their approach, tailoring treatments to individual needs, while being aware of benefits, adverse effects, and costs. The prompt recognition and treatment of respiratory infections, heart failure, and other complications of COPD likely reduce mortality, avoid the need for hospitalization, and lengthen survival time. Knowledge of community resources, particularly with regard to social services, disability compensation, and vocational rehabilitation, is of particular importance to the disabled patient.

Comprehensive care programs and specialized respiratory care clinics have been enthusiastically endorsed by some physicians and many patients. Many patients undoubtedly derive some medical and psychological benefits from these programs, but the programs are expensive, and whether the advantages outweigh their greater

Fig. 39-6. The potential benefits of therapy in patients with established COPD. A 50-year-old man (*X*) has mild COPD with an FEV_1 of 1.5 liters/s. If he continues to sustain annual FEV_1 losses of 100 ml/s/year, death is likely within 10 years (*A*). However, if by therapeutic intervention, annual FEV_1 losses revert to normal (27 ml/s/year), death from COPD is unlikely to occur for at least 30 years (*B*).

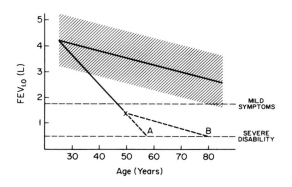

costs is uncertain. Since structured comprehensive care and rehabilitation programs are unavailable to most patients, most patients with COPD will continue to receive individual care from their primary physicians. Further discussion of rehabilitation in the treatment of COPD patients is found in Chapter 47.

Smoking Cessation

Since cigarette smoking is the principal cause of COPD, it is self-evident that patients with this disorder should stop smoking. There is now good scientific data showing that the course of COPD is favorably influenced by smoking cessation, although the evidence for this is better established in patients with milder disease.

Smoking cessation does not result in appreciable improvements in lung function in most patients. McCarthy and associates [135] carried out detailed studies of pulmonary function over a 49-week period in persons who stopped smoking. Most subjects had only mild impairment in lung function that was closely related to lifetime cigarette consumption. Improvement in lung function was detected by spirometry and by the single-breath nitrogen test after both reduction and cessation of smoking. While statistically significant, the average magnitude of the change was quite small. These findings were confirmed in another study of similar design [34], and they indicate that the reversible component of cigarette smoke–induced lung injury is relatively slight, even in the earlier stages of COPD.

While patients with mild COPD do not regain much lung function after smoking cessation, they no longer suffer accelerated losses as they get older. Evidence that ex-smokers revert to normal aging losses in ventilatory function has been provided from population studies showing that average levels of ventilatory function in ex-smokers consistently lie midway between those of lifelong nonsmokers and those of current smokers [38,222]. The best documentation of the beneficial effects of smoking cessation on age-related decreases in ventilatory capacity is provided by the studies of Fletcher and associates [72]. They observed that the decline in ventilatory function among ex-smokers was no greater than for those who had never smoked, even though average values were lower. Thus, it is clear that in mild COPD, smoking cessation slows or completely stops progressive lung damage.

The effects of smoking cessation on the subsequent course of advanced COPD is less clear. Burrows and Earle [36] observed a tendency toward a more favorable course in patients who stopped smoking, but patients with more severe disease were more likely to quit their cigarette habit, so that meaningful comparisons were difficult to make. Johnston and associates [103] did not observe a correlation between smoking status and the decline in the FEV_1 in 54 patients with advanced COPD. They did observe that the D_LCO did not deteriorate as steeply in ex-smokers, and this suggests that the development of emphysema might have slowed.

Although the benefits of smoking cessation on lung function have not been demonstrated conclusively in patients with advanced COPD, it has been shown that smoking cessation does cause improvement in certain respiratory symptoms. Cough and sputum production lessen appreciably in patients with COPD who are able to quit smoking, at all stages of the disease [10,34].

While smoking cessation is imperative in patients with COPD, all physicians are well aware of the highly addictive nature of this habit and of the difficulties most patients experience in attempting to quit. Patients with COPD should be forcefully and repeatedly warned by their physicians of the particular dangers they face from continued cigarette use. Referral to hospital- and community-based smoking cessation and support groups may be helpful in well-motivated patients. There is also evidence that nicotine chewing gum is a helpful adjunctive measure in some patients, but only if it is employed in conjunction with ongoing support from physicians or other health care professionals [24].

Antibiotic Treatment

Despite considerable evidence that recurrent bronchial infection has no causal significance in the development of COPD, purulent exacerbations of bronchitis cause significant morbidity in many patients and these exacerbations may be life-threatening in patients with severe COPD. It is suspected that acute exacerbations of bronchitis are usually infectious in origin, but it has been difficult to identify specific etiologic agents. Clinical studies revealed an association between bronchial inflammation and the presence of bacteria, particularly *H. influenzae* and *S. pneumoniae*, in the sputum and lower respiratory tract [132]. Various viral and mycoplasmal agents also have been isolated from sputum during acute episodes [83]. However, many of these same microorganisms are also found in the sputum during quiescent periods, which suggests that they may colonize the lower respiratory tract without necessarily causing inflammation. It was concluded that no clear-cut causal role has been definitely established for any infective organism in acute exacerbations of bronchitis [207].

At one time, many physicians favored the prophylactic use of antibiotics in patients with COPD, particularly those prone to purulent bronchitis, with the belief that suppression of infection might slow the course of COPD. Clinical trials have not shown this to be the case [30,65,103], so there is rarely justification for the chronic administration of antibiotics to patients with COPD.

Acute bronchitis occurring in patients with COPD is one of the most common conditions for which antibiotics are prescribed, and they are given with the widely held presumption that they lessen morbidity and shorten the duration of the illness. However, the putative benefits of antibiotics for this condition have been difficult to demonstrate in controlled clinical trials. Some controlled studies demonstrated a significant advantage from antibiotics, whereas others did not, even though a favorable trend was frequently evident in the latter trials [63,163,170,171]. In a more recent and better-designed clinical trial involving larger numbers of patients, it was clearly demonstrated that a broad-spectrum antibiotic was superior to placebo [6]. The average effect was relatively small in that that antibiotic treatment was associated with a success rate of 68 percent versus a 55 percent success rate in those patients who received placebo.

Despite the modest overall impact of antibiotics on the course of bronchitis exacerbations in COPD, it is appropriate to prescribe a broad-spectrum antibiotic for this condition because therapy is definitely beneficial for a few patients, and the costs and adverse effects of the treatment are acceptably small. In the absence of roentgenographic or clinical evidence of pneumonia, there is no reason to obtain bacterial or viral cultures of the sputum prior to treatment. Choice of a broad-spectrum antibiotic should be based primarily on considerations of cost and toxicity, as there are no good data to support the use of one agent over another. A 7- to 10-day course of tetracycline, ampicillin, or sulfamethoxazole-trimethoprim appears to be the safest and most cost-effective therapy.

Bronchodilator Therapy

COPD is frequently described as *irreversible* to distinguish it from the *reversible* airflow obstruction of asthma, but this distinction is a relative one. Nearly all patients with COPD exhibit at least a small improvement in ventilatory function acutely and chronically after receiving a bronchodilator [62,122,160,208], and this is associated with modest improvements in exercise tolerance and dyspnea [60,85,128]. It is not known whether regular bronchodilator use influences the natural history of COPD, as long-term controlled studies have not been performed.

Acute spirometric responses to bronchodilators are useful in gauging the degree of airflow reversibility and in distinguishing patients with COPD from those with asthma. However, such testing is of limited value in guiding bronchodilator therapy. Most patients with COPD exhibit an improvement in the FEV_1 of between 5 and 20 percent after receiving a bronchodilator. Because the treatment response is small in relation to background test variations, some patients, particularly those with less reversible disease, will on some occasions appear to have no bronchodilator response. In most instances this phenomenon is due to chance variation, and if the subject is tested repeatedly, improvement with bronchodilator therapy can be detected. Therefore, a trial of bronchodilator therapy is indicated in all patients with symptomatic COPD, irrespective of the apparent spirometric response, and the subjective response of the patient must serve as the principal guide for adjusting therapy.

Beta-adrenergic agonists, delivered by aerosol inhalation, remain a mainstay of bronchodilator therapy in COPD. Isoproterenol is the prototype of this class of agents, and it was widely used for many years. Its use has now been largely supplanted by a family of more selective beta$_2$-adrenergic agonists, such as metaproterenol, albuterol, and terbutaline. Compared to isoproterenol, these agents have greater activity toward bronchial smooth muscle and less cardiac effect [114], but their principal clinical advantage resides in their longer duration of action. Beta-adrenergic agonists can be delivered to the respiratory tract from either a metered-dose canister or a constant-flow nebulizer device [43]. In patients with stable disease, the two modes of drug administration provide equivalent therapeutic effects, with the metered-dose canister by far the more convenient. A number of beta$_2$-adrenergic agonists are also available in oral dosage forms, but these preparations appear to be less effective than aerosols while producing substantially more severe side effects [172].

A few patients may experience difficulties in coordinating the metered-dose inhaler so as to ensure delivery of drug to the lower respiratory tract, but these problems can usually be corrected with adequate instruction [187]. Spacers and reservoir systems may marginally improve drug delivery [181], but in the case of the beta$_2$-adrenergic agonists, this small advantage usually does not outweigh the disadvantages. Spacers may be helpful in severely dyspneic patients, as may constant-flow nebulizer devices. Inhalation of single puffs of a drug at intervals of 1 minute or more appears to be more effective than if the same amount of drug is taken in rapid sequence [87]. In the usually recommended doses (2 puffs every 3 to 6 hours), beta$_2$-adrenergic agonists rarely cause any systemic side effects. Many patients benefit from more frequent dosing, and this practice need not be discouraged, as there appears to be a wide margin of safety with inhaled beta agonists [11].

Anticholinergics now represent a second option for inhaled bronchodilator therapy in COPD. The bronchodilator properties of atropine and other anticholinergic agents have been known for many years. However, even when given by inhalation, substantial amounts of atropine sulfate are absorbed systemically, and the attendant side effects, tachycardia, blurred vision, urinary retention, and disorientation, were a practical limit to its clinical use. Ipratropium bromide, a quaternary ammonium derivative of atropine, is now available for inhalational administration from metered-dose canisters [157]. Side effects from this drug are negligible, as there is very little absorption from the gastrointestinal tract, and it does not cross the blood-brain barrier to any appreciable extent. It is an effective bronchodilator in the treatment of COPD, and while its onset of action is somewhat slower, its peak effect is equivalent or slightly better than that achieved with beta-adrenergic agonists [82]. If either ipratropium bromide or a beta-adrenergic agonist is administered in optimally effective doses, addition of the second agent achieves little additional benefit [61]. Hence, there is not a sound rationale for the simultaneous administration of both classes of drugs, even though this is common practice. Ipratropium bromide should be considered as a first-line bronchodilator in the treatment of COPD, as an alternative to beta-adrenergic therapy.

Over the past two decades, xanthine derivatives, particularly theophylline, have enjoyed a resurgence of popularity in the treatment of COPD and other bronchospastic disorders. Much new information has become available concerning theophylline pharmacokinetics, and the relationships among dosing schedules, serum drug levels, and ventilatory function responses have been carefully worked out [62,102,142]. The availability of sustained-release preparations has simplified treatment schedules and improved patient compliance. Theophylline does produce modest bronchodilation in patients with COPD, both acutely and chronically, and these increases in ventilatory function are associated with correspondingly small improvements in exercise tolerance and dyspnea [62,128,208]. Some, but not all reports suggest that theophylline may improve respiratory muscle function [110,146]. If this effect is present, its clinical significance has yet to be determined.

Balanced against its proved bronchodilator activity, theophylline does have some serious disadvantages, principally related to its narrow therapeutic index. Dose-dependent improvements in lung function are observed with serum theophylline levels of between 10 and 20 μg/ml [62]. A few patients may experience significant adverse effects within this therapeutic range, and with levels above 25 μg/ml, there is a rapidly increasing incidence of convulsions, cardiac arrhythmias, and severe gastrointestinal symptoms [220]. The daily dose required to achieve safe therapeutic levels varies considerably in normal subjects, and it may be further affected by age, cigarette smoking status, diet, intercurrent illnesses, and interactions with many different drugs [102]. Serum theophylline levels must be measured periodically to ensure that drug levels are therapeutic, and the prescribing physician must be aware of the many factors that may affect theophylline metabolism. Literature reports confirm an impression that serious theophylline toxicity is not an uncommon problem, particularly among older patients [185,220].

The proper role for theophylline in the treatment of COPD remains a controversial subject. Simplicity of administration, proved efficacy, and wide margin of safety make inhaled bronchodilators, either anticholinergics or beta-adrenergic agonists, the agents of choice. The important question is whether theophylline should be used in conjunction with an inhaled bronchodilator and other standard therapies. In acute exacerbations of COPD, theophylline appears to have no role [179]. In chronic therapy for patients with stable COPD, theophylline may produce some benefits beyond those provided by inhaled bronchodilators alone [60,85,208]. It bears emphasizing that the average improvement is so small as to be indiscernible to many patients, and that theophylline does carry with it a small risk of a serious adverse effect. For the most seriously disabled patients, a therapeutic trial of theophylline can be justified. For those patients with less severe COPD, the disadvantages probably outweigh the benefits.

Corticosteroid Therapy

Numerous clinical studies indicate that most patients with stable COPD do not benefit from systemic corticosteroids [16,17,68]. Despite these generally negative results, there is evidence that a few patients with COPD may experience substantial spirometric and symptomatic benefit from corticosteroids [16,17]. Mendella and associates [138] reported that 8 of 44 patients with a clinical diagnosis of COPD experienced a 29 percent or greater increase in their FEV_1 after taking 32 mg of methylprednisolone daily for 2 weeks. Patients who responded to methylprednisolone could not be distinguished in terms of age, smoking history, duration of symptoms, presence of wheezing, or blood or sputum eosinophilia. Corticosteroid-responsive patients had larger average responses to bronchodilators, but there was much overlap between the two groups.

This small subset of patients with apparently corticosteroid-responsive COPD is variably described as having occult asthma, bronchospastic COPD, or asthmatic bronchitis. It is unclear whether this poorly defined entity is a variant form of COPD, or whether it merely represents the simultaneous occurrence of COPD and asthma, both of which are relatively common diseases. It is important that these patients be identified, because their response to appropriate treatment may be substantial, and their prognosis correspondingly better. It is also important to identify those patients who do not benefit from long-term oral corticosteroids, because of the serious adverse effects. Since clinical criteria and bronchodilator responses are not entirely reliable predictors, some experienced clinicians advise that most patients with severe COPD should be given a carefully controlled therapeutic trial with oral corticosteroids. If this is done, careful spirometric measurements should be obtained before and after the patient is given 40 to 60 mg of prednisone, or its equivalent, daily for 1 to 2 weeks. If the FEV_1 increases by 25 percent or greater, the patient can be considered to be corticosteroid-responsive. Therapy with one of the inhaled corticosteroid preparations should be instituted immediately, and the dose of oral corti-costeroids should be discontinued or tapered to the minimum level that allows reasonable control of the patient's symptoms. While inhaled corticosteroids are not an adequate replacement for oral corticosteroids in many steroid-responsive patients with COPD [188], they can be substituted in some, and maximally effective doses (4 to 8 puffs four times daily) usually allow a reduction in the doses of oral corticosteroid in most patients.

Alpha₁-Protease Inhibitor Replacement Therapy

As discussed previously, severely depressed serum alpha₁-protease inhibitor levels place affected individuals at great risk for developing COPD, particularly if they also smoke. Since the development of emphysema seems clearly to be related to low blood and lung levels of a single protein, replacement therapy should logically be effective in preventing COPD.

The feasibility of such therapy has been demonstrated. Intravenous infusion of alpha₁-protease inhibitor at weekly or monthly intervals results in sustained, protective levels of alpha₁-protease inhibitor in both the blood and the lower airways [96]. Treatment over periods of several months appears to be safe. Due to the anticipated high costs of such a trial, no controlled study of clinical efficacy has been performed, nor is one planned. Nonetheless, an alpha₁-protease inhibitor replacement product isolated from pooled blood has been licensed under the Orphan Drug Law and is now commercially available (Prolastin, Cutter Laboratories). The license is specifically restricted to those patients with severe deficiency states, most commonly the ZZ phenotype, and the annual cost of replacement therapy for one patient is presently in excess of $50,000.

The dilemma as to which affected individuals should receive such treatment has not been resolved. Patients with severe alpha₁-protease inhibitor deficiency and end-stage COPD are unlikely to benefit appreciably from replacement therapy. It is also known that nonsmokers are at a relatively lower risk for developing severe emphysema, despite being severely deficient in alpha₁-protease inhibitor [100,190]. Available evidence also suggests that smoking cessation appreciably slows the rate of lung damage in those who are alpha₁-protease inhibitor–deficient. Hence, the most logical recipients of replacement therapy are largely those deficient persons who also smoke. Whether such inordinately expensive therapy, the long-term efficacy and safety of which have not been conclusively shown, should be offered to those persons is open to conjecture. Most experts do agree that replacement therapy should be considered in alpha$_1$-protease inhibitor–deficient nonsmokers and ex-smokers who have moderate impairment in lung function and who continue to exhibit deterioration in lung function during a period of observation.

Chronic Oxygen Therapy

Hypoxemia is a characteristic feature of more advanced COPD. This has important consequences both for systemic oxygen delivery and for the development of pulmonary hypertension. It is important to recognize hypoxemia in COPD, as its correction through long-term oxygen supplementation has a significant effect on the natural history of the disorder.

The uneven distribution of ventilation in lungs affected by COPD is thought to be the primary abnormality responsible for arterial hypoxemia. Underventilation with intact perfusion is termed a *low* $\dot{V}/\dot{Q}$ *abnormality*, and blood flowing through such areas is not fully oxygenated. The admixture of poorly oxygenated blood from low $\dot{V}/\dot{Q}$ regions causes some degree of hypoxemia in arterial blood. $\dot{V}/\dot{Q}$ mismatches also impair the ability of the lung to clear carbon dioxide. Alveolar hypoventilation is an important contributing factor in the causation of hypoxemia and hypercapnia in patients with more severe COPD. Mild arterial hypoxemia is frequently detectable even in patients with mild COPD; in severe COPD it may be profound. In acute respiratory failure from COPD, hypoxemia may cause life-threatening tissue hypoxia. In chronic respiratory failure secondary to COPD, the systemic effects of hypoxemia are less profound, but chronic lack of oxygen may contribute to exercise limitation, weight loss, and neuropsychological dysfunction. Adverse effects of chronic hypoxemia may be partly compensated by a secondary erythrocytosis and perhaps by other poorly understood mechanisms.

Additionally, alveolar hypoxia elicits a local pulmonary vasoconstrictor response. This may be advantageous in maintaining regional $\dot{V}/\dot{Q}$ ratios near unity, since it tends to reduce blood flow through those regions that are underventilated. However, sustained hypoxic vasoconstriction eventually causes hypertrophy of pulmonary vascular smooth muscle and widespread obliterative changes in the pulmonary vascular bed. Increases in pulmonary vascular resistance result in pulmonary hypertension and eventually to failure of the right ventricle.

Supplemental oxygen is universally accepted as beneficial for patients with COPD who develop respiratory failure acutely. There is also now firm scientific evidence that selected patients with chronic respiratory failure secondary to COPD are also benefited by long-term, continuous oxygen therapy.

Multicenter, prospective, and randomized trials to evaluate chronic oxygen therapy in hypoxemic patients with COPD have been conducted in the United Kingdom and in North America [137,154]. The British administered either no oxygen or oxygen at a rate of 2 liters/min for 15 hours each day, including the sleeping hours. In the North American study, patients were randomized to receive oxygen sufficient to maintain PaO$_2$ above 65 mmHg for either 12 or 19 hours each day, sleeping hours being included in both groups. In both studies, patients entering the study had a PaO$_2$ persistently less than 55 to 60 mmHg and/or they had polycythemia, edema, or an electrocardiogram consistent with right ventricular enlargement. Mortality among the patients receiving 12 hours of oxygen daily was nearly double that of the other group at the end of 3 years in the North American study. Results of the United Kingdom study were complementary in showing that mortality in patients receiving oxygen for 15 hours daily was substantially better than in those patients who received no oxygen. Thus, it is clear that chronic oxygen therapy improves survival in hypoxemic patients with COPD and that survival is best among those patients who receive the more continuous therapy.

The mechanisms by which chronic oxygen therapy improves patient survival are not entirely clear. In both the American and British studies, average treatment-related changes in spirometry, hematocrit, arterial blood gases while breathing room air, and pulmonary hemodynamics were relatively slight in most patients, and it has been questioned whether these differences are sufficient to explain the effects of oxygen on mortality. Smaller earlier studies suggested that chronic oxygen therapy caused more substantial decreases in red blood cell mass and in pulmonary vascular pressures and resistance [1,23,117,118].

The impact of chronic oxygen therapy on patient well-being, apart from prolonged survival, has been difficult to assess. Heaton and associates [86] examined variables related to neuropsychological function in a subset of patients who participated in the North American oxygen trial described above. After 12 months of therapy, patients receiving continuous oxygen registered slightly better neuropsychological function than did patients who received nocturnal oxygen only. However, none of the patients reported substantial improvements in emotional state or overall quality of life.

Increased activity levels and improved exercise tolerance also are claimed for many patients receiving long-term oxygen therapy [118], but there may be a large placebo effect when effort-dependent variables are tested. Lilker and associates [123] reported that patients felt better when given liquid air, and no improvements in activity levels could be detected when patients were given low-flow oxygen continuously during waking hours. Others also observed a significant placebo effect from the administration of room air through a nasal cannula [1]. Oxygen therapy may permit some improvement in exercise capacity [137], but the effect is modest at best, and it is unlikely to make major differences in the quality of life for most patients.

Based on the information obtained in controlled studies, it is now recommended that chronic oxygen therapy be considered in all patients with COPD who consistently have a PaO_2 of less than 55 mmHg while in a stable clinical state. Oxygen should also be considered for patients who have polycythemia, electrocardiographic evidence of right ventricular hypertrophy, or clinical signs of cor pulmonale, even though the PaO_2 is greater than 55 mmHg. Some patients may have adequate arterial oxygen while awake and at rest, but experience periods of desaturation with exercise or sleep. These abnormalities are considered sufficient indication for oxygen therapy by some physicians, but a fuller appreciation of their clinical significance awaits long-term controlled studies. Patients who qualify should receive oxygen for a minimum of 15 to 18 hours daily, and as close to 24 hours/day as is practical. Oxygen should be administered in amounts to raise the PaO_2 to between 65 and 80 mmHg, or to an arterial oxygen saturation of at least 88 to 90 percent if treatment response is assessed by pulse oximetry. It may be desirable to increase the oxygen flow by 1 liter/min when patients are sleeping or exercising.

Oxygen can be supplied from steel cylinders, liquid systems, or concentrators. For the fully ambulatory patient, liquid systems are the most portable, but they are also the most expensive and they are probably unnecessary for most patients. Oxygen concentrators are the most economic when oxygen demands are large, but they suffer the disadvantage of being the least portable. Oxygen is ordinarily delivered through nasal prongs. Oxygen-saving devices, which deliver oxygen only during inspiration, have been developed but are not in widespread use [210]. The administration of oxygen through transtracheal catheters has been advocated, since this method also conserves oxygen supply, but the advantages of this delivery system appear marginal and it has not gained widespread acceptance [45]. The hazards and complications of chronic oxygen therapy are minimal. Patients should be reassessed at intervals to determine whether their oxygen requirements have changed.

Measures To Alter Sputum

In advanced stages of COPD, many patients have difficulty in coughing up what appears to be abnormally sticky and tenacious sputum. Numerous measures have been evaluated in an effort to find methods for decreasing the viscosity of sputum and allowing it to be cleared more easily. Aggressive systemic hydration and inhalation of droplet aerosols have been advocated in the past. However, there is no evidence that water intake beyond normal daily requirements improves bronchial toilet, and excessive water loads may be detrimental in patients with cor pulmonale. Droplet aerosols are of no proved benefit and may result in an acute worsening of lung function [166].

A variety of mucolytic agents, including iodides, acetylcysteine, bromhexine, glyceryl guaiacolate, and proteolytic enzymes, have some demonstrated capability for liquefying tenacious sputum, but their clinical efficacy is, for the most part, marginal or unproved. Acetylcysteine has been shown to have a slight beneficial effect, but it may also cause pulmonary function to deteriorate acutely in some patients [145]. A recent multicenter trial demonstrated that iodinated glycerol provided significant improvement in selected symptoms, including cough frequency and severity, but several hundred study subjects were required to demonstrate the effect, so that the clinical significance of the result is uncertain [165]. No clinical trial has shown a significant long-term effect from mucolytic therapy on lung function. Selected patients in whom sticky sputum is a particularly prominent feature of their disease might benefit from a therapeutic trial of a mucolytic agent.

Intermittent Positive-Pressure Breathing

For many years, intermittent positive-pressure breathing (IPPB), usually with a nebulized bronchodilator, was widely employed in the treatment of patients with COPD. Assisted ventilation does acutely decrease the work of breathing, so that it may briefly relieve dyspnea in patients with severe disease. Many patients also claim that it is helpful in raising bronchial secretions. However, a multicenter trial in North America failed to identify any objective benefits of IPPB in terms of mortality, need for hospitalization, change in pulmonary function, or quality of life [98]. Hence, this rather cumbersome and expensive treatment is no longer recommended and it has fallen into disuse.

Physical Therapy and Exercise Training

Physical therapy measures, consisting of chest-wall percussion and postural drainage, have been advocated and widely used in the treatment of COPD. While they may have some role in the treatment of acute respiratory failure associated with copious and tenacious bronchial secretions, clinical trials have not shown any prolonged objective benefits from these forms of therapy in patients with stable COPD or those with infective episodes, and there is no justification for their regular use [7,163].

Because of their impaired ventilatory capacity and resulting exercise-induced dyspnea, patients with advanced COPD frequently avoid physical activities and assume an increasingly sedentary existence. Due to their inactivity, many patients also develop secondary deconditioning effects related to their cardiovascular and muscular systems. Various exercise programs have been employed in efforts to rehabilitate severely disabled patients with COPD. These have included general conditioning programs as well as more specific measures directed at the respiratory muscles.

It has been demonstrated repeatedly that exercise programs of only a few weeks' duration have a favorable impact on the general sense of well-being and exercise tolerance in patients with COPD [13,44,168]. The physiologic basis for these improvements is not fully understood. Most studies have failed to show changes in lung function or cardiovascular performance, and it is suspected that poorly understood adaptive changes

in skeletal muscle metabolism and nonspecific motivational factors are largely responsible. Respiratory muscle training, specifically inspiratory resistance breathing and isocapnic hyperventilation, has also been investigated as a method for improving disability in COPD [158,223]. While some improvements in respiratory muscle function can be achieved, it has been more difficult to show that these changes translate into better exercise tolerance or a decrease in dyspnea.

Some programs are highly structured and are conducted under close supervision, but the need for such effort-intensive and costly programs is debatable. Unsupervised programs, which include daily 15- to 20-minute periods of walking, stair climbing, calisthenics, or stationary cycling, appear to work equally as well. The key factor appears to be one of motivation in that the patient must be convinced that such programs are worthwhile when they are followed on a regular basis.

Variant Forms

Bullous Emphysema

Bullous emphysema is considered separately because it has certain distinctive pathologic and roentgenographic features and because it is one instance where surgery may benefit the patient with COPD. As described in Chapter 37, a *bulla* is an abnormally enlarged airspace, measuring more than 1 cm in diameter, that results from destruction of alveolar walls. Bullae are thought to represent a variant form of emphysema, in which the destructive changes are exaggerated within focal areas. Most patients with bullae also have some evidence of anatomic emphysema in other lung regions, but extensive bullous disease may be present with few other pathologic changes.

Small bullae, occurring singly or in clusters, are sometimes seen at the apices of otherwise normal lungs, particularly in tall young adults. They may spontaneously rupture into the pleural space and cause a pneumothorax. Whether these small apical bullae are the forerunners of more extensive bullous disease in older patients is not known. Giant bullae may occur singly, but they are more commonly multiple and frequently involve both lungs. They are located immediately below the pleural surface and occur more commonly in the upper portions of the lung. It has been suggested that the predilection for bullae to be located in lung apices might be explained by gravitational effects which result in greater tissue stresses in the more cephalad lung regions [218]. However, bullae occur in all parts of the lung, and a basal location is more frequently observed in patients with severe alpha$_1$-protease inhibitor deficiency [80].

Bullous disease, when extensive, can usually be recognized on the plain chest roentgenogram as regions of absent or decreased vascular markings demarcated by curving hair-thin shadows. These thin lines represent the walls of the bullae and when visible are virtually pathognomonic. Bullae are visualized much better by tomography, particularly CT, and this is the preferred method if their location and extent need to be carefully defined. The displacement of the pulmonary vasculature away from areas of bullous involvement can be demonstrated very elegantly by pulmonary angiography, but this procedure is rarely necessary. Radioisotope scanning can also be utilized to assess the location and severity of bullous disease, as the involved areas have markedly diminished ventilation and perfusion [12].

It is difficult to judge the extent of functional disturbance that can be directly attributed to bullae. Bullae are largely avascular, and since they also are underventilated, they contribute little to overall gas exchange [173]. Patients with bullae frequently have reduced maximal expiratory flow rates; an increase in TLC, FRC, and RV; and a reduction of the DlCO. To what extent bullous disease is responsible for these functional disturbances is usually uncertain, because patients usually have coexisting diffuse emphysema and airways disease.

Bullae are frequently viewed as enclosed airspaces, which because of pressure differentials, particularly during expiration, compress and impair function in more normal adjacent lung regions. However, careful pathologic examination reveals that most bullae have some communications with surrounding airspaces, and it therefore seems improbable that large pressure differentials could exist across the walls of the bullae. Bullae probably impair lung function merely as space-occupying structures that do not permit more normal areas of the lung to expand fully.

The suspicion that bullae may directly contribute to impaired lung function and exercise intolerance in affected patients has led to repeated surgical efforts for their removal or ablation [22,84,173,202]. In general, these efforts have not yielded encouraging results; only a few patients experience appreciable objective improvement and subjective benefits are usually not sustained. Furthermore, the surgery is hazardous in patients whose underlying lung function is severely impaired. Despite the overall disappointing results, surgery clearly offers a substantial advantage for selected patients, and the problem is in knowing how to identify those individuals who are likely to benefit.

Pride and coworkers [173] carefully studied 18 patients before and 6 to 9 months after surgical ablation of large bullae. On average, there were small but significant increases in the FEV$_1$ and in the PaO$_2$ and decreases in TLC and FRC after surgery. Improvements were nonuniformly distributed in that large changes were observed in a few patients while very small changes were seen in the majority. Only 6 of the 18 patients had an increase in the FEV$_1$ of greater than 300 ml. Only 7 of the 18 had an improvement in the PaO$_2$ of more than 10 mmHg. As might be expected, the largest improvements in lung function tended to be associated with the greatest symptomatic benefit.

Based on the case analysis from that study and other experience, certain general guidelines can be offered to predict the response to surgery. The larger and more localized the bullae, the more likely there will be a favorable result from surgical ablation. Patients with the worst preoperative pulmonary function have the poorest chance of appreciable objective improvement. The presence of diffuse severe emphysema, as indicated by a very low DlCO, is associated with a particularly poor surgical success rate. However, if bullae are localized, if they involve at least one-third to one-half of a hemithorax, if the patient is severely disabled from dyspnea, and if overall lung function is reasonably well preserved, then consideration should be given to surgical ablation.

Unilateral Hyperlucent Lung Syndrome

Swyer and James [204] first described the unilateral hyperlucent lung syndrome in 1953; this report was followed shortly by descriptions of similar cases by MacLeod [126]. Since then, many other cases have been recognized, and the clinical features, pathology, physiology, and cause of this interesting entity are now quite well understood.

The diagnosis is principally a roentgenographic one, and many cases are first recognized from routine chest roentgenograms in asymptomatic persons. The principal feature is an abnormal degree of radiolucency involving one lung or one lobe within a lung that is due to attenuated vascular markings and not to overexpansion. In addition, there is ordinarily a smaller-than-normal hilar shadow on the affected side.

There is severe airflow obstruction on the affected side which is evident with fluoroscopy or with inspiratory and expiratory chest roentgenograms. With inspiration, the mediastinum shifts toward the affected lung, and there is only minimal movement of the rib cage and diaphragm on the involved side. On expiration, the mediastinum shifts toward the normal lung as it empties, while the volume of the affected lung changes little or not at all. Pulmonary angiograms show a relatively small pulmonary artery on the affected side, with marked attenuation in the number and size of the smaller arterial branches. The decrease in ventilation and perfusion in the radiolucent lung can also be readily appreciated by radioisotope scans.

Originally it was thought that this syndrome represented a congenital or acquired vascular abnormality similar to hypoplastic pulmonary artery, but it is now known that diffuse obstruction in the peripheral airways is the primary lesion, with the vascular changes being secondary. Roentgenographic and pathologic studies by Reid and Simon [175] demonstrated the severe bronchiolar disease responsible for airflow obstruction and air trapping. Bronchograms of affected lungs showed largely normal proximal bronchi but there was dilatation and beading more distally, and many of the terminal airways failed to fill completely with contrast material. The clubbed and tapered peripheral airways were described as having a "broken bough" appearance. Pathologic studies of these same lungs revealed widespread inflammation and fibrosis of the nonalveolated bronchioles with narrowing or complete obliteration of their lumina. Emphysema of varying severity was present in the parenchyma of some of the affected lungs. Small pulmonary arterioles, although narrowed, were not occluded by thrombi and were not involved by an endarteritis. The large pulmonary arteries were normal by histologic examination.

Many patients with the unilateral hyperlucent lung syndrome have a history of severe childhood pneumonia. MacPherson and associates [127] reported the occurrence of this syndrome in children following adenoviral infections, and it has also been observed following *Mycoplasma pneumoniae* infection, measles, pertussis, tuberculosis, radiation, foreign-body aspiration, and hydrocarbon pneumonia [19,129,175,200,219]. The clinical and pathologic observations are consistent with the notion that severe inflammation in the small airways, induced by infection or toxin, causes severe airflow obstruction. Hypoperfusion occurs only secondarily due to relative alveolar hypoxia.

The physiologic abnormalities associated with the hyperlucent lung syndrome have been described in some detail [52,105,148]. The affected lung receives some ventilation (atelectasis would occur if it did not), but minute volume and oxygen uptake on that side are usually less than 25 percent of the total and may be much less. Mixing time for inert gases is greatly prolonged, because of the marked disparities in the amounts of ventilation received by the two lungs. Because perfusion is reduced roughly in proportion to ventilation, the $\dot{V}/\dot{Q}$ of the involved lung remains near unity, and severe arterial oxygen desaturation does not usually occur. Patients may experience some arterial desaturation with exercise. Spirometry characteristically shows a modest reduction in the VC and a modest impairment of expiratory flow rates. If the opposite lung is relatively free of disease, pulmonary function test results may be surprisingly normal.

Unilateral hyperlucent lung syndrome usually presents few difficulties in differential diagnosis, provided that fluoroscopy or inspiratory and expiratory roentgenograms are obtained. Most patients have no symptoms directly attributable to the disorder, so that no specific treatment is required. If the opposite lung is also involved, but to a lesser degree, severe airflow obstruction and a clinical picture indistinguishable from COPD may be present, and the treatment is the same as for COPD. Rarely, recurrent infections in the affected lung may be an indication for surgical removal.

References

1. Abraham AS, Cole RB, Bishop JM. Reversal of pulmonary hypertension by prolonged oxygen administration to patients with chronic bronchitis. *Circ Res* 23:147, 1968.
2. American College of Chest Physicians–American Thoracic Society. Report of the Joint Committee on Pulmonary Nomenclature. *Chest* 67:583, 1974.
3. American Thoracic Society, Committee on Diagnostic Standards for Nontuberculous Respiratory Diseases. Definitions and classifications of chronic bronchitis, asthma, and pulmonary emphysema. *Am Rev Respir Dis* 85:762, 1962.
4. Anderson AE Jr, et al. Pulmonary emphysema: Prevalence, severity and anatomical patterns in

macrosections, with respect to smoking habits. *Arch Environ Health* 12:569, 1966.

5. Anthonisen NR, et al. Regional lung function in patients with chronic bronchitis. *Clin Sci* 35:495, 1968.

6. Anthonisen NR, et al. Antibiotic therapy in exacerbations of chronic obstructive pulmonary disease. *Ann Intern Med* 106:196, 1987.

7. Anthonisen P, Riise P, Sogaard-Andersen T. The value of lung physiotherapy in the treatment of acute exacerbations in chronic bronchitis. *Acta Med Scand* 175:715, 1964.

8. Ashley R. Pulmonary function: Relation to aging, cigarette habit, and mortality. The Framingham Study. *Ann Intern Med* 82:739, 1975.

9. Auerbach O, et al. Relation of smoking and age to emphysema: Whole-lung section study. *N Engl J Med* 286:853, 1972.

10. Baker TR, et al. Screening and treatment program for mild chronic obstructive pulmonary disease. *JAMA* 214:1448, 1970.

11. Barclay J, Whiting B, Aadis GJ. The influence of theophylline on maximal response to salbutamol in severe chronic obstructive pulmonary disease. *Eur J Clin Pharmacol* 22:289, 1983.

12. Barter CE, et al. Radiology compared with xenon-133 scanning and bronchoscopic lobar sampling for assessing regional lung function in patients with emphysema. *Thorax* 28:29, 1973.

13. Bass H, Whitcomb JF, Forman R. Exercise training: Therapy for patients with chronic obstructive pulmonary disease. *Chest* 57:116, 1970.

14. Bates DV. The fate of the chronic bronchitic: A report of the ten-year follow-up in the Canadian Department of Veterans' Affairs Coordinated Study of Chronic Bronchitis (The J. Burns Amberson Lecture). *Am Rev Respir Dis* 108:1043, 1973.

15. Bates DV, Christie RV. Intrapulmonary mixing of helium in health and in emphysema. *Clin Sci* 9:17, 1950.

16. Beerel F, Jick H, Tyler JM. A controlled study of the effect of prednisone on airflow obstruction in severe pulmonary emphysema. *N Engl J Med* 268:226, 1963.

17. Beerel F, Vance JW. Prednisone treatment for stable pulmonary emphysema. *Am Rev Respir Dis* 104:264, 1971.

18. Begin R, et al. Flow and age dependence of airway closure and dynamic compliance. *J Appl Physiol* 38:199, 1975.

19. Berdon WE, Baker DH, Boyer J. Unusual benign and malignant sequelae to childhood radiation therapy, including "unilateral hyperlucent lung." *AJR* 95:545, 1965.

20. Bergin C, et al. The diagnosis of emphysema. A computer tomographic-pathologic correlation. *Am Rev Respir Dis* 133:541, 1986.

21. Berglund E, et al. Spirometric studies in normal subjects: I. Forced expirograms in subjects between 7 and 70 years of age. *Acta Med Scand* 173:185, 1963.

22. Billing DM, Boushy SF, Kohen R. Surgical treatment of bullous emphysema. *Arch Surg* 97:744, 1968.

23. Block AJ, Castle JR, Keitt AS. Chronic oxygen therapy: Treatment of chronic obstructive pulmonary disease at sea level. *Chest* 65:279, 1974.

24. Blum A. Nicotine chewing gum and the medicalization of smoking (editorial). *Ann Intern Med* 101:121, 1984.

25. Boren HG, Kory RC, Syner JC. The Veterans Administration-Army Cooperative Study of Pulmonary Function: II. The lung volume and its subdivisions in normal men. *Am J Med* 41:96, 1966.

26. Bouhuys A, et al. Chronic respiratory disease in hemp workers. *Am J Med* 46:526, 1969.

27. Bouhuys A, et al. Epidemiology of chronic lung disease in a cotton mill community. *Lung* 154:167, 1977.

28. Boushy SF, et al. Lung recoil pressure, airway resistance and forced flow related to morphologic emphysema. *Am Rev Respir Dis* 104:551, 1971.

29. Boushy SF, et al. Prognosis in chronic obstructive pulmonary disease. *Am Rev Respir Dis* 108:1373, 1973.

30. British Medical Research Council. Value of chemoprophylaxis and chemotherapy in early chronic bronchitis: A report to the Medical Research Council by their working party on trials of chemotherapy in early chronic bronchitis. *Br Med J* 1:1317, 1966.

31. British Ministry of Health. *Mortality and Morbidity during the London Fog of December, 1952*. Ministry of Health report on public health no 95. London: Her Majesty's Stationery Office, 1954.

32. Bruce RM, et al. Collaborative study to assess risk of lung disease in Pimz phenotype subjects. *Am Rev Respir Dis* 130:386, 1984.

33. Buist AS, Ross BB. Predicted values for closing volumes using a modified single breath nitrogen test. *Am Rev Respir Dis* 107:744, 1973.

34. Buist AS, et al. The effect of smoking cessation and modification on lung function. *Am Rev Respir Dis* 114:115, 1976.

35. Buist AS, van Fleet DL, Ross BB. A comparison of conventional spirometric tests and the test of closing volume in an emphysema screening center. *Am Rev Respir Dis* 107:735, 1973.

36. Burrows B, Earle RH. Course and prognosis of chronic obstructive lung disease: A prospective study of 200 patients. *N Engl J Med* 280:397, 1969.

37. Burrows B, et al. Patterns of cardiovascular dysfunction in chronic obstructive lung disease. *N Engl J Med* 286:912, 1972.

38. Burrows B, et al. Quantitative relationships be-

tween cigarette smoking and ventilatory function. *Am Rev Respir Dis* 115:195, 1977.

39. Burrows B, et al. A reexamination of risk factors for ventilatory impairment. *Am Rev Respir Dis* 138:829, 1988.

40. Burrows B, Knudson RJ, Lebowitz MD. The relationship of childhood respiratory illness to adult obstructive airway disease. *Am Rev Respir Dis* 115:751, 1977.

41. Burrows B, Lebowitz MD, Barbee RA. Respiratory disorders and allergy skin-test reactions. *Ann Intern Med* 84:134, 1976.

42. Campbell EJM, Howell JBL. The sensation of breathlessness. *Br Med Bull* 19:36, 1963.

43. Chester EH, et al. Bronchodilator therapy: Comparison of acute response to three methods of administration. *Chest* 62:394, 1972.

44. Christie D. Physical training in chronic obstructive lung disease. *Br Med J* 2:150, 1968.

45. Christopher KL, et al. Program for transtracheal oxygen delivery: Assessment of safety and efficacy. *Ann Intern Med* 107:802, 1987.

46. Ciba Guest Symposium Report. Terminology, definitions, and classification of chronic pulmonary emphysema and related conditions. *Thorax* 14:286, 1959.

47. Cole TJ. The influence of height on the decline in ventilatory function. *Int J Epidemiol* 3:145, 1974.

48. Collier AM, et al. Spirometric changes in normal children with upper respiratory infections. *Am Rev Respir Dis* 117:47, 1978.

49. Cooper DM, et al. Lung function in alpha₁-antitrypsin heterozygotes (Pi type MZ). *Am Rev Respir Dis* 110:708, 1974.

50. Cotes JE, et al. Average normal values for the forced expiratory volume in white Caucasian males. *Br Med J* 1:1016, 1966.

51. Cox DW, Hoeppner VH, Levison H. Protease inhibitors in patients with chronic obstructive pulmonary disease: The alpha₁-antitrypsin heterozygote controversy. *Am Rev Respir Dis* 113:601, 1976.

52. Darke CS, Chrispin AR, Snowden BS. Unilateral lung transradiance: A physiological study. *Thorax* 15:74, 1960.

53. Detels R, et al. The UCLA population studies of chronic obstructive respiratory disease. 9. Lung function changes associated with chronic exposure to photochemical oxidants; a cohort study among never-smokers. *Chest* 92:594, 1987.

54. do Pico GA, et al. Respiratory abnormalities among grain handlers: A clinical, physiologic, and immunologic study. *Am Rev Respir Dis* 115:915, 1977.

55. Doll R, Hill AB. Mortality in relations to smoking: Ten years' observation of British doctors. *Br Med J* 1:1399, 1964.

56. Dosman J, et al. The use of a helium-oxygen mixture during maximum expiratory flow to demonstrate obstruction in small airways in smokers. *J Clin Invest* 55:1090, 1975.

57. Dosman J, et al. The relationship between symptoms and functional abnormalities in clinically healthy cigarette smokers. *Am Rev Respir Dis* 114:297, 1976.

58. Dubois AB, Botelho SY, Comroe JH Jr. A new method for measuring airway resistance in man using a body plethysmograph: Values in normal subjects and in patients with respiratory disease. *J Clin Invest* 3335:327, 1956.

59. Dubois AB, et al. A rapid plethysmographic method for measuring thoracic gas volume: A comparison with a nitrogen washout method for measuring functional residual capacity in normal subjects. *J Clin Invest* 35:322, 1956.

60. Dullinger D, Kronenberg R, Niewoehner DE. Efficacy of inhaled metaproterenol and orally administered theophylline in patients with chronic airflow obstruction. *Chest* 89:171, 1986.

61. Easton PA, et al. A comparison of the bronchodilating effects of a beta-2 adrenergic agent (albuterol) and an anticholinergic agent (ipratropium bromide) given by aerosol alone or in sequence. *N Engl J Med* 315:735, 1986.

62. Eaton ML, et al. Efficacy of theophylline in "irreversible" airflow obstruction. *Ann Intern Med* 92:758, 1980.

63. Elmes PC, et al. Value of ampicillin in the hospital treatment of exacerbations of chronic bronchitis. *Br Med J* 2:904, 1965.

64. Emirgil C, Sobol BJ. Long-term course of chronic obstructive pulmonary disease: A new view of the mode of functional deterioration. *Am J Med* 51:504, 1971.

65. Emirgil C, et al. A study of the long-term effect of therapy in chronic obstructive pulmonary disease. *Am J Med* 47:367, 1969.

66. Eriksson S. Pulmonary emphysema and alpha₁-antitrypsin deficiency. *Acta Med Scand* 175:197, 1964.

67. Eriksson S. Studies in alpha₁-antitrypsin deficiency. *Acta Med Scand Suppl* 432:6, 1965.

68. Evans JA, Morrison IM, Saunders KB. A controlled trial of prednisone, in low dosage, in patients with chronic airways obstruction. *Thorax* 23:401, 1974.

69. Ferris BG Jr, Anderson DO. The prevalence of chronic respiratory disease in a New Hampshire town. *Am Rev Respir Dis* 86:165, 1962.

70. Ferris BG Jr, Anderson DO. Epidemiological studies related to air pollution: A comparison of Berlin, New Hampshire, and Chilliwack, British Columbia. *Proc R Soc Med* 57:979, 1964.

71. Ferris BG Jr, Anderson DO, Zickmantel R. Prediction values for screening tests of pulmonary function. *Am Rev Respir Dis* 91:252, 1965.

72. Fletcher C, et al. *The Natural History of*

Chronic Bronchitis and Emphysema: An Eight-Year Study of Early Chronic Obstructive Lung Disease in Working Men in London. Oxford, England: Oxford University Press, 1976.

73. Fletcher CM. Chronic bronchitis: Its prevalence, nature and pathogenesis. *Am Rev Respir Dis* 80:483, 1959.

74. Fletcher CM. The clinical diagnosis of pulmonary emphysema: An experimental study. *Proc R Soc Med* 45:577, 1952.

75. Fletcher CM, Horn D. Smoking and health. *WHO Chron* 24:3445, 1970.

76. Fowler WS. Lung function studies: III. Uneven pulmonary ventilation in normal subjects and in patients with pulmonary disease. *J Appl Physiol* 2:283, 1949.

77. Frank NR, Mead J, Ferris BG Jr. The mechanical behavior of the lungs in healthy elderly persons. *J Clin Invest* 36:1680, 1957.

78. Godfrey S, et al. Repeatability of physical signs in airways obstruction. *Thorax* 24:4, 1969.

79. Gould GA, et al. Measurements of lung density in life can quantitate distal air space enlargement—An essential defining feature of human emphysema. *Am Rev Respir Dis* 137:380, 1988.

80. Greenberg SD, et al. The lungs in homozygous alpha$_1$-antitrypsin deficiency. *Am J Clin Pathol* 60:581, 1973.

81. Gregg I. A Study of the Causes of Progressive Airway Obstruction in Chronic Bronchitis. In *Current Research in Chronic Respiratory Disease: Proceedings of the Eleventh Aspen Emphysema Conference.* Public Health Service publication no 1879. Washington, DC: US Public Health Service, 1968. Pp 235–246.

82. Gross NJ, Skorodin MS. Role of the parasympathetic system in airway obstruction due to emphysema. *N Engl J Med* 311:421, 1984.

83. Grump DW, et al. Role of infection in chronic bronchitis. *Am Rev Respir Dis* 113:465, 1976.

84. Gunstensen J, McCormack RJM. The surgical management of bullous emphysema. *J Thorac Cardiovasc Surg* 65:920, 1973.

85. Guyatt GH, et al. Bronchodilators in chronic airflow limitation. Effects on airway function, exercise capacity, and quality of life. *Am Rev Respir Dis* 135:1069, 1987.

86. Heaton RK, et al. Psychologic effects of continuous and nocturnal oxygen therapy in hypoxemic chronic obstructive pulmonary disease. *Arch Intern Med* 143:1941, 1983.

87. Heimer D, Shim C, Williams MH Jr. The effect of sequential inhalation of metaproterenol aerosol in asthma. *J Allergy Clin Immunol* 66:75, 1980.

88. Hepper NG, et al. The prevalence of alpha$_1$-antitrypsin deficiency in selected groups of patients with chronic obstructive lung disease. *Mayo Clin Proc* 44:697, 1969.

89. Higgins MW, Keller J. Familial occurrence of chronic respiratory disease and familial resemblance in ventilatory capacity. *J Chronic Dis* 28:239, 1975.

90. Higgins MW, Keller JB, Metzner HL. Smoking, socioeconomic status, and chronic respiratory disease. *Am Rev Respir Dis* 116:403, 1977.

91. Higgins MW, Thom T. Incidence, prevalence, and mortality: Intra- and intercountry differences. In MJ Hensley, NA Saunders (Eds), *Clinical Epidemiology of Chronic Obstructive Pulmonary Disease.* New York: Marcel Dekker, 1989. Pp 23–29.

92. Higgins MW, et al. An index of risk for obstructive airways disease. *Am Rev Respir Dis* 125:144, 1982.

93. Holland WW, Reid DD. The urban factor in chronic bronchitis. *Lancet* 1:445, 1965.

94. Howard P. Evolution of the ventilatory capacity in chronic bronchitis. *Br Med J* 3:392, 1967.

95. Howard P, Astin TW. Precipitous fall of the forced expiratory volume. *Thorax* 24:492, 1969.

96. Hubbard RC, et al. Biochemical efficacy and safety of monthly augmentation therapy for α_1-antitrypsin deficiency. *JAMA* 260:1259, 1988.

97. Ingram RH Jr, O'Cain CF. Frequency dependency of compliance in apparently healthy smokers versus nonsmokers. *Bull Physiopathol Respir* 7:195, 1971.

98. The Intermittent Positive-Pressure Breathing Trial Group. Intermittent positive-pressure breathing therapy of chronic obstructive pulmonary disease: A clinical trial. *Ann Intern Med* 99:612, 1983.

99. Jamal K, et al. Chronic bronchitis: Correlation of morphologic findings to sputum production and flow rates. *Am Rev Respir Dis* 129:719, 1984.

100. Janus ED, Phillips NT, Carrell RW. Smoking, lung function, and alpha 1-antitrypsin deficiency. *Lancet* 1:152, 1985.

101. Jenne JW, et al. The course of chronic *Hemophilus* bronchitis treated with massive doses of penicillin and penicillin combined with streptomycin. *Am Rev Respir Dis* 101:907, 1970.

102. Jenne JW, et al. Pharmacokinetics of theophylline: Application to adjustment of the clinical dose of aminophylline. *Clin Pharmacol Ther* 13:349, 1972.

103. Johnston RN, et al. Chronic bronchitis: Measurements and observations over 10 years. *Thorax* 31:25, 1976.

104. Jones NL, Burrows B, Fletcher CM. Serial studies of 100 patients with chronic airway obstruction in London and Chicago. *Thorax* 22:327, 1967.

105. Kent DC. Physiologic aspects of idiopathic unilateral hyperlucent lung, with a review of the literature. *Am Rev Respir Dis* 90:202, 1964.

106. Klayton R, Fallat R, Cohen AB. Determinants of chronic obstructive pulmonary disease in patients with intermediate levels of alpha$_1$-antitrypsin. *Am Rev Respir Dis* 112:71, 1975.

107. Knudson RJ, Burrows B, Lebowitz MD. The maximal expiratory flow-volume curve: Its use in the detection of ventilatory abnormalities in a population study. *Am Rev Respir Dis* 14:871, 1976.

108. Knudson RJ, Lebowitz MD. Comparison of flow-volume and closing volume variables in a random population. *Am Rev Respir Dis* 116:1039, 1977.

109. Knudson RJ, et al. The maximal expiratory flow-volume curve: Normal standards, variability, and effects of age. *Am Rev Respir Dis* 113:587, 1976.

110. Kongragunta VR, Druz WS, Sharp JT. Dyspnea and diaphragmatic fatigue in patients with chronic obstructive pulmonary disease. Responses to theophylline. *Am Rev Respir Dis* 137:662, 1988.

111. Koren HS, et al. Ozone-induced inflammation in the lower airways of human subjects. *Am Rev Respir Dis* 139:407, 1989.

112. Kory RC, et al. The Veterans Administration-Army Cooperative Study of Pulmonary Function: I. Clinical spirometry in norman men. *Am J Med* 30:243, 1961.

113. Kueppers F, Black LF. State of the art: Alpha$_1$-antitrypsin and its deficiency. *Am Rev Respir Dis* 110:176, 1974.

114. Lands AM, et al. Differentiation of receptor systems activated by sympathomimetic amines. *Nature* 214:597, 1967.

115. Larson RK, et al. Genetic and environmental determinants of chronic obstructive pulmonary disease. *Ann Intern Med* 72:627, 1970.

116. Laurell CB, Eriksson S. The electrophoretic alpha$_1$-globulin pattern of serum in alpha$_1$-antitrypsin deficiency. *Scand J Clin Lab Invest* 15:132, 1963.

117. Leggett RJ, et al. Long-term domiciliary oxygen therapy in cor pulmonale complicating chronic bronchitis and emphysema. *Thorax* 31:414, 1976.

118. Levine BE, et al. The role of long-term continuous oxygen administration in patients with chronic airway obstruction and hypoxemia. *Ann Intern Med* 66:639, 1967.

119. Levine G, et al. Gas-exchange abnormalities in mild bronchitis and asymptomatic asthma. *N Engl J Med* 282:1277, 1970.

120. Lewis BM, et al. Effect of uneven ventilation on pulmonary diffusion capacity. *J Appl Physiol* 16:679, 1961.

121. Ligas JR, et al. A comparison of measures of forced expirations. *J Appl Physiol* 42:607, 1977.

122. Light RW, Summer WR, Luchinger PC. Response of patients with chronic obstructive lung disease to the regular administration of nebulized isoproterenol: A double-blind crossover study. *Chest* 67:634, 1975.

123. Lilker ES, Karnick AD, Lerner L. Portable oxygen in chronic obstructive lung disease with hypoxemia and cor pulmonale: A controlled double-blind crossover study. *Chest* 68:236, 1975.

124. Linn WS, et al. Respiratory function and symptoms in urban office workers in relation to oxidant air pollution exposure. *Am Rev Respir Dis* 114:477, 1976.

125. Linn WS, et al. Short-term respiratory effects of 0.12 ppm ozone exposure in volunteers with chronic obstructive pulmonary disease. *Am Rev Respir Dis* 125:658, 1982.

126. MacLeod WW. Abnormal transradiancy of one lung. *Thorax* 9:147, 1954.

127. MacPherson RI, Cumming GR, Chernick V. Unilateral hyperlucent lung: A complication of viral pneumonia. *J Can Assoc Radiol* 20:225, 1969.

128. Mahler DA, et al. Sustained-release theophylline reduces dyspnea in nonreversible obstructive airways disease. *Am Rev Respir Dis* 131:22, 1985.

129. Margolin HN, et al. Idiopathic unilateral hyperlucent lung: A roentgenologic syndrome. *AJR* 82:63, 1959.

130. Martin AE. Mortality and morbidity statistics and air pollution. *Proc R Soc Med* 57:969, 1964.

131. Martin CJ, Kasura S, Cochran TH. The relationship of chronic bronchitis to the diffuse obstructive pulmonary syndrome. *Am Rev Respir Dis* 102:362, 1970.

132. May JR. The bacteriology of chronic bronchitis. *Lancet* 2:534, 1953.

133. May JR. Antibodies to *Haemophilus influenzae* in the sera of patients with chronic bronchitis. *J Pathol Bacteriol* 90:163, 1965.

134. May JR, et al. A study of *Hemophilus influenzae* precipitins in the serum of working men in relation to smoking habits, bronchial infection, and airway obstruction. *Am Rev Respir Dis* 108:460, 1973.

135. McCarthy DS, Craig DB, Cherniack RM. Effect of modification of the smoking habit on lung function. *Am Rev Respir Dis* 114:103, 1976.

136. Mead J, Lindgren I, Gaensler EA. The mechanical properties of the lung in emphysema. *J Clin Invest* 343:1005, 1955.

137. Medical Research Council Working Party. Long term domiciliary oxygen therapy in chronic hypoxia and cor pulmonale complicating chronic bronchitis and emphysema. *Lancet* 1:681, 1981.

138. Mendella LA, et al. Steroid response in stable chronic obstructive pulmonary disease. *Ann Intern Med* 96:17, 1982.

139. Meneely GR, Kalreider NL. The volume of the lung determined by helium dilution: Description of the method and comparison with other procedures. *J Clin Invest* 28:129, 1949.

140. Mitchell RS, Filley GF. Chronic obstructive bronchopulmonary disease: I. Clinical features. *Am Rev Respir Dis* 89:360, 1964.

141. Mitchell RS, et al. The morphologic features of the bronchi, bronchioles, and alveoli in chronic airway obstruction: A clinicopathologic study. *Am Rev Respir Dis* 114:137, 1976.

142. Mitenko PA, Ogilvie RI. Rational intravenous doses of theophylline. *N Engl J Med* 289:609, 1973.

143. Morgan WKC, Lapp NL. State of the art: Respiratory disease in coal miners. *Am Rev Respir Dis* 113:531, 1976.

144. Morris JF, Koski A, Johnson LC. Spirometric standards for healthy nonsmoking adults. *Am Rev Respir Dis* 103:57, 1971.

145. Moser KM, Rhodes PG. Acute effects of aerosolized acetylcysteine upon spirometric measurements in subjects with and without obstructive pulmonary disease. *Dis Chest* 49:370, 1966.

146. Murciano D, et al. Effects of theophylline on diaphragmatic strength and fatigue in patients with chronic obstructive pulmonary disease. *N Engl J Med* 311:349, 1984.

147. Musk AW, et al. Pulmonary function in granite dust exposure: A four-year follow up. *Am Rev Respir Dis* 115:769, 1977.

148. Nairn JR, Prime FJ. A physiological study of MacLeod's syndrome. *Thorax* 22:148, 1967.

149. National Center for Health Sciences. Limitation of activity due to chronic conditions, United States, 1969–1970. *Vital and Health Statistics*, series 10, no 80. Washington: US Government Printing Office, 1973.

150. Nicklaus TM, et al. The accuracy of the roentgenologic diagnosis of chronic pulmonary emphysema. *Am Rev Respir Dis* 93:889, 1966.

151. Nicklaus TM, et al. Roentgenologic, physiologic, and structural estimations of the total lung capacity in normal and emphysematous subjects. *Am J Med* 42:547, 1967.

152. Niewoehner DE, Kleinerman J, Rice DB. Pathologic changes in the peripheral airways of young cigarette smokers. *N Engl J Med* 291:755, 1974.

153. Nishimoto Y, et al. Chronic obstructive lung disease in Japanese poison gas workers. *Am Rev Respir Dis* 102:173, 1970.

154. Nocturnal Oxygen Therapy Trial Group. Continuous or nocturnal oxygen therapy in hypoxemic chronic obstructive lung disease: A clinical trial. *Ann Intern Med* 93:391, 1980.

155. O'Connor GT, Sparrow D, Weiss ST. The role of allergy and nonspecific airway hyperresponsiveness in the pathogenesis of chronic obstructive pulmonary disease. *Am Rev Respir Dis* 140:225, 1989.

156. Oxhoj H, Bake B, Wilhelmsen L. Ability of spirometry, flow-volume curves and the nitrogen closing volume test to detect smokers: A population study. *Scand J Respir Dis* 58:80, 1977.

157. Pakes GE, et al. Ipratropium bromide: A review of its pharmacological properties and therapeutic efficacy in asthma and chronic bronchitis. *Drugs* 20:237, 1980.

158. Pardy RL, et al. The effects of inspiratory muscle training on exercise performance in chronic airflow obstruction. *Am Rev Respir Dis* 123:426, 1981.

159. Park SS, et al. Relationship of bronchitis and emphysema to altered pulmonary function. *Am Rev Respir Dis* 102:927, 1970.

160. Payne CB Jr, Chester EH, Hsi BP. Airway responsiveness in chronic obstructive pulmonary disease. *Am J Med* 42:554, 1967.

161. Peters JM. Cumulative pulmonary effects in workers exposed to toluene diisocyanate. *Proc R Soc Med* 63:372, 1970.

162. Peters JM, Ferris BG Jr. Smoking, pulmonary function, and respiratory symptoms in a college-age group. *Am Rev Respir Dis* 95:774, 1967.

163. Petersen ES, et al. A controlled study of the effect of treatment on chronic bronchitis: An evaluation using pulmonary function tests. *Acta Med Scand* 182:293, 1967.

164. Peto R, et al. The relevance in adults of air-flow obstruction, but not mucus hypersecretion, to mortality from chronic lung disease. *Am Rev Respir Dis* 128:491, 1983.

165. Petty TL. The National Mucolytic Study. Results of a randomized, double-blind, placebo-controlled study of iodinated glycerol in chronic obstructive bronchitis. *Chest* 97:75, 1990.

166. Pflug AE, Cheney FW Jr, Butler J. The effects of an ultrasonic aerosol on pulmonary mechanics and arterial blood gases in patients with chronic bronchitis. *Am Rev Respir Dis* 101:710, 1970.

167. Picken JJ, Niewoehner DE, Chester EH. Prolonged effects of viral infections of the upper respiratory tract upon small airways. *Am J Med* 52:738, 1972.

168. Pierce AK, et al. Response to exercise training in patients with emphysema. *Arch Intern Med* 113:228, 1964.

169. Pierce JA, Ebert RV. The barrel deformity of the chest, the senile lung, and obstructive pulmonary emphysema. *Am J Med* 25:13, 1958.

170. Pines A, et al. Antibiotic regimens in moderately ill patients with purulent exacerbations of chronic bronchitis. *Br J Dis Chest* 66:107, 1972.

171. Pines A, et al. Antibiotic regimens in severe and acute purulent exacerbations of chronic bronchitis. *Br Med J* 2:735, 1968.

172. Popa VT. Clinical pharmacology of adrenergic drugs. *J Asthma* 21:183, 1984.

173. Pride NB, Barter CE, Hugh-Jones P. The ventilation of bullae and the effect of their removal on thoracic gas volumes and tests of overall

pulmonary function. *Am Rev Respir Dis* 107:83, 1973.

174. Reid L. Measurement of the bronchial mucous gland layer: A diagnostic yardstick in chronic bronchitis. *Thorax* 15:132, 1960.

175. Reid L, Simon G. Unilateral lung transradiance. *Thorax* 17:230, 1962.

176. Reid LM. Pathology of chronic bronchitis. *Lancet* 1:275, 1954.

177. Renzetti AD Jr, McClement JH, Litt BD. Veterans Administration Cooperative Study of Pulmonary Function: III. Mortality in relation to respiratory function in chronic obstructive pulmonary disease. *Am J Med* 41:115, 1966.

178. Report of a National Heart, Lung, and Blood Institute, Division of Lung Diseases, Workshop. The definition of emphysema. *Am Rev Respir Dis* 132:182, 1985.

179. Rice KL, et al. Aminophylline for acute exacerbations of chronic obstructive pulmonary disease—A controlled trial. *Ann Intern Med* 107:305, 1987.

180. Robertson JS, Siri WE, Jones HB. Lung ventilation patterns determined by analysis of nitrogen elimination rates: Use of mass spectrometer as a continuous gas analyzer. *J Clin Invest* 29:577, 1950.

181. Sackner MA, Kim CS. Auxiliary MDI aerosol delivery systems. *Chest* 88(Suppl 2):161S, 1985.

182. Schneider IC, Anderson AE Jr. Correlation of clinical signs with ventilatory function in obstructive lung disease. *Ann Intern Med* 62:477, 1965.

183. Seely JE, Zuskinn E, Bouhuys A. Cigarette smoking: Objective evidence for lung damage to teenagers. *Science* 172:741, 1971.

184. Seltzer CC, et al. Differences in pulmonary function related to smoking habits and race. *Am Rev Respir Dis* 110:598, 1974.

185. Shannon M, Lovejoy FH Jr. The influence of age vs peak serum concentrations on life-threatening events after chronic theophylline intoxication. *Arch Intern Med* 150:2045, 1990.

186. Sharp JT, et al. A longitudinal study of bronchitic symptoms and spirometry in a middle-aged, male, industrial population. *Am Rev Respir Dis* 108:1066, 1973.

187. Shim C, Williams MH Jr. The adequacy of inhalation of aerosol from canister nebulizers. *Am J Med* 69:891, 1980.

188. Shim C, Williams MH Jr. Aerosol beclomethasone in patients with steroid-responsive chronic obstructive pulmonary disease. *Am J Med* 78:655, 1985.

189. Sidor R, Peters JM. Fire fighting and pulmonary function: An epidemiologic study. *Am Rev Respir Dis* 109:249, 1974.

190. Silverman EK, et al. Variability of pulmonary function in alpha-1-antitrypsin deficiency: Clinical correlates. *Ann Intern Med* 111:982, 1989.

191. Simon G, et al. Relation between abnormalities in the chest radiograph and changes in pulmonary function in chronic bronchitis and emphysema. *Thorax* 28:15, 1973.

192. Smith TJ, et al. Pulmonary impairment from chronic exposure to sulfur dioxide in a smelter. *Am Rev Respir Dis* 116:31, 1977.

193. Smylie HC, Blendis LM, Armitage P. Observer disagreement in physical signs of the respiratory system. *Lancet* 2:412, 1965.

194. Sobol BJ. Assessment of ventilatory abnormality in the asymptomatic subject: An exercise in futility. *Thorax* 21:445, 1966.

195. Spain DM, Siegel H, Bradess VA. Emphysema in apparently healthy adults: Smoking, age, and sex. *JAMA* 224:322, 1973.

196. Sparrow D, et al. The influence of age and level of pulmonary function on nonspecific airway responsiveness. The Normative Aging Study. *Am Rev Respir Dis* 143:978, 1991.

197. Spektor DM, et al. Effects of ambient ozone on respiratory function in active normal children. *Am Rev Respir Dis* 137:313, 1988.

198. Spektor DM, et al. Effects of ambient ozone on respiratory function in healthy adults exercising outdoors. *Am Rev Respir Dis* 138:821, 1988.

199. Stebbings JH Jr. A survey of respiratory disease among New York City postal and transit workers. *Environ Res* 6:147, 1973.

200. Stokes D, et al. Unilateral hyperlucent lung (Swyer-James syndrome) after severe *Mycoplasma pneumoniae* infection. *Am Rev Respir Dis* 117:145, 1978.

201. Stuart-Harris CH. Shortness of breath. *Br Med J* 1:1203, 1964.

202. Sung DT, Payne S, Black LP. Surgical management of giant bullae associated with obstructive airway disease. *Surg Clin North Am* 53:913, 1973.

203. Sutinen S, et al. Roentgenologic criteria for the recognition of nonsymptomatic pulmonary emphysema: Correlation between roentgenologic findings and pulmonary pathology. *Am Rev Respir Dis* 91:69, 1965.

204. Swyer PR, James GCW. A case of unilateral pulmonary emphysema. *Thorax* 8:13, 1953.

205. Tager IB, et al. Household aggregation of pulmonary function and chronic bronchitis. *Am Rev Respir Dis* 114:485, 1976.

206. Tager IB, Seizer FE. Risk estimates for chronic bronchitis in smokers: A study of male-female differences. *Am Rev Respir Dis* 113:619, 1976.

207. Tager IB, Speizer FE. Role of infection in chronic bronchitis. *N Engl J Med* 292:563, 1975.

208. Taylor DB, et al. The efficacy of orally administered theophylline, inhaled salbutamol, and a combination of the two as chronic therapy in the management of chronic bronchitis with reversible air-flow obstruction. *Am Rev Respir Dis* 131:747, 1985.

209. Thurlbeck WM, et al. Chronic obstructive lung disease: A comparison between clinical, roentgenologic, functional, and morphologic criteria in chronic bronchitis, emphysema, asthma, and bronchiectasis. *Medicine* 49:81, 1970.
210. Tiep BL, et al. Low-concentration oxygen therapy via a demand delivery system. *Chest* 87:636, 1985.
211. Tockman M, et al. A comparison of pulmonary function in male smokers and nonsmokers. *Am Rev Respir Dis* 114:711, 1976.
212. Toyama T. Air pollution and its health effects in Japan. *Arch Environ Health* 8:153, 1964.
213. Turner J, Mead J, Wohl ME. Elasticity of human lungs in relation to age. *J Appl Physiol* 25:664, 1968.
214. US Public Health Service. *Smoking and Health: Report of the Advisory Committee to the Surgeon General of the Public Health Service.* Public Health Service publications no 1103. Washington, DC: US Department of Health, Education and Welfare, 1964.
215. US Public Health Service. *The Health Consequences of Smoking: Chronic Obstructive Lung Disease. A Report of the Surgeon General.* Rockville, MD: US Department of Health and Human Services, Office on Smoking and Health, 1984.
216. Valic F, Beritic-Stahnijak D, Mark B. A follow-up study of functional and radiological lung changes in carbon black exposure. *Int Arch Occup Environ Health* 34:51, 1975.
217. Wagner PD, et al. Ventilation-perfusion inequality in chronic obstructive pulmonary disease. *J Clin Invest* 59:203, 1977.
218. West JB. Distribution of mechanical stress on the lung, a possible factor in localization of pulmonary disease. *Lancet* 1:839, 1971.
219. Wiseman DH. Unilateral pseudoemphysema. A case report. *Pediatrics* 35:300, 1965.
220. Woodcock AA, Johnson MA, Geddes DM. Theophylline prescribing, serum concentrations, and toxicity. *Lancet* 2:610, 1983.
221. Woodcock AJ, Colman MH, Blackburn CRB. Factors affecting normal values for ventilatory lung function. *Am Rev Respir Dis* 106:692, 1972.
222. Woolf CR, Suero JT. The respiratory effects of regular cigarette smoking in women. *Am Rev Respir Dis* 103:26, 1971.
223. Zack M, Palang A. Oxygen-supplemented exercise of ventilatory and non-ventilatory muscles in pulmonary rehabilitation. *Chest* 88:669, 1985.

40

Interstitial (Diffuse Parenchymal) Lung Disease: Etiologic, Clinical, and Roentgenologic Considerations

Michael S. Bernstein   Michael S. Stulbarg

The interstitial lung diseases (ILDs) are a heterogeneous group of disorders that affect predominantly the lung parenchyma with minimal airway involvement. Detection is at times difficult and diagnosis challenging. While this chapter provides an overview of the diagnostic approach to ILDs, others discuss staging, diagnostic procedures, and treatment as well as some of the specific diseases. Initial consideration of ILD may occur because of findings on the chest x-ray film or because of symptoms (e.g., dyspnea, cough) of unexplained cause. When confronted by an individual patient with possible ILD, the categories of disease to be considered depend greatly on the clinical presentation (e.g., acute fever and cough versus insidious dyspnea), but clinicians are often misled by this category of disease (e.g., idiopathic pulmonary fibrosis [IPF] with a normal-appearing chest x-ray film or left-sided heart failure presenting as a chronic interstitial disease). It is therefore important to have a comprehensive concept of the diseases that may involve the interstitium to help guide diagnostic and therapeutic decisions. For example, appropriate treatment for one of the diseases (e.g., corticosteroids for sarcoidosis) might be catastrophic for another (e.g., alveolar proteinosis, disseminated infection).

The guiding principle in approaching ILD is that a diagnosis should be sought in any patient with evidence of ILD. Specific diagnoses are occasionally suggested by a clear history of exposure (e.g., bird fanciers' lung), from specific extrapulmonary physical findings (e.g., skin involvement in dermatomyositis), from a "classic" radiologic finding (e.g., bamboo spine of ankylosing spondylitis), or from a laboratory abnormality (e.g., peripheral eosinophilia). Special physiologic studies may give great insight into the physiologic dysfunction, but in many cases, examination of tissue is often required to establish a specific diagnosis. The value of traditional clinical methods (i.e., history, physical examination, laboratory and radiologic evaluation) is discussed in considerable detail. Physiologic testing and diagnostic procedures are discussed elsewhere.

Anatomy

The pulmonary interstitium provides the connective-tissue structure that supports the lung. It extends in a continuous compartment from the mediastinum to the pleura. The interstitium has two major compartments in continuity with each other—the peribronchovascular interstitium, which surrounds the airways and blood vessels, and the alveolar interstitium [107]. The alveolar interstitium is the nearly invisible space separating the alveolar epithelial and the capillary endothelial cell membranes (Fig. 40-1). It is across this space that gas exchange occurs. In some areas the boundaries of the space are actually comprised of two epithelial cells back to back, and in fact the space may disappear with apparent fusion of the basement membranes of the cells. This space is filled with amorphous ground substance containing proteoglycans which are comprised of the connective-tissue components (collagen, elastic fibers) that provide much of the "backbone" of the lung. A small population of cells can be identified in the nor-

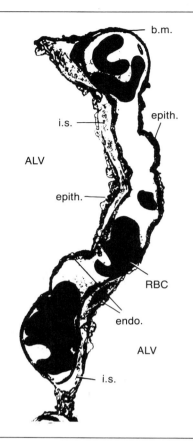

Fig. 40-1. Normal morphology of the interstitial space as shown by transmission electron microscopy (b.m. = basement membrane; i.s. = interstitial space; epith. = type I alveolar epithelial cell; ALV = lumen of the alveolus; RBC = red blood cell; endo. = capillary endothelial cell). (Courtesy of Dr. H. Benfer Kaltreider.)

mal interstitium (fibroblasts, pericytes, occasional smooth muscle cells, macrophages, and iflammatory cells), though the numbers and relative predominance of cell types as indicated by analysis of bronchoalveolar lavage or lung biopsy specimens change drastically in response to various disease processes.

Possible responses of the lung to widely varying insults to the alveolar interstitium are limited. Spencer [90] described four steps that might result in chronic interstitial disease following an initial insult: (1) organization of alveolar exudate, (2) damage to alveolar epithelium, (3) persistent lymphedema of alveolar walls (by hydrostatic pressure or active lymphatic obstruction), and (4) injury to the capillary endothelium. The inter-

stitium may be swollen passively by fluid (e.g., left ventricular failure) or actively by accumulation of proteins and infiltration of cells (e.g., immune effector cells, tumor cells) from the circulation. Since inflammation is often present in ILD, there may be progression to fibrosis, though the time course may vary from several weeks to many years [3]. Therefore, *pulmonary fibrosis* is sometimes used as a synonym for ILD. In fact, this term should be reserved for those patients with pathologic evidence of fibrosis because even noninflammatory diseases (e.g., chronic left ventricular failure, lymphangitic spread of cancer) can mimic pulmonary fibrosis and the assumption that fibrosis is present may hinder the search for specific treatable diseases. The variety of diseases capable of producing these insults is very large, but the effects on the interstitium—edema and cellular infiltration—are remarkably similar, especially before structural reorganization occurs.

The term *interstitial disease* is a misnomer in the sense that the disease process is rarely restricted to the interstitium. In fact, the alveolar wall, comprised of both alveolar epithelium and capillary endothelium, is usually considered the initial site of the chronic inflammation of ILDs [37]. The airways, arteries, veins, and pleura are often caught up in the processes as well [21]. Exudation of fluid and cells into the alveoli is variable, but widening of the interstitial space, whether by fluid or cells, is a constant finding pathologically in the early phases of the diseases under discussion. Far-advanced disease results in reorganization of the lung, often with such destruction that normal lung anatomy is no longer identifiable in some areas. Advanced destruction of the lung with bands of fibrosis is known as *end-stage lung*, while the term *honeycomb lung* should be reserved for those lungs that have small cysts (4 to 10 mm in diameter) with common walls [47]. Such findings make etiologic diagnosis almost impossible. Early diagnosis before such widespread destruction occurs or biopsy of less involved areas is thus critical for making an etiologic diagnosis as well as understanding the pathogenesis of the individual diseases.

Epidemiology

ILDs are far more common than is generally appreciated. It has been estimated that more than 10 million people in the United States are affected by one of them. A 1972 task force report suggested that ILD constitutes 15 percent of non-infectious problems seen by pulmonary physicians [83]. A subsequent report suggested that nearly 100,000 patients are admitted to the hospital each year with chronic interstitial fibrosis [99].

Etiologic Classification

More than 150 distinct entities that produce or are associated with chronic ILD have been described [21]. These may be grouped as diseases of known etiology (Table 40-1) and those of unknown etiology (Table 40-2) [21,64,65]. New causes are reported regularly (e.g., see [22,24, 28,30,57,58,92,96]). The long list of occupational exposures underlines the importance of an adequate occupational history in the patient presenting with ILD of unknown cause. Unfortunately, despite the length of the list of known causes of ILD, in approximately 75 percent of cases no specific etiologic factor can be identified [37].

Table 40-1. **Interstitial lung diseases of known etiology**

Inorganic dusts
  Silica (variants of silicon dioxide)
  Silicates
    Asbestos (hydrated sodium, iron, calcium, and magnesium silicates)
    Talc (hydrated magnesium silicates)
    Kaolin ("China clay," hydrated aluminum silicate)
    Sillimanite (anhydrous aluminum silicate)
    Diatomaceous earth ("Fuller's earth," aluminum silicate with iron and magnesium)
    Nepheline (hard rock containing mixed silicates)
    Mica (potassium and magnesium aluminum silicates)
  Aluminum
    Powdered aluminum
    Bauxite ("Shaver's disease," aluminum oxide)
  Antimony (oxides and alloys)
  Carbon (with or without silica)
    Coal dust
    Graphite
  Beryllium
  Mixed dusts (predominantly oxides of iron with silica, silicates, and other inorganic compounds)
  Hard-metal dusts
    Titanium oxide
    Tungsten, titanium, hafnium, and niobium carbides
    Cadmium
Organic dusts
  Living sources
    Aspergillosis
    Bagassosis
    Bird breeders' lung
    Cheese workers' lung
    Chicken or turkey handlers' lung
    Coffee workers' lung
    Coptic disease
    Detergent workers' lung
    Dove handlers' disease
    Duck fever
    Farmers' lung
    Fish meal workers' lung
    Furriers' lung
    Humidifier or air conditioner lung
    Japanese "summer type"
    Lycoperdonosis
    Maple bark strippers' lung
    Malt workers' lung
    Mouldy lichen handlers' disease
    Mushroom workers' lung
    New Guinea lung
    Paprika splitters' lung
    Pituitary snuff lung
    Sauna-takers' disease
    Sequoiosis
    Smallpox handlers' lung
    Suberosis
    Tea growers' lung
    Thatched roof lung
    Tobacco farmers' lung
    Wheat weevil disease (a.k.a. millers' lung)
    Wood-pulp or wood-dust workers' disease
  Chemical sources
    Bakelite workers' lung
    Synthetic-fiber lung
Gases, fumes, vapors, aerosols
  Gases
    Chlorine gas
    Oxygen
    Sulfur dioxide
  Fumes
    Oxides of zinc, copper, manganese, cadmium, iron, magnesium, nickel, brass, selenium, tin, and antimony
  Vapors
    Mercury
    Thermosetting resins
    Toluene diisocyanate
  Aerosols
    Copper sulfate neutralized with hydrated lime ("Bordeaux mixture")

Table 40-1. (continued)

Fats	Nonsteroidal antiinflammatory drugs
Pyrethrum	Pentolinium
Hydrogen peroxide	Penicillamine
Drugs	Propranolol
Chemotherapeutic agents	Tocainamide
Bleomycin	Poisons
Busulfan	Paraquat
Chlorambucil	Radiation
Cyclophosphamide	External
Cytosine arabinoside	Inhaled
Melphalan	Infectious agents
Mercaptopurine	Viral pneumonia (e.g., cytomegalovirus, influenza, respiratory syncytial virus, herpes simplex virus, adenovirus)
Methotrexate	
Mitomycin	
Nitrosoureas (BCNU, CCNU)	Psittacosis (*Chlamydia psittaci*)
Procarbazine	Miliary tuberculosis
Vinblastine	Fungal pneumonia (e.g., coccidioidomycosis, histoplasmosis)
Antibiotics	
Nitrofurantoin	Pneumocystosis
Penicillin	Residue of active infection of any type
Sulfonamides	Schistosomiasis
Others	Neoplasms
Aminosalicylic acid	Bronchoalveolar cell carcinoma
Amiodarone	Lymphangitic or hematogenous carcinomatosis
Carbamazepine	Kaposi's sarcoma
Chlorpropamide	Interstitial disease caused by nonpulmonary disorders
Diphenylhydantoin	
Drugs inducing lupus-like syndrome (e.g., hydralazine, procainamide)	Chronic pulmonary edema
	Left atrial hypertension (e.g., congestive failure, mitral stenosis)
Gold salts	
Hexamethonium	Pulmonary veno-occlusive disease
Hydrochlorothiazide	Chronic uremia
Lidocaine	Chronic gastric aspiration
Mecamylamine	
Methysergide	
Mineral oil (as oral stool softener or nose drops)	

Source: Modified from RG Crystal et al. Interstitial lung disease: Current concepts of pathogenesis, staging and therapy. *Am J Med* 70:542, 1981.

Presentation

The typical patient with ILD presents with insidious onset of dyspnea on exertion, often associated with fatigue and cough; physical examination reveals bilateral end-inspiratory crackles and the chest x-ray film shows diffuse or bibasilar reticular densities. Although emphasis is usually given to this most common presentation of the patient with ILD, it is critical to recognize the variability of clinical presentations. Dyspnea is a virtually constant finding in patients with IPF, but it is by no means so consistent in other ILDs. Less common but important and sometimes misleading presentations include the following:

1. Fatigue in the absence of dyspnea
2. Cough without other respiratory symptoms [94]
3. Predominant systemic symptoms (e.g., fever, weight loss)
4. Abnormal-appearing chest x-ray film in the absence of symptoms
5. Incidental abnormalities of pulmonary function studies

When confronted with a patient with unexplained shortness of breath, the differential diagnosis is immense. Pulmonary, cardiac, hematologic, renal, neuromuscular, and even endocrine

Table 40-2. **Interstitial lung diseases of unknown etiology**

Miscellaneous (common)
    Idiopathic pulmonary fibrosis (cryptogenic fibrosing alveolitis, usual interstitial pneumonia)
    Sarcoidosis
    Bronchiolitis obliterans and organizing pneumonia (BOOP)
    Eosinophilic granuloma/histiocytosis X
Interstitial diseases associated with the collagen-vascular disorders
    Rheumatoid arthritis
    Progressive systemic sclerosis
    Systemic lupus erythematosus
    Polymyositis dermatomyositis
    Mixed connective-tissue disease
    Sjögren's syndrome
    Giant cell arteritis
Pulmonary granulomatoses
    Wegener's granulomatosis
    Bronchocentric granulomatosis
Vasculitides
    Churg-Strauss syndrome (allergic angiitis and granulomatosis)
    Polyarteritis nodosa
    Hypersensitivity vasculitis
    Relapsing polychondritis
    Behçet's syndrome
    Takayasu's arteritis
    Chronic intravenous drug abuse (foreign-body granulomatosis)

Lymphoproliferative disorders
    Lymphomatoid granulomatosis
    Lymphocytic interstitial pneumonia (LIP)
    Immunoblastic lymphadenopathy
    Pseudolymphoma
    Non-Hodgkin's lymphoma
Inherited disorders
    Tuberous sclerosis
    Neurofibromatosis
    Familial pulmonary fibrosis
    Cystic fibrosis
Miscellaneous (uncommon)
    Idiopathic pulmonary hemosiderosis
    Immune complex deposition with diffuse alveolar hemorrhage
    Pulmonary veno-occlusive disease
    Ankylosing spondylitis
    Diffuse amyloidosis of lung
    Chronic eosinophilic pneumonia
    Lymphangioleiomyomatosis
    Whipple's disease
    Weber-Christian disease
    Hermansky-Pudlak syndrome
    Bone marrow transplantation lung
    Post–adult respiratory distress syndrome
    Goodpasture's syndrome
    Alveolar microlithiasis
    Respiratory bronchiolitis
    Pulmonary alveolar proteinosis

Source: Modified from RG Crystal et al. Interstitial lung disease: Current concepts of pathogenesis, staging and therapy. *Am J Med* 70:542, 1981.

diseases may present with exercise intolerance or dyspnea. A step-by-step approach beginning with the history and physical examination and followed by chest x-ray films, screening laboratory studies, pulmonary function studies, and exercise testing is usually sufficient to identify the presence of ILD. However, in only a minority of cases will this approach be adequate to make an etiologic diagnosis. This discussion emphasizes the usefulness and limitations of each part of this organized approach to the patient with possible ILD.

History

The patient with ILD usually presents with insidious but progressive dyspnea on exertion. The symptom is usually persistent so that variability in intensity or spontaneous remission should suggest another process (e.g., asthma, congestive heart failure). If dyspnea is not related to exer-

tion, then ILD is an unlikely explanation. When assessing patients' exercise limitations, it is critical to understand what actually limits them. As patients may confuse dyspnea and fatigue, exercise limitation by fatigue may have equal significance. Questions aimed at the sensations experienced by the patient during exercise are often helpful. Inability to get enough air in or dyspnea may suggest lung disease while chest pain or claudication suggests disease in other organ systems. Sometimes it is only with exercise testing that one can really understand what limits a patient's activities. There is increasing interest in actually measuring respiratory symptoms using visual analogue scales during exercise testing [13]. These techniques can also give insights into what limits a patient during his or her normal daily activities.

The mechanism of dyspnea usually relates to the effort associated with breathing [11,13]. As discussed in greater detail in the section on exercise physiology, dyspnea in patients with ILD is due to increased work of breathing caused primarily by the "stiffness" (i.e., decreased distensibility) of the lungs, by excessive minute ventilation (i.e., from hypoxemia, lactic acidosis, and wasted ventilation), and possibly by stimulation of extrapulmonary receptors [11]. Hypoxemia, often aggravated by exercise, may amplify the sensation of dyspnea by carotid body stimulation. If the interstitial disease is associated with muscle dysfunction (e.g., polymyositis), then the perception of dyspnea will be increased because of decreased respiratory muscle reserve.

Dyspnea is more common in IPF than it is in other interstitial pulmonary disorders. Jackson reviewed the symptoms associated with IPF in 180 patients in six series reported between 1957 and 1976 [52]. Dyspnea occurred in nearly all patients (97 percent) and cough in most (82 to 90 percent). Chest pain, weight loss, and fever were less common, occurring in up to 50 percent, while arthralgias were distinctly unusual (5 to 11 percent).

There is less information about the occurrence of symptoms in other groups of patients with interstitial disorders. Gaensler and colleagues [38] described 369 patients seen from 1950 to 1970 with a variety of interstitial disorders documented on open lung biopsy. The largest single group of patients (167) would have fit with the above-described IPF group but findings in the rest were distributed among viral infections (9), radiation pneumonitis (20), drug toxicity (2), chronic eosinophilic pneumonia (13), collagen-vascular diseases (69), pneumoconiosis (72), gas exposure (5), and chronic left-sided heart failure (12). Among this heterogeneous group of patients, dyspnea was by far the most frequent symptom (61 percent). Cough, usually nonproductive, was the next most common (13.4 percent). Less common complaints were joint pain (5 percent), fatigue or exhaustion (4.2 percent), chest pain (4.2 percent), hemoptysis (2.5 percent), and leg edema (1.7 percent). Fifteen patients (4.2 percent) had no symptoms but had undergone lung biopsy because of an abnormal-appearing chest x-ray film.

Once ILD is suspected, an appropriate history may play a vital role in diagnosis. Table 40-1 emphasizes the long list of possible occupational exposures that may result in lung disease. The temporal relationship to the exposure may be obvious in some cases, but in others a low-grade exposure may provoke chronic illness without acute flares after exposure (e.g., hypersensitivity

pneumonitis may present either as acute or as chronic disease). The latency may be extremely long (e.g., more than 20 years for asbestosis) so that it is mandatory to take a detailed occupational history, including summer jobs and hobbies, in all patients with suspected ILD. Unfortunately, individuals will not always know what toxins they were exposed to and exposures to toxins may be easily overlooked so that considerable sleuthing may be required. For example, fungi in cooling systems or birds in the home may be a source of allergens that can elicit hypersensitivity pneumonitis. History of medication use is also critical to diagnosing ILD. Patients who have been using drugs for years (e.g., nitrofurantoin) may not report them as medications on routine questioning. Mineral oil taken as a laxative or as nose drops may not be considered medicines either.

As diseases in other organs may present as ILD, a detailed review of systems is important. Occult chronic heart disease, for example, may present as ILD with dyspnea, cough, crackles, and interstitial-type abnormalities on the chest x-ray film. Malignancies of virtually any organ system may spread to the lungs and present as interstitial disease. The protean manifestations of the collagen-vascular diseases may give important clues on history taking (e.g., rashes, Raynaud's phenomenon, fevers, arthralgias, muscle weakness). Dysphagia or regurgitation may relate to either recurrent aspiration or collagen-vascular disease, especially scleroderma. Patients with acquired immunodeficiency syndrome (AIDS) complicated by pneumocystosis or lymphocytic interstitial pneumonia may first present with an insidious onset of shortness of breath and fatigue as do patients with other ILDs. Therefore sexual preference and other possible risk factors for AIDS (e.g., blood transfusion) should be identified.

Physical Examination

Although often helpful, the findings on physical examination may be misleadingly benign in patients with ILD. Subtle increases in respiratory rate may not be noticed at rest, though tachypnea or even respiratory distress may become evident with mild exertion such as walking with the patient in the corridor or up a few stairs. Tachycardia may be present in patients who have progressed to pulmonary hypertension or who have underlying cardiac disease.

Although inspiratory crackles are considered

the hallmark of ILD, they are sometimes absent. In one review, only 80 percent of patients with established IPF had crackles [52]. Epler and colleagues [27] prospectively studied 272 patients with biopsy-proved diffuse infiltrative lung disease and showed that crackles varied in frequency from less than 20 percent in eosinophilic granuloma to 80 percent in usual interstitial pneumonia (UIP), which is equivalent to IPF. Examination of patients with sarcoidosis, the most common ILD, revealed crackles in less than 40 percent.

In advanced forms of ILD, decreased respiratory expansion may be evident, but this is unusual in the early stages. Clubbing is often mentioned as a physical finding in patients with ILD, but it too usually occurs only in advanced forms of the disease. Jackson [52] found that it occurred in 72 percent of the patients with IPF in the multiple series he reviewed, with a range from 53 to 83 percent. Cyanosis reflects even more advanced disease and has been found in 23 to 53 percent of patients.

Progression of interstitial diseases may be marked by evidence of pulmonary hypertension including a palpable pulmonary artery impulse, second heart sound, or right ventricular heave. Cardiac auscultation may reveal accentuation of the pulmonic component of the second heart sound even when it is not palpable. A flow murmur, usually accentuated with inspiration, may be heard in the pulmonic region. As right ventricular failure supervenes, physical examination may reveal jugular venous distension, hepatic enlargement, or tenderness and pedal edema [48].

Laboratory Tests

With the exception of finding unsuspected peripheral eosinophilia, laboratory tests have proved particularly unhelpful in the evaluation of the patient with suspected ILD. Routine hematologic, chemistry, and urine screenings are certainly justifiable, as Tables 40-1 and 40-2 indicate the large number of systemic illnesses that may present with clinical and radiologic findings of ILD. Such screenings may, for example, uncover occult malignancies (e.g., hematuria). A need for more specialized studies might be suggested by other symptoms (e.g., serologic studies for mixed connective-tissue disease in a patient with Raynaud's phenomenon, esophagoscopy in a patient with reflux) but discussion of these is beyond the scope of this chapter.

While elevation of the erythrocyte sedimentation rate (ESR) may support the suspicion of an inflammatory process in the lung [102], it is too nonspecific to help either in localization of the process to the lungs or in determination of the diagnosis. In fact, the ESR is often normal despite active ILD [102]. Serologic determinations of antinuclear antibody (ANA) or rheumatoid factor may support the suspicion of collagen-vascular disease, but elevations of these substances are also found in patients with IPF in the absence of collagen-vascular disease. Turner-Warwick and colleagues [102] found that more than a third of their patients with IPF had elevation of the ESR (37 percent) and elevation of globulins (37 percent) while more than a fourth had elevation of the ANA (26 percent). Crystal and associates [20] considered these to be epiphenomena without pathogenetic or diagnostic importance.

In sarcoidosis, the finding of elevated levels of angiotensin-converting enzyme (ACE) supports the diagnosis and may be useful in following responses to therapy [24], but there are too many false-positive and false-negative results for it to be diagnostic in itself [84]. Unexpected hypercalcemia/hypercalciuria, especially in the absence of hypophosphatemia, would raise the suspicion of sarcoidosis in a patient with unexplained ILD, but could also be explained by metastatic carcinoma.

Immunologic testing is sometimes helpful. The presence of serum precipitins directed against specific antigens is strong supportive evidence of hypersensitivity pneumonitis in the proper clinical setting. Unfortunately, many exposed individuals (e.g., bird breeders) will have precipitins in the absence of any clinical illness. If specific granulomatous infection is suspected, a positive result on skin testing would support the diagnosis but a negative result would by no means exclude it, especially in the presence of miliary infection. In the case of a fungal disease, the presence of specific complement-fixing antibodies (also bands on immunodiffusion) is diagnostically suggestive.

Radiology

Abnormalities on the chest x-ray film may be the first clue to the presence of ILD, and radiographs can strongly suggest this diagnosis even in asymptomatic patients [41]. However, since patients without symptoms are only rarely subjected to open lung biopsy (4 percent in one series [38]), it is difficult to know how many patients with diffuse abnormalities on their x-ray films actually have pathologic evidence of ILD.

On the other hand, despite the prominent role of the chest x-ray in the recognition of the presence of ILD, it is clear that patients may have normal-appearing chest films despite symptomatic ILD [22,29,31,59]. In a study of 458 patients with biopsy-proved diffuse infiltrative lung disease, Epler and associates [29] found that 10 percent of their patients had normal-appearing chest films. Presumably this is an underestimation, as many physicians would be reluctant to consider open lung biopsy in the absence of radiologic abnormalities. Several investigators have demonstrated parenchymal densities by computed tomographic (CT) scanning of patients with occupational lung disease that were missed on standard chest x-ray films [22,59].

Descriptions of these abnormalities have been variable and some noted authorities have pleaded for a more uniform approach to their description based on the radiologic pattern rather than on the presumed pathologic abnormalities [32]. One of several radiologic patterns is usually present [32,46]: (1) "ground glass," (2) reticular, (3) nodular, and (4) honeycombing. These patterns have important, albeit imperfect clinical, pathologic, and diagnostic implications. Felson [32] stated that the term *interstitial pattern* is to be strongly avoided. He preferred the term *irregular shadows* to emphasize the radiologic findings quite apart from any presumed pathologic abnormality [32].

Clinicopathologic studies have shown that there is not always a clear correlation between the x-ray and the pathologic findings [32,46,61]. To some extent, the apparent location of the process in either the alveoli or the interstitium is due to the extent of the process; a very diffuse interstitial process may silhouette the airways much as lobar consolidation does [46] and an interstitial process that has spread to the alveoli may mask the major interstitial component [32].

As the early changes on the chest x-ray films of patients with ILD may be subtle (e.g., haziness or faint reticulation), comparison with old films may be critical. A decrease in lung volumes may be the earliest radiologic findings in ILD but is often unapparent without comparison to prior films. The prior finding of hilar adenopathy is suggestive of sarcoidosis. The finding of a reticular infiltrate on past films can drastically affect the interpretation about the differential diagnosis and aggressiveness of a current reticular infiltrate. Since many of the ILDs have an exudative phase that begins in or extends into the alveoli, it is not uncommon to have a diffuse ground-glass or hazy appearance as the earliest radiologic abnormality. As noted, comparison with prior films will make assessment of such soft abnormalities more reliable. In many cases, this exudative phase does not occur or is not picked up radiologically except perhaps by change in lung volumes.

The development of fine reticular densities on the radiographs of patients with ILD is thought to be the result of edema, infiltration, or fibrosis of the septa in the periphery of the lung. Because of lack of pathologic confirmation, Kerley used letters (A, B, C) when he first described these reticular densities or lines that bear his name. They have all been shown by postmortem clinicopathologic correlation to be due to thickening of the interlobular septa [46]. The widely recognized Kerley B lines, well seen in the periphery of the lower lung fields, represent single horizontal septa thickened by fluid, cells, or collagen. The less well-recognized A lines occur diagonally in the upper and central lung fields and also represent individual thickened septa. The C lines, seen in the commonly described reticular pattern, are thought to reflect an abundance of thickened individual septa seen en face and superimposed on each other. Heitzman [46] believes that the C line or reticular pattern is equivalent to the small irregular opacities commonly used in the UICC radiographic classification of the pneumoconioses [103].

Among patients with chronic disease, definite thickening of the septal lines is most commonly due to bronchogenic or lymphangitic malignancy, pneumoconioses, or chronic left atrial hypertension (e.g., rheumatic heart disease), though virtually all of the diseases listed in Tables 40-1 and 40-2 can present with a reticular infiltrate [32]. As the interstitial compartments communicate freely, the same conditions that produce Kerley lines may extend into the axial or bronchovascular portion of the interstitium. This may result in the radiologic appearance of peribronchial cuffing, best seen if a large airway is seen end on, or indistinctness of the central pulmonary vessels.

Another important pattern is that of diffuse nodules. These may vary in diameter from miliary (about 1 mm) to as large as 5 mm. Though radiologic summation of these nodules may simply appear as patchy consolidation, careful analysis of the periphery of the lung where there is less superimposition of abnormalities should allow determination of the nodular character. Although some authors have argued that this nodular character may be artifactual, related to summation of many thickened septa [16,101] or to misinterpretation of a primarily alveolar process (e.g., alveolar proteinosis, alveolar microlithiasis), newer information from CT scanning has emphasized the importance of the nodular pattern [4–6,76]. Finding of nodules is particularly important in narrowing the differential diagnosis of ILD. Such nodules are most commonly found in granulomatous diseases (e.g., sarcoidosis, miliary tuberculosis, or mycosis), hypersensitivity pneumonitis, lymphangitic spread of malignancy, eosinophilic granuloma (histiocytosis X), and silicosis. Though such nodules may be seen in bronchiolitis obliterans with organizing pneumonia, patchy infiltrates may also be seen and, in the appropriate clinical setting, may actually suggest this diagnosis [44].

Eventually, with persistent edema and inflammation, fibrosis develops, with subsequent distortion of the lung parenchyma. Fibrosis pathologically similar to that occurring in IPF may occur in a few weeks in patients with the adult respiratory distress syndrome [3] or over many years in patients with UIP or desquamative interstitial pneumonia (DIP) [15]. It is still unclear whether this is associated with reorganization of collagen in the lung or the actual laying down of new collagen [20].

Progression of inflammation and fibrosis eventually results in the most characteristic radiologic finding in interstitial disease, honeycombing, in which normal lung is replaced by small, rounded, cystlike spaces varying from 4 to 10 mm in diameter and with walls 0.5 to 1.0 mm in thickness [69]. This radiologic finding has been associated with end-stage lung in which no diagnostic pattern can be identified on pathologic examination. It is associated with destruction and reorganization of lung. The normal alveolar cells (type I epithelial cells, type II pneumonocytes) disappear and are replaced by cells normally found only along the airways (e.g., columnar epithelium). Unfortunately by the time this is evident on x-ray film, the patient has far-advanced disease. Nonetheless, the finding of honeycombing does not necessarily preclude consideration of an aggressive diagnostic and therapeutic approach because the disease process is often patchy, with more cellular and reversible disease present in other areas. However, if lung biopsy is to be performed, it is important to avoid the honeycombed areas as no meaningful information can be obtained about either the diagnosis or the degree and kind of inflammatory cells present.

Besides the possibility of a normal-appearing x-ray film, there are several pitfalls that may make radiologic recognition of ILD difficult [46]. Some pathologically interstitial diseases (e.g., DIP) have a major alveolar component on radiographs that may obscure the more classic reticular appearance (i.e., recognition of the large interstitial component may be impossible on the radiograph when there is no air in the alveoli to contrast with the thickened interstitial septa). Congestive heart failure may serve as a dramatic example of this. In its chronic phase, congestive failure presents symptomatically, physiologically, and radiologically like an ILD. However, when acute pulmonary edema supervenes, the interstitial pattern is attenuated or disappears as the thickened septa are no longer silhouetted by air in the alveoli. On the other hand, when interstitial disease is extensive, it can mimic alveolar disease. Replacement of lung by sheets of cells (e.g., lymphocytic interstitial pneumonia) or granulomas (e.g., sarcoid) may also give an alveolar appearance to the x-ray film with loss of the reticular pattern and silhouetting of the airways.

Another problem that may make radiologic recognition of ILD or interpretation of parenchymal changes difficult is the presence of preexisting lung disease. For example, either congestive heart failure or acute pneumonia may suggest the presence of honeycombing when superimposed on emphysema. This may seriously delay recognition of an acute process.

With these comments as background, there are clues on the chest radiograph that may help guide clinical decision making and narrow the differential diagnosis in a minority of patients (Table 40-3). Upper-zone predominance is suggestive of the conditions shown but is not specific enough to preclude the need for a diagnostic procedure. Eggshell calcification is nearly pathognomonic for silicosis, though it has been observed in sarcoidosis as well [24]. Eosinophilic pneumonia may present with marked peripheral location of infiltrates, which has been described as the negative or reverse of cardiogenic pulmonary edema. Spontaneous pneumothorax is a potential complication of any of the ILDs but is particularly common in patients with eosinophilic granuloma (histiocytosis X). Pleural effusions are uncommon in ILD but if present, suggest common entities such as congestive heart failure or lymphangitic spread of malignancy or very rarely lymphangioleiomyomatosis. In a patient at risk

Table 40-3. **Radiologic clues for diagnosis of interstitial lung diseases**

Upper-zone predominance
  Histiocytosis X
  Silicosis
  Cystic fibrosis
  Sarcoidosis
  Granulomatous infection
Peripheral predominance
  Eosinophilic pneumonia
Hilar adenopathy
  Sarcoidosis
  Berylliosis
  Kaposi's sarcoma
Hilar "eggshell" calcification
  Silicosis
  Sarcoidosis
Pneumothorax
  Eosinophilic granuloma (histiocytosis X)
  Lymphangioleiomyomatosis
Pleural effusion
  Congestive heart failure
  Kaposi's sarcoma
  Lymphangioleiomyomatosis (chylous)
  Lymphangitic spread of malignancy
Pleural calcification
  Asbestosis

for AIDS, the finding of pleural effusion in combination with radiologic findings of ILD is somewhat suggestive of Kaposi's sarcoma [78]. Another specific finding that is helpful if present is the finding of calcified pleural plaques, which are virtually pathognomonic of prior asbestos exposure. Though insufficient for the diagnosis of parenchymal asbestosis, this finding would raise the suspicion of this diagnosis in a patient with a reticular infiltrate or honeycombing.

Computed Tomographic Scanning

The disappointing sensitivity and specificity of routine chest radiography in ILD [32,38] have led to a search for better techniques for detecting and diagnosing these disorders. CT scanning of the chest has substantially improved the ability to detect subtle ILD, with a number of studies demonstrating that routine CT scanning is considerably more sensitive for identification of interstitial abnormalities than are routine chest x-ray films [5,22,59,62].

Bergin and Muller [5,6] attempted to classify the pattern of interstitial abnormalities detected by CT scanning to aid in the diagnosis of specific diseases. The pulmonary interstitium is divided into three compartments: axial (central), parenchymal (midlung), and peripheral. Axial abnormalities were most commonly due to sarcoidosis or neoplastic lesions (lymphoma or lymphangitic carcinomatosis). The peripheral compartment was most often affected in IPF and ILD associated with connective-tissue diseases (rheumatoid arthritis and scleroderma) [6] as has been described pathologically [90]. Interstitial abnormalities in the parenchymal compartment were the least specific and were seen in many diseases, but most notably in drug toxicity states, granulomatous diseases, and extrinsic allergic alveolitis. Nodules were seen particularly in silicosis, sarcoidosis, lymphangitic metastases, and other granulomatous diseases [5,6]. The combination of compartment involvement and presence or absence of nodularity makes it possible to limit diagnostic possibilities.

While it is clear that CT scanning can better determine the extent of interstitial abnormalities in the lung, its clinical reliability has been questioned. In recent years, several studies confirmed the superiority of CT over chest x-ray films in diagnosing and assessing disease severity in ILD. Staples and colleagues [91] demonstrated in 23 patients with UIP that CT scans closely correlated with extent of disease as assessed by clinical symptoms and diffusing capacity, while chest x-ray findings correlated poorly. Comparative studies by Bergin and coworkers [4] and Mathieson and associates [67] showed that CT is superior to chest radiography in making specific diagnoses in chronic ILD.

High-Resolution Computed Tomography

While conventional CT represented a major advance in chest imaging, the standard thickness (1 cm) of conventional CT sections results in blurring of much of the fine detail of the interstitium [71,76]. Thin-section or high-resolution CT scans with 1.0- to 2.0-mm collimation (slice thickness) utilize image reconstruction algorithms that enhance interfaces between adjacent structures, providing finer detail of high-contrast anatomy such as the pulmonary interstitium. This provides a spatial resolution of less than 1 mm [50]. High-resolution CT of the thorax can resolve the secondary pulmonary lobule at the periphery of the lung. The interlobular septum that borders the lobule is about 100-μ thick and can be visualized as smooth lines extending to the pleural surface or as polygonal lines centrally, but is more easily seen when abnormally thickened [70]. Bronchioles and arterioles within the secondary pulmonary lobule appear as small dots or short branching structures in the center of lobules [106]. (See Chap. 11.)

Several signs of ILDs may be noted on high-resolution CT. Most common are *interface signs*—the thickened and irregular appearance of the normally smooth interface of lung parenchyma with bronchi, blood vessels, and visceral pleura. Interstitial nodules as small as 1 mm in diameter are detectable and are distinguished from airspace nodules by their sharp margination and lack of coalescence into larger opacities. Several reticular patterns of varying lattice size have been described. Large 15- to 25-mm polyhedrons centered on pulmonary arteries are thickened secondary lobular septa, seen in interstitial pulmonary edema and lymphangitic carcinomatosis. A medium-size pattern of 6- to 10-mm units may reflect primary lobules and is seen along with cystic changes with a honeycomb appearance. This pattern is typically seen in IPF and other diseases caused by infiltration of the interstitium. These changes are most apparent in the periphery of the lung, particularly in the subpleural areas. Finally, a very fine, diffuse pattern of 2- to 3-mm reticulation may occasionally be seen in miliary tuberculosis and methotrexate toxicity states [112]. It is important to understand that pseudoreticulation and apparent interstitial abnormalities are frequently seen in gravity-dependent regions of normal lungs, caused by physiologic fluid shifts and atelectasis. For this reason, high-resolution CT scans of the chest often include images obtained with the patient in both supine and prone positions, to distinguish these normal findings from true abnormalities. Other signs of interstitial disease include architectural distortions due to fibrosis, seen in sarcoidosis or silicosis, and multifocal areas of fine, granular, hazy, increased density, which represent thickened alveolar interstitial areas or incomplete filling of alveolar spaces.

A number of studies supported by clinico-pathologic data suggest that the sensitivity of high-resolution CT in diagnosing ILD is superior to that of standard CT scanning [71,76] (Figs. 40-2, 40-3, and 40-4). In a study of nine patients undergoing open lung biopsy for ILD subsequently shown to be fibrosing alveolitis (IPF), excellent correlation was found between thin-section CT images and open lung biopsy specimens from the same region of lung [71]. Conventional CT correlated far less well with biopsy specimens than did high-resolution CT. Kerley B lines, which are not seen on standard CT scans, may be dramatically evident on a thin-section study done at the same time.

In a subsequent study, Muller and associates [72] reviewed CT scans in 12 patients with IPF who had undergone open lung biopsy. A close correlation was found between CT identification of airspace consolidation and pathologic indicators of active inflammation including alveolar

Fig. 40-2. High-resolution CT scan (1.5 mm) of normal lungs at a level just below the carina. Note the central branching vessels and the lack of peripheral markings.

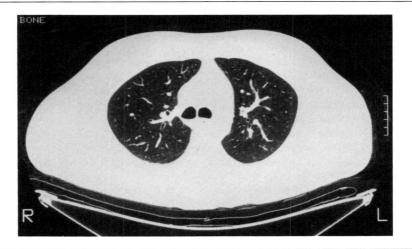

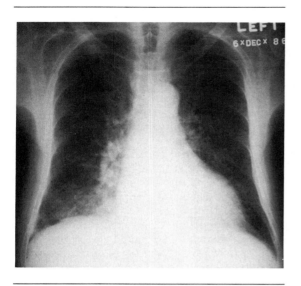

Fig. 40-3. Plain chest x-ray from a patient with biopsy-proved IPF demonstrates a diffuse, nonspecific increase in radiographic density.

septal inflammation and alveolar cell desquamation. This correlation with the disease activity was best seen on high-resolution scans. Webb and coworkers [106] performed high-resolution CT scans on 12 isolated, inflated lungs obtained fresh from autopsies and compared the scans with histologic sections of the lungs obtained from the same levels. In normal lungs, high-resolution CT was able to resolve anatomic structures to the level of normal interlobular septa. In diseased lungs, high-resolution CT was particularly good at detecting honeycombing, which could be easily distinguished from emphysema.

The sensitivity and diagnostic accuracy of high-resolution CT have been studied in several specific disorders. Schurawitzki and associates [85] found high-resolution CT to be highly sensitive in detecting early disease in progressive systemic sclerosis (PSS). High-resolution CT detected disease in 91 percent of patients with PSS, less than half (39 percent) of whom had chest x-ray abnormalities. The most common findings on high-resolution CT were subpleural lines. Aberle and colleagues [2] found high-resolution CT to be highly sensitive and superior to conventional CT in detecting pleural and parenchymal abnormalities in patients with asbestos exposure and clinical asbestosis. High-resolution CT detected pleural abnormalities in 100 percent of patients and parenchymal abnormalities in 96 percent, compared to 83 percent by conventional CT. This study also reported that high-resolution scans performed with the patients in a prone position allowed abnormalities in the basal lung segments to be distinguished from gravity-related findings. The sensitivity of high-resolution CT in diagnosing sarcoidosis is unknown. Preliminary study suggests that it may be useful in sarcoidosis in identifying unsuspected parenchymal disease, quantifying the degree of pulmonary fibrosis, following patients receiving therapy, and selecting sites for lung biopsy [66].

With the increasing use of lung transplantation for the treatment of end-stage lung disease, the efficiency of high-resolution CT in distinguishing between allograft rejection and other abnormalities has been evaluated. Hruban and coworkers [49] studied seven inflation-fixed transplanted lung specimens by high-resolution CT. Unfortunately, high-resolution CT could not reliably distinguish between lung allograft rejection and infection. In particular, acute rejection was characterized by only minimal changes on high-resolution CT scans. Chronic rejection was characterized by severe bronchiectasis, but this was not specific for rejection. In addition, bronchiolitis obliterans, a finding invariably present in chronic rejection, could not be identified on high-resolution CT scans [49]. Therefore, it appears that high-resolution CT is disappointing in its failure to identify early ILD in the diagnosis of rejection of transplanted lungs.

There are several other specific diseases where high-resolution CT, in combination with clinical information, may make specific diagnoses. Lymphangitic spread of tumor may be detected as increased number and thickness of interlobular septa or nodularity present along thickened septa. High-resolution CT is highly sensitive in detecting lucencies representing parenchymal destruction in emphysema before the destruction is identified by other modalities. It appears to be very accurate in diagnosing bronchiectasis and has largely replaced bronchography in delineating the extent of focal bronchiectasis [43]. High-resolution CT provides a relatively specific cystic pattern in lymphangioleiomyomatosis [80].

Although high-resolution CT is proving to be an exceptional new tool for the evaluation of parenchymal lung disease, it is important to note its limitations. It cannot be used practically to study the entire thorax; conventional CT must be used to avoid missing abnormalities between images.

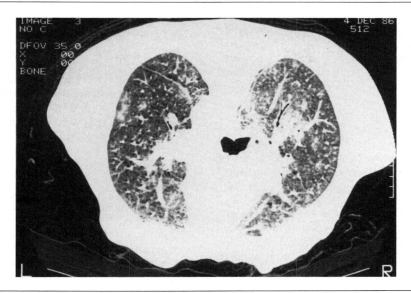

Fig. 40-4. High-resolution CT scan (1.5 mm) of the patient in Fig. 40-3 shows peripheral interlobular thickening as well as a patchy increase in density.

Some high-resolution CT findings may be difficult to interpret without a conventional CT image to use for reference. Although CT scanning is considered too expensive for routine screening, it is possible to do a few thin sections at a cost approaching that of a routine chest x-ray film. The value of this procedure in the diagnosis, staging, and serial study of patients with ILD is likely to increase as additional clinicopathologic studies are performed.

Magnetic Resonance Imaging

Preliminary data suggest that magnetic resonance imaging (MRI) may be useful in assessing disease activity in ILD, but few patients have been studied to date and additional data are needed before the usefulness of this modality can be ascertained [39]. MRI may be useful in differentiating radiation fibrosis from recurrent pulmonary tumor [40].

Major Disease Syndromes of Unknown Etiology

Tables 40-1 and 40-2 illustrate the vast differential diagnosis of ILD. Many ILD syndromes are

Table 40-4. **Interstitial lung diseases of unknown etiology: Common clinical entities**

Idiopathic pulmonary fibrosis
Collagen-vascular–associated ILD
    Rheumatoid arthritis, progressive systemic sclerosis, systemic lupus erythematosus, polymyositis dermatomyositis, mixed connective-tissue disease
Sarcoidosis
Systemic granulomatous vasculitides
    Wegener's granulomatosis, Churg-Strauss syndrome, lymphomatoid granulomatosis
Goodpasture's syndrome
Bronchiolitis obliterans organizing pneumonia
Eosinophilic granuloma/histiocytosis X
Chronic eosinophilic pneumonia
Respiratory bronchiolitis–associated ILD
Pulmonary alveolar proteinosis

caused by occupational and environmental exposures, drug toxicity, or other toxic exposures such as radiation or chemotherapy. These diagnoses are usually apparent if a thorough history is obtained. The most common remaining clinical entities are diseases of unknown etiology that may be characterized as distinctive syndromes or disease groups, and are briefly reviewed here (Table 40-4).

Idiopathic Pulmonary Fibrosis

Despite an unexplained etiology, wide variability in clinical progression of disease, and substantial histologic heterogeneity in pathologic findings, IPF is a well-recognized disease. An immunologic pathogenesis is highly suspected as the disease is most responsive to immunosuppressive therapy. IPF typically presents in an older patient with the insidious and persistent progression of dyspnea and nonproductive cough. Lung examination usually reveals crackles in the lower lung zones. Clubbing may be present. Chest x-ray films most often demonstrate diffuse reticulonodular infiltrates that may be most apparent peripherally; a honeycomb pattern may be present in advanced disease. Findings in bronchoalveolar lavage and transbronchial biopsy specimens may suggest the diagnosis, but open lung biopsy is necessary to establish firmly the diagnosis and exclude other causes. Nonetheless, in severely ill or elderly patients, a clinical diagnosis may be preferred to the risks of thoracotomy. A number of distinct histologic patterns may be seen, but are not particularly helpful in prognosticating, and all have been described to coexist in a single patient [109]. A careful history must exclude asbestosis and other exposure or drug-induced diseases. Therapy consists of trials of high-dose corticosteroids, to which about 15 to 20 percent of patients respond. Cyclophosphamide and azathioprine have been used as adjunctive therapy, but firm data supporting added benefit of these agents are lacking [56].

Collagen-Vascular Diseases Associated with ILD

SYSTEMIC LUPUS ERYTHEMATOSUS

Systemic lupus erythematosus is a multisystem disease predominantly affecting young women who may present with pleural or pulmonary manifestations. Diffuse ILD may be seen but is relatively uncommon. The most common thoracic manifestations are pleural disease and acute lupus pneumonitis with alveolar infiltrates. Opportunistic infections due to immunosuppressive therapy, alveolar hemorrhage, and pulmonary edema due to renal or cardiac disease may all present with interstitial infiltrates. Basilar atelectasis and reduced lung volumes are commonly seen and may be due to respiratory muscle weakness. Although chronic diffuse ILD is less common, patients with systemic lupus erythematosus have been reported to die of pulmonary fibrosis

[108]. Most lupus-related lung disease responds to immunosuppressive treatment with corticosteroids and cytoxan [26].

RHEUMATOID ARTHRITIS

Only 1 to 2 percent of patients with rheumatoid arthritis demonstrate evidence of ILD on chest x-ray films. As many as 30 to 40 percent, however, will have abnormal pulmonary function with reduced diffusing capacity and restrictive mechanics. Pathologic evaluation often reveals mild interstitial fibrosis [35].

Other abnormalities seen include pleural disease, parenchymal nodules, bronchiolitis obliterans, bronchiolitis obliterans with organizing pneumonia [82], and very rarely pulmonary vasculitis. Caplan described a distinct form of pneumoconiosis seen in coal workers and rheumatoid patients of other occupations in whom rapidly cavitating nodules develop. Rheumatoid lung disease responds very poorly to drug therapy; a trial of prednisone is usually given but less than 10 percent of patients have a measurable response.

PROGRESSIVE SYSTEMIC SCLEROSIS

PSS or scleroderma is a disease of multiorgan sclerosis that afflicts middle-aged individuals with a 3 : 1 female predominance. All patients suffer from skin disease with frequent involvement of joints, blood vessels, esophagus, or lungs. About 50 to 60 percent of patients with PSS will develop lung disease, which may consist of interstitial fibrosis, pulmonary arterial hypertension, or recurrent aspiration pneumonia caused by esophageal dysfunction. Pulmonary hypertension is usually the result of vascular injury due to the underlying disease rather than secondary to pulmonary fibrosis. Renal involvement, particularly in association with severe hypertension, may progress rapidly and be accompanied by pulmonary edema. When PSS is also associated with Sjögren's syndrome, respiratory complaints are more common and may be due to an increased incidence of lymphocytic alveolitis [10].

Dyspnea is the most common symptom. Physical examination frequently reveals bibasilar crackles and decreased thoracic expansion. The interstitial disease appears on chest x-ray films as diffuse bilateral infiltrates that are most dense at the bases and may progress to honeycombing at advanced stages. High-resolution CT may reveal abnormalities, such as subpleural lines, early in the course of disease before changes are evident on chest films [85,105]. A reduced diffusing capacity is a sensitive screening parameter for lung involvement. Lung volumes are usually reduced if fibrosis is present. A decreased diffusing capacity of carbon monoxide with normal lung volumes is highly suggestive of pulmonary vascular disease [79]. Barium swallow and cineesophagram may be used to assess esophageal motility and the presence of aspiration. Pulmonary disease in PSS is often poorly responsive to therapy. Corticosteroids are of no benefit and only a few patients respond to D-penicillamine [23,110].

POLYMYOSITIS DERMATOMYOSITIS

Polymyositis dermatomyositis is a degenerative inflammatory disease of striated muscle that leads to symmetric weakness and atrophy of proximal skeletal muscle groups, including the limb girdle, neck, and pharynx. Polymyositis dermatomyositis is twice as common in women as in men and has a bimodal age distribution with an early peak in the first decade and a later peak around the age of 50 years. The three types of lung disease classically described with polymyositis dermatomyositis are interstitial pneumonitis, aspiration pneumonia due to esophageal dysmotility, and pneumonia secondary to hypoventilation as a result of respiratory muscle involvement. More than a third of patients have symptoms of cough and dyspnea preceding their development of skin and muscle disease by up to 2 years [86]. The clinical presentation of the interstitial pneumonitis is variable and does not correlate with the degree of muscle involvement. It may present as a severe acute pneumonitis or as an asymptomatic radiographic finding. In a patient with pulmonary infiltrates and rash or weakness, creatine phosphokinase measurements, electromyography, or muscle biopsy specimens should be obtained. Several serum antibodies, including anti-Jo-1 and anti-KJ, are found frequently in patients with polymyositis and ILD [97]. Histopathologic findings on lung biopsy specimens are often similar to those of IPF. There is nothing specific about the interstitial disease associated with polymyositis dermatomyositis to distinguish it pathologically. Lung biopsy should nonetheless be considered to rule out other causes of ILD if clinically appropriate. A recent study of open lung biopsy specimens from these patients showed three major histologic findings: bronchiolitis obliterans with organizing pneumonia, interstitial pneumonia, and diffuse alveolar damage. Patients with bronchiolitis obliterans with organizing pneumonia had the most favorable prognosis while those with diffuse alveolar damage did very poorly [98]. The interstitial pneumonitis associated with polymyositis dermatomyositis responds to corticosteroids about 50 percent of the time. Cyclophosphamide has also been used with some success. Recurrent aspiration must always be excluded in patients with pharyngeal involvement.

MIXED CONNECTIVE-TISSUE DISEASE

Mixed connective-tissue disease is an overlap syndrome with clinical features of systemic lupus erythematosus, rheumatoid arthritis, progressive systemic sclerosis, and polymyositis. Typical features include polyarthritis, Raynaud's phenomenon, sclerodactyly, myopathy, esophageal dysmotility, and pulmonary involvement. There is no particular peak age of occurrence; women are affected four times more frequently than men. Pulmonary disease occurs in as many as 85 percent of patients with mixed connective-tissue disease, but may not cause symptoms until late in its course. Patients most commonly complain of exertional dyspnea. Chest radiographs typically demonstrate fine interstitial infiltrates, more evident in the lower lung fields but diffuse in up to 30 percent [95]. All patients with mixed connective-tissue disease have positive ANA at high titer with a speckled pattern and very high titers of antibody against the ribonucleoprotein (RNP) component of extractable nuclear antigen. The most common pulmonary function aberration is a reduced diffusing capacity. A patient with compatible clinical features and these specific serologic abnormalities does not require a tissue diagnosis of the pulmonary disease, although bronchoalveolar lavage may be indicated in some circumstances to rule out other processes such as infection. When available, lung pathology reveals fibrosis and chronic inflammation. Pulmonary disease in patients with mixed connective-tissue disease may remain stable or may progress. About half of patients treated with steroids for progressive disease will improve clinically; those refractory to steroids may respond to cyclophosphamide.

Sarcoidosis

Sarcoidosis is a multisystem syndrome of unknown etiology that most frequently affects the lung. It appears to result from an unbridled cellular immune response to an unknown antigen stimulus. Pathologic manifestations are the result of organ infiltration by inflammatory cells: helper T lymphocytes, mononuclear phagocytes, and granulomas [100]. The lung is the most common organ affected, followed by lymph node, skin, and ocular involvement. In the United States, sarcoidosis is seen in blacks about 10 times more frequently than in whites. The most common presenting symptom is insidious onset of dyspnea on exertion. About 10 to 20 percent of cases are discovered by chest x-ray in asymptomatic individuals, occurring as hilar adenopathy and/or ILD. Lung examination is usually normal but may reveal dry crackles. Pulmonary function tests are most likely to show a reduction in diffusing capacity. Diagnosis is made by tissue biopsy specimens demonstrating characteristic granulomas, and may also be supported by an elevated ACE level and positive findings on gallium-67 scan. Many patients will improve spontaneously. For those with progressive disease or extrapulmonary involvement, a trial of steroids is indicated [54].

Systemic Granulomatous Vasculitides

WEGENER'S GRANULOMATOSIS

Wegener's granulomatosis is characterized by a triad of (1) necrotizing granulomatous vasculitis of the upper and lower respiratory tracts, (2) glomerulonephritis, and (3) variable degrees of vasculitis of small arteries and veins. The etiology of this disease is unknown. Wegener's granulomatosis may appear at any age, with a mean age of onset of 40 years. Clinical presentation is highly variable and the vast majority of patients present with both upper and lower respiratory tract lesions. Upper respiratory tract lesions include sinusitis, otitis media, and nasal septal ulceration. Pulmonary manifestations vary from focal granulomatous vasculitis to diffuse alveolitis and capillaritis that may present as alveolar hemorrhage [74]. Renal disease also varies from focal glomerulitis to fulminant necrotizing glomerulonephritis. Renal involvement develops in 85 percent of patients but may not be apparent at presentation. Generalized symptoms of fever, weight loss, arthralgias, and fatigue are common. Pulmonary infiltrates occur in about 70 percent of patients and are quite variable [1]. Characteristic findings are nodular densities or infiltrates, often with cavitation. Diffuse infiltrates may be seen in more fulminant disease and in alveolar hemorrhage. Pulmonary function tests may reveal a restrictive pattern, although airway obstruction due to granulomatous lesions of large airways may occur. Definitive diagnosis generally requires tissue biopsy. Autoantibodies directed at cytoplasmic components of neutrophils (antineutrophil cyto-

plasmic antibodies [ANCA]) were recently demonstrated to be highly specific for Wegener's granulomatosis [77,89,104]. Specific diagnosis is important, because cyclophosphamide is highly effective, inducing remission in up to 90 percent of patients. High-dose steroids are also indicated early in the treatment of disease but can usually be discontinued within a few months while cyclophosphamide is continued for a year or longer.

LYMPHOMATOID GRANULOMATOSIS

Lymphomatoid granulomatosis is a systemic disease consisting of angiocentric lymphomatoid granulomatous vasculitis primarily of the lungs, with frequent involvement of the kidneys and skin. It most likely represents a vasculitis associated with a lymphoproliferative disorder, often behaving as an indolent lymphoma. Most patients present in early middle age. Presenting symptoms are typically respiratory (cough or dyspnea) but may also include systemic complaints (fever, weight loss). Chest x-ray findings are usually multiple, bilateral, ill-defined, or nodular densities that may cavitate. Upper airway disease is not present and glomerulonephritis is not seen, distinguishing it from Wegener's granulomatosis. Recent studies showed that regimens including cyclophosphamide and high-dose steroids, similar to those used for Wegener's granulomatosis, result in a high rate of remission [63].

ALLERGIC GRANULOMATOSIS AND ANGIITIS (CHURG-STRAUSS SYNDROME)

This entity is a rare disorder characterized by necrotizing angiitis of the lungs, heart, skin, and central nervous system, with involved organs containing infiltration with eosinophils. Patients typically have an allergic history, particularly bronchial asthma. Peripheral eosinophilia is common and appears to correlate with disease activity. Chest x-ray abnormalities may range from evanescent patchy densities to large bilateral nodular infiltrates. High-resolution CT scans may be relatively specific, demonstrating enlarged, irregular, stellate-shaped arteries and small patchy opacities [12]. Unlike in Wegener's granulomatosis, cavitation is rare. There are no controlled studies of therapy, but the disease appears to respond favorably to moderate or high doses of corticosteroids [18].

Goodpasture's Syndrome

Goodpasture's syndrome refers to the clinical entity of diffuse alveolar hemorrhage and glomerulonephritis associated with antibodies directed against pulmonary alveolar and glomerular basement membranes (anti-GBM antibodies). Young adult males account for the majority of cases, but the disease may be seen in women and adults of all ages. The most common initial symptom is hemoptysis, which eventually occurs in most patients, although alveolar hemorrhage may occur in the absence of gross hemoptysis. Dyspnea, cough, fever, and chest pain may accompany bleeding. Renal insufficiency usually follows pulmonary symptoms, but it can occur first. Gross or microscopic hematuria, proteinuria, and red cell casts are frequently present. Patients with episodes of pulmonary hemorrhage present with fluffy, bilateral alveolar filling densities on chest x-ray films. Between episodes, chest x-ray films may appear normal, although with chronic hemorrhage, permanent reticulonodular infiltrates may develop. Evidence of alveolar hemorrhage and a positive anti-GBM antibody assay are usually sufficient to confirm the diagnosis. Iron stains of bronchoalveolar lavage fluid can establish alveolar hemorrhage by demonstrating hemosiderin-laden macrophages. The differential diagnosis of pulmonary hemorrhage with glomerulonephritis includes a number of other disorders including systemic lupus erythematosus, Wegener's granulomatosis, other forms of vasculitis, and drug reactions [8]. Tissue obtained from the kidneys or lungs demonstrates linear basement membrane staining on immunofluorescence. Although controlled studies are few, small series support the use of early plasmapheresis in conjunction with steroids and cyclophosphamide [55].

Bronchiolitis Obliterans with Organizing Pneumonia

Bronchiolitis obliterans with organizing pneumonia is a disease characterized by patchy organizing pneumonia without apparent cause. Pathologically there are masses of granulation tissue in the lumina of small airways and in alveolar ducts, with organizing pneumonia distal to these obstructions. Patients typically present with a 1- to 2-month history of cough or symptoms suggestive of viral or upper respiratory tract infection. Physical examination reveals inspiratory crackles or inspiratory squeaks. Chest x-ray films show patchy alveolar infiltrates, often with a ground-glass appearance [28]. Neutrophils or occasionally lymphocytes are prominent in bronchoalveolar lavage fluid. Restrictive ventilatory defects and impaired diffusing capacity are frequently

present. The disease has been associated with connective-tissue diseases, infection, marrow or organ transplantation, and toxic fume inhalation. Definitive diagnosis requires tissue examination. Clinically, bronchiolitis obliterans with organizing pneumonia may be difficult to distinguish from IPF, although symptoms are usually of much shorter duration in the former [44]. Corticosteroids may be effective in as many as 65 percent of patients, leading at times to complete clinical recovery [28].

Eosinophilic Granuloma/Histiocytosis X

Eosinophilic granuloma can affect the bones, pituitary gland, and multiple organs including the lungs, where it is a cause of IPF. Pulmonary involvement may occur alone or as part of generalized disease, and is associated with skeletal lesions in more than 20 percent of patients. Pulmonary eosinophilic granuloma affects all ages, from infancy to old age, but is most often seen in younger adults aged 20 to 40 years, and may be more common among individuals who smoke. Presenting symptoms or signs may be insidious with cough, dyspnea, or constitutional symptoms or abrupt onset of spontaneous pneumothorax. Chest pain may be due to pneumothorax or rib lesions. Physical findings may be normal, with rales occurring in only about 20 percent of patients. Chest x-ray findings typically reveal a micronodular or interstitial infiltrate, especially in the upper lobes, that may progress to a cystic honeycomb pattern. Lung biopsy specimens reveal typical stellate granulomas comprised of histiocytes and eosinophils. Specific cellular markers can identify the pathologic histiocytosis X cells and distinguish them from normal histiocytes. The diagnosis can be made by careful examination of bronchoalveolar lavage cells [17]. Peripheral eosinophilia is not present. A bone scan is recommended to identify bone lesions. The course of eosinophilic granuloma is quite variable, ranging from rapid progression to spontaneous resolution, the latter being more common [36]. Patients may suffer from recurrent spontaneous pneumothoraces. Prognosis is usually better for patients with focal lung disease than for those with wide dissemination. There are no controlled studies demonstrating efficacy of steroids, but it is accepted practice to use steroids if patients are deteriorating. There is no role for cytotoxic drugs or radiation therapy. The disease is more common among smokers and cessation of smoking is strongly recommended [36,45].

Chronic Eosinophilic Pneumonia

Chronic eosinophilic pneumonia can present as a severe respiratory illness with fever, night sweats, dyspnea, and weight loss. This illness is more common in women. Wheezing or rales may be evident on lung examination. Peripheral blood eosinophilia is variable and may not be present. The chest x-ray film may demonstrate a unique pattern of dense peripheral infiltrates that spare the central portions of the lungs, often called the reverse image of pulmonary edema. Infiltrates may appear and remit spontaneously, as the disease may wax and wane over months. Other disorders that should be considered in the differential diagnosis include filariasis and other parasitic infections, hypersensitivity pneumonitis, and eosinophilic granuloma. Chronic eosinophilic pneumonia is remarkably sensitive to corticosteroids, with clinical response usually evident within a few days. As therapy is tapered, the pneumonia may reappear, requiring close follow-up. Persistent disease can lead to interstitial fibrosis and honeycombing [87].

Respiratory Bronchiolitis–Associated ILD

Respiratory bronchiolitis is a pathologic lesion observed in asymptomatic young cigarette smokers, characterized by an accumulation of pigmented macrophages in respiratory bronchioles, alveolar ducts, and alveoli with thickening of adjacent interstitium. Recent reports suggested a possible association with ILD that may abate with cessation of smoking and/or steroid therapy. Patients are typically young (mean age, 36 years) with an average 30 to 40 pack-year smoking history. Presenting symptoms consist of cough, dyspnea, and sputum production. Chest x-ray films appear abnormal in the majority of patients, usually showing a diffuse, fine reticular, or reticulonodular pattern; however, the chest x-ray can appear normal. Pulmonary function tests may show mild to moderate restriction and decreased diffusing capacity; mild obstruction is also occasionally observed. Prognosis in this disorder is generally good. Patients who abstain from smoking have resolution of symptoms. Even those who continue to smoke do not develop progressive fibrotic lung disease when followed for several years. It may be important to establish this diagnosis because of its significantly better prognosis than other chronic ILDs, and to avoid unnecessary treatment with potentially toxic medications [75,111].

Pulmonary Alveolar Proteinosis

Pulmonary alveolar proteinosis is characterized by the accumulation within distal air spaces of periodic acid–Schiff (PAS)–positive, lipid-rich, proteinaceous material. It is an intraalveolar disease, but because of similar symptoms and diffuse radiographic findings, pulmonary alveolar proteinosis is usually grouped with ILDs. The peak age of onset is between 30 and 50 years, but it is seen in all age groups. Males are affected more often than females by a ratio of 3 : 1. The onset of symptoms is usually insidious, beginning with dyspnea on exertion and cough, and progressing to dyspnea at rest. Lung examination will reveal coarse crackles over affected areas. Clubbing of fingers and toes may develop. Chest x-ray findings consist of a diffuse alveolar filling pattern that may include patchy, confluent, or nodular infiltrates. In extensive disease, lung fields may be uniformly infiltrated, giving a ground glass appearance. Pulmonary function tests typically show a restrictive ventilatory pattern with a reduced diffusing capacity.

The etiology of pulmonary alveolar proteinosis is unknown. The intraalveolar material is composed of surfactant phospholipid, surfactant-specific apoproteins, and other serum proteins also found in alveolar lining fluid. A similar pathologic picture may be seen in acute exposure to silica or aluminum dust. The diagnosis usually requires open lung biopsy, but when suspected, PAS staining and electron microscopy of bronchoalveolar lavage fluid can be diagnostic. Alveolar macrophages from patients with pulmonary alveolar proteinosis have numerous lamellar inclusions, rich in phospholipid, within their cytoplasm. It is unclear whether this accumulation of alveolar material is due to overproduction by type II pneumonocytes or impaired clearance by macrophages. Alveolar macrophage chemotactic and intracellular killing functions have been shown to be abnormal in patients with pulmonary alveolar proteinosis [42]. Perhaps for this reason, pulmonary infections, particularly with *Nocardia*, are the most common complication of this disease.

Pulmonary alveolar proteinosis is usually a progressive disease, although about 25 percent of patients may recover spontaneously. Some patients have been reported to respond to aerosolized agents that can thin the alveolar filling fluid, such as trypsin [53], streptokinase [88], and potassium iodide [34], but small numbers and the possibility of spontaneous recovery hamper interpretation of these reports. In progressive disease, whole-lung lavage can produce dramatic improvements. The procedure is performed under general anesthesia with large-volume (20 liters) irrigation of one lung while the contralateral lung is ventilated. The procedure may be repeated in the contralateral lung at a later date [19]. Lavage of individual lobes using the bronchoscope may also result in improvement of both clinical and pulmonary function indices [7,9]. Corticosteroids are contraindicated because of the increased risk of infectious complications, emphasizing the importance of making a specific diagnosis and not treating empirically.

References

1. Aberle DR, Gamsu G, Lynch D. Thoracic manifestations of Wegener granulomatosis: Diagnosis and course. *Radiology* 174:703, 1990.
2. Aberle DR, et al. Asbestos-related pleural and parenchymal fibrosis: Detection with high-resolution CT. *Radiology* 166:729, 1988.
3. Ashbaugh DG, Maier RV. Idiopathic pulmonary fibrosis in adult respiratory distress syndrome. *Arch Surg* 120:530, 1985.
4. Bergin CJ, et al. Chronic lung diseases: Specific diagnosis by using CT. *AJR* 152:1183, 1989.
5. Bergin CJ, Muller NL. CT in the diagnosis of interstitial lung disease. *AJR* 145:505, 1985.
6. Bergin CJ, Muller NL. CT of interstitial lung disease: A diagnostic approach. *AJR* 148:8, 1987.
7. Bernstein MS, et al. Fiberoptic bronchoscopic lavage in alveolar proteinosis and analysis of protein component. *Am Rev Respir Dis* 137(4 Part 2):182, 1988.
8. Boyce NW, Holdsworth SR. Idiopathic Goodpasture's syndrome. Fatal pulmonary hemorrhage and crescentic glomerulonephritis in the absence of immune-reactant deposition. *Nephron* 44:22, 1986.
9. Brach BB, Harrell JH, Moser KM. Alveolar proteinosis, lobar lavage by fiberoptic bronchoscopic technique. *Chest* 69:224, 1976.
10. Breit SN, et al. The presence of Sjogren's syndrome is a major determinant of the pattern of interstitial lung disease in scleroderma and other connective tissue diseases. *J Rheumatol* 16:1043, 1989.
11. Burki NK. Dyspnea. *Clin Chest Med* 1:47, 1980.
12. Buschman DL, Waldron JA, King TE. Churg-Strauss pulmonary vasculitis. High-resolution computed tomography scanning and pathologic findings. *Am Rev Respir Dis* 142:458, 1990.
13. Carrieri VK, Janson-Bjerklie SJ, Jacobs S. The sensation of dyspnea: A review. *Heart Lung* 13:436, 1984.
14. Carrington CB. Organizing interstitial pneumonia: Definition of the lesions and attempts to devise an experimental model. *Yale J Biol Med* 40:352, 1968.
15. Carrington CB, et al. Natural history and treated course of usual and desquamative interstitial pneumonia. *N Engl J Med* 298:801, 1978.
16. Carstairs LS. The interpretation of shadows in a restricted area of a lung field on the chest radiograph. *Proc R Soc Med* 54:978, 1961.
17. Chollet S, et al. Diagnosis of pulmonary histiocytosis X by immunodetection of Langerhans cells in bronchoalveolar lavage fluid. *Am J Pathol* 115:225, 1984.
18. Chumbley LC, Harrison EG Jr, Remee RA. Allergic granulomatosis and angiitis (Churg-Strauss syndrome): Report and analysis of 30 cases. *Mayo Clin Proc* 52:477, 1977.
19. Claypool W, Rogers R, Matuschak G. Update on clinical diagnosis, management, and pathogenesis of pulmonary alveolar proteinosis (phospholipidosis). *Chest* 85:550, 1984.
20. Crystal RG, et al. Interstitial lung disease of unknown cause. *N Engl J Med* 310:154, 235, 1984.
21. Crystal RG, et al. Interstitial lung disease: Current concepts of pathogenesis, staging and therapy. *Am J Med* 70:542, 1981.
22. Davison AG, et al. Interstitial lung disease and asthma in hard-metal workers: Bronchoalveolar lavage, ultrastructural, and analytical findings and results of bronchial provocation tests. *Thorax* 38:119, 1983.
23. DeClerck LS, et al. D-Penicillamine therapy and interstitial lung disease in scleroderma. A long-term follow-up study. *Arthritis Rheum* 30:643, 1987.
24. DeRemee RA, Gracey DR. Diffuse interstitial lung disease. *Dis Mon* 29:1, 1983.
25. DeRemee RA, Rohrbach MS. Serum angiotensin-converting enzyme activity in evaluating the clinical course of sarcoidosis. *Ann Intern Med* 92:361, 1980.
26. Eisenberg H. The interstitial lung diseases associated with the collagen-vascular disorders. *Clin Chest Med* 3:565, 1982.
27. Epler GR, Carrington CB, Gaensler EA. Crackles (rales) in the interstitial pulmonary diseases. *Chest* 73:333, 1978.
28. Epler GR, et al. Bronchiolitis obliterans organizing pneumonia. *N Engl J Med* 312:152, 1985.
29. Epler GR, et al. Normal chest roentgenograms in chronic diffuse infiltrative lung disease. *N Engl J Med* 298:934, 1978.
30. Feldman C, et al. Diffuse interstitial pulmonary fibrosis and spontaneous pneumothorax associated with *Schistosoma haematobium* infestation of the lungs. A case report. *S Afr Med J* 69:138, 1986.
31. Felson B. Disseminated interstitial diseases of the lung. *Ann Radiol* 9:325, 1966.
32. Felson B. A new look at pattern recognition of diffuse pulmonary disease. *AJR* 133:183, 1979.
33. Fisher MR. Magnetic resonance for evaluation of the thorax. *Chest* 95:166, 1989.
34. Fraimow W, et al. Pulmonary alveolar proteino-

sis. A correlation of pathological and physiological findings in a patient followed up with serial biopsies of the lung. *Am J Med* 28:458, 1960.

35. Frank ST, et al. Pulmonary dysfunction in rheumatoid disease. *Chest* 63:27, 1973.

36. Friedman PJ, Liebow AA, Sokoloff J. Eosinophilic granuloma of the lung. Clinical aspects of primary pulmonary histiocytosis in the adult. *Medicine* 60:385, 1981.

37. Fulmer JD, Crystal RG. Interstitial lung disease. *Curr Pulmonol* 11:1, 1979.

38. Gaensler EA, Carrington CB, Coutu RE. Chronic interstitial pneumonias. *Clin Notes Respir Dis* Spring:3, 1972.

39. Gamsu G, Sostman D. Magnetic resonance imaging of the thorax. *Am Rev Respir Dis* 139:254, 1989.

40. Glazer HS, et al. Differentiation of radiation fibrosis from recurrent pulmonary neoplasm by MRI. *AJR* 143:729, 1984.

41. Glossary of terms for thoracic radiology: Recommendations of the nomenclature committee of the Fleischner Society. *AJR* 143:509, 1984.

42. Golde DW, et al. Defective lung macrophages in pulmonary alveolar proteinosis. *Ann Intern Med* 85:304, 1976.

43. Grenier P, et al. Bronchiectasis: Assessment by thin-section CT. *Radiology* 161:95, 1986.

44. Guerry-Force ML, et al. A comparison of bronchiolitis obliterans with organizing pneumonia, usual interstitial pneumonia and small airways disease. *Am Rev Respir Dis* 135:705, 1987.

45. Hance AJ, et al. Smoking and interstitial lung disease: The effect of cigarette smoking on the incidence of pulmonary histiocytosis X and sarcoidosis. *Ann NY Acad Sci* 465:643, 1986.

46. Heitzman E. *The Lung: Radiologic-Pathologic Correlations.* St. Louis: Mosby, 1984. Pp 79–92, 98–105.

47. Heppleston AG. The pathology of honeycomb lung. *Thorax* 11:77, 1956.

48. Hill NS. The cardiac exam in lung disease. *Clin Chest Med* 8:273, 1987.

49. Hruban RH, et al. Inflation-fixed lungs: Pathologic-radiologic (CT) correlation of lung transplantation. *J Comp Assist Tomogr* 14:329, 1990.

50. Huang HK (Moderator UCLA Conference). Advances in medical imaging. *Ann Intern Med* 112:203, 1990.

51. Irwin RS, Curley FJ, French CL. Chronic cough: The spectrum and frequency of causes, key components of the diagnostic evaluation, and outcome of specific therapy. *Am Rev Respir Dis* 141:640, 1990.

52. Jackson LK. Idiopathic pulmonary fibrosis. *Clin Chest Med* 3:579, 1982.

53. Jay SJ. Pulmonary alveolar proteinosis. Successful treatment with aerosolized trypsin. *Am J Med* 66:348, 1979.

54. Johns CJ, Scott PP, Schonfeld SA. Sarcoidosis. *Annu Rev Med* 40:353, 1989.

55. Johnson JP, et al. Therapy of anti-glomerular basement membrane antibody disease. An analysis of prognostic significance of clinical, pathologic, and treatment factors. *Medicine (Baltimore)* 64:219, 1985.

56. Johnson MA, et al. Randomized controlled trial comparing prednisone alone with cyclophosphamide and low dose prednisone in combination in cryptogenic fibrosing alveolitis. *Thorax* 44:280, 1989.

57. Kaelin RM, Kapanci Y, Tschopp JM. Diffuse interstitial lung disease associated with hydrogen peroxide inhalation in a dairy worker. *Am Rev Respir Dis* 137:1233, 1988.

58. Karam GH, Fulmer JD. Giant cell arteritis presenting as interstitial lung disease. *Chest* 82:781, 1982.

59. Katz D, Kreel L. Computed tomography in pulmonary asbestosis. *Clin Radiol* 30:207, 1979.

60. Keogh BA, Crystal RG. Alveolitis: The key to the interstitial lung disorders. *Thorax* 37:1, 1982.

61. Kerr IH. Interstitial lung disease: The role of the radiologist. *Clin Radiol* 35:1, 1984.

62. Kreel L. Computed tomography of interstitial pulmonary disease. *J Comput Assist Tomogr* 6:181, 1982.

63. Leavitt RY, Fauci AS. Pulmonary vasculitis. *Am Rev Respir Dis* 134:149, 1986.

64. Liebow AA. Pulmonary angiitis and granulomatosis. *Am Rev Respir Dis* 1108:1, 1973.

65. Liebow AA, Carrington CB. The Interstitial Pneumonias. In M Simon, EJ Potchen, M LeMay (Eds). *Frontiers of Pulmonary Radiology.* New York: Grune & Stratton, 1969.

66. Lynch DA, et al. Computed tomography in pulmonary sarcoidosis. *J Comp Assist Tomogr* 13:405, 1989.

67. Mathieson JR, et al. Chronic diffuse infiltrative lung disease: Comparison of diagnostic accuracy of CT and chest radiography. *Radiology* 171:111, 1989.

68. McLoud T, Gaensler EA, Carrington CB. Chronic diffuse infiltrative lung disease: Newer approaches. *Clin Chest Med* 5:329, 1984.

69. Meyer EC, Liebow AA. The relationship of interstitial pneumonia, honeycombing, and atypical epithelial proliferation to cancer. *Cancer* 18:322, 1965.

70. Muller NL, Miller RA. Computed tomography of chronic diffuse infiltrative lung disease. Parts 1 and 2. *Am Rev Respir Dis* 142:1206, 1440, 1990.

71. Muller NL, et al. Fibrosing alveolitis: CT-pathological correlations. *Radiology* 160:585, 1986.

72. Muller NL, et al. Disease activity in idiopathic pulmonary fibrosis: CT and pathologic correlation. *Radiology* 165:731, 1987.

73. Murata K, et al. Centrilobular lesions of the

lung: Demonstration by high-resolution CT and pathologic correlation. *Radiology* 161:641, 1986.

74. Myers J, Katzenstein A. Wegener's granulomatosis presenting with massive pulmonary hemorrhage and capillaritis. *Am J Surg Pathol* 11:895, 1987.

75. Myers JL, et al. Respiratory bronchiolitis causing interstitial lung disease. *Am Rev Respir Dis* 135:880, 1987.

76. Nakata H, et al. Diffuse peripheral lung disease: Evaluation by high-resolution computed tomography. *Radiology* 157:181, 1985.

77. Nolle B, et al. Anticytoplasmic autoantibodies: Their immunodiagnostic value in Wegener granulomatosis. *Ann Intern Med* 111:28, 1989.

78. Ognibene FP, et al. Kaposi's sarcoma causing pulmonary infiltrates and respiratory failure in the acquired immunodeficiency syndrome. *Ann Intern Med* 102:471, 1985.

79. Owens GR, Follansbee WP. Cardiopulmonary manifestations of systemic sclerosis. *Chest* 91:118, 1987.

80. Rappaport DC, et al. Pulmonary lymphangioleiomyomatosis: High-resolution CT findings in four cases. *Am J Radiol* 152:961, 1989.

81. Reed JC, Madewell JE. The air bronchogram in interstitial disease of lungs. *Radiology* 116:1, 1975.

82. Rees JH, et al. Rheumatoid arthritis and cryptogenic organising pneumonitis. *Respir Med* 85:243, 1991.

83. Respiratory Diseases Task Force. *Report on Problems, Research Approaches and Needs.* DHEW publication no NIH 76-432. Washington, DC: US Government Printing Office, 1972.

84. Rohrbach MS, DeRemee RA. Pulmonary sarcoidosis and serum angiotensin-converting enzyme. *Mayo Clin Proc* 57:64, 1982.

85. Schurawitzki H, et al. Interstitial lung disease in progressive systemic sclerosis: High resolution CT versus radiography. *Radiology* 176:755, 1990.

86. Schwarz MI, et al. Interstitial lung disease in polymyositis and dermatomyositis: Analysis of 6 cases and a review of the literature. *Medicine* 55:89, 1976.

87. Sederlinic PJ, Sicilian L, Gaensler EA. Chronic eosinophilic pneumonia: A report of 19 cases and a review of the literature. *Medicine* 67:154, 1988.

88. Slutzker B, Perryman PH. Pulmonary alveolar proteinosis. Response to nebulized enzyme therapy. *Arch Intern Med* 109:406, 1962.

89. Specks U, et al. Anticytoplasmic autoantibodies in the diagnosis and follow-up of Wegener's granulomatosis. *Mayo Clin Proc* 64:28, 1989.

90. Spencer H. *Pathology of the Lung* (4th ed). Oxford: Pergamon, 1985. Pp 788–802.

91. Staples CA, et al. Usual interstitial pneumonia: Correlation of CT with clinical, functional, and radiologic findings. *Radiology* 162:377, 1987.

92. Stein MG, et al. Computed tomography: Pathologic correlation in lung disease due to tocainamide. *Am Rev Respir Dis* 137:458, 1988.

93. Stein MG, et al. Pulmonary lymphangitic spread of carcinoma: Appearance on CT scans. *Radiology* 162:371, 1987.

94. Stulbarg M. Evaluation and treatment of intractable cough. *West J Med* 143:223, 1985.

95. Sullivan WD, et al. A prospective evaluation emphasizing pulmonary involvement in patients with mixed connective tissue disease. *Medicine* 63:92, 1984.

96. Takimoto CH, Lynch D, Stulbarg MS. Pulmonary infiltrates associated with sulindac therapy. *Chest* 97:230, 1990.

97. Targoff IN, et al. Anti-KJ: A new antibody associated with the syndrome of polymyositis and interstitial lung disease. *J Clin Invest* 84:162, 1989.

98. Tazelaar HD, et al. Interstitial lung disease in polymyositis and dermatomyositis. *Am Rev Respir Dis* 141:727, 1990.

99. *The Hospital Record Study: Commission on Professional and Hospital Activities.* Ambler, PA: IMS American 1977.

100. Thomas PD, Hunninghake GW. Current concepts of the pathogenesis of sarcoidosis. *Am Rev Respir Dis* 135:747, 1987.

101. Trapnell DH. Radiological appearances of lymphangitis carcinomatosa of the lung. *Thorax* 19:251, 1964.

102. Turner-Warwick M, Burrows B, Johnson A. Cryptogenic fibrosing alveolitis: Clinical features and their influence on survival. *Thorax* 35:171, 1980.

103. UICC-Cincinnati classification of the radiographic appearance of the pneumoconioses. *Chest* 58:57, 1970.

104. Van der Woude F, et al. Autoantibodies against neutrophils and monocytes: Tool for diagnosis and marker of disease activity in Wegener's granulomatosis. *Lancet* 1:425, 1985.

105. Warrick JH, et al. High-resolution computed tomography in early scleroderma lung disease. *J Rheumatol* 18:1520, 1991.

106. Webb WR, et al. Normal and diseased isolated lungs: High-resolution CT. *Radiology* 166:81, 1988.

107. Weibel ER, Gil J. Structure-Function Relationships at the Alveolar Level. In JB West (Ed), *Bioengineering Aspects of the Lung.* New York: Marcel Dekker, 1971.

108. Weinrib L, Sharma OP, Quismorio FP. A long-term study of interstitial lung disease in systemic lupus erythematosus. *Semin Arthritis Rheum* 20:48, 1990.

109. Winterbauer RH, et al. Diffuse interstitial pneumonitis: Clinicopathologic correlations in 20

patients treated with prednisone/azathioprine. *Am J Med* 65:661, 1978.

110. Wolheim FA, Akesson A. Treatment of systemic sclerosis in 1988. *Semin Arthritis Rheum* 18: 181, 1989.

111. Yousem SA, Colby TV, Gaensler EA. Respiratory bronchiolitis-associated interstitial lung disease and its relationship to desquamative interstitial pneumonia. *Mayo Clin Proc* 64:1373, 1989.

112. Zerhouni E. Computed tomography of the pulmonary parenchyma. An overview. *Chest* 95: 901, 1989.

41

Interstitial (Diffuse Parenchymal) Lung Disease: Physiology

Jeffrey A. Golden

The functional correlate of abnormal alveolar-capillary wall structure is restrictive lung disease, that is, reduced ventilable lung volume. Classically, patients with infiltrative or interstitial lung disease (ILD) have diminished or restricted lung volumes in association with decreased diffusing capacity, decreased lung distensibility or compliance, and preserved air flow rates. With exercise, such patients have inappropriate hyperventilation with rapid, shallow breaths and progressive arterial hypoxemia [99,411].* It should be stressed that diseases of the lung parenchyma comprise only one of several categories of processes that result in lung restriction which include lung resection, pleural disease, neuromuscular and/or thoracic skeletal abnormalities, as well as obesity [36].

Lung Volumes

Interest in detecting restricted lung volumes began with Hutchison's attempt to show that a decreased forced vital capacity predicted the presence of tuberculosis [199]. In general, the pattern of lung volume abnormalities suggests the cause of restriction (Table 41-1). In interstitial or parenchymal processes, the volumes are normal with early disease [99]. With progressive parenchymal involvement, patients usually present with decreased vital capacity, and if the total lung capacity is decreased, it is primarily because of this vital capacity reduction [45,64,429]. Because the vital capacity is decreased in ILD, it is important to be aware of the determinants of this measurement. The *vital capacity* is the difference between total lung capacity and the residual volume, so factors determining these volumes are also relevant in understanding the cause of a diminished vital capacity. The *total lung capacity* is that volume at which maximal tension, generated by the diaphragm and other muscles of inspiration, is balanced by the inward recoil of the lungs and chest wall. Therefore, the total lung capacity may be restricted by abnormalities of the bony thorax, inspiratory muscles, or pleura, as well as loss of functioning alveoli, as in ILD. Similarly, during pulmonary function assessment, poor effort, fatigue, and chest pain all may prevent maximal effort and a diminution of total lung capacity [106,158,222,432].

The *residual volume* is the volume at which maximal expiratory force is balanced by the outward recoil of the chest wall and the effect of airway narrowing and/or closure on limiting further exhalation. The outward recoil of the chest-wall determinant of residual volume is more important in children, whereas in normal adults, airway closure in dependent lung regions due to decreased lung elastic recoil is a relatively more important factor [130]. In the presence of diseases that obstruct airflow, the residual volume will be abnormally increased and, in the setting of a relatively preserved total lung capacity, impinge on or restrict the vital capacity.

Further, in the presence of obstructive lung disease, the measurement of total lung capacity will be artifactually decreased, further complicating the interpretation of a restricted vital capacity. The assessment of total lung capacity requires either gas dilution or plethysmographic measurement of the volume of gas remaining after exhalation, that is, the functional residual capacity. In the context of obstructive disease, there are lung

*References for this chapter appear at the end of Chapter 42.

Table 41-1. Patterns of lung volume changes in restrictive lung disease

	VC	TLC	FRC	RV
Alveolar filling/loss disease	↓	↓	↓	↓
Interstitial diseases (↓ compliance)	↓	↓	↘	N/↘
Neuromuscular*				
Selective inspiratory	↓	↓	N	N
Selective expiratory	↓	N	N	↑
Both	↓	↓	N	↑
Thoracic cage				
E.g., kyphoscoliosis	↓	↓	↓	↘
E.g., ankylosing spondylitis	↓	↓	↑	↑
Pleural disease	↓	↓	↓	↓
Pulmonary vascular disease	N/↓	N/↓	N/↓	N/↓

VC = vital capacity; TLC = total lung capacity; FRC = functional residual capacity; RV = residual volume; N = normal; ↓ = decreased; ↘ = slightly decreased; ↑ = increased.
*These patterns are for pure neuromuscular disease. Associated complications such as atelectasis and pneumonia will produce concomitant reduction in lung volumes related to alveolar filling.
Source: From AL Ries, JL Clausen. Lung Volumes. In AF Wilson (Ed), *Pulmonary Function Testing: Indications and Interpretations.* Orlando, FL: Grune & Stratton, 1985.

regions in poor communication with airways which will not be adequately measured by gas-dilution techniques. This is especially true of the single-breath helium-dilution test, where there is only 10 seconds for gas distribution. In one study, this dilution test underestimated the total lung capacity by 20 percent in the presence of moderate disease and 38 percent in patients with severe obstructive disease [56]. The plethysmographic technique gives a better estimate of the true lung volume. However, in the setting of airway obstruction, this test artifactually increases the total lung capacity unless the frequency of panting is kept low (less than 1 Hz) [364].

In contrast to the decreased vital capacity and total lung capacity, infiltrative parenchymal diseases have minimal impact on the residual volume. The residual volume in ILD is relatively preserved, so that the residual volume to total lung capacity ratio (RV/TLC) is often increased. The mechanism of the preserved or relatively increased residual volume in ILD is unknown. However, morphologic evidence of small peripheral airways disease correlates with the increased RV/TLC ratio in patients with ILD and was noted on pathologic examination of the original patients with ILD described by Hamman and Rich [170]. Perhaps such peripheral airways disease results in airway closure and limits further exhalation, resulting in a relatively preserved re-

sidual volume [45,143,158,287]. Another explanation for the preserved residual volume in ILD is that the determinants of residual volume, unlike vital capacity and total lung capacity, are less affected by processes that affect lung compliance. Finally, an alternative explanation is that at end expiration in ILD, the noncompliant or stiff lung is relatively fixed in position and resists further decreases in volume with further expiratory effort [336,420].

The functional residual capacity is determined by a balance between the outward recoil of the chest wall and the inward recoil of the lung parenchyma. Therefore, the functional residual capacity will be decreased by diseases causing lung infiltration or alveolar filling, resulting in decreased compliance (i.e., increased recoil). Similarly, the functional residual capacity will be decreased by skeletal-wall diseases such as kyphoscoliosis where there is less outward recoil, and increased in other skeletal-wall diseases such as ankylosing spondylitis where there is increased outward recoil of the chest [36]. Functional residual capacity is unaffected by neuromuscular diseases unless there is chronic atelectasis and scarring. Finally, although controversial, it has been stated that pulmonary vascular disease such as recurrent pulmonary emboli or primary pulmonary hypertension is associated with a decrease in all lung volumes in about 40 percent of cases [186].

Pressure-Volume Characteristics of the Lung: Increased Elastic Recoil

In addition to restricted lung volumes, the other major physiologic hallmark of infiltrative parenchymal disease is the presence of increased lung recoil or decreased distensibility. Along with airway diameter, which it also influences by providing a distending force, elastic recoil is a major determinant of maximal airflow, ventilatory capacity, and distribution of ventilation. Further, the elastic recoil of the lung is a major determinant of the work of breathing as well as the total lung capacity [154,228,232,252].

Like a rubber balloon, the lung is an elastic structure that is held inflated at a specific volume by the pressure difference between the inside (alveolar airspace) and the outside (pleural space) [154]. This transpulmonary pressure can be calculated by simultaneously measuring the pressures in the alveoli and the pleural space at multiple lung volumes between total lung capacity and residual volume during an interrupted expiration. The pressure in the pleural space can be estimated by careful placement of an esophageal catheter whose distal tip is protected by a balloon [157,252]. Alveolar pressure is identical to mouth pressure when there is no airflow. With no flow in the airway, the pressure difference between mouth (alveolar) pressure and esophageal (pleural) pressure (i.e., the transpulmonary pressure) is due to the elastic recoil of the lung (Pst) [154]. Therefore, elastic recoil is measured during a breath hold (static airflow) with the glottis held open [252].

The static pressure-volume curve of the lung is the relationship between lung volume and recoil or transpulmonary pressure [252]. As can be seen in Figure 41-1, recoil pressure varies with lung volume. Lung recoil is determined by the stress-strain properties of collagen and elastin and their arrangement in the lung's connective-tissue fiber network, by alveolar lining fluid surface tension, and by the number of alveoli sharing a particular lung volume [154].

Interpretation of the Pressure-Volume Curve

The clinical and research value of pressure-volume assessment is limited by the traditional use of linear approximations of the curve (chord compliance) or arbitrary indices such as recoil pressure at various volumes. *Lung compliance* is the change in volume per change in lung trans-

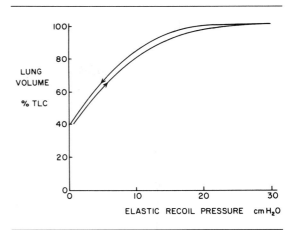

Fig. 41-1. Normal pressure-volume curve of the lung. At any specific lung volume, the elastic recoil pressure is slightly greater on inflation than it is on deflation. The lung volume is expressed as percent total lung capacity (*TLC*). (From P Macklem. New tests to assess lung function. *N Engl J Med* 293:339, 1975.)

pulmonary distending or elastic recoil pressure, that is, the slope of the pressure-volume curve. As can be seen from Figures 41-1 and 41-2, the pressure-volume curve in the normal or various disease states reveals that the slope changes at different lung volumes. The traditional chord compliance is measured over the volume range between the functional residual capacity and the functional residual capacity plus 500 cc. However, this value is influenced by determinants of the functional residual capacity as well as by the shape and/or position of the pressure-volume curve [159,252]. Instead of compliance, other authors report the lung's maximal recoil pressure (Pst_{max}) at total lung capacity. But this value is very sensitive to small changes in lung volume, especially in the setting of increased recoil; further, Pst_{max} depends on patient cooperation and effort [45,99,252].

Instead of describing only portions of the curve, it has been recommended that the entire pressure-volume curve be evaluated—shape, position, and slope. For example, in Figure 41-2, as Macklem elucidates, in both interstitial pulmonary fibrosis and pulmonary vascular congestion there is a similar decrease in slope, but there is much more displacement down and to the right in interstitial pulmonary fibrosis. It is the shift to the right and the downward displacement that reflect increased recoil or decreased distensibility

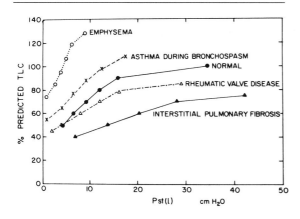

Fig. 41-2. Static deflation pressure-volume curves in various diseases. On the ordinate, the lung volume is expressed as percent predicted total lung capacity (*TLC*), and on the abscissa, it is expressed as elastic recoil pressure (*PstL*) in centimeters of water. (From P Macklem. New tests to assess lung function. *N Engl J Med* 293:339, 1975.)

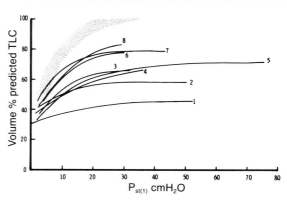

Fig. 41-3. Static expiratory pressure-volume curves for eight patients with fibrosing alveolitis. Volume is expressed as percent predicted total lung capacity (*TLC*); lung elastic recoil pressure (*PstL*) is expressed as centimeters of water. Numbers refer to specific individual patients. Stippled area represents normal range for subjects more than 45 years old. (From GJ Gibson, NB Pride. Pulmonary mechanics in fibrosing alveolitis: The effects of lung shrinkage. *Am Rev Respir Dis* 116:637, 1977.)

that is fundamental to ILDs in contrast to the decreased elastic recoil in the setting of emphysema, where the curve is shifted upward and to the left.

Traditionally, recoil is related to percent predicted total lung capacity to compensate for differences in patient (but not lung) size (Fig. 41-3). As pointed out by Gibson and Pride, the decreased slope (compliance) and abnormal position (i.e., shift downward and to the right) were originally said to reflect stiffness of the alveolar wall due to an infiltrating pulmonary process [137,157]. However, pathologic evaluation in ILD revealed a patchy distribution of disease with some alveoli replaced by fibrous tissue and others that were normal. The total number of air-containing alveoli was reduced. To understand the mechanism of the alterations in the pressure-volume curve, it is necessary to control for this decreased alveolar volume. As noted in Figure 41-1, compliance is critically dependent on lung (alveolar) volume [45,158].

If there is a decreased number of alveoli, the remaining alveoli are more distended (the same lung volume shared among fewer alveoli) and the *net* elastic recoil pressure of the lung is increased. Thus, the pressure-volume curve is shifted downward and to the right, and the slope is decreased [154]. Further, with decreased lung volume, the maximum force generated by the

muscles of inspiration is increased because at a particular lung volume the muscles are longer (force-length properties) and are at a greater mechanical advantage. Therefore, in the presence of a decreased lung volume, the overdistension of functioning alveolar units and mechanical advantage of the muscles of inspiration will decrease the slope and shift downward and to the right the pressure-volume relationship despite the presence of normal elastic properties of the surviving functioning alveoli [159]. Similarly, in the setting of pneumonectomy, plotting transpulmonary pressure or recoil (Pst) against predicted total lung capacity results in a shift downward and to the right in the pressure-volume curve despite normal elastic properties of the remaining lung [45,252].

To determine if lung smallness rather than lung stiffness is the cause of the decreased lung compliance in ILD, lung elastic recoil has been plotted against percent actual or observed lung volume, rather than predicted volume (Figs. 41-3 and 41-4). As in Figure 41-4, although recoil at full inflation remains increased, compliance is normal at lower lung volumes when recoil is plotted against percent of measured total lung capacity. Thus, relating the recoil to observed rather than

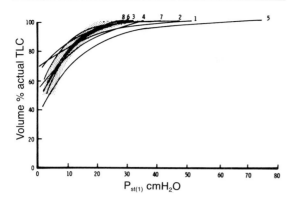

Fig. 41-4. Static expiratory pressure-volume curves for eight patients with fibrosing alveolitis. Volume is expressed as percent measured total lung capacity (*TLC*), same as for Figure 41-3. (From GJ Gibson, NB Pride. Pulmonary mechanics in fibrosing alveolitis: The effects of lung shrinkage. *Am Rev Respir Dis* 116:637, 1977.)

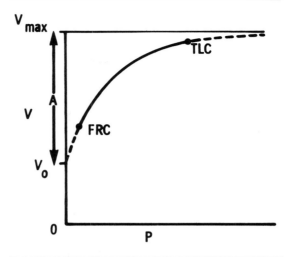

Fig. 41-5. Equation of exponential pressure-volume (*PV*) curve fitted to data between total lung capacity (*TLC*) and functional residual capacity (*FRC*) (*solid line*). V_{max} and V_o represent volumes extrapolated (*broken lines*) to P = infinity and P = 0, respectively. (From GJ Gibson et al. Exponential description of the static pressure-volume curve of normal and diseased lungs. *Am Rev Respir Dis* 120:799, 1979.)

predicted total lung capacity allows a first approximation of the role of volume loss alone as a cause of increased recoil, but it does not correct for the maximal recoil at total lung capacity resulting from the improved mechanical advantage of the inspiratory muscles [158,287].

Therefore, to describe the lung's elastic properties totally independent of lung size, it is useful to describe the entire curve by a single exponential expression. By describing the entire curve over a wide range of volumes and pressures, this exponential expression is more accurate than measuring linear approximations over a small range of transpulmonary pressures near functional residual capacity or maximal recoil at total lung capacity [81,158,159]. In one such approach (Fig. 41-5), data points were fitted according to the equation

$$V = V_{max} - Ae^{-KP}$$

where V_{max} represents the extrapolated volume at infinite transpulmonary pressure and A is a constant related to the intercept on the volume axis. The parameter K is related to the incremental compliance (dV/dP):

$$dV/dP = AKe^{-KP} = K(V_{max} - V)$$

If P is measured in centimeters of water (cmH_2O), K has the dimensions of cmH_2O^{-1} [159].

In the setting of increased recoil, the effects of lung shrinkage could be differentiated from increased tissue stiffness due to a thickened alveolar wall by analyzing the extrapolated theoretical maximum lung capacity. If the compliance is decreased because the alveoli are stiff, the extrapolated volume at a limitless distending pressure should be normal. If the lung compliance is reduced due to loss of alveoli, then this extrapolated maximal volume should be decreased; that is, compliance is diminished because fewer, not stiffer, alveoli are available to expand at a specific transpulmonary pressure [159].

In a series of patients with infiltrative lung disease, increased elastic recoil was due primarily to lung shrinkage and not alveolar wall stiffness. That these patients with sarcoidosis and idiopathic pulmonary fibrosis have normal values for K in the presence of restrictive ventilatory defects supports the hypothesis that decreased distensibility or increased elastic recoil is primarily due to loss of lung units. However, in those patients with the most severely restricted ventilatory defect, there were abnormally low values for K consistent with increased tissue elasticity or stiffness. In brief, the exponential description provides a mathematic expression of the visual inspection of the entire pressure-volume curve between total lung capacity and functional residual capacity, including a description of the position, shape, and slope of the entire curve. This analysis suggests that alveolar number may be quantitatively more important than alveolar wall thickening in causing the mechanical abnormalities in ILD, that is, decreased compliance or increased recoil [45,159].

Utility of Pressure-Volume Assessment

In terms of research, the analysis of pressure-volume characteristics of the lung has contributed to a better understanding of pulmonary physiology in terms of the mechanism of increased recoil, maximal airflow, and small airways function associated with certain ILD such as asbestosis or lymphangioleiomyomatosis [31, 53]. Clinically, there is only a limited utility in obtaining pressure-volume analysis. Performance of the maneuver is invasive, uncomfortable, and technically difficult, and it requires patient cooperation. There are insufficient normal values [137,372,397]. Obtaining a pressure-volume curve in restrictive disease of obscure cause is useful in differentiating muscle weakness (low recoil or distending pressure) from a parenchymal process (high recoil) [137,252]. Decreased compliance may precede conventional at-rest indices of lung restriction [31,206]. It has been stated that a shift downward and to the right of the curve or an increased value for the maximal recoil divided by the total lung capacity (coefficient of retraction) correlates with the degree of interstitial fibrosis [99,137]. However, simple measurement of lung volumes may be as informative as the more involved pressure-volume curve analysis. In one study, when the vital capacity was normal, there was normal compliance. Conversely, when the vital capacity was restricted, there was increased compliance on pressure-volume curve analysis [45,420].

Determinants of Maximal Airflow and ILD

Theory

The increased lung recoil associated with ILD, whether due to lung stiffness or lung smallness, maintains normal or supernormal maximal airflow rates [158,387]. Maximal airflow is determined by lung recoil and airway geometry (di-

ameter as well as airway compressibility or compliance). The fundamental role of recoil in determining maximal flow is based on the equal-pressure point (EPP) theory [253,273]. During a forced exhalation, the driving pressure to expel air from the lung (alveolar pressure, P_A) is the sum of static recoil pressure (P_{st}), which is lung volume–dependent, and pleural pressure (P_{PL}), which is effort-dependent:

$$P_A = P_{PL} + P_{st} \qquad (41\text{-}1)$$

As simplified in Figure 41-6, on expiration, the intraluminal pressure in the airways falls progressively (downstream) from the alveoli until a point is reached, the *equal-pressure point* (EPP), where the intraluminal pressure equals the pleural pressure. At this point, increased expiratory effort (increased P_{PL}) further compresses the large intrathoracic airways, resulting in proportionate increases in expiratory resistance such that airflow cannot be further increased (i.e., greater force is met with greater resistance) and maximum airflow becomes effort-independent. Maximal expiratory airflow at lung volumes below two-thirds of vital capacity is determined

Fig. 41-6. The upstream and downstream segments of the tracheobronchial tree on forced expiration. On expiration, pressure is most positive in the alveoli and steadily falls until it reaches atmospheric pressure at the mouth. Alveolar pressure is the sum of pleural pressure (P_{pl}) and elastic recoil pressure (P_{el}) at any specified lung volume. At some point along the airway, the intraluminal pressure must be equal to the pleural pressure. This is the equal-pressure point (*EPP*), which divides the tracheobronchial tree into upstream airways on the alveolar side and downstream airways on the mouth side of the EPP. (From NB Pride. The assessment of airflow obstruction, role of measurements of airways resistance and tests of forced expiration. *Br J Dis Chest* 65:135, 1971.)

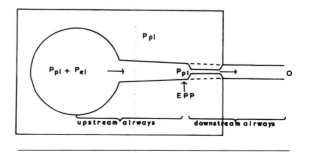

by elastic recoil of the lungs and airway geometry (resistance and compressibility), independent of effort [321]. As in Figure 41-6, the airways can be divided into segments that are "upstream" and "downstream" from the EPP. During exhalation, the position of the EPP changes with lung volume and moves upstream toward the alveolus at progressively lower lung volumes as elastic recoil commensurately decreases and airways resistance increases. At high lung volumes, the EPP is in large extrapulmonary airways, whereas at volumes about 25 percent of vital capacity, the EPP moves to segmental bronchi and further upstream toward the alveoli at progressively lower volumes [253,431].

As pointed out by Mead and associates [273], the pressure drop from the alveoli to the EPP approximates the static recoil pressure of the lungs (Pst). Therefore, maximal expiratory airflow is set by lung recoil pressure and the flow resistance of the uncompressed airways upstream from these points (upstream airways resistance, Rus). Thus, the maximal flow through the upstream segment and for the lung as a whole (V_{max}), at a given lung volume, can be derived from the equation

$$V_{max} = Pst/Rus \qquad (41\text{-}2)$$

where Rus is the resistance of the upstream airway during forced exhalation. Recoil pressure (Pst) diminishes and airways resistance becomes greater with decreasing lung volumes, so flow progressively decreases as forced expiration continues toward residual volume. The configuration of the maximal expiratory flow-volume curve is the clinical counterpart to this theory [253,273].

Increased Airflow

The presence of increased recoil in ILD has fundamental effects on maximal airflow; the forced expired volume in 1 second as a percent of the forced vital capacity ($FEV_1/FVC\%$) and flows on a maximal expiratory flow-volume maneuver are increased. Increased recoil also increases flows by tethering or dilating airways, thereby lowering airway resistance. Further, airway resistance is also minimized in the setting of ILD because the increased recoil at a particular lung volume moves the EPP downstream to less collapsible airways where dynamic airway compression is opposed [273]. Among patients with ILD, there is a direct relationship between the degree of increased recoil and the increased flows corrected

for lung volume [158]. In my experience, the presence of an elevated $FEV_1/FVC\%$ indicates the presence of an interstitial process early, before progression to lung volume restriction or radiographic abnormality [164]. Further, normal subjects with experimental restrictive disease induced by chest strapping have increased recoil. These subjects develop increased flows on the maximal expiratory flow-volume maneuver and have decreased airways resistance. The increased flows and the decreased resistance are uniquely determined by the increased recoil consequent to chest strapping and restriction. Such experiments give credence to the EPP theory that increased lung elastic recoil has a fundamental role in determining increased expiratory flows in ILD [387].

Small Airways Disease

Although flow rates are increased in ILD, pathologic and physiologic abnormalities of peripheral airways have been documented. Large central airways have normal morphology and function [124]. Sarcoid is an exception in which there may be granulomatous inflammation in central airways associated with hyperreactivity [29,299]. In contrast, more peripheral or so-called small airways dysfunction seems common. In the series from Fulmer's group of patients with idiopathic pulmonary fibrosis, 17 of 18 patients had small airways pathology, including peribronchiolar fibrosis and inflammation and bronchiolitis. Although some of their subjects were smokers with a known potential for similar small airways pathology, their findings were evident among nonsmokers with ILD and were confirmed by others [287]. In their original pathologic description of idiopathic pulmonary fibrosis, Hamman and Rich described narrowing and stenosis of small airways [170]. Similarly, morphologic small airways abnormalities have been noted in hypersensitivity pneumonitis, eosinophilic granuloma, scleroderma, and asbestos-exposed workers [215,269, 301].

The physiologic assessment of small airways function is controversial [89,154]. Ostrow and Cherniack documented increased upstream airway resistance (Rus) as a possible manifestation of small airways dysfunction in patients with ILD. They determined upstream airways resistance by measuring lung elastic recoil and maximal expiratory flow in patients with a variety of ILD [301] (see Eq. 41-2). Although controversial, similar morphologic and physiologic abnormalities of small airways have been documented in other groups of patients. However, determining upstream airways resistance requires an esophageal balloon and is not clinically practical, and furthermore, it has not always been found to be abnormal in patients with ILD with known pathologic involvement of the peripheral airways [143].

A more practical but still controversial way to assess small airways function is the maximal expiratory flow-volume curve, especially examining flow rates at low lung volumes. Since different regions of normal lung empty almost synchronously, the shape of the curve for maximal expiratory flow has a linear relationship to lung volume. If different regions empty asynchronously, this is reflected by an abnormal shape of the curve. The proportion of airways resistance determined by small airways relative to large airways increases at progressively lower lung volumes. It has been speculated that abnormalities of peripheral airways result in low flow rates that would be especially apparent, therefore, at low lung volumes [106,143,154].

In the study from Fulmer's group, none of their patients with idiopathic pulmonary fibrosis had an abnormal $FEV_1/FVC\%$ or airways resistance; however, half had abnormal flows at low lung volumes on maximal expiratory flow-volume curve assessment. Other tests of small airways disease, including dynamic compliance, closing volume, comparison of flow rates while breathing air and less-dense gas mixtures such as helium, and flows in the midvolume range (forced expired flow between 25 and 75 percent of expired vital capacity, $FEF_{25-75\%}$), are inadequate for one of several reasons: poor reproducibility, technical difficulty, clinical impracticality, and wide variation among normal values. Ultimately, the topic of small airways disease is controversial because there have been too few structure-function correlations [89].

Significance of Small Airways Disease

The presence and significance of small airways disease are unclear [74]. However, hypoxia may relate to ventilation-perfusion mismatching due to increased resistance in peripheral small airways [254]. In the experience of Fulmer and coworkers, improvement of small airways function with therapy correlated with lessening of hypoxia on progressive exercises [143]. Ostrow and Cherniack similarly suggested that small airways dysfunction may respond to therapeutic intervention [301].

The Diffusing Capacity

A decrease in the pulmonary diffusing capacity (D_L), like restricted lung volumes and increased elastic recoil, is an additional physiologic correlate of abnormal alveolar wall structure. In brief, D_L is defined as the rate at which an inhaled test gas such as carbon monoxide enters the blood per unit of driving pressure of that gas across the alveolar-capillary membrane (partial pressure difference of the gas between alveoli and pulmonary capillaries) [20]. A detailed review of the methods employed to measure D_L is provided in Chapter 6.

D_L describes the amount of functioning capillary bed in contact with ventilated alveoli and reflects the intactness of the alveolar-capillary membrane. D_L is decreased in ILD due to obliteration or distortion of the alveolar-capillary bed and not due to an increased distance for gas diffusion consequent to alveolar wall thickening by inflammation or fibrosis [116,384]. Alveolar proteinosis may be the one exception where an increased distance for gas diffusion causes a decreased D_L [21].

Interpretation of a Decreased Diffusing Capacity

D_L relates directly to the alveolar-capillary membrane surface area. This surface is dependent on the size of the subject's lungs, which relates to body size, especially height [97,154]. Therefore, D_L is affected by the simultaneously measured alveolar volume (V_A). However, in a specific individual, a decrease in alveolar volume results in a similar but disproportionately less diminution in D_L. For example, a normal subject's D_L decreases only 12 percent when assessed at roughly half total lung capacity (half alveolar volume) [276]. Similarly, in lung restriction due to chest-wall and/or neuromuscular disease or poor patient effort, the decrease in D_L is much less than the decrease in alveolar volume. If D_L is interpreted on the basis of an observed restricted lung volume, D_L as a percent of predicted may be artificially elevated. This is so because the observed absolute value for D_L will be compared to that of a shorter person with smaller lungs and concomitantly less alveolar-capillary surface area available for diffusion. Therefore, some authors suggest that it is useful to relate the measured D_L both to the simultaneously determined lung volume and to the D_L predicted for a given patient's age, sex, and height [21,151]. In fact, to understand the mechanism of a decreased D_L in the context of possible ILD, it has been recommended that the measured D_L be expressed per unit of alveolar volume (D_L/V_A), the specific diffusing capacity [21].

In interstitial pulmonary fibrosis, the reduced D_L is associated with a normal D_L/V_A ratio, suggesting that there is parallel loss of both capillaries and alveoli (i.e., alveolar units). Similarly, in lung resection there is a decreased D_L in relation to predicted age and height of a subject. However, the D_L/V_A ratio is normal following lung resection because there are equal decrements of alveolar-capillary bed and alveolar volume. In contrast, in chronic pulmonary vascular disease such as pulmonary emboli or vasculitis, the decreased D_L is associated with a normal alveolar volume, so there is a decreased D_L/V_A ratio [290]. Similarly, in patients with emphysema who have dilated peripheral airspaces and reduction in gas-exchange surface area, D_L is decreased more than alveolar volume, so the D_L/V_A ratio is decreased [21].

Significance of a Decreased Diffusing Capacity

A decreased D_L is considered a common finding in ILD [99]. In ILD, the D_L may be decreased before the chest x-ray film appears abnormal [99,131,132]. Also, a decrease in D_L may be present prior to lung volume restriction in various ILDs: sarcoid [257], asbestosis [426], scleroderma [68], and systemic lupus erythematosus [162]. In sarcoid, D_L is more useful than vital capacity in predicting overall severity of lung pathology [436]. Finally, in detecting severe ILD as subsequently documented by invasive exercise testing, a decrease in D_L to less than 40 percent of predicted was more sensitive than lung volume assessment [132]. A reduced D_L may not necessarily imply the presence of ILD. Abnormalities in diffusion are associated with pulmonary emboli, chronic congestive heart failure among candidates for heart transplantation, and advanced liver disease, and as has been described, isolated low D_L with normal flow rates can indicate the presence of emphysema [187,188,227]. It should be stressed, however, that a decreased D_L does not imply a defect in oxygen diffusion, but simply signifies a reduction of available alveolar-capillary membrane. In fact, there is a lack of correlation between D_L and hypoxia in ILD [99].

Limitation of Conventional Tests of ILD: Lung Volumes and Diffusing Capacity

General Limitation

Classic tests of pulmonary function may be inadequate in the assessment of ILD. First, it is not the role of such tests to be diagnostic. Tests of lung volume and D_L are a functional assessment of the alveolar structures. Fundamentally, pulmonary function testing is an attempt to evaluate respiration, that is, gas exchange between an organism and its environment. Conventional at-rest analysis of lung volumes, D_L, airflow rates, and arterial blood gases do not adequately assess the components of respiratory function: ventilation, blood flow, diffusion of oxygen and carbon dioxide (between inspired gas and alveolar-capillary blood), and control of breathing [288].

The other fundamental problem with pulmonary physiologic assessment is the unavailability of adequate structure-function data. In the context of ILD, patients usually have an initial single-lung biopsy, and morphology is correlated to pulmonary function. All structure-function correlations are drawn from groups of such patients, with each patient representing a single data point. The known potential for even an open lung biopsy specimen to be nonrepresentative of the entire lung further complicates structure-function analysis [148,149,292].

Also, despite their alleged value in screening for lung disease, these tests can fail to detect the presence of ILD [88]. In some series, the vital capacity can be normal in up to half the patients with biopsy-proved interstitial disease associated with significant exercise hypoxemia and impairment; up to a third of patients can have both normal lung volumes and D_L [45,99].

Even when restriction is present on conventional at-rest physiologic assessment, this decrease in vital capacity and/or D_L does not correlate with the degree of histologic abnormality or predict the future course of the interstitial process in terms of natural history of the disease or therapeutic responsiveness. It is generally held that a more cellular process signifies a relatively early stage in the disease at a time when therapy would be more likely to be effective than in later stages when fibrosis develops [64]. Tests of lung volume or D_L, however, do not distinguish between fibrosis and cellularity of the alveolar wall [99,144].

The complex basis for the frequent inadequacy of lung volume and D_L assessment, as outlined by Butler, involves problems with equipment, technique, and interpretation of results [58]. Lung volume assessment by flow-integrating spirometers has been disappointing. Similarly, the failure of some laboratories to make BTPS (body temperature, ambient pressure, saturated with water vapor) corrections can erroneously lead to a 10 percent decrease in lung volume measurements. The most common measurement of D_L, the single-breath carbon monoxide test ($D_{LCO_{sb}}$), is associated with an interlaboratory variation of up to almost 13 percent [78]. In an individual patient, the absolute value for the $D_{LCO_{sb}}$ varied up to 100 percent between five London hospitals [353]. Technical issues such as the type of gas analyzer employed [324], test-gas inspiration time, and conditions of breath hold such as Valsalva or Mueller maneuver all affect the D_{LCO}. In the setting of restrictive lung volumes, D_L can be artifactually lowered by contamination of the expired gas sample with anatomic dead-space gas [96]. Finally, D_L relates to various potentially fluctuating patient factors, including the presence of congestive heart failure, anemia, acute cigarette use, and diurnal variation of the measurement [76,93,139].

The adequacy of pulmonary assessment is also limited by problems of interpretation. The normal reference standards themselves involve wide ranges of variation; predicted D_L varies up to 20 percent among three published sets of normal data [20]. Similarly, there is large variation between predicted normal lung volumes; the residual volume varied up to 100 percent among published series [77]. The wide variation in predicted normal values is due to various factors such as study population (including race) and history of cigarette consumption, as well as factors relating to the particular laboratory, such as equipment, technique, or altitude [81,97].

In addition to the variations in specific technical standards and normal reference population among laboratories, there is disagreement as to what constitutes abnormal. The traditional definition of abnormal as a measured value below 20 percent of predicted mean value has neither scientific nor statistical merit [371,372]. Instead, the accepted statistical definition of an abnormal value is the measured value that statistically would be expected in less than 95 percent of normal subjects. Therefore, if the normal data follow a normal (Gaussian) distribution, for a one-tailed t test, the lower limit of normal values at a confidence level of 95 percent is the mean minus the product of 1.65 times the standard deviation [97,309]. Normal values above this 95 percent confidence limit may be less than 20 percent of the mean and may be erroneously defined as abnormal. As stated by Crapo and Morris, the common practice of designating normal as predicted minus 20 percent of the mean may lead to large errors in predicting normal because the 95 percent confidence limits are relatively constant over the entire range of predicted values rather than fluctuating by a fixed 20 percent of the entire range of mean values [97]. Finally, the common practice of reporting abnormalities of pulmonary function as mild, moderate, or severe also suffers from the lack of uniformity among pulmonary function laboratories. For restrictive lung diseases, such clinical staging of the degree of abnormality is associated with disagreement among laboratories in at least a third of the patients studied.

Limitation of Pulmonary Function Assessment in Specific ILD: Sarcoid and Idiopathic Pulmonary Fibrosis

The traditional tests of pulmonary function, such as lung volume, airflow rates, and D_L, are difficult to uniformly characterize among the wide variety of processes that involve the pulmonary parenchyma. For example, in contrast to most ILDs, sarcoid may result in granulomatous obstruction of proximal airways with or without associated airway hyperreactivity [239]. Assessing the presence of infiltrative pulmonary processes among patients with systemic lupus erythematosus is confounded by the presence of pleuritis or diaphragmatic myopathy, the presence of which also will result in lung restriction. Similarly, D_L may decrease in scleroderma by disease localized to the capillary bed without alveolar wall thickening, whereas pulmonary hemorrhage, a manifestation of vascular involvement by Wegener's granulomatosis, may increase D_L.

Evaluating the utility of pulmonary function testing in specific processes such as sarcoid depends on which aspect of the study is examined—detection of disease, severity of disease, prediction of subsequent clinical course—and the value of serial testing in assessing the natural history or therapeutic response. In terms of disease detection, even among sarcoid patients with hilar adenopathy alone on chest x-ray films, there is near-universal presence of parenchymal involvement. However, the majority of such patients have normal lung volumes and DL [429]. Even with more extensive disease resulting in parenchymal abnormalities on the chest radiograph, a third of sarcoid patients have normal lung volume and DL [114,217,429].

In staging the severity of lung involvement, lung volume and DL assessments have only a general overall correlation with open-biopsy histology: Minimal histologic changes could be separated functionally from severe pathologic abnormalities, but moderate disease could not be distinguished from severe on the basis of lung volume and DL [65,189,429,436]. Furthermore, there is sufficient overlap that in any one individual it is not possible to assess the degree of pathologic severity on the basis of observed lung volume and DL. In contrast, gas exchange with exercise correlated with severity of histologic involvement, but could not distinguish alveolitis (alveolar wall inflammation) from fibrosis [217]. Finally, pulmonary function at one point in time does not provide information on the future course of disease. In Colp's study, patients with sarcoid were grouped into those whose lung volume and/or DL were more or less than 65 percent of predicted. There was a similar subsequent pattern of spontaneous variation in disease [84,86].

Sequential pulmonary function assessment in an individual patient is of some benefit in assessing changes in disease course. There is a general relation between the changes in the chest radiograph and those in pulmonary function. Seventy percent of patients with chest x-ray improvement have improvement in the vital capacity, and about half these patients will show an improvement in DL. No patient with a decrease in vital capacity had an improved chest x-ray appearance, and patients with persistently abnormal or worsening chest x-rays will, in general, have a decrement in their lung volume and DL.

Similarly, sequential pulmonary function in the individual patient has benefit in assessing therapeutic response. Winterbauer and Hutchinson evaluated patients with improved pulmonary function coincident with corticosteroid therapy from seven published series [429]. Sixty percent of the 291 patients with parenchymal sarcoid had a 10 percent or greater improvement in vital capacity coincident with therapy; DL was improved (by greater than 20 percent) in half these patients, while 20 percent improved their arterial oxygen tension at rest (by more than or equal to 5 mmHg). Therefore, among those patients with improvement in some pulmonary function parameter coincident with steroid therapy, the vital capacity was the most sensitive index of response. In summary, with the important exception of serial follow-up in an individual patient, routine tests of pulmonary function have a limited utility in sarcoid [217,429].

In idiopathic pulmonary fibrosis, the assessment of resting parameters of pulmonary function is even less useful than for sarcoid. Lung volume, DL, and resting arterial oxygen tension do not even generally relate to severity of pathologic abnormalities in idiopathic pulmonary fibrosis. These parameters can be normal, even with a significant degree of fibrosis; the degree of fibrosis is an important determinant in the progression of the disease and the response to therapy [99,217]. Yet these physiologic tests are commonly employed to stage and monitor disease activity [64,99,150]. According to Fulmer and associates, the explanation for the lack of correlation between vital capacity and histology is speculative [144]. Total lung capacity, as noted, is determined by maximal inspiratory muscle strength and chest-wall and lung compliance. Interstitial fibrosis only affects lung recoil, and in the setting of decreased lung volumes, the muscles of inspiration are at a mechanical advantage, so that even a fibrotic lung can be relatively overdistended at total lung capacity [144]. Alternatively, postmortem morphometric assessment reveals that even in the setting of severe alveolar wall thickening, the actual amount of excess pathologic tissue displacing normal gas volume is only about 20 percent of normal lung volume. Given the noted wide variations in quantitating lung volume among laboratories, it is not surprising that even in the setting of severe ILD, the presence of lung restriction could be obscured [37].

Exercise Testing

The importance of assessing pulmonary function during exercise is becoming increasingly recognized, especially for patients with possible ILD. The evaluation of patients during exercise, although not constituting a direct measurement of respiration, gives more information than static measurements of lung volume or DL regarding ventilation, blood flow, gas exchange, and control of breathing.

In comparison to static physiologic assessment of lung volume and DL, gas exchange with exercise appears to be the most sensitive functional test of overall interstitial histology. Worsening gas exchange with exercise parallels worsening interstitial pathology [64,65,99,217,268]. Fulmer and colleagues [144] showed that relating the decrease in arterial oxygen tension (or increase in the difference between alveolar and arterial oxygen tension) between rest and exercise to liters of oxygen consumption at maximum work loads has good correlation with overall interstitial pathology. Data presented by Carrington and coworkers [64,65] suggest that the absolute measurement of alveolar minus arterial oxygen tension at maximal exercise is the work-related gas-exchange parameter that most closely correlates with overall histologic severity. Whichever measurement is used, however, the degree of fibrosis cannot be distinguished from the degree of cellular involvement of the alveolar wall [99,217].

Classically, patients with early ILD initially complain of shortness of breath only with exertion. Therefore, it is intuitive that such patients should be evaluated physiologically during exercise [411]. Exercise testing is important in detecting the presence of ILD, since such patients often have normal at-rest measurements of lung volume and DL [45,99]. Further, exercise testing provides information regarding the degree of pulmonary impairment, in contrast to static lung volumes. Exercise assessment provides information regarding the presence and degree of pulmonary impairment in employment-related lung disorders such as among workers exposed to asbestos, not afforded by the symptom of dyspnea and conventional assessment of lung function at rest [95,226,308,369,388]. Serial analysis of exercise physiology is useful in assessing therapeutic benefit, because, as noted, exercise gas-exchange abnormalities correlate with the degree of alveolar wall pathology [99,144]. Finally, in patients with dyspnea on exertion, the pattern of gas-exchange and ventilatory abnormalities with exercise can distinguish between cardiac and pulmonary disease and, among patients with lung dysfunction, often identifies the presence of obstructive, restrictive, or primary vascular disease [6,411].

Exercise Ventilatory Abnormalities

Patients with ILD of diverse etiology have characteristic abnormalities in ventilation and gas exchange with exercise. A major factor contributing to dyspnea and reduced exercise capacity among patients with ILD is abnormally elevated ventilation in the setting of decreased lung distensibility [52]. Patients with ILD hyperventilate at rest and during exercise; ventilation at maximum work rate approaches the maximum voluntary ventilation. Further, patients with ILD increase their minute ventilation with exercise by increasing respiratory rate rather than their restricted tidal volume (Fig. 41-7). Normal subjects increase their minute ventilation with exercise by increasing tidal volume until they reach a level of exercise that is about 60 percent of their maximal obtainable work load, above which further increases in minute ventilation are achieved by increases in respiratory rate. Also, at maximal work load, a normal person employs a tidal volume that does not exceed about 60 percent of his or her resting inspiratory capacity. Although the absolute tidal volume is decreased during exercise in patients with ILD, it is a relatively larger fraction of their inspiratory capacity; at maximal exercise, the tidal volume approaches 90 percent of the inspiratory capacity (Fig. 41-8). In summary, on exercise, patients with ILD hyperventilate and adopt a rapid, shallow pattern of ventilation which nonetheless results in a tidal volume at their maximal work load that is a relatively larger percent of their inspiratory capacity than what is seen in normal individuals [114,247,271,411].

The characteristic rapid, shallow breathing pattern during exercise in ILD is consequent to decreased pulmonary distensibility or compliance [232,247]. There is increased work of breathing in patients with ILD because the increased elasticity of the lung parenchyma imposes an impedance to

Fig. 41-7. Relationship between tidal volume and minute ventilation during incremental work. The dashed lines are responses of patients with restrictive lung disease working to their maximum level of exercise. Normal responses are noted as indicated in the legend. (From K Wasserman, BJ Whipp. Exercise physiology in health and disease. *Am Rev Respir Dis* 112:219, 1975.)

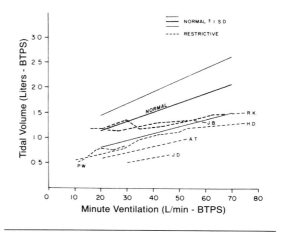

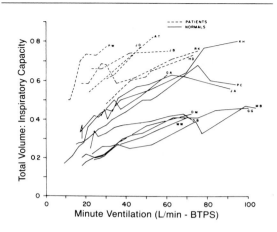

Fig. 41-8. The fraction of the resting inspiratory capacity used during tidal breathing at various levels of ventilation during an incremental work test. The solid lines represent normal responses, and the dashed lines represent patients with restrictive lung defects. (From K Wasserman, BJ Whipp. Exercise physiology in health and disease. *Am Rev Respir Dis* 112:219, 1975.)

inspiratory muscle function that becomes progressively more severe at higher tidal volumes [94,138,323]. Thus, patients with ILD have an increased oxygen cost of breathing [420].

The depth and rate of breathing are linked to maintain gas exchange at minimal cost in terms of respiratory muscle force and work [52,271]. The maintenance of a given tidal volume in the setting of high elasticity requires a large peak intensity of inspiratory muscle force that would result in diaphragmatic fatigue. Instead, by adopting a smaller tidal volume and an increased respiratory rate to meet the increased ventilatory demands of exercise, patients minimize the peak force required by the muscles of inspiration and thereby decrease the work of breathing. However, these patients still hyperventilate in relation to the metabolic demands of exercise, as indicated by a low arterial carbon dioxide tension. The mechanism for the breathlessness and the ventilatory limitation with exercise is not understood [232] (see Chap. 10).

Control of Breathing

The receptors which signal the increased respiratory muscle activity that results in a high minute ventilation with a rapid, shallow ventilatory pattern are unknown. It appears that mechanical factors consequent to decreased compliance, and not chemical factors, influence respiratory control in ILD. Administering oxygen to patients with ILD at rest and normalizing their oxygen saturation do not alter the increased minute ventilation [52,109,247,396].

Mechanical abnormalities alone can increase ventilatory drive. Two human models have been employed to simulate the decreased compliance of ILD: chest strapping and inspiratory external elastic loading. Placing an elastic harness around the chest restricts chest expansion [113,167,232]. In the other model, normal subjects inspire from a rigid container such that end-inspiratory effort becomes more negative, reflecting increased muscular effort [59]. In both models, these normal subjects develop increased minute ventilation with a shallow, rapid ventilatory pattern. The perceived magnitude of the elastic load increases as both elasticity and tidal volume increase; this perception, as well as the sensation of dyspnea, is related directly to the inspiratory muscle tension to overcome the elastic load [52,54,410].

To understand the mechanism of the observed hyperventilation with rapid, shallow breathing pattern in these models of ILD, as well as spontaneous disease, neural ventilatory drive has been assessed by measurement of mouth occlusion pressure. The mouth occlusion pressure 0.1 second after initiation of inspiration ($P_{0.1}$) is a measure of the negative pressure generated by muscles of inspiration when inspiratory flow is almost immediately transiently prevented. Although potentially flawed, the mouth occlusion pressure ($P_{0.1}$) is said to reflect inspiratory neural drive. In normal subjects given an external elastic load, as well as in children and adults with ILD, there is increased neural drive to ventilate as determined by the $P_{0.1}$. This increased neural drive relates directly to both increased elasticity and perceived magnitude of the load [54,410,423].

It is unclear how increased elasticity enhances neural drive to ventilate. Because patients with ILD and subjects given elastic loads have similar sensory responses, it has been speculated that the increased drive to ventilate with a rapid, shallow pattern of breathing may be a normal *behavioral* response adopted to reduce peak inspiratory muscle force and minimize respiratory distress. The sensation of dyspnea with elastic loading may be conscious awareness of inspiratory motor neuron output [19,46,54,410].

Alternatively, the ventilatory and sensory responses to increased elastic loads may be due to a reflex arising from afferent receptors in the respiratory system: airway, lung, and/or chest wall. A vagal reflex is probably involved. Cats given an elastic load developed medullary inspiratory neuron activity that was abolished by sectioning the vagus nerve [141,251]. Phillipson and coworkers showed that vagal blockade decreased exercise-related hyperventilation and associated rapid, shallow breathing in dogs with experimentally induced ILD [312]. Finally, Guz and associates showed that sectioning of the vagus nerve decreased the respiratory frequency and increased the tidal volume in two of three humans with ILD [168].

Although the distinctive ventilatory response to decreased distensibility is probably due to a reflex, it is not known which afferent receptors stimulate the drive to ventilation in the setting of increased elastic work. Airway vagal afferent irritant and/or stretch receptors might be stimulated by high transpulmonary pressure in the setting of noncompliant lungs. However, blocking these afferent receptors with airway anesthesia did not alter the ventilatory pattern in patients with ILD [354].

Alternatively, lung rather than airway vagal receptors may be involved, such as the so-called J or juxtapulmonary receptor, and pulmonary C-type endings [232]. In the setting of parenchymal inflammation and/or fibrosis, perireceptor pathology itself may stimulate lung receptors [83,392]. Mediators of inflammation such as histamine and prostaglandins have a direct effect on lung receptors.

Chest-wall or respiratory muscle afferent receptors may be involved in the increased drive to ventilate associated with decreased lung compliance. Phillipson's experiments with vagal blockade suggested that nonvagal pathways also were potentially involved [312]. Mechanoreceptors in the chest wall are stimulated by changes in muscle tension, muscle length, or velocity of muscle shortening. Respiratory reflexes originating in sensory receptors in respiratory muscles or the chest wall respond to external elastic loading [19,189,251]. For example, intercostal muscle spindle receptors can be stimulated to increase ventilation by an effect on higher respiratory centers in the presence of increased elastic loading or restriction of chest-wall expansion among other stimuli [19,59,184,403].

Gas Exchange at Rest and Exercise

In addition to the increased drive to ventilate and the pattern of rapid, shallow breathing, patients with ILD also have characteristic gas-exchange abnormalities. Although these patients are often minimally hypoxic at rest, the development of hypoxia with exercise is universal. Impaired gas exchange is a hallmark of alveolar disorders [52,99,383].

At rest, oxygen tension may be normal, but there is usually an increased alveolar-arterial oxygen tension difference. This is associated with a decreased alveolar and arterial carbon dioxide tension resulting from the increased stimulation to breathe. The alveolar-arterial oxygen tension difference is the best indicator of the adequacy of pulmonary gas exchange. Further, unlike normal subjects, rising from the supine to the sitting position results in worsened hypoxia in 20 percent of patients with ILD, presumably due to increased perfusion of more involved and less well-ventilated basilar lung regions [99]. In severe cases of ILD, there is pronounced hypoxia at rest, although carbon dioxide retention is rare [411].

Finally, although the object of only a few studies, it is clear that restrictive lung disease results in a wide range of breathing and oxygenation abnormalities during sleep. As fibrotic lung disease progresses, the degree of nocturnal desaturation and breathing dysrhythmias progress. More research in sleep and ILD is needed [156].

The cause of hypoxia in ILD is controversial. Initially, hypoxia at rest was said to result from an increased path length for oxygen diffusion across the thickened alveolar wall, that is, alveolar-capillary block [18]. Subsequently, it was determined that hypoxia was due to ventilation-perfusion abnormalities. Finley and coworkers calculated that to result in hypoxia, the path length for gas exchange would have to be so large as to actually obliterate the alveolus [136,384]. It should be stressed that measurement of a reduced D_L does not correlate with hypoxia. The decrease in D_L does not imply a defect in oxygen diffusion, but rather a reduction of available alveolar-capillary bed [169,268,384]. In addition to ventilation-perfusion abnormalities, physiologic shunting as assessed by breathing 100% oxygen can be the cause of significant hypoxia in severe ILD. This complicates the efficacy of oxygen therapy in relieving hypoxia in late disease [99,136].

With progressive exercise, a normal subject maintains an alveolar-arterial oxygen tension difference that is relatively unchanged from baseline resting values until very high exercise levels are achieved [208]. In contrast, exercise characteristically induces hypoxia in patients with ILD. Exercise-induced hypoxia is primarily due to ventilation-perfusion inequalities. Although these patients have decreased total lung compliance, there are regional differences in lung tissue distensibility or compliance. With exercise, there is increased ventilation to more compliant lung regions already hyperventilated at rest and progressively increased perfusion to relatively hypoventilated, noncompliant lung regions. In addition to regional differences in compliance, peripheral airways disease and pulmonary circulatory alterations also create ventilation-perfusion abnormalities [143,144,268]. At a given degree of volume restriction, gas-exchange abnormalities are less severe in sarcoidosis than in idiopathic pulmonary fibrosis [121]. Although the major cause of hypoxia with exercise is ventilation-perfusion inequality, there is some evidence implicating diffusion limitation as a potential component of exercise-related hypoxia. With increased work and commensurate increased cardiac output, there is progressively decreased red blood cell transit time through alveolar capillaries. A thickened alveolar-capillary membrane, especially in the presence of lung regions with low alveolar oxygen tension, slows diffusion of oxygen sufficiently that there is insufficient time for equilibration of oxygen between alveoli and the capillary blood [7,204,404].

Exercise Limitation

Patients with ILD have limitation of exercise secondary to ventilatory and gas-exchange abnormalities. In the setting of ILD and decreased pulmonary compliance, exercise is limited by an abnormal ventilatory response to exercise and not desaturation [52]. There is no relation between maximum exercise capacity and either absolute level or exercise-related fall in oxygen saturation. However, gas-exchange factors during exercise are additive to the ventilatory limitation to increased work [52].

Patients with ILD have an increase in nonperfused alveoli, that is, dead space. The vasculature is compromised in such patients by distortion or obliteration due to alveolar wall disease, vasculitis, or both. In addition to the increased drive to ventilate and consequent increased work of respiratory muscles, the increase in dead space to tidal volume ratio characteristic of patients with ILD further limits their ability to exercise [383,411]. With progressive exercise, normal subjects have a decrease in their dead space to tidal volume ratio which results in a reduction in the amount of ventilation required to affect appropriate alveolar ventilation for progressively increased carbon dioxide production consequent to work [208]. In ILD, 60 percent of patients have an increased dead space to tidal volume ratio at rest (greater than 0.4; normal less than 0.33), and in 90 percent of these patients, the dead space to tidal volume ratio fails to fall or may actually rise with progressive exercise. Such patients have inefficient ventilation in terms of alveolar ventilation and gas exchange; perfused alveoli must be ventilated more to compensate for the nonperfused alveoli [99,181,383,411].

There are additional mechanisms wherein characteristic gas-exchange abnormalities in ILD have an impact on ventilation and exercise limitation. Hypoxia itself stimulates carotid chemoreceptors, resulting in increased drive to breathe [232]. Further, hypoxia may be sufficient to result in pulmonary arterial hypertension. An increase in pulmonary artery pressure stimulates ventilation by a vagal reflex that may involve vagal afferent pressure receptors in the pulmonary artery itself [209]. Further, an increased pulmonary artery pressure secondary to progressive hypoxia may result in a decreased stroke volume and decreased cardiac output. Pulmonary vascular congestion (without extravasation of lung water) itself results in rapid, shallow breathing mediated by the vagus nerve [258,326,418]. Finally, hypoxia-induced increased pulmonary artery pressure may result in shunting through a patent foramen ovale, further complicating gas exchange.

42

Interstitial (Diffuse Parenchymal) Lung Disease: Tissue Diagnosis and Therapy

Jeffrey A. Golden

Pathologic Diagnosis

The fundamental approach to identifying the specific cause of interstitial lung disease (ILD) in an individual patient should begin with the noninvasive clinical evaluation, including careful history and physical examination. If the clinical workup is negative and the interstitial lung process is established as chronic (more than 1 month), a more invasive approach involving obtaining lung tissue must be considered. Ultimately, based on a review of large series, 30 to 40 percent of patients require lung biopsy of some type for diagnosis [148,149]. The history is especially important in making a specific diagnosis in occupationally and/or environmentally related diseases (including hobbies), especially in the case of hypersensitivity pneumonitis. History is also crucial in drug-related disease (see Table 40-1). Physical examination may be helpful in suggesting a systemic process with lung involvement, such as in the case of collagen-vascular diseases. Similarly, routine laboratory data, including results of urinalysis and serologic evaluation, may be helpful in suggesting a systemic process with pulmonary manifestations. Finally, the chest roentgenogram, although primarily important for determining the presence and temporal pace of an interstitial process, can confirm historical information. However, the chest x-ray film may appear normal in 10 percent of patients with ILD [131].

If no diagnosis is made after a noninvasive clinical evaluation, lung tissue should be obtained [149,405]. Initially, percutaneous or closed procedures were employed to obtain tissue or cytologic diagnosis: fine-needle aspiration [262], needle biopsy procedures [434], cutting-needle biopsy [437], punch biopsy [407], high-speed tre-phine drill biopsy, and pleuroscopic lung biopsy with various flexible fiberoptic devices [35]. However, closed procedures have been abandoned because of diagnostic failure and unacceptable complication rates. In 25 percent of closed procedures, either no lung tissue or only normal lung tissue was obtained. Further, even if abnormal tissue or cytology was obtained, it was insufficient or unrepresentative of the lung pathology [325]. Finally, these techniques resulted in a 50 percent complication rate, primarily hemoptysis and pneumothorax [262,295,434,438], air embolism [421,434], and death [295,307].

Transbronchial Lung Biopsy

Performance of transbronchial biopsy through the flexible fiberoptic bronchoscope is the first invasive diagnostic lung procedure after an unrevealing clinical evaluation. If the transbronchial biopsy is not helpful or is contraindicated, an open biopsy should be performed [149]. Transbronchial biopsy was originally performed with the rigid bronchoscope, but this required general anesthesia. Further, even with use of a relatively large forceps, insufficient tissue was obtained in 20 percent of procedures [12,13]. Transbronchial biopsy is now performed with the fiberoptic bronchoscope [171,229,238,358]. Complications of transbronchial biopsy include pneumothorax (5 percent) and hemorrhage (1 to 9 percent). In one series of 200 transbronchial biopsies through the fiberoptic bronchoscope employing fluoroscopic guidance, there were no pneumothoraces [438]. Certain subsets of patients such as those with uremia have as high as a 45 percent incidence of hemorrhage [176].

Contraindications include bullae, blebs, pulmonary artery hypertension, respiratory failure, and the use of positive airway pressure associated with ventilator support, as well as poor patient cooperation [405].

The far less invasive bronchoalveolar lavage (BAL) utilizing the fiberoptic bronchoscope can itself be diagnostic for certain relatively uncommon causes of ILD. Lavage provides an opportunity, not possible in most other organs, to sample and examine repetitively soluble constituents and cells of the injured or inflamed lung. In fact, lavage may be a better diagnostic modality than open biopsy in some situations such as berylliosis where lung lymphocytes can be analyzed for their immune or functional response to beryllium salts [104]. In other situations, different specific tests on lavage-derived material can obviate tissue diagnosis. Lavage that reveals large acellular eosinophilic bodies against a background of small eosinophilic granules with periodic acid–Schiff staining of the proteinaceous material (without alcian blue staining) is pathognomonic for alveolar proteinosis [165,260]. Also, BAL can be diagnostic of eosinophilic granuloma if electron microscopic evaluation reveals histiocytosis X cells, as shown by their cleft nuclei and the X bodies throughout the cell cytoplasm [23]. However, similar Langerhans cells, as identified by electron microscopy or monoclonal antibody staining (T6 antigen), have also been identified in lavage fluid from cigarette smokers [67,165]. In my experience, the diagnosis of eosinophilic granuloma in men can be confirmed by the characteristic high-resolution computed tomographic (CT) finding of geographic cysts (also seen in women with lymphangioleiomyomatosis) [385].

The diagnostic yield of transbronchial biopsy is highest in diffuse disease with a specific recognizable histologic pattern, such as sarcoid or lymphangitic carcinoma [35,231,316]. The diagnostic yield for sarcoid is as high as 90 percent because this process involves peribronchial and bronchiolar tissue [149]. The diagnostic yield of transbronchial biopsy in sarcoid is independent of the radiographic pattern, and positive biopsies are as likely with normal-appearing x-rays as with radiographically abnormal lung fields [405]. Of note, the findings on transbronchial biopsy are likely to be positive even if the high-resolution CT scan reveals a normal lung parenchyma in patients presenting with hilar adenopathy [284]. It has been recommended that if a patient with suspected sarcoid has a negative bronchoscopy, the procedure should be repeated [316,317]. Although other diffuse processes such as Wegener's granulomatosis, rheumatoid lung disease, lymphangiomyomatosis, eosinophilic granuloma, eosinophilic pneumonia, pulmonary alveolar proteinosis, and silicosis can be recognized by characteristic lesions, diagnostic sensitivity of transbronchial biopsy is low [405].

The diagnostic yield of transbronchial biopsy in unselected patients with diffuse ILD is about 50 percent [405]. Lung samples provided by transbronchial biopsy are small, unselected, and subject to crush artifact. In 25 percent of cases, inadequate or normal tissue is obtained. The transbronchial biopsy samples only peribronchial tissue and may lead to a false-positive diagnosis of ILD in cases of chronic bronchitis, since inflammation and fibrosis in this location may be misinterpreted as representing diffuse lung parenchymal disease [149].

There are few transbronchial biopsy–open lung biopsy correlations [238,405]. Although such studies suggest a specific diagnostic yield for transbronchial biopsy in as many as 67 percent of patients, these authors and others who describe an even higher diagnostic yield for transbronchial biopsy include nonspecific inflammation and/or fibrosis on the transbronchial biopsy specimen as being a specific histologic diagnosis of idiopathic fibrosis. However, nonspecific findings on transbronchial biopsy occur in the range of 31 to 59 percent of procedures [12,134,316,317,405,427]. Some authors justify a pathologic diagnosis of idiopathic pulmonary fibrosis (IPF) (when such a nonspecific transbronchial biopsy specimen is obtained) only if subsequent clinical follow-up is consistent with that diagnosis [427]. However, clinical follow-up is too varied in IPF to justify defining a nonspecific transbronchial biopsy as being diagnostic.

Using strict diagnostic criteria for tumor or sarcoid, Wall and colleagues showed that the transbronchial biopsy resulted in a specific diagnosis in 20 (38 percent) of 53 patients [405]. In the 33 patients without a specific transbronchial biopsy diagnosis, an open lung biopsy led to a specific diagnosis in 91 percent of cases (30 of 33). In 8 patients with an open lung biopsy diagnostic of IPF, the transbronchial biopsy specimen was positive in only 4. Conversely, in only 2 of 4 patients with IPF suggested by the transbronchial specimen was this diagnosis confirmed by open lung biopsy [405] (Fig. 42-1). Patients with nonspecific transbronchial biopsy specimens, interpreted as being consistent with IPF, subsequently proved to have tuberculosis, tumor, actinomy-

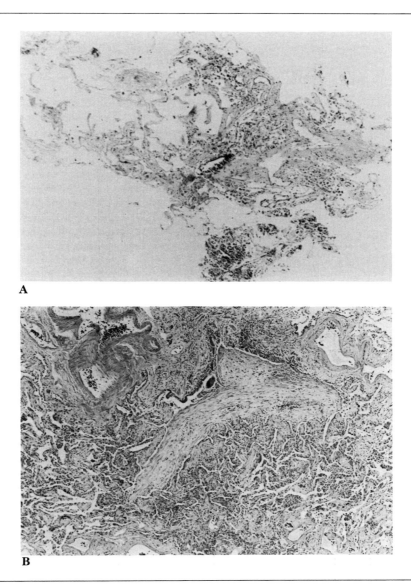

Fig. 42-1. A 35-year-old woman with restrictive lung disease underwent a fiberoptic transbronchial biopsy which suggested fibrotic or usual interstitial pneumonia (*A*). The subsequent open biopsy (*B*) showed active interstitial inflammation and bronchiolitis obliterans (bronchiolitis obliterans organizing pneumonia). The patient had a clear steroid response, as anticipated, given the cellular infiltration noted on the open biopsy in contrast to the end-stage–appearing interstitial fibrosis noted on the small transbronchial biopsy specimen.

cetes, etc. Therefore, nonspecific chronic inflammation and/or fibrosis on a transbronchial biopsy specimen can be unreliable and misleading [134, 149,405].

Open Lung Biopsy

Given the limited sampling capacity of transbronchial biopsy and the patchy distribution of chronic ILD, it is not surprising that about half of such patients requiring a tissue diagnosis eventually come to open biopsy. Although the processes causing ILD are diffuse, there is interlobar and intralobar variation [149,428]. In view of this regional inhomogeneity, open lung biopsy is likely to yield a specific diagnosis by virtue of larger and multiple tissue samples [152,223,356, 405]. Further, the open procedure provides the opportunity to select appropriate lung regions for biopsy. Normal lung and regions of end-stage honeycombing can be avoided. Instead, lung regions with average involvement or, in the cases of advanced disease, the area with active and characterizable histology can be selected [1,149]. Although open biopsy may reveal normal lung or nonspecific pathology, there are fewer false-negative results than with the smaller transbronchial biopsy specimens. The diagnostic yield of open lung biopsy among more than 2200 patients from combined series is between 92 and 100 percent [149]. Furthermore, nonspecific pathology on a large open biopsy sample is more confidently diagnosed as IPF than is chronic inflammation and/or fibrosis on a small transbronchial biopsy sample [325,405].

The technique of open lung biopsy has undergone revision since first introduced by Klassen and colleagues in 1949 [224]. Gaensler recommends a small anterior exploratory thoracotomy in the fourth to fifth or second to third interspace (modified Chamberlain technique), which affords easy access to all lobes and the mediastinum [71,148,149]. The length of the incision has no effect on morbidity [148,149]. Chest tube placement for 24 hours is imperative to obliterate the pleural space so as to avoid hemorrhage and tension pneumothorax [149]. The lingula, like the right middle lobe, should be avoided because it may not be representative of the rest of the lung. Because of its unique anatomy, the lingula is subjected to more inflammation and/or fibrosis than other lung segments [149,237]. In one autopsy study, there was statistically more fibrosis and vasculopathy and a trend toward more chronic inflammation in the lingula than in other lung regions [292]. Further, to maximize diagnostic yield, there must be scrupulous care of the biopsy sample; the sample should not be excessively handled to avoid hemorrhage and atelectasis. The specimen should be resected while the lung is fully inflated, followed by immediate fixation [148,149].

In general, open lung biopsy is a safe procedure, even among severely impaired patients. The overall mortality for open lung biopsy in general among combined series of over 2200 patients is less than 1.8 percent, and more than half of these deaths are due to the underlying lung disease, such as terminal lung cancer. Deaths due to the procedure per se were 0.3 percent (2 of 416) in one series, and both patients had severe pulmonary hypertension [148,149,325].

Therapy

Although a comprehensive review of the specific treatment of each process that afflicts the lung parenchyma is beyond the scope of this chapter, there are fundamental therapeutic points that can be illustrated by important specific examples. First, cessation of known inimical exposure, as in hypersensitivity pneumonitis or adverse pulmonary drug reactions, constitutes the most effective therapeutic modality; the best chance for therapeutic success begins with the correct diagnosis. Second, effective therapy is often unavailable because the etiology or mechanism of disease is unknown, as in sarcoidosis or IPF. Third, where specific medication is employed, such as prednisone or cytotoxic agents, there is usually suppression rather than cure of the primary process. There is a wide spectrum of therapeutic benefit from agents such as prednisone. The dramatic response to prednisone in chronically ill patients with eosinophilic pneumonia is itself considered a diagnostic modality [63,339]. In contrast, the long-term benefit of steroid therapy for the majority of ILDs, such as sarcoid and IPF, is unproved, but it is probably beneficial in selected cases. Fourth, there are very few processes consistently amenable to specific therapeutic modalities. For example, it has been shown that subsegmental flexible fiberoptic bronchoscopic lavage in alveolar proteinosis is effective therapy (Fig. 42-2). Finally, where curative and/or suppressive therapy fails, supportive care is very important. Patients should be followed for signs of infection, pneumothorax [313], or development of lung cancer, which occurs in 5 to 10 percent of patients [377,382,395,401]. Most impor-

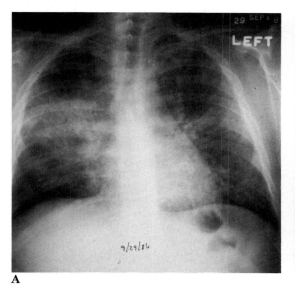
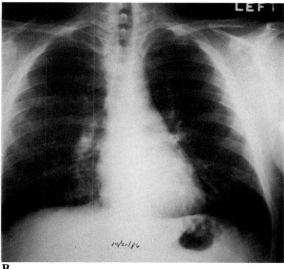

A **B**

Fig. 42-2. Treatment of alveolar proteinosis by fiberoptic bronchoscopy. Following selective segmental serial bronchoscopic lavage, this patient experienced dramatic relief of dyspnea and clearing of the chest x-ray associated with normalization of his restricted physiology (*A*: chest radiograph before bronchoscopy; *B*: following lavage).

tant, in view of exercise-related hypoxia, patients should be assessed for benefit of supplemental oxygen during exercise and perhaps sleep [14,310]. ILD patients who have significant desaturation with exercise were shown to have increased exercise endurance with supplemental oxygen associated with decreased minute ventilation and reduced hypoxic drive [214,249,389, 405,424].

Therapy of ILD of Known Cause

HYPERSENSITIVITY PNEUMONITIS
Although cessation of exposure is a potentially effective therapeutic modality, diseases such as hypersensitivity pneumonitis or pulmonary drug reactions can result in chronic ILD. The development of permanent fibrosis in hypersensitivity pneumonitis depends on the intensity and chronicity of exposure to organic antigen. Insidious exposure to humidifiers contaminated by *thermophilic actinomycetes* in home, office, or car can result in chronic ILD. Such chronic exposure

is less obvious than the classic systemic reactions (dyspnea, fever, chills, and malaise) 4 to 8 hours after exposure to antigens in farmers' lung or pigeon breeders' disease. Delayed cessation of exposure may result in irreversible restrictive disease [135,179,324]. However, steroids are generally effective in hypersensitivity pneumonitis because an immune mechanism is involved in this disease. In part, antigen exposure results in a suppressor T-cell alveolitis [90,235]. Similarly, possible beryllium exposure, such as occurs among dental technicians or aerospace industry employees, should be evaluated because berylliosis is a steroid-responsive hypersensitivity disease with systemic manifestations simulating sarcoid in every way but for uveitis [382].

DRUG TOXICITY
Drug-related pulmonary toxicity is another category of ILD where exposure history is fundamental to diagnosis and therapeutic results. Prior reviews document the broad categories of drugs that result in diffuse lung injury [63,160,342]. Deleterious reexposure to drugs known to have possibly caused prior lung toxicity is well established, such as in the case of lung diseases related to gold, naproxen, or cephalosporin [57,117,177]. Although frequently employed, the benefit of steroid therapy is unclear. This may be an expres-

sion of our lack of understanding regarding the mechanism of a particular drug's toxicity.

The treatment and prevention of drug toxicity are complicated by several factors. In the case of antineoplastic medications, there is reputedly a dose-related toxicity. However, in the case of bleomycin, an idiosyncratic lung reaction can develop at a very low dose [160]. Nevertheless, predictive formulas for the likelihood of drug toxicity have been developed to prevent ILD. From such analyses it has been shown that preexisting lung disease itself should preclude the use of agents such as BCNU [16]. The mechanism of bleomycin lung toxicity involves oxidant lung injury; therefore, minimizing supplemental oxygen reduces the incidence of this event [264]. Another issue in preventing drug toxicities due to antineoplastic agents is that one compound is often synergistic with another drug or treatment modality, such as radiation therapy [160]. In addition, chemotherapy-related lung disease can simulate the disease being treated as well as intercurrent infection. Bleomycin can cause nodular infiltrates that resemble metastatic lesions, and lung pathology in methotrexate-related lung toxicity may reveal granulomatous changes [115,160,289]. Finally, therapeutic response to steroids is variable and often negative in established disease. Lung disease due to methotrexate resolves only with cessation of the drug, although steroid therapy may hasten resolution [160]. It should be stressed that although steroids are generally ineffective in treating bleomycin lung toxicity, there is a subset of patients with bleomycin hypersensitivity lung disease associated with eosinophilia who dramatically improve with prednisone [183].

As in the case of ILD in general, treatment of drug-induced lung diseases is most likely to be successful when the drug is discontinued and steroid therapy is initiated early, when there is cellular rather than fibrotic histology. Even chronic lung toxicity due to nitrofurantoin or phenytoin (Dilantin) is reversible when there is lavage or transbronchial biopsy documentation of active lymphocytic alveolitis. Therefore, lavage may be useful in the early detection and follow-up of established disease after cessation of the culpable drug and/or institution of steroid therapy [50,70].

Therapeutic dilemmas arise because discontinuation of such drugs as tocainide or amiodarone may result in life-threatening arrhythmias. Initially, it was thought that amiodarone resulted in toxic lung injury manifested by an accumulation within the alveolar macrophages of phospholipid

lamellar bodies. However, this histologic finding is a reflection of exposure to the drug and not an expression of toxicity [17]. Amiodarone lung toxicity may be an immune-mediated process with similarities to hypersensitivity pneumonitis [90,235,334,352]. By developing techniques to monitor the alveolitis, perhaps by serial BAL, steroid therapy can be undertaken while amiodarone is continued, thus affording protection against life-threatening arrhythmias.

Therapy of ILD of Unknown Cause

IDIOPATHIC PULMONARY FIBROSIS
Therapy for relatively common ILD, such as sarcoidosis and IPF, is controversial. There is no controlled trial demonstrating long-term efficacy of steroid therapy in ILD [98]. Assessing benefit of steroid therapy in sarcoid or IPF is confounded by clinical and morphologic variability; the course of either of these diseases is unpredictable in the individual patient [428]. In the case of IPF, untreated patients or those with steroid unresponsiveness have a duration of survival following the onset of symptoms of about 4 years. Of note, the Denver group considers stabilization of IPF, or a decrease in the rate of functional decline, to be a favorable response to treatment [302]. Unfortunately, even after steroid improvement, late relapse of desquamative interstitial pneumonia has been observed as long as 12 years after prior therapeutic remission [245].

There is some evidence that steroids are effective. Certain patients improve dramatically with steroid therapy, and some investigators found that patients with IPF treated with steroids ultimately did better than untreated patients. Without therapy, for example, Carrington and coauthors stated that no case of fibrotic IPF (usual interstitial pneumonitis) spontaneously improved, whereas with steroids, 12 percent improved [64]. Without therapy in the more cellular form of IPF (desquamative interstitial pneumonitis), 22 percent spontaneously improved, whereas with steroid therapy, over 60 percent improved. Further support for a beneficial role for steroid therapy in IPF is the observation that relapse occurs with cessation of therapy and can be successfully retreated with reapplication of steroids [399]. Steroid therapy results in improved gas exchange with exercise [256]. Steroid therapy has resulted in histologic improvement in serial samples of lung taken following therapy. However, in contrast to the initial open lung biopsy, the follow-up specimen after steroid treatment was uniformly obtained with a needle biopsy [166]. The mechanism of possible steroid benefit is unknown. Apparently steroids do not cause suppression of alveolar macrophage release of fibronectin or fibroblast growth factor [233]. Steroids may directly affect fibroblasts and inhibit collagen synthesis [92,101].

The specific steroid regimen varies. In general, steroid therapy is initiated with 1 mg/kg of prednisone for 6 to 8 weeks, and then it is slowly tapered over about 4 months to 0.25 mg/kg of prednisone [98]. Because the *same* patient may have pathologic evidence of cellular disease as well as less cellular, fibrotic disease, all patients should get a trial of steroids [49,395]. It is unknown if every-other-day therapy or inhaled steroids is effective or could lower oral steroid requirements [244].

The best predictor of ultimate steroid responsiveness and a better prognosis is early benefit following the initial 1 to 2 months of steroid therapy [382,395,399]. In general, about half the treated patients improve subjectively. However, only about 15 to 17 percent have significant benefit from steroids when benefit is defined as decreased dyspnea on exertion, improved chest x-ray appearance, and an increase in the vital capacity by at least 10 percent [382,399]. There is increased survival in steroid responders. Such patients with a measurable steroid response have a 5-year survival rate of 67 percent, while those with less or no response have a 5-year survival rate of 20 percent. Nevertheless, Turner-Warwick pointed out that there is a late mortality that is similar between the steroid responders and nonresponders. Perhaps, as she suggested, even in responders in whom there is decreased inflammation, there is nevertheless a relentless progression of the fibrotic changes that eventually results in mortality. Thus, steroid response may not ultimately change mortality [398].

Another predictor of steroid responsiveness is lung pathology. A fibrotic biopsy specimen, especially associated with honeycombing, suggests less responsiveness, while more cellularity suggests earlier disease and likely steroid responsiveness [64,382,395,399,428]. Additional factors implying steroid responsiveness include less physiologic derangement [99,382,395], shorter duration of symptoms (less than 1 year as opposed to more than 2 years) [395,428], younger age (under 50 years old) [395], female gender, and perhaps presence of circulating immune complexes [118]. The degree of radiologic abnormality does not appear to relate to steroid responsiveness.

The benefit of cytotoxic therapy in IPF has not been proved. Single case reports or small series suggest that cytotoxic agents may permit decreased steroid dosage in successfully treated patients with intolerable steroid side effects [49,395,416,428]. Other reports have suggested that these agents by themselves or with prednisone provide better therapeutic response than steroids alone [49,90,275,360]. One preliminary controlled double-blind study suggested that therapy with cyclophosphamide (Cytoxan) is better than steroids; however, after 2 years of therapy, cyclophosphamide frequently needed to be discontinued because of bone marrow toxicity. Also, the benefit of agents such as cyclophosphamide may require up to 6 months of therapy to appear [398]. Obviously, the benefits of cytotoxic agents must be balanced against risks, including the development of secondary cancers [11]. Both cyclophosphamide and chlorambucil have been implicated themselves as causes of ILD [161,210,390,399]. In contrast to steroids, colchicine can suppress the production of macrophage-derived growth factors for fibroblasts and this drug may have a role in the treatment of IPF [226,330]. Finally, lung transplantation or heart-lung transplantation have become useful modalities in patients with IPF [391].

In evaluating clinical deterioration in patients with IPF, disease progression should be distinguished from disease-associated complications and adverse effects of therapy. Recently, the Denver group reviewed the reported causes of clinical deterioration from six studies involving 550 patients with IPF [302]. The mean duration of survival varied from 3.2 to 5.0 years. These authors noted that disease progression was difficult to distinguish from disease-associated complications or adverse effects of therapy. Mortality was most frequently due to respiratory failure due to worsening disease (39 percent); other causes of death included heart failure (14 percent), bronchogenic carcinoma (10 percent), ischemic heart disease (10 percent), infection (7 percent), and pulmonary embolism (5 percent). Other nonfatal disease-associated complications included pneumothorax, steroid myopathy, and complications of therapy-related immunosuppression. The authors stressed that the cause of clinical deterioration should be carefully determined as a guide to therapeutic intervention; disease progression should not be accepted as the problem until other processes are evaluated [302].

SARCOIDOSIS

The treatment of pulmonary sarcoid is one of the most controversial topics in medicine [109]. Although there are no controlled trials establishing long-term benefit, steroid therapy for pulmonary sarcoid has been employed for almost 40 years [373]. In part, the lack of documentation of long-term steroid benefit is due to the varied and unpredictable course of this syndrome. Although spontaneous resolution within 2 to 3 years occurs in at least 75 percent of patients [200,202], there exists a subgroup of sarcoid patients, perhaps up to 30 percent of patients seen in referral centers, who develop permanent respiratory impairment and/or respiratory failure and death [109,200,202].

There are only two points regarding prednisone therapy for pulmonary sarcoid for which there is general agreement. First, steroids do *not* cure sarcoid [109]. Second, at best, steroids suppress the pulmonary granulomatous reaction only during the time this therapy is actively employed. Evidence for short-term steroid suppression of sarcoid includes randomized studies showing that patients while on therapy do better than patients without therapy, especially if treated early [105,201,203]. Also, about half the patients with resolution of pulmonary sarcoid on steroids relapse when steroids are stopped but subsequently respond to retreatment [206]. Finally, the common knowledge that brief therapy with steroids, even if effective, has no lasting benefit years later after cessation of therapy has been misinterpreted to imply that chronic steroid therapy has no long-term benefit [109,201,435]. Although the long-term benefit of such chronic steroid therapy in a subgroup of patients with persistent and progressive pulmonary disease has never been documented in a carefully randomized control study, benefit is suggested by several large long-term series. At this time, it is the experience of several investigators that steroids are effective if constantly applied [109,206].

The lack of unanimity regarding the long-term benefit of steroid therapy parallels the controversy regarding indication, dose, duration, and follow-up for such therapy. In 1952, Siltzbach recommended that steroids should be used in pulmonary sarcoid "where the extent of the involvement portends dire consequences" [365]. Although up to 30 percent of sarcoid patients in some series require steroid therapy, the precise indications for such therapy are no clearer today than in the early 1950s. Some authors recommend therapy if the chest x-ray evidence of parenchymal sarcoid worsens or is without improvement over 1 year [110,203], while others treat only if there are symptoms referable to parenchymal involvement. Other investigators base their therapeutic decisions on pulmonary function test abnormalities independent of chronic stable radiographic findings [85,86]. It is thought that delaying therapy until symptoms arise may be too late, since steroids are most effective with early cellular histology [85,86]. Although it is unclear if chest x-ray or pulmonary function abnormalities constitute the criteria for steroid therapy, it seems wise to follow patients with both modalities, especially if the chest radiographic changes during follow-up are equivocal [109].

The dose and duration of therapy are also unclear, although all authors agree that prednisone should be given in the lowest effective dose. It appears that every-other-day therapy is effective [44,109,363,380]. When therapy is discontinued, about half the patients relapse but respond to retreatment [85,206]. There is controversy as to how to assess disease activity while progressively lowering steroid dosage: Symptoms [206], chest x-ray, pulmonary function tests [86], serum angiotensin-converting enzyme [102,111,240,241], or a combination of chest radiograph and pulmonary physiology is used [86,109]. It has been suggested that the disease activity is best assessed with periodic probing by discontinuing steroids and observing subsequent changes in pulmonary physiology and/or chest radiographs. For example, if a patient is off steroids for 1 year without changes in these parameters, the disease can be considered "arrested"; otherwise, steroids would be reintroduced and discontinued at some further date when the underlying unknown stimulus hopefully wanes [109]. Although no control data support long-term benefit, this does not imply that there is no place for steroid therapy in the subset of patients with progressive parenchymal changes due to sarcoid.

Case reports of the patients with progressive pulmonary sarcoid who cannot tolerate prednisone therapy, suggest that cytotoxic agents as well as chloroquine may be effective. All are associated with toxicity [73,201,211,282,298,349, 355]. Methotrexate has been shown to improve lung function in association with a decrease in posttherapy lavage lymphocytosis and macrophage activation as assessed by hydrogen peroxide and spontaneous release of tumor necrosis factor [27]. Inhaled steroid therapy may permit reduction or discontinuation of systemic oral prednisone [280,362,378]. In a placebo-controlled study, budesonide for 16 weeks, 800 μg twice daily with a spacer device, resulted in clinical and radiologic improvement associated with a decrease in follow-up lavage lymphocytosis and macrophage activation [95]. Of note, cyclosporine was not useful despite its known effect on helper T-cell function and evidence that this drug can suppress the spontaneous release of interleukin-2 from T cells recovered from the lungs of patients with active sarcoid. Perhaps cyclosporine failed in clinical trials because of dose-related issues [261]. It would appear that nebulized cyclosporine should be tried.

PULMONARY MANIFESTATIONS OF COLLAGEN-VASCULAR DISEASES

For several reasons, it is difficult to summarize the treatment of the pulmonary expressions of the various collagen-vascular diseases. First, there are few controlled therapeutic studies [193,359]. The diseases themselves often defy categorization and have overlapping clinical manifestations. Further, there are multiple and complex thoracic manifestations of these processes that result in lung volume restriction: interstitial disease, primary pulmonary vascular disease and hemorrhage, pleural effusion, respiratory muscle weakness, recurrent aspiration due to pharyngeal and/or esophageal dysfunction, as well as infection and/or pulmonary toxicity consequent to therapy.

In general, therapy is successful where immune mechanisms of lung injury are best documented, where therapy is undertaken early, and when histology is cellular rather than fibrotic [360]. Benefit from immunosuppressive therapy with prednisone and/or cytotoxic agents has been noted in this context [22,193]. Cytotoxic agents may work where steroids fail and are of unquestioned benefit in the treatment of Wegener's granulomatosis [425,430]. However, their use is associated with significant toxicity, including infection among patients with collagen-vascular diseases [272], secondary malignancies, and ILD itself [305,375,376,417].

Systemic Lupus Erythematosus. Lung dysfunction may be the first manifestation of systemic lupus erythematosus (SLE) [267]. The presence of ILD is relatively uncommon in SLE, and other secondary processes must be excluded: congestive heart failure, uremia, drug reactions, and most commonly, infection [61]. Acute lupus pneumonitis may present as unilateral or bilateral alveolar infiltrates or with more of an interstitial pattern on chest radiograph. Such primary

lupus involvement of the interstitium can result in life-threatening hemorrhage with or without hemoptysis; vasculitis is rare [3]. Although the pathologic basis of lupus ILD is unclear because patients are usually on prior therapy, the presence of an immune process has been documented [75,122], and steroids are usually of benefit. In some cases, cyclophosphamide has been required owing to steroid unresponsiveness [265,266]. Confounding the presence of an interstitial process in the context of lung restriction, there may be weakness of inspiratory muscles and/or pleural effusions in SLE patients [72,259]. It should be stressed that lupus patients are at risk of pulmonary embolus independent of the activity of their systemic disease. The presence of a circulating lupus anticoagulant may be a useful marker of thromboses. Finally, pulmonary hypertension is unusual in lupus, but when it occurs, therapy with vasodilating medication is ineffective [255].

Rheumatoid Arthritis. In rheumatoid arthritis, lung disease also may precede systemic manifestations. Physiologic evidence may reveal subclinical pulmonary restrictive disease in up to 40 percent of patients with normal chest x-ray appearance and absence of symptoms. ILD may be mild to severe with honeycombing. Although there are no control trials, steroids are of benefit in treating the ILD associated with rheumatoid arthritis [107,193,306]. Cytotoxic agents such as cyclophosphamide or methotrexate also have been of benefit. Although effective for arthritis, penicillamine has not been shown to be effective in ILD associated with rheumatoid arthritis [360,361].

Dermatomyositis and Polymyositis. ILD in dermatomyositis may be mild or have a fulminate course leading to death [112,414]. ILD may commonly precede skin or muscle manifestations by months or years [119,140,359]; dyspnea may mask muscle weakness [415]. Physiologic evidence of restriction is three times more likely than radiographic interstitial changes. Respiratory muscle weakness itself results in restriction and respiratory failure [175]. Atelectasis results from decreased tone of the chest-wall muscles, which leaves the elastic recoil of the lung relatively unopposed, resulting in small resting lung volumes [112]. Infection is likely in such patients, especially where aspiration frequently occurs secondary to pharyngeal muscle dysfunction [222,283]. Infection is also likely in these patients because of an ineffective cough secondary to decreased respiratory muscle strength [172].

Prednisone therapy in doses of 1.0 mg/kg/day or greater is effective, especially if the ILD is mainly cellular and the patient is young [350, 359,415]. Cyclophosphamide, in the case of steroid failure, has been used [315]. However, in one controlled study, azathioprine (Imuran) did not provide added benefit to steroid therapy [51]. Failure of steroid therapy is a bad prognostic sign. Patients with respiratory muscle dysfunction should be monitored by serial measurements of vital capacity [320] or maximal inspiratory pressure or maximal expiratory pressure [42]. These patients may be benefited by use of intermittent positive-pressure breathing [367]. Further, assisted ventilation at night has been effectively employed [293,346].

SCLERODERMA

Scleroderma lung disease is notoriously unresponsive to therapy [87,193], perhaps owing to the paucity of evidence for an immune and/or inflammatory mechanism of disease [123,343,366]. Postmortem studies show virtually all scleroderma patients to have a fibrotic pulmonary interstitium [193]. Clinically, almost all patients have increased pulmonary vascular resistance secondary to sclerosis or intimal proliferation of small pulmonary blood vessels with or without abnormal pulmonary function [348]. Such vascular changes may be present without inflammation or fibrosis of the alveolar wall. There is only a transient benefit of vasodilator therapy [142]. In the setting of Raynaud's phenomenon, it was once speculated that there is a pulmonary vascular spasm to cold exposure. However, elevation of pulmonary artery pressure is due to increased pulmonary capillary wedge pressure and cardiac dysfunction resulting from such exposure [129, 296]. Clinically, patients with scleroderma have abnormal distal esophageal function which results in chronic aspiration, another cause of ILD [300]. Thoracic skin tightening does not impinge on pulmonary function [4,348]. However, chest-wall muscle weakness does cause restriction due to a noninflammatory myopathy which is generally steroid-unresponsive [72,80].

Staging

Staging patients with disorders of the lung parenchyma involves determination of the presence and severity of impairment as well as an assessment of the degree of disease activity, that is, cellularity versus fibrosis. Although the specific etiologic agent is usually unknown, the pathogenesis of ILD is generally understood. Disorders such as sarcoid or IPF are associated with chronic inflammation that begins with an accumulation of the inflammatory cells in the alveolar walls referred to as *alveolitis*. Crystal and associates stated that although it is the dysfunction of alveolar capillary units that causes symptoms and impairment in the patient, it is the chronic alveolitis that leads to injury and fibrosis [98]. Two patients can have equivalent exercise impairment with fundamentally different histologic findings. A patient with a more active or cellular process is more likely to respond to therapy than another patient with similar exercise impairment but whose histology reveals fibrosis and honeycombing [64,99,217].

Staging of Impairment

Quantifying the presence and degree of impairment in ILD is important in terms of prognosis and documenting subsequent therapeutic benefit. However, assessing the severity of impairment due to ILD is controversial because it is not clear on what basis this estimate should be made, that is, symptoms, chest x-ray, pulmonary function, or histology [98,398]. If impairment is based on histology, it is clear that grading systems for dyspnea or radiographic changes only roughly quantify the extent of the abnormalities of the alveolar structures. The chest x-ray can be normal in 10 percent of patients with substantial physiologic impairment due to ILD. Similarly, it is well known that patients with histiocytosis X or sarcoidosis can have dramatic radiographic findings with minimal functional impairment [65,99,112,389]. Similarly, for the reasons discussed in Chapter 41, conventional pulmonary function measurements of lung volume, diffusing capacity, and arterial blood gases at rest are often inadequate for determining the presence and extent of the histologic abnormality in the *individual* patient with a parenchymal process [47,99,100,217,361]. Instead, evaluating exercise-related gas exchange is the best estimate of the overall histologic abnormality [98,99,143,217]. To better quantify the clinical status of an individual patient with ILD, some authors suggest a scoring system reflecting a composite of clinical, radiographic, and physiologic variables. In this composite analysis, gas exchange with exercise as related to oxygen consumption was the most important factor in determining the clinical status of the patient. In this study, the less invasive ear oximetry measurement of oxygen saturation paralleled the changes in the alveolar-arterial oxygen tension difference with progressive exercise [143,150, 412].

Exercise testing has been particularly helpful in determining the presence of ILD, especially in the context of medical-legal evaluation of asbestos-exposed individuals. In one study of 120 asbestos workers with complaints of dyspnea, assessment of exercise testing determined that there was no physiologic limitation in half the patients and that the majority of those with impairment on exercise had cardiac dysfunction [6].

Staging Disease Activity

Ideally, assessment of disease activity should provide predictive information regarding clinical course and, by serial evaluation, benefit of therapeutic intervention. Disease activity is defined by the cellularity of the interstitial process. Although not universally accepted [398,422], it is generally held that a more cellular process is indicative of relatively early disease where impairment is likely to progress, but therapy may be more successful in comparison to more fibrotic changes [64,99,100,120,125,195,216,350,357, 415]. However, most biopsy specimens in ILD reveal both cellular and fibrotic elements, which make prognostic statements difficult. Nevertheless, new modalities such as monoclonal antibody and flow cytometric analysis of lymphocyte and alveolar macrophage populations may provide important insights into disease activity [281, 304,398].

Presently, there is no accepted way to assess disease activity. The history of dyspnea on exertion, chest x-ray abnormalities, and measurements of lung volumes, diffusing capacity, and arterial blood gas at rest do not correlate with the degree of overall parenchymal abnormality. Although gas exchange with exercise or abnormal pulmonary distensibility on pressure-volume analysis can detect early disease and do relate to the degree of overall parenchymal pathology, these modalities cannot distinguish between fibrosis and cellularity [99,100,144,150,205]. Although the open biopsy can allow initial evaluation of parenchymal cellularity, this procedure is performed only once and is itself potentially flawed by sampling error [47,144,149,398]. After the initial open lung biopsy, noninvasive tests of disease activity that can be serially repeated are needed [327]. BAL and gallium lung scanning are two such modalities that have been used to assess the intensity of the inflammatory and/or effector cell alveolar wall infiltration or alveolitis [195,344]. It is still unproved, however, that results of gallium scanning or lavage can be used to make clinical decisions [98,153,216,422].

BRONCHOALVEOLAR LAVAGE

The attraction of lavage in ILD is that the procedure provides direct access to the cellular and noncellular constituents of the alveolar wall and airspace, as well as being well tolerated by patients [163,386]. The fact that the lung can function as an independent immune organ makes direct evaluation of the pulmonary parenchyma as afforded by lavage important for research and clinical approaches to ILD [163]. The lung can be the site of a compartmentalized inflammatory response as in hypersensitivity pneumonitis where the disease is restricted to the lung. In other systemic disorders, the inflammatory response that evolves in the lung may not be reflected in the peripheral blood. Notably, in sarcoidosis the immunologic abnormalities that occur within the lung parenchyma are opposite to those in peripheral blood [104].

However, it must be stressed that cells derived from lavage fluid may not be representative of cells in the pulmonary interstitium. Cells obtained by lavage have already passed out of the interstitium and are not subjected to the same microenvironment as cells within the alveolar walls [304]. Based on observations in experimental animals, the inflammatory response in the alveolar airspace may not be in phase with that in the interstitium [248].

The first studies validating the use of lavage in ILD compared cells in lavage fluid with an extract of the open lung biopsy specimen, not the histology itself. Such an extract may cause cell damage or loss and may not be representative of the actual lung tissue [173,174,196,198]. Also, inflammatory reactions within the peripheral airways, such as those caused by smoking and infection, may confound interpretation of the results of BAL [104]. Fractional processing of sequential lavage specimens to separate bronchial from alveolar samples will minimize the artifact of airway inflammation [331]. Improved techniques of handling lavage cells may account for better correlation with biopsy results [153, 173,304]. New technologies have improved analysis of lavage fluid in ILD. As stated by Daniele and colleagues [104], an essentially technical advance can accelerate inquiries into the pathogenesis of pulmonary disease. For example, the fluorescent-activated cell sorter and monoclonal antibodies have increased our knowledge of basic immune mechanisms and the pathogenesis of immune disease [104,180,246,328,374]. As summarized by Reynolds [335], although interpretation and standardization of lavage need to be better understood before clinical application can be recommended, it should be stressed that this direct pulmonary sampling technique may yield more relevant information than remote specimens such as blood.

Lavage and Sarcoidosis. Lavage has provided important research insights into the pathogenesis of sarcoidosis [163]. The alveolar wall cellular infiltration or alveolitis is made up of T lymphocytes. These effector cells are primarily activated helper T cells that spontaneously release interleukin-2 and monocyte chemotactic factor [69,195–197,261,314,341]. Lavage has established a key role for the alveolar macrophage. Although the proportion of alveolar macrophages is less than in normal persons, the actual total number is greater than normal. Furthermore, there is morphologic and functional evidence of macrophage activation [104]. Alveolar macrophages derived by lavage from patients with sarcoidosis spontaneously release interleukin-1 or T-lymphocyte growth factor, further developing the alveolitis of sarcoid [190,261]. Of note, interleukin-1-beta gene expression by alveolar macrophages is not different in sarcoid patients as compared to normals. This does not mean that there is a low or normal level of interleukin-1 protein production but that its increased elaboration is the result of changes in the posttranscriptional regulation of interleukin-1-beta and/or changes in interleukin-1-beta transcription occurring at some time point in the disease [221]. Alveolar macrophages from patients with sarcoidosis spontaneously produce fibronectin [329]. This macromolecule appears to play an important role in attracting fibroblasts to the lung and provides a scaffold for cells and extracellular matrix proteins, resulting in excess accumulation of collagen in the interstitial space [329].

As reviewed by Daniele and coauthors [104], the major lesson derived from lavage studies in sarcoid patients is the difference in distribution and function of lymphocytes derived from the lung compared to circulating cells from the peripheral blood in these same patients. In contrast to lavage fluid, in the peripheral blood there is a generalized lymphopenia and a decrease in T cells; functionally, the response to mitogens is impaired and B-cell function is depressed as well

[103]. In vitro studies of lung lymphocytes show enhanced activation of T cells. In fact, lung T cells from patients with active sarcoidosis induce B cells from normal persons to secrete immunoglobulin [104,192]. This finding is particularly interesting because it provides insight into the occurrence of hypergammaglobulinemia in sarcoidosis [104].

In terms of diagnosis, finding an increased number of lymphocytes in lavage fluid is not specific for sarcoidosis, as hypersensitivity pneumonitis and berylliosis may have the same cell population profile. Analysis of lymphocyte subsets (helper and suppressor T cells), however, may aid in distinguishing sarcoidosis from hypersensitivity pneumonitis. In hypersensitivity pneumonitis, in contrast to sarcoidosis, there is an increased suppressor population and a decreased ratio of helper to suppressor T cells [91,236,381]. Further, in patients with more chronic and fibrotic sarcoidosis, there may be increased neutrophils rather than lymphocytes in the lavage fluid [345].

Clinically, lavage may be useful as a staging procedure by virtue of direct assessment of the lymphocytic alveolitis. Patients with active disease have a higher percentage of lymphocytes in their lavage differential, and experience functional deterioration over a subsequent 6-month period, unlike sarcoid patients with a lower-intensity lymphocytic alveolitis whose course is more benign. In contrast to lavage lymphocyte assessment, conventional radiographs and pulmonary function testing cannot distinguish these two groups of patients at the time of initial evaluation [215,216,219]. Other studies suggest that finding higher percentages of lymphocytes or helper T cells in lavage material consistent with active disease predicted improvement in the lung function subsequent to medication with steroids, a therapy known to decrease helper T-cell activity; no other parameter (gallium scanning, serum angiotensin-converting enzyme level) had similar prognostic significance [25,182,322,368]. Perhaps monoclonal antibody and flow cytometry evaluation of serial lavage samples will be found clinically useful to monitor disease activity [24,69, 90,281,368].

Other studies do not indicate that an elevated lavage lymphocyte percentage suggests subsequent deterioration [297,409]. The apparent disagreement among authors as to the significance of an initially elevated lymphocyte percentage in lavage material may relate to the type of sarcoid patients studied based on symptoms at the time of initial presentation. Patients with an acute onset manifested by erythema nodosum or acute uveitis invariably have a higher T-lymphocyte count and a greater elevation of helper to suppressor T-cell ratio in lavage analysis than do patients with a pulmonary presentation or those studied after resolution of erythema nodosum. Patients with an acute onset have a better prognosis than those with a more insidious presentation despite the markedly abnormal lavage cell population profile in the former patients. Differences in the clinical syndrome at the time of presentation and bronchoscopy could relate to the disagreement regarding the meaning of an initial elevated lymphocyte count and predicting the subsequent clinical course [409].

In addition to lavage cell population, quantitation and monitoring of cell function (such as release of interleukin-2 by activated lung T lymphocytes derived from lavage) may be of benefit in monitoring therapeutic intervention [8,191,286, 314]. Similarly, assessment of alveolar macrophage–derived collagenase was found to correlate with disease activity, suggesting a role in assessing sarcoid disease activity [55]. The presence of lavage collagenase on initial evaluation was associated with more severe disease and predicted an adverse outcome [408]. Lavage assessment of extracellular matrix components also has potential as a marker of disease activity. Procollagen III peptide, a precursor of type III collagen, is produced by pulmonary fibroblasts and is potentially a marker of fibroblast activity; both lavage and serum levels of this marker have correlated with disease activity and outcome [43,319]. Similarly, other serum tests such as spontaneous expression of the interleukin-2 receptor gene and the presence of functional interleukin-2 receptors on T lymphocytes in the blood may obviate lavage analysis of these markers of active disease [230].

Lavage and Idiopathic Pulmonary Fibrosis. As described by Gadek, the quantum leap in our understanding of IPF was made possible by BAL, which provides cellular and noncellular lung samples from patients that could be analyzed with new techniques of cell biology. From serial lavage analysis of patients with IPF, it is clear that pulmonary fibrosis is a consequence of chronic progressive lung parenchymal injury. This chronic inflammatory injury or alveolitis is the prelude to subsequent fibrotic morphologic and functional abnormalities. Today, the principal area of controversy is precisely which

cell is the fundamental cause of lung injury in IPF [10,212,370].

In contrast to sarcoidosis, IPF is associated with an increased percentage of polymorphonuclear leukocytes in lavage fluid [173,174,196]. This finding does not diminish the key role of the alveolar macrophage in the pathogenesis of IPF. In IPF there is an influx of peripheral blood monocytes into the interstitium and alveoli where they complete their differentiation [185]. Research utilizing lavage has suggested that the alveolar macrophage, perhaps after becoming activated by immune complexes, spontaneously releases neutrophil chemotactic factor, which leads to the accumulation of leukocytes in the alveolar wall and subsequent tissue damage [146,147,196]. The mechanism by which the alveolar macrophage recruits neutrophils to the lung is an important area of research. For example, using a quantitative assay employing reverse transcription of messenger RNA (mRNA) and the polymerase chain reaction, interleukin-8 derived from lavaged alveolar macrophages has been shown to contribute to neutrophil involvement in the development of IPF [62].

The active secretory products of neutrophils, including neutral proteases (elastase and collagenase) and oxygen radicals, may injure the lung's structure. This possibility is supported by the presence of neutral proteases (collagenase) in lavage fluid from patients with IPF but not from patients with sarcoidosis or normal subjects. It is likely that destructive cystic changes in lung parenchyma are related to this neutrophil activity [145,147].

In addition to providing chemotaxis for neutrophils, the alveolar macrophage in IPF spontaneously releases two mediators that stimulate fibroblast replication and subsequent fibrosis: fibronectin and alveolar macrophage–derived fibroblast growth factor [39,40,332,333]. Activated macrophages have been found to produce platelet-derived growth factor (PDGF). PDGF is a potent mitogen and chemoattractant for fibroblasts and smooth muscle cells and a stimulator of collagen synthesis. Unlike normals, lung tissue from patients with IPF reveals in situ evidence for hybridization of PDGF mRNA gene expression accompanied by the presence of PDGF-like proteins in the epithelial cells and macrophages of fibrotic tissue [15,41,128].

There are important enigmas regarding the clinical application of lavage in IPF [398]. Although lavage fluid contains increased percentages of leukocytes and/or eosinophils and less often an increased lymphocyte percentage, the neutrophils and eosinophils are far outnumbered by lymphocytes and plasma cells on histologic evaluation of the open lung biopsy specimen [398]. In terms of predicting therapeutic responsiveness, it is the presence of an increased percentage of lymphocytes, and not neutrophils, that correlates with subsequent steroid benefit. In several studies, the finding of an initially increased eosinophil percentage in lavage material consistently implied a downhill course and prednisone unresponsiveness [9,174,347,400,413]. Despite the support for a central role of the neutrophil in the pathogenesis of IPF, other cells are clearly important.

Nevertheless, the neutrophil must still be considered a key factor in the lung injury associated with IPF. Successful amelioration of IPF with cyclophosphamide therapy was associated with a reduction of the chronic neutrophil alveolitis [400]. Further support for the role of the neutrophil in the lung injury preceding fibrosis in IPF comes from animal work where a specific neutrophil product, myeloperoxidase, produced lung injury that resulted in pulmonary fibrosis [207]. Most likely more than one specific cell is important in the pathogenesis of IPF: B lymphocytes (immune complexes), alveolar macrophages (chemotactic activity for neutrophils, fibroblasts), eosinophils (markers of aggressive disease), and lung fibroblasts. As Allen and Gadek suggest [10], the better the process of lung injury and repair are understood in diseases like IPF, the more complex the process becomes.

Serially performed lavage may document a clinical trend in an individual patient. Patients in whom the percentage of neutrophils decreases with therapy undergo clinical improvement, whereas continued elevation of lavage neutrophil count correlates with therapeutic failure [104]. The patients with persistently elevated lavage neutrophils who had the worst prognosis were characterized clinically as having a productive cough [178]. By following serial neutrophil counts in lavage fluid, it may be possible to identify the lowest possible effective dose of steroids [398,400]. There is a small subgroup of patients with IPF whose lavage cell counts return to normal and who may then be able to have the prednisone discontinued [225].

The presence of increased neutrophils in lavage fluid occurs in other interstitial lung processes such as asbestosis and lung dysfunction associated with collagen-vascular disease [163]. In fact, elevation of lavage neutrophils may pre-cede the onset of symptoms or chest x-ray abnormalities in these conditions [108,406].

Presently, other markers identified in lavage are being investigated for clinical utility in staging the activity of ILD. Neutrophil myeloperoxidase and alveolar macrophage–derived oxygen metabolites, both of which likely relate to lung injury, have been shown to correlate with disease activity and response to therapy [34,79,226]. Mast cells are increased in lavage fluid from patients with sarcoidosis and IPF. Stimulated mast cells release a number of potent vasoactive, chemotactic, and proteolytic mediators with potential for lung injury. Markers of local mast cell degranulation such as histamine have been shown to correlate with disease activity and prognosis [66].

Another approach to assess disease activity is to measure connective-tissue components in lavage fluid. Extracellular matrix molecules such as fibronectin, vitronectin, and hyaluronan that contribute to the repair or exaggeration of interstitial pathologic changes seem to correlate with ongoing inflammation but not fibrosis itself [127,318,319]. Other authors, such as Begin and colleagues [32], have shown both in animal models and in asbestos workers that fibronectin and procollagen III peptide in lavage correlate with fibrotic activity and could be useful markers to predict fibrosis. In asbestos workers, these markers may be used as a means of early detection of asbestos-induced pulmonary injury [32].

Lipid alterations in BAL fluid may have utility in assessing activity of disease. Abnormalities of surfactant may promote organ dysfunction. Alterations in surface-active material may contribute to the pathogenesis of IPF both by increasing the elastic recoil due to surface forces and by promoting alveolar collapse. One hypothesis for the loss of gas-exchange units after lung injury is the irreversible fusion of denuded alveolar basement membranes. Lavage levels of phosphatidylglycerol are reduced in untreated IPF and return to normal in patients responding to prednisone but not in nonresponders. Similarly, the decreased levels of surfactant protein A in IPF correlate with subsequent outcome. Such surfactant abnormalities may reflect the extent of damage to the alveolar epithelium in IPF [270].

Abnormalities in lavage fluid that are consistent with concepts of lung injury and fibrosis are interesting but their clinical application has yet to be substantiated. There are many factors that confound the ultimate utility of lavage in ILD. Cigarette consumption and bronchitis affect the neutrophil count in lavage fluid independent of parenchymal lung disease. Lavage results vary in relation to stage of a particular disease [345], the lobe of the lung assessed [60,152,311], and the technique employed in performing lavage differential cell counts [279,351]. Presently, there is no way to control for the dilution factor of lung-lining fluid by the lavage procedure itself [25,26]. Thus, the utility of lavage in assessing activity of disease is still a matter of major controversy [398,427].

GALLIUM LUNG SCANNING

The radioactive nuclide gallium-67 (^{67}Ga) localizes to neoplastic tissue as well as areas of acute or chronic inflammation. Lung scans are obtained 48 hours after intravenous injection of [67]Ga (50 μCi/kg of body weight). Although the scan of normal lung does not demonstrate gallium uptake, ^{67}Ga can be detected in the cellular component of lavage fluid from normal subjects [47].

Pulmonary inflammation, infectious or noninfectious, results in increased ^{67}Ga uptake on the lung scan. The intensity of the ^{67}Ga uptake relates to the degree of inflammation; the activity of pulmonary tuberculosis, for example, can be assessed by serial gallium lung scanning [31]. Similarly, the presence of lung inflammation on biopsy or lavage due to sarcoidosis, IPF, and asbestosis correlates with the degree of gallium uptake [31,242,243,294]. In assessing lung inflammation, ^{67}Ga has two advantages over lavage: First, the entire lung is sampled [26]; and second, unlike lavage, a gallium scan is not affected by cigarette smoking or bronchitis [242].

The mechanism of ^{67}Ga uptake in pulmonary inflammatory disorders is unclear. Various inflammatory and/or immune effector cells have been reported to take up gallium: lymphocytes [133,274], polymorphonuclear leukocytes [55,274, 393], and activated macrophages [2,31,98,198]. Alternatively, ^{67}Ga uptake may reflect increased vascular permeability due to inflammation, as experimentally induced by intramuscular histamine [394,402]. After intravenous injection, ^{67}Ga is bound to serum proteins such as transferrin. Lung inflammation results in increased vascular permeability for such proteins that could result in gallium accumulation [263,278,379]. After leaking out of the vascular compartment at sites of inflammation, protein-bound ^{67}Ga could then be phagocytized by alveolar macrophages [31,402].

There are some data supporting a potential role for gallium lung scanning in staging the alveolitis of various interstitial lung processes. In sarcoid, gallium scanning is more sensitive than the chest roentgenogram in detecting parenchymal disease [338]. In patients with abnormalities of the lung parenchyma, gallium scanning, unlike the radiograph, can distinguish between fibrosis and active inflammation [28]. Therefore, in patients with chronic sarcoid (defined as parenchymal involvement for more than a 2-year period), gallium scanning can determine which patients still have active disease, which is both more likely to progress and be more amenable to prednisone therapy than fibrosis [340,433]. It has been suggested that gallium scanning and lavage together give the best overview of disease activity [216]. Patients with persistently positive findings on gallium lung scans and lavage lymphocytosis are more likely to subsequently deteriorate functionally than patients with negative results on gallium lung scans and without a similar lymphocytosis in their lavage differential [2,28,126, 216]. Similarly, active disease, as defined by increased gallium uptake and increased helper to suppressor T-cell ratio in lavage fluid, is predictive of a favorable subsequent functional response to steroids [26].

In IPF, the degree of gallium uptake correlates with interstitial cellularity on open biopsy [242]. After 1 year of prednisone therapy, patients with persistent elevation of neutrophils above 10 percent in the lavage fluid and persistent positive findings on gallium scans were more likely to have functional deterioration than patients with neutrophil differential counts below 10 percent and negative findings on gallium scan [220]. Such patients with persistent disease activity after 1 year of prednisone therapy may be candidates for alternative therapy. For example, intermittent high-dose prednisone therapy was more likely to decrease the uptake of gallium in patients with IPF than were conventional prednisone daily dosages. The clinical and functional implication of intermittent, high-dose prednisone therapy has not been ascertained, however [200]. Alternatively, patients with persistent active disease, as defined by gallium lung scanning and lavage neutrophil differential counts despite prednisone, may be candidates for chemotherapeutic agents [398].

Gallium lung scanning has been shown to be more sensitive than the chest x-ray in other interstitial processes such as asbestosis [105]. In a sheep model of asbestosis, Begin and colleagues showed that gallium detected parenchymal inflammation months before the chest x-ray [31]. Increased gallium lung uptake in some asbestos workers predicted the subsequent development of asbestosis years before such conventional modalities as the chest radiograph or determinations of lung volume [30,31,33,234]. As Bisson and coworkers suggested, gallium lung scanning may detect early, active, environmental lung disease [38]. Unfortunately, there are problems with gallium lung scanning in terms of clinical utility. Gallium uptake is nonspecific. The cost is substantial. Although the radiation dose has been described as comparable to that in radiographic studies [99], this dose has been calculated to be 600 mrads per examination [277,291].

Fundamentally, the major difficulty in the clinical application of gallium lung scanning is the absence of a uniform, quantifiable method of interpretation [398]. In general, gallium scans are described by the area of lung involved and the intensity of the uptake. Although this approach has been effective in some parenchymal processes, such as *Pneumocystis carinii* pneumonia [82], such qualitative assessment is not useful for the majority of interstitial processes, which are associated with more subtle gallium uptake [133]. The semiquantitative index developed at the National Institutes of Health, derived from estimates of lung involvement, intensity of uptake, and texture (patchy versus diffuse gallium uptake), has been shown to correlate with alveolar and interstitial cellularity on open biopsy [242]. However, this gallium index relies on a visual approach that is too subjective [419]. Various computer-assisted techniques are now being developed to quantitate gallium interpretation [31, 38,419]. Finally, measuring the amount of gallium contained in lavage fluid from patients with sarcoid is being investigated as a potentially objective method to stage disease activity [48]. At the present time, the precise utility of gallium lung scanning and lavage is unknown. Assessment of impairment and disease activity presently involves a composite of serially performed modalities, including the history (especially related to dyspnea on exertion), chest radiograph, and pulmonary physiology.

NEWER IMAGING TECHNIQUES

There are newer imaging techniques that have potential for assessment of disease activity. The clearance of small solutes from the lungs has been used to detect alterations in the permeability of the tissues separating the air from blood. Clearance of aerosolized radionuclides such as technetium-99m diethylenetriaminepentaacetate (^{99m}Tc-DTPA) was greater in patients with ILD

consistent with the presence of increased epithelial injury [155,337]. In one study, clearance of ^{99m}Tc-DTPA correlated with pulmonary inflammation as detected by lavage as well as clinical status but did not correlate with the subsequent clinical course [303]. Positron emission tomography (PET) detected increased utilization of glucose in IPF and sarcoidosis, which correlated with the subsequent clinical course. If glucose uptake was normal or normalized with therapy, the patient's condition remained stable or improved; if glucose utilization was elevated or increased during this prospective study, the patient's condition deteriorated [302].

As further discussed in Chapter 41, high-resolution CT is useful in suggesting tissue cellular activity (i.e., haze or patchy opacification of peripheral airspaces) in sarcoid and less so in IPF in patients with more inflamed disease [285]. Lynch and coworkers have been able to show that sarcoid patients with haze on high-resolution CT scans, suggesting active inflammation, subsequently respond to therapy, even with disease of many years' duration [250].

References

1. Aaron BL, et al. Open lung biopsy: A strong stand. *Chest* 59:18, 1971.
2. Abe S, et al. Gallium-67 scintigraphy, bronchoalveolar lavage, and pathologic changes in patients with pulmonary sarcoidosis. *Chest* 85: 650, 1984.
3. Abud-Mendoza C, Diaz-Jouanen E, Alarcon-Segovia D. Fatal pulmonary hemorrhage in systemic lupus erythematosus: Occurrence without hemoptysis. *J Rheumatol* 12:558, 1985.
4. Adhakari PK, et al. Pulmonary function in scleroderma: Its relation to changes in the chest roentgenogram and the skin in the thorax. *Am Rev Respir Dis* 86:823, 1962.
5. Agostini C, et al. Pulmonary alveolar macrophages from patients with active sarcoidosis express type IV collagenolytic proteinase. *J Clin Invest* 84:605, 1989.
6. Agostoni P, et al. Evaluation of breathlessness in asbestos workers: Results of exercise testing. *Am Rev Respir Dis* 135:812, 1987.
7. Agusti AGN, et al. Mechanisms of gas-exchange impairment in idiopathic pulmonary fibrosis. *Am Rev Respir Dis* 143:219, 1991.
8. Ainslie GM, Poulter LW, duBois RM. Relation between immunocytological features of bronchoalveolar lavage fluid and clinical indices in sarcoidosis. *Thorax* 44:501, 1989.
9. Allen JN, Davis B, Pacht ER. Diagnostic significance of increased bronchoalveolar lavage

fluid eosinophils. *Am Rev Respir Dis* 142:642, 1990.

10. Allen JN, Gadek JE. Concepts of the pathogenesis of idiopathic pulmonary fibrosis. *Pulmon Perspect* 5:2, 1988.

11. Ambrus JL Jr, Fauci AS. Diffuse histiocytic lymphoma in a patient treated with cyclophosphamide for Wegener's granulomatosis. *Am J Med* 76:745, 1984.

12. Andersen HA. Transbronchoscopic lung biopsy for diffuse pulmonary diseases: Results in 939 patients. *Chest* 73 (Suppl):734, 1978.

13. Andersen H, Fontana R. Transbronchoscopic lung biopsy for diffuse pulmonary diseases: Technique and results in 450 cases. *Chest* 62:125, 1972.

14. Anderson SD, Bye PTB. Exercise testing in the evaluation of diffuse interstitial lung disease. *Aust NZ J Med* 14:762, 1984.

15. Antoniades HN, et al. Platelet-derived growth factor in idiopathic pulmonary fibrosis. *J Clin Invest* 86:1055, 1990.

16. Aronin PA, et al. Prediction of BCNU pulmonary toxicity in patients with malignant gliomas: An assessment of risk factors. *N Engl J Med* 303:183, 1980.

17. Aubas P, et al. Amiodarone induced pulmonary disease: Lipidosis or fibrosing alveolitis (abstract)? *Am Rev Respir Dis* 131:A79, 1985.

18. Austrian R, et al. Clinical and physiologic features of some types of pulmonary diseases with impairment of alveolar-capillary diffusion: The syndrome of "alveolar-capillary block." *Am J Med* 11:667, 1951.

19. Axen K, Bergofsky E. Thoracic reflexes stabilizing loaded ventilation in normal and cord-injured man. *J Appl Physiol* 43:339, 1977.

20. Ayers LN. Carbon Monoxide Diffusing Capacity. In AF Wilson (Ed), *Pulmonary Function Testing and Interpretations: A Project of the California Thoracic Society.* Orlando, FL: Grune & Stratton, 1985. Pp 137–150.

21. Ayers LN, et al. Diffusing capacity, specific diffusing capacity and interpretation of diffusion defects. *West J Med* 123:255, 1975.

22. Balow JE, Austin HA III, Muenz LR. Effect of treatment on the evolution of renal abnormalities in lupus nephritis. *N Engl J Med* 311:491, 1984.

23. Basset F, Corrin B, Spencer H. Pulmonary histiocytosis X. *Am Rev Respir Dis* 118:811, 1978.

24. Bauer W, et al. T-lymphocyte subsets and immunoglobulin concentrations in bronchoalveolar lavage of patients with sarcoidosis and high and low intensity alveolitis. *Am Rev Respir Dis* 132:1060, 1985.

25. Baughman RP, et al. Quantitation of bronchoalveolar lavage with methylene blue. *Am Rev Respir Dis* 128:266, 1983.

26. Baughman RP, et al. Comparison of gallium-67 scanning, bronchoalveolar lavage, and serum angiotensin-converting enzyme levels in pulmonary sarcoidosis. *Am Rev Respir Dis* 129:676, 1984.

27. Baughman RP, Lower EE. The effect of corticosteroid or methotrexate therapy on lung lymphocytes and macrophages in sarcoidosis. *Am Rev Respir Dis* 142:1268, 1990.

28. Beaumont D, et al. Gallium-67 in the evaluation of sarcoidosis: Correlations with serum angiotensin-converting enzyme and bronchoalveolar lavage. *Thorax* 37:11, 1982.

29. Bechtel JJ, et al. Airway hyperreactivity in patients with sarcoidosis. *Am Rev Respir Dis* 124:759, 1981.

30. Begin R, et al. Early gallium-67 uptake in the lung of asbestos exposed sheep: Association with enhanced macrophage-derived fibronectin accumulation. *J Nucl Med* 27:538, 1986.

31. Begin R, et al. Pulmonary uptake of gallium-67 in asbestos-exposed humans and sheep. *Am Rev Respir Dis* 137:623, 1983.

32. Begin R, et al. Fibronectin and procollagen 3 levels in bronchoalveolar lavage of asbestos-exposed human subjects and sheep. *Chest* 89:237, 1986.

33. Begin R, et al. Asbestos exposure and retention as determinants of airway disease and asbestos alveolitis. *Am Rev Respir Dis* 134:1176, 1986.

34. Behr J, et al. Pathogenetic significance of reactive oxygen species in diffuse fibrosing alveolitis. *Am Rev Respir Dis* 144:146, 1991.

35. Ben-Isaac FE, Simmons DH. Flexible fiberoptic pleuroscopy: Pleural and lung biopsy. *Chest* 67:573, 1975.

36. Bergofsky EH. Respiratory failure in disorders of the thoracic cage. *Am Rev Respir Dis* 119:643, 1979.

37. Bignon J, Herr B, Molinier B. Morphometric and Angiographic Studies in Diffuse Interstitial Pulmonary Fibrosis. In H Herzog (Ed), *Progress in Respiration Research.* Basel: Karger, 1975.

38. Bisson G, et al. Computer-based quantitative analysis of gallium-67 uptake in normal and diseased lungs. *Chest* 84:513, 1983.

39. Bitterman PB, Adelberg S, Crystal RG. Mechanisms of pulmonary fibrosis: Spontaneous release of the alveolar macrophage–derived growth factor in the interstitial lung disorders. *J Clin Invest* 72:1801, 1983.

40. Bitterman PB, et al. Human alveolar macrophage growth factor for fibroblasts. *J Clin Invest* 70:806, 1982.

41. Bitterman PB, et al. Modulation of alveolar macrophage–derived fibroblast proliferation by alternative macrophage mediators. *J Clin Invest* 77:700, 1986.

42. Black LF, Hyatt RE. Maximal static respiratory pressures in generalized neuromuscular disease. *Am Rev Respir Dis* 103:641, 1971.

43. Blaschke E, Eklund A, Hernbrand R. Extracellular matrix components in bronchoalveolar lavage fluid in sarcoidosis and their relationship to signs of alveolitis. *Am Rev Respir Dis* 141:1020, 1990.

44. Block AJ, Light RW. Alternate-day steroid therapy in diffuse pulmonary sarcoidosis. *Chest* 63:495, 1973.

45. Boushy SM, North LB. Pulmonary function in infiltrative lung disease. *Chest* 64:448, 1973.

46. Bowie DM, et al. Can the intensity of breathlessness be predicted from the inspiratory flow rate (abstract)? *Am Rev Respir Dis* 129:239, 1984.

47. Braude AC, Chamberlain DW, Rebuck AS. Pulmonary disposition of gallium-67 in humans: Concise communication. *J Nucl Med* 23:574, 1982.

48. Braude AC, et al. An in vitro gallium-67 lung index for the evaluation of sarcoidosis. *Am Rev Respir Dis* 130:783, 1984.

49. Brown CH, Turner-Warwick M. The treatment of cryptogenic fibrosing alveolitis with immunosuppressant drugs. *Q J Med* 158:289, 1971.

50. Brutinel WM, Martin WJ II. Chronic nitrofurantoin reaction associated with T-lymphocyte alveolitis. *Chest* 89:150, 1986.

51. Bunch TW, et al. Azathioprine with prednisone for polymyositis: A controlled, clinical trial. *Ann Intern Med* 92:365, 1980.

52. Burdon JGW, Killian KJ, Jones NL. Pattern of breathing during exercise in patients with interstitial lung disease. *Thorax* 38:778, 1983.

53. Burger CD, Hyatt RE, Staats BA. Pulmonary mechanics in lymphangioleiomyomatosis. *Am Rev Respir Dis* 143:1030, 1991.

54. Burki NK. Detection of added respiratory loads in patients with restrictive lung disease. *Am Rev Respir Dis* 132:1210, 1985.

55. Burleson RL, Johnson MC, Head H. Scintigraphic demonstration of experimental abscesses with intravenous ^{67}Ga citrate and ^{67}Ga labeled blood leukocytes. *Ann Surg* 178:446, 1973.

56. Burns CB, Scheinhorn DJ. Evaluation of single-breath helium dilution total lung capacity in obstructive lung disease. *Am Rev Respir Dis* 130:580, 1984.

57. Buscaglia AJ, Cowden FE, Brill H. Pulmonary infiltrates associated with naproxen. *JAMA* 251:65, 1984.

58. Butler J. The pulmonary function test: Cautious overinterpretation. *Chest* 79:498, 1981.

59. Campbell EJM, Dinnick OP, Howell JBL. The immediated effects of elastic loads on the breathing of man. *J Physiol* 156:260, 1961.

60. Cantin A, et al. Heterogeneity of bronchoalveolar lavage. *Am Rev Respir Dis* 124:1, 1981.

61. Carette S, et al. Severe, acute pulmonary disease in patients with systemic lupus erythematosus: Ten years of experience at the National Institutes of Health. *Semin Arthritis Rheum* 14:52, 1984.

62. Carre PC, et al. Increased expression of the interleukin-8 gene by alveolar macrophages in idiopathic pulmonary fibrosis. *J Clin Invest* 88:1802, 1991.

63. Carrington CB, et al. Chronic eosinophilic pneumonia. *N Engl J Med* 280:787, 1969.

64. Carrington CB, et al. Natural history and treated course of usual and desquamative interstitial pneumonia. *N Engl J Med* 298:801, 1978.

65. Carrington CB, et al. Structure and Function in Sarcoidosis. In LE Siltzbach (Ed), *Seventh International Conference on Sarcoidosis and Other Granulomatous Disorders. Ann NY Acad Sci* 1976. Pp 265–284.

66. Casale TB, et al. Bronchoalveolar lavage fluid histamine levels in interstitial lung diseases. *Am Rev Respir Dis* 138:1604, 1988.

67. Casolaro MA, et al. Accumulation of Langerhans' cells on the epithelial surface of the lower respiratory tract in normal subjects in association with cigarette smoking. *Am Rev Respir Dis* 137:406, 1988.

68. Catterall M, Rowell NR. Respiratory function in progressive systemic sclerosis. *Thorax* 18:10, 1963.

69. Ceuppens JL, et al. Alveolar T-cell subsets in pulmonary sarcoidosis: Correlation with disease activity and effect of steroid treatment. *Am Rev Respir Dis* 129:563, 1984.

70. Chamberlain DW, Hyland H, Ross DJ. Diphenylhydantoin-induced lymphocytic interstitial pneumonia. *Chest* 90:458, 1986.

71. Chamberlain JM. Discussion of "mediastinoscopy." *J Thorac Cardiovasc Surg* 2:532, 1965.

72. Chausow AM, et al. Reversible hypercapnic respiratory insufficiency in scleroderma caused by respiratory muscle weakness. *Am Rev Respir Dis* 130:142, 1984.

73. Chaves AD, et al. Treatment of sarcoidosis: A statement by the Committee on Therapy. *Am Rev Respir Dis* 103:433, 1971.

74. Churg A. Asbestos fiber content of the lungs in patients with and without asbestos airways disease. *Am Rev Respir Dis* 127:470, 1983.

75. Churg A, et al. Pulmonary hemorrhage and immune-complex deposition in the lung. *Arch Pathol Lab Med* 104:388, 1980.

76. Cinkotai FF, Thomson ML. Diurnal variation in pulmonary diffusing capacity for carbon monoxide. *J Appl Physiol* 21:539, 1977.

77. Clausen JL. Prediction of Normal Values. In JL Clausen (Ed), *Pulmonary Function Testing Guidelines and Controversies.* New York: Academic Press, 1982. Pp 49–59.

78. Clausen JL, Crapo R, Gardner R. Interlaboratory comparisons of pulmonary function testing (abstract). *Am Rev Respir Dis* 129:A37, 1984.

79. Clement A, et al. A controlled study of oxygen metabolite release by alveolar macrophages from children with interstitial lung disease. *Am Rev Respir Dis* 136:1424, 1987.

80. Clements PJ, et al. Muscle disease in progressive systemic sclerosis. *Arthritis Rheum* 21:62, 1978.

81. Colebatch HJH, Greaves IA, Ng CKY. Exponential analysis of elastic recoil and aging in healthy males and females. *J Appl Physiol* 47:683, 1979.

82. Coleman DL, et al. Correlation between gallium lung scans and fiberoptic bronchoscopy in patients with suspected *Pneumocystis carinii* pneumonia and the acquired immune deficiency syndrome. *Am Rev Respir Dis* 130:1166, 1984.

83. Coleridge HM, et al. Comparison of the Effects of Histamine and Prostaglandin on Afferent C-Fiber Endings and Irritant Receptors in the Intrapulmonary Airways. In RS Fitzgerald, H Gautier, S Lahiri (Eds), *The Regulation of Respiration during Sleep and Anesthesia*. New York: Plenum Press 1978. Pp 291–305.

84. Colp C. Sarcoidosis: Course and treatment. *Med Clin North Am* 61:1267, 1977.

85. Colp C, Park SS, Williams MH Jr. Pulmonary function follow-up of 120 patients. *Ann NY Acad Sci* 278:301, 1976.

86. Colp CR. Treatment of pulmonary sarcoidosis. *Chest* 72:547, 1977.

87. Colp CR, Riker J, William MH. Serial changes in scleroderma and idiopathic interstitial lung disease. *Arch Intern Med* 132:506, 1973.

88. Comroe JH Jr, Nadel JA. Current concepts: Screening tests of pulmonary function. *N Engl J Med* 282:1249, 1970.

89. Cosio M, et al. The relations between structural changes in small airways and pulmonary-function tests. *N Engl J Med* 298:1277, 1978.

90. Costabel V, et al. Prognostic value of helper cell counts in bronchoalveolar lavage fluid of pulmonary sarcoidosis (abstract). *Am Rev Respir Dis* 127:62, 1983.

91. Costabel V, et al. T-lymphocytosis in bronchoalveolar lavage fluid of hypersensitivity pneumonitis: Changes in profile of T-cell subsets during the course of the disease. *Chest* 85:514, 1984.

92. Costabel U, Matthys H. Different therapies and factors influencing response to therapy in idiopathic diffuse fibrosing alveolitis. *Respiration* 42:141, 1981.

93. Cotes JE, et al. Iron-deficiency anaemia; Its effect on transfer factor for the lung (diffusing capacity) and ventilation and cardiac frequency during submaximal exercise. *Clin Sci* 42:325, 1972.

94. Cotes JE, Johnson GR, McDonald A. Breathing Frequency and Tidal Volume: Relationship to Breathlessness. In R Porter (Ed), *Breathing: Hering-Breuer Centenary Symposium*. London: Churchill, 1970. Pp 297–314.

95. Cotes JE, Zejda J, King B. Lung function impairment as a guide to exercise limitation in work-related lung disorders. *Am Rev Respir Dis* 137:1089, 1988.

96. Crapo RO, et al. Preliminary recommendations for standard technique: Single-breath carbon monoxide diffusing capacity (transfer factor). *ATS News* (Spring): 6, 1986.

97. Crapo RO, Morris AH. Standardized single-breath normal values for carbon monoxide diffusing capacity. *Am Rev Respir Dis* 123:185, 1981.

98. Crystal RG, et al. Interstitial lung diseases of unknown cause: Disorders characterized by chronic inflammation of the lower respiratory tract. *N Engl J Med* 310:155; 310:235, 1984.

99. Crystal RG, et al. Idiopathic pulmonary fibrosis: Clinical, histologic radiographic, physiologic, scintigraphic, cytologic, and biochemical aspects. *Ann Intern Med* 85:769, 1976.

100. Crystal RG, et al. Interstitial lung disease: Current concepts of pathogenesis, staging, and therapy. *Am J Med* 70:542, 1981.

101. Cutroneo KR, Rokowski R, Counts DF. Glucocorticoids and collagen synthesis: Comparison of in vivo and cell culture studies. *Collagen Rel Res* 1:557, 1981.

102. Daniele RP. Sarcoidosis: Diagnosis and management. *Hosp Pract* 113, 1983.

103. Daniele RP, Dauber JH, Rossman MD. Immunologic abnormalities in sarcoidosis. *Ann Intern Med* 92:406, 1980.

104. Daniele RP, et al. Bronchoalveolar lavage: Role in the pathogenesis, diagnosis, and management of interstitial lung disease. *Ann Intern Med* 102:93, 1985.

105. Davies J, Nellen M, Goodwin JF. Reversible pulmonary hypertension in sarcoidosis. *Postgrad Med J* 58:282, 1982.

106. Dawson A. Spirometry. In AF Wilson (Ed), *Pulmonary Function Testing and Interpretations: A Project of the California Thoracic Society*. Orlando, FL: Grune & Stratton, 1985. Pp 9–31.

107. DeHoratius RJ, Abruzzo JL, Williams RC Jr. Immunofluorescent and immunologic studies of rheumatoid lung. *Arch Intern Med* 129:441, 1972.

108. Delclos GL, et al. Bronchoalveolar lavage analysis and quantitative gallium lung scanning in asbestosis (abstract). *Am Rev Respir Dis* 135: A22, 1987.

109. DeRemee RA. The present status of treatment of pulmonary sarcoidosis: A house divided. *Chest* 71:388, 1977.

110. DeRemee RA, Andersen HA. Sarcoidosis: A correlation of dyspnea with roentgenographic stage and pulmonary function changes. *Mayo Clin Proc* 49:742, 1974.

111. DeRemee RA, Rohrbach MS. Serum angiotensin-converting enzyme activity in evaluating the clinical course of sarcoidosis. *Ann Intern Med* 92:361, 1980.

112. Dickey BF, Myers AF. Pulmonary disease in polymyositis/dermatomyositis. *Semin Arthritis Rheum* 14:60, 1984.

113. Dimarco AF, et al. Effect on breathing of selective restriction of movement of the rib cage and abdomen. *J Appl Physiol* 50:412, 1981.

114. Dimarco AF, et al. Occlusion pressure and breathing pattern in patients with interstitial lung disease. *Am Rev Respir Dis* 127:425, 1983.

115. Dineen MK, Englander LS, Huben RP. Bleomycin-induced nodular pulmonary fibrosis masquerading as metastatic testicular cancer. *J Urol* 136:473, 1986.

116. Divertie MB, et al. Fine structural morphometry of diffuse lung disease with abnormal blood-air gas transfer. *Mayo Clin Proc* 51:42, 1976.

117. Dreis DF, et al. Cephalosporin-induced interstitial pneumonitis. *Chest* 86:138, 1984.

118. Dreisin RB, et al. Circulating immune complexes in the idiopathic interstitial pneumonias. *N Engl J Med* 298:353, 1978.

119. Dubowitz LM, Dubowitz V. Acute dermatomyositis presenting with pulmonary manifestations. *Arch Dis Child* 39:293, 1964.

120. Duncan PE, et al. Fibrosing alveolitis in polymyositis: A review of histologically confirmed cases. *Am J Med* 57:621, 1974.

121. Dunn TL, et al. Gas exchange at a given degree of volume restriction is different in sarcoidosis and idiopathic pulmonary fibrosis. *Am J Med* 85:221, 1988.

122. Eagen JW, et al. The composition of pulmonary immune deposits in systemic lupus erythematosus. *Clin Immunol Immunopathol* 12:204, 1979.

123. Edelson JD, et al. Lung inflammation in scleroderma: Clinical, radiographic, physiologic and cytopathological features. *J Rheumatol* 12:957, 1985.

124. Edwards CW, Carlile A. The larger bronchi in cryptogenic fibrosing alveolitis: A morphometric study. *Thorax* 37:828, 1982.

125. Eisenberg H. The interstitial lung diseases associated with the collagen-vascular disorders. *Clin Chest Med* 3:565, 1982.

126. Eisentrout C, Baughman RP. Predictive value of gallium scanning, bronchoalveolar lavage and angiotensin converting enzyme in two-year follow-up of pulmonary sarcoidosis (abstract). *Am Rev Respir Dis* 4:A23, 1986.

127. Eklund AG, Siguradardottir O, Ohrn M. Vitronectin and its relationship to other extracellular matrix components in bronchoalveolar lavage fluid in sarcoidosis. *Am Rev Respir Dis* 145:646, 1992.

128. Elias JA, Gustilo K, Freundlich B. Human alveolar macrophage and blood monocytes inhibition of fibroblast proliferation. *Am Rev Respir Dis* 138:1595, 1988.

129. Ellis WM, et al. Left ventricular dysfunction induced by cold exposure in patients with systemic sclerosis. *Am J Med* 80:385, 1986.

130. Engel LA, Grassino A, Anthonisen NR. Demonstration of airway closure in man. *J Appl Physiol* 38:1117, 1975.

131. Epler GR, et al. Normal chest roentgenograms in chronic diffuse infiltrative lung disease. *N Engl J Med* 298:934, 1978.

132. Epler GR, Saber FA, Gaensler EA. Determination of severe impairment (disability) in interstitial lung disease. *Am Rev Respir Dis* 131:647, 1980.

133. Fajman WA, et al. Assessing the activity of sarcoidosis: Quantitative ^{67}Ga-citrate imaging. *AJR* 142:682, 1984.

134. Fechner RE, et al. Evaluation of transbronchial biopsy of the lung. *Am J Clin Pathol* 68:17, 1977.

135. Fink JN, et al. Interstitial lung disease due to contamination of forced air systems. *Ann Intern Med* 84:406, 1976.

136. Finley TN, Swenson EW, Comroe JH Jr. The cause of arterial hypoxemia at rest in patients with "alveolar-capillary block syndrome." *J Clin Invest* 41:618, 1962.

137. Finucane KE. Lung volumes and distensibility. *Aust NZ J Med* 14:790, 1984.

138. Fitting JW, et al. Resting energy expenditure in interstitial lung disease. *Am Rev Respir Dis* 142:631, 1990.

139. Frans A, et al. Smoking and pulmonary diffusing capacity. *Scand J Respir Dis* 56:165, 1975.

140. Frazier AR, Miller RD. Interstitial pneumonitis in association with polymyositis and dermatomyositis. *Chest* 65:403, 1974.

141. Frazier DT, Shannon R, Zechman FW. Response of Medullary Respiratory Neurones to Mechanical Loads. In LD Pengelly, AS Rebuck, EJM Campbell (Eds), *Loaded Breathing*. Edinburgh: Churchill-Livingstone, 1974. Pp 165–171.

142. Fudman EJ, Kelling DG Jr. Transient effect of nifedipine on pulmonary hypertension of systemic sclerosis. *J Rheumatol* 12:1191, 1985.

143. Fulmer JD, et al. Small airways in idiopathic pulmonary fibrosis: Comparison of morphologic and physiologic observations. *J Clin Invest* 60:595, 1977.

144. Fulmer JD, et al. Morphologic-physiologic correlates of the severity of fibrosis and degree of cellularity in idiopathic pulmonary fibrosis. *J Clin Invest* 63:665, 1979.

145. Gadek JE, et al. A role for oxidative products of neutrophils in both fibrotic and destructive lung diseases (abstract). *Clin Res* 30:429A, 1982.

146. Gadek JE, Hunninghake GW, Zimmerman RL.

Regulation of the release of alveolar macro-phage-derived neutrophil chemotactic factor. *Am Rev Respir Dis* 121:723, 1980.

147. Gadek JE, et al. Collagenase in the lower respiratory tract of patients with idiopathic pulmonary fibrosis. *N Engl J Med* 301:737, 1979.

148. Gaensler EA. Open and Closed Lung Biopsy. In MA Sackner (Ed), *Diagnostic Technique in Pulmonary Diseases*, Part II. New York: Marcel Dekker, 1980. Pp 579–622.

149. Gaensler EA, Carrington CB. Open biopsy for chronic diffuse infiltrative lung disease: Clinical, roentgenographic, and physiological correlations in 502 patients. *Ann Thorac Surg* 30:411, 1980.

150. Gaensler EA, Carrington CB, Coutu RE. Radiographic-physiologic-pathologic correlations in interstitial pneumonias. *Prog Respir Res* 8:223, 1975.

151. Gaensler EA, Smith AA. Attachment for automated single-breath diffusing capacity measurement. *Chest* 63:136, 1973.

152. Garcia JGN, et al. Assessment of interlobar variation of bronchoalveolar lavage cellular differential in interstitial lung diseases. *Am Rev Respir Dis* 133:444, 1986.

153. Gelb AF, et al. Immune complexes, gallium lung scans, and bronchoalveolar lavage in idiopathic interstitial pneumonitis-fibrosis: A structure-function clinical study. *Chest* 84:148, 1983.

154. Gelb AF, Zamel N Simplified diagnosis of small-airway obstruction. *N Engl J Med* 288:395, 1973.

155. Gellert AR, et al. Clearance of 99m-technetium-labelled DTPA in asbestos-exposed subjects without clinical or radiologic evidence of interstitial lung disease. *Br J Dis Chest* 79:37, 1985.

156. George CF, Kryger MH. Sleep in restrictive lung disease. *Sleep* 10:409, 1987.

157. Gibson GJ, Pride NB. Lung distensibility: The static pressure-volume curve of the lungs and its use in clinical assessment. *Br J Dis Chest* 70:143, 1976.

158. Gibson GJ, Pride NB. Pulmonary mechanics in fibrosing alveolitis: The effects of lung shrinkage. *Am Rev Respir Dis* 116:637, 1977.

159. Gibson GJ, et al. Exponential description of the static pressure-volume curve of normal and diseased lungs. *Am Rev Respir Dis* 120:799, 1979.

160. Ginsberg SJ, Comis RL. The pulmonary toxicity of antineoplastic agents. *Semin Oncol* 9:34, 1982.

161. Godard P, Marty JP, Michel FB. Interstitial pneumonia and chlorambucil. *Chest* 76:471, 1979.

162. Gold WM, Jennings B. Pulmonary function in patients with systemic lupus erythematosus. *Am Rev Respir Dis* 93:556, 1966.

163. Golden J. Bronchoalveolar lavage: Medical Staff Conference, University of California, San Francisco. *West J Med* 145:362, 1986.

164. Golden JA. Pulmonary Complications of AIDS.

In JA Levy (Ed), *AIDS Pathogenesis and Treatment*. New York: Marcel Dekker, 1989. Pp 403–447.

165. Goldstein RA, et al. Clinical role of bronchoalveolar lavage in adults with pulmonary disease. *Am Rev Respir Dis* 142:481, 1990.

166. Gracey DR, Divertie MB. Corticosteroid treatment of diffuse interstitial pulmonary fibrosis. *JAMA* 211:495, 1979.

167. Green M, Mead J, Sears TA. Muscle activity during chest wall restriction and positive pressure breathing in man. *Respir Physiol* 35:283, 1978.

168. Guz A, et al. Experimental Results of Vagal Block in Cardiopulmonary Disease. In R Porter (Ed), *Breathing: Hering-Breuer Centenary Symposium.* London: Churchill, 1970. Pp 315–329.

169. Hamer J. Cause of low arterial oxygen saturation in pulmonary fibrosis. *Thorax* 19:507, 1964.

170. Hamman L, Rich AR. Fulminating diffuse interstitial fibrosis of the lungs. *Trans Am Clin Climatol Assoc* 51:154, 1935.

171. Hanson RR, et al. Transbronchial lung biopsy via flexible fiberoptic bronchoscopy: Results in 164 patients. *Am Rev Respir Dis* 114:67, 1976.

172. Harrison BD, et al. Respiratory failure in neuromuscular diseases. *Thorax* 26:579, 1971.

173. Haslam PL, et al. Bronchoalveolar lavage in pulmonary fibrosis: Comparison of cells obtained with lung biopsy and clinical features. *Thorax* 35:9, 1980.

174. Haslam PL, et al. Bronchoalveolar lavage fluid cell counts in cryptogenic fibrosing alveolitis and their relation to therapy. *Thorax* 35:328, 1980.

175. Hepper NG, Ferguson RH, Howard FM. Three types of pulmonary involvement in polymyositis. *Med Clin North Am* 48:1031, 1964.

176. Herf SM, Suratt PM, Arora NS. Deaths and complications associated with transbronchial lung biopsy. *Am Rev Respir Dis* 115:708, 1977.

177. Heyd J, Simmerman A. Gold-induced lung disease. *Postgrad Med J* 59:368, 1983.

178. Hiwatari N, et al. Prognosis of idiopathic pulmonary fibrosis in patients with mucous hypersecretion. *Am Rev Respir Dis* 143:182, 1991.

179. Hodges GR, Fink JN, Schlueter DP. Hypersensitivity pneumonitis caused by a contaminated cool-mist vaporizer. *Ann Intern Med* 80:501, 1974.

180. Hoffman RA, et al. Simple and rapid measurement of human T-lymphocytes and their subclasses in peripheral blood. *Proc Natl Acad Sci USA* 77:4914, 1980.

181. Holland RAB. Physiologic dead space in the Hamman-Rich syndrome: Physiologic and clinical implications. *Am J Med* 28:61, 1960.

182. Hollinger WM, et al. Prediction of therapeutic response in steroid-treated pulmonary sarcoidosis: Evaluation of clinical parameters, bron-

choalveolar lavage, gallium-67 lung scanning, and serum angiotensin-converting enzyme levels. *Am Rev Respir Dis* 132:65, 1985.

183. Holoye PY, et al. Bleomycin hypersensitivity pneumonitis. *Ann Intern Med* 88:47, 1978.

184. Homma I, et al. Effect of chest wall vibration on ventilation in patients with spinal cord lesion. *J Appl Physiol* 50:107, 1981.

185. Hoogsteden HC, et al. Phenotype of blood monocytes and alveolar macrophages in interstitial lung disease. *Chest* 95:574, 1989.

186. Horn M, et al. Restrictive ventilatory pattern in precapillary pulmonary hypertension. *Am Rev Respir Dis* 128:163, 1983.

187. Hosenpud JD, et al. Abnormal pulmonary function specifically related to congestive heart failure: Comparison of patients before and after cardiac transplantation. *Am J Med* 88:493, 1990.

188. Hourani JM, et al. Pulmonary dysfunction in advanced liver disease: Frequent occurrence of an abnormal diffusing capacity. *Am J Med* 90:693, 1991.

189. Huang CT, et al. Pulmonary sarcoidosis. *Respiration* 37:335, 1979.

190. Hunninghake GW. Release of interleukin 1 by alveolar macrophages of patients with acute pulmonary sarcoidosis. *Am Rev Respir Dis* 129:569, 1984.

191. Hunninghake GW, et al. Role of interleukin-2 release by lung T-cells in active pulmonary sarcoidosis. *Am Rev Respir Dis* 128:634, 1983.

192. Hunninghake GW, Crystal RG. Mechanism of hypergammaglobulinemia in pulmonary sarcoidosis: Site of increased antibody production and role of T-lymphocytes. *J Clin Invest* 67:6786, 1981.

193. Hunninghake GW, Fauci AS. Pulmonary involvement in the collagen-vascular diseases. *Am Rev Respir Dis* 119:471, 1979.

194. Hunninghake GW, et al. Localization of the immune response in sarcoidosis. *Am Rev Respir Dis* 120:49, 1979.

195. Hunninghake GW, et al. Inflammatory and immune processes in the human lung in health and disease: Evaluation by bronchoalveolar lavage. *Am J Pathol* 97:149, 1979.

196. Hunninghake GW, et al. Mechanisms of neutrophil accumulation in the lungs of patients with idiopathic pulmonary fibrosis. *J Clin Invest* 68:259, 1981.

197. Hunninghake GW, et al. Maintenance of granuloma formation in pulmonary sarcoidosis by T-lymphocytes within the lung. *N Engl J Med* 302:594, 1980.

198. Hunninghake GTW, et al. Characterization of inflammatory and immune effector cells in the lung parenchyma in patients with interstitial lung disease. *Am Rev Respir Dis* 123:407, 1981.

199. Hutchison J. On the capacity of the lungs and on the respiratory functions with a view of establishing a precise and easy method of detecting disease by the spirometer. *Trans Med Chir Soc Lond* 29:137, 1846.

200. Israel HL. Prognosis of sarcoidosis. *Ann Intern Med* 73:1038, 1970.

201. Israel HL, Fouts DW, Beggs RA. A controlled trial of prednisone treatment of sarcoidosis. *Am Rev Respir Dis* 107:609, 1973.

202. James DG. Course and prognosis of sarcoidosis: London. *Am Rev Respir Dis* 84:66, 1961.

203. James DG, et al. Treatment of sarcoidosis: Report of a controlled therapeutic trial. *Lancet* 2:526, 1967.

204. Jernudd-Wilhelmsson Y, Hornblad Y, Hedenstierna G. Ventilation-perfusion relationships in interstitial lung disease. *Eur J Respir Dis* 68:39, 1986.

205. Jodoin G, et al. Early effects of asbestos exposure on lung function. *Am Rev Respir Dis* 105:525, 1971.

206. Johns CJ, et al. Extended Experience in the Long-Term Corticosteroid Treatment of Sarcoidosis. In *Proceedings of the Seventh International Conference on Sarcoidosis and Other Granulomatous Disorders. Ann NY Acad Sci*, 1976. Pp 722–731.

207. Johnson KJ, et al. In vivo damage of rat lungs by oxygen metabolites. *J Clin Invest* 67:983, 1981.

208. Jones NL, et al. Physiological dead space and alveolar-arterial gas pressure differences during exercise. *Clin Sci* 31:19, 1966.

209. Kan WO, Ledsome JR, Botter CP. Pulmonary arterial distension and activity in phrenic nerve of anesthetized dogs. *J Appl Physiol* 46:625, 1979.

210. Karim FWA, et al. Pulmonary fibrosis after prolonged treatment with low-dose cyclophosphamide: A case report. *Oncology* 40:174, 1983.

211. Kataria YP. Chlorambucil in sarcoidosis. *Chest* 78:36, 1980.

212. Kelley J. Cytokines of the lung. *Am Rev Respir Dis* 141:765, 1990.

213. Kelley MA, et al. When to order the pulmonary angiogram: A clinical predictive model for diagnosing pulmonary embolism. *Am Rev Respir Dis* 121:155, 1980.

214. Kennedy JI, Fulmer JD. Pulmonary hypertension in the interstitial lung diseases. *Chest* 87:558, 1985.

215. Kennedy SM, et al. Pulmonary function and peripheral airway disease in patients with mineral dust or fume exposure. *Am Rev Respir Dis* 132:1294, 1985.

216. Keogh BA, et al. Effect of intermittent high-dose parenteral corticosteroids on the alveolitis of idiopathic pulmonary fibrosis. *Am Rev Respir Dis* 127:18, 1983.

217. Keogh BA, Crystal RG. Clinical significance of

pulmonary function tests: Pulmonary function testing in interstitial pulmonary disease. What does it tell us? *Chest* 78:856, 1980.

218. Keogh BA, Crystal RG. Alveolitis: The key to the interstitial lung disorders. *Thorax* 37:1, 1982.

219. Keogh BA, et al. The alveolitis of pulmonary sarcoidosis: Evaluation of natural history and alveolitis-dependent changes in lung function. *Am Rev Respir Dis* 128:256, 1983.

220. Keogh B, et al. Clinical staging of patients with idiopathic pulmonary fibrosis (abstract). *Am Rev Respir Dis* 123:89, 1981.

221. Kern JA, et al. Interleukin-1-beta gene expression in human monocytes and alveolar macrophages from normal subjects and patients with sarcoidosis. *Am Rev Respir Dis* 137:1180, 1988.

222. Kilman WJ, Goyal RK. Disorders of pharyngeal and upper esophageal sphincter motor function. *Arch Intern Med* 136:592, 1976.

223. Klassen KP, Andrews NC. Biopsy of diffuse pulmonary lesions: A 17-year experience. *Ann Thorac Surg* 4:117, 1967.

224. Klassen KP, Anlyan AJ, Curtis GM. Biopsy of diffuse pulmonary lesions. *N Engl J Med* 59:694, 1949.

225. Klech H, Hutter C. Clinical guidelines and indications for bronchoalveolar lavage (BAL): Report of the European Society of Pneumology Task Group on BAL. *Eur Respir J* 3:937, 1990.

226. Klech H, Pohl W. Technical recommendations and guidelines for bronchoalveolar lavage (BAL). *Eur Respir J* 2:561, 1989.

227. Klein J, et al. High resolution computerized tomography diagnosis of emphysema in symptomatic patients after normal chest x-ray and isolated low diffusing capacity. *Radiology* 182:817, 1992.

228. Knudson RJ, et al. Effect of aging alone on mechanical properties of normal adult human lung. *J Appl Physiol* 43:1054, 1977.

229. Koerner SK, et al. Transbronchial lung biopsy for the diagnosis of sarcoidosis. *N Engl J Med* 293:268, 1975.

230. Konishi K, et al. Spontaneous expression of the interleukin 2 receptor gene and presence of functional interleukin 2 receptors on T lymphocytes in the blood of individuals with active pulmonary sarcoidosis. *J Clin Invest* 82:775, 1988.

231. Koontz CH, Joyner LR, Nelson RA. Transbronchial lung biopsy via the fiberoptic bronchoscope in sarcoidosis. *Ann Intern Med* 85:64, 1976.

232. Kornbluth RS, Turino GM. Respiratory control in diffuse interstitial lung disease and diseases of the pulmonary vasculature. *Clin Chest Med* 1:91, 1980.

233. Lacronique JG, et al. Alveolar macrophages in idiopathic pulmonary fibrosis have glucocorticoid receptors, but glucocorticoid therapy does not suppress alveolary macrophage release of fibronectin and alveolar macrophage derived growth factor. *Am Rev Respir Dis* 130:450, 1984.

234. Lambert R, et al. Gallium-67 thoracic scan and pleural disease in asbestos workers. *J Nucl Med* 26:600, 1985.

235. Leatherman JW, et al. Lung T-cells in hypersensitivity pneumonitis. *Ann Intern Med* 100:390, 1984.

236. Lecossier D, et al. Antigen-induced proliferative response of lavage and blood T lymphocytes. *Am Rev Respir Dis* 144:861, 1991.

237. Lemberskaya EY. Morphological changes in the areas of the lingual segment of the lung, biopsied during mitral commissurotomy. *Arkh Patol* 29:20, 1967.

238. Levin DC, Wicks AB, Ellis JH Jr. Transbronchial lung biopsy via the fiberoptic bronchoscope. *Am Rev Respir Dis* 110:4, 1974.

239. Levinson RS, et al. Airway function in sarcoidosis. *Am J Med* 62:51, 1977.

240. Lieberman J. The Specificity and Nature of Serum Angiotensin-Converting Enzyme (ACE) Elevations in Sarcoidosis. In *Proceedings of the Seventh International Conference on Sarcoidosis and Other Granulomatous Disorders. Ann NY Acad Sci*, 1976. Pp 488–497.

241. Lieberman J, et al. Serum ACE (angiotensin-converting enzyme) for diagnosis and therapeutic evaluation of sarcoidosis. *Am Rev Respir Dis* 120:329, 1979.

242. Line BR, et al. Gallium-67 citrate scanning in the staging of idiopathic pulmonary fibrosis: Correlation with physiologic and morphologic features and bronchoalveolar lavage. *Am Rev Respir Dis* 118:355, 1978.

243. Line BR, et al. Gallium-67 scanning to stage the alveolitis of sarcoidosis: Correlation with clinical studies, pulmonary function studies, and bronchoalveolar lavage. *Am Rev Respir Dis* 123:440, 1981.

244. Linklater JPT. Beclomethasone aerosol in treatment of nonspecific pulmonary fibrosis. *Br Med J* 1:672, 1974.

245. Lipworth B, et al. Late relapse of desquamative interstitial pneumonia. *Am Rev Respir Dis* 136:1253, 1987.

246. Loken MR, Stall AM. Flow cytometry as an analytical and preparative tool in immunology. *J Immunol Methods* 50:R85, 1982.

247. Lourenco RV, et al. The regulation of ventilation in diffuse pulmonary fibrosis. *Am J Med* 38:199, 1965.

248. Lugano EM, Dauber JH, Daniele RP. Acute experimental silicosis: Lung morphology, histology, and macrophage chemotaxis secretion. *Am J Pathol* 109:27, 1982.

249. Lupi-Herrera E, et al. Hemodynamic effect of

hydralazine in interstitial lung disease patients with cor pulmonale. *Chest* 87:564, 1985.

250. Lynch DA, et al. High resolution CT in sarcoidosis. *J Comput Assist Tomogr* 13:405, 1989.

251. Lynne-Davies P, et al. Partitioning of immediate ventilatory stability to added elastic loads in cats. *J Appl Physiol* 30:814, 1971.

252. Macklem PT. Medical intelligence: Current concepts. New tests to assess lung function. *N Engl J Med* 293:339, 1975.

253. Macklem PT, Mead J. Factors determining maximum expiratory flow in dogs. *J Appl Physiol* 25:149, 1968.

254. Macklem PT, Thurlbeck MB, Fraser, MD. Chronic obstructive disease of small airways. *Ann Intern Med* 74:167, 1971.

255. Mahowald ML, et al. Pulmonary hypertension in systemic lupus erythematosus: Effect of vasodilators on pulmonary hemodynamics. *J Rheumatol* 12:773, 1985.

256. Malmberg R, Berglund E, Ander L. Idiopathic interstitial fibrosis of the lungs: II. Reversibility of respiratory disturbances during steroid administration. *Acta Med Scand* 178:59, 1965.

257. Marshall R, et al. Pulmonary function in sarcoidosis. *Thorax* 13:48, 1958.

258. Marshall R, Widdicombe JG. The activity of pulmonary stretch receptors during congestion of the lungs. *Q J Exp Physiol* 43:320, 1958.

259. Martens J, et al. Respiratory muscle dysfunction in systemic lupus erythematosus. *Chest* 84:170, 1983.

260. Martin RJ, et al. Pulmonary alveolar proteinosis: The diagnosis by segmental lavage. *Am Rev Respir Dis* 121:819, 1980.

261. Martinet Y, et al. Evaluation of the in vitro and in vivo effects of cyclosporine on the lung T-lymphocytes alveolitis of active pulmonary sarcoidosis. *Am Rev Respir Dis* 138:1242, 1988.

262. Martinez O, et al. An evaluation of needle punch biopsy specimens in the diagnosis of diffuse lung disease. *Am Rev Respir Dis* 107:209, 1973.

263. Mason GR, et al. Accelerated solute clearance in *Pneumocystis carinii* pneumonia. *Am Rev Respir Dis* 135:864, 1987.

264. Matalon S, et al. Modification of pulmonary oxygen toxicity by bleomycin treatment. *J Appl Physiol* 58:1802, 1985.

265. Matthay RA, Hudson LD, Petty TL. Acute lupus pneumonitis: Response to azathioprine therapy. *Chest* 63:117, 1973.

266. Matthay RA, Petty TL. Treatment of acute lupus pneumonitis with azathioprine. *Chest* 66:219, 1974.

267. Matthay RA, et al. Pulmonary manifestations of systemic lupus erythematosus: Review of twelve cases of acute lupus pneumonitis. *Medicine* 54:397, 1975.

268. McCarthy D, Cherniack RM. Regional ventilation-perfusion and hypoxia in cryptogenic fibrosing alveolitis. *Am Rev Respir Dis* 107:200, 1973.

269. McCarthy DS, Ostrow DN, Hershfield ES. Chronic obstructive pulmonary disease following idiopathic pulmonary fibrosis. *Chest* 77:473, 1980.

270. McCormack FX, et al. Idiopathic pulmonary fibrosis—Abnormalities in the bronchoalveolar lavage content of surfactant protein A. *Am Rev Respir Dis* 144:160, 1991.

271. McIlroy MB, Marshall R, Christie RV. The work of breathing in normal subjects. *Clin Sci* 13:127, 1954.

272. McNeely DJ, et al. Acute respiratory failure due to strongyloidiasis in polymyositis. *J Rheumatol* 7:745, 1980.

273. Mead J, et al. Significance of the relationship between lung recoil and maximum expiratory flow. *J Appl Physiol* 22:95, 1967.

274. Merz T, et al. The mechanism of ^{67}Ga association with lymphocytes. *Cancer Res* 34:2495, 1974.

275. Meuret G, Fueter R, Gloor F. Early stage of fulminant idiopathic pulmonary fibrosis cured by intense combination therapy using cyclophosphamide, vincristine, and prednisone. *Respiration* 36:228, 1978.

276. Miller JM, Johnson RL Jr. Effect of lung inflation on pulmonary diffusing capacity at rest and exercise. *J Clin Invest* 45:493, 1966.

277. MIRD. Dose Estimate Report 2: Summary of current radiation dose estimates to humans from ^{66}Ga, ^{67}Ga, and ^{72}Ga-citrate. *J Nucl Med* 14:755, 1973.

278. Montgomery AB, et al. Pulmonary extravascular protein accumulation is not affected by continuous positive airway pressure (CPAP) (abstract). *Am Rev Respir Dis* 135:A7, 1987.

279. Mordelet-Dambrine M, et al. Processing of lung lavage fluid causes variability in bronchoalveolar cell counts. *Am Rev Respir Dis* 130:305, 1984.

280. Morgan AD, et al. The action of inhaled corticosteroids as a steroid sparing agent in chronic pulmonary sarcoidosis. *Am Rev Respir Dis* 135:349, 1987.

281. Mornex JF, et al. Pulmonary sarcoidosis: Flow cytometry measurement of lung T-cell activation. *J Lab Clin Med* 105:70, 1985.

282. Morse SI, et al. The treatment of sarcoidosis with chloroquine. *Am J Med* 30:779, 1961.

283. Mukhopadhyay AK, Graham DY. Esophageal motor dysfunction in systemic diseases. *Arch Intern Med* 136:583, 1967.

284. Muller NL, Miller RR. Computed tomography of chronic diffuse infiltrative lung disease. *Am Rev Respir Dis* 142:1440, 1990.

285. Muller NL, et al. Disease activity in idiopathic pulmonary fibrosis: CT and pathologic correlation. *Radiology* 165:731, 1987.

286. Muller-Quernheim J, et al. Staging the alveolitis of sarcoidosis: Dichotomy of the spontaneous release of interleukin 2 and the extent of the T-cell alveolitis (abstract). *Am Rev Respir Dis* 135:A305, 1987.

287. Murphy DMF, et al. The effect of diffuse pulmonary fibrosis on lung mechanics. *Bull Eur Physiopathol Resp* 17:27, 1981.

288. Murray JF. The Limitations of Pulmonary Function Testing. In AF Wilson (Ed), *Pulmonary Function Testing and Interpretations: A Project of the California Thoracic Society.* Orlando, FL: Grune & Stratton, 1985. Pp 1–8.

289. Nachman JB, et al. Bleomycin-induced pulmonary fibrosis mimicking recurrent metastatic disease in a patient with testicular carcinoma: Case report of the CT scan appearance. *Cancer* 47:236, 1981.

290. Nadel J, Gold W, Burgess J. Early diagnosis of chronic pulmonary vascular obstruction: Value of pulmonary function tests. *Am J Med* 44:16, 1968.

291. Nelson B, et al. Distribution of gallium in human tissues after intravenous administration. *J Nucl Med* 13:92, 1972.

292. Newman SL, Michel RP, Wang, N-S. Lingular lung biopsy: Is it representative? *Am Rev Respir Dis* 132:1084, 1985.

293. Newson-Davis J, et al. Diaphragm function and alveolar hypoventilation. *Q J Med* 45:87, 1976.

294. Niden AH, Mishkin FS, Khurana MML. ^{67}Gallium citrate lung scans in interstitial lung disease. *Chest* 69:266, 1976.

295. Norenberg R, Claxton CP Jr, Takaro T. Percutaneous needle biopsy of the lung: Report of two fatal complications. *Chest* 66:216, 1974.

296. Ohar JM, et al. Increased pulmonary artery pressure in association with Raynaud's phenomenon. *Am J Med* 81:361, 1986.

297. Okada M, et al. Correlative analysis of longitudinal changes in bronchoalveolar lavage, gallium scanning, serum angiotensin-converting enzyme activity, chest x-ray, and pulmonary function tests in pulmonary sarcoidosis. *Jpn J Med* 26:360, 1987.

298. O'Leary TJ, et al. The effects of chloroquine on serum 1,25-dihydroxyvitamin D and calcium metabolism in sarcoidosis. *N Engl J Med* 315:727, 1986.

299. Olsson T, Bjornstad-Pettersen H, Stjernberg NL. Bronchostenosis due to sarcoidosis: A case of atelectasis and airway obstruction simulating pulmonary neoplasm and chronic obstructive pulmonary disease. *Chest* 75:663, 1979.

300. Opie LH. The pulmonary manifestations of generalized scleroderma (progressive systemic sclerosis). *Dis Chest* 28:665, 1955.

301. Ostrow D, Cherniack RM. Resistance to airflow in patients with diffuse interstitial lung disease. *Am Rev Respir Dis* 108:205, 1973.

302. Panos RJ, et al. Clinical deterioration in patients with idiopathic pulmonary fibrosis: Causes and assessment. *Am J Med* 88:396, 1990.

303. Pantin CF, et al. Measures of the inflammatory response in cryptogenic fibrosing alveolitis. *Am Rev Respir Dis* 138:1234, 1988.

304. Paradis IL, Dauber JH, Rabin BS. Lymphocyte phenotypes in bronchoalveolar lavage and lung tissue in sarcoidosis and idiopathic pulmonary fibrosis. *Am Rev Respir Dis* 133:855, 1986.

305. Patel AR, et al. Cyclophosphamide therapy and interstitial pulmonary fibrosis. *Cancer* 38:1542, 1976.

306. Patterson CD, Harville WE, Pierce JA. Rheumatoid lung disease. *Ann Intern Med* 62:685, 1965.

307. Pearce JG, Patt NL. Fatal pulmonary hemorrhage after percutaneous aspiration lung biopsy. *Am Rev Respir Dis* 110:346, 1974.

308. Pearle J. Exercise performance and functional impairment in asbestos-exposed workers. *Chest* 80:701, 1981.

309. Pennock BE, Rogers RM, McCaffree DR. Changes in measured spirometric indices: What is significant? *Chest* 80:97, 1981.

310. Perez-Padilla R, et al. Breathing during sleep in patients with interstitial lung disease. *Am Rev Respir Dis* 132:224, 1985.

311. Peterson MW, et al. Uniformity of bronchoalveolar lavage in patients with pulmonary sarcoidosis. *Am Rev Respir Dis* 137:79, 1988.

312. Phillipson EA, et al. Role of vagal stimuli in exercise ventilation in dogs with experimental pneumonitis. *J Appl Physiol* 39:76, 1975.

313. Picado C, et al. Spontaneous pneumothorax in cryptogenic fibrosing alveolitis. *Respiration* 48:77, 1985.

314. Pinkston P, Bitterman PB, Crystal RG. Spontaneous release of interleukin 2 by lung T-lymphocyte in active pulmonary sarcoidosis. *N Engl J Med* 308:793, 1983.

315. Plowman PN, Stablefort DE. Dermatomyositis with fibrosing alveolitis: Response to treatment with cyclophosphamide. *Proc R Soc Med* 70:738, 1977.

316. Poe RH, et al. Sensitivity and specificity of the nonspecific transbronchial lung biopsy. *Am Rev Respir Dis* 119:25, 1979.

317. Poe RH, et al. Probability of a positive transbronchial lung biopsy result in sarcoidosis. *Arch Intern Med* 139:761, 1979.

318. Pohl WR, et al. Vitronectin in bronchoalveolar lavage fluid is increased in patients with interstitial lung disease. *Am Rev Respir Dis* 143:1369, 1991.

319. Pohl WR, et al. Serum procollagen III peptide levels in subjects with sarcoidosis. *Am Rev Respir Dis* 145:412, 1992.

320. Pontoppidan H, Geffin B, Lowenstein E. Acute

respiratory failure in the adult. *N Engl J Med* 287:743, 1972.

321. Pride NB. The assessment of airflow obstruction: Role of measurements of airways resistance and of tests of forced expiration. *Br J Dis Chest* 65:135, 1971.

322. Prior C, et al. Lavage versus serum measurements of lysozyme, angiotensin converting enzyme and other inflammatory markers in pulmonary sarcoidosis. *Eur Respir J* 3:1146, 1990.

323. Rahn H, et al. The pressure-volume diagram of the thorax and lung. *Am J Physiol* 146:161, 1946.

324. Rankin J, et al. Pulmonary granulomatoses due to inhaled organic antigens. *Med Clin North Am* 51:459, 1967.

325. Ray JF III, et al. Open pulmonary biopsy: Nineteen-year experience with 416 consecutive operations. *Chest* 69:43, 1976.

326. Reed JW, Ablett M, Cotes JE. Ventilatory responses to exercise and to carbon dioxide in mitral stenosis before and after valvulotomy: Causes of tachypnoea. *Clin Sci* 54:9, 1978.

327. Refvem O. Long-Term Corticosteroid Treatment of Pulmonary Sarcoidosis. In K Iwai, Y Hosoda (Eds), *Proceedings of the Sixth International Conference on Sarcoidosis.* Baltimore: University Park Press, 1974. Pp 547–550.

328. Reinherz EL, Schlossman SF. Current concepts in immunology: Regulation of the immune response: Inducer and suppressor T-lymphocyte subsets in human beings. *N Engl J Med* 303:370, 1980.

329. Rennard S, et al. Alveolar macrophage fibronectin: A possible mediator of tissue remodeling in fibrotic lung disease (abstract). *Clin Res* 29:374A, 1981.

330. Rennard SI, et al. Colchine suppresses the release of fibroblast growth factors from alveolar macrophages in vitro. *Am Rev Respir Dis* 137:181, 1988.

331. Rennard SI, et al. Fractional processing of sequential bronchoalveolar lavage to separate bronchial and alveolar samples. *Am Rev Respir Dis* 141:208, 1990.

332. Rennard SI, et al. Production of fibronectin by the human alveolar macrophage: Mechanism for the recruitment of fibroblasts to sites of tissue injury in interstitial lung diseases. *Proc Natl Acad Sci USA* 78:7147, 1981.

333. Rennard SI, Crystal RG. Fibronectin in human bronchopulmonary lavage fluid. *J Clin Invest* 69:113, 1981.

334. Reynolds HY. Hypersensitivity pneumonitis. *Clin Chest Med* 3:503, 1982.

335. Reynolds HY. Bronchoalveolar lavage. *Am Rev Respir Dis* 135:250, 1987.

336. Ries AL, Clausen JL. Lung Volumes. In AF Wilson (Ed), *Pulmonary Function Testing and Interpretations: A Project of the California Thoracic Society.* Orlando, FL: Grune & Stratton, 1985. Pp 69–85.

337. Rinderknecht J, et al. Accelerated clearance of small solutes from the lungs in interstitial lung disease. *Am Rev Respir Dis* 121:105, 1980.

338. Rizzato G, et al. Assessment of sarcoidosis activity by ^{67}gallium lung scan: A study with follow-up. *Respiration* 44:360, 1983.

339. Rogers RM, et al. Eosinophilic pneumonia: Physiologic response to steroid therapy and observations on light and electron microscopic findings. *Chest* 68:665, 1975.

340. Rohatgi PK, Kuzmowych TV. Assessment of activity in chronic sarcoidosis: Usefulness of serum angiotensin-converting enzyme and gallium scan. *Respiration* 49:140, 1986.

341. Rosen Y, et al. Nongranulomatous interstitial pneumonitis in sarcoidosis: Relationship to development of epithelioid granulomas. *Chest* 74:122, 1978.

342. Rosenow EC III. The spectrum of drug-induced pulmonary disease. *Ann Intern Med* 77:977, 1972.

343. Rossi GA, et al. Evidence for chronic inflammation as a component of the interstitial lung disease associated with progressive systemic sclerosis. *Am Rev Respir Dis* 131:612, 1985.

344. Rossi GA, Hunninghake GW, Crystal RG. Evaluation of Inflammatory and Immune Processes in the Interstitial Disorders: Use of Bronchoalveolar Lavage. In G Cumming, G Bonsignore (Eds), *Cellular Biology of the Lung.* New York: Plenum Press, 1982. Pp 107–139.

345. Roth C, et al. Bronchoalveolar cells in advanced pulmonary sarcoidosis. *Am Rev Respir Dis* 124:9, 1981.

346. Roussos C, Macklem PT. The respiratory muscles. *N Engl J Med* 307:786, 1982.

347. Rudd RM, Haslam PL, Turner-Warwick M. Cryptogenic fibrosing alveolitis: Relationships of pulmonary physiology and bronchoalveolar lavage in response to treatment and prognosis. *Am Rev Respir Dis* 124:1, 1981.

348. Sackner MA, et al. The pathophysiology of scleroderma involving the heart and respiratory system. *Ann Intern Med* 60:611, 1964.

349. Sahgal SM, Sharma OP. Fatal herpes simplex infection during chlorambucil therapy for sarcoidosis. *J R Soc Med* 77:144, 1984.

350. Salmeron G, Greenberg SD, Lidsky MD. Polymyositis and diffuse interstitial lung disease: A review of the pulmonary histopathologic findings. *Arch Intern Med* 141:1005, 1981.

351. Saltini C, et al. Accurate quantification of cells recovered by bronchoalveolar lavage. *Am Rev Respir Dis* 130:650, 1984.

352. Sandron D, et al. Immunoglobulin abnormalities in bronchoalveolar lavage specimens from amiodarone-treated subjects. *Chest* 89:617, 1986.

353. Saunders KB. Current practice in six London lung function laboratories. *Proc R Soc Med Lond* 70:162, 1977.
354. Savoy J, Dhingra S, Anthonisen R. Role of vagal airway reflexes in control of ventilation in pulmonary fibrosis. *Clin Sci* 61:781, 1981.
355. Scadding JG. Chloroquine in the treatment of sarcoidosis: A report from the Research Committee of the British Tuberculosis Association. *Tubercle* 48:257, 1967.
356. Scadding JG. Lung biopsy in the diagnosis of diffuse lung disease. *Br Med J* 2:557, 1979.
357. Scadding, JG, Hinson, KFW. Diffuse fibrosing alveolitis (diffuse interstitial fibrosis of the lungs): Correlations of history at biopsy with prognosis. *Thorax* 22:291, 1967.
358. Scheinhorn DJ, Joyner LR, Whitcomb ME. Transbronchial forceps lung biopsy through fiberoptic bronchoscope in *Pneumocystis carinii* pneumonia. *Chest* 66:294, 1974.
359. Schwarz MI, et al.Interstitial lung disease in polymyositis and dermatomyositis: Analysis of six cases and review of the literature *Medicine* 55:89, 1976.
360. Scott DGI, Bacon PA. Response to methotrexate in fibrosing alveolitis associated with connective tissue disease. *Thorax* 35:725, 1980.
361. Scott DGI, Bacon PA. Intravenous cyclophosphamide plus methylprednisolone in treatment of systemic rheumatoid vasculitis. *Am J Med* 76:377, 1984.
362. Selroos OB. Relapsing pulmonary stage II–III sarcoidosis can be treated with inhaled budesonide (abstract). *Am Rev Respir Dis* 135:A349, 1987.
363. Selroos O, Sellergren TL. Corticosteroid therapy of pulmonary sarcoidosis: A prospective evaluation of alternate day and daily dosage in stage II disease. *Scand J Respir Dis* 60:215, 1979.
364. Shore SA, et al. Impact of panting frequency on plethysmographic determination of thoracic gas volume in chronic obstructive pulmonary disease. *Am Rev Respir Dis* 128:54, 1983.
365. Siltzbach LE. Effects of cortisone in sarcoidosis: A study of thirteen patients. *Am J Med* 12:139, 1952.
366. Silver RM, Metcalf JF, LeRoy EC. Interstitial lung disease in scleroderma: Immune complexes in sera and bronchoalveolar lavage fluid. *Arthritis Rheum* 29:525, 1986.
367. Sinha R, Bergofsky EH. Prolonged alteration of lung mechanics in kyphoscoliosis by positive pressure hyperinflation. *Am Rev Respir Dis* 106:47, 1972.
368. Slade JD, Hepburn B. Prednisone-induced alterations of circulating human lymphocyte subsets. *J Lab Clin Med* 101:479, 1983.
369. Smith DD, Agostoni PG. The discriminatory value of the $P(A-a)O_2$ during exercise in the detection of asbestosis in asbestos exposed workers. *Chest* 95:52, 1989.
370. Snider GL. Interstitial pulmonary fibrosis—Which cell is the culprit? *Am Rev Respir Dis* 127:535, 1983.
371. Sobol BJ, Sobol PG. Percent of predicted as the limit of normal in pulmonary function testing: A statistically valid approach. *Thorax* 34:1, 1979.
372. Sobol BJ, Weinheimer B. Assessment of ventilatory abnormality in the asymptomatic subject: An exercise in futility. *Thorax* 21:445, 1966.
373. Sones M, et al. Effect of cortisone in sarcoidosis. *N Engl J Med* 244:209, 1951.
374. Songcharoen S, Raju SF, Pennebaker JB. Interstitial lung disease in polymyositis and dermatomyositis. *J Rheumatol* 7:353, 1980.
375. Sostman HD, Matthay RA, Putman CE. Cytotoxic drug-induced lung disease. *Am J Med* 62:608, 1977.
376. Sostman HD, et al. Methotrexate-induced pneumonitis. *Medicine* 55:371, 1976.
377. Spain DM. The association of terminal bronchiolar carcinoma with chronic interstitial inflammation and fibrosis of the lungs. *Am Rev Tuberc* 76:559, 1967.
378. Spiteri MA, et al. Inhaled corticosteroids can modulate the immunopathogenesis of pulmonary sarcoidosis. *Eur Respir J* 2:218, 1989.
379. Spragg RG, Smith RM, Harrell JH III. Evidence of lung inflammation in patients with AIDS and *P. carinii* pneumonia (abstract). *Am Rev Respir Dis* 135:A169, 1987.
380. Spratling L, et al. Daily vs. alternate-day prednisone therapy for stage II sarcoidosis. *Chest* 88:687, 1985.
381. Sprince NL, Kazemi H, Hardy HL. Current (1975) problem of differentiating between beryllium disease and sarcoidosis. *Ann NY Acad Sci* 278:654, 1976.
382. Stack BHR, Choo-Kang YFJ, Heard BE. The prognosis of cryptogenic fibrosing alveolitis. *Thorax* 27:535, 1972.
383. Stanek V, et al. The pulmonary gas exchange during exercise in patients with pulmonary fibrosis. *Scand J Respir Dis* 48:11, 1967.
384. Staub NC. Alveolar-arterial oxygen tension due to diffusion. *J Appl Physiol* 18:673, 1963.
385. Stern EJ, et al. Cystic lung disease associated with eosinophilic granuloma and tuberous sclerosis: Air trapping at dynamic ultrafast high-resolution CT. *Radiology* 182:325, 1992.
386. Strumpf IJ, et al. Safety of fiberoptic bronchoalveolar lavage in evaluation of interstitial lung disease. *Chest* 80:268, 1981.
387. Stubbs SE, Hyatt RE. Effect of increased lung recoil pressure on maximal expiratory flow in normal subjects. *J Appl Physiol* 32:325, 1972.
388. Sue DY, et al. Lung function and exercise performance in smoking and nonsmoking asbes-

tos-exposed workers. *Am Rev Respir Dis* 132: 612, 1985.

389. Todisco T, Cegla UH, Matthys H. Oxygen breathing during exercise in patients with diffuse interstitial lung fibrosis. *Bull Eur Physiopathol Respir* 13:387, 1977.

390. Topilow AA, Rothenberg SP, Cottrell TS. Interstitial pneumonia after prolonged treatment with cyclophosphamide. *Am Rev Respir Dis* 108:114, 1973.

391. Toronto Lung Transplant Group (Cooper JD, et al.). Unilateral lung transplantation for pulmonary fibrosis. *N Engl J Med* 314:1140, 1986.

392. Trenchard D, Gardner D, Guz A. Role of pulmonary vagal afferent nerve fibres in the development of rapid, shallow breathing in lung inflammation. *Clin Sci* 42:251, 1972.

393. Tsan MF, et al. Studies on gallium accumulation in inflammatory lesions: I. Gallium uptake by human polymorphonuclear leukocytes. *J Nucl Med* 19:36, 1978.

394. Tsan MF, Scheffel U. Gallium-67 accumulation in inflammatory lesions. *J Nucl Med* 20:173, 1979.

395. Tukiainen P, et al. Prognosis of cryptogenic fibrosing alveolitis. *Thorax* 38:349, 1983.

396. Turino GM, et al. The control of ventilation in patients with reduced pulmonary distensibility. *Ann NY Acad Sci* 109:932, 1963.

397. Turner M, Mead J, Wohl ME. Elasticity of human lungs in relation to age. *J Appl Physiol* 25:664, 1968.

398. Turner-Warwick M. Staging and therapy of cryptogenic fibrosing alveolitis. *Chest* 89:148S, 1986.

399. Turner-Warwick M, Burrows B, Johnson A. Cryptogenic fibrosing alveolitis: Response to corticosteroid treatment and its effect on survival. *Thorax* 35:593, 1980.

400. Turner-Warwick M, Haslam PL. The value of serial bronchoalveolar lavages in assessing the clinical progress of patients with cryptogenic fibrosing alveolitis. *Am Rev Respir Dis* 135:26, 1987.

401. Turner-Warwick M, et al. Cryptogenic fibrosing alveolitis and lung cancer. *Thorax* 35:496, 1980.

402. Tzen KY, et al. Role of iron-binding proteins and enhanced capillary permeability on the accumulation of gallium-67. *J Nucl Med* 21:31, 1980.

403. Von Euler C, Fritts HW Jr. Quantitative aspects of respiratory reflexes from the lungs and chest walls of cats. *Acta Physiol Scand* 57:284, 1963.

404. Wagner PD, et al. Distribution of ventilation-perfusion ratios in patients with interstitial lung disease. *Chest* 69(Suppl):256, 1976.

405. Wall CP, et al. Comparison of transbronchial and open biopsies in chronic infiltrative lung diseases. *Am Rev Respir Dis* 123:280, 1981.

406. Wallaert B, et al. Subclinical pulmonary involvement in collagen-vascular diseases assessed by bronchoalveolar lavage: Relationship between alveolitis and subsequent changes in lung function. *Am Rev Respir Dis* 133:574, 1986.

407. Walton M, Skeoch T. Diagnosis of asbestosis by needle lung biopsy. *Thorax* 23:556, 1968.

408. Ward K, et al. Pulmonary disease progress in sarcoid patients with and without bronchoalveolar lavage collagenase. *Am Rev Respir Dis* 142:636, 1990.

409. Ward K, et al. Prognostic value of bronchoalveolar lavage in sarcoidosis: The critical influence of disease presentation. *Thorax* 44:6, 1989.

410. Ward ME, Stubbing DG. Effect of chronic lung disease on the perception of added inspiratory loads. *Am Rev Respir Dis* 132:652, 1985.

411. Wasserman K, Whipp BJ. Exercise physiology in health and disease. *Am Rev Respir Dis* 112:219, 1975.

412. Watters LC, et al. A clinical, radiographic, and physiologic scoring system for the longitudinal assessment of patients with idiopathic pulmonary fibrosis. *Am Rev Respir Dis* 133:97, 1986.

413. Watters LC, et al. Idiopathic pulmonary fibrosis—Pretreatment bronchoalveolar lavage cellular constituents and their relationships with lung histopathology and clinical response to therapy. *Am Rev Respir Dis* 135:696, 1987.

414. Weaver AL, et al. Pulmonary involvement in polymyositis: Report of a case with response to corticosteroid therapy. *Arthritis Rheum* 11:765, 1968.

415. Webb DR, Currie GD. Pulmonary fibrosis masking polymyositis: Remission with corticosteroid therapy. *JAMA* 222:1146, 1972.

416. Weese WC, Levine BW, Kazemi I. Interstitial lung disease resistant to corticosteroid therapy: Report of three cases treated with azathioprine or cyclophosphamide. *Chest* 67:57, 1975.

417. Weiss RB, Muggia FM. Cytotoxic drug-induced pulmonary disease: Update 1980. *Am J Med* 68:259, 1980.

418. Weitzenblum E, et al. Pulmonary hemodynamics in idiopathic pulmonary fibrosis and other interstitial pulmonary diseases. *Respiration* 44:118, 1983.

419. Wesselius LJ, et al. Computer-assisted versus visual lung gallium-67 index in normal subjects and in patients with interstitial lung disorders. *Am Rev Respir Dis* 128:1084, 1983.

420. West JR, Alexander JK. Studies on respiratory mechanics and the work of breathing in pulmonary fibrosis. *Am J Med* 27:529, 1959.

421. Westcott JL. Air embolism complicating percutaneous needle biopsy of the lung. *Chest* 62:484, 1972.

422. Whitcomb ME, Dixon GF. Gallium scanning, bronchoalveolar lavage, and the national debt. *Chest* 85, 719, 1984.

423. Whitelaw WA, Derenne J, Milic-Emili J. Occlu-

sion pressure as a measure of respiratory center output in conscious man. *Respir Physiol* 23:181, 1975.

424. Widimsky J, Riedel M, Stanek V. Central haemodynamics during exercise in patients with restrictive pulmonary disease. *Bull Eur Physiopathol Respir* 13:369, 1977.

425. Wiener-Kronish JP, et al. Severe pulmonary involvement in mixed connective-tissue disease. *Am Rev Respir Dis* 124:499, 1981.

426. Williams R, Hugh-Jones P. The significance of lung function changes in asbestosis. *Thorax* 15:109, 1960.

427. Wilson RK, et al. Clinical implications of a "nonspecific" transbronchial biopsy. *Am J Med* 65:252, 1978.

428. Winterbauer RH, et al. Diffuse interstitial pneumonitis: Clinicopathologic correlations in 20 patients treated with prednisone/azathioprine. *Am J Med* 65:661, 1978.

429. Winterbauer RH, Hutchinson JF. Clinical significance of pulmonary function tests: Use of pulmonary function tests in the management of sarcoidosis. *Chest* 78:640, 1980.

430. Wolff SM, et al. Wegener's granulomatosis. *Ann Intern Med* 81:513, 1974.

431. Woolcock AJ. Airflow limitation. *Aust NZ J Med* 14:794, 1984.

432. Woolcock AJ, Colman MH, Blackburn CRB. Factors affecting normal values for ventilatory lung function. *Am Rev Respir Dis* 106:692, 1972.

433. Wurm K, Rosner R. Prognosis of chronic sarcoidosis. *Ann NY Acad Sci* 278:732, 1976.

434. Youmans CR Jr, et al. Needle biopsy of the lung in diffuse parenchymal disease: An analysis of 151 cases. *Am J Surg* 120:637, 1970.

435. Young RL, et al. Pulmonary sarcoidosis: A prospective evaluation of glucocorticoid therapy. *Ann Intern Med* 73:207, 1970.

436. Young RL, et al. Pulmonary sarcoidosis: I. Pathophysiologic considerations. *Am Rev Respir Dis* 97:997, 1968.

437. Zavala DC. Pulmonary hemorrhage in fiberoptic transbronchial biopsy. *Chest* 70:584, 1976.

438. Zavala DC, Bedell GN. Percutaneous lung biopsy with a cutting needle: An analysis of 40 cases and comparison with other biopsy techniques. *Am Rev Respir Dis* 106:186, 1972.

43

Sleep Apnea Syndrome and Sleep-Disordered Breathing

Kingman P. Strohl

Sleep-disordered breathing comprises a collection of syndromes characterized by breathing abnormalities during sleep, by intermittent disruptions in gas exchange, and by sleep interruption. According to cross-sectional studies, sleep apnea is relatively common in the population, and 1.2 percent of the population could be candidates for treatment on the basis of excessive daytime sleepiness, cardiac arrhythmias, cognitive abnormalities, and/or behavioral abnormalities [25,27,46]. In addition, there are epidemiologic data to suspect that snoring (partial upper airway obstruction during sleep) is associated with systemic hypertension and stroke and, possibly, myocardial infarction and premature sudden death [8,34,42]. Finally, a positive association between sleep apnea and motor vehicle accidents exists, affecting morbidity and mortality in the general population [2,14,21,37]. Clearly, sleep-disordered breathing has a medical and social impact on the community.

The purpose of this chapter is to describe the pathophysiology and clinical management issues for respiratory disorders of sleep.

Definitions Used in Describing Sleep-Disordered Breathing

Sleep apnea syndrome is a disorder characterized by the association of apnea and/or hypoventilation during sleep with a constellation of symptoms and signs related to sleep fragmentation and hypoxic exposure. The syndrome will resolve when the sleep-induced respiratory disturbance is eliminated [1,17,19,25,46].

Three patterns of apnea can be observed during sleep. These are schematically shown in Figure 43-1. A *central apnea* occurs when both airflow and respiratory efforts are absent. Other terms used in the literature that are equivalent to a central apnea are *diaphragmatic* or *arrhythmic apnea*. These terms imply that there is a cessation of respiratory effort by the muscles of the chest. During an *obstructive apnea*, respiratory efforts persist, although airflow is absent at the nose and mouth. Other terms for obstructive apnea are *upper airway* and *peripheral apnea*. Obstructive and central apneas are not necessarily unrelated. Many adult patients exhibit apneas in which both central and obstructive patterns occur, which are termed *mixed apneas*. In a single apneic episode there may be a period of absent airflow in which no efforts occur, followed by the appearance of respiratory efforts, also without airflow. In addition, in the same night, patients may have central, mixed, and obstructive apneas.

Hypoventilation during sleep may arise by mechanisms similar to that producing apnea. *Hypoventilation* (hypopnea) leads to increased carbon dioxide and decreased oxygen levels in arterial blood and, like apneas, may be the result of an overall reduction in respiratory efforts or of partial upper airway obstruction. Snoring is a form of partial airway obstruction. While in most instances snoring is of mild severity, patients who snore heavily may present with symptomatic features of sleep apnea syndrome even if complete cessation of airflow (apnea) never occurs during sleep; moreover, these patients may exhibit abnormal sleep and cardiorespiratory changes as well.

Epidemiology of Sleep-Disordered Breathing

Subjects without clinical problems may exhibit obstructive or central apneas at sleep onset or

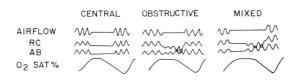

CENTRAL   OBSTRUCTIVE   MIXED

AIRFLOW
RC
AB
O_2 SAT %

Fig. 43-1. Shown in diagrammatic form are the three patterns of apnea identified during sleep in human subjects. In each, airflow at the nose and mouth is absent, indicating apnea. In central apneas, respiratory efforts, indicated in this instance by rib cage (*RC*) and abdominal (*AB*) displacement, are absent. During an obstructive apnea, efforts by the chest-wall muscles are present throughout the entire episode of apnea. In mixed apneas, both central and obstructive patterns are present in the same apnea. Oxygen saturation (O_2 *SAT %*) will fall according to the general level of oxygen saturation and the length of the apnea. (Reproduced from KP Strohl et al. Physiologic basis for therapy of sleep apnea. *Am Rev Respir Dis* 134:791, 1986.)

during periods of rapid eye movement (REM) sleep [46]. Apneic episodes are usually less than 10 to 15 seconds in duration and are not repetitive. Occasionally, longer periods of apnea lasting up to 30 seconds are seen in normal subjects, particularly during REM sleep. These episodes are not usually accompanied by arousal or sleep-state changes. Whether there are sex differences in the appearance of sleep apneas in healthy subjects is unclear. In healthy young subjects, some studies have shown that more males than females have frequent apneas during sleep, while others report little sex difference in the occurrence of apneas. Study differences may be confounded by small numbers of subjects, subject selection, and the effect of obesity. After the sixth decade, however, respiratory disturbances during sleep seem to increase in number and occur with equal frequency in males and females [46]. Patients with a clinically important sleep apnea may be distinguished from normal (1) by the existence of repetitive apneas of greater than 10 seconds' duration during stages I and II and REM sleep, (2) by evidence that oxygen saturation falls with each apnea and carbon dioxide levels increase through the night, and (3) by improvement in daytime symptoms and general performance with treatment of sleep-disordered breathing.

Using symptom questionnaires, it is estimated that 5 to 10 percent of the population in industrial societies may have a breathing disturbance dur-

ing sleep. In a sample of 1500 factory workers, it was found that at least 2 percent had symptomatic sleep apnea [27]. These studies also suggest that these subjects have higher accident rates and substantial disability.

Snoring is believed to be a predisposing feature in the development of disease. Snoring increases markedly with age, so that approximately 45 percent of males and 30 percent of females over age 65 are said to snore. Hypertension is twice as common among persons who snore, even after age and obesity are taken into account.

Reports from sleep clinics suggest that sleep apnea should be considered in any patient referred for disorders of initiating and maintaining sleep (DIMS) or disorders of excessive somnolence (DOES) [9]. The incidence of sleep apnea in patients presenting to sleep centers ranges from 7 to 33 percent [9].

There is increasing evidence that sleep apnea has a familial distribution. Symptoms relating to apnea are present with two to six times greater frequency in family members of affected patients than in a control population [46]. Sleep apneic activity itself is present more often in first-degree relatives of patients than in age-, sex-, and socioeconomic-matched control families. These family studies also suggest that the frequency of sleep apnea is underestimated in the community and that the symptomatic sequelae of multiple apneas are quite variable. The differential impact of genetics versus environmental factors that explain the familial and symptomatic expression of this disease remains to be determined.

Clinical Features of Sleep Apnea

Patients will often have five or more of the traits listed in Table 43-1. Signs and symptoms in a particular patient may be associated with central, obstructive, or mixed apneas during sleep [46].

Patients with obstructive sleep apnea may be obese and physically resemble patients described as suffering with pickwickian syndrome, exhibiting obesity, cardiopulmonary failure, polycythemia, and hypersomnolence [7]. Yet nearly half of patients with the sleep apnea syndrome are not obese, and the suspicion that the syndrome is present should not be limited to the fat patient or to those with characteristics previously called the pickwickian syndrome [48].

Restless sleep and sleep disturbances are associated with the recurrent apneas. Sleep complaints include either excessive daytime sleepiness or insomnia. Both are related to the number

***Table 43-1.* Clinical problems associated with sleep-disordered breathing**

Historical data	Clinical signs
Altered sleep: snoring, thrashing	Cardiac arrhythmias
Excessive daytime sleepiness	Systemic hypertension
Dyspnea, especially on exercise	Edema
Morning headaches	Polycythemia
Insomnia	Pulmonary hypertension
Fatigue	
Intellectual deterioration	Reduced sleep latency by EEG
Personality changes	
Hallucinations, automatic behavior	Reddened uvula; pharyngeal crowding
Family history of sleep apnea	

and type of nocturnal arousals [41]. Patients with insomnia generally have fewer and shorter, primarily central, apneas with little hypoxemia, whereas patients with excessive daytime sleepiness have more and longer, primarily mixed and obstructive, apneas with greater hypoxemia.

Since bradyarrhythmias during sleep are also commonly found in patients with sleep apnea [35,51], Holter monitoring can be the first clue to the presence of apneas during sleep. An example of bradyarrhythmia during sleep apnea is shown in Figure 43-2. During obstructive apneas, the depressive effects of the carotid body on heart rate predominate, while quickening of heart rate occurs when ventilation occurs. Patients with sleep apnea who exhibit bradycardia during sleep may have normal findings on His bundle studies and otherwise normal cardiac function during wakefulness. Other cardiac arrhythmias include ventricular ectopy and escape rhythms, but in addition, reflexes elicited by forceful respiratory efforts against a closed airway and the resulting swings in pleural pressure probably have significant effects on circulatory function. Arrhythmias in patients with sleep apnea disappear when the apneas are relieved.

Less than a fourth of patients with sleep apnea associated with sleep disturbances will present with signs of hypoxic exposure–polycythemia and/or cor pulmonale [6]. Biochemical markers of hypoxic exposure are, however, present in many patients who do not have physical signs of

hypoxic stress [13,28]. In some patients, however, a disturbance in sleep or hypersomnolence is not noticeably symptomatic, and these signs of hypoxic exposure may be the first indication of the presence of sleep apnea. The presence of hypoxemia during both wakefulness and sleep probably contributes to the progression of signs for hypoxic exposure. Signs of hypoxic exposure more often are present in patients with concomitant obstructive lung disease [6]. Pulmonary artery pressure has been observed to rise over the course of repetitive apneas during sleep, and reversal of pulmonary hypertension occurs with treatment of sleep apnea. It is unknown, however, what levels of hypoxemia for what length of time are needed for the development of cor pulmonale. It is clear, however, that patients with repetitive sleep apnea experience hypoxemia more profoundly during sleep than during wakefulness and that treatment of sleep apnea is associated with improved oxygenation, particularly during sleep.

Often it is the family members, rather than the patient, who first recognize the sleep disturbance—periods of absent breathing, loud snoring, or thrashing movements during sleep [24]. The symptoms of sleep apnea can develop insidiously over many years and may infrequently present only with complaints of fatigue or decreased alertness or with apparently unexplained polycythemia. In addition, sleep apnea is part of the differential diagnosis of sexual dysfunction, personality changes, and morning headache [22,41].

Routine laboratory examinations are not helpful screening tools. Likewise, pulmonary function tests also may reveal no abnormality except those caused by associated obesity (somewhat diminished lung capacities, with greater reduction in the expiratory reserve volume). While patients with lung diseases also may have the sleep apnea syndrome, there is no evidence that sleep apnea occurs more frequently in patients with pulmonary impairment.

The sleep apnea syndrome should be considered as a possibility in patients with hypercapnia that is disproportionate to abnormalities in mechanical function of the lungs. Hypercapnia rarely occurs with obstructive lung disease unless forced expiratory volume in 1 second (FEV_1) is reduced to less than 50 percent of predicted. Carbon dioxide elevation occurs in patients with asthma and fibrotic pulmonary disease only with even more severe reduction in the FEV_1. Patients with unexplained right-sided heart failure or pulmonary hypertension likewise should be exam-

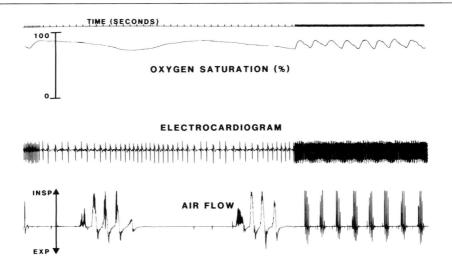

Fig. 43-2. Shown is the relationship between oxygen saturation, heart rate (indicated by an ECG rhythm strip), and ventilation (measured from a face mask). Cyclic changes in heart rate found on Holter monitoring of a patient can indicate the presence of apneas during sleep. *INSP* = inspiration; *EXP* = expiration.

ined for the presence of sleep-disordered breathing. Finally, some patients with the sleep apnea syndrome may be mistakenly treated for primary heart disease because cardiac arrhythmias have been detected during sleep, while the respiratory disturbances have not.

Laboratory Diagnosis

Sleep Studies

Definitive study can be made by polysomnography, in which continuous measurements are made to assess sleep stages, breathing, and gas exchange. Figure 43-3 shows the elements of sleep and breathing that can be monitored in patients.

Sleep staging requires monitoring of the electroencephalogram (EEG) (usually with two or three leads), the chin electromyogram (activity decreases in REM), and the electro-oculogram (EOG) to detect REMs. It is also useful to record the electrocardiogram (ECG) to see if arrhythmias occur with the apneic episodes.

To distinguish central from obstructive apneas, both respiratory efforts and some index of airflow must be measured.

Oxygenation can be assessed most accurately during sleep by sampling from indwelling arterial catheters. However, intermittent sampling may miss some of the most dramatic falls in oxygen tension and saturation that occur during apneas. PO_2 can be assessed transcutaneously using elec-

trodes applied to the skin, which is heated to increase blood flow, but these electrodes probably have too long a response time to be useful in sleep apnea. Noninvasive oximeters that spectrophotometrically and continuously measure the level of oxygenated hemoglobin are ideal for use in sleep studies. These instruments are reliable and accurate to ±2 to 4 percent in the range of oxygen saturations from 70 to 99 percent, although anemia or pigment in the skin may affect their readings.

Nonpolysomnography Monitoring Techniques

Given the expense and time commitment involved in performing polysomnography, there have been three approaches to reduce the cost or performance of this diagnostic procedure. First, questionnaires have been proposed that could serve to screen individuals, thereby improving the diagnostic yield and reducing the number of subjects that need polysomnography [10,48]. Second, equipment has been developed to allow performance of a study equivalent to polysomnography in the home setting. In some instances, a van brings equipment and a technician to the pa-

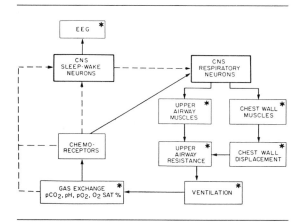

Fig. 43-3. This schematic diagram shows the general relationships between the respiratory system (CNS respiratory neurons, upper airway and chest-wall muscles, ventilation, chemoreceptors, etc.) and the CNS sleep-wake process. The boxes designated by the asterisks indicate the respiratory variables and the electroencephalogram (*EEG*) that can be measured in human subjects and are used in the diagnosis and assessment of treatment in patients with sleep apnea. Note that the basic mechanisms in respiration or sleep can be measured only indirectly. (Reproduced from KP Strohl et al. Physiologic basis for therapy of sleep apnea. *Am Rev Respir Dis* 134:791, 1986.)

tient. Third, simplified unattended monitoring of selected, crucial variables could be used to assess therapeutic efficacy [31].

For the last purpose, a number of approaches have been suggested. Some include use of tracheal sound recordings, for which automated computer techniques can be used to detect apneas and hypopneas. A computer has also been employed with a carbon dioxide detector to monitor for apnea. Analysis of oximetry data alone can be used to detect apneas and hypopneas associated with desaturations and has some utility in monitoring sleep states. However, the predictive value with respect to apneas is low. Screening studies that combine continuous measurement of arterial oxygen saturation and ventilatory effort may be adequate for the presumptive diagnosis of sleep apnea if cyclic breathing and saturation abnormalities are detected and then abolished by the application of nasal continuous positive airway pressure (CPAP). However, the absence of abnormalities in such screening tests does not prove that the

patient is free of sleep apnea, that the amount and quality of sleep are not directly monitored, and that other sleep disorders which can produce similar symptoms are not assessed.

Several approaches to unattended simultaneous monitoring of several variables have been developed recently, using both digital and analogue recording techniques [31]. Such devices are being continuously upgraded, as is the software for detection of respiratory events. Many devices employ signals from the chest and abdomen to detect apneas and hypopneas. In some instances, tidal volume changes can be estimated from the phase relationship between the rib cage and abdomen. Simultaneous with the respiratory measurements, recordings are made of other important variables, for example, ear oximetry, heart rate determined by the R-R interval of the ECG, tibialis electromyogram, and body movement with an activity monitor strapped to subject's wrist. The latter is used in an attempt to estimate sleep time.

At the present stage of development, the number of apneas detected by these instruments shows a good correlation with those detected by simultaneous polysomnography. Thus, in general, the instruments correctly identify persons who have sleep apnea. However, the devices are not as proficient in classifying apneas as being obstructive or central. In particular, with current digital systems, central apneas are frequently classified as obstructive. Improvements to obviate these and other problems will be made since the costs of polysomnography limit access to diagnosis and management.

Interpretation of Polysomnographic Measurements

Sleep apnea is often considered to be present if there are at least 30 apneas or hypopneas (each more than 10 seconds) occurring in both non-REM (NREM) and REM sleep in a sleep recording lasting 6 hours. There are reports, however, of patients who have more than 200 apneas per night yet are relatively asymptomatic, and many otherwise normal, healthy aging subjects would be classified as having sleep apnea syndrome based on currently used criteria, which depend on numbers of apneas. Definitive prospective longitudinal data on the risks associated with only the number of respiratory events during sleep are currently not available. Retrospective studies suggest mortality increases as the apneic index (number of apneas per hour of sleep) increases

[34,37,42]. Controversy on the predictive value of polysomnography still exists [3,5,45].

Levels of oxygen saturation during wakefulness and sleep may be clinically more important than the number of abnormal respiratory events, however defined. Using continuous monitoring of oxygen saturation, the fraction of the sleep period spent at each level of oxygen saturation can be determined to quantify hypoxemic exposure (Fig. 43-4). Minimum levels of oxygen saturation are important, since severe hypoxia can trigger cardiac arrhythmias, but mean levels may be even more important. Recently, methods of quantitatively describing the profile of oxygen saturation throughout sleep and wakefulness have been developed and should prove valuable in diagnosis and in evaluating the effects of treatment [3,4].

Some sleep investigators believe that sleep studies should be performed on at least two nights, since it has been shown that the distribution of sleep stages may be altered by unfamiliar surroundings. In patients with lung disease, however, ventilatory changes within a given sleep stage can usually be accurately assessed during a single night's examination. Because all night studies are costly, attempts have been made

to diagnose sleep apnea and its severity with shorter examinations of sleep. The specificity and sensitivity of such studies are unknown.

It is proposed that any diagnostic study for sleep apnea should include periods of both NREM and REM sleep for the reason that it is during REM sleep that severe changes in respiration often occur [3,46]. While this approach is reasonable, correlation of sleep events with clinical symptoms is currently imprecise, and furthermore, the relative importance of abnormal respiration occurring in REM and NREM sleep is unknown.

Figure 43-5 typifies one viewpoint of the spectrum of disease. Those with severe disease could be defined as individuals who have active daytime sleepiness interfering with normal daily activities and associated with signs of cardiopulmonary failure, polycythemia, and cor pulmonale. Such an individual would be now easily recognized as having a treatable disease. Once the apneic episodes during sleep are eliminated, excessive daytime sleepiness would resolve and signs of hypoxic stress, such as polycythemia and cor pulmonale, would resolve or not progress. Noted is a correlation between the number of arousals, the number of respiratory events during sleep, and sleepiness as measured by multiple sleep latency testing. Patients fall asleep during the day,

Fig. 43-4. The effect of treatment on oxygen saturation over time in two patients, one treated with tracheostomy and one with oxygen, progesterone, and associated weight loss. Studies in both patients were performed on room air. Treatment in both cases reversed hypersomnolence, an increased hematocrit, pedal edema, and signs of right-sided heart failure. S = sleep; W = wakefulness.

Fig. 43-5. Degrees of pathophysiology that exist in sleep apnea syndrome. Although this figure illustrates the spectrum of disease, it should be considered a hypothesis. For instance, the population at risk is presumed to be those who snore heavily, somewhere in the vicinity of 50 percent of males and 30 percent of females. Also, the natural progression of the disease is not known.

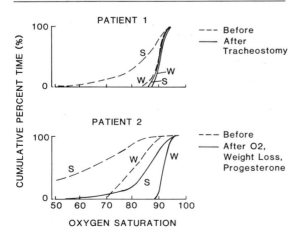

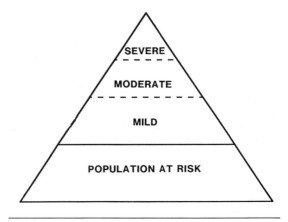

in a sitting posture, and are at extreme risk for accidental injury. Clinical studies have shown that reversal of sleep-related hypoxemia can improve sleepiness, hypertension, and abnormalities associated with hypoxemia, such as reversal of the polycythemic state, and resolution of edematous states associated with cor pulmonale. The category of severe disease includes patients with more than 45 apneas per hour of sleep and hypoxemia that exceeds lower thresholds of 85 percent saturation for at least 15 percent of the time during sleep.

A second category would be that of moderate disease. This would include daytime sleepiness of which the patient is aware and takes steps to avoid falling asleep at times that might be inappropriate. One example might be the patient who often takes a nap in the middle of the day or avoids driving for fear of falling asleep. These individuals are less disabled by their daytime sleepiness than those with severe disease and often are able to continue their daily activity. These individuals may or may not have daytime signs and symptoms of hypoxemic stress; however, they often have hypertension. Detailed studies of pulmonary vascular resistance or of cognitive studies in these individuals have not been performed; however, this group has an increased incidence of motor vehicle violations or accidents. Generally in these patients the apneic/hypopneic index is between 25 and 45, but positionally induced or positionally altered apneic indices could be common and a high hypopneic index may be present. Sleep fragmentation is observed, but the progression of sleep stages is apparent. This category is distinguished from severe disease by the absence of disabling sleepiness, of cor pulmonale, and of hypercapnic respiratory failure.

A third category is that of mild disease. In these individuals there is sleepiness that is manifested by a regular tendency to fall asleep under circumstances of inactivity such as reading the newspaper, going to movies, or watching television shows. This "passive" sleepiness may not be recognized by the patient, and the patient does not take steps to avoid activities that might make him or her sleepy. Indeed, sleepiness may be recognized only by family members and be noticed only in retrospect after direct treatment of apnea or of improvement by weight loss or alcohol abstinence. Respiratory disturbance indices in these individuals are generally in the range of 10 to 25 per hour. There may be no signs of hypoxic stress, and oxygen saturation levels during sleep are generally confined to less than 90 percent for

only 5 to 100 percent of the time. Sleep stages and stretches of stage III and IV sleep are preserved. These individuals are distinguished from those with moderate disease to the extent that their sleepiness does not intrude on daily activity or behavior, and the absence of problems ascribed to hypoxic stress.

The substrate for development of disease related to sleep apnea is considered to be those individuals who snore on a regular basis and do not have observed apneas. People with simple snoring generally are not sleepy, although perhaps more susceptible to behavioral influences and morbidity from alcohol or sedatives than individuals who do not snore at all. This group would comprise half of the male and a third of the female population. Respiratory disturbance indices are usually low, certainly no more than 15 per hour, and a positional component to snoring and apnea may be present. Aspects of the association between snoring and other common diseases and the distinction between heavy snoring and mild snoring have been reviewed in other sections of this chapter. The major epidemiologic associations with hypertension, cardiovascular disease, myocardial infarction, and stroke possibly include these individuals as well as those with mild or moderate disease severity.

Currently I set the therapeutic threshold for the elimination of obstructive apneas during sleep in those individuals with moderate to severe disease. It is clear that in the case of the excessively sleepy individual with cor pulmonale, carbon dioxide retention, and a polycythemia, elimination of apneas during sleep by tracheostomy or by nasal CPAP is desirable and leads to clinical remission, and as indicated by retrospective studies, reduces mortality. The same studies suggest that elimination of apneas in those with moderate disease can reduce mortality; perhaps more importantly, therapy will improve symptoms of sleepiness to the extent that there may be less morbidity from complications such as automobile or industrial accidents.

It is not clear what to do for patients with mild disease or those who snore heavily. The natural history is unclear and therapy is not well developed. However, this is a large population, and untried and unproved therapies abound. These include antisnoring pillows, devices that attach to the glasses that keep one alert, dental prostheses, or other sorts of antisnoring devices. Some may have merit. However, prospective randomized trials are needed to assess beneficial effect not only in terms of patient and/or bed partner satisfaction, but also in terms of physiologic and objective criteria that may relate to morbidity and mortality.

The pyramid shown in Figure 43-5 really relates to that individual with uncomplicated obstructive sleep apnea, that is, those individuals who do not have other concomitant illness. It is known that sleep apnea can complicate other diseases, as outlined in other chapters; hence, distinguishing the effects of sleep apnea from other sorts of diseases that promote sleepiness and/or hypoxic complications is one major task of the clinician.

Studies during Wakefulness

The patient with sleep-disordered breathing should undergo a complete medical examination specifically looking for the presence of cardiovascular, respiratory, or metabolic disturbances that may predispose the patient to or cause repetitive apneas during sleep [48]. Drug addiction or depression may masquerade as sleep apnea, especially in the elderly subject in whom a number of apneas during sleep may be considered "normal." In addition, some patients with sleep apnea (10 percent) may have concomitant narcolepsy, as suggested by family history, and/or evidence for cataplexy. A careful history is the key to recognizing these diseases [24]. Certain diagnostic tests, such as arterial blood gases, thyroid function testing, pulmonary function tests, the ECG, and chest roentgenogram, are routinely indicated to determine the potential cause, presence, or severity of signs of hypoxic exposure occurring as the result of repetitive apneas during sleep.

If the predominant pattern of apnea during sleep consists of repetitive obstructive or mixed apneas, a more detailed examination is indicated to determine the presence of anatomic or pathologic narrowing of the upper airway. Physical examination will exclude pathologic processes. In the patient without pathology, the flow-volume loop may be abnormal and can reveal a pattern consistent with variable extrathoracic obstruction, that is, a decreased inspiratory flow relative to expiratory flow at 50 percent of vital capacity.

Specialized assessment of upper airway structure or function can be performed in the patient without obvious anatomic or pathologic narrowing of the pharynx. Computed tomography has shown nasopharyngeal and pharyngeal narrowing in obese patients; of interest, this narrowing

does not appear to be caused by fat deposition [18]. Measurements of the bony structures and alignment of the jaw to the head and neck (cephalometrics) have revealed individual and familial traits of a relatively shortened mandible; the degree of such trait correlates with the development of sleep apnea. Electromyography of upper airway muscles has shown a correlation between a decrease in muscle activation and the onset of apnea [33,38], yet this finding is universal in patients. The usefulness of nasoendoscopy during wakefulness and sleep is currently being explored as a way of selecting patients for surgical therapy directed at enlarging the airway. Preliminary studies suggest that those patients who exhibit the tendency to obstruct at the level of the nasopharynx, as opposed to the oropharynx, have a greater likelihood of success with uvulopalatopharyngoplasty [23]. Acoustic imaging of the extrathoracic airway has shown that patients with sleep apnea have a smaller and more compliant pharyngeal airway than age- and weight-matched controls. While all these special studies have given insight into potential mechanisms causing sleep apnea, none has shown sufficient specificity or reliability to dictate one or another therapeutic approach. Therefore, none can be recommended in the routine testing of patients.

Multiple sleep latency testing consists of repetitive, hourly observations of the time to sleep onset and REM [41]. Healthy subjects will generally be unable to reproducibly initiate sleep or exhibit REM sleep at hourly intervals during periods of usual wakefulness. Patients with sleep apnea or narcolepsy will fall asleep and even exhibit REMs within 10 minutes of each hourly trial. This test is useful in the laboratory documentation of excessive daytime sleepiness, but its specificity and ability to predict daytime performance in the workplace have not been systematically demonstrated.

Natural History of Sleep Apnea

The natural history of sleep apnea syndrome is largely unknown. While there appear to be clinical categories of disease such as mild, moderate, and severe (see Interpretation of Polysomnographic Studies and Fig. 43-4), there is little evidence showing that progression from health to severe disease occurs according to these categories. There are few longitudinal studies in untreated patients with sleep apnea syndromes; those available have one or two subjects studied

4 to 8 years apart and show little change in the quantitative determination of breathing patterns during sleep. If this is the case, the disease progression is either slower than this time interval or sporadic.

It is proposed that snoring in early life leads to the insidious development of hypersomnolence and cardiovascular disease in patients with obstructive sleep apnea [46]. In support of these suggestions are the findings that a history of heavy snoring is reported in greater than 70 percent of adult patients with obstructive sleep apnea syndrome. Patients and family members often report minor symptoms of hypersomnolence occurring 10 to 20 years prior to diagnosis. Most clinical reports have emphasized the recognition of sleep apnea syndrome in the middle-aged male. Little is known about the natural history of these disorders in women, in the elderly, or in children. However, it is likely that in all groups, symptoms will increase abruptly with the appearance of increased hypoxemia and cardiopulmonary complications.

Death and sleep apnea are associated, but the nature of the association and extent of causality have not been satisfactorily explained [34,37,42]. Early reports of patients with the pickwickian syndrome noted a high in-hospital mortality due to cardiorespiratory failure, pulmonary embolus, and renal failure. Death has been reported to result from sedative drug use, particularly preoperative medications. However, it is the impression of many investigators that automobile accidents related to excessive daytime sleepiness may have a greater impact on morbidity and mortality than cardiovascular complications or other nonaccidental sudden death [14,21].

Pathophysiology

In few patients is there one cause found for sleep apnea [18]. This may not be surprising, since a variety of functional and anatomic factors can interact and produce repetitive apneas during sleep. These include sleep state, changes in respiratory control or mechanics with sleep, body habitus, body position, circulation time and cardiac output, and hereditary factors of respiratory control and upper airway morphology. Certain diseases of the cardiovascular and respiratory system are associated with respiratory disturbances during sleep, but in these instances, it is the disease rather than sleep-disordered breathing that dominates the clinical picture.

Neurophysiology

The rhythmic cycle of a breath depends on interactions between groups of neurons located in the medulla: a dorsal group located in the vicinity of the nucleus tractus solitarius and a ventral group consisting of neurons in the nucleus retro- and para-ambigualis, the nucleus retrofacialis, and nucleus ambigualis (NA). Efferent activity of the cranial nerves which supply upper airway muscles is adjusted by NA activity and the neural discharge to the chest-wall muscles by dorsal medullary nuclei. The activity of these medullary groups of respiratory neurons can be altered by descending pathways from pontine and suprapontine areas and can be affected by the sleep-wake cycle [44,47].

It is difficult to produce apnea by hyperventilation in awake humans, but in anesthetized and sleeping animals and humans there seems to be some threshold level of carbon dioxide that is required to initiate breathing. This threshold level of PCO_2 is decreased by hypoxia in certain subjects, possibly by excitation caused by miscellaneous nonchemical stimuli [11].

The respiratory controller also can influence the activity of the upper airway as well as the muscles of the chest wall [46]. The electrical activity of upper airway muscles often seems to be entrained to the respiratory rhythm, and phasic increases and decreases in the activity of many upper airway muscles can be discerned. The amplitude of these phasic changes can be altered by the same chemical stimuli (carbon dioxide and hypoxia) that affect diaphragm and intercostal muscle activity. Sleep may depress the sensitivity of upper airway muscles to chemical stimulation even more than the diaphragm.

The cardinal feature of sleep apnea syndrome in adults is this presence of recurrent apneas during sleep. Apneas may be central, obstructive, or mixed, but all are repetitively present. Theoretically, the causes of an apneic event include (1) reduced excitatory stimulation; (2) active suppression of breathing from inhibitory reflexes arising from the cardiovascular system, the lungs, and the chest wall or via other somatic and visceral afferents; and (3) loss of the mechanisms that normally ensure the maintenance of ventilation and do not depend on chemical drives.

Two other explanations for repetitive apneas during sleep are (1) that sleep apnea patients have more pronounced ventilatory oscillations during wakefulness and sleep, and (2) that these oscillations have the same amplitude as in normal individuals, but nonspecific excitatory stimuli contribute to a larger extent to sleep apnea patients' total respiratory drive. Apnea occurs rather than just swings in ventilation during sleep because sleep, in addition to reducing the respiratory stimulatory effects of hypoxia and hypercapnia, also depresses metabolic rate and the overall level of respiratory excitatory input.

An alternative idea is that recurrent apneas result from instability in the feedback control of breathing which causes ventilation to cycle rather than maintain a constant level. Instability of feedback control or a spontaneous oscillatory phenomenon could cause central, obstructive, or mixed apneas if in response to the cyclic changes in drive, the mechanical outputs of chest-wall muscles and upper airway muscles are not identical either in phase or in amplitude [46].

Mechanical Properties of the Respiratory System

Significant changes occur in chest-wall and lung mechanics during sleep and can affect ventilation and later the efficiency of gas-exchange and upper airway resistance increases during sleep. For instance, in NREM sleep the ratio of rib cage to abdominal displacement is greater than during wakefulness, while in REM sleep it is less. These changes in movement may affect the distribution of ventilation in the lungs, increasing ventilation-perfusion mismatching, and so contribute to hypoxia, necessitating changes in respiratory output and possibly initiating an unstable breathing pattern.

Negative pressures produced by the chest-wall muscles during inspiration tend to collapse the semirigid structure of the tissues forming the neck and pharynx. The degree of upper airway rigidity can depend both on the morphologic features of the upper airway and on the level of activity in upper airway muscles. Studies suggest that the mechanical features of small airstream size and collapsible airway wall are essential in the pathogenesis of obstructive apneas [46]. Furthermore, the spectrum of disease could relate to graded differences in these mechanical properties.

Obesity

The initial reports emphasized the association between obesity and sleep apnea, but larger clinical series report that only 60 to 70 percent of patients with excessive daytime sleepiness and sleep apnea are obese, as defined by a body weight greater than 120 percent predicted lean body weight for height. Several factors could predispose the obese patient to apneas during sleep. Hypoxemia occurs in the supine posture as a result of decreased functional residual capacity. Patients with obesity can show a decreased ability to respond with increased respiratory muscle output to added loading of the respiratory system. Another factor could be narrowing of the upper airway. Yet the fact remains that many obese people do not have sleep apnea or a history of snoring; neither can it be shown that sleep apneas cause obesity. Thus, the association between obesity and sleep apnea is quite indirect.

Aging and Sex Influences

In the adult population, the peak incidence of sleep apnea syndrome appears to be in the fifth decade of life, and the male-to-female ratio is 3 to 5 : 1. The reason for this is unknown. Referral patterns to sleep centers and the confounding variables of physician recognition and diagnostic standards may contribute to make this association more apparent than real. It is thought that after the sixth decade of life there is an equal incidence of sleep apnea syndrome in males and females, and as already discussed, the incidence of apneas during sleep in apparently healthy subjects generally increases with age. Considerable work is proceeding over the role of sex hormones in influencing respiratory control during both wakefulness and sleep. In support of this approach, several case reports have described an association between androgen administration and the development of the sleep apnea syndrome. Hence it is likely that the level and interplay between sex hormones could have a role in the development of the disease.

Heredity

Sleep apnea syndrome has been shown to exhibit familial clustering, and if snoring is considered as a variant of sleep apnea, the familial incidence of snoring and sleep apnea is quite striking. There is some evidence from cephalometric measurements that the structural arrangement of the jaw to the head and neck is familially determined. Conceivably, individuals with a certain structural framework would be predisposed to apneas. It is also known that there are familial traits in hypercapnic and hypoxic sensitivity; these could relate to the tendency to breathe periodically during sleep. It is not known if there is a familial trait involving the respiratory coordination of muscles of the chest wall and upper airway. In addition, obesity and alcoholism can be family traits, and to the extent that they are causally related to apneas, they could be the basis for familial clustering of subjects with sleep apnea.

Respiratory Depressants: Exogenous or Endogenous

Patients with unrecognized sleep apnea may already be given hypnotic medications on the basis of their sleep complaint. However, studies using flurazepam on breathing during sleep have produced conflicting results on whether or not these agents produce apneas in healthy subjects. No study has shown that these drugs produce a syndrome of sleep apnea with associated daytime symptoms, yet it is best to avoid prescribing these medications to patients with sleep apnea.

On the other hand, alcohol has consistently been shown to promote apnea and, in particular, obstructive apneas during sleep in asymptomatic subjects and in patients. In one study it was shown that the number of episodes of respiratory disturbance during sleep doubled and that the effect of alcohol ingestion may even persist to the subsequent night's sleep. The mechanism by which alcohol promotes apneas may be through a relatively selective reduction in the respiratory output to the genioglossus muscle. What role alcohol has in the development of sleep apnea syndrome is unclear, but patients can benefit from abstinence from alcohol as a therapeutic intervention.

Do endogenous substances produce this syndrome? Naloxone has been given to patients with sleep apnea on the basis of speculation that opiate-like substances produce the problem, yet opiate receptor blockade does not affect apneas during sleep. There are sleep-promoting substances, but their role in sleep apnea has not been defined.

Treatment of Sleep Apnea

General Measures

Therapy is directed at sleep fragmentation and hypoxic exposure. Simple measures may be efficacious in many patients with sleep apnea. Initially, there should be a review of the patient for the presence of anatomic or medical conditions that, if reversed, would ameliorate or eliminate breathing disturbances during sleep. Since respiratory depressants seem to increase the appearance of respiratory disturbances during sleep, perhaps by elevating PCO_2 threshold, withdrawal of respiratory depressants such as major tranquilizers, antihistamine, or alcohol is indicated. There are prophylactic measures on which to advise the patient. Since preoperative sedation has been reported to be accompanied by a risk of lethal respiratory disturbances, the patient should be advised to inform the anesthesiologist of his or her diagnosis prior to any elective surgical procedure. In addition, the excessively sleepy patient should not operate a motor vehicle or engage in activities during which sleep attacks would be hazardous. The risk of serious injury or death from accidents is possibly greater than that of the disease itself.

Metabolic diseases such as hypothyroidism may be associated with sleep apnea syndrome. Treatment with replacement hormones reverses the sleep apnea and clinical symptoms. Patients with sleep apnea and heart or respiratory disease, such as congestive heart failure or asthma, should be placed on maximal therapy for the concomitant disease [46]. Of interest, treatment of hypertension will decrease apneic activity [29]. Decreased circulation time and/or increased oxygenation may reduce the tendency for periodic behavior during sleep and decrease the incidence or severity of respiratory disturbances during sleep [26]. Consequently, therapy is indicated for renal failure or congestive heart failure. In the patient with recent stroke or cerebrovascular disease, time may be all that is needed before respiratory stability will be restored [44]. Treatment should be tailored to the individual patient and to the degree to which he or she is disabled by the breathing disturbances during sleep.

Surgical Procedures

TRACHEOSTOMY

Tracheostomy bypasses the site of obstruction during sleep and is the most effective therapeutic maneuver for obstructive apnea [19]. The procedure of choice is a semipermanent tracheal stoma, using skin flaps leading down to the edges of the tracheal fenestration. However, the tracheostomy may be technically difficult owing to morphologic features such as obesity, a short neck, or a short mandible. Problems with stomal infection and granulation tissue often occur, and it may take a year or more before the tracheal site is well healed.

Tracheostomy is often not well tolerated because it can interfere with speech, exercise, and social interactions. Chronic cough, irritation from cold dry air, and positional pain or dyspnea are also common complaints. In some patients, revision of the tracheal stoma or custom-fit tracheostomy tubes are needed. Considerable education and counseling are advised both before and after the operation.

PLASTIC PROCEDURES

Surgical correction of pathologic narrowing of the upper airway caused by enlarged tonsils, nasal polyps, macroglossia, or micrognathia is reported to improve signs and symptoms of sleep apnea. In prospective studies in which tonsillectomy has been performed for sleep apnea, it has been shown that obstructive apneas may persist, but their frequency is greatly diminished.

There are case reports to suggest that surgical intervention for a deviated nasal septum or for redundant nasal mucosa will reduce the symptoms and signs of sleep apnea [32]. The rationale for these procedures lies in the association between increased nasal resistance and inspiratory pharyngeal occlusion. It should be noted that surgical manipulation of the posterior nasal cavity at the level of the velopharyngeal sphincter may in fact result in airway narrowing and precipitate the development of sleep apnea.

Extensive excision of soft tissue in the oropharynx, termed *uvulopalatopharyngoplasty*, was developed to improve pharyngeal function during sleep [50]. The procedure involves a submucosal resection of redundant tissue from the tonsillar pillars to the arytenoepiglottic folds. The indications for the procedure are the same as for a tracheostomy. In the series of patients reported in the literature, the success rate was approximately 60 percent, but success varied considerably from center to center. Most patients report symptomatic improvement; however, objective improvement of a reduction in the number or magnitude of respiratory disturbances during sleep is often absent. Patients with massive obesity or with anatomic narrowing of the airway may not show success with uvulopalatopharyngoplasty, whereas patients who snore but do not have frank obstructive apneas may do well. Potential complications of the procedure include speech and swallowing difficulties, in particular regurgitation of food. Some patients may have an increased number of respiratory disturbances during sleep after the procedure, but their recognition is obscured because snoring is absent.

These "silent obstructions" may be as severe as apneas prior to surgical intervention.

Recently, new surgical procedures directed at increasing the size of the hypopharynx have been developed. *Expansion hyoidplasty* is a procedure directed at moving the hyoid arch forward by placing a prosthetic device in the hyoid arch [40]. Other procedures include mandibular advancement, mandibular osteotomy, sectioning the hyoid, and midline glossectomy [16,40]. With all these procedures, success in large series of patients remains to be determined.

Medical Treatment

NASAL SPRAYS

There are case reports of successful treatment of obstructive apneas during sleep using nasal vasoconstrictive sprays. Apneas and arousals during sleep are more frequent when the nasal passage is occluded than when it is unoccluded. It is probable that an increase in baseline nasal resistance increases negative pharyngeal pressure on inspiration, thus magnifying the collapsing forces on oropharyngeal soft-tissue structures and promoting pharyngeal obstruction. Consequently, a trial of nasal decongestants is warranted in the patient in whom nasal obstruction is present.

WEIGHT LOSS

Even a 5 to 10 percent decrease in body weight can be accompanied by clinical and objective remission of sleep apnea syndrome in obese subjects. Few investigators, however, are enthusiastic about the long-term efficacy of dietary strategies, perhaps because adherence to dietary restrictions is difficult in the hypersomnolent patient.

Studies have documented that major surgical intervention (ileal bypass or gastric partitioning) for weight loss in obesity can reduce the number and severity of apneas and alleviate signs and symptoms of sleep apnea syndrome. It is interesting that with surgical treatment, large amounts of weight loss, on the order of 150 to 200 lb, may be needed before a beneficial effect of weight loss can be demonstrated.

OXYGEN THERAPY

Studies of oxygen therapy in sleep apnea show inconsistent results [46]. Certainly, in the patient with resting hypoxemia and cor pulmonale, 24-hour oxygen therapy can improve symptoms and cardiovascular performance, alleviating heart failure. Oxygen therapy appears to be effective in reducing or eliminating *central* apneas and hypopneic events. This relatively selective effect on central apneas occurs with oxygen therapy in patients who also have obstructive apneas. However, a beneficial effect of oxygen on upper airway obstruction during sleep cannot be found in every patient. Indeed, in some patients with obstructive sleep apnea syndrome, oxygen administration provokes respiratory acidosis. At the present time, one cannot predict which patient will respond to oxygen therapy.

DRUG THERAPY

General. Various drugs have been used in an attempt to specifically stimulate upper airway muscles in order to prevent obstructive apneas or to increase respiratory neural drive in general in order to alleviate central apneas or increase both upper airway and chest-wall muscle activation. While this kind of therapy would seem optimal, it has had the least success and surprisingly has generated little interest in organized research. The efficacy of most proposed medical therapies has not been demonstrated. However, certain classes of medications have been used with moderate success.

Respiratory Stimulants. Good results have been reported in clinical demonstrations with acetazolamide and progesterone in patients with central apneas during sleep [46]. Studies have shown that respiratory rhythmogenesis may be restored to some degree, thereby eliminating a need for other therapeutic measures. Patients who present with primarily central apneas during sleep are, however, in the minority of adult patients with sleep apnea syndromes. As a consequence, few large series have employed adequate clinical drug trials.

Agents with a progesterone-like activity have been tried in obstructive sleep apnea because of their apparent effectiveness in improving daytime sleepiness, cor pulmonale, and polycythemia in patients presenting with obesity, hypoventilation syndromes, and chronic mountain sickness [46]. It is still unclear how progesterone specifically stimulates breathing. The two clinical demonstrations of progesterone usefulness in sleep apnea have suggested that if patients are considered as a group, progesterone has little effect on obstructive sleep apnea. Yet each study has shown that certain patients may respond with a reduction in obstructive apneas and an amelioration of symptoms. This subclass of patients appears to be those who present with hy-

percapnic respiratory failure. Both studies, however, lacked adequate control trials and were not intended to be adequate clinical trials of efficacy.

There are reports of the use of nicotine, acting both as a central and as a peripheral respiratory stimulant, in the management of obstructive apneas during sleep. While effective, nicotine has a very short half-life, and it is probably not a clinically practical drug. Drugs directed only at stimulation of the carotid body have met with only partial success. These drugs include the dopamine-blocking agent prochlorperazine and the orally administered almitrine. A third medication, strychnine, a glycine antagonist, reduces the threshold for activation of the motor neuron and has been tried in selected patients with obstructive sleep apnea. This report suggested that the beneficial effects of strychnine were produced by elevating tonic activity in upper airway muscles rather than by altering their respiratory-related activation. In summary, respiratory stimulants appear to be more efficacious in patients with primarily central apneas, and use in patients with obstructive sleep apnea may be restricted to those with hypercapnic respiratory failure. A most likely candidate for a trial of progesterone, for instance, would be a patient who presents with obesity hypoventilation syndrome, in whom the drug might be given solely on the basis of daytime signs of polycythemia and cardiopulmonary failure.

Antidepressants. The tricyclic medications protriptyline and clomipramine have been used in the therapy of obstructive sleep apnea. The rationale for their use is that they suppress REM sleep, a sleep stage in which apneas occur frequently and the stage of sleep in which there is often intermittent inhibition of chronic activity in postural muscles, including those of the upper airway. Several uncontrolled trials with protriptyline have suggested that it may have some use in diminishing the number of apneas or in improving oxygenation. The one double-blind trial in the literature found that both 2-week and 6-month administrations were associated with a mild reduction in daytime sleepiness and an unexplained increase in oxygenation associated with a diminished time in REM sleep. Side effects of the drug include drying of the mouth, urine retention, and increased cardiac arrhythmias, including ventricular arrhythmias, and these may limit its use.

More recently, more specific agents, such as the serotonin receptor antagonist fluoxetine, have been shown to reduce apneic activity [20]. The precise role of these agents in the management of sleep apnea remains to be determined.

Hypnotic Drugs. While it may seem odd to suggest that sleep apneic patients be given a drug that promotes sleep, the argument could be made that these agents might increase the tendency for sleep and could, at least theoretically, reduce arousals and sleep fragmentation. It is known that apneas infrequently occur at deep stages of sleep (stages III to IV) and that in healthy subjects apneas appear only in early sleep stages I or II or in the transition between light and deep sleep. There is one report that found that the sleep-promoting substance L-tryptophan can decrease the number of obstructive, but not central, apneas during sleep. A mechanism of action of this drug was presumed to depend on central neural serotonergic transmitters and was related to its ability to promote sleep. There are no large clinical trials of this medication.

Other Agents. A variety of other agents have been tried without success. Bromocryptine, theophylline, and naloxone are three that have been tried in a small number of patients with sleep apnea and have not shown immediate success; therefore, they cannot be recommended even for clinical trials.

The enthusiasm for medical therapy is thus quite moderate at this particular time. It is hoped that with greater understanding of the neurophysiologic basis of respiration in sleep, newer pharmacologic agents can be developed. It should be noted that perhaps one of the reasons for the mixed success of respiratory stimulant drugs in the treatment of apneas in general could be their relative unselectiveness in stimulating muscles. For instance, an increase in chest-wall muscle activity without a corresponding increase in upper airway muscle activity might actually worsen obstructive apneas. Indeed, in some of the clinical trials with progesterone, this actually may have occurred.

MECHANICAL DEVICES

Electrical pacing of the phrenic nerve can achieve adequate ventilation in the absence of spontaneous respiration in the patients with C2–3 spinal injuries. Phrenic nerve pacing at the level of the thoracic inlet also has been successfully attempted in treating patients with only central sleep apnea. Yet stimulation of the diaphragm without upper airway muscle activation may lead to inward collapse of the upper airway and chest wall, producing upper airway obstruction and hypoventilation. Hence a tracheostomy is necessary when the phrenic nerves are paced. Problems inherent with phrenic pacing result from the direct damage to the phrenic nerve occurring with operative handling or with postoperative infection or inflammation around the electrode. Experience and careful surgical technique will minimize these complications. Pacing with electrodes placed directly in the muscle may achieve equal or greater respiratory output in the diaphragm than phrenic pacing.

Ventilatory support also can be achieved by placing the patient with central apneas on mechanical ventilation during sleep. A ventilator attached to a tracheostomy is tolerated well by both children and adults. Other measures such as rocking beds, the iron lung, or a cuirass can effectively accomplish adequate gas exchange in patients with central apneas. However, the creation of negative pressures in the chest by an iron lung or cuirass may cause upper airway obstruction by a mechanism identical to that occurring with phrenic nerve pacing.

Two newer approaches include the use of a dental prosthesis [43] and of electrical stimulation of submental muscles [30]. At present these approaches should be considered experimental demonstrations rather than clinical devices.

NASAL CPAP

Continuous positive pressure applied to the nose (nasal CPAP) may eliminate obstructive apneas during sleep in adult patients with sleep apnea syndrome. Nasal CPAP seems to act as a pneumatic splint, preventing airway collapse [25,46].

Nasal CPAP is effective in the long-term treatment of obstructive sleep apnea and in the prevention of snoring [36,39]. The effect is dependent on the level of positive pressure applied to the upper airway, and the optimal levels of pressure differ among patients. In general, though, at lower levels of pressure (3 to 6 cmH_2O), apneas are eliminated, but episodes of partial upper airway obstruction (snoring) persist. At higher levels of pressure (5 to 15 cmH_2O), regular breathing tends to be restored. An example of the effect of nasal CPAP in eliminating apneas is shown in Figure 43-6. The effect of different levels of nasal CPAP on oxygenation over time is shown in Figure 43-7. Most reports suggest that positive pressures must be present over the entire respiratory cycle for nasal CPAP to be effective.

Some patients can use their device every second or third night and remain free of apnea on

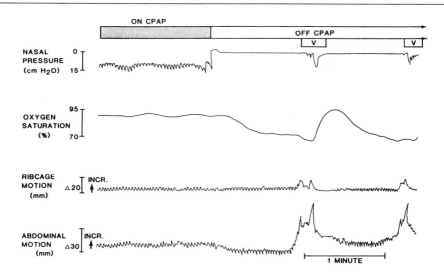

Fig. 43-6. The effects of approximately 14 cmH$_2$O positive pressure applied to the nose (nasal CPAP) on oxygen saturation and rib cage and abdominal motion during sleep. On CPAP, oxygen saturation was stable and approximately 90 percent. Respiratory efforts by the rib cage and abdomen were regular. When CPAP was abruptly discontinued, episodic upper airway obstruction interrupted by periods of ventilation (V) occurred, accompanied by hypoxemia. The patient is in REM sleep.

the intervening nights. Symptoms always recur if CPAP is completely withdrawn, but this may take several days and occurs gradually, so that short interruptions of therapy for surgery or acute medical illnesses are usually well tolerated. Late failures of nasal CPAP occur occasionally. Some are due to poor application of the mask, so that pressure is lost; some are due to too low a pressure being initially prescribed; and some are due to an increase in the pressure required to prevent apnea. Factors such as alcohol use, hypothyroidism, and obesity may worsen airway stability.

There are no contraindications to nasal CPAP therapy. Patients generally accept CPAP therapy fairly well, but in most large series there are some patients who do not [15,49]. Minor side effects of therapy include feelings of suffocation, nasal drying or rhinitis, ear pain, and conjunctivitis. Inner ear and eye problems are said to resolve spontaneously and do not recur with continued CPAP therapy. Pulmonary function does not deteriorate with nasal CPAP, and in patients with lung disease there have been no adverse effects.

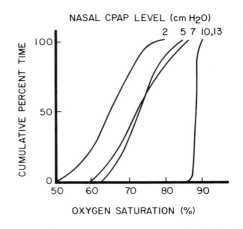

Fig. 43-7. The changes in oxygen saturation over time in one patient in different levels of nasal CPAP during a single study. Levels of 2 and 5 or 7 cmH$_2$O were accompanied by repetitive obstructive apneas and partial upper airway obstruction, respectively. At 10 or 13 cmH$_2$O, apneas and upper airway obstruction were eliminated.

Psychosocial Factors in Treatment

Sleep apnea has a profound effect on the personal and family life of the patient because excessive sleepiness compromises the patient's ability to solve problems at work or at home or to perform even simple tasks. Family members may suffer injury from automobile accidents caused by the patient falling asleep at the wheel. In some instances, chronic delinquency may result from absent parental authority. Patients who are excessively sleepy limit social activities out of embarrassment. These and other family conflicts may result in personal and financial losses before a diagnosis is sought or made.

Treatment of the respiratory disturbance during sleep also entails psychological and social adjustments. Tracheostomy may change a patient's body image. Fears of inviting social ridicule or limitations in sexual activity are frequently present in patients facing the possibility of a tracheostomy. If the patient and family feel reasonably informed of therapeutic alternatives, they will be better able to cope with a tracheostomy. Supervised meetings between patient and family with other patients and their families who have faced the same problem may be of help in this process.

Also, after effective treatment, changes in family dynamics may occur as the patient becomes a more active person. The health team can be helpful in assessing how both the patient and the family are adapting to treatment. Furthermore, employer education is often necessary before the patient can return fully to work.

Need for Basic Research

Unfortunately, our knowledge of respiratory disorders of sleep is at a descriptive level and, as a consequence, the management is not based on a detailed understanding of the sequence of pathophysiologic events. At the present time, clinical indications for treatment are clear only for those with severe disease, as indicated by signs of hypoxic stress (polycythemia and right ventricular hypertrophy), cardiac arrhythmias, and disabling daytime sleepiness. There is, however, a large group of asymptomatic subjects (30 to 50 percent of the population) who snore heavily and have occasional apneas, and this large group of people is considered at risk for development of overt sleep apnea syndrome as well as being the population in whom qualitative traits of sleep apnea are associated with cognitive dysfunction, stroke, hypertension, and sudden death.

If one could better define the relationship between quantifiable physiologic or biochemical measures and the qualitative symptoms and signs of morbidity, one could begin to track or identify those patients at risk for developing disease from sleep-disordered breathing and to specify the need for, the time for, and the type of therapeutic intervention in an individual patient. Current clinical and physiologic evidence suggests that consequences of sleep-disordered breathing represent the effect of chronic intermittent disruptions in normal oxygenation and sleep. Given this conceptual framework, the basic humoral, neural, mechanical, and biochemical mechanisms by which physiologic systems respond to changes in state (e.g., wakefulness to sleep, or to hypoxemia and sleep interruption) are not well understood.

In the past 10 years, independent investigators in pulmonary medicine, cardiology, neurology, and psychiatry have begun to form new collaborations to focus on the basis of the pathophysiology of sleep-disordered breathing so that insights gathered in basic physiology and clinical practice can be applied to the problems encountered in the recognition, treatment, and ultimately prevention of sleep apnea syndrome and related sleep-disordered cardiorespiratory events. The economy of the current funding climate has promoted greater interdependence of models and techniques among these different disciplines as well as with the national community at large.

The pathophysiology of sleep apnea allows us to address, in a multidisciplinary manner, aspects of cellular and organ-system physiology relevant to understanding events related to sleep, sleep hypoxemia, and sleep interruption. The major systems currently being examined are in the broad categories of control and mechanical function of the upper airway, control of cardiorespiratory function during sleep, and brain neurophysiology and neuropharmacology. Investigation of these systems will begin to elucidate interactions between sleep and breathing and the mechanisms for sleep-disordered breathing. Another approach is to study the adaptations to sleep-disordered breathing on the assumption that the basis of the clinical syndromes may relate to the disruptions in complementary homeostatic systems rather than to a definable lesion such as a genetic defect. These themes would include the competition of central and peripheral influences on upper airway and cardiovascular responses and the interactions between hypoxic adaptations affecting hematocrit, neuroendocrine function, and brain blood flow. Understanding the time course and impact of these adaptations also requires communication of investigators from various disciplines. As a result, new perspectives will develop and new information on pathophysiology will be useful in designing and evaluating therapeutic interventions in patients.

A primary theme is the hypothesis that the development of morbidity in sleep apnea is dependent on the response to hypoxic exposure. Hypoxia is known to influence all cells to one degree or another; however, the pattern of cellular responses and subsequent organ dysfunction in response to hypoxic exposure varies from transient cognitive effects of mild hypoxia to long-term sequelae, like polycythemia and pulmonary hypertension. It is assumed that patients with sleep apnea experience the complications of hypoxia, yet there are other events in sleep apnea (airway occlusion, arousal, hypercapnia, etc.) that could modify, by amplification or attenuation, hypoxic effects. Alternatively, these other events would be more important than hypoxia. In addition, if any of these factors explain the behavioral, hematologic, and autonomic complications of sleep apnea, then the paradigm for understanding disease should be based on chronic intermittent events during sleep (rather than wakefulness) and during brief exposure (seconds to minutes rather than hours at a time). It may be that the intermittent nature of sleep-disordered breathing results in different patterns of cellular and organ dysfunction than the more common paradigm of steady-state exposure.

It is recognized that the pattern of sleep disruption in sleep apnea syndrome is chaotic and intermittent; hence, the usual model of general sleep deprivation is not precisely applicable to the pathophysiologic state. Rather the paradigm is one that is better categorized as sleep interruption or, as in the case of apneas only during REM sleep, selective interruption of sleep. How these factors influence daytime sleepiness, cognitive and affective dysfunction, and autonomic imbalance is poorly understood. It may be that the symptoms of sleep apnea relate to an individual's tolerance for sleep interruption. Alternatively, experiences in early life that link sleep with respiratory rhythm could be important in determining the impact or, more speculatively, the incidence of sleep-disordered breathing in the adult. Certainly, behavioral as well as genetic substrates could play a role in disease expression.

One crucial area of research likely to provide direction to this field is that of epidemiologic investigations. Many factors and mechanisms are identified in the study of patients; however, the insight into general mechanisms and into disease control from this approach is limited because of the adaptive and maladaptive responses that occur in disease. Rather, longitudinal studies in nonselected general populations will provide data needed to measure disease and attempts at prevention.

Last but not least is the issue of the medical significance of sleep. First, the impact of sleep in health and disease has garnered more speculation than data. From the patient point of view, sleep quality is a measure of satisfaction in the treatment of medical illness. From the physician point of view, sleep-wake cycles can and will alter disease progression, disease manifestation, and in regard to circadian changes in metabolism, the optimization of therapy. Hence, consideration of the sleep is an issue relevant for internal medicine. Second is the issue of the function and mechanisms for sleep itself. This is an essential issue related closely to many of the concerns discussed above.

Cardiopulmonary disorders of sleep are common and important health problems in need of better therapy and disease prevention. In addition, the understanding required to solve these disorders requires broad knowledge in human physiology and common communication among disparate medical and surgical specialties. Prevention and management of these disorders may be achieved by fostering interdependence rather than independence among investigators in basic science and clinical practice.

Variant Presentations of Sleep-Disordered Breathing

Upper Airway Disease

Patients with disease of the nose, larynx, and pharynx present with two major classes of sleep problems—sleep apnea and aspiration. Aspiration of secretions may occur because of excessive production of mucus, as exemplified by chronic allergic rhinitis, or because of inadequate neuromuscular tone, as in bilateral recurrent laryngeal nerve paralysis. In both instances, there occur frequent arousals from sleep associated with cough and/or a choking sensation. In sleep, and, in particular, in REM sleep, the cough response is less than during wakefulness. As a result, greater amounts of secretions are tolerated before a cough ensues. After awakening, this larger amount of material may precipitate paroxysmal cough. It is important to recognize that in these cases the disturbed sleep and what might sound like apnea result from problems with secretions or aspiration. Treatment with hypnotic medications may be particularly harmful, since greater amounts of secretions may be tolerated before arousal from sleep, increasing the likelihood of aspiration injury to the lungs. In the patient with allergic rhinitis, nasal decongestants given before bedtime may be helpful. In the patient with neuromuscular impairment, elevation of the bed may diminish the tendency to aspirate pharyngeal contents.

Chronic Obstructive Pulmonary Disease

Patients with chronic obstructive pulmonary disease (COPD) may present with a variety of sleep problems [12]. Nocturnal cough can be related to bronchitis. Insomnia may be the consequence of therapy with drugs such as aminophylline. Hypoxemia during sleep may occur as a consequence of mechanical impairment of the airways already present during wakefulness but exacerbated by the normal changes in gas exchange during sleep. There seems to be an association between the occurrence of hypoxemia only during sleep and the development of cor pulmonale in the patient with moderately severe COPD. Recognition of these individuals occurs when it is noticed that features of hypoxemia and hypercapnia are not associated with a severe mechanical defect on pulmonary function testing. Certainly other diagnostic entities such as recurrent pulmonary emboli or chest-wall muscle weakness also should be explored. Hypoventilation will occur during sleep not only because of sleep apnea, but also because of changes in ventilation-perfusion matching and a decrease in respiratory drive, especially during REM sleep. If the problem is sleep apnea, usually there is historical evidence for snoring and restless sleep, and the patient should be treated appropriately (see above). If apneas are not the problem, treatment with supplemental oxygen only during sleep may be indicated.

Patients with severe COPD recently have been shown to improve their arterial blood gases and lung function after brief periods of time in a negative-pressure cuirass ventilator. These changes are associated with improved indices of respiratory muscle strength and endurance. It is thought that these patients may experience chronic muscle fatigue because of their severe mechanical lung function and that the time in the cuirass serves as a brief rest period for the muscles of the chest wall. These observations suggest a role for the use of negative-pressure ventilators, perhaps even during sleep, in the management of patients with COPD.

Asthma

The most common sleep problem associated with asthma is cough. Cough and arousals from sleep with cough may be the presenting complaints of the patient with asthma and increased airway reactivity. Cough may result from changes in airway smooth-muscle tone during sleep and of bronchoconstriction during REM sleep. There is some indication that gastroesophageal reflux may precipitate bronchoconstriction; however, patients with reflux are usually symptomatic during wakefulness as well as sleep. Cough occurring in the patient with uncomplicated asthma may indicate inadequate therapeutic effect of medication throughout the night or exacerbation of airway disease.

A related clinical problem is that of "morning dipping," which refers to the fall in lung function that occurs in the early morning hours. Morning dipping has been reported in severe asthmatic attacks and has been held somewhat responsible for deaths from asthma. Morning dipping represents an extreme form of diurnal variation in lung function present in most patients with airway reactivity. Reports describing morning dipping emphasize that lung function measured some hours later during the day may be normal, while values during the night may show moderately severe airway obstruction. Symptoms suggestive of morning dipping are an indication that additional treatment is needed. If nocturnal symptoms are persistently bothersome, instruction of the patient in the use of a peak-flow measurement device and in the frequent recording of values of peak flow at night may be helpful in identifying changes in lung function throughout the day and in monitoring the effectiveness of medications over the course of a night's sleep.

Neuromuscular Disorders

Respiratory disturbances due to obstructive apneas during sleep may occur because upper airway muscles such as the genioglossus are affected by the underlying disease process. Inadequate respiratory activation of upper airway muscles makes the upper airway vulnerable to collapse during inspiratory efforts by the muscles of the chest wall. Indeed, respiratory failure in the patient with neuromuscular disease may be due to upper airway muscle disease and not have as dire prognostic consequences as primary involvement of the chest-wall muscles such as the diaphragm.

Disturbances of sleep and respiration during sleep may be the first indication of involvement of the respiratory system in the patient with neuromuscular disease. Occasionally, sleep fragmentation and the effects of sleep deprivation dominate the clinical presentation of the patient with neuromuscular disease. After treatment for sleep-disordered breathing, the clinical manifestations of the primary neuromuscular disorder may not appear so severe.

Kyphoscoliosis

Severe kyphoscoliosis is associated with restrictive lung disease and cor pulmonale; however, recently it has been shown that treatment of hypercapnic respiratory failure by tracheostomy with or without positive-pressure ventilator support during sleep can reverse cor pulmonale and improve the appearance of the chest roentgenogram.

Interstitial Diseases

Restrictive lung disease also can be associated with respiratory disturbances during sleep due to cough or hypoxemia. Patients also may have a concomitant sleep apnea. Sleep hypoxemia may be a factor in the development of pulmonary hypertension. Treatment of sleep hypoxemia is directed at apneas, or if apneas are not present, a trial of oxygen therapy may be indicated.

A restrictive defect on pulmonary function testing and interstitial fibrosis on the chest roentgenogram can reflect a history of chronic aspiration. There are ongoing investigations on aspiration during sleep and its acute and chronic effect on lung function. During sleep, the tone of the gastroesophageal junction relaxes, allowing stomach contents to regurgitate to the level of the pharynx. In patients in whom such a phenomenon is suspected, it may be useful to measure pH levels in the pharynx and esophagus during sleep in order to document gastroesophageal reflux during sleep as a potential cause for aspiration pneumonitis.

References

1. Aldrich MS. Neurologic aspects of sleep apnea and related respiratory disturbances. *Otolaryngol Clin North Am* 23:761, 1990.
2. Ancoli-Israel S, et al. Sleep apnea in female patients in a nursing home. Increased risk of mortality. *Chest* 96:1054, 1989.
3. ATS Consensus Conference. Indications and standards for cardiopulmonary sleep studies. *Am Rev Respir Dis* 139:559, 1989.
4. Bedard MA, et al. Nocturnal hypoxemia as a determinant of vigilance impairment in sleep apnea syndrome. *Chest* 100:367, 1991.
5. Block AJ. Polysomnography: Some difficult questions (editorial). *Ann Intern Med* 95:644, 1981.
6. Bradley TD, et al. Role of daytime hypoxemia in the pathogenesis of right heart failure in the obstructive sleep apnea syndrome. *Am Rev Respir Dis* 131:835, 1985.
7. Burwell C, et al. Extreme obesity associated with alveolar hypoventilation: A pickwickian syndrome. *Am J Med* 21:811, 1956.
8. Chan HS, et al. Obstructive sleep apnea presenting with nocturnal angina, heart failure, and near-miss sudden death. *Chest* 99:1023, 1991.
9. Coleman RM, et al. Sleep-wake disorders based on polysomnographic diagnosis (A National Cooperative Study). *JAMA* 247:997, 1982.
10. Crocker BD, et al. Estimation of the probability of disturbed breathing during sleep before a sleep study. *Am Rev Respir Dis* 142:14, 1990.
11. Dempsey JA, Skatrud JB. A sleep-induced apneic threshold and its consequences. *Am Rev Respir Dis* 133:1163, 1986.
12. Douglas NJ, Flenley DC. State of the art. Breathing during sleep in patients with obstructive lung disease. *Am Rev Respir Dis* 141:1055, 1990.
13. Ehlenz K, et al. Reduction of nocturnal diuresis and natriuresis during treatment of obstructive sleep apnea (OSA) with nasal continuous positive air pressure (nCPAP) correlates to cGMP excretion. *Med Klin* 86:294, 1991.
14. Findley LJ, Weiss JW, Jabour ER. Drivers with untreated sleep apnea. A cause of death and serious injury. *Arch Intern Med* 151:1451, 1991.
15. Fletcher EC, Luckett RA. The effect of positive reinforcement on hourly compliance in nasal continuous positive airway pressure users with obstructive sleep apnea. *Am Rev Respir Dis* 143:936, 1991.
16. Fujita S, et al. Laser midline glossectomy as a treatment for obstructive sleep apnea. *Laryngoscope* 101:805, 1991.
17. Gastaut H, Tassinari CA, Duron B. Polygraphic study of the episodic diurnal and nocturnal (hypnic and respiratory) manifestations of the Pickwick syndrome. *Brain Res* 1:167, 1966.
18. Guilleminault C, Mondini S. Need for multidiagnostic approaches before considering treatment in obstructive sleep apnea. *Bull Eur Physiopathol Respir* 19:583, 1983.
19. Guilleminault C, et al. Obstructive sleep apnea syndrome and tracheostomy: Long-term follow-up experience. *Arch Intern Med* 141:985, 1981.
20. Hanzel DA, Proia NG, Hudgel DW. Response of

obstructive sleep apnea to fluoxetine and pro-triptyline. *Chest* 100:416, 1991.

21. Haraldsson PO, et al. Clinical symptoms of sleep apnea syndrome and automobile accidents. *ORL J Otorhinolaryngol Relat Spec* 52:57, 1990.

22. Hudgel DW. Neuropsychiatric manifestations of obstructive sleep apnea: A review. *Int J Psychiatry Med* 19:11, 1989.

23. Hudgel DW, et al. Uvulopalatopharyngoplasty in obstructive sleep apnea. Value of preoperative localization of site of upper airway narrowing during sleep. *Am Rev Respir Dis* 143:942, 1991.

24. Kales A, Soldatos CR, Kales JD. Taking a sleep history. *Am Fam Physician* 22:101, 1980.

25. Kaplan J, Staats BA. Obstructive sleep apnea syndrome. *Mayo Clin Proc* 65:1087, 1990.

26. Kimmel PL, Miller G, Mendelson WB. Sleep apnea syndrome in chronic renal disease. *Am J Med* 86:308, 1989.

27. Lavie P. Incidence of sleep apnea in a presumably healthy working population: A significant relationship with excessive daytime sleepiness. *Sleep* 6:312, 1983.

28. Maillard D, et al. Decreased oxyhemoglobin affinity in patients with sleep apnea syndrome. *Am Rev Respir Dis* 143:486, 1991.

29. Mayer J, et al. Influence of metoprolol and cilazapril in blood pressure and on sleep apnea activity. *J Cardiovasc Pharmacol* 16:952, 1990.

30. Miki H, et al. Effects of submental electrical stimulation during sleep on upper airway patency in patient with obstructive sleep apnea. *Am Rev Respir Dis* 140:1285, 1989.

31. Miles LE, Broughton RJ (Eds), *Medical Monitoring in the Home and Work Environment.* New York: Raven, 1990.

32. Olsen KD, Kern EB. Nasal influences on snoring and obstructive sleep apnea. *Mayo Clin Proc* 65:1095, 1990.

33. Onal E, Lopata M, O'Connors T. Pathogenesis of apneas in hypersomnia-sleep apnea syndrome. *Am Rev Respir Dis* 125:167, 1982.

34. Partinen M, Guilleminault C. Daytime sleepiness and vascular morbidity at seven-year follow-up in obstructive sleep apnea patients. *Chest* 97:27, 1990.

35. Podszus TE. Hemodynamics in sleep apnea. *Prog Clin Biol Res* 345:353, 1990.

36. Rauscher H, et al. Acceptance of CPAP therapy for sleep apnea. *Chest* 100:1019, 1991.

37. Remmers JE. Sleep apnea. In *Proceedings of the Annual Meeting of the Medical Section of the American Council of Life Insurance.* 1990. P 75.

38. Remmers JE, et al. Pathogenesis of upper airway occlusion during sleep. *J Appl Physiol* 44:931, 1978.

39. Remmers JE, et al. Nasal positive airway pressure in patients with occlusive sleep apnea. *Am Rev Respir Dis* 130:1152, 1984.

40. Riley RW, Powell NB, Guilleminault C. Maxillary, mandibular, and hyoid advancement for treatment of obstructive sleep apnea: A review of 40 patients. *J Oral Maxillofac Surg* 48:20, 1990.

41. Roehrs T, et al. Sleep-wake complaints in patients with sleep-related respiratory disturbances. *Am Rev Respir Dis* 132:520, 1985.

42. Roth T, Roehrs T, Kryger M. Mortality in obstructive sleep apnea. *Prog Clin Biol Res* 345:347, 1990.

43. Schmidt-Nowara WW, Meade TE, Hays MB. Treatment of snoring and obstructive sleep apnea with a dental orthosis. *Chest* 99:1378, 1991.

44. Skatrud JB, Dempsey JA. Interaction of sleep state and chemical stimuli in sustaining rhythmic ventilation. *J Appl Physiol* 55:813, 1983.

45. Stoohs R, Guilleminault C. Obstructive sleep apnea syndrome or abnormal upper airway resistance during sleep? *J Clin Neurophysiol* 7:83, 1990.

46. Strohl KP, Cherniack NS, Gothe B. Physiologic basis for therapy of sleep apnea. *Am Rev Respir Dis* 134:791, 1986.

47. Sullivan CE, et al. Ventilatory control in sleep apnea: A search for brain neurochemical defects. *Prog Clin Biol Res* 345:325, 1990.

48. Viner S, Szalai JP, Hoffstein V. Are history and physical examination a good screening test for sleep apnea? *Ann Intern Med* 115:356, 1991.

49. Waldhorn RE, et al. Long-term compliance with nasal continuous positive airway pressure therapy of obstructive sleep apnea. *Chest* 97:33, 1990.

50. Zorick F, et al. Effects of uvulopalatopharyngoplasty on the daytime sleepiness associated with sleep apnea syndrome. *Bull Eur Physiopathol Respir* 19:600, 1983.

51. Zwillich C, et al. Bradycardia during sleep apnea: Characteristics and mechanism. *J Clin Invest* 60:1286, 1982.

44

Adaptation and Maladaptation to High Altitude

Robert B. Schoene

Oxygen delivery to the tissues depends on an adequate supply of oxygen at each step of the oxygen transport chain from the inspired air to the mitochondria. The inspired partial pressure of oxygen is approximately 21 percent of the atmospheric pressure, which decreases predictably at altitudes above sea level (Table 44-1). Humans at high altitude, therefore, must overcome the disadvantage of ambient hypoxia by making a number of adaptations to optimize the availability of oxygen to the tissues.

For the sojourner, easy access to high altitude for work or recreation requires that the body must undergo rapid changes to overcome the disadvantage of hypoxia; for the nearly 30 million people who live at a high altitude in Asia, Africa, and North and South America, their bodies have had generations to adapt to the hypoxic stress. A large majority of travelers and high-altitude dwellers are successful in overcoming this stress, but some do not adapt well and suffer from acute and chronic altitude illness. This chapter, therefore, first reviews what is known about both acute and chronic adaptation to high altitude and then reviews the illnesses that occur when the body maladapts.

Adaptation

Abrupt exposure to high altitude (more than 3000 m) can result in illness and even death. This lesson was tragically learned in 1875 when two of three scientists died while exploring altitudes of over 8000 m in their hot-air balloon, the Zenith. Gradual ascent to these same heights, on the other hand, permits a number of physiologic adaptations to take place that allow some exceptional humans to function quite well. Populations have lived for centuries as high as 5000 m, while brief forays above 8000 m, where the atmospheric pressure is a third that at sea level, are well documented and are a tribute to the resiliency of human physiology.

In order to optimize oxygen delivery, important compensations take place at each step of the oxygen cascade, which has a number of components: ventilation, matching of ventilation with blood flow, diffusion of oxygen from the air to the blood, circulation of the blood, diffusion of oxygen from the red blood cell to the tissue, and oxidative metabolism in the cell. The first portion of this chapter reviews each of these steps, beginning with the lung.

Pulmonary

VENTILATION

Acute Ventilatory Response. An increase in alveolar ventilation occurs immediately upon ascent to a high altitude. The partial pressures of oxygen and carbon dioxide in the alveolus reflect the degree of hyperventilation that attempts to preserve oxygen partial pressure [21,91,120,181]. For instance, at an extreme altitude (summit of Mt. Everest, 8848 m, 253 mmHg), alveolar ventilation in a climber increases to maintain an alveolar partial pressure of oxygen of about 32 mmHg and of carbon dioxide of about 8 to 10 mmHg [238]. Lower altitudes have a proportionately lower degree of ventilation.

The increase in ventilation is a result of a complex interaction of physiologic events, mediated largely by the hypoxic stimulus to the carotid body. The course of the ventilatory response is what constitutes ventilatory acclimatization. There is individual variation in this response, but

Table 44-1. **U.S. standard atmosphere: Altitude, barometric pressure, and inspired partial pressure of oxygen***

Altitude		Barometric pressure (mmHg)	Inspired PO_2 (mmHg)
Meters	Feet		
0	0	760.0	159.1
1000	3280	674.4	141.2
2000	6560	596.3	124.9
3000	9840	525.8	110.1
4000	13,120	462.8	96.9
5000	16,400	405.0	84.8
6000	19,680	354.0	79.1
8000	26,240	267.8	56.1
8848	29,028	253.0	43.1

*Values except 8848 are taken for midlatitude (45°N). There is greater variation at higher latitudes.
SOURCE: Modified from PL Altman, DS Dittmer (Eds), *Respiration and Circulation*. Bethesda, MD: Federation of American Societies for Experimental Biology, 1971. Pp 12–13.

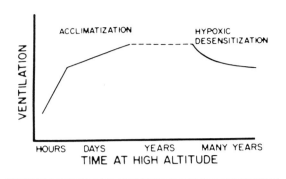

Fig. 44-1. The time course of ventilatory adaptation to high-altitude exposure. (From JV Weil. Ventilatory Control at High Altitude. In *Handbook of Physiology: The Respiratory System*, Vol 2: *Control of Breathing*, Part 2. Bethesda, MD: American Physiological Society, 1986. Chap 21.)

essentially the pattern of any given level of high altitude is one of an abrupt increase in ventilation followed by a more gradual increase over the next 10 to 14 days to a plateau (Fig. 44-1). The carotid body plays a primary role in this acute ventilatory response [4,35,154,169], which may be blunted in part by the resulting alkalosis. The classic explanation for the subsequent ventilatory events goes as follows: Excretion of bicarbonate by the kidneys over days in compensation for the respiratory alkalosis partially restores the acid-base status, resulting in further respiratory stimulation.

An arterial alkalemia is still present, however, and Severinghaus and colleagues [205] presented data showing a cerebrospinal fluid (CSF) acidosis which they claimed was the central stimulus for ventilation. Subsequent investigators [20, 42–44,62,139,234] at altitudes from 3000 to 4000 m documented that in humans and animals, both blood and CSF alkalosis developed in parallel during acclimatization. Additionally, a lower but persistent hyperventilation continued upon descent [16,41,60,173,234]. In light of the loss of hypoxic stimulus upon descent and a blood and CSF alkalosis, a further explanation was sought.

The CSF may not reflect the actual milieu around the chemosensors. Data from brain interstitial and intercellular fluid in animals show an acidosis during hypoxic exposure, which may account for stimulation of ventilation [56,175]. Recent data [168] may shed light on the ongoing re-

spiratory stimulation in the face of blood and CSF alkalosis. Ventilation is stimulated by hypoxia, leading to a degree of hypocapnia that is proportional to the magnitude of ventilation. Hypocapnia decreases cerebral blood flow, which in addition to a leftward shift of the oxygen-hemoglobin dissociation curve by the respiratory alkalemia, may result in a decreased delivery of oxygen to the brain and subsequent anaerobic metabolism and tissue acidosis. A study in humans which used nuclear magnetic resonance (NMR) spectroscopy before and after a 7-day exposure to a simulated 4300-m altitude in a hypobaric chamber, however, failed to document brain tissue acidosis.

A further increase in ventilation is inhibited by a central suppression of ventilation. After 15 to 25 minutes of acute hypoxic exposure, ventilation decreases 25 to 30 percent [101], which is thought to be secondary to the action of neurotransmitters and a decrease in the metabolic rate in the brain [172,187], even though ventilation is elevated to a greater degree than the decrease in the metabolic rate alone would dictate. Acutely, however, true depression of ventilation with hypoxia does not occur when the partial pressure of arterial oxygen falls below 20 mmHg. A full understanding of the ventilatory adaptation to altitude is clearly lacking.

A further stay at a high altitude for the sojourner results in an improvement in arterial oxygen saturation, secondary to a gradual increase in ventilation over a fortnight or so [181]. At extreme altitude, ventilatory adaptation may take weeks or months or may never be complete [24]. The mechanism of this subsequent adaptation is not understood, but an increased sensitivity of the carotid body has been observed in humans [61,198,227] and animals [16,36,169] and must play an important role in the progressive hyperventilation. Carbon dioxide sensitivity, which is mediated primarily in the central chemosensors, has also been shown to increase with time at a high altitude [49,154,198] and may, therefore, interact with input from the carotid body to effect an increase in ventilation.

Upon descent, even after the hypoxic stimulus has been removed, ventilation is greater for at least a couple of days than it was prior to ascent [41,198]. This phenomenon may be secondary to the rise in carbon dioxide that occurs as the hypoxic stimulus is removed [69].

Chronic Ventilatory Response. Alveolar ventilation and hypoxic chemosensitivity decrease in most lifelong residents of high-altitude regions [21,33,47,107,133,135,136,139,157,203,209,223,233] (see Fig. 44-1). This decrease in hypoxic drive occurs in spite of a hypertrophy of the carotid bodies [4,94] and is proportional to both the altitude and the duration of habitation [61,134,135,233]. The relative hypoventilation of the high-altitude native compared to sojourners may predispose some populations to chronic mountain sickness (CMS), which involves excessive hypoxemia and hypoventilation, pulmonary hypertension, polycythemia, and decreased cerebral function (see Chronic Mountain Sickness). Natives of the Tibetan and Nepal Himalayas, in whom CMS is very rare, are reported to have less blunted alveolar ventilation and hypoxic chemosensitivity [80, 81,107] than other high-altitude dwellers, especially those in the Andes of South America, where CMS is much more common, but this issue is not fully resolved. This intriguing difference suggests an evolutionary influence wherein the Tibetans who have lived at a high altitude much longer than the South Americans have physiologic characteristics that have led to more successful tolerance of high altitude. A genetic factor is also theoretically possible.

FUNCTIONAL AND STRUCTURAL CHANGES
Lung mechanics are affected at least transiently upon ascent to a high altitude. Increased blood flow and central blood volume and a possible increase in interstitial fluid may lead to a decreased vital capacity [31,47,117,140,152,223], an increased residual volume [31], and decreased

lung compliance [152]. Increased lung water, which usually resolves upon acclimatization, also has been noted [102,117]. High-altitude dwellers in South America, on the other hand, have large chests on physical examination [112,160], accompanied by larger vital capacities, compared to low-altitude dwellers [22,64,65]. The younger the age that the subjects begin living at a high altitude, the more pronounced is this characteristic.

GAS EXCHANGE
The increased ventilation upon ascent to a high altitude results in an increased alveolar partial pressure of oxygen, but the arterial oxygen content depends on the transfer of oxygen from the alveolus to the capillary and red blood cells. This step requires matching of ventilation ($\dot{V}A$) to perfusion ($\dot{Q}$) and the diffusion of oxygen to hemoglobin in the red blood cell.

The increase in ventilation is matched in part by an increase in cardiac output and pulmonary blood flow [66,127,228,232,238]. Alveolar hypoxia leads to pulmonary vasoconstriction [59,189], which at rest improves the $\dot{V}A/\dot{Q}$ match primarily by increasing blood flow to the apical portions of the lung, which are usually areas of high $\dot{V}A/\dot{Q}$ [37,38,66,92,219]. This redistribution of blood flow results in greater homogeneity of $\dot{V}A/\dot{Q}$.

The next step in gas exchange relies on diffusion of oxygen to the blood. This transfer depends on a pressure gradient for oxygen from the alveolus to the capillary, diffusion capacity of the alveolar-capillary interface (DM), capillary blood volume (VC), and the surface area for gas exchange. A true diffusion limitation for oxygen transfer exists at high altitudes. This phenomenon occurs for several reasons. With increasing altitude, the lower alveolar partial pressure of oxygen results in a lower alveolar-capillary oxygen pressure gradient. Full equilibration of oxygen to the blood is also dependent on the transit time of the red blood cell across the pulmonary capillary, usually requiring at sea level about 0.25 second (one-third) of the estimated 0.75-second normal transit time. At high altitude, this estimated resting pulmonary transit time may not allow enough time for full equilibration. This problem is accentuated during exercise, when an increased cardiac output shortens transit time. For example, the circumstances at the summit of Mt. Everest, where the barometric pressure is about 250 mmHg are expressed by a model for this diffusion limitation with given values for hemoglobin concentration, oxygen face area consumption

($\dot{V}O_2$), diffusion capacity (D_M), acid-base status, and capillary transit time as shown in Figure 44-2 [204].

An important factor in this process at extreme altitude may be relatively high oxygen-hemoglobin affinity secondary to respiratory alkalosis found in some high-altitude animals and in climbers at extreme altitudes [235]. The diffusion capacity of the lung (D_L) may be more optimal in high-altitude natives secondary to either an increased capillary surface area (D_M) or pulmonary blood volume (V_C) [25,40,45,77,113,129,185,199, 225,226], which may compensate for the slightly lower level of ventilation at rest and during exercise.

Cardiovascular Adaptation

CARDIAC RESPONSE
The cardiac response to high altitude also counteracts the stress of hypoxia and optimizes oxygen transport. To maintain a viable oxygen consumption in light of a decreased arterial oxygen content at a high altitude, heart rate increases, which results in a greater cardiac output [123, 151,212,228,230]. An accompanying elevation of catecholamines suggests that they mediate the increase in chronotropic effect on the heart [34,151,155,170,182]. Subsequently, over the next few days, resting heart rate decreases as other compensatory mechanisms are invoked. Stroke volume decreases secondary to either a lower

plasma volume or an increased pulmonary vascular resistance [2].

During exercise at high altitudes, the relationship between cardiac output and work is maintained [230], but both maximal work rates and cardiac output achieved at sea level are not reached at high altitudes [26,48,66,180,210,212,216, 231,237,239]. Both stroke volume and maximal heart rate are lower at high altitudes. The lower maximal heart rate is more marked in sojourners [180,237]; may be secondary to hypervagal tone, hypoxic myocardial depression, or dysfunction of electrical conduction; and may be a major factor in the decrease in maximal exercise at high altitude. There are, however, few data in sojourners to support these possibilities, and it is now generally thought that the cardiac response is appropriate for the amount of work that is being done which is limited by other factors. Studies in a few high-altitude natives suggest that they may not have a limitation to maximal heart rate at high

Fig. 44-2. Comparison of the calculated time course of partial pressure of oxygen in the pulmonary capillary of a climber at rest at sea level (*left*) (P_B = 760 mmHg) and the summit of Mt. Everest (*right*) (P_B = 250 mmHg). Adequate time for equilibration is available at sea level, while at 8848 full equilibration is not possible. *PB* = barometric pressure; $\dot{V}O_2$ = oxygen consumption; D_MO_2 = diffusion capacity of oxygen at the alveolar-capillary interface. (From JB West, PD Wagner. Predicted gas exchange on the summit of Mt. Everest. *Respir Physiol* 42:1, 1980.)

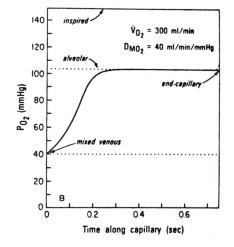

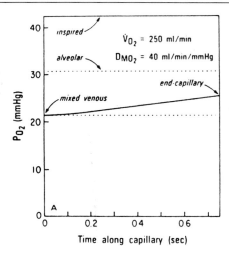

levels of exercise [74,139], but further work is needed to elucidate this question.

Acute exposure to high altitudes results in an increase in systemic blood pressure and systemic vascular resistance both at rest and during exercise, whereas the dweller at a high altitude may actually develop a lower systemic blood pressure, perhaps secondary to microcirculatory vasodilation [176].

PULMONARY VASCULAR RESPONSE

Pulmonary artery pressure and pulmonary vascular resistance increase acutely at high altitudes, and this is secondary to the hypoxic pulmonary vascular response (HPVR). This initially results in improved $\dot{V}A/\dot{Q}$ matching [37–39,59, 66,79,92,127,141,189,219,228,238], but may progress to $\dot{V}A/\dot{Q}$ heterogeneity and possible interstitial edema [232].

HPVR does not become marked until an alveolar partial pressure of oxygen (PAO_2) of 60 mmHg or less is reached, and as with the ventilatory response to hypoxia, there is individual and interspecies variation of HPVR [184]. Prolonged exposure to hypoxia may lead to pulmonary hypertension [96,147,189]. Sojourners may have a more reactive HPVR than high-altitude natives [32]. Smooth muscle hypertrophy occurs at the pulmonary arteriolar level and may be the mechanism of HPVR [6,95,118]. Fibrosis of the intima, which may not be reversible, was found in high-altitude dwellers [18,96,108,147,184], suggesting a more fixed pulmonary vascular resistance. There is evidence that some high-altitude natives who have adapted well to the high altitude may have normal pulmonary artery pressures [75] and no hypertrophy of the smooth muscle of the pulmonary arterioles [78].

Hematologic Adaptations

The purpose of optimizing $\dot{V}A/\dot{Q}$ matching is to make oxygen available to hemoglobin in the red blood cell, which then carries oxygen in the vascular compartment to tissues where it is consumed. At high altitudes, two major adaptations of the carrier mechanism take place to facilitate delivery: (1) The number of red blood cells is increased by the process of erythropoiesis, and (2) the configuration of the hemoglobin molecule changes to alter the affinity of hemoglobin for oxygen in order to optimize the loading and unloading of oxygen [98,99,242,243].

ERYTHROPOIESIS

The decrease in arterial oxygen partial pressure and subsequently oxygen content that occurs with progressive hypobaria at high altitude is counterbalanced in part by an increase in hemoglobin concentration, and subsequent oxygen-carrying capacity. The rise over the first day or so is secondary to hemoconcentration from a diuresis, whereas the continued rise over the ensuing 2 to 3 weeks is a result of increased red blood cell production, which is stimulated by a humoral substance secreted in the kidney cell, erythropoietin [51,52,116]. Erythropoietin levels increase rapidly according to the hypoxic stimulus and then decline a bit in the face of a continued rise in hemoglobin [1,55,156]. Erythropoiesis stops abruptly upon descent [186], and hemoglobin concentrations return to sea-level values in approximately 3 weeks [156].

A striking feature of the erythropoietic response is the variability between individuals and between different highland populations, which may reflect less-than-optimal adaptations to comparable hypoxic stress [131,243,245,251]. For instance, in the Himalayas at 3600 m, hemoglobin levels of 16.1 ± 1.2 gm/dl have been documented [13], whereas in the Andes at the same altitude, the values are 18.2 to 19.0 gm/dl [7]. Although the increase in hemoglobin concentration augments arterial oxygen content, an actual decrease in oxygen delivery may ensue if hyperviscosity of the blood limits perfusion to the microvasculature of the exercising muscle [23,53]. Climbers on Mt. Everest undergoing isovolemic phlebotomy to decrease their hematocrits from 60 to 50 percent had an increase in psychometric function while not experiencing a decrease in aerobic capacity [193]. Hemodilution in high-altitude natives of the Andes achieved by decreasing the hematocrit 20 percent resulted in an improved exercise performance [14]. Excessive polycythemia in the highland dweller is discussed later.

OXYGEN-HEMOGLOBIN AFFINITY

The role of oxygen-hemoglobin affinity in oxygen delivery is not fully understood. Conditions of stress, such as fever and acidemia, are associated with a rightward shift of the oxygen-hemoglobin dissociation curve, or low oxygen and hemoglobin affinity, presumably to facilitate the unloading of oxygen to the tissues [58], whereas conditions such as hypothermia and alkalosis have opposite effects. At sea level, where there is an excess of oxygen in healthy individuals, shifts in the oxygen-hemoglobin curve make little difference in oxygen delivery, but at a high altitude, shifts in the curve may have a significant effect.

Upon acute ascent to a high altitude, hypoxia and the resultant hypocapnic alkalosis stimulate production of 2,3-diphosphoglycerate (2,3-DPG) within the red blood cell, which shifts the curve to the right [8,30,106,114,122,162]. At the tissue level, production of carbon dioxide and hydrogen ions also improves the unloading of oxygen from hemoglobin, the Bohr effect [8]. This shift was thought to be an advantage to acute high-altitude adaptation, but in subjects at 4300 m who had the curve shifted experimentally to the right, performance was not improved [162]. Andean high-altitude natives both with [171] and without [114] evidence of polycythemia and pulmonary hypertension also were found to have right-shifted curves.

At moderate altitude, the rightward shifts may be an advantage [192], but the ease of unloading oxygen must be weighed against the potential disadvantage at higher altitudes of loading oxygen onto hemoglobin at the pulmonary capillary level. A leftward shift would theoretically convey an advantage to loading oxygen at altitudes where the partial pressure of the inspired oxygen is so low that the diffusion gradient from air to blood is also very low. High-altitude animals and birds, such as the bar-headed goose, that migrate over the Himalayas have left-shifted curves, presumably from the marked hypocapnic alkalosis [17,54,177,217]. Other experimental animal models bear out the advantage of a leftward shift during acute exposure. An optimal model may exist in the llamas and alpacas of the Andes, who have a left-shifted curve at the lung level and a right-shifted curve at the peripheral tissues [13].

Humans, on the other hand, have not lived long enough at high altitudes to evolve a characteristic hemoglobin that would be most suitable for high-altitude survival. A number of workers have found a modest leftward shift of the curve in humans living at high altitudes [143]. Increased levels of 2,3-DPG have been found in these humans [175], but a leftward shift of the oxygen-hemoglobin curve was found probably because of the countereffect of the respiratory alkalosis. A group of climbers after 2 months at 6300 m or higher on Mt. Everest was found to have respiratory alkalosis, a modest polycythemic response (mean hematocrit of 54.4 ± 4.01 percent), and a persistently left-shifted curve, despite an increased level of 2,3-DPG [242] (Fig. 44-3). The advantages of a left-shifted curve at extreme altitudes, therefore, are at least suggested by the

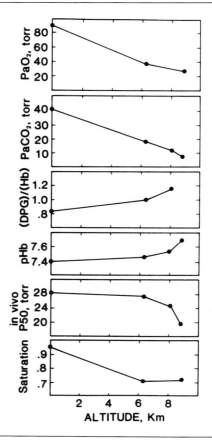

Fig. 44-3. Effect of altitude on oxygen-hemoglobin affinity. *P50* = oxygen half–saturation pressure of hemoglobin; *DPG* = diphosphoglycerate. (From RM Winslow. Red Cell Function at Extreme Altitude. In JB West, S Lahiri (Eds), *High Altitude and Man.* Bethesda, MD: American Physiological Society, 1984. Pp 59–72.)

preceding data, but further work is necessary to elucidate the underlying mechanisms.

Tissue Alterations

The final stages of oxygen delivery involve the diffusion of oxygen from the blood across the muscle capillary and muscle cell membrane to the cytoplasm and ultimately to the mitochondrion, where oxidative phosphorylation takes place. This process depends on a critical pressure gradient and radial distance for diffusion of oxygen from the blood to the cell. The critical pressure gradient is probably about 10 to 12 mmHg [128], and certain adaptations that may optimize cellular transport and metabolism of oxygen take place.

MORPHOLOGIC CHANGES

The purpose of structural changes is presumably to decrease the distance for diffusion of oxygen from the blood to the mitochondrion. Formation of new capillaries and a recruitment of preexisting capillaries in response to a hypoxic stimulus are strategies that can achieve that goal. Experimental animals exposed to hypoxia [10] and guinea pigs native to high altitudes had an increased capillary density in the lung. Quantification of this response is difficult since muscle cell atrophy also occurs during prolonged (weeks, months) stays at high altitudes [19,188].

The adaptation of the mitochondria to hypoxia is not well defined. Mitochondria have been found to be increased [174] as well as unchanged [68,114,148,221] at high altitudes. Human studies at very high altitudes, on the other hand, have shown a decrease in mitochondrial concentration [114,148]. Whatever the final verdict, theoretically, an increase in both capillary and mitochondrial density would result in a facilitation of oxygen transport by decreasing the diffusion distance for oxygen from the blood to the mitochondria.

BIOCHEMICAL ADAPTATIONS

Several biochemical mechanisms occur and improve oxygen metabolism. Myoglobin, an intracellular protein that binds oxygen at a very low tissue partial pressure of oxygen, facilitates diffusion of oxygen to muscle mitochondria and is increased in animals exposed to [68] and native to [221] hypoxia. The enzymes of oxidative metabolism also upgrade their function in response to exposure to and living at high altitudes. Succinic and lactate dehydrogenase, part of the glycolytic pathway, increase at high altitudes [93,100,149,167,178,222], but the changes in these studies were not consistent and depended on the degree of exposure, the tissue involved, and the stress itself. In human studies, the results suggest that fatty acid metabolism, which contributes to exercise endurance, is enhanced while glycolytic metabolism, which is responsible for high levels of aerobic work, is decreased. Further work is necessary to clarify this area of cellular adaptation to hypoxia.

Central Nervous System

The brain is the organ most sensitive to hypoxic stress. The historic flight of the Zenith in 1875, a hot-air balloon that carried three Italian scientists to over 8000 m, during which two of the scientists died, is a testament to the catastrophic effects of acute severe hypoxia on the brain. Less vivid but impressive examples of the effect of hypoxia on the brain are found throughout the medical and mountaineering literature.

The brain's defenses to the stress of hypoxia are both acute and chronic. The initial decrease in cerebral blood flow that occurs with hypocapnia secondary to hypoxia secondary to the respiratory alkalosis is outweighed by the increase in cerebral blood flow from the hypoxic stimulus [121,126,204]. Blood flow increased 33 percent after 12 hours at 3800 m and decreased as respiratory adaptation continued, but still was 13 percent greater than control values after 5 days [204]. The net result is that oxygen supply to the brain is probably well preserved despite profound hypoxemia. Tibetans, a well adapted high-altitude population, maintain cerebral blood flow during exercise better than sojourners [250].

In spite of augmented blood flow, varying degrees of cerebral dysfunction occur, depending on the acuity, duration, and degree of hypoxic stress [24,29,63,103,125,190,202,206,207]. The higher one goes, the more that motor, sensory, and complex cognitive abilities are affected. Learning is impaired at 3000 m, and at 6000 m sensation, perception, and motor skills are diminished [24,125].

Acute elevation to 3500 m results in cortical depression of the electroencephalographic (EEG) pattern that is not apparent in inhabitants of that altitude [202]. Correlation of the changes in the EEG with the symptoms of acute mountain sickness (AMS) at 4300 m was noted [63].

Several studies have addressed the question of prolonged or permanent effects of hypoxic exposure on central nervous system function. Some investigators found no residual psychometric deficits in climbers who had been above 5100 m in the Himalayas [29], while two other studies of individuals who had been at a high altitude for 10 months found residual motor incoordination and impaired speech which resolved within a year [206,207]. There was individual variation in these findings, which was also documented in a study of Polish alpinists who had climbed to 5500 m [190]. All had some impairment noted by psychological testing, and 11 of 30 had EEG abnormalities. A later study [103] showed transient deficits in learning, memory, and verbal expression in two groups of individuals, one of which had been on an expedition to Mt. Everest while the other had been exposed to a simulated similar altitude for 40 days in a hypobaric chamber. Fine-motor skills remained abnormal for up to 1 year in many. Unexpectedly, individuals with a high ventilatory response to hypoxia who are better oxygenated and who usually perform better physically had the greatest deficits. The authors speculated that those who hyperventilated more had greater hypocapnic cerebral vasoconstriction and thus lower oxygen delivery to the brain.

Sleep

Periodic breathing, which was described as far back as 1886 [165], occurs during early exposure to high altitudes but decreases as acclimatization ensues [14,214]. The degree of periodic breathing varies among individuals and may be a function of individual hypoxic chemosensitivity. Findings in both sojourners and high-altitude natives during sleep when cortical input is minimized suggest that individuals with high hypoxic chemosensitivity have ventilatory overshoot, resulting in hypocapnic alkalosis, suppression of ventilation, and periodicity of respiration [9,14,138,240]. These oscillations persist throughout sleep and can result in profound arterial oxygen desaturation during the hypopneic and apneic phases. The resulting hypoxemia may contribute to some of the aspects of altitude illness.

Carbonic anhydrase inhibitors eradicate periodic breathing [214,215,218], which may be a result of drug-induced tissue acidosis and subsequent ventilatory stimulation. Discussion of their therapeutic efficacy follows in the section on altitude illness.

Exercise

Although a number of observations of the effect of hypoxia on oxygen transport during exercise have been made, an understanding of exercise limitation at high altitudes remains elusive. One thing is certain: Oxygen consumption and, subsequently, exercise performance predictably decrease with ascent to high altitudes [26,48,180, 210,212,216,231,237,252] (Fig. 44-4).

VENTILATION

The increased metabolic rate of exercise and hypoxia of high altitude interact synergistically to augment exercise hyperpnea. The increase in exercise ventilation is proportional to the degree of hypoxia [194] (Fig. 44-5). The degree of exercise

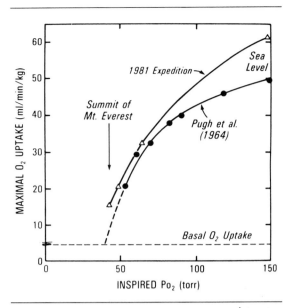

Fig. 44-4. Maximal oxygen consumption ($\dot{V}O_{2max}$) against inspired partial pressure of oxygen. There is a predictable decrease in $\dot{V}O_{2max}$ at higher altitudes. The more recent data demonstrate that a low amount of work is possible on the summit of Mt. Everest. (From JB West, et al. Maximal exercise at extreme altitudes on Mount Everest. *J Appl Physiol* 55:688, 1983.)

hyperpnea is also influenced by the individual's hypoxic ventilatory response, measured at sea level or a high altitude [196]. The study on Mt. Everest demonstrated that climbers with higher hypoxic chemosensitivity had greater exercise ventilation, less arterial oxygen desaturation, and better climbing performance. These data supported studies suggesting that climbers to extreme altitudes (higher than 7500 m) benefited from a brisk high ventilatory response [153,171, 195]. It is, therefore, the ventilatory response at high altitudes that is primarily responsible for the preservation of alveolar and arterial oxygen partial pressure. On the other hand, in the high-altitude dweller, a lower exercise ventilation is accompanied by a lower alveolar-arterial gradient, suggesting a genetic or adaptive increase in diffusion capacity of the lungs for oxygen which results in improved gas exchange [45,137,199].

GAS EXCHANGE

Arterial oxygen saturation in sojourners decreases with exercise at high altitude [216,224,

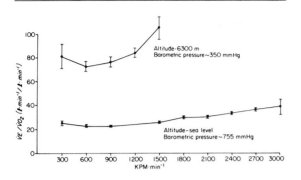

Fig. 44-5. The ventilatory equivalent ($\dot{V}E/\dot{V}O_2$) for given work loads in a group of climbers at sea level (*lower line*) and at 6300 m (*upper line*). The data demonstrate the stimulation to ventilation from hypoxia. (From RB Schoene. Hypoxic Ventilatory Response and Exercise Ventilation at Sea Level and High Altitude. In JB West, S Lahiri (Eds), *Man at High Altitude*. Bethesda, MD: American Physiological Society, 1984. Pp 19–30.)

231,237,239]. This desaturation is largely secondary to a diffusion limitation for oxygen from the air to the blood, but some $\dot{V}/\dot{Q}$ heterogeneity contributes to this phenomenon [66,224,231,232]. This $\dot{V}/\dot{Q}$ heterogeneity may be secondary to interstitial lung water, while the diffusion limitation is a result of a decreased driving pressure of oxygen from air to blood compounded by a decrease in transit time of blood across the alveolar-capillary membrane.

CARDIAC RESPONSE
At submaximal work loads during acute exposure, cardiac output is moderately higher than at sea level, while after prolonged exposure, heart rate and cardiac output are matched for comparable sea-level work loads [230]. Upon acute high-altitude exposure, maximum cardiac output is the same as at sea level, but it decreases 20 to 30 percent after 2 months above 4300 m [191]. This decrease is a result of a decrease in both maximum heart rate and stroke volume [230]. The decrease in maximum heart rate is more pronounced in sojourners than high-altitude natives [74,139,180,230,237]. On the other hand, cardiac output remains appropriate for oxygen consumption, and myocardial contractility, as measured by echocardiography, is preserved even at extreme altitudes [183]. Although pulmonary artery pressures are very high during exercise at extreme al-

titudes, the increase in pulmonary vascular resistance is not a limiting factor [76].

HEMATOLOGIC CHANGES
A modest increase in hemoglobin secondary to the erythropoietic response may improve oxygen transport, but polycythemia and its accompanying hyperviscosity may result in a decrease in microperfusion of the muscle tissue and a subsequent decrease in oxygen extraction. A study on Mt. Everest showed that isovolemic hemodilution of mountaineers from hematocrits of 60 percent to the low 50 percent range did not decrease maximum exercise capabilities [193]. In fact, data from Himalayan highlanders suggest that the optimal hematocrit may be somewhat lower than previously thought [13].

TISSUE
Muscle tissue undergoes some morphologic and chemical changes, the net result of which is that oxidative capacities are reduced. For instance, in climbers returning from 2 months at an extreme altitude, muscle mass decreased, capillary density was unchanged, mitochondrial density increased, and muscle succinic dehydrogenase (a marker for aerobic metabolism) decreased—all of which resulted in impaired aerobic functioning [27]. It is not clear from other studies what effect a decrease in muscle fiber size has on the relationship of capillary and mitochondrial density and subsequent oxygen extraction.

In summary, exercise at modest altitude results in a number of cardiopulmonary changes that optimize gas exchange, while the blood and peripheral vasculature also undergo certain changes that may improve oxygen transport. At extreme altitude, on the other hand, the tissue adaptations may impose limitations on both submaximal and maximal exercise.

ATHLETIC PERFORMANCE AND TRAINING AT HIGH ALTITUDES
Much of the work on athletic performance at high altitudes was done during the Mexico City Olympics [48,179,210]. In middle-distance running events (at 2270-m elevation), times were about 8 percent slower on arrival and approached but did not reach previous best sea-level performances [179]. These findings correlated with measurements of maximum oxygen consumption. Performances in short-distance events (less than 2 minutes) are not impaired and in fact may be better than at sea

level because of decreased air resistance. On the other hand, for prolonged work activities, endurance is improved by training and living at high altitude [150].

There is controversy over the benefits of training for athletic events at moderate altitudes. After the success in the Mexico City Olympics of the Africans who lived at an altitude of approximately 2000 m, it became quite fashionable for middle- and long-distance athletes to live and train at these altitudes. The results of studies to document this presumed benefit were mixed [73,126]. The benefits of living at these altitudes (e.g., increased level of hemoglobin) may be outweighed by the fact that training schedules cannot be as intense. A recent study tried to address this controversy by studying four groups of athletes: individuals living and training at a low altitude, ones living and training at a high altitude (3000 m), those living at a high altitude and training at a low altitude, and a final group living at a low altitude and training at a high altitude [144]. The results were not striking but suggested that those who lived at a high altitude and trained at a low altitude had a slight edge over the others. These findings may be explained by the slight elevation in hemoglobin.

Maladaptation

Overview

Modern travel and recreation permit rapid ascent to high altitudes, which is the major cause of acute mountain illnesses. On the other hand, millions of people reside at altitudes above 2500 m, and a certain percentage of those individuals develop chronic altitude disorders. In both of these groups, mounting evidence [70,84,132,163] suggests that failure of the body to respond to hypoxic stress with an adequate ventilatory response results in greater hypoxemia, pulmonary hypertension, increased intracranial pressure, fluid retention, and erythropoietic response—all of which may lead to clinical illnesses at high altitudes. Hypoventilation, therefore, may be one of the crucial factors underlying all altitude illnesses. With the previous notes on formal adaptation as a guide, it therefore is the purpose of this section to deal with both acute and chronic mountain sicknesses.

Illnesses of Sojourners to High Altitudes

As was so tragically demonstrated by nineteenth-century balloonists, acute ascent above 8000 m can lead to death, whereas, as has been repeatedly achieved in the twentieth century, climbers can gradually ascend to these altitudes and live and work for short periods of time quite effectively. Failure of the body to adapt to the hypoxic stress leads to acute mountain illnesses that can be fatal. These disorders are classified as AMS, high-altitude pulmonary edema (HAPE), and high-altitude cerebral edema (HACE). Although there is a great deal of individual variability and overlap in these disorders, this section deals with them separately.

ACUTE MOUNTAIN SICKNESS

Clinical Picture. Historically, AMS was described many centuries ago, and one consistently described symptom is headache. The headache usually begins shortly after ascent, is more severe in the morning, and is usually treatable with mild analgesics. Other symptoms can include anorexia, lassitude, insomnia, nausea, and vomiting, and some subjects show signs of fluid retention [83,161,208]. Sojourners with AMS may be tachycardic and tachypneic but are not febrile. All these signs and symptoms usually abate over several days as acclimatization ensues and rarely requires more than rest, hydration, and mild analgesics. The severity and duration of AMS are a function of the altitude and the rapidity of ascent. For instance, on Mt. Rainier (4400 m), nearly two-thirds of climbers who routinely ascend from sea level over 1 to 3 days develop AMS [140], and in Summit County, Colorado (2880 m), 25 percent of travelers from low altitude have AMS [249]. In both of these cases, the symptoms usually resolve in 1 to 3 days without sequelae. AMS can progress, however, to HAPE and/or HACE, which can be life-threatening.

In many subjects with AMS, hypoventilation [70,82,84,115,163], gas-exchange abnormalities, and pulmonary mechanical dysfunction [72] occur. Fluid retention [84], weight gain, proteinuria, and increased CSF pressure and brain swelling [90,124,146] also have been documented. Individuals who are susceptible to AMS have an exaggerated aldosterone and antidiuretic hormone (ADH) response upon ascent that is different from well-acclimatizing individuals who have low ADH and a diuresis [12]. A shift of fluid from the extracellular space to the interstitial and intracellular compartments occurs normally during the initial few days at high altitude, but it may be accentuated and prolonged in persons with hypoventilation and AMS. Fluid shifts also may explain the pulmonary dysfunctions of relative hypoxemia and mechanical dysfunction, which may be precursors of overt HAPE. Evidence that dexamethasone, a medication commonly used for the treatment of many forms of edema, is effective in preventing and treating AMS supports the concept that extravascular fluid extravasation plays a role in altitude illnesses [57,89,145].

Why do some individuals get AMS and others not? Although the answer is not known, mounting evidence suggests that individuals with a blunted hypoxic ventilatory response are more predisposed to AMS and fluid retention [140,163]. It is probably safe to say that the individual who does not mount sufficient ventilatory response is more hypoxemic and susceptible to the ill effects thereof and will, therefore, be predisposed to all forms of altitude illness, the first of which is AMS.

Treatment. Successful management of AMS involves recognition and appropriate treatment. If the awareness of and suspicion for AMS are keen enough, then AMS usually will not progress and can be treated with conservative measures, such as rest and mild analgesics (aspirin, acetaminophen, codeine, prochlorperazine). Sedatives, narcotics, and alcohol should be avoided, since they may suppress ventilation and mask worsening symptoms. If the subject seems more ill with worsening headache or any other clear neurologic signs, especially ataxia, then this situation should be considered serious, and the patient should descend as quickly as possible. Even a few hundred meters may be helpful. If conditions do not permit descent, then oxygen, if available, is a good temporizing measure.

Few medications have been found to be helpful in either the prevention or the treatment of AMS. Acetazolamide, a carbonic anhydrase inhibitor, is effective in preventing and treating AMS, although its mechanism of action is unknown [15,50,71,72,140,248]. Acetazolamide eradicates periodic breathing and arterial oxygen desaturation during sleep at high altitudes [87,214,218], which may improve overall oxygen delivery. The drug also stimulates ventilation at rest and during exercise; induces a renal excretion of bicarbonate, which may facilitate acclimatization; and lowers CSF pressure by decreasing CSF formation. Which of these effects is responsible for the drug's efficacy is not known, but it is effective and safe. Its side effects are minimal and include peripheral, self-limited paresthesias and mild gastrointestinal upset. The present recommendations are that sojourners who frequently get AMS should take acetazolamide upon ascent to mini-mize the chances of illness; otherwise, those who go high quickly should begin therapy only after the first signs of illness. Individuals who are allergic to sulfa drugs should not take acetazolamide.

Dexamethasone has been shown to be effective in treating and preventing AMS [57,89,145] and should be used in situations where treatment is imperative to aid a sojourner's descent. Since there are no data to suggest that the drug facilitates acclimatization, a person who stops taking the drug while still at a high altitude may suffer a rebound of altitude illness. Individuals progressing to more severe signs suggestive of cerebral edema should use dexamethasone immediately.

Recently, a portable hyperbaric chamber has been used for treatment of altitude illnesses in the field [86,119,220]. This equipment is lightweight and is effective in treating illness. This manually operated chamber can lower the altitude by 1500 m with a pressure of 2 psi, which after several hours is enough to improve symptoms such that a victim can descend under his or her own power. In remote areas, the hyperbaric bag provides an excellent, reusable alternative to oxygen. Whether it is more effective than oxygen alone has not been established.

The best treatment is prevention, and slow, gradual ascent is still the best preventive measure. Maintenance of fluids to ensure a normal urine output and adequate calories in carbohydrates are time-honored tactics. A number of other drugs (morphine, furosemide, spironolactone, phenytoin) have been used, but none is effective and most have potentially deleterious side effects.

HIGH-ALTITUDE PULMONARY EDEMA

Clinical Picture. HAPE was thought for many years to be pneumonia or heart failure at a high altitude. It was not until the 1960s that HAPE was described as a noncardiogenic form of pulmonary edema [104,110]. HAPE affects healthy sojourners of all ages, usually within several days of ascent above 3000 m, although it can occur later and at lower altitudes. It also is more common at higher altitudes with quick ascent. Symptoms and signs of AMS may precede those of HAPE, and often HAPE and HACE occur simultaneously with varying degrees of each. Dyspnea on exertion, fatigue, and dry cough are early symptoms, with cyanosis, tachypnea, and tachycardia as accompanying signs. Crackles are universally present, although pink frothy sputum is present only in severe cases. Many victims have a low-grade fever, and all will have fluffy infiltrates without cardiomegaly on chest radiograph (Fig. 44-6). If symptoms are recognized early enough, while the patient is still ambulatory, descent is very effective as a treatment. Most patients recover fully, and many have been able to reascend to very high altitude within a fortnight. This observation is important, since it implies that the lung architecture is preserved.

HAPE may be an extension of the normal process of accumulation of lung water that occurs upon acute ascent to altitude [31,33,67,102,117, 152]. Additionally, many asymptomatic individuals have crackles on chest auscultation that resolve with further acclimatization. These findings suggest either that those who go on to develop HAPE are not able to compensate for the normal fluid accumulation or that their fluid shift is overwhelming.

Pathophysiology. Both autopsy and bronchoalveolar lavage (BAL) data demonstrate that HAPE is a high-protein/high-permeability leak (Fig. 44-7). Over 20 autopsies demonstrated a proteinaceous alveolar exudate with hyaline membrane forma-

Fig. 44-6. Chest x-ray film from a victim of high-altitude pulmonary edema with bilateral infiltrates and normal cardiac silhouette. (From Hackett, personal communication, 1987.)

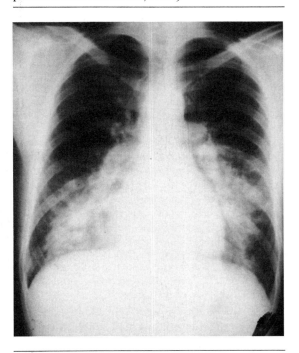

tion [5,46,166]. Neutrophils were present and capillary and arteriolar thrombi and fibrin deposition were found. These data are from those individuals who did not survive and thus are not representative of the early pathophysiologic process.

BAL at 4400 m on Mt. McKinley characterized the cellular and biochemical responses in subjects with HAPE [200]. The protein content was higher than that of patients with adult respiratory distress syndrome (ARDS), and the fluid also was very cellular, but unlike the fluid found in ARDS, which contains primarily neutrophils, BAL fluid from subjects with HAPE consisted largely of alveolar macrophages. Additionally, there was evidence of inflammation with complement activation and leukotriene B_4 production, but inhibition of neutrophil chemotaxis was present, suggesting a mechanism protecting against parenchymal destruction. Thromboxane B_2 also was present, suggesting a vasoactive process. These findings provide important insight into the underlying mechanism of HAPE, although the picture is not complete.

Other physiologic observations may provide further understanding of this high-permeability lung leak. A number of subjects with HAPE have a blunted ventilatory response to hypoxia [88] that presumably leads to a more profound degree of hypoxemia, especially during sleep, and subsequent higher pulmonary artery pressures mediated by the HPVR. In addition, studies have shown that subjects with HAPE had very elevated pulmonary artery pressures [109,247]. In a number of patients with HAPE, congenital absence of a pulmonary artery has also been demonstrated [109]. These findings suggest that the pulmonary vascular endothelium undergoes extraordinary stress from an increased cardiac output from exercise at high altitudes, which is being directed through an either globally or patchily vasoconstricted and compromised pulmonary vascular bed. An animal model for capillary stress and failure has been described [241]. Could high shear forces lead to a mechanical stretching of endothelial pores and subsequent permeability leak [211] or are other biochemical mechanisms responsible? Clearly, high intravascular pressures play a role in the development of HAPE but are not the entire story.

The BAL data showed that biochemical mediators are present [200]. These findings suggest that stress on the endothelium may lead to release of inflammatory mediators, which may affect permeability. It would seem reasonable, therefore, not to classify pulmonary edema as due to either pure increased permeability or pure increased hydrostatic pressure. This arbitrary division has led to some misunderstanding of some clinical illnesses which may have a number of contributory factors. It is conceivable that the pathophysiologic process in HAPE begins with high hydrostatic forces, which may lead to leak of protein into the interstitial and alveolar spaces and/or to biochemical mediators that affect pulmonary vascular integrity. This latter scenario suggests mechanisms that would violate the traditional separation of causes of lung leak but that may be more realistic.

Treatment. The guidelines for field treatment that have been outlined for AMS are applicable to HAPE, except that it is important to emphasize that HAPE can be fatal. Early recognition is essential to avoid catastrophe. Descent is still the most important step, and avoidance of any medications that may suppress ventilation, especially sleeping pills, is mandatory. Oxygen, if available,

Fig. 44-7. Protein concentration in bronchoalveolar lavage fluid in patients (left to right) with high altitude pulmonary edema (HAPE), acute mountain sickness with mild arterial oxygen saturation, adult respiratory distress syndrome (ARDS) and two control populations. (From Schoene RB, et al. The lung at high altitude: Bronchoalveolar lavage in acute mountain sickness and pulmonary edema. *J Appl Physiol* 64:2605, 1988.

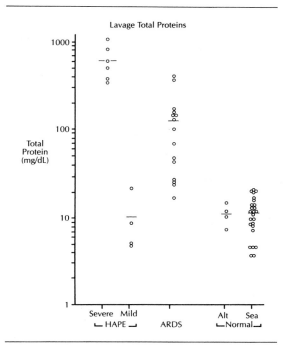

is very effective, but it should be regarded only as a temporizing measure. Since HAPE and HACE often occur together to varying degrees, the victim may be more or less incapacitated, and rescue units should have oxygen and/or a portable hyperbaric bag available, since they improve oxygenation and decrease pulmonary artery pressure. Victims usually improve enough within 12 to 24 hours of descent to safer altitudes. Recent studies have shown end-positive airway pressure (EPAP) masks to be effective in improving oxygenation, and these may be useful until the victim can descend or be evacuated [197].

A number of medications have been used, but no data are available to validate their efficacy. The low incidence of HAPE and the lack of an animal model make a drug trial very difficult. Acetazolamide is certainly safe and may be effective in preventing or treating HAPE, but no studies have been done to prove this point. Potent diuretics are potentially dangerous. Morphine sulfate may improve symptoms, but it suppresses ventilation. Drugs that decrease pulmonary artery pressures have been shown to be efficacious [11]. In a field study in the Alps, Bartsch and colleagues [11] pretreated HAPE-susceptible climbers with nifedipine and placebo. There was a decrease in pulmonary artery pressure and no HAPE occurred in the nifedipine group.

HIGH-ALTITUDE CEREBRAL EDEMA
Since the symptoms of AMS are similar yet milder than those of HACE, it is reasonable to assume that HACE is merely an extension of AMS. HACE usually, but not always, follows AMS and is marked by severe headache and papilledema with deterioration of mental status in the presence of objective neurologic signs, especially ataxia. This usually is seen after recent ascent [85,105,208]. The symptoms may rapidly progress to coma and death. HACE usually occurs at higher altitudes (higher than 4000 m) and is less common than HAPE (approximately 1 percent). If a severe headache cannot be relieved by analgesics, then HACE should be suspected, especially if other neurologic signs or symptoms develop. HAPE and HACE often occur simultaneously with differing degrees of severity.

Autopsies have shown gross cerebral edema with herniation and small petechial hemorrhages in seven of eight HACE victims [46,105]. The underlying pathophysiologic mechanism is unclear, but it probably involves high cerebral vascular pressures with filtration of plasma proteins and water into the interstitial spaces.

Recognition is absolutely essential, because HACE more than any other altitude illness can progress rapidly to death. Recovery occurs with descent, although oxygen and dexamethasone may give symptomatic relief until descent can be achieved. Hyperbaric therapy may also be helpful but should never delay descent if the patient is ambulatory or transportable.

OPHTHALMOLOGIC SYNDROMES

A number of ophthalmologic changes have been noted at high altitudes. As the window of the brain, the retina may offer some interesting insight into the effect of altitude on the brain. Retinal hemorrhages are common (more than 50 percent) in sojourners above 4500 m [82] and were recently observed in all eight subjects who underwent a 40-day simulated ascent of Mt. Everest. Rarely are visual changes encountered, and the hemorrhages resolve within a fortnight and deserve no treatment per se. Other funduscopic changes include papilledema, vitreous hemorrhages, and vascular tortuosity and engorgement [208]. The hemorrhages are similar to those found in necropsies of the brain at high altitude, and one can only speculate if these are concomitant processes in the eye and brain.

Visual changes, including visual blurring and intermittent blindness, also occur. This latter phenomenon is probably cortical in origin secondary to global hypoxia and/or decreased perfusion secondary to hypocapnic vasospasm. Visual field impairment also has been described and is vascular in origin.

Illnesses of High-Altitude Residents

SUBACUTE MOUNTAIN SICKNESS

Recently, a syndrome has been found in Indian soldiers who lived for longer than 3 months at an altitude of 5800 m [3]. It is characterized by fluid retention, cor pulmonale, polycythemia, and left ventricular dysfunction. The mortality rate was high in these individuals unless they moved to a low altitude. An infantile counterpart has been observed in Han Chinese infants who have moved to Lhasa, Tibet [213]. Investigators are presently trying to understand the underlying mechanisms of this newly described entity.

CHRONIC MOUNTAIN SICKNESS

Human habitation at high altitudes is limited both by prolonged hypoxic stress and by the harsh nature of the environment. Nevertheless, millions of

people live between 3000 and 5000 m. Some environments might permit living at higher altitudes, but anecdotally, civilizations have settled below 5000 m, suggesting that chronic deterioration occurs above this altitude such that populations tend not to thrive.

Some insight into this phenomenon can be gained by observing some individuals in populations residing at high altitudes who develop deleterious manifestations of chronic hypoxic stress—polycythemia, pulmonary hypertension, mental slowing, and cor pulmonale. This disease is termed *chronic mountain sickness* (CMS) and was first described by Monge in 1928 who noted the sickness in high-altitude natives of the South American Andes [159]. Interestingly, although CMS has been observed in all mountain ranges, some populations, especially inhabitants of the Tibetan plateau and women, do not seem very susceptible to CMS. Populations of lowland natives who move to high altitudes develop CMS over the ensuing years. An interesting study on the Tibetan plateau showed a 13 percent incidence of CMS in relocated Chinese males, 1.6 percent incidence in Chinese females, and a 1 percent incidence in Tibetan men [246]. One could speculate that the Tibetans, who have lived at high altitudes for over 250,000 years, have evolved more successful mechanisms to improve oxygen transport and cope with the hypoxic stress than have Andean natives, who have lived at high altitudes for less than 30,000 years.

Clinical Picture. Andean villages have many individuals suffering from CMS. The plethoric, sometimes obese male with both mental and physical torpor is classic. Neurologic findings include mental dullness, lethargy, and poor memory. The subjects have polycythemia and cyanosis and resemble in many respects the sea-level dweller with cor pulmonale, polycythemia, and sleep disorders with marked nocturnal oxygen desaturation [130,132,158,164,244,253]. There may be underlying lung disease as well.

Most of the clinical manifestations can be attributed to hypoventilation, which is associated with a blunted hypoxic chemosensitivity and subsequent relatively greater hypoxemia. Worse pulmonary hypertension may lead to right-sided heart failure and cor pulmonale. A high-frequency, low-tidal-volume pattern of ventilation may contribute to a low $\dot{V}/\dot{Q}$ ratio, contributing further to the hypoxemia [33]. An increase in red cell mass relative to plasma volume results in a true hyperviscous polycythemia. Hematocrit levels as high as 80 percent have been described. Hypoventilation, therefore, may be one of the key factors that allows CMS to develop. Other underlying problems, such as lung disease and an inordinate erythropoietic response, may contribute to the development of CMS.

Treatment. The mainstay of treatment is improvement of arterial oxygenation, which should decrease the polycythemia, improve pulmonary hypertension, and improve cerebral function. If possible, the individual should move to a lower altitude and stop cigarette smoking. Often a relocation is not logistically or culturally possible, and most victims of CMS languish away in remote high-altitude villages. On the other hand, some therapeutic interventions are beneficial. Phlebotomy improves cor pulmonale and increases cardiac output and oxygen transport, but the erythropoiesis eventually returns. Low-flow oxygen, especially at night, is also helpful but not always logistically feasible. Medications that stimulate ventilation and result in a marked improvement in nocturnal oxygen saturation are also beneficial [130,132]. Acetazolamide is particularly effective, as is medroxyprogesterone acetate, although to a lesser degree. Other respiratory stimulants have not been tried.

REENTRY PULMONARY EDEMA
Long-time residents at high altitudes may be more susceptible to high-altitude pulmonary edema if they descend to a low altitude and reascend [111,201]. Young people (children and teenagers) may be more susceptible, especially if descent and ascent are rapid. Cases have been reported from South America (6.4 percent incidence [111]) and Leadville, Colorado [201], but none from Asia. The reasons for this difference are not clear, but it may be secondary to the logistic imposition of a slower ascent in the Himalayas or to the overall better adaptive capabilities of the Tibetan descendants. The cause of reentry HAPE is not known, but it may be secondary to a hypermuscularization and subsequent hyperreactivity of the pulmonary vasculature to hypoxia on reascent [110].

References

1. Abbrecht PH, Littell JK. Plasma erythropoietin in men and mice during acclimatization to different altitudes. *J Appl Physiol* 32:54, 1972.
2. Alexander JK, Grover RF. Mechanism of reduced stroke volume at high altitude. *Clin Cardiol* 6:301, 1983.
3. Anand IS, et al. Adult subacute mountain sickness—A syndrome of congestive heart failure in man at very high altitude. *Lancet* 335:561, 1990.
4. Arias-Stella J. Human carotid body at high altitude. *Am J Pathol* 55:82a, 1969.
5. Arias-Stella J, Kruger H. Pathology of high altitude pulmonary edema. *Arch Pathol Lab Med* 76:4353, 1963.
6. Arias-Stella J, Saldana M. The terminal portion of the pulmonary vascular tree in people native to high altitude. *Circulation* 28:915, 1963.
7. Arnaud J, et al. Methemoglobin and erythrocyte reducing systems in high-altitude natives. *Ann Hum Biol* 6:585, 1979.
8. Aste-Salazar H, Hurtado A. The affinity of hemoglobin for oxygen at sea level and high altitude. *Am J Physiol* 142:733, 1944.
9. Badr MS, et al. Effect of hypercapnia on total pulmonary resistance during wakefulness and during NREM sleep. *Am Rev Respir Dis* 144:406, 1991.
10. Banchero N. Capillary density of skeletal muscle in dogs exposed to simulated altitude. *Proc Soc Exp Biol Med* 148:435, 1975.
11. Bartsch P, et al. Prevention of high-altitude pulmonary edema by nifedipine. *N Engl J Med* 325:1284, 1991.
12. Bartsch P, et al. Enhanced exercise-induced rise of aldosterone and vasopressin preceding mountain sickness. *J Appl Physiol* 711:136, 1991.
13. Beall CM, Reischman AB. Hemoglobin levels in a Himalayan high altitude population. *Am J Phys Anthropol* 63:301, 1984.
14. Berssenbrugge A, Dempsey J, Skatrud J. Hypoxic versus Hypocapnic Effects on Periodic Breathing during Sleep. In JB West, S Lahiri (Eds), *High Altitude and Man.* Bethesda, MD: American Physiological Society, 1984. Pp 115–128.
15. Birmingham Medical Research Expeditionary Society Mountain Sickness Study Group. Acetazolamide in control of acute mountain sickness. *Lancet* 1:180, 1981.
16. Bisgard GE, Busch MA, Forster HV. Ventilatory acclimatization to hypoxia is not dependent on cerebral hypocapnic alkalosis. *J Appl Physiol* 60:1011, 1986.
17. Black CP, Tenney SM. Oxygen transport during progressive hypoxia in high altitude and sea-level waterfowl. *Respir Physiol* 39:217, 1980.
18. Blount SG Jr, Vogel JHK. Altitude and the pulmonary circulation. *Adv Intern Med* 13:11, 1967.
19. Bontellier U, et al. Human muscle adaptation to chronic hypoxia. *Prog Clin Biol Res* 136:273, 1983.
20. Bouverot P, Bureau M. Ventilatory acclimatiza-

tion and CSF acid-base balance in carotid chemodenervated dogs at 3550 m. *Pflugers Arch* 361:17, 1975.

21. Boycott AE, Haldane JS. The effects of low atmospheric pressure on respiration. *J Physiol* 37:355, 1908.

22. Brody JS, et al. Lung elasticity and airway dynamics in Peruvian natives to high altitude. *J Appl Physiol* 42:245, 1977.

23. Buick FJ, et al. Effect of induced erythrocythemia on aerobic work capacities. *J Appl Physiol* 48:636, 1980.

24. Cahoon PL. Simple decision making at high altitude. *Ergonomics* 14:157, 1972.

25. Cerny FC, Dempsey JA, Reddan WG. Pulmonary gas exchange in non-native residents of high altitude. *J Clin Invest* 52:2993, 1973.

26. Cerretelli P. Limiting factors to oxygen transport on Mount Everest. *J Appl Physiol* 40:658, 1976.

27. Cerretelli P, di Prampero PE. Aerobic and anaerobic metabolism during exercise at altitude. *Med Sport Sci* 19:1, 1985.

28. Chiodi H. Respiratory adaptations to chronic high altitude hypoxia. *J Appl Physiol* 10:81, 1957.

29. Clark CF, Heaton RK, Wiens AN. Neuropsychological functioning after prolonged high altitude exposure in mountaineering. *Aviat Space Environ Med* 54:202, 1983.

30. Clench J, Ferrell RE, Schull WJ. Effect of chronic altitude hypoxia on hematologic and glycolytic parameters. *Am J Physiol* 242:R447, 1982.

31. Coates G, et al. Changes in lung volume, lung density, and distribution of ventilation during hypobaric decompression. *J Appl Physiol* 46:752, 1979.

32. Coudert J. La circulation pulmonaire du natif de la haute altitude a La Paz (3700 m). In *Anthropologie des Populations Andines*, Vol 63. Paris: Inserm, 1976. P 305.

33. Cruz JC. Mechanics of breathing in high altitude and sea level subjects. *Respir Physiol* 17:146, 1973.

34. Cunningham WL, Becker EJ, Krueger F. Catecholamines in plasma and urine at high altitude. *J Appl Physiol* 20:607, 1965.

35. Daristotle L, et al. The effects of carotid body hypocapnia on ventilation in goats. *Respir Physiol* 79:123, 1990.

36. Daristotle L, et al. Ventilatory effects and interactions with change in PaO_2 in awake goats. *J Appl Physiol* 71:1254, 1991.

37. Dawson A. Regional pulmonary blood flow in sitting and supine man during and after acute hypoxia. *J Clin Invest* 48:301, 1969.

38. Dawson A. Regional lung function during early acclimatization to 3100 m altitude. *J Appl Physiol* 33:218, 1972.

39. Dawson A, Grover RF. Regional lung function in natives and long-term residents at 3100 m altitude. *J Appl Physiol* 36:294, 1974.

40. DeGraff AC Jr, et al. Diffusing capacity of the lung in Caucasians native to 3100 m. *J Appl Physiol* 29:71, 1970.

41. Dempsey JA, et al. Role of cerebrospinal fluid in ventilatory deacclimatization from chronic hypoxia. *J Clin Invest* 64:199, 1979.

42. Dempsey JA, et al. Regulation of CSF [HCO_3^-] during long-term hypoxic hypocapnia in man. *J Appl Physiol* 44:175, 1978.

43. Dempsey JA, Forster HV, doPico GA. Ventilatory acclimatization to moderate hypoxemia in man: The role of spinal fluid. *J Clin Invest* 53:1091, 1974.

44. Dempsey JA, et al. Effects of moderate hypoxemia and hypocapnia on CSF and ventilation in man. *J Appl Physiol* 38:665, 1975.

45. Dempsey JA, et al. Effects of acute through life-long hypoxic exposure in exercise pulmonary gas exchange. *Respir Physiol* 13:62, 1971.

46. Dickinson JD, et al. Altitude-related deaths in seven trekkers in the Himalayas. *Thorax* 38:646, 1983.

47. Dill DB, Hillyard SD, Miller J. Vital capacity, exercise performance, and blood gases at altitude related to age. *J Appl Physiol* 48:6, 1980.

48. Dill DB, et al. Work capacity in acute exposures to altitude. *J Appl Physiol* 21:1168, 1966.

49. Eger EI II, et al. Influence of CO_2 on ventilatory acclimatization to altitude. *J Appl Physiol* 24:607, 1968.

50. Ellsworth AJ, Larson EB, Strickland D. A randomized trial of dexamethasone and acetazolamide for acute mountain sickness prophylaxis. *Am J Med* 83:1024, 1987.

51. Erslev A. Erythropoietin coming of age. *N Engl J Med* 316:101, 1987.

52. Erslev AJ. Humoral regulation of red cell production. *Blood* 8:349, 1953.

53. Fan FC, et al. Effect of hematocrit variations on regional hemodynamics and oxygen transport in the dog. *Am J Physiol* 238:H545, 1980.

54. Faraci FM, Kilgore DL Jr, Feddle MR. Oxygen delivery to the heart and brain during hypoxia: Peking duck vs. bar-headed goose. *Am J Physiol* 247:R69, 1984.

55. Faura J, et al. Effect of altitude on erythropoiesis. *Blood* 33:668, 1969.

56. Fencl V, Gabel R, Wolfe D. Composition of cerebral fluids in goats adapted to high altitude. *J Appl Physiol* 47:508, 1979.

57. Ferrazzini G, et al. Successful treatment of acute mountain sickness with dexamethasone. *Br Med J* 294:1380, 1986.

58. Finch CA, Lenfant C. Oxygen transport in man. *N Engl J Med* 296:407, 1972.

59. Fishman AP. Hypoxia and the pulmonary cir-

culation: How and where it acts. *Circ Res* 38:221, 1976.

60. Forster HV, et al. Role of intracranial receptor in physiologic regulation of ventilation in ponies. *Chest* 73 (Suppl):253, 1978.

61. Forster HV, et al Effects of chronic exposure to hypoxia on ventilatory response to CO_2 and hypoxia. *J Appl Physiol* 31:586, 1971.

62. Forster HV, Dempsey JA, Chosy LW. Incomplete compensation of CSF in man during acclimatization to high altitude (4300 m). *J Appl Physiol* 38:1067, 1975.

63. Forster HV, et al. Effect of sojourn at 4300 meters altitude on electroencephalogram and visual evoked response. *J Appl Physiol* 39:109, 1975.

64. Frisancho AR. Functional adaptation to high altitude hypoxia. *Science* 187:313, 1975.

65. Frisancho AR, Velasquez T, Sanchez J. Influence of developmental adaptation on lung function at high altitude. *Hum Biol* 45:583, 1973.

66. Gale GE, et al. Ventilation-perfusion inequality in normal humans during exercise at sea level and simulated altitude. *J Appl Physiol* 58:978, 1985.

67. Gautier H, et al. Mechanical properties of the lungs during acclimatization to altitude. *J Appl Physiol* 52:1407, 1982.

68. Gimenz M, et al. Effects of altitude on myoglobin and mitochondrial protein in canine skeletal muscle. *Respiration* 34:171, 1977.

69. Goldberg S, et al. Brain tissue pH and ventilatory acclimatization to high altitude. *J Appl Physiol* 72:58, 1991.

70. Gray GW, et al. Control of acute mountain sickness. *Aerospace Med* 1:81, 1971.

71. Greene MK, et al. Acetazolamide in prevention of acute mountain sickness: A double blind controlled cross-over study. *Br Med J* 283:811, 1981.

72. Grissom CK, et al. Acetazolamide in the treatment of acute mountain sickness: Clinical efficacy and effect on gas exchange. *Ann Intern Med* 116:461, 1992.

73. Grover RF, Reeves JT. Exercise performance of athletes at sea level and 3100 meters altitude. *Med Thorac* 23:129, 1966.

74. Grover RF, et al. Muscular exercise in young men native to 3100 meters altitude. *J Appl Physiol* 22:555, 1967.

75. Groves BM, et al. Minimal hypoxic pulmonary hypertension in normal Tibetans at 3658 m. *J Appl Physiol* 74:312–318, 1993.

76. Groves BM, et al. Operation Everest II: Elevated high altitude pulmonary resistance unresponsive to oxygen. *J Appl Physiol* 63:521, 1987.

77. Guleria JS, et al. Pulmonary diffusing capacity at high altitude. *J Appl Physiol* 31:536, 1971.

78. Gupta ML, et al. Lack of smooth muscle in the small pulmonary arteries of the native Ludakhi:

Is the Himalayan highlander adapted? *Am Rev Respir Dis* 145:1201, 1992.

79. Haab P, et al. Ventilation perfusion relationships during high altitude adaptation. *J Appl Physiol* 26:77, 1969.

80. Hackett PH, et al. Ventilation in Human Populations Native to High Altitude: In JB West, S Lahiri (Eds), *High Altitude and Man.* Bethesda, MD: American Physiological Society, 1984. Pp 179–191.

81. Hackett PH, et al. Control of breathing in Sherpas at low and high altitude. *J Appl Physiol* 49:374, 1980.

82. Hackett PH, Rennie ID. Rales, peripheral edema, retinal hemorrhage and acute mountain sickness. *Am J Med* 67:214, 1979.

83. Hackett PH, Rennie D. Acute mountain sickness. *Semin Respir Med* 5:132, 1983.

84. Hackett PH, et al. Fluid retention and relative hypoventilation in acute mountain sickness. *Respiration* 43:321, 1982.

85. Hackett PH, Rennie D, Levine HD. The incidence, importance, and prophylaxis of acute mountain sickness. *Lancet* 2:1149, 1976.

86. Hackett PH, et al. A Portable, Fabric Hyperbaric Chamber for Treatment of High Altitude Pulmonary Edema (abstract). In JR Sutton, G Coates, JE Remmers (Eds), *Hypoxia: The Adaptations.* Philadelphia: BC Dekker, 1990. P 291.

87. Hackett PH, et al. Respiratory stimulants and sleep periodic breathing at high altitude. Almitrine versus acetazolamide. *Am Rev Respir Dis* 135:896, 1987.

88. Hackett PH, et al. Abnormal control of ventilation in high-altitude pulmonary edema. *J Appl Physiol* 64:1268, 1988.

89. Hackett PH, et al. Dexamethasone for prevention and treatment of acute mountain sickness. *Aviat Space Environ Med* 59:950, 1988.

90. Hackett PH, Yarnell P, Hill RP. MRI in High Altitude Cerebral Edema: Evidence for Vasogenic Edema (abstract). In JR Sutton, G Coates, JE Remmers (Eds), *Hypoxia: The Adaptations.* Philadelphia: BC Dekker, 1990. P 295.

91. Haldane JS, Priestley JG. The regulation of lung ventilation. *J Physiol* 32:225, 1905.

92. Hansen TN, LeBlanc AL, Gest AL. Hypoxia and angiotensin II infusion redistribution lung blood flow in lambs. *J Appl Physiol* 58:812, 1985.

93. Harris P, et al. Succinic and lactic dehydrogenase activity in myocardial homogenates from animals at high and low altitude. *J Mol Cell Cardiol* 1:189, 1970.

94. Heath D, Edwards C, Harris P. Post mortem size and structure of the human carotid body: Its relation to pulmonary disease and cardiac hypertrophy. *Thorax* 25:129, 1970.

95. Heath D, et al. Small pulmonary arteries in

some natives of La Paz, Bolivia. *Thorax* 36:599, 1981.

96. Heath D, Williams DR. Pulmonary hypertension. In *Man at High Altitude: The Pathophysiology of Acclimatization and Adaptation.* Edinburgh: Churchill-Livingstone, 1977. Pp 75–88.

97. Heath D, Williams DR. Circulation. In *Man at High Altitude: The Pathophysiology of Acclimatization and Adaptation.* Edinburgh: Churchill-Livingstone, 1977. Pp 61–63.

98. Heath D, Williams DR. The Blood. In *Man at High Altitude: The Pathophysiology of Acclimatization and Adaptation.* Edinburgh: Churchill-Livingstone, 1977. Pp 39–53.

99. Hlastala MP. Interactions between O_2 and CO_2: The Blood. In JR Sutton, NL Jones, CS Houston (Eds), *Hypoxia: Man at Altitude.* New York: Thieme-Stratton, 1982. Pp 17–23.

100. Hochachka PW, et al. Metabolic meaning of elevated levels of oxidative enzymes in high altitude adapted animals: An interpretive hypothesis. *Respir Physiol* 52:303, 1982.

101. Holtby JG, Berezanski DJ, Anthonisen NR. Effect of 100% O_2 on hypoxic eucapnic ventilation. *J Appl Physiol* 65:1157, 1988.

102. Hoon RS, et al. Changes in transthoracic electrical impedance at high altitude. *Br Heart J* 39:61, 1977.

103. Hornbein TF, Townes B, Houston CS. The cost to the central nervous system of climbing to extremely high altitude. *N Engl J Med* 321:1714, 1989.

104. Houston CS. Acute pulmonary edema of high altitude. *N Engl J Med* 263:478, 1960.

105. Houston CS, Dickinson JD. Cerebral form of high altitude illness. *Lancet* 2:758, 1975.

106. Hoyt RW, et al. Effects of long distance running at high altitude on the standard oxygen-hemoglobin dissociation curve and red cell 2,3 DPG. *Eur J Appl Physiol* 51:175, 1983.

107. Huang SY, et al. Ventilatory Control in Tibetan Highlanders. In *Geological and Ecological Studies of Qinghai-Xizang Plateau.* New York: Gordon and Breach, 1981. Pp 1363–1369. [*Proc. Symp. Qinghai-Xizang (Tibet) Plateau Beijing, China,* Vol 2.]

108. Hultgren HN, Grover RF. Circulatory adaptation to high altitude. *Annu Rev Med* 19:119, 1968.

109. Hultgren HN, Grover RF, Hartley LH. Abnormal circulatory responses to high altitude in subjects with a previous history of high altitude pulmonary edema. *Circulation* 44:759, 1971.

110. Hultgren HN, et al. Physiologic studies of pulmonary edema at high altitude. *Circulation* 29:393, 1964.

111. Hultgren HN, Marticorena EA. High altitude pulmonary edema: Epidemiologic observations in Peru. *Chest* 74:372, 1978.

112. Hurtado A. Respiratory adaptations in the Indian natives of the Peruvian Andes. *Am J Phys Anthropol* 17:137, 1932.

113. Hurtado A. Animals in High Altitude: Man above 5000 Meters—Mountain Exploration. In DB Dill (Ed), *Handbook of Physiology,* sect 4: *Adaptation to the Environment.* Washington, DC: American Physiological Society, 1964. Pp 843–860.

114. Green HJ, et al. Altitude acclimatization and energy metabolic adaptations in skeletal muscle during exercise. *J Appl Physiol* 73:2701, 1992.

115. Hyers TM, et al. Accentuated hypoxemia at high altitude in subjects susceptible to high altitude pulmonary edema. *J Appl Physiol* 46:41, 1979.

116. Jacobson LO, et al. Role of kidney in erythropoiesis. *Nature* 179:633, 1957.

117. Jaeger JJ, et al. Evidence for increased intrathoracic fluid volume in man at high altitude. *J Appl Physiol* 47:670, 1979.

118. Jaenke RS, Alexander AF. Fine structural alterations of bovine peripheral pulmonary arteries in hypoxia-induced hypertension. *Am J Pathol* 73:377, 1973.

119. Kasic JF, et al. Treatment of acute mountain sickness: Hyperbaric versus oxygen therapy. *Ann Emerg Med* 20:1109, 1991.

120. Kellogg RH. Effect of altitude on respiratory regulation. *Ann NY Acad Sci* 109:815, 1963.

121. Kety SS, Schmidt CF. The effects of altered arterial tensions of carbon dioxide and oxygen on cerebral blood flow and cerebral oxygen consumption of normal young men. *J Clin Invest* 27:484, 1948.

122. Keys A, Hall FG, Barron ES. The position of the oxygen dissociation curve of human blood. *Am J Physiol* 115:292, 1936.

123. Klausen K. Cardiac output in man in rest and work during and after acclimatization to 3800 m. *J Appl Physiol* 21:609, 1966.

124. Kobayashi T, et al. Clinical features of patients with high altitude pulmonary edema in Japan. *Chest* 92:814, 1987.

125. Kobrick JL. Effects of hypoxia on peripheral visual response to dim stimuli. *Percept Mot Skills* 41:467, 1975.

126. Kogure K, et al. Mechanisms of cerebral vasodilation in hypoxia. *J Appl Physiol* 29:223, 1970.

127. Kontos HA, et al. Comparative circulatory responses to systemic hypoxia in man and in unanesthetized dog. *J Appl Physiol* 23:281, 1967.

128. Krogh A. Number and distribution of capillaries in muscles with calculations of the oxygen pressure head necessary to supply the tissue. *J Physiol (Lond)* 52:409, 1919.

129. Krueger F, et al. Alveolar-arterial oxygen gradient in Andean natives at high altitude. *J Appl Physiol* 19:13, 1964.

130. Kryger MH, Grover RF. Chronic mountain sickness. *Semin Respir Med* 5:164, 1983.
131. Kryger M, et al. Treatment of excessive polycythemia of high altitude with respiratory stimulant drugs. *Am Rev Respir Dis* 117:455, 1978.
132. Kryger M, et al. Excessive polycythemia of high altitude: Role of ventilatory drive and lung disease. *Am Rev Respir Dis* 118:659, 1978.
133. Lahiri S. Alveolar gas pressures in man with lifetime hypoxia. *Respir Physiol* 4:373, 1968.
134. Lahiri S. Respiratory Control in Andean and Himalayan High-Altitude Natives. In JB West, S Lahiri (Eds), *High Altitude and Man.* Bethesda, MD: American Physiological Society, 1984. Pp 147–162.
135. Lahiri S, et al. Relative role of environmental and genetic factors in respiratory adaptation to high altitude. *Nature* 261:133, 1976.
136. Lahiri S, et al. Irreversible blunted respiratory sensitivity to hypoxia in high altitude natives. *Respir Physiol* 6:360, 1969.
137. Lahiri S, et al. Respiration of man during exercise at high altitude: Highlanders vs. lowlanders. Respir. Physiol. 8:361–375, 1970.
138. Lahiri S, Maret K, Sherpa MG. Dependence of high-altitude sleep apnea on ventilatory sensitivity to hypoxia. *Respir Physiol* 52:281, 1983.
139. Lahiri S, et al. Respiration and heart rate of Sherpa highlanders during exercise. *J Appl Physiol* 23:545, 1967.
140. Larson EB, et al. Acute mountain sickness and acetazolamide: Clinical efficacy and effect on ventilation. *JAMA* 248:328, 1982.
141. Lechner AJ, Banchero N. Lung morphometry in guinea pigs acclimated to hypoxia during growth. *Respir Physiol* 42:155, 1980.
142. Lenfant C, et al. Effect of altitude on oxygen binding by hemoglobin and on organic phosphate levels. *J Clin Invest* 47:2652, 1968.
143. Lenfant C, Torrance JD, Reynafarje C. Shift of the O$_2$-Hb dissociation curve at altitude: Mechanism and effect. *J Appl Physiol* 305:625, 1971.
144. Levine BD, Roach RC, Houston CS. Work and Training at High Altitude. In JR Sutton, G Coates, CS Houston (Eds), *Hypoxia and Mountain Medicine.* Burlington, VT: Queen City Printers, 1992. Pp 192–201.
145. Levine BD, et al. Dexamethasone in the treatment of acute mountain sickness. *N Engl J Med* 321:1707, 1989.
146. Levine BD, et al. Dexamethasone in the treatment of acute mountain sickness. *N Engl J Med* 321:1707, 1989.
147. Lockhart A, Saiag B. Altitude and the human pulmonary circulation. *Clin Sci* 60:599, 1981.
148. MacDougall JD, et al. Operation Everest II: Structural adaptations in skeletal muscle in response to extreme simulated altitude. *Acta Physiol Scand* 142:421, 1991.
149. Mager M, et al. Effect of high altitude on lactic dehydrogenase isozymes of neonatal and adult rats. *Am J Physiol* 215:5, 1968.
150. Maher JT, Jones LG, Hartley LH. Effects of high altitude exposure on submaximal endurance capacity of men. *J Appl Physiol* 37:895, 1974.
151. Manchander SC, Maher JT, Cymerman A. Cardiac performance during graded exercise in acute hypoxia. *J Appl Physiol* 38:858, 1975.
152. Mansell A, Poules A, Sutton JR. Changes in pulmonary PV characteristics of human subjects at an altitude of 5366 m. *J Appl Physiol* 49:79, 1980.
153. Masuyama S, et al. Control of ventilation in extreme-altitude climbers. *J Appl Physiol* 61:500, 1986.
154. Mathew L, et al. Chemoreceptor sensitivity in adaptation to high altitude. *Aviat Space Environ Med* 54:121, 1983.
155. Meerson FZ, Pshennikava MG. Effects of adaptation to high altitude hypoxia on the contractile function and adrenoreactivity of the heart. *Basic Respir Cardiol* 74:142, 1979.
156. Milledge JS, Coates PM. Serum erythropoietin in humans at high altitude and its relation to plasma renin. *J Appl Physiol* 59:360, 1985.
157. Milledge JS, Lahiri S. Respiratory control in lowlanders and Sherpa highlanders at altitude. *Respir Physiol* 2:310, 1967.
158. Monge CC. *Natural Acclimatization to High Altitudes: Clinical Conditions in Life at High Altitudes.* Scientific publication no 140. Washington, DC: Pan American Health Organization, 1966. Pp 46–52.
159. Monge MC. La enfermedad de los Andes. Sindromes eritremicos. *Ann Fac Med Univ San Marcos (Lima)* 11:1, 1928.
160. Monge MC, Monge CC. In *High Altitude Diseases: Mechanism and Management.* Springfield, IL: Charles C Thomas, 1966. P 14.
161. Montgomery AB, Mills J, Luce JM. Incidence of acute mountain sickness at intermediate altitude. *JAMA* 261:732, 1989.
162. Moore LG, Brewer GJ. Beneficial effect of rightward hemoglobin-oxygen dissociation curve shift for short-term high altitude adaptations. *J Lab Clin Med* 98:145, 1981.
163. Moore LG, et al. Low acute hypoxic ventilatory response and hypoxic depression in acute altitude sickness. *J Appl Physiol* 60:1407, 1986.
164. Moore LG, Sun SF. Physiologic Adaptation to Hypoxia in Tibetan and Acclimatized Han Residents of Lhasa. In JR Sutton, G Coates, JE Remmers (Eds), *Hypoxia: The Adaptations.* Philadelphia: BC Decker, 1990. Pp 66–71.
165. Mosso A. La respiration periodique et la respiration superflue ou de luxe. *Arch Ital Biol* 7:48, 1886.
166. Nayak NC, Roy S, Narayaran TK. Pathologic

features of altitude sickness. *Am J Pathol* 45:381, 1964.

167. Nelson BD, Highman B, Altland PD. Oxidative phosphorylation during altitude acclimation in rats. *Am J Physiol* 213:1414, 1967.

168. Neubauer JA, Simone A, Edelman NH. Role of brain lactic acidosis in hypoxic depression of respiration. *J Appl Physiol* 65:1324, 1988.

169. Nielsen AM, Bisgard GE, Vidruk EH. Carotid chemoreceptor activity during acute and sustained hypoxia in goats. *J Appl Physiol* 65:1796, 1988.

170. Novikova NA, Gorina MS, Kapel'Ko VI. Contractile function of the heart and its reactivity to noradrenaline in the process of the body's adaptation to moderate altitude. *Buill Eksp Biol Med* 84:5, 1977.

171. Oelz O, et al. Physiological profile of world-class high-altitude climbers. *J Appl Physiol* 60:1734, 1986.

172. Olson EB Jr, Dempsey JA. Rat as a model for humanlike ventilatory adaptation to chronic hypoxia. *J Appl Physiol* 44:763, 1978.

173. Orr JA, et al. Cerebrospinal fluid alkalosis during high altitude sojourn in unanesthetized ponies. *Respir Physiol* 25:23, 1975.

174. Ou LC, Tenney SM. Properties of mitochondria from hearts of cattle acclimatized to high altitude. *Respir Physiol* 8:151, 1970.

175. Pelligrino DA, Musch TI, Dempsey JA. Interregional differences in brain intracellular pH and water compartmentation during acute normoxic and hypoxic hypocapnia in the anesthetized dog. *Brain Res* 214:387, 1981.

176. Penaloza D, et al. The heart and pulmonary circulation in children at high altitude: Physiological, anatomical and clinical observations. *Pediatrics* 34:568, 1964.

177. Petschow D, et al. Causes of high blood O_2 affinity of animals living at high altitude. *J Appl Physiol* 42:139, 1977.

178. Pickett CB, Cascarano J, Wilson MA. Acute and chronic hypoxia in rats. *J Exp Zool* 210:49, 1979.

179. Pugh LGCE. Athletes at altitude. *J Physiol* 192:619, 1967.

180. Pugh LGCE. Cardiac output in muscular exercise at 5800 m (19,000 feet). *J Appl Physiol* 19:441, 1964.

181. Rahn H, Otis AB. Man's respiratory response during and after acclimatization to high altitude. *Am J Physiol* 157:445, 1946.

182. Rapin JR, et al. Uptake of noradrenaline in high altitude native hearts. *Experientia* 33:739, 1977.

183. Reeves JT, et al. Operation Everest II: Preservation of cardiac function at extreme altitude. *J Appl Physiol* 63:531, 1987.

184. Reeves JT, et al. Physiological Effects of High Altitude on the Pulmonary Circulation. In D Robertshaw (Ed), *International Review of Phys-iology, Environmental Physiology III.* Baltimore: University Park Press, 1979.

185. Remmers JE, Mithoefer JC. The carbon monoxide diffusing capacity in permanent residents at high altitude. *Respir Physiol* 6:233, 1969.

186. Reynafarje C, et al. Humoral control of erythropoietic activity in man during and after high altitude exposure. *Proc Soc Exp Biol Med* 116:649, 1964.

187. Robinson KA, Hayner EM. Metabolic effects of exposure to hypoxia plus cold at rest and during exercise in human. *J Appl Physiol* 68:720, 1990.

188. Rose MS, et al. Operation Everest II: Nutrition and body composition. *J Appl Physiol* 65:2545, 1988.

189. Rotta A, et al. Pulmonary circulation at sea level and at high altitudes. *J Appl Physiol* 9:328, 1956.

190. Ryn Z. Psychopathology in alpinism. *Acta Med Pol* 12:453, 1976.

191. Saltin B, et al. Maximal oxygen uptake and cardiac output after two weeks at 4300 meters. *J Appl Physiol* 25:400, 1968.

192. Samaja M, Veicsteinas A, Cerritelli P. Oxygen affinity of blood in altitude Sherpas. *J Appl Physiol* 47:337, 1979.

193. Sarnquist FH, Schoene RB, Hackett PH. Exercise tolerance and cerebral function after acute hemodilution of polycythemic mountain climbers. *Aviat Space Environ Med* 57:313, 1986.

194. Schoene RB. Hypoxic Ventilatory Response and Exercise Ventilation at Sea Level and High Altitude. In JB West, S Lahiri (Eds), *Man at High Altitude.* Bethesda, MD: American Physiological Society, 1984. Pp 19–30.

195. Schoene RB. The control of ventilation in climbers to extreme altitude. *J Appl Physiol* 53:886, 1982.

196. Schoene RB, et al. Relationship of hypoxic ventilatory response to exercise performance on Mount Everest. *J Appl Physiol* 56:1478, 1984.

197. Schoene RB, et al. High altitude pulmonary edema and exercise at 4400 meters on Mount McKinley: Effect of expiratory positive airway pressure. *Chest* 87:330, 1985.

198. Schoene RB, et al. Operation Everest II: Ventilatory adaptation during gradual decompression to extreme altitude. *Med Sci Sports Exerc* 22:804, 1990.

199. Schoene RB, et al. Increased diffusion capacity maintains arterial saturations during exercise in the Quechua Indians of the Chilean Altiplano. *Am J Hum Biol* 2:663, 1990.

200. Schoene RB, et al. The lung at high altitude: Bronchoalveolar lavage in acute mountain sickness and pulmonary edema. *J Appl Physiol* 64:2605, 1988.

201. Scoggin CH, et al. High altitude pulmonary edema in the children and young adults of Leadville, Colorado. *N Engl J Med* 297:1269, 1977.

202. Selvamurthy W, et al. Changes in EEG pattern during acclimatization to high altitude (3500 meters) in man. *Aviat Space Environ Med* 49:968, 1968.
203. Severinghaus JW, Bainton CR, Carcellen A. Respiratory insensitivity to hypoxia in chronically hypoxic man. *Respir Physiol* 1:308, 1966.
204. Severinghaus JW, et al. Cerebral blood flow in man at high altitude. Role of cerebrospinal fluid pH in normalization of flow in chronic hypocapnia. *Circ Res* 19:274, 1966.
205. Severinghaus JW, et al. Respiratory control at high altitude suggesting active transport regulation of CSF pH. *J Appl Physiol* 18:1155, 1963.
206. Sharma VM, Malhotra MS. Ethnic variations in psychological performance under altitude stress. *Aviat Space Environ Med* 47:248, 1976.
207. Sharma VM, Malhotra MS, Baskoran AS. Variations in psychomotor efficiency during prolonged stay at high altitude. *Ergonomics* 18:511, 1975.
208. Singh I, et al. Acute mountain sickness. *N Engl J Med* 280:175, 1969.
209. Sorensen SC, Severinghaus JW. Irreversible respiratory insensitivity to acute hypoxia in men born at high altitude. *J Appl Physiol* 25:217, 1968.
210. Squires RW, Buskirk ER. Aerobic capacity during acute exposure to simulated altitude 914 to 2286 m. *Med Sci Sports Exerc* 14:36, 1982.
211. Staub NC. Overperfusion edema. *N Engl J Med* 302:1085, 1980.
212. Stenberg J, Ecblom B, Messin R. Hemodynamic response to work at simulated altitude, 4000 m. *J Appl Physiol* 21:1589, 1966.
213. Sui GJ, et al. Subacute infantile mountain sickness. *J Pathol* 155:161, 1988.
214. Sutton JR, et al. Effects of duration at altitude and acetazolamide in ventilation and oxygenation during sleep. *Sleep* 3:455, 1980.
215. Sutton JR, et al. Effect of acetazolamide on hypoxia during sleep at high altitude. *N Engl J Med* 301:1329, 1979.
216. Sutton JR, et al. Operation Everest II: Oxygen transport during exercise at extreme simulated altitude. *J Appl Physiol* 64:1309, 1988.
217. Swan LW. Goose of the Himalaya. *Nat Hist* 79:68, 1970.
218. Swenson ER, et al. Renal carbonic anhydrase inhibition reduces high altitude periodic breathing. *Respir Physiol* 86:333, 1991.
219. Sylvester JT, et al. Components of alveolar-arterial O_2 gradient during rest and exercise at sea level and high altitude. *J Appl Physiol* 50:1129, 1981.
220. Taber RL. Protocols for the use of a portable hyperbaric chamber for the treatment of high altitude disorders. *J Wilderness Med* 1:181, 1990.
221. Tappan DV, Reynafarje B. Tissue pigment man-
ifestations of adaptation to high altitudes. *Am J Physiol* 190:99, 1957.
222. Tappan DV, et al. Alterations in enzymes and metabolites resulting from adaptation to low oxygen tensions. *Am J Physiol* 190:93, 1957.
223. Tenney SM, et al. Adaptation to high altitude: Changes in lung volumes during the first seven days at Mt. Evans, Colorado. *J Appl Physiol* 5:607, 1953.
224. Torre-Bueno JR, et al. Diffusion limitation in normal humans during exercise at sea level and simulated altitude. *J Appl Physiol* 58:989, 1985.
225. Vargas E, et al. Pulmonary diffusing capacity in young Andean highland children. *Respiration* 43:330, 1982.
226. Vincent J, et al. Pulmonary gas exchange, diffusing capacity in natives and newcomers at high altitude. *Respir Physiol* 34:219, 1978.
227. Vizek M, Pickett CK, Weil JV. Increased carotid body hypoxic sensitivity during acclimatization to hypobaric hypoxia. *J Appl Physiol* 63:2403, 1987.
228. Vogel JA, Harris CW. Cardiopulmonary responses of resting man during early exposure to high altitude. *J Appl Physiol* 22:1124, 1967.
229. Vogel JA, Hartley H, Cruz JC. Cardiac output during exercise in altitude natives at sea level and high altitude. *J Appl Physiol* 36:173, 1974.
230. Vogel JA, et al. Cardiac output during exercise in sea-level residents at sea level and high altitude. *J Appl Physiol* 36:169, 1974.
231. Wagner PD, et al. Pulmonary gas exchange in humans exercising at sea level and simulated altitude. *J Appl Physiol* 61:280, 1986.
232. Wagner PD, et al. Operation Everest II: Pulmonary gas exchange during simulated ascent of Mt. Everest. *J Appl Physiol* 63:2348, 1987.
233. Weil JV, et al. Acquired attenuation of chemoreceptor function in chemically hypoxic man at high altitude. *J Clin Invest* 50:186, 1971.
234. Weiskopf RB, Gabel RA, Fencl V. Alkaline shift in lumbar and intracranial CSF in man after 5 days at high altitude. *J Appl Physiol* 41:93, 1976.
235. West JB, Wagner PD. Predicted gas exchange on the summit of Mt. Everest. *Respir Physiol* 42:1, 1980.
236. West JB. Rate of ventilatory acclimatization to extreme altitude. *Respir Physiol* 74:323, 1988.
237. West JB, et al. Maximal exercise at extreme altitudes on Mount Everest. *J Appl Physiol* 55:688, 1983.
238. West JB, et al. Pulmonary gas exchange on the summit of Mt. Everest. *J Appl Physiol* 55:678, 1983.
239. West JB, et al. Arterial oxygen saturation during exercise at high altitude. *J Appl Physiol* 17:617, 1962.
240. West JB, et al. Nocturnal periodic breathing at altitudes of 6300 and 8050 meters. *J Appl Physiol* 61:280, 1987.

241. West JB, et al. Stress failure in pulmonary capillaries. *J Appl Physiol* 70:1731, 1991.

242. Winslow RM. Red Cell Function at Extreme Altitude. In JB West, S Lahiri (Eds), *High Altitude and Man.* Bethesda, MD: American Physiological Society, 1984. Pp 59–72.

243. Winslow RM. High Altitude Polycythemia. In JB West, S Lahiri (Eds), *High Altitude and Man.* Bethesda, MD: American Physiological Society, 1984. Pp 163–172.

244. Winslow RM. Relationship between Erythropoiesis and Ventilation in High Altitude Natives. In S Lahiri, NS Cherniack, RS Fitzerland (Eds), *Response and Adaptation to Hypoxia. Organ to Organelle.* New York: Oxford University Press, 1991. Pp 143–156.

245. Winslow RM, Carlos Monge C. *Hypoxia, Polycythemia, and Chronic Mountain Sickness.* Baltimore: Johns Hopkins University Press, 1987.

246. Xie C-F, Pei S-X. Some Physiological Data on Sojourners and Native Highlanders at Three Different Altitudes in Xizang. In LD Shang (Ed), *Proceedings of Symposium on Tibet Plateau.* New York, Gordon and Breach Science, 1981. Pp 1449–1452.

247. Yagi H, et al. Doppler assessment of pulmonary hypertension induced by hypoxic breathing in subjects susceptible to high altitude pulmonary edema. *Am Rev Respir Dis* 142:796, 1990.

248. Zell SC, Goodman PH. Acetazolamide and dexamethasone in the prevention of acute mountain sickness. *West J Med* 148:541, 1988.

249. Honigman B, et al. Acute mountain sickness in a general tourist population at moderate altitudes. *Ann Intern Med* 118:587, 1993.

250. Huang S, et al. Internal carotid arterial velocity during exercise in Tibetan and Han Chinese residents of Lhasa. *J Appl Physiol* 73:2638, 1992.

251. Knaupp W, Khilnani, Sherwood J. Erythropoietin response to acute normobaric hypoxia in humans. *J Appl Physiol* 73:837, 1992.

252. Serebrovskaya TV, Ivashkevich AA. Effect of a 1-year stay at altitude on ventilation, metabolism and work capacity. *J Appl Physiol* 73:1749, 1992.

253. Zhuang J, et al. Hypoxic ventilatory responsiveness in Tibetan compared to Han residents at 3658 M. *J Appl Physiol* 74:303, 1993.

45

Near-drowning and Diving Accidents

Tom S. Neuman

Epidemiology

Drowning and near-drowning are common clinical problems, and pulmonary physicians and internists should be well versed in the management of such victims. By definition, *drowning* is meant to imply that death occurred due to the effects of submersion in a fluid medium, whereas *near-drowning* implies that the individual survived the immediate effects of the event. The term *secondary drowning* is sometimes used to refer to individuals who died after a prolonged course and in other cases, the term is used to describe individuals who only demonstrate significant symptoms several hours after the submersion incident. In any event, the term is not well defined, and therefore, it is probably of little clinical utility.

Drowning is responsible for 7000 to 8000 deaths per year in the United States and there are estimated to be over 90,000 near-drowning incidents that occur annually [17,161]. From a strictly numerical point of view, drownings and near-drownings are predominantly a problem of the pediatric age group. Until recently, motor vehicle accidents were the chief cause of death of children aged 4 to 14 years [68]; however, as more and more states have legislated mandatory child restraint laws, drowning has replaced motor vehicle accidents as the leading cause of death among children in those states [30,179].

The risk factors that lead to drowning and near-drowning incidents are quite variable. About 20 percent of the annual number of fatalities are related to boating accidents. In the majority of those cases, death could have been prevented had the victim been wearing a personal flotation device [60]. Another 5 to 10 percent of victims are individuals trapped in submerged motor vehicles [170].

Most drownings occur in fresh water (swimming pools, lakes, ponds, etc.) and under conditions where victims are not supervised. Indeed, 80 percent of all drownings occur at sites that have not been designated for swimming [6,31, 109,143,182]. Thus, it is not clear whether there is an inherently greater risk in these bodies of water or whether it is the lack of supervision per se that plays a greater role.

In the toddler age group, the majority of drownings occur in residential pools [124,130,131, 134,151]. There is no question that inadequate safety measures play a major role in these deaths [40,131], and in areas with legislated safety requirements (fences with height requirements, self-latching gates, etc.), the incidence of pediatric drownings is lower than in areas without such legislation [95,132,133].

Demographically, drowning is more common in males than females, and in boating-related incidents, this ratio is more than 10 to 1, whereas for all groups, the overall ratio is 5 to 1 [124]. For males, the risk is greatest among toddlers, peaking at age 2, with a second rise in incidence occurring during adolescence, with a peak at age 18 [127]. For females, toddlers are also at greater risk; however, there is no rise in incidence during adolescence [6,187].

Several studies suggest that race is a risk factor for drowning as well. Blacks drown almost twice as frequently as whites, and black males drown almost three times as frequently as white males [31,162]. It seems reasonable to assume that these differences are related to underlying socioeconomic conditions; however, this is a phenomenon that has not been studied.

As with fatal motor vehicle accidents, the single greatest risk factor for drowning in adults and teenagers appears to be alcohol consumption [63,64]. Multiple different studies, done in widely disparate geographic locations around the world, indicate that alcohol plays a role in approximately 50 percent of the fatal immersion incidents [15,17,27,31,139,140]. In boating accidents that result in fatalities, this figure is even higher [110,186].

Special Circumstances Associated with Drowning

Scuba Diving

Drowning appears to be the leading cause of the approximately 100 deaths that occur annually in the population of recreational scuba divers. These drowning and near-drowning incidents are most frequently due to the exhaustion of the diver's air supply at depth which may be associated with entanglement in kelp or a wreck or simply being lost in a cave. A smaller percentage of these accidents are due to exhaustion and/or panic on the surface at the end of a dive. The second most common cause of death among scuba divers is arterial gas embolism (AGE) (see section on diving accidents later in this chapter) and drowning or near-drowning incidents frequently complicate this entity even when it does not yield a fatal result [86–90,156–160].

Shallow-Water Blackout

Intentional hyperventilation prior to underwater swimming activities can result in unconsciousness, which then results in either a drowning or a near-drowning episode. Hyperventilation reduces the PCO_2 in the arterial blood, and therefore, allows a longer period for $PaCO_2$ to reach the breath-hold breakpoint. Although hyperventilation increases the PaO_2, it does not appreciably increase the amount of oxygen (oxygen content) dissolved in the blood. As a result, the PO_2 falls in the arterial blood at much the same rate whether or not there was prior hyperventilation. By and large, a swimmer's decision to return to the surface is dependent on $PaCO_2$ and thus, hyperventilation prior to underwater swimming activities can allow an individual to remain underwater to the point where hypoxia occurs before the breath-hold breakpoint (which is as noted above, dependent on $PaCO_2$) and unconsciousness ensues [23,24,168] (Table 45-1). This situation is further aggravated by two other aspects of underwater swimming: First, the $PaCO_2$ at the breath-hold breakpoint is higher during exercise than rest; and second, ascent in the water column at the end of a breath-hold dive further reduces

the alveolar PO_2 on the basis of the reduction in total barometric pressure [24]. Indeed, the combination of a prolonged breath-hold dive and the reduction in barometric pressure can lower alveolar PO_2 below that of mixed venous PO_2 and cause a reversal of the alveolar-arterial oxygen gradient [62].

Hypothermia

Although it has been written about extensively, hypothermia per se is rarely the actual cause of death in immersion victims. Long before an individual succumbs to the direct effects of hypothermia, lowered body temperature interferes with a person's ability to function appropriately in the water. Ultimately, unconsciousness ensues and the victim drowns. Historically, the sinking of the Titanic is probably the most striking example. Although assistance was only a few hours away and the sea was calm, there were no survivors among the people in the water whereas there were no fatalities among those in lifeboats [94]. Similarly, when the Lakonia sank in 16°C water, more than 200 passengers were immersed. In less than 3 hours, 113 of those died of the combination of drowning and hypothermia [84]. It is important, however, to realize that hypothermia can have a profound effect on the prognosis of near-drowning victims, and should an individual's core temperature drop rapidly enough, the hypothermia can have a significant protective effect [164,166,184,190].

Trauma

Although most drownings and near-drownings occur under circumstances where trauma does not complicate the issue, there exists a subset of victims for whom trauma was the initiating factor that ultimately led to the near-drowning event. This can be due to either loss of consciousness or inability to remain afloat secondary to an injury. Obviously, a swimmer can be struck by a boat and either suffer a head injury or sustain direct propeller injuries, and surfers (as well as body surfers) are at risk for neck and back injuries that can result in paralysis. Of the approximately 2000 spinal cord injuries that occur in the United States each year, approximately half of them are due to diving into shallow water and striking the bottom [12,53,73,77,135]. Many of these incidents are complicated by near-drowning.

Table 45-1. **Effects of hyperventilation on the breath-holding (BH) time and alveolar gas pressure at the breaking point in resting and exercising humans**

Measurements	Resting		Exercising	
	Without hyperventilation	With hyperventilation	Without hyperventilation	With hyperventilation
BH time (s)	87	146	62	85
End-tidal PCO_2 (mmHg)				
Before BH	40	21	38	22
Breaking point	51	46	54	49
End-tidal PO_2 (mmHg)				
Before BH	103	131	102	130
Breaking point	73	58	54	43

Source: Reproduced from AB Craig Jr, Causes of loss of consciousness during underwater swimming. *J Appl Physiol* 16:583–586, 1961.

Child Abuse

The intentional immersion of a child underwater in a bathtub is a well-recognized form of child abuse [129]. Although a complete discussion of the nature of child abuse is beyond the scope of this chapter, it is worthwhile to be aware of the situation, which should make a treating physician extremely suspicious that direct abuse rather than simple neglect has occurred. Bathtub incidents that are not frank abuse (although one might argue this degree of neglect constitutes abuse) typically occur when a child under the age of 12 to 18 months is left in a tub either completely unsupervised or under the care of an older sibling (e.g., when the caretaker goes to answer the phone or door). In this setting, when the child submerges, the toddler is too young or physically not adequately developed to either stand or even get up out of the water. An incident where an older child who is normally developed (i.e., without a seizure disorder) and who should have been physically capable of getting up unassisted is said to have suffered such an incident should raise the suspicion of child abuse [7,59,145]. In any event, it is probably wise to inform a child advocacy team about any child who suffers an immersion incident in a bathtub.

Pathophysiology

When a person is initially immersed in water, the first response is panic followed by violent struggling. Reflex swallowing and attempts at breathing then occur, with resultant aspiration of varying amounts of water [81,121]. Aspiration of fluid, however, does not appear to occur universally, as it appears that as many as 15 percent of victims do not have evidence of aspiration. The mechanism that protects the tracheobronchial tree in this setting is presumed to be laryngospasm [22,98]; however, there is no direct evidence that this actually occurs. Nonetheless, the lung is clearly the target organ insofar as immersion incidents are concerned, and it has been clearly established that the underlying mechanism of the pathophysiologic processes involved in drowning and near-drowning is hypoxemia [61,97,101,147, 163]. Whether this occurs as a consequence of aspiration or laryngospasm, the immediate results are largely the same. Hypoxemia eventually leads to unconsciousness and finally to cardiac arrest [61]. When aspiration does not occur, the period of hypoxemia is generally only limited to the period of immersion and the time of inadequate ventilation. As soon as normal ventilation is reestablished, hypoxemia is corrected, and as long as the victim did not develop circulatory collapse, oxygenation is quickly reestablished. Assuming irreversible cardiac or cerebral damage did not occur during the period of hypoxemia, the recovery should be relatively rapid and complete. When aspiration does occur, the pathophysiologic processes involved are markedly different, although the effect on the victim is still mediated through hypoxemia. Unlike the victim who does not aspirate, the victim who has aspirated remains hypoxemic even after being rescued from the water and this hypoxemia persists long after normal ventilation is reestablished. Consequently, the period of hypoxemia is potentially much longer with a much higher likelihood for the development of secondary problems. The mechanisms of continued hypoxemia in the face of fluid aspiration have not been completely elucidated. Clearly, one mechanism may be concomitant aspiration of stomach contents, as drowning victims often swallow large amounts of the water in which they are immersed. In the case of freshwater aspiration, there is evidence to suggest that surface-active agents are washed out of the lung and Type II pneumocytes are sufficiently injured to prevent, at least temporarily, the production of surfactants. This, in turn, leads to focal areas of atelectasis and collapse, which results in areas of low ventilation-perfusion ($\dot{V}A/\dot{Q}$) ratio and hypoxemia. In the case of saltwater aspiration, it has been postulated that the aspiration of hypertonic materials (sand, diatom algae, etc.) leads to the production of a reactive exudate, and this in turn also leads to surfactant loss and results in areas of low $\dot{V}A/\dot{Q}$ ratio. In either situation, the result is a persistent $\dot{V}A/\dot{Q}$ mismatch, which leads to prolonged hypoxemia. Although these simplistic explanations are satisfying, they by no means fully explain the processes involved in lung dysfunction secondary to near-drowning. Such syntheses do not explain the hypoxemia associated with bronchopulmonary lavage; the progressive nature of the alterations of gas exchange, which may not reach their maximum for as much as 6 to 8 hours; or the delay in the onset of symptoms, which can take as much as 24 hours. Indeed, there is some evidence that the initial injury is to the vascular endothelium rather than to the pneumocytes. In any event, whatever the exact mechanism of hypoxemia, it appears to make no difference to the outcome whether an individual aspirates seawater, fresh water, brackish water, or water with 1 to 2 ppm of chlorine, in spite of the evidence in animal models which suggests that pure water produces the greatest amount of pulmonary injury [18,48,54,56,58,104,105].

In addition to the hypoxemia that occurs on the basis of a $\dot{V}/\dot{Q}$ mismatch, other abnormalities of gas exchange also take place. As previously noted, many victims of near-drowning swallow large quantities of the water in which they are submerged. This results in gastric distension (Fig. 45-1) and elevation of the diaphragm. Coupled with loss of consciousness from hypoxemia and potential partial or complete upper airway obstruction from flaccid musculature or foreign bodies, this leads to significant alveolar hypoventilation. As a result, varying degrees of carbon dioxide retention are frequently found in near-drowning victims and varying degrees of respi-

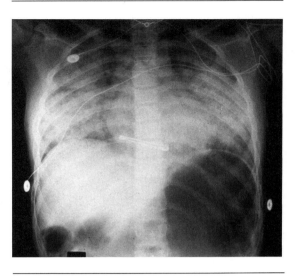

Fig. 45-1. Radiograph of a near-drowning victim on arrival at the hospital. Note the bilateral diffuse infiltrates and pattern of pulmonary edema. The stomach is distended secondary to reflex swallowing and resuscitation efforts.

ratory acidosis ensue. In addition to the respiratory acidosis due to alveolar hypoventilation, a metabolic acidosis that results from the accumulation of lactic acid frequently occurs. Lactic acid accumulation is thought to be secondary to both hypoxemia and the antecedent struggle before the victim loses consciousness underwater. The metabolic component of the acidosis is usually more significant than the respiratory component and it is not unusual to see base deficits greater than -15 mEq/liter in near-drowning victims, with initial pH levels less than 7.20 [97] (Table 45-2). As the above-mentioned abnormalities progress, the likelihood of circulatory collapse and cardiac arrest increases. If hypoxemia and decreased cardiac output persist for long enough, irreversible anoxic brain damage occurs.

Abnormalities of serum electrolytes associated with near-drowning appear to be neither a consistent nor a significant problem in most victims. In the past, it was believed that a major portion of the physiologic abnormalities associated with near-drowning were due to electrolyte imbalance. These beliefs were based on animal work where varying quantities of either fresh or salt water were instilled into the endotracheal tubes of anesthetized dogs. When ocean water, which has an average potassium concentration of 11 mEq/liter

[189], was instilled (at 10 ml/lb), hypernatremia, hyperchloremia, and hyperkalemia ensued [174–176]. This then appeared to produce fatal electrolyte abnormalities. When fresh water was instilled instead, hyponatremia, hypochloremia, and hyperkalemia (presumably on the basis of red cell lysis) occurred, resulting in ventricular fibrillation and death. It is clear, however, from repeated observations of human victims that clinically significant electrolyte abnormalities do not occur except under very unusual conditions (Table 45-3). It appears that the amount of fluid aspirated during either a drowning or a near-drowning episode is simply insufficient to cause the changes seen in the previously described dog model [7,38,56,59,61,102,106,163,185]. Furthermore, the hyperkalemia seen in the dog model was more than likely due to acidosis rather than red cell lysis, as the major intracellular cation in the dog erythrocyte is sodium rather than potassium [147]. There is, however, one exception to this situation. Victims who have near-

Table 45-2. Arterial blood gas and pH values found on admission to the hospital after near-drowning

pH	PaCO$_2$ (mmHg)	Base excess (mEq/liter)	PaO$_2$ (mmHg)	FiO$_2$
In fresh water				
6.95	64	−19	245	1.0
7.01	38	−22	28	0.2
7.05	59	−16	40	1.0 R
7.13	30	−19	67	0.2
7.14	45	−14	68	0.2
7.18	33	−15	110	1.0
7.19	29	−16	108	+0.8 R
7.21	37	−13	175	1.0
7.22	54	−7	123	1.0 R
7.28	54	−3	35	0.4
7.33	41	−4	127	1.0
7.40	32	−4	103	0.2
7.44	32	−2	76	0.2
7.45	35	1	84	0.2
In seawater				
7.03	36	−21	58	1.0
7.08	58	−14	21	1.0 R
7.20	46	−10	27	0.2
7.29	49	−4	364	1.0 R
7.31	35	−8	85	0.8 R
7.35	47	−1	45	0.2
7.46	25	−5	71	0.2
7.47	26	−3	82	0.4

R = mechanical ventilation.
Source: Reproduced from JH Modell, *The Pathophysiology and Treatment of Drowning and Near-Drowning.* Springfield, IL: CC Thomas, 1971. Pp. 44–45.

Table 45-3. Serum electrolytes in human near-drowning victims

	Na$^+$ (mEq/liter)			Cl$^-$ (mEq/liter)			K$^+$ (mEq/liter)		
	No.	Mean	Range	No.	Mean	Range	No.	Mean	Range
Freshwater victims	22	137	126–146	25	101	88–116	21	4.4	3.0–6.3
Seawater victims	26	147	132–160	28	111	96–127	25	4.2	3.2–5.4

Source: Reproduced from JH Modell, *The Pathophysiology and Treatment of Drowning and Near-Drowning.* Springfield, IL: CC Thomas, 1971. Pp. 17–18.

Table 45-4. **Electrolyte abnormalities in Dead Sea near-drowning victims**

	On admission	Maximum
Ca^{2+} (7 patients)	12.0 mg/dl	16.7 mg/dl
Mg^{2+} (5 patients)	7.2 mg/dl	8.2 mg/dl

Source: Adapted from Y Yagil et al. Near drowning in the Dead Sea: Electrolyte imbalances and therapeutic implications. *Arch Intern Med* 145:50, 1985.

drowning episodes in the Dead Sea do have major abnormalities of electrolyte concentration (Table 45-4). In this unique environment the concentration of salts is so high that aspiration of even small volumes of water have been thought to induce electrolyte changes that may have been responsible for fatal arrhythmias [3,189].

Pneumonia can of course be a direct consequence of aspiration, and it occurs with some frequency in near-drowning victims; however, other consequences of near-drowning appear by and large to be due to the hypoxemia and acidosis secondary to the event. Thus, the renal failure, hemoglobinuria, and diffuse intravascular coagulation that have been reported in association with near-drowning appear to be nonspecific responses to hypoxemia, hypotension, and acidosis. Similarly there appears to be nothing unique about the cerebral anoxia associated with near-drowning episodes [52,108,111,141,150,181]. There is a small amount of evidence to suggest that the cardiac arrest associated with near-drowning episodes and subsequent cardiac dysfunction may in part be due to very high levels of circulating catecholamines during the incident itself [35,71]; however, whether cardiac arrest is due solely to hypoxia, acidosis, and hypotension or some combination of these with high levels of catecholamines is of little clinical relevance.

General Clinical Presentation and Complications

The clinical presentation of patients after near-drowning episodes can vary considerably, and as should be evident from the preceding section, much of the presentation depends on the degree and duration of the hypoxemia immediately surrounding the incident. Patients can be nearly asymptomatic or they can present in cardiac arrest, requiring total ventilatory and cardiovascular support. Equally importantly, the appearance a patient has on presentation to the hospital may be quite dissimilar from the patient's appearance at the time of rescue. Since the status of the patient can vary so tremendously, it is easiest to describe the clinical presentation of each of the major organ systems of victims involved in near-drowning episodes.

Cardiovascular System

It is not unusual for near-drowning victims to suffer cardiac arrest. Frequently, the cardiac arrest can be successfully treated by appropriate resuscitative measures in the field; however, patients are all too frequently brought to the emergency department still requiring cardiopulmonary resuscitation or advanced cardiac life support. Supraventricular tachycardias are the most frequent rhythms seen in both patients who never suffer a cardiac arrest and those in whom the cardiac arrest is successfully treated. These rhythms are predominantly due to hypoxia and acidosis [72,136]. Other arrhythmias are unusual and should suggest an etiology other than simple near-drowning. Generally patients do not develop cardiac dysfunction subsequent to a near-drowning episode, and under most circumstances the patient is able to maintain his or her blood pressure and cardiac output without hemodynamic support once a stable rhythm has been reestablished. In some patients, however, shock persists in spite of an adequate volume status and oxygenation. In these cases, careful hemodynamic monitoring and support are indicated [61,99]. (Treatment is discussed in the next section.)

Pulmonary System

Near-drowning victims who do not aspirate any water generally do not have significant pulmonary complications, and as mentioned previously, once adequate ventilation and oxygenation have been reestablished, they should have a relatively uneventful recovery, assuming some form of irreversible injury did not occur during the period of hypoxemia. On the other hand, victims who aspirate usually have ongoing respiratory signs or symptoms. These problems may be so mild as to cause few if any complaints, or patients may present in pulmonary edema. Almost all patients who have aspirated water will present with a widened alveolar-arterial oxygen gradient and they can be either mildly to profoundly hypoxemic, depending on the severity of the lung injury and the inspired oxygen concentration (FIO_2) [78]. $PaCO_2$ can be low or elevated depending on alveolar ventilation, which may be affected by gastric distension or the adequacy of artificial ventilation (see Table 45-2). Pulmonary edema, when it occurs, is noncardiac in nature and is a form of adult respiratory distress syndrome (ARDS) [39]. The respiratory failure associated with severe drowning is similar to the respiratory failure associated with other forms of ARDS (see Chap. 46 on ARDS). Abnormalities on chest radiographs are extremely common in near-drowning victims and frequently include patchy infiltrates that are predominantly in the basilar regions, although as mentioned previously, the appearance of frank, pulmonary edema may be present [66,112,149] (Figs. 45-1 to 45-5). Pneumonias, empyemas, and lung abscesses are infrequent complications and generally represent hospital-acquired infections [61,65,102,188]; however, victims of near-drownings in heavily contaminated waters (such as hot tubs) can develop pulmonary infections related to the bacteriology of the water they aspirate.

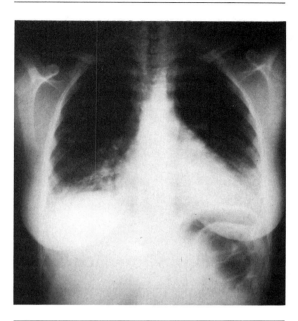

Fig. 45-3. Radiograph of a patient who almost drowned while scuba diving. There are bibasilar infiltrates, which cleared over several days.

Fig. 45-2. Radiograph of the same victim as in Figure 45-1 12 hours later after being treated with 5 cmH$_2$O of positive end-expiratory pressure. Note the presence of a nasogastric tube used to decompress the stomach.

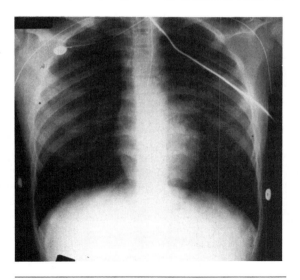

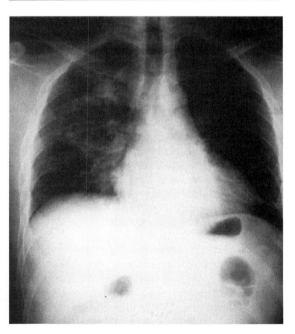

Fig. 45-4. Patchy infiltrate associated with a near-drowning episode.

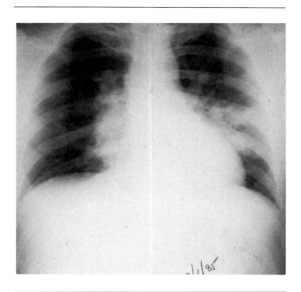

Fig. 45-5. Perihilar infiltrates associated with a near-drowning episode.

Central Nervous System

The neurologic status of the near-drowning victim tends to vary more than the status of any other major organ system. Patients can be fully conscious and alert or they can be unconscious, unresponsive, and without motor function. Once again, the severity of the neurologic presentation generally parallels the degree and duration of hypoxemia and/or hypotension attendant to the near-drowning episode. A classification system has been proposed to try to categorize patients and to help predict their prognosis. In this system, patients are placed into categories A, B, or C depending on their neurologic status at the time of presentation to the hospital. Patients classified in category A are awake, patients in category B have some blunting of their neurologic status, and patients in category C are comatose. The C group is further subdivided into C1, C2, and C3 patients depending on their motor response to a noxious stimulus. Patients in group C1 manifest decorticate behavior; patients in group C2, a decerebrate response; and those in group C3, no response at all [20]. This classification system is being used less frequently as mounting evidence indicates that different treatment modalities aimed at the different neurologically defined groups do not alter the eventual outcome.

Treatment

The major thrust of the treatment of any near-drowning patient must be correction of the underlying disorder of gas exchange. Victims of cardiac arrest should be treated aggressively as the cardiac arrest is invariably due to hypoxemia and acidosis. Recovery with completely normal neurologic function even after prolonged cardiac arrest is well documented [164,166,184,190]. The first goal of therapy must be to establish a reliable airway and administer the highest FIO_2 possible until the results of blood gas analysis are available. In an alert patient who is capable of protecting his or her own airway, simple supplemental oxygen may be appropriate. On the other hand, the comatose or even lethargic patient who is not capable of protecting his or her airway should probably be intubated, both to supply an appropriate FIO_2 and to protect the airway from the consequences of further aspiration of stomach contents. Aspiration of stomach contents is a constant risk in near-drowning victims as they swallow reflexively during the incident. In addition, many providers of emergency care use a bag valve mask or Elder valve system to provide artificial ventilation, which causes further risk of aspiration should reflex vomiting occur. Endotracheal intubation, however, carries certain risks in this setting. Obviously, reflex vomiting as described above is quite likely, but victims of near-drowning can also have unstable neck fractures and therefore, care must be taken to provide adequate stabilization until the presence of an occult neck fracture has been ruled out.

Near-drowning patients presenting in cardiac arrest often have a profound metabolic acidosis. Currently, the American Heart Association has lowered the recommended doses of bicarbonate for the treatment of the victim of a cardiac arrest. However, in the setting of a sudden and unexpected cardiac arrest from coronary artery disease, the precipitating event is generally not acidosis or hypoxemia, but rather those factors are secondary to the cardiac arrest. Promptly resuscitated victims of cardiac arrest from coronary artery disease can and often do have only small degrees of acidosis and hypoxemia. This is not necessarily true for the near-drowning victim in cardiac arrest. Thus, dosing of bicarbonate to reverse the metabolic acidosis of near-drowning should ideally be determined by blood gas measurements. Recent evidence suggests that the indiscriminate use of bicarbonate can worsen the physiologic derangement it is attempting to correct; however, these conclusions are based on as equally incomplete and flawed data as the original American Heart Association recommendations [171,172]. The exact role of bicarbonate in this setting remains to be determined. Clearly, it seems reasonable to attempt to correct a metabolic acidosis associated with a cardiac arrest that has failed to respond to adequate oxygenation and ventilation.

Concomitant with the above-mentioned measures, other emergency steps should be taken as well. If not already in place, a nasogastric tube should be inserted to reduce the likelihood of aspiration. A nasogastric tube will also assist a victim who is having trouble ventilating secondary to elevation of the diaphragm (see Figs. 45-1 and 45-2). Body temperature should also be measured to rule out hypothermia. A significantly lowered body temperature can occur in near-drowning victims, particularly in children, and can tremendously alter the cerebral oxygen demands. As a result, there are several well-documented cases of victims submerged in cold water for periods up to 45 minutes who have had complete recoveries [164,166,184,190]. These victims may appear clinically dead upon rescue; thus, such a patient should not be declared dead until active rewarming procedures have been attempted. The management of the profoundly hypothermic victim is beyond the scope of this chapter; however, there are several excellent review articles that address the appropriate management of this condition [19,50,85,183,191].

As soon as a stable airway has been obtained and spontaneous cardiac activity has been achieved, the next step is to ensure adequate oxygen delivery to the tissues. This is generally achieved merely by obtaining an adequate arterial concentration of oxygen, as hemodynamic stability is usually relatively easy to obtain in most near-drowning victims. On occasion, however, there are patients with reduced blood pressure and low cardiac outputs. Although in most circumstances the initial treatment for hypotension is a trial of volume infusion, in severely nearly drowned patients, this may not be appropriate as these patients often have pulmonary edema as well. This subset of patients is best managed in an intensive care unit with invasive hemodynamic monitoring (i.e., a Swan-Ganz catheter). With knowledge of pulmonary artery pressures, wedge pressures, vascular resistance, and cardiac output, more rational decisions concerning fluid administration and ventilator settings can be made [177]. It is important to realize

that in this unstable group of patients, simple monitoring techniques such as the measurement of the central venous pressure are unreliable and potentially misleading as well. In noncardiac pulmonary edema of any cause, the central venous pressure is not a reliable indicator of fluid status, even in patients with normal cardiac function, let alone those who have abnormal function. Similarly, changes in central venous pressure, whether up or down, do not reliably reflect changes in pulmonary artery wedge pressures or ventricular filling pressures, and thus this measurement is of extremely limited utility to assess either volume status or oxygen delivery to tissues. Direct measurement of critical hemodynamic parameters such as pulmonary artery wedge pressure, mean pulmonary artery pressure, cardiac output, and vascular resistance is the most effective method to manage the hypotensive victim with pulmonary edema.

In order to achieve a level of oxygenation adequate to provide sufficient oxygen to the tissues, positive end-expiratory pressure (PEEP) has been shown in animal models and in human trials to reverse the basic abnormalities of $\dot{V}_A/\dot{Q}$ distribution, and thus most effectively reverses hypoxemia [10,100,123,152,180]. In most circumstances the pulmonary injury associated with near-drowning is modest compared to the injury seen in other forms of ARDS, and as a result, only modest levels of PEEP are usually necessary to dramatically alter the abnormalities of gas exchange associated with near-drowning (see Figs. 45-1 and 45-2). PEEP does not reverse the course of the underlying pulmonary injury but rather reverses the underlying physiologic derangement and thus allows for adequate tissue oxygenation while the lung is recovering from the submersion incident. It also allows tissue oxygenation to take place at an FIO_2 that is not, in and of itself, toxic to the lungs [80]. Notwithstanding the development of a complicating pneumonia, pulmonary injury usually resolves over a period of 48 to 72 hours and from a purely ventilatory point of view, respiratory support can, under most circumstances, be relatively brief [100]. It is tempting to speculate whether the course of near-drowning victims can be modified by the use of inhaled surfactants as has been experimentally attempted in other forms of ARDS and in the respiratory distress syndrome of the newborn. Although this method of treatment might actually alter the course of the pulmonary injury [44,93], as noted above, in most circumstances the near-drowning victim is easily managed by the use of conventional amounts of PEEP. The PEEP can be administered either via intermittent mandatory ventilation (IMV) in the intubated patient, or in the less severely affected patients (particularly children) for whom support is only briefly anticipated, a continuous positive airway pressure (CPAP) mask can be used [100,126].

The most common secondary pulmonary complication of near-drowning is pneumonia. However, most pneumonias that develop appear to be hospital-acquired rather than from direct aspiration of organisms from the environment [102]. The one exception to this appears to be near-drowning incidents that occur in hot tubs. These tubs are frequently heavily contaminated with *Pseudomonas* species, and as a result, expectant therapy for *Pseudomonas* pneumonia appears to be appropriate. In other cases, the use of prophylactic antibiotics does not seem to improve mortality or decrease morbidity [61,65]. Indeed, their use seems associated with the appearance of more resistant organisms [102]; thus, the use of antibiotics should be reserved for those victims who develop purulent sputum or new infiltrates or who become febrile [76]. An elevated white blood cell count is generally not an indication for the use of antibiotics, as leukocytosis is quite common in victims at the time of presentation [47,49]. Should a leukocytosis occur later in the course of hospitalization, infection should be suspected [45,96,147]. The use of steroids to assist in the management of the pulmonary injury associated with near-drowning is also not indicated [16,32]. Although one series of four cases suggests that high-dose methylprednisolone may be beneficial for victims presenting in pulmonary edema [167], the bulk of experimental evidence suggests that neither outcome nor short-term morbidity is affected by the use of steroids, either in near-drowning or in other forms of aspiration pneumonia. Well-done controlled trials, however, have not been performed. In other forms of aspiration pneumonia the tracheobronchial tree can become contaminated with large particulate matter, but in most cases of near-drowning the only aspiration that takes place during the incident is the aspiration of the fluid in which the victim is submerged. Although there is evidence that the aspiration of particulate matter such as sand, mud, algae, and vomitus occurs in as many as 70 percent of drowning victims [45,46], there is no experience to suggest that routine bronchoscopy is warranted to search for foreign bodies. Long-term evaluation of near-drowning victims via assessment of pulmonary function and arterial blood gases suggests there are no clinically distinct abnormalities after clinical recovery [14].

The remaining area of treatment that must be addressed early in the management of the near-drowning victim is injury to the central nervous system. Clearly the most significant long-term morbidity associated with near-drowning is the damage associated with an anoxic insult to the brain; however, it has been extremely difficult to assess the incidence of such damage following near-drowning episodes. Different studies have had differing entrance criteria, differing treatments, and differing degrees of follow-up. Estimates have ranged from 0 percent to as high as 25 percent for clinically relevant long-term neurologic disability following significant near-drowning episodes [38,102,125,128,134]. In one study, it was suggested that the occurrence of this sort of problem could be reduced by aggressive attention to the central nervous system early in the course of the injury. This treatment regimen included barbiturate coma, paralysis with controlled hyperventilation, intentional hypothermia, diuretics, and steroid therapy. The rationale for this therapy was to control cerebral edema, lower intracranial pressures (ICPs), improve cerebral perfusion pressure, lower cerebral oxygen demand, and thereby improve long-term neurologic outcome, assuming further neurologic damage occurs after the initial hypoxic event [21]. Unfortunately, with almost two decades of experience with this mode of therapy it is not clear if the neurologic outcome has changed appreciably. The most recent large series of patients treated in this manner demonstrated a long-term incidence of neurologic injury of 7 percent [20] and this is not appreciably different from studies published earlier not using these forms of treatment [38,102,125,128,134,136]. Additionally, it has been demonstrated that although high ICPs are associated with poor neurologic outcome [28], normal ICPs do not guarantee a good neurologic result. The described therapy does not necessarily prevent elevations of ICP [122]. It appears that the elevation of ICP seen in the near-drowning victim is the result of anoxic damage rather than the cause of it, and interventions after the event are of little clinical utility [153]. There seems to be little risk to an elevated head position, hyperventilation to reduce $PaCO_2$, and the judicious use of osmotic diuretics; however, the more aggressive aspects of cerebral resuscitation should probably be reserved for centers well versed in their use and only for victims in whom the ICP cannot be controlled by more usual methods [42,103,148].

The decision to admit the less severely affected victim of a near-drowning episode for observation is usually straightforward. As the nadir of pulmonary dysfunction may not be evident for several hours after the incident [61,144], any victim who has symptoms referable to the respiratory tract, an abnormal arterial blood gas measurement, an abnormal-appearing chest radiograph, or a history of a period of unconsciousness should be observed to ensure that gas exchange does not deteriorate further.

The prognosis of the near-drowning victim depends almost entirely on the duration of immersion, the length of the anoxic period, and the degree of damage secondary to the initial period of anoxia. Patients who arrive at the hospital neurologically intact have an excellent prognosis [4,29,103,125]. In general, patients who arrive at the hospital still requiring cardiopulmonary resuscitation do poorly [136]. Cardiopulmonary resuscitation at the scene of the accident does not in and of itself indicate a poor prognosis. Whether this is because individuals who respond to treatment at the scene are less severely injured or because the true need for bystander cardiopulmonary resuscitation is not documented cannot be determined. In any event, the return of spontaneous ventilatory efforts in the field following cardiopulmonary resuscitation is a good prognostic sign [69]. Other good prognostic signs for children are an estimation that the submersion time was less than 5 minutes, that on-scene advanced or basic life support was administered, and as mentioned previously, that there was a good response to initial therapy [128]. Bad prognostic signs include age of less than 3 years, estimated submersion time of longer than 5 minutes, coma, the requirement for cardiopulmonary resuscitation on admission to the emergency department, or an initial arterial blood pH of less than 7.10 [125].

Diving Accidents

There are currently estimated to be over 2.5 million divers in the United States, and approximately 200,000 additional divers are trained each year [92]. This group, in addition to caisson workers, scientific divers, commercial divers, and aviators, is subject to a group of disorders that are extremely rare in the course of a normal medical practice. However, as drowning may be the leading cause of death among scuba divers [91,92], a pulmonary physician treating a scuba diver for a near-drowning episode may be faced with treating a less common injury specific to diving activity in conjunction with the near-drowning. The following section deals with two general forms of injury that may be encountered in a patient hospitalized for near-drowning: barotrauma and decompression sickness (DCS). A variety of other conditions can also affect a diver, and the interested reader is referred to a number of recent texts and review articles [8,11,34,113,165].

Barotrauma

Barotrauma is probably the most common injury that affects divers. It is due to the expansion or the contraction of gas that occurs due to changes in barometric pressure. Boyle's law states that pressure and volume are inversely related ($P_1V_1 = P_2V_2$) and thus, the changes in barometric pressure due to either ascent or descent in the water column result in a change in the volume of any gas-containing space on which that pressure change is exerted. Conditions that occur as a diver descends in the water column (i.e., as the atmospheric pressure increases) are called *squeeze* or *barotrauma of descent*. Conditions that occur as the atmospheric pressure decreases are called *barotrauma of ascent*. Barotrauma of descent most frequently affects the ears and sinuses. As a diver descends in the water column and the atmospheric pressure increases, the gas within the middle ear, which is compressible, suffers a loss in volume. Under normal circumstances a diver will cause additional air to enter the middle ear by a variety of maneuvers in order to reduce the deforming force acting on the tympanic membrane (Fig. 45-6). Should a diver not be able to accomplish this, damage to the tympanic membrane, the middle ear, or even the inner ear may result. Injury to the inner ear can be brought about by rupture of either the round or oval window and produces a picture characterized by vertigo, tinnitus, and hearing loss [33,41]. Increased barometric pressure also requires that additional air enter the sinuses. If, however, the sinuses are blocked for some reason, compression of the gas space within them can cause injury to the epithelial lining or the vascular bed of the mucosal membranes of the sinuses [37].

For the pulmonologist, the most interesting air-containing space the diver brings into the water is the lungs. In theory, if the lungs were to be compressed below their residual volume, injury to the lung would occur, since further reductions

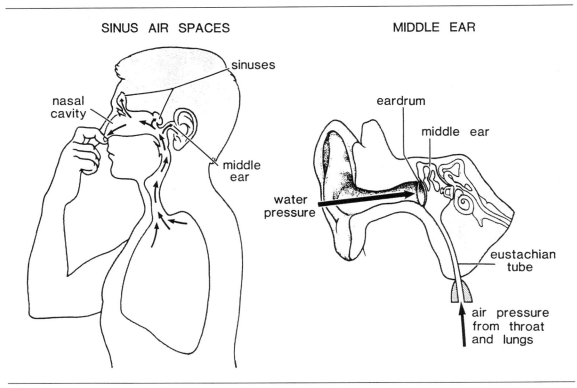

SINUS AIR SPACES

sinuses

nasal cavity

middle ear

MIDDLE EAR

eardrum

middle ear

water pressure

eustachian tube

air pressure from throat and lungs

Fig. 45-6. Middle ear and sinuses. (Reproduced from TS Neuman. Unusual Forms of Trauma. In WG Baxt (Ed), *Trauma: The First Hour.* Norwalk, CT: Appleton-Century-Crofts, 1985. P 270.)

in volume could only be accomplished by bleeding or edema in the lungs. As average lungs contain about 6 liters of air and the average residual volume is 25 percent of that, any breath-hold dive below 30 m should compress the lungs beyond their residual volume and produce this condition. In practice, lung squeeze is a condition so rare that it has only been reported once, and the circumstances surrounding that case suggest that near-drowning may have been the underlying cause of the pulmonary injury [173]. During deep breath-hold dives, it has been shown that the pulmonary vascular bed dilates and pressure gradients are equalized by the presence of an increased intrathoracic blood volume [25,154]. Additionally, the chest wall itself is compliant, allowing further reductions in residual volume to occur [2,26]. As a result, extremely deep breath-hold dives, some to as much as 100 m, take place without pulmonary injury.

Barotrauma of ascent also occurs due to pressure gradients across tissues, with resultant deformation and damage; however, in these circumstances, the pressure is decreasing and injury

generally occurs due to overdistension of the air-containing space. In the middle ear and sinuses, significant injury on ascent is rare [37,67,82] because the anatomy is such that expanding gas can usually gain egress and large pressure differentials do not generally occur. However, gas expanding within the lungs, due to the presence of intrinsic obstruction of the airways or more commonly the diver holding his or her breath during an episode of panic, can create a variety of pulmonary injuries. In general, one of four syndromes may result:

1. *Overdistension with local injury.* This is generally the mildest form of pulmonary barotrauma. The most common finding is hemoptysis with or without mild chest pain. On occasion there is a small pleural effusion. Rarely, massive hemoptysis occurs with blood loss significant enough to cause hemodynamic compromise (Fig. 45-7). In the absence of significant blood loss

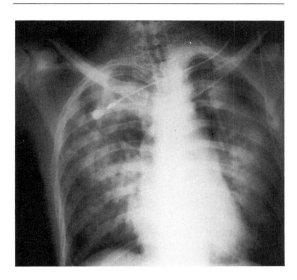

Fig. 45-7. Radiograph of a victim who had an episode of panic during a dive and suffered severe pulmonary barotrauma. This victim had at least 800 ml of hemoptysis.

and/or complications of blood aspiration, only symptomatic treatment is required.

2. *Interstitial emphysema.* This injury is caused by air rupturing into the interstitial space after disruption of alveoli [70,155]. The air can dissect to the root of the lung along intrapulmonary tissue planes and cause mediastinal emphysema or even subcutaneous emphysema at the root of the neck. This is one of the more common forms of pulmonary barotrauma and may be asymptomatic. The radiographic appearance of this form of pulmonary barotrauma may be extremely subtle, and even experienced physicians looking specifically for evidence of barotrauma have been reported to overlook the signs of this injury [117]. Abnormalities of this sort most easily missed are best appreciated by a careful examination of the mediastinum, paying special attention to the aortic arch, the left cardiac border, the descending aorta, and the hilar vessels (Fig. 45-8).

3. *Pneumothorax.* When overdistended alveoli rupture into the pleural space, or when air that has dissected to the mediastinum ruptures the parietal pleura, a pneumothorax results. Although intuitively this might seem to be a common injury, it is in fact the rarest of the overinflation syndromes [107].

4. *Arterial gas embolism.* Should the gas from overdistended and ruptured alveoli enter the pulmonary venous circulation, arterial (systemic) gas embolization can result (Fig. 45-9). AGE is generally thought to be the second most common cause of fatal scuba diving accidents after drowning [91,92]. It was originally believed that the brain was the target organ for gas embolization [79] because divers are generally in an upright position and because of the buoyancy of the gas. However, a growing body of evidence suggests that embolization is a more generalized phenomenon and that the bubbles distribute more according to flow than to buoyancy [13]. Experimental evidence suggests that alveolar rupture can occur with as little as 80 mmHg of overpressure; however, overpressurization alone without overdistension requires much higher pressures before embolization occurs [155]. The most common symptoms of AGE are sudden loss of consciousness, blindness, seizures, hemiparesis, and any neurologic presentation compatible with occlusion of part of the cerebral circulation within minutes of surfacing from a dive [36]. The onset is usually sudden and dramatic. It is important that the practitioner not be misled by what appears to be multiple lesions, since many vessels can be embolized simultaneously. Less than 50 percent of patients with AGE have evidence of some sort of barotrauma on their chest radiograph [36,117]. Although in some cases the evidence for barotrauma will be straightforward (Fig. 45-10), as noted above, in a significant percentage of cases the radiographic signs of barotrauma will be quite subtle.

Treatment should be directed at transferring the patient to a recompression facility as quickly as possible. Additionally, the highest FIO_2 possible should be delivered. One hundred percent oxygen has been shown to reduce bubble size in animal models [55]; however, there is no strong clinical or experimental evidence that nasal prong or mask oxygen alters the clinical outcome. Recent evidence suggests that hemoconcentration can be clinically significant in patients with AGE so adequate fluid intake should be maintained [118].

Decompression Sickness

Although the clinical symptomatology of DCS and AGE can overlap, and therefore the differential diagnosis between the two can be difficult,

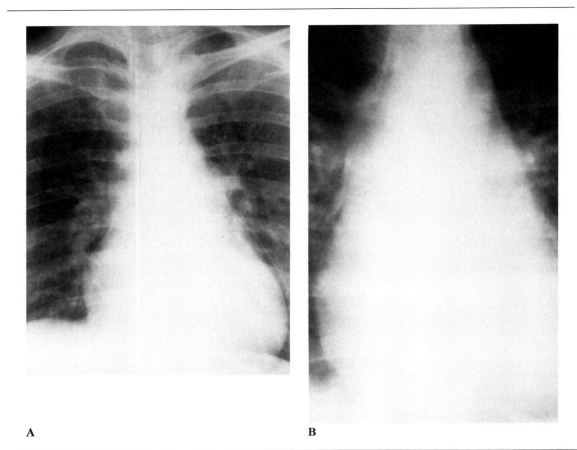

A   B

Fig. 45-8. (*A*) Subtle pneumomediastinum initially misinterpreted as pneumopericardium. (*B*) Pneumomediastinum that is easily confused with pneumopericardium.

the pathophysiology of the two conditions is different and in most cases the syndromes are distinct. DCS is due to the evolution and growth of a gas phase in the tissues of the body (due to supersaturation), whereas AGE is due to the introduction of gas directly into the vascular space. When a diver descends in the water column, atmospheric pressure increases as described previously. At increased atmospheric pressure, the tissues of the body are able to dissolve larger amounts of inert gas. As the atmospheric pressure is reduced, that gas must come out of solution. If the reduction in atmospheric pressure occurs at too fast a rate, the liberated gas cannot be excreted without the formation of a gas phase, and as a result, bubbles form within the tissues. The bubbles in turn can cause a variety of secondary biochemical and mechanical effects, which eventually reach the clinical horizon as symptomatic DCS. In order for sufficient gas to be dissolved in the body to produce DCS, a diver

not only must be exposed to an elevated pressure but also must be exposed to that elevated pressure for a period of time long enough to absorb a sufficient quantity of gas to allow DCS to occur. Thus, the occurrence of DCS depends on both the depth to which a diver goes (i.e., the magnitude of pressure exposure) and the time spent there (the duration of the exposure). The greater the depth (pressure), the shorter the period of time (duration) necessary to absorb a sufficient quantity of gas to produce DCS.

The clinical features of DCS are quite varied; however, for purposes of classification, a system first used to describe DCS in caisson workers has gained wide acceptance and is generally used by most workers in the field [51]. Type I DCS is characterized by deep boring pains in the joints. The

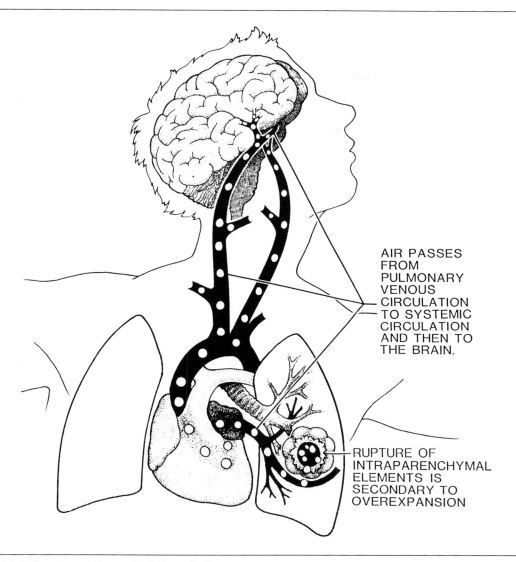

AIR PASSES
FROM
PULMONARY
VENOUS
CIRCULATION
TO SYSTEMIC
CIRCULATION
AND THEN TO
THE BRAIN.

RUPTURE OF
INTRAPARENCHYMAL
ELEMENTS IS
SECONDARY TO
OVEREXPANSION

Fig. 45-9. Barotraumatic cerebral air embolism.
(Reproduced from TS Neuman. Unusual Forms of
Trauma. In WG Baxt (Ed), *Trauma: The First
Hour.* Norwalk, CT: Appleton-Century-Crofts, 1985.
P 274.)

pain is not affected by motion and there are usually no objective signs. In caisson workers and
military divers, type I DCS accounts for approximately 80 percent of the cases [146,178]. In centers treating sport divers, however, type I symptoms account for only about 50 percent of the
cases [55]. Whether this represents a true difference in the incidence of type I DCS or merely reporting bias is not clear and there are hypotheses
to support both concepts. Type II DCS is the
more serious form of the disease and symptoms
most often involve the spinal cord. Typically, the
first symptoms are paresthesias, which over varying periods of time can progress to complete paralysis. Bladder problems are also common [75].
There are several other, less common forms of
type II DCS as well; cerebral symptoms occur
rarely, most often seen in aviators, and rarely
patients present with respiratory symptoms
(chokes), which consist of substernal chest pain,
dyspnea, and cough [146]. After decades of research, the pathophysiology of DCS remains

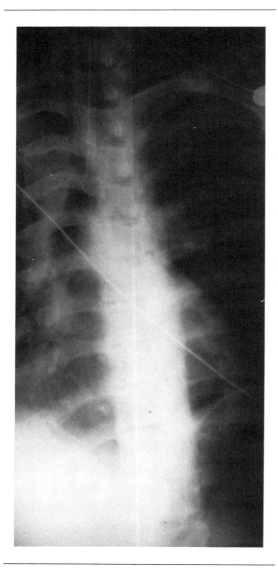

Fig. 45-10. Radiograph of a victim of massive arterial gas embolism who did not survive. Note the presence of air in the left ventricle, the aorta, the carotid arteries, and the subclavian vessels.

poorly understood. Although the presence of bubbles seems to be a requirement for the development of most forms of DCS, many studies have demonstrated the presence of large numbers of bubbles (by Doppler systems) in patients without any symptoms [9,115,142,169]. In the spinal cord, bubbles can occlude the epidural plexus (Battson's plexus) and produce a picture of venous in-

farction of the spinal cord [57]. However, other studies have suggested that in situ bubbles are the primary process, and still other reports have suggested that DCS can be precipitated by AGE [114]. Numerous other hematologic, circulatory, and rheologic abnormalities have been observed in patients with DCS [1,5,83,116,119,120,137,138]. However, once again, what role these factors play in its pathogenesis remains to be elucidated.

As with AGE, emergency management of a patient with DCS must be directed toward arranging for recompression therapy as rapidly as possible. Once again, a high FiO_2 should be administered and adequate urine output maintained. The use of steroids has been advocated by some authorities but there are few data to support this [77]. There are proponents of the use of aspirin, other nonsteroidal agents, and heparin [43,74], but as with steroids there are no firm data to demonstrate their efficacy.

References

1. Ackles KN (Ed), *Blood-Bubble Interaction in Decompression Sickness: An International Symposium.* Report no 73-CP-960. Toronto: Defense and Civil Institute of Environmental Medicine, 1973.
2. Agostoni E, et al. Respiratory mechanics during submersion and negative pressure breathing. *J Appl Physiol* 21:251, 1966.
3. Alkan ML, et al. Near drowning in the Dead Sea. *Isr J Med Sci* 13:290, 1977.
4. Allman FD, et al. Outcome following cardiopulmonary resuscitation in severe pediatric near drowning. *Am J Dis Child* 140:571, 1986.
5. Anderson JC, Vann RD, Dick A. Correlation of hematologic alterations with Doppler bubble scores and clinical bends following shallow closed circuit nitrogen oxygen dives. *Undersea Biomed Res* 8(Suppl):43, 1981.
6. Baker SP, O'Neill B, Karpf RS. *The Injury Fact Book.* Lexington, MA: Lexington Books, 1984.
7. Barrett O, Martin CM. Drowning and near drowning: A review of 10 years experience in a large Army hospital. *Mil Med* 136:439, 1971.
8. Baxt W. *Trauma, the First Hour.* Norwalk, CT: Appleton-Century-Crofts, 1985.
9. Bayne CG, Hunt WS, Bray PG. Doppler diagnosis: A prospective clinical trial in human decompression sickness. *Undersea Biomed Res* 6(Suppl):17, 1979.
10. Berquist RE, et al. Comparison of ventilatory patterns in the treatment of fresh-water near drowning in dogs. *Anesthesiology* 52:142, 1980.

11. Bove AA, David JC. *Diving Medicine* (2nd ed). Philadelphia: Saunders, 1990.
12. Burke DC. Spinal cord injuries from water sports. *Med J Aust* 2:1190, 1972.
13. Butler BD, et al. Effect of Trendelenburg position on the distribution of arterial air emboli in dogs. *Ann Thorac Surg* 45:198, 1988.
14. Butt MP, et al. Pulmonary function after resuscitation from near drowning. *Anesthesiology* 32:275, 1970.
15. Cairns FJ, Koelmeyer TD, Smeeton WM. Deaths from drowning. *NZ Med J* 97:65, 1984.
16. Calderwood HW, Modell JH, Ruiz BC. The ineffectiveness of steroid therapy for treatment of fresh-water near drowning. *Anesthesiology* 43:642, 1975.
17. Centers for Disease Control. Aquatic deaths and injuries: United States. *MMWR* 31:417, 1982.
18. Colebatch HJ, Halmagyi DF. Lung mechanics and resuscitation after fluid aspiration. *J Appl Physiol* 16:684, 1961.
19. Collis ML. Survival Behaviour in Cold Water Immersion. In *Proceedings of the Cold Water Symposium.* Toronto: Royal Life-Saving Society of Canada, 1976.
20. Conn AW, Barker GA. Fresh water drowning and near drowning: An update. *Can Anaesth Soc J* 31:538, 1984.
21. Conn AW, Edmonds JF, Barker GA. Cerebral resuscitation in near drowning. *Pediatr Clin North Am* 26:691, 1979.
22. Cot C. Asphyxia from drowning: Treatment based on experimental findings. *Bull Acad Natl Med (Paris)* 105:758, 1931.
23. Craig AB. Causes of loss of consciousness during underwater swimming. *J Appl Physiol* 16:583, 1961.
24. Craig AB. Underwater swimming and loss of consciousness. *JAMA* 176:255, 1961.
25. Craig AB. Depth limits of breath-hold diving (an example of fennology). *Respir Physiol* 5:14, 1968.
26. Craig AB, Ware DE. Effect of immersion in water on vital capacity and residual volume of the lungs. *J Appl Physiol* 23:423, 1967.
27. Davis S, Smith LS. Alcohol and drowning in Cape Town. *S Afr Med J* 62:931, 1982.
28. Dean JM, McComb JG. Intracranial pressure monitoring in severe pediatric near drowning. *Neurosurgery* 9:627, 1981.
29. Dean MJ, Kaufman ND. Prognostic indicators in pediatric near drowning: The Glasgow Coma Scale. *Crit Care Med* 9:536, 1981.
30. Decker MD, et al. The use and efficacy of child restraint devices: The Tennessee experience, 1982 and 1983. *JAMA* 252:2571, 1984.
31. Dietz PE, Baker SP. Drowning: Epidemiology and prevention. *Am J Public Health* 64:303, 1974.
32. Downs JB, et al. An evaluation of steroid therapy in aspiration pneumonitis. *Anesthesiology* 40:129, 1974.
33. Edmonds C, Freeman P, Tonkin J. Fistula of the round window in diving. *Trans Am Acad Ophthalmol Otol* 78:444, 1974.
34. Edmonds C, Lowery C, Penneyfather J. *Diving and Subaquatic Medicine.* Mosman, NSW Australia: Diving Medical Center, 1981.
35. Eliot RS, Todd GL, Pieper GM. Pathophysiology of catecholamine-mediated myocardial damage. *J SC Med Assoc* 75:513, 1979.
36. Elliott DH, Harrison JAB, Barnard EEP. Clinical and Radiographical Features of 88 Cases of Decompression Barotrauma. In CW Shilling, MW Beckett (Eds), *Proceedings of the Sixth Symposium on Underwater Physiology.* Bethesda, MD: Federation of American Societies for Experimental Biology, 1978. Pp 527–535.
37. Fagan P, McKenzie B, Edmonds E. Sinus barotrauma in divers. *Ann Otol Rhinol Laryngol* 85:61, 1976.
38. Fandel I, Bancalari E. Near drowning in children: Clinical aspects. *Pediatrics* 58:573, 1976.
39. Fine NL, et al. Near drowning presenting as the adult respiratory disease syndrome. *Chest* 65:347, 1974.
40. Flood TJ, et al. Child drownings and near drownings associated with swimming pools. Maricopa County, Arizona, 1988 and 1989. *MMWR* 39:441, 1990.
41. Freeman P, Edmonds C. Inner ear barotrauma. *Arch Otolaryngol* 95:556, 1972.
42. Frewen TC, et al. Cerebral resuscitation therapy in pediatric near drowning. *J Pediatr* 106:615, 1985.
43. Fructus X. Treatment of Serious Decompression Sickness. In *Treatment of Serious Decompression Sickness and Arterial Gas Embolism.* UMS publication no 34. Bethesda, MD: Undersea Medical Society, 1979. Pp 37–44.
44. Fujiwara T, et al. Artificial therapy in hyaline membrane disease. *Lancet.* 1:55, 1980.
45. Fuller RH. The clinical pathology of human near drowning. *Proc R Soc Med* 56:33, 1963.
46. Fuller RH. Drowning and the postimmersion syndrome. A clinico-pathologic study. *Mil Med* 128:22, 1963.
47. Gauto A, Majeski JA, Alexander JW. Drowning and near drowning: Current concepts and neutrophil function studies. *South Med J* 72:690, 1979.
48. Giammona ST, Modell JH. Drowning by total immersion: Effects on pulmonary surfactant of distilled water, isotonic saline and sea water. *Am J Dis Child* 114:612, 1967.
49. Gilfoil MP, Carvajal HF. Near drowning in children. *Tex Med* 73:39, 1977.

50. Golding FC. Accident hypothermia. *R Naval Med Serv* 58:196, 1972.

51. Golding FC, Griffiths P, Hempleman HV. Decompression sickness during construction of the Dartford Tunnel. *Br J Ind Med* 17:167, 1960.

52. Grausz H, Amend WJC, Earley LE. Acute renal failure complicating submersion in sea water. *JAMA* 217:207, 1971.

53. Green BA, et al. Analysis of swimming pool accidents resulting in spinal cord injury. *Paraplegia* 18:94, 1980.

54. Greenberg MI, et al. Effects of endotracheally administered distilled water and normal saline on arterial blood gases of dogs. *Ann Emerg Med* 11:600, 1982.

55. Grulke DC, Hills BA. Experimental Cerebral Air Embolism and Its Resolution. In CW Shilling, MW Beckett (Eds), *Proceedings of the Sixth Symposium on Underwater Physiology.* Bethesda, MD: Federation of American Societies for Experimental Biology, 1978. Pp 587–594.

56. Haglund P, et al. Biological disturbances during drowning in sea water. *Resuscitation* 3:121, 1974.

57. Hallenbeck JM, Bove AA, Elliot DG. Mechanisms underlying spinal cord damage in decompression sickness. *Neurology* 25:308, 1975.

58. Halmagyi DF, Colebatch HJ. Ventilation and circulation after fluid aspiration. *J Appl Physiol* 16:35, 1961.

59. Hasan S, et al. Near drowning in humans: A report of 36 patients. *Chest* 59:191, 1971.

60. Hedberg K, et al. Drownings in Minnesota 1980–1985: A population based study. *Am J Public Health* 80:1071, 1990.

61. Hoff BH. Multisystem failure: A review with special reference to drowning. *Crit Care Med* 7:310, 1979.

62. Hong SK, et al. Diving pattern, lung volumes and alveolar gas of the Korean diving woman (Ama). *J Appl Physiol* 18:457, 1963.

63. Howland J, Hingson R. Alcohol as a risk factor for drownings: A review of the literature (1950–1985). *Accid Anal Prev* 20:19, 1988.

64. Howland J, et al. A pilot survey of aquatic activities and related consumption of alcohol with implications for drowning. *Public Health Rep* 105:415, 1990.

65. Hughs JA. Drowning—An overview. *JACEP* 6:172, 1977.

66. Hunter TB, Whitehouse WM. Fresh-water near drowning: Radiological aspects. *Radiology* 112:51, 1974.

67. Idicula J. Perplexing case of maxillary sinus barotrauma. *Aerospace Med* 43:891, 1972.

68. Immersion and drowning in children (editorial). *Br Med J* 2:146, 1977.

69. Jacobsen WK, et al. Correlation of spontaneous respiration and neurologic damage in near drowning. *Crit Care Med* 11:487, 1983.

70. James RE. *Extra-alveolar Air Resulting from Submarine Escape Training: A Post-training Roentgenographic Survey of 170 Submariners.* Navy Submarine Medical Research Lab report no 550. Groton, CT: NSMRL, 1968.

71. Karch SB. Pathology of the heart in near drowning. *Arch Pathol Lab Med* 109:176, 1985.

72. Kaukinen L. Clinical course and prognostic signs in near drowned patients. *Ann Chir Gynaecol* 73:34, 1984.

73. Kewalramani LS, Kraus JF. Acute spinal cord lesions from diving: Epidemiological and clinical features. *West J Med* 126:353, 1977.

74. Kindwall E. Adjunctive Treatment Methods. In *Treatment of Serious Decompression Sickness and Arterial Gas Embolism.* UMS publication no 34. Bethesda, MD: Undersea Medical Society, 1979. Pp 45–49.

75. Kizer KW. Delayed treatment of decompression sickness: A retrospective review of 50 cases. *JAMA* 247:2555, 1982.

76. Kizer KW. Resuscitation of submersion casualties. *Emerg Med Clin North Am* 1:643, 1983.

77. Kizer KW. Dysbaric Diving Accidents. In RF Edlich, DA Spyker (Eds), *Current Emergency Medicine Therapy.* Norwalk, CT: Appleton-Century-Crofts, 1984. Pp 219–226.

78. Lheureux P, Vincent JL, Brimioulle S. Fulminant pulmonary edema after near drowning: Remarkably high colloid osmotic pressure in tracheal fluid. *Intensive Care Med* 10:205, 1984.

79. Liebow AA, et al. Intrapulmonary air trapping in submarine escape casualties. *US Armed Forces Med J* 10:265, 1959.

80. Lindner KH, Dick W, Lotz P. The delayed use of positive end expiratory pressure (PEEP) during respiratory resuscitation following near drowning with fresh or salt water. *Resuscitation* 10:197, 1983.

81. Lougheed DW, James JM, Hall GE. Physiological studies in experimental asphyxia and drowning. *Can Med Assoc J* 40:423, 1939.

82. Lundgren CEG. Alternobaric vertigo—A diving hazard. *Br Med J* 2:511, 1965.

83. Martin KJ, Nichols GN. Observations in platelet changes in man after simulated diving. *Aerospace Med* 43:827, 1972.

84. Martin TG. Near drowning and cold water immersion. *Ann Emerg Med* 13:263, 1984.

85. Matz R. Hypothermia: Mechanisms and counter measures. *Hosp Pract* 21:45, 1986.

86. McAniff JJ. *United States Underwater Fatality Statistics, 1970–78.* Report no URI-SSR-80-13. Kingston, RI: National Underwater Accident Data Center, University of Rhode Island, September 1980.

87. McAniff JJ. *United States Underwater Fatality Statistics, 1970–79.* Report no URI-SSR-80-14. Kingston, RI: National Underwater Accident

Data Center, University of Rhode Island, August 1981.

88. McAniff JJ. *United States Underwater Fatality Statistics, 1970–80, Including a Preliminary Assessment of 1981 Fatalities.* Report no URI-SSR-82-15. Kingston, RI: National Underwater Accident Data Center, University of Rhode Island. December 1982.

89. McAniff JJ. *United States Underwater Fatality Statistics, 1970–81, Including a Preliminary Assessment of 1982 Fatalities.* Report no URI-SSR-83-16. Kingston, RI: National Underwater Accident Data Center, University of Rhode Island, 1983.

90. McAniff JJ. *United States Underwater Fatality Statistics, 1970–82, Including a Preliminary Assessment of 1983 Fatalities.* Report no URI-SSR-84-17. Kingston, RI: National Underwater Accident Data Center, University of Rhode Island, 1984.

91. McAniff JJ. *United States Underwater Diving Fatality Statistics, 1985.* US Department of Commerce, NOAA, U.S. Government Printing Office report no URI-SSR-87-19. Washington, DC: US Government Printing Office, 1987.

92. McAniff JJ. *United States Underwater Diving Fatality Statistics, 1988.* US Department of Commerce, NOAA, US Government Printing Office report no URI-SSR-90-21. Washington, DC: US Government Printing Office, 1990.

93. Merritt TA, et al. Reduction of lung injury by human surfactant treatment in respiratory distress syndrome. *Chest* 83:275, 1983.

94. Mersey L (Wreck Commissioner). *Report of a Formal Investigation into the Circumstances Attending the Foundering on 15th April 1912 of the British Steamship Titanic of Liverpool after Striking Ice in or near Latitude 41° 46' N, Longitude 50° 14'W, North Atlantic Ocean, Whereby Loss of Life Ensued.* London: His Majesty's Stationery Office, 1912.

95. Millner N, Pearn J, Guard R. Will fenced pools save lives? *Med J Aust* 2:510, 1980.

96. Modell JH. Resuscitation after aspiration of chlorinated freshwater. *JAMA* 185:651, 1963.

97. Modell JH. Blood Gas and Acid Base Changes. In *The Pathophysiology and Treatment of Drowning and Near Drowning.* Springfield, IL: CC Thomas, 1970. Pp 13–18.

98. Modell JH. Biology of drowning. *Annu Rev Med* 29:1, 1978.

99. Modell JH. Near Drowning. In ML Callaham (Ed), *Current Therapy in Emergency Medicine,* St. Louis: Mosby, 1986.

100. Modell JH, et al. Effects of ventilatory patterns on arterial oxygenation after near drowning in sea water. *Anesthesiology* 46:376, 1974.

101. Modell JH, et al. Blood gas and electrolyte changes in human near drowning victims. *JAMA* 203:337, 1968.

102. Modell JH, Graves SA, Ketover A. Clinical course of 91 consecutive near drowning victims. *Chest* 70:231, 1976.

103. Modell JH, Graves SA, Kuck EJ. Near drowning: Correlation of level of consciousness and survival. *Can Anaesth Soc J* 27:211, 1980.

104. Modell JH, Moya F. Effects of volume of aspirated fluid during chlorinated fresh-water drowning. *Anesthesiology* 27:662, 1966.

105. Modell JH, et al. The effects of fluid volume in sea water drowning. *Ann Intern Med* 67:68, 1967.

106. Modell JH, Wiebley TC, Ruiz BC. Serum electrolyte concentrations after fresh-water aspiration. *Anesthesiology* 30:421, 1969.

107. Moses J. *Casualties in Individual Submarine Escape.* Navy Submarine Medical Research Lab report no 438. Groton, CT: NSMRL, 1964.

108. Munroe WD. Hemoglobinuria from near drowning. *J Pediatr* 64:57, 1964.

109. National Safety Council. *Accident Facts, 1984.* Chicago: National Safety Council, 1984.

110. National Transportation Safety Board Safety Study. *Recreational Boating Safety and Alcohol.* Washington, DC: National Transportation Safety Board, publication no SS 83-02, 1983.

111. Neale TJ, et al. Acute renal failure following near drowning in salt water. *NZ Med J* 97:319, 1984.

112. Neuman TS. Near Drowning. In KM Moser, RS Spragg (Eds), *Respiratory Emergencies* (2nd ed). St. Louis: Mosby, 1982. Pp 282–284.

113. Neuman TS. Diving medicine. *Clin Sports Med* 6:647, 1987.

114. Neuman TS, Bove AA. Combined arterial gas embolism and decompression sickness following no-stop dives. *Undersea Biomed Res* 17:429, 1990.

115. Neuman TS, Hall D, Linweaver PG. Gas phase separation during decompression in man: Ultrasound monitoring. *Undersea Biomed Res* 3:121, 1976.

116. Neuman TS, Harris M, Linaweaver PG. Blood viscosity in man following decompression: Correlations with hematocrit and venous gas emboli. *Aviat Space Environ Med* 47:803, 1976.

117. Neuman TS, Jacoby I, Olson L. Clinical nature of AGE III (radiographic features). *Undersea Biomed Res* 19(Suppl): 45, 1992.

118. Neuman TS, Smith RM. Clinical nature of AGE (hemoconcentration). *Undersea Biomed Res* 19(Suppl): 43–44, 1992.

119. Neuman TS, et al. Cardiopulmonary consequences of decompression stress. *Respir Physiol* 41:143, 1980.

120. Neuman TS, Spragg RG, Wohl H. Platelet aggregates following decompression. *Undersea Biomed Res* 8(Suppl):42, 1981.

121. Noble CS, Sharp N. Drowning: Its mechanism and treatment. *Can Med Assoc J* 89:402, 1963.

122. Nussbaum E, Galant SP. Intracranial pressure monitoring as a guide to prognosis in the nearly drowned, severely comatose child. *J Pediatr* 102:215, 1983.

123. Oaks DD, et al. Prognosis and management of victims of near drowning. *J Trauma* 22:544, 1982.

124. O'Carroll PW, Alkon E, Weiss B. Drowning mortality in Los Angeles County 1976–1984. *JAMA* 260:380, 1988.

125. Orlowski JP. Prognostic factors in pediatric cases of drowning and near drowning. *JACEP* 8:176, 1979.

126. Orlowski JP. Drowning, near drowning and ice-water submersions. *Pediatr Clin North Am* 34:75, 1987.

127. Orlowski JP. *Pediatr Ann* 17:125, 1987.

128. Pearn J. Neurologic and psychometric studies in children surviving fresh-water immersion incidents. *Lancet* 1:7, 1979.

129. Pearn J, et al. Bathtub drownings: Report of seven cases. *Pediatrics* 60:68, 1979.

130. Pearn J, Hsia EY. Swimming pool drownings and near drownings involving children: A total population study from Hawaii. *Mil Med* 190:15, 1980.

131. Pearn J, Nixon J. Prevention of childhood drowning accidents. *Med J Aust* 1:616, 1977.

132. Pearn J, Nixon J, Wilkey I. Freshwater drowning and near drowning accidents involving children. *Med J Aust* 2:942, 1976.

133. Pearn J, Thompson J. Drowning and near drowning in the Australian Capital territory: A 5 year total population study of immersion accidents. *Med J Aust* 1:130, 1977.

134. Pearn J, et al. Drowning and near drowning involving children: A five year total population study from the City and County of Honolulu. *Am J Public Health* 69:450, 1979.

135. Perspectives in disease prevention and health promotion. *MMWR* 31:417, 1982.

136. Peterson B. Morbidity of childhood near drowning. *Pediatrics* 59:364, 1977.

137. Philp RB. A review of blood changes associated with compression-decompression: Relationship to decompression sickness. *Undersea Biomed Res* 1:117, 1974.

138. Philp RB, Inwood MJ, Warren BA. Interactions between gas bubbles and components of the blood: Implications in decompression sickness. *Aerospace Med* 43:946, 1972.

139. Plueckhahn VD. The aetiology of 134 deaths due to "drowning" in Geelong during the years 1957–1971. *Med J Aust* 2:1183, 1972.

140. Plueckhahn VD. Alcohol and accidental drowning. *Med J Aust* 2:22, 1984.

141. Ports TA, Deuel TF. Intravascular coagulation in fresh-water submersion. *Ann Intern Med* 87:60, 1977.

142. Powell MR, Johanson DC. Ultrasound Monitoring and Decompression Sickness. In CW Shilling, MW Beckett (Eds), *Proceedings of the Sixth Symposium on Underwater Physiology*. Bethesda, MD: Federation of American Societies for Experimental Biology, 1978. Pp 503–510.

143. Press E, Walker J, Crawford I. An interstate drowning study. *Am J Public Health* 12:2275, 1968.

144. Putman CE. Drowning: Another plunge. *Am J Roentg Radium Ther Nucl Med* 125:543, 1975.

145. Quan L, et al. Ten year study of pediatric drownings and near drownings in King County, Washington: Lessons in injury prevention. *Pediatrics* 83:1035, 1989.

146. Rivera JC. Decompression sickness amongst divers: An analysis of 935 cases. *Mil Med* 129:314, 1963.

147. Rivers JF, Orr G, Lee HA. Drowning: Its clinical sequelae and management. *Br Med J* 2:157, 1970.

148. Rogers MC. Near drowning: Cold water on a hot topic? *J Pediatr* 106:603, 1985.

149. Rosenbaum HT, Thompson WL, Fuller RH. Radiographic pulmonary changes in near drowning. *Radiology* 83:306, 1964.

150. Rosenthal S, Zuger JH, Apollo E. Respiratory colonization with *Pseudomonas* putrefaciens after near drowning in salt water. *Am J Clin Pathol* 64:382, 1975.

151. Rowe MI, Arango A, Allington G. Profile of pediatric drowning victims in a water-oriented society. *J Trauma* 17:587, 1977.

152. Rutledge RR, Flor RJ. The use of mechanical ventilation with positive end expiratory pressure in the treatment of near drowning. *Anesthesiology* 38:194, 1973.

153. Sarnaik AP, et al. Intracranial pressure and cerebral perfusion pressure in near drowning. *Crit Care Med* 13:224, 1985.

154. Schaefer KE, et al. Pulmonary and circulatory adjustment determining the limits of depths in breath-hold diving. *Science* 162:1020, 1968.

155. Schaefer KE, et al. Mechanisms in development of interstitial emphysema and air embolism on decompression from depth. *J Appl Physiol* 13:15, 1958.

156. Schench HV, McAniff JJ. *United States Underwater Fatality Statistics, 1972*. US Department of Commerce, NOAA, US Government Printing Office report no URI-73-8. Washington, DC: US Government Printing Office, December 1973.

157. Schench HV, McAniff JJ. *United States Underwater Fatality Statistics, 1973*. US Department of Commerce, NOAA, US Government Printing Office report no URI-SSR-75-9. Washington, DC: US Government Printing Office, May 1975.

158. Schench HV, McAniff JJ. *United States Underwater Fatality Statistics, 1974*. US Depart-

ment of Commerce, NOAA, US Government Printing Office report no URI-SSR-75-10. Washington, DC: US Government Printing Office, April 1976.

159. Schench HV, McAniff JJ. *United States Underwater Fatality Statistics, 1975.* US Department of Commerce, NOAA, US Government Printing Office report no URI-SSR-77-11. Washington, DC: US Government Printing Office, March 1977.

160. Schench HV, McAniff JJ. *United States Underwater Fatality Statistics, 1976.* US Department of Commerce, NOAA, US Government Printing Office report no URI-SSR-78-12. Washington, DC: US Government Printing Office, December 1978.

161. Schuman SH, Rowe JR, Glazer HM. Risk of drowning: An iceberg phenomenon. *JACEP* 6:139, 1977.

162. Schuman SH, et al. The iceberg phenomenon of near drowning. *Crit Care Med* 4:127, 1976.

163. Segarra F, Redding RA. Modern concepts about drowning. *Can Med Assoc J* 110:1057, 1974.

164. Sekar TS, et al. Survival after prolonged immersion in cold water without neurologic sequelae. *Arch Intern Med* 140:775, 1980.

165. Shilling CW, Carlston CB (Eds), *Physicians Guide to Diving Medicine.* San Pedro, CA: RA Mathias Best, 1984.

166. Siebke H, et al. Survival after 40 minutes submersion without cerebral sequelae. *Lancet* 1:1275, 1975.

167. Sladen A, Zauder HL. Methyl prednisolone therapy for pulmonary edema following near drowning. *JAMA* 215:1793, 1971.

168. Snively WD, Thuerbach J. Voluntary hyperventilation as a cause of needless drowning. *WV Med J* 68:153, 1972.

169. Spencer MP, Johanson DC. *Investigations of New Principles for Human Decompression Schedules Using the Doppler Ultrasonic Blood Bubble Detector.* Technical report. Seattle: Seattle Institute of Applied Physiology and Medicine, 1974.

170. Spyker DA. Submersion injury: Epidemiology, prevention, management. *Pediatr Clin North Am* 32:113, 1985.

171. Stacpoole PW. Lactic acidosis: The case against bicarbonate therapy (editorial). *Ann Intern Med* 105:276, 1986.

172. Standards and guidelines for cardiopulmonary resuscitation (CPR) and emergency cardiac care (ECG). *JAMA* 255:2905, 1986.

173. Strauss MB, Wright PW. Thoracic squeeze diving casualty. *Aerospace Med* 42:673, 1971.

174. Swann HG, Brucer M. The cardiorespiratory and biochemical events during rapid anoxic death. VI. Fresh-water and sea-water drowning. *Tex Rep Biol Med* 7:604, 1949.

175. Swann HG, et al. Fresh-water and sea-water drowning: A study of the terminal cardiac and biochemical events. *Tex Rep Biol Med* 5:423, 1947.

176. Swann HG, Spafford NR. Body salt and water changes during fresh and sea-water drowning. *Tex Rep Biol Med* 9:356, 1951.

177. Tabeling BB, Modell JH. Fluid administration increases oxygen delivery during continuous positive pressure ventilation after fresh-water near drowning. *Crit Care Med* 11:693, 1983.

178. Thalman ED. Air tables revisited: Development of a decompression computer algorithm. *Undersea Biomed Res* 12(Suppl):45, 1985.

179. United Press International. More tots in state killed by drowning. *San Diego Union,* May 23, 1985.

180. Van Haeringen JR, et al. Treatment of the respiratory distress syndrome following nondirect pulmonary trauma with positive end expiratory pressure with special emphasis on near drowning. *Chest* 66(Suppl):30S, 1974.

181. Vieira DF, Van Saene HKF, Miranda DR. Invasive pulmonary aspergillosis after near drowning. *Intensive Care Med* 10:203, 1984.

182. *Vital Statistics Monthly Report.* Richmond, VA: Virginia Department of Health, Bureau of Vital Records and Health Statistics. 1978.

183. Webb P. Afterdrop of body temperature during rewarming. *J Appl Physiol* 60:385, 1986.

184. Wolford JP. Cold water near drowning response. *JEMS* Spring, 1984.

185. Wong LL, McNamara JJ. Salt-water drowning. *Hawaii Med J* 43:208, 1984.

186. Wright SJ. SOS: Alcohol, drugs and boating. *Alcohol Health Res World* 9:28, 1985.

187. Wurtemute GJ. Childhood drowning and near drowning in the United States. *Am J Dis Child* 144:663, 1990.

188. Wynne JW, Modell JH. Respiratory aspiration of stomach contents. *Ann Intern Med* 87:466, 1977.

189. Yagil Y, et al. Near drowning in the Dead Sea: Electrolyte imbalances and therapeutic implications. *Arch Intern Med* 145:50, 1985.

190. Young RSK, Zaineraitis ED, Dooling EO. Neurologic outcome in cold water drowning. *JAMA* 244:1233, 1980.

191. Zell SC, Kurtz KJ. Severe exposure hypothermia. *Ann Emerg Med* 14:339, 1985.

46

Critical Care for Acute Respiratory Failure

Michael A. Matthay   Philip C. Hopewell

The need for critical care in managing patients with respiratory disorders usually arises when the abnormalities of gas exchange are sufficiently severe to threaten or actually impair function of critical organs. Occasionally, patients are observed and monitored in critical care units to enable early detection and prompt treatment of anticipated severe respiratory dysfunction. Critical care units offer the facilities, equipment, and personnel for close observation of patients, cardiorespiratory monitoring, airway management, vigorous respiratory care, including mechanical ventilation, and frequent or continuous administration of pharmacologic agents [120]. Generally speaking, none of these modalities can be consistently and effectively applied on general hospital wards. However, the determination of which patients are to be managed in critical care units cannot be based exclusively on their diagnostic and/or therapeutic requirements, but rather on an assessment of each individual patient in the context of the capabilities of the particular hospital. In order to use critical care appropriately in the management of patients with respiratory disorders, the physician must be aware of the principles of pathophysiology and management of the various disorders that may cause respiratory failure and the benefits that a critical care unit may offer. It is equally important to understand how to assess an individual patient to determine the severity of respiratory dysfunction and to evaluate the response to therapy. Finally, the physician must, whenever possible, incorporate knowledge of the individual patient, the specific effects and prognosis of the process for which critical care is being considered, and the patient's wishes into the decision concerning admission to a critical care unit [120].

This chapter reviews the means for assessment of respiratory failure in severely ill patients, describes the major elements of supportive care and monitoring available in critical care units, and discusses the pathophysiology and management of the major categories or processes that result in acute respiratory failure. The disorders covered in this chapter are dealt with more comprehensively in other chapters. Insofar as possible, only those aspects of the illness that relate to critical care are considered in this chapter.

Assessment of the Severity of Respiratory Dysfunction

From the perspective of a critical care physician, acute respiratory failure can be defined as any rapidly developing clinical disorder that leads to severe arterial hypoxemia or hypercapnia, either of which may be associated with metabolic or respiratory acidosis. In most of these patients, monitoring and treatment in an intensive care unit is indicated. If the patient's respiratory failure is sufficiently severe to require support with mechanical ventilation, then admission to a critical care unit is mandatory in order to monitor the mechanical ventilation and to treat the underlying cause of the acute respiratory failure. In the initial evaluation, an accurate assessment of the severity of the patient's acute respiratory failure is very important. This assessment should include a careful history and physical examination (clinical evaluation) as well as relevant laboratory and radiographic studies.

Clinical Evaluation

The course of acute respiratory failure may evolve slowly, developing during a period of days, or quite rapidly, in minutes to a few hours. The clinical manifestations of the process and the ways in which they are perceived by the patient will vary depending on the nature of the process itself and on its course. In most instances, the symptomatic hallmark of respiratory failure is dyspnea. The presence of this symptom, as with any subjective manifestation of disease, requires that the patient be sufficiently alert to be aware of the sensation and be able to convey that awareness to observers [6]. Thus, for example, patients who have taken overdoses of sedative-hypnotic drugs or narcotic agents, even if awake, may not be dyspneic in the presence of marked gas-exchange abnormalities. Also, dyspnea tends to be more intense when it develops rapidly. In respiratory failure that develops more slowly, dyspnea may appear at first only with exertion or with assumption of the supine position (orthopnea), but as the process becomes more severe, the dyspnea becomes constant and even may be present at rest. Patients with chronic airways obstruction commonly have chronic dyspnea; in these patients, relatively minor changes from the baseline level of dyspnea may represent a major worsening of gas exchange. Progressive hypoxemia, hypercapnia, or both may blunt the sensation of dyspnea and occasionally result in a misleading symptomatic assessment. In spite of its frequency as a symptom, dyspnea is poorly defined, is virtually impossible to quantify, and correlates very poorly with the severity of respiratory failure [175]. For these reasons, more objective assessments are essential in evaluating dyspneic patients.

Other symptoms such as cough, sputum production, and chest pain are important manifestations of processes that may be associated with respiratory failure but are less helpful than dyspnea as an indicator of respiratory dysfunction. In the initial evaluation of a patient, however, these ancillary symptoms may provide valuable clues that guide early diagnostic and therapeutic interventions.

In addition to the symptoms that usually are directly associated with respiratory or cardiac disease, other less specific subjective manifestations may be of importance. Patients with progressive hypoxemia or hypercapnia may report alterations in mental functioning. These include headache, visual disturbances, memory loss, confusion, excessive somnolence or insomnia, hallucinations, and transient loss of consciousness. When possible, confirmation of these symptoms

by a mental status examination serves as an important part of the evaluation.

The physical examination also may provide important information in patients with respiratory failure. Perhaps the most important evaluation rests on the general assessment of the severity of illness from the patient's appearance, including the degree of respiratory distress and the patient's mental status. Both these assessments help guide the initial approach to management by indicating the degree of cooperation that can be anticipated. Cyanosis, especially central cyanosis, is helpful as an indication of hypoxemia, but it may not be detectable. The respiratory rate, although influenced by a large number of factors, may serve as an indicator of the severity of respiratory distress, and measuring the respiratory rate also can be used as a monitoring technique to judge response to therapy. As described for the symptom of dyspnea, tachypnea may not be present in patients whose ventilatory drive is blunted. The degree of respiratory failure may be roughly quantified by noting the patient's ability to speak. Severely distressed patients will be able to speak only a few words at a time. As the respiratory failure becomes less severe, longer phases and sentences are possible. Stridorous breathing represents an important finding that suggests severe upper airway obstruction. An inability to phonate may be associated with marked obstruction at the larynx or above. Retraction of the sternum and supraclavicular, suprasternal, and intercostal spaces constitutes evidence of respiratory distress and increased resistance to lung inflation, generally caused by airways obstruction or an infiltrative process. These findings have been correlated with the severity of airways obstruction in patients with asthma [106] and with pneumonia in children [87]. The decrease in arterial systolic blood pressure that occurs with inspiration (pulsus paradoxus) also correlates with the severity of airways obstruction, especially in asthma [134]. Changes in the magnitude of the pulsus paradoxus also can be used to evaluate the response to therapy.

Examination of the lungs per se does not provide much information concerning the severity of respiratory dysfunction but may be helpful in determining the cause of respiratory failure. The findings associated with specific processes are discussed in other chapters, but several points are worth emphasizing. First, although wheezing is the characteristic feature of severe airways obstruction, the absence of wheezing may be an even more important finding. In patients with very severe airways obstruction, airflow may be so reduced that it is inadequate to produce the turbulence required for wheezing. Second, unilateral absence of breath sounds in a patient with respiratory distress may be associated with pneumothorax or mucous plugging of a main bronchus. Physical findings suggestive of pneumothorax are especially important in a mechanically ventilated patient because of the greater likelihood of a tension pneumothorax. Subcutaneous emphysema and a systolic crunch heard with systole (Hamman's sign) indicate pneumomediastinum with or without pneumothorax. The finding of digital clubbing in a person with respiratory failure suggests a chronic process. This finding may be helpful, for example, in distinguishing chronic interstitial fibrosis, in which clubbing is common, from a diffuse infiltrative process caused by an acute infection or left ventricular failure.

Because pulmonary edema may be the cause of acute respiratory failure, it is important to search for evidence of heart failure, although in patients who are critically ill the physical findings of left ventricular failure may be difficult to appreciate [38]. The presence of right ventricular failure usually implies a chronic pulmonary process usually with long-standing hypoxemia, although in some patients acute right ventricular failure may be associated with pulmonary embolism.

General Laboratory Evaluations

Routine hematologic studies and blood chemistries have limited relevance in assessing patients with respiratory failure, although clues to the acuteness or chronicity of the process may be provided. For example, an elevated hemoglobin and hematocrit implies the presence of chronic hypoxemia leading to secondary polycythemia. Hypercapnia may be inferred to be chronic if the plasma bicarbonate concentration is increased. Renal compensation for respiratory acidosis requires several days to occur; hence, an increase in bicarbonate concentration does not occur as a result of acute respiratory failure of short duration [25]. Patients who have long-standing elevations in $PaCO_2$ also are likely to be hypochloremic and hypokalemic. These abnormalities are likely to be more marked in patients who have been taking diuretics or adrenal corticosteroids. Hypokalemia and hypophosphatemia may be as-

sociated with weakness of the respiratory muscles that on occasion can lead to respiratory failure or can complicate underlying lung disease [121,159]. These electrolyte abnormalities also can be a cause for difficulties in weaning a patient from mechanical ventilation.

As with the physical examination of the chest, the chest radiograph cannot assist in quantifying the severity of respiratory dysfunction. It is, however, of crucial importance in determining the etiology of the respiratory disorder and is an essential component of the initial evaluation. Likewise, the electrocardiogram is essential to detect arrhythmias, myocardial ischemia, injury, or infarction, and chamber enlargement.

Pulmonary Evaluation

ARTERIAL BLOOD GAS AND pH MEASUREMENTS

The single most useful test in evaluating the severity of respiratory dysfunction is the measurement of arterial blood gas tensions (PaO_2, $PaCO_2$) and pH. These provide an indication of the status of integrated cardiorespiratory function and acid-base balance. Although these measurements are not particularly sensitive to early cardiorespiratory abnormalities and are not specific for the kind of abnormality present, they provide valuable information in patients with severe dysfunction. This section focuses on the interpretation of arterial blood gas and pH values in the assessment of severely ill patients and discusses how these interpretations can be used to infer the pathophysiology of acute respiratory failure and to guide the general approach to treatment.

Hypoxemia. The mechanisms by which clinically significant reductions in PaO_2 are produced include alveolar hypoventilation ($PaCO_2 > 40$ mmHg), mismatching of ventilation to perfusion, and right to left intrapulmonary or intracardiac shunting of blood. It is important to determine which of these mechanisms is operative in a given patient. Hypoxemia caused purely by hypoventilation implies that the lung itself is normal and that the only necessary therapeutic goal is to improve ventilation. This type of hypoxemia is characterized by a normal alveolar-to-arterial PO_2 difference [$P(A-a)O_2$]. The $P(A-a)O_2$ can be determined using the alveolar gas equation [Eq. (46-5)] to calculate PaO_2 and measuring PaO_2. In young patients breathing room air, the difference should not be greater than 10 mmHg, and it may increase to 16 mmHg in older persons [103]. With an increased fractional concentration of oxygen in inspired gas (FIO_2) sufficient to cause a PaO_2 of 200 mmHg or greater, the $P(A-a)O_2$ should not be greater than 40 mmHg.

The distinction between ventilation-perfusion mismatching and shunting can be made by measuring the response to administration of 100% oxygen. The PaO_2 will increase normally to values of nearly 600 mmHg if the hypoxemia is due purely to mismatching, whereas with a shunt the increase may be markedly reduced depending on the magnitude of the shunt flow. Figure 46-1 shows the relationship between PaO_2 and FIO_2 with different shunt fractions. Figure 46-2 demonstrates the effect of increasing amounts of mismatching of ventilation to perfusion on PaO_2 with different FIO_2 values. The approach to treatment of acute respiratory failure varies considerably depending on whether the hypoxemia is caused primarily by shunting or ventilation-perfusion mismatching. With ventilation-perfusion mismatching, relatively small amounts of supple-mental oxygen can increase the PaO_2 sufficiently, whereas with shunting, mechanical ventilation is much more likely to be necessary.

Hypercapnia. Alveolar hypoventilation is the only mechanism by which hypercapnia occurs. The amount of alveolar ventilation necessary to eliminate carbon dioxide and maintain a normal $PaCO_2$ varies depending on carbon dioxide production, as indicated by Equation (46-1). Alveolar ventilation will in turn be influenced by the amount of wasted ventilation, as shown in Equation (46-2). Thus, alveolar hypoventilation can occur because of increased production of carbon dioxide, a decrease in minute ventilation, or an increase in wasted ventilation.

The relationship between $PaCO_2$ and plasma bicarbonate concentrations ($[HCO_3^-]$) determines the arterial pH, as shown in the Henderson-Hasselbalch equation [Eq. (46-11)]. The relationship between $PaCO_2$ and arterial pH varies, however, depending on the time over which the $PaCO_2$ has increased. Thus, by examining the relationships among $PaCO_2$, arterial pH, and

Fig. 46-1. The relationship between inspired oxygen concentration and PaO_2 for lungs with varying degrees of shunt. The increase in PaO_2 is small for lungs with large shunts. (Reproduced from DR Dantzker. Gas exchange in the adult respiratory distress syndrome. *Clin Chest Med* 3:57, 1982.)

Fig. 46-2. The relationship of PaO_2 to FIO_2 with increasing amounts of ventilation to perfusion mismatching (0 = standard deviation of log-normal distribution of ventilation and perfusion). Note that even with marked mismatching the PaO_2 increases to nearly normal values with a very high FIO_2. (Reproduced from JB West. *Pulmonary Pathophysiology: The Essentials.* Baltimore: Williams & Wilkins, 1977.)

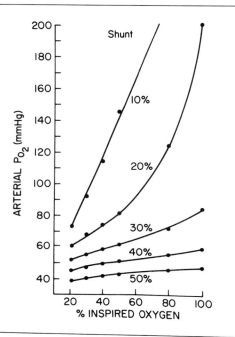

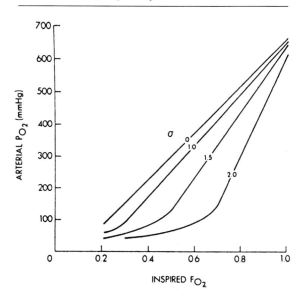

[HCO$_3^-$], the acuity or chronicity of the carbon dioxide elevation can be inferred (Fig. 46-3). Acute increases in PaCO$_2$ are accompanied by only small increases in [HCO$_3^-$], and arterial pH changes in a nearly linear fashion with PaCO$_2$. For every 1 mmHg change in PaCO$_2$, there is approximately a 0.008 pH unit change in the opposite direction [24]. An acute rise in PaCO$_2$ from 40 to 60 mmHg would be expected to cause a decrease in arterial pH to 7.25. Over a period of 1 to 3 days, however, renal conservation of bicarbonate causes the [HCO$_3^-$] to increase and buffer the pH change. Thus, for a given change in PaCO$_2$, the change in pH is much less than when the change occurs quickly. Obviously, the therapeutic implications of an acute versus a chronic change in PaCO$_2$ make this an important distinction.

Acid-Base Abnormalities. In addition to respiratory acidosis, metabolic acidosis and metabolic and respiratory alkalosis are important problems in some patients with serious respiratory dysfunction. One of the several causes of metabolic acidosis is an imbalance between oxygen delivery and metabolic oxygen needs leading to an-

aerobic metabolism and lactic acid production. In patients with severe respiratory disorders, such as severe asthma, this imbalance may occur because the work of breathing increases the demand for oxygen in the presence of hypoxia caused by the lung disease. Metabolic acidosis in this setting is a particularly ominous finding, suggesting that rapid deterioration is imminent and that prompt therapeutic interventions are necessary [4].

Both respiratory and metabolic alkalosis have important nonrespiratory effects in critically ill patients. Alkalosis predisposes to arrhythmias, decreases cardiac output, and reduces the threshold for seizures [83]. Hypocapnia with or without alkalosis reduces cerebral blood flow and may depress the level of consciousness [82]. For these reasons, alkalosis should be recognized as an important acid-base disturbance, and corrective measures should be taken.

MEASUREMENTS OF LUNG FUNCTION

The lung function studies that can be used in severely ill patients are rather limited. Depending on the nature and severity of the illness and the patient's ability to cooperate, one may measure vital capacity (VC), timed forced expiratory volume (FEV$_1$), peak expiratory flow rate (PEFR), and maximal inspiratory pressure (MIP). The VC is the maximal volume of air that can be exhaled after maximal inspiration and provides an indication of the patient's ventilatory capability. Because the VC is influenced by the respiratory neuromuscular system, the chest wall, the elastic properties of the lung, and the caliber of the airways, it cannot be used to identify specific abnormalities. Nevertheless, it is particularly helpful in assessing and following patients with neuromuscular illnesses and in evaluating patients being ventilated mechanically to determine if it is feasible to consider weaning from the ventilator. The minimal acceptable VC in most instances is 10 to 15 ml/kg of body weight. This value must, however, be interpreted in light of the patient's clinical condition.

Measurement of MIP provides some of the same information as the VC, and it is influenced by most of the same factors. However, the ability to generate an acceptable inspiratory pressure, less than -20 cmH$_2$O, does not necessarily imply that the VC will be acceptable.

The timed forced expiratory volume, which is usually expressed as the FEV$_1$ divided by the forced vital capacity (FVC), is used as a measure

Fig. 46-3. Effects of acute and chronic variations in PaCO$_2$ on plasma [HCO$_3^-$] and pH. The line connecting points *A* and *C* represents the effects of an acute change in PaCO$_2$ to a value above or below 40 mmHg. Renal compensation over time results in a shift of the relationship to that represented by the line connecting points *B* and *D*, as is indicated by the arrows. (Reproduced from JF Murray. *The Normal Lung.* Philadelphia: Saunders, 1976.)

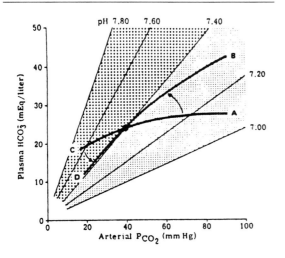

of the severity of airways obstruction in patients with asthma or chronic airways obstruction. The measurement may not be possible in severely obstructed patients who have marked tachypnea; the maneuver itself may even transiently worsen airways obstruction. However, the FEV_1 provides the best objective indicator of the degree of airways obstruction and, when measured serially, the response to therapy. Absolute FEV_1 values of less than 0.75 liter or less than 25 percent of the predicted value are commonly associated with increased $PaCO_2$ values [135].

Measurement of the PEFR provides information similar to the FEV_1 in patients with airways obstruction. The PEFR has the distinct advantage, however, of not requiring a full inhalation followed by a full forced exhalation. It is measured by having the patient slowly inhale and then blow a short, forced puff through the flowmeter, a maneuver similar to a cough. Values below 60 liters/min indicate severe obstruction.

Calculations of Respiratory Variables

A number of equations and calculations are helpful in the assessment of respiratory function. The use of these equations is discussed later in this chapter in the section that considers specific cases of acute respiratory failure. Descriptions of the physiologic principles involved with the equations were presented in the preceding section. Representative normal values for selected cardiorespiratory variables are listed in Table 46-1.

EQUATIONS RELATED TO ARTERIAL CARBON DIOXIDE TENSION

$PaCO_2$ is related directly to carbon dioxide production (VCO_2, in milliliters per minute — $\dot{V}CO_2$) and inversely to alveolar ventilation ($\dot{V}A$, in liters per minute — $\dot{V}A$) as follows:

$$PaCO_2 = K \frac{\dot{V}CO_2}{\dot{V}A} \qquad (46\text{-}1)$$

where K is a constant.

The $\dot{V}A$ is the difference between the tidal volume (VT in liters) and the wasted or dead-space ventilation (VD) multiplied by the respiratory rate (F, in breaths per minute):

$$\dot{V}A = (VT - VD) \times F \qquad (46\text{-}2)$$

Table 46-1. Representative normal values for selected respiratory and hemodynamic values

Normal	
PaO_2	95 mmHg
$PaCO_2$	40 mmHg
pH (arterial)	7.40
$P(A\text{-}a)O_2$	<10 mmHg
O_2 saturation	98%
CaO_2	19.8 ml/100 ml
$P\bar{v}O_2$	40 mmHg
$\dot{V}O_2$	240 ml/min
$\dot{V}CO_2$	192 ml/min
R	0.8
Respiratory rate	12
$\dot{V}E$	6 liters/min
VD	150 ml
VT	450 ml
VD/VT	0.33
$\dot{Q}_t$	5 liters/min
$\dot{Q}_s/\dot{Q}_t$	7%
PVR	50–150 dyn · s/cm^5
SVR	800–1200 dyn · s/cm^5

Total minute ventilation (VE in liters per minute, — $\dot{V}E$) is the product of VT and F:

$$\dot{V}E = VT \times F \qquad (46\text{-}3)$$

From these three equations, it can be seen that the factors determining the $PaCO_2$ are VT, VD, F, and $\dot{V}CO_2$.

The volume of dead-space or wasted ventilation can be calculated from a modification of the Bohr equation:

$$VD = \frac{PaCO_2 - PeCO_2 \times VT}{PaCO_2} \qquad (46\text{-}4)$$

where $PeCO_2$ is the partial pressure of carbon dioxide in mixed expired air. The VD so derived is commonly expressed as a fraction of VT. Normal values for the VD/VT are 0.30 to 0.35.

EQUATIONS RELATED TO OXYGENATION

The partial pressure of oxygen in the alveolus (PAO_2) can be calculated from the alveolar gas equation as follows:

$$PAO_2 = FIO_2 (P_b - 47 \text{ mmHg}) - PaCO_2/R \qquad (46\text{-}5)$$

where R is the respiratory exchange ratio ($\dot{V}CO_2/\dot{V}O_2$), P_b is barometric pressure, and 47 is the partial pressure of water vapor in millimeters of mercury in fully saturated air at body temperature. The value of R is usually assumed to be 0.8. Having calculated the PAO_2, the $P(A\text{-}a)O_2$ can then be determined, enabling a more quantitative assessment of the degree of hypoxemia and the mechanisms responsible for it. For example, a normal $P(A\text{-}a)O_2$ indicates that hypoxemia is secondary to alveolar hypoventilation alone. On the other hand, an increased $P(A\text{-}a)O_2$ indicates either an intrapulmonary or intracardiac right-to-left shunt or mismatching of ventilation and perfusion.

Oxygen consumption ($\dot{V}O_2$, in liters per minute – $\dot{V}O_2$) can be estimated fairly accurately from the relationship

$$\dot{V}O_2 = (FIO_2 - FeO_2) \times \dot{V}E \qquad (46\text{-}6)$$

where FeO_2 is the fractional concentration of oxygen in expired air.

Oxygen delivery to the tissues depends not only on PaO_2, but also on arterial oxygen content (CaO_2) and cardiac output. The CaO_2 (milliliters of oxygen per 100 ml of blood) is calculated as follows:

$$CaO_2 = 1.34\,[Hb] \times \frac{\text{percent saturation}}{100} + (0.003 \times PaO_2) \qquad (46\text{-}7)$$

where 1.34 is the milliliters of oxygen carried by each gram of hemoglobin, [Hb] is the hemoglobin concentration in grams per 100 ml of blood, and percent saturation is the saturation of hemoglobin with oxygen in arterial blood. The saturation is usually determined from the oxyhemoglobin dissociation curve. The constant, 0.003, is the amount of dissolved (unbound) oxygen in blood in milliliters per millimeter of mercury PaO_2.

Systemic oxygen transport (SO_2T) in milliliters per minute is calculated as follows:

$$SO_2T = CaO_2 \times \dot{Q}_t \qquad (46\text{-}8)$$

where $\dot{Q}_t$ is cardiac output in liters per minute.

Thus, oxygen delivery to the tissues depends not only on PaO_2, but also on [Hb] and $\dot{Q}_t$ as well. In evaluating and managing patients with severe respiratory dysfunction, all these factors need to be taken into account.

The balance between oxygen supply and systemic oxygen demands can be evaluated by cal-

culating the difference between CaO_2 and the content of oxygen in mixed venous blood ($C\bar{v}O_2$). The $C\bar{v}O_2$ is calculated in the same manner as the CaO_2, but the oxyhemoglobin saturation value in mixed venous (pulmonary artery) blood is used.

Using the $\dot{V}O_2$ and the $C(a\text{-}\bar{v})O_2$, the cardiac output can be calculated according to the Fick principle:

$$\dot{Q}_t = \frac{\dot{V}O_2}{CaO_2 - C\bar{v}O_2} \qquad (46\text{-}9)$$

The contribution of right-to-left shunting of blood to hypoxemia can be quantitated in patients receiving an FIO_2 of 1.0 using the following equation:

$$\frac{\dot{Q}_s}{\dot{Q}_t} = \frac{Cc'O_2 - CaO_2}{Cc'O_2 - C\bar{v}O_2} \qquad (46\text{-}10)$$

where $\dot{Q}_s$ is the volume of shunted blood and $Cc'O_2$ is an approximation of end-capillary blood oxygen content, assuming the $Pc'O_2$ to be the same as PAO_2 and calculating the $Cc'O_2$ based on this assumption.

The effect of the percent shunt on PaO_2 as calculated from this equation is shown in Figure 46-1, which illustrates the lack of responsiveness of PaO_2 to increases in FIO_2 (PAO_2) once the $\dot{Q}_s/\dot{Q}_t$ exceeds 30 percent.

ACID-BASE EQUATIONS

The essential relationships among the factors controlling arterial blood pH are described in the Henderson-Hasselbalch equation:

$$pH = pK - \frac{\log\,[HCO_3^-]}{[H_2CO_3]} \qquad (46\text{-}11)$$

where pK, the dissociation constant, is 6.1 for plasma at 37°C. Because

$$[H_2CO_3] = PaCO_2 \times 0.0301 \qquad (46\text{-}12)$$

where 0.0301 is the solubility constant of carbon dioxide in plasma at 37°C, Equation (46-13) can be substituted as follows:

$$pH = 6.1 + \frac{\log\,[HCO_3^-]}{PaCO_2 \times 0.0301} \qquad (46\text{-}13)$$

The relationships among these variables under acute and chronic conditions are shown in Figure 46-3.

EQUATIONS FOR LUNG MECHANICS

The stiffness (resistance to inflation) of the lung and chest wall is termed the *compliance* of the respiratory system (C_{rs}). In patients being mechanically ventilated, it is expressed by the following formula:

$$C_{rs} = V_t/P_{plateau} - P_{ee} \qquad (46\text{-}14)$$

where V_t is the tidal volume delivered by the ventilator, $P_{plateau}$ is the inspiratory plateau pressure, and P_{ee} is the end-expiratory pressure read from the manometer of the ventilator. The effect of airways resistance can be included in the measurement by using the peak inspiratory pressure (P_{peak}) rather than $P_{plateau}$. This is termed the *effective compliance* (C_{eff}):

$$C_{eff} = V_t/P_{peak} - P_{ee} \qquad (46\text{-}15)$$

Assuming that the compliance of the chest wall is stable, changes in C_{rs} reflect changes in lung mechanical properties, whereas changes in C_{eff} may indicate changes in airways resistance (if inspiratory flow is unchanged) as well as lung compliance.

General Aspects of Supportive Care for Acute Respiratory Failure

Supplemental Oxygen

The administration of supplemental oxygen is frequently necessary in patients with any cardiorespiratory disorder that results in hypoxemia or in which hypoxemia may be expected. Generally speaking, it is not prudent to rely on external oxygen delivery devices for patients with hypoxemia sufficient to require an FIO_2 of 0.6 or greater or who could be expected to suffer serious consequences should the device not be positioned properly.

There are a variety of types of external oxygen delivery systems that can be used to provide supplemental oxygen. The choice of a particular device depends on at least four factors: (1) the amount of oxygen needed, (2) the need for precise control of the FIO_2, (3) the need for humidification, and (4) the patient's comfort. Nasal prongs are the simplest and most comfortable delivery device. However, the FIO_2 provided cannot be quantified reliably and humidification is poor. Open face masks or face tents provide a high flow of well-humidified gas with a moderately reliable FIO_2 usually set by a Venturi device

in a humidifier/mixer. Tight-fitting face masks provide higher concentrations of oxygen, and the same sort of tight mask fitted with a nonbreathing valve and a reservoir bag can be used to provide even higher concentrations of oxygen, perhaps up to an FIO_2 of 0.7 for short periods. One version of this system incorporates a valve for providing positive end-expiratory pressure (PEEP) [26]. However, such devices are generally uncomfortable, and the oxygen may be poorly humidified. The FIO_2 is controlled much more precisely by the Venturi mask, which uses a calibrated Venturi device in the delivery line to provide high flows of gas containing 24, 28, 35, or 40% oxygen [123]. This sort of mask is used for patients with chronic airways obstruction and chronic hypercapnia in whom uncontrolled high oxygen concentrations may cause further hypoventilation.

External Ventilatory Assist Devices

A variety of devices have been used to provide temporary ventilatory assistance without resorting to an endotracheal airway and mechanical ventilation. These devices are generally of limited usefulness in the acute setting. The devices of this sort that are employed most frequently are simple pressure-limited ventilators used to provide intermittent positive-pressure ventilation (IPPV) via a mouthpiece. These devices only transiently increase alveolar ventilation and for this reason are of limited value [57]. External negative-pressure devices, such as the cuirass ventilator, which fits over the chest wall and augments ventilation by lowering the pressure around the chest causing it to expand, may be of value in patients with chronic neuromuscular diseases even in the presence of acute deterioration [141]. Other ventilatory assist devices include the rocking bed and surgically implanted phrenic nerve pacemakers; however, these are of little applicability in acute respiratory failure.

Airway Management

Definitive, unambiguous indications for endotracheal intubation that apply to all situations are difficult to define. Some patients require endotracheal intubation because of progressive arterial hypercapnia and respiratory acidosis, as in acute exacerbations of chronic obstructive pulmonary disease or in status asthmaticus. These patients may also have a decreased level of consciousness, which indicates that they will not be able to cooperate with inhaled bronchodilator therapy, cough effectively, or protect their airway from aspiration of gastric or pharyngeal contents. Other patients may require intubation because of progressive muscle fatigue in association with exacerbation of a primary neurologic disease such as myasthenia gravis. Other patients may have severe hypoxemia even when given high-flow supplemental oxygen therapy. Most commonly, this pattern of severe hypoxemia is secondary to acute lung injury from sepsis, aspiration, or primary pneumonia, although cardiogenic pulmonary edema and intravascular volume overload need to be excluded also. Once acute respiratory failure has been recognized, the decision to proceed to endotracheal intubation and support with mechanical ventilation is based in part on observation of the patient's clinical course including the acid-base status, arterial oxygenation, alveolar ventilation (as reflected by the $PaCO_2$), vital signs, level of consciousness, and clinical evidence of respiratory muscle fatigue. Regardless of the situation, the potential reversibility of the patient's underlying disorder must be taken into account in determining whether intubation is indicated.

Endotracheal tubes may be passed through either the mouth or the nose. The oral route has the advantage of accepting a larger-diameter tube and is easier under emergency circumstances. Because direct laryngoscopy is required, sedation and often muscle-relaxing agents are needed in awake patients. Semielective tube placement in a spontaneously ventilating patient may be accomplished via the nose without direct visualization of the vocal cords; however, direct visualization may be necessary to guide the tube into the larynx. Topical anesthesia is necessary, but systemic agents are not usually required. In difficult situations, such as when the neck is immobilized, placement of either an oral or a nasal tube may be accomplished over a fiberoptic bronchoscope. In any case, intubation should be done only by physicians experienced with the procedure who are familiar with intravenous anesthetics and muscle-relaxing agents.

Nasal endotracheal tubes are generally more comfortable for the patient and are more acceptable for long-term management. In addition, oral hygiene can be better maintained. Nasal tubes have the disadvantage of being more difficult to suction through compared with oral tubes because of their smaller diameter. For the same reason, it may be difficult or impossible to perform fiberoptic bronchoscopy through a nasal tube.

The effective lumen may be further narrowed by compression or kinking within the nose or nasopharynx.

Immediately after the tube is placed, the lungs should be auscultated to determine if air is entering both hemithoraces. Because of the relatively obtuse angle of the right main bronchus, positioning of the tip of the tube in the right main airway is quite common (Fig. 46-4). If the tube seems to be in good position as determined by auscultation, it should be taped securely in place and its position should be confirmed by a chest radiograph. The ideal location is when the tip of the tube is midway between the thoracic inlet, indicated by the sternoclavicular joints, and the carina on a standard frontal view of the chest. Even with secure taping, the tip of the tube can move and may enter a main bronchus or migrate in retrograde fashion to a position very high inside or outside the trachea. After the correct position of

Fig. 46-4. Right mainstem intubation. The endotracheal tube is in the right mainstem bronchus (carina = *arrowhead*). There is complete opacification of the left lung with marked atelectasis. (Reproduced from LR Goodman, CE Putman. Radiological evaluation of patients receiving assisted ventilation. *JAMA* 245:858, 1981.)

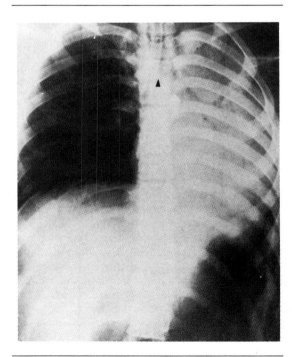

the endotracheal tube has been confirmed radiographically, the length of the tube that is external should be measured in reference to the patient's nose or teeth and the measurement should be recorded and displayed on the patient's bedside data flow chart.

All endotracheal tubes should be fitted with a bonded high-volume, low-pressure cuff that will occlude the trachea around the tube, enabling positive-pressure ventilation and preventing aspiration of oropharyngeal contents. Care should be taken to avoid overinflation of the cuff. An overinflated cuff (>20 mmHg) may cause pressure necrosis of the adjacent tracheal mucosa and predispose to the development of a tracheoesophageal fistula or subsequent tracheal stenosis [19,70,160].

Nasal or, occasionally, oral endotracheal tubes can be left in place for long periods of time in patients who continue to require mechanical ventilation or airway protection. There is no absolute time limit for endotracheal intubation beyond which tracheostomy is indicated [70,160]. Tracheostomy may be necessary, however, because of complications, such as infection or soft-tissue necrosis in the upper air passages, including the nose. Occasionally, tracheostomy facilitates removal of secretions more effectively than an endotracheal tube. In addition, patients may find a tracheostomy more comfortable and may be able to eat and talk with a tracheostomy tube in place [70].

Because endotracheal and tracheostomy tubes bypass the normal humidifying mechanisms in the upper airway, all inspired gas must be fully humidified. Removal of pulmonary secretions using a suction catheter should be done at regular intervals as determined by the volume of secretions present. Sterile technique must be used for suctioning. Likewise, all gas-delivery circuits in direct communication with the airway should be sterile when connected and changed at least at 48-hour intervals [85].

It is important to realize that once an endotracheal or tracheostomy tube is in place, complete responsibility for the airway rests with the persons caring for the patient. The patient can no longer humidify inspired air, cough effectively, or defend the lower airways against airborne microorganisms. Perhaps more important, he or she cannot call for help or unblock the tube should it become obstructed. For all these reasons, in addition to the gravity of the illness for which the tube was placed, patients with artificial airways should nearly always be managed in a critical care unit.

Mechanical Ventilation

Through the use of mechanical ventilation, patients who have severe derangements of gas exchange may be supported until the underlying process has resolved. Thus, nearly always, mechanical ventilation is a temporary life support technique, although in some situations the need for ventilatory support may not be temporary but lifelong. This is the case for patients with chronic, progressive neuromuscular diseases that preclude effective spontaneous ventilation.

The general clinical situations in which mechanical ventilation is most commonly used include (1) hypoxemia, usually due to intrapulmonary shunting of blood wherein external devices cannot provide a sufficiently high FIO_2, and (2) progressive hypoventilation with respiratory acidosis. Other indications include (3) prophylactic mechanical ventilation in patients in whom respiratory support is needed, such as after cardiac, thoracic, or upper abdominal surgery, and (4) patients who are barely maintaining adequate gas exchange at the cost of expending energy with a high work of breathing. Finally, mechanical ventilation is necessary in patients who require general anesthesia or heavy sedation to allow diagnostic or therapeutic interventions.

FEATURES OF MECHANICAL VENTILATORS
The most common feature used to categorize mechanical ventilators is the mechanism that determines the point at which the changeover from the inspiratory phase to the expiratory phase takes place. This point may be determined by the volume of gas delivered (volume-cycled), the airway pressure achieved (pressure-cycled), or the elapsed time of inspiration (time-cycled). Both time-cycled and pressure-cycled ventilators have the disadvantage of not necessarily delivering a constant tidal volume. For this reason, volume-cycled ventilators are most commonly used. Many ventilators, however, have options that allow the device to be pressure- or time-cycled in addition to a volume-cycling mode.

To be of optimal usefulness in providing adequate ventilatory support in patients with different types of respiratory disorders, mechanical ventilators must have certain essential features. The most important of these is the need to deliver a wide range of tidal volumes (100 to 2000 ml), with an adjustable respiratory frequency (5 to 60), and an accurate, adjustable FIO_2 (0.21 to 1.00). Also, controls for adjusting the inspiration-expiration ratio (or the inspiratory flow rate) and the inspiratory pressure limit are important. The device should be capable of operating in an assist (patient-triggered) mode, a controlled (machine-triggered) mode, and an assist-control combination mode. It is also essential that the ventilator be equipped with devices that monitor exhaled tidal volume, inspiratory pressure, and FIO_2 and have battery-operated alarms that signal loss of exhaled tidal volume, excessive inspiratory pressure, and reduction in FIO_2. In addition, it is necessary that the temperature of the inspired gas be monitored.

Although not essential to their basic operation, it is desirable that ventilators have built-in controls for adjusting PEEP, for allowing intermittent mandatory ventilation (IMV), and for providing continuous positive airway pressure (CPAP) in spontaneously breathing patients. The effects on airway and pleural pressures of the different general modes of respiratory support are compared to spontaneous ventilation in Figure 46-5.

TYPES OF VENTILATORY SUPPORT

Two basic modes of ventilatory support are usually employed in the management of patients with respiratory failure. These are IPPV and IMV. The obvious difference between these two modes is that there is no allowance for spontaneous ventilation with IPPV, whereas with IMV a portion of respiration is spontaneous. The use of one or the other of these two modes is often a matter of the physician's personal preference; however, some guidelines can be provided. The use of IPPV is clearly indicated in patients who do not breathe spontaneously. In addition, in patients who have severe pain with respiration and/or an unstable chest wall, IPPV should be used. Also for patients whose work of breathing is substantial, IMV is of limited value.

On the other hand, IMV may offer an advantage by maintaining the condition of the respiratory muscles. For this reason, IMV may be more useful in patients who have acute processes without preexisting deconditioned muscles [92]. In addition, some patients may find IMV more comfortable than IPPV. IMV also may be useful for patients who develop significant reductions of cardiac output with mechanical ventilation, especially with PEEP, in that it may allow greater amounts of PEEP to be used. In patients who are

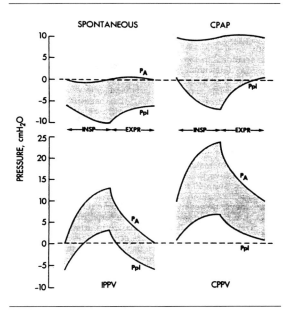

Fig. 46-5. Schematic representations of airway and pleural pressures with spontaneous respiration, spontaneous respiration with continuous positive airway pressure (*CPAP*), intermittent positive-pressure ventilation (*IPPV*), and continuous positive-pressure ventilation (*CPPV*). Note that with CPAP and CPPV, the pressure gradient between the airway and the pleural space is increased compared to spontaneous respiration and IPPV, respectively. *Ppl* = pleural pressure; *PA* = alveolar pressure. (Reproduced from HC Hinshaw, JF Murray (Eds), *Diseases of the Chest.* Philadelphia: Saunders, 1980.)

not capable of synchronizing their inspiratory efforts with the ventilator, IMV may provide adequate ventilation without the need for sedation or muscle-relaxing agents. It also may be a useful weaning technique in some situations.

It is also possible to provide a patient with a certain pressure-limited support ventilation in between the regular cycling of the ventilator at the preset rate and tidal volume. This mode is called *pressure-support*. When the patient exerts negative pleural pressure, he or she receives a tidal volume generated by preset pressure levels (perhaps 20 cmH_2O), which therefore relieves the patient of some of the work of breathing. This mode of ventilation is often used along with IMV once the patient's respiratory failure has stabilized. Some authorities believe that pressure-support is useful for weaning some patients from mechanical ventilation, but its superiority over current T-piece on standard IMV weaning remains to be demonstrated [93].

POSITIVE END-EXPIRATORY PRESSURE

PEEP may be added to IPPV to produce continuous positive-pressure ventilation (CPPV) or it may be added to IMV. In addition, it can be used in spontaneously ventilating patients to produce CPAP. By increasing the distending pressure across the walls of the airways and alveoli, PEEP increases the volume of gas in the lung [178]. This is most beneficial in disorders characterized by pulmonary edema (usually noncardiogenic in origin) with consequent loss of functioning gas-exchange units because of fluid filling or atelectasis. PEEP tends to increase the functional residual capacity by reexpanding collapsed units and allowing more gas exchange, thereby reducing intrapulmonary shunting of blood and improving PaO_2.

PEEP generally is not beneficial and in fact may be harmful in patients with other types of respiratory failure, especially those caused by airway obstruction in which the lungs are already overinflated. In such cases, further increases in lung volume may be hazardous. This caution applies not only to CPPV but also to IMV with PEEP and to CPAP. Levels of PEEP that are commonly used range from 3 to 20 cmH_2O. Higher levels are occasionally used with IMV, but the indications for and the value of the high levels of PEEP have not been clearly defined.

Because PEEP increases intrathoracic pressure, return of blood from the venous circulation to the right ventricle may be impaired and as a consequence cardiac output may be reduced [55]. Even though PaO_2 may be increased by PEEP, this apparently beneficial effect may be offset by the fall in cardiac output with a consequent decrease in systemic oxygen transport [178]. Application of PEEP may cause generalized overdistension of the lungs in patients with airway obstruction or focal overdistension in patients with infiltrative processes. Such overdistension may predispose to the development of pneumothorax, the second major complication of PEEP. Finally, when infiltrative processes are unevenly distributed, PEEP may decrease blood flow to the more normal alveoli and increase flow to the fluid-filled or collapsed alveoli. This will be manifested as a decrease in a PaO_2 when PEEP is applied [178].

EMERGENCIES IN THE VENTILATED PATIENT

Mechanically ventilated patients are at risk for several potentially disastrous complications that can occur suddenly and may be related either to the underlying disorder or to malfunction of the ventilator or artificial airway. Because such occurrences may be rapidly fatal, it is important that personnel caring for critically ill patients develop a routine for assessment and management of these situations.

When a patient is not being adequately ventilated, the problem may be manifested by patient distress, by sounding of either the high-pressure limit alarm or the low-V_T alarm, or by sudden hemodynamic changes. When the high-pressure limit is exceeded, the differential diagnosis includes obstruction of the endotracheal or tracheostomy tube by kinking, mucus, or a blood clot; obstruction in the patient's airways; or pneumothorax. Occasionally, migration of the tip of the tube into a mainstem bronchus (usually the right; see Fig. 46-4) will cause the high-pressure limit to be exceeded. When the high-pressure limit is exceeded and the patient is not being ventilated adequately, the patient should be immediately disconnected from the ventilator and hand ventilation begun using an FIO_2 of 1.0. At nearly the same time as hand ventilation begins, the artificial airway should be checked for correct position and for evidence of external obstruction, such as kinking between the ventilator tubing connection and the nose, mouth, or hypopharynx. If there is no external obstruction, the tube position seems correct, and compression of the bag is still difficult, a suction catheter should be passed through the tube to check its patency and/or to remove mucous plugs or blood clots that may be causing the problem. Assuming the suction catheter can be passed, failure of these maneuvers to relieve the apparent obstruction indicates that the problem is within the thorax and may be caused by major airway obstruction that was not removed by suctioning, sudden severe peripheral airways obstruction, or pneumothorax. These can usually be distinguished from one another by a rapid physical examination of the chest. Tracheal obstruction is manifested by the finding of no or markedly reduced entry of air into the lungs. Main bronchial obstruction is indicated by the absence of entry of air into the lung distal to the obstruction causing a rocking motion of the chest with the affected side not expanding with inspiration and the unobstructed side being overinflated. Peripheral airways obstruction may be suspected from the patient's history and is usually indicated by wheezing, although with severe bronchoconstriction there may be little air movement and thus little or no wheezing. Nearly always, a pneumothorax that occurs in a patient being mechanically ventilated quickly becomes a tension pneumothorax. This is indicated by difficulty with ventilation and usually by a reduction in systemic arterial blood pressure and an increase in central venous pressure. In addition, examination of the chest shows no entry of air on the affected side. In contrast to the findings of mainstem bronchial obstruction, the affected side is hyperinflated and hyperresonant to percussion. If the clinical situation allows, a chest roentgenogram (Fig. 46-6) will allow a definitive diagnosis; often, however, there is not sufficient time to take a chest x-ray film and a presumptive diagnosis of pneumothorax must be acted on.

Fig. 46-6. In a patient who was being mechanically ventilated, a right pneumothorax developed during mechanical ventilation. Note that there is an endotracheal tube in place as well as a nasogastric tube in the stomach. There is some evidence of radiographic tension with depression of the right hemidiaphragm. (Courtesy of Dr. Gordon Gamsu, University of California at San Francisco.)

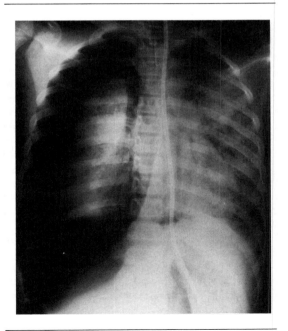

Management of each of these situations is obviously different. Vigorous chest physical therapy and suctioning of the airway usually will remove obstructing mucous plugs or clots. Occasionally, emergency fiberoptic bronchoscopy may be necessary to visualize and remove mucus. A tension pneumothorax requires prompt intervention to reduce the intrathoracic pressure; a No. 14 gauge needle can be placed in the second anterior intercostal space and air may be removed by suction. Relief of the tension will restore the hemodynamic status and ability to ventilate the patient. A chest tube should always be placed. Even if the diagnosis of pneumothorax was mistaken, a chest tube must be placed because of the high probability of lung puncture with the needle.

When inadequate ventilation is noted and the high-pressure limit is not being exceeded, the possible problems to be considered are (1) leaks in the ventilator tubing or around the cuff of the artificial airway, (2) ventilator malfunction, or (3) a tracheoesophageal fistula. Again, the first step is to disconnect the ventilator and begin manual ventilation using an FIO_2 of 1.0. At the same time, the position of the tube and the degree of cuff inflation should be checked. If the external pilot balloon is deflated, more air should be added. Cuff leakage may be detected by air escaping from the mouth with each ventilator inflation. The leaks may be caused by breaks in the cuff itself or in the external pilot balloon. Occasionally, an endotracheal tube may be positioned too high in the airway with the cuff at the level of the vocal cords or higher, causing air to leak around the cuff. If the cuff itself is leaking, the tube must be replaced. With some kinds of tubes, the outer balloon may be replaced without changing the tube. Leaks also may be caused by enlargement of the trachea at the site of the cuff because of pressure on the tracheal wall. If this is the cause of the leak, the problem may be solved by adding air to the cuff within the trachea. If air is added, care should be taken not to exceed a measured intracuff pressure of 20 mmHg [70,160].

Tracheal dilatation is often the precursor of a much more serious problem, formation of a tracheoesophageal fistula. This usually can be prevented by maintaining the intracuff pressures at less than 20 to 25 mmHg [160]. When a fistula does develop, however, it is often catastrophic. Patients with fistulas can sometimes be managed temporarily by placing the tube at a lower level in the trachea with the cuff below the fistula. Definitive management is surgical correction of the fistula.

WEANING FROM MECHANICAL VENTILATION

Patients being ventilated mechanically should be evaluated frequently to determine if their lung function has improved sufficiently to begin weaning from the ventilator.

Both the techniques of weaning and the rapidity of the process may vary considerably depending on the nature of the underlying disorder that caused the need for mechanical ventilation. There are, however, some basic criteria that are generally applicable in determining if it is feasible to initiate weaning [131]. First, the patient should be reasonably alert. Second, the underlying medical problem that necessitated mechanical ventilation must be improving. For example, hemodynamic abnormalities associated with sepsis or cardiac failure must be stabilized before weaning can begin. Lung function should be adequate, as indicated by the ability of the patient to generate a VC of greater than 10 ml/kg of body weight. This ability also may be inferred by the generation of a MIP of less (more negative) than -20 cmH$_2$O. In addition, the patient should not require an F$_{IO_2}$ greater than 0.6. Recently, it was reported that a ratio of the respiratory rate to the tidal volume can predict successful weaning in medical patients, with a positive predictive value of 78 percent [184]. Additional criteria that may be useful include a resting minute ventilation of less than 10 liters, the ability to double this volume voluntarily, a P(A-a)O$_2$ less than 350 mmHg, and a V$_D$/V$_T$ of less than 0.55. It must be kept in mind, however, that many patients with severe chronic airways obstruction will never meet these criteria [131]. Decisions to initiate weaning in these patients generally are based more on subjective than objective criteria. However, independent of meeting acceptable pulmonary criteria for weaning, it is equally important that the patient's nonpulmonary problems be considered before weaning from mechanical ventilation is initiated. For instance, anemia, fluid overload, electrolyte imbalance, impaired cardiovascular function, or altered mental status can prevent successful weaning, even if the primary problem, respiratory failure [95], seems well enough controlled to proceed.

The techniques used in weaning include progressive lengthening of periods of spontaneous ventilation with the endotracheal tube attached to a T-piece or a similar arrangement with CPAP.

Weaning by IMV can be accomplished with a progressive reduction in the number of breaths delivered by the ventilator. Patients whose lungs were previously normal and who have required only a short period of mechanical ventilation usually can be quickly weaned and extubated. The process is often much longer in patients who have required an extended period of ventilatory support. The physiologic bases for failure to wean are categorized in Table 46-2 into the clinical manifestations, and the usual clinical disorders associated with failure to wean [131].

Cardiorespiratory Monitoring

In this section a wide range of techniques for monitoring the hemodynamic and respiratory status of critically ill patients with respiratory failure is considered. In the last two decades many invasive techniques for monitoring the systemic and pulmonary circulation have been developed. More recently, however, there has been increasing interest in developing noninvasive methods for monitoring important physiologic variables with the goal of reducing the risk and expense of invasive measurements whenever possible.

Systemic Arterial Catheterization

Systemic arterial catheters are widely used in a variety of critically ill patients. They are most useful for monitoring systemic arterial blood pressure in patients who are hemodynamically unstable, including patients with severe, uncontrolled hypertension as well as patients with hypotension and clinical shock. In addition, systemic arterial catheters are useful as a means of obtaining repeated blood samples from patients, thus obviating the need for repeated percutaneous venous or arterial puncture. In general, systemic arterial catheters are well tolerated, although there are a few important concerns regarding insertion technique and complications that need to be remembered.

INSERTION TECHNIQUES FOR SYSTEMIC ARTERIAL CATHETERS

Peripheral arterial cannulation is accomplished most frequently by percutaneous insertion of a No. 18 or 20 gauge catheter using sterile technique. When percutaneous insertion is not possible, a surgical cutdown may be necessary. The radial artery is usually chosen because of its accessibility and because there is generally good

Table 46-2. **Physiologic and clinical bases for failure to wean from mechanical ventilation**

Mechanisms	Clinical manifestations	Implication	Causes
Hypoxemia	$P(A-a)O_2 > 300–350$ mmHg (FIO_2 1.0) $PaO_2/FIO_2 < 200$ mmHg $\dot{Q}_s/\dot{Q}_t > 20–25\%$	Continued severe acute respiratory dysfunction	Diffuse process (ARDS; cardiogenic pulmonary edema) Localized process (pneumonia; extensive atelectasis)
Insufficient ventilatory drive	Absent or minimal spontaneous ventilation (pH > 7.40)	Appropriate response to alkalosis	Respiratory alkalosis (hyperventilation, either absolute or in relation to patient's baseline) Metabolic alkalosis (nasogastric suction; diuretics; bicarbonate administration)
	Acute respiratory acidosis (pH < 7.30) when taken off ventilator	Inadequate output from respiratory center in medulla	Sedatives; narcotics; other analgesics Malnutrition Primary central nervous system disorder Myxedema
High ventilation requirement	$\dot{V}E$ needed to keep $PaCO_2$ 40 > 12 liters/min $\dot{V}E > 50\%$ of MVV $VD/VT > 0.6$	Ventilatory demand exceeds patient's capability	Excessive CO_2 production (sepsis; fever; other hypermetabolic states; agitation; shivering; excessive carbohydrate intake) High dead-space ventilation (ARDS; pulmonary embolism; bronchospasm; COPD)
Respiratory muscle weakness	VC < 10 ml/kg MIF < 20 cmH$_2$O	Patient is not strong enough to keep up with ventilatory needs	Malnutrition Primary neuromuscular disorder Drugs (pancuronium; curare; aminoglycoside antibiotics) Hypophosphatemia; hypomagnesemia; hypokalemia
Excessive work of breathing	Respiratory rate > 30–30 breaths/min VT < 4–5 ml/kg	Work of spontaneous breathing exceeds patient's capability	Airway obstruction (bronchospasm; secretions; foreign body; kinked endotracheal tube) Endotracheal tube too small (7-mm ID or less in average-size adult) Chest restriction (bandages; body cast; restraints; positioning) Pain; anxiety

FIO_2 = fraction of inspired oxygen; $\dot{Q}_s/\dot{Q}_t$ = right-to-left intrapulmonary shunt; ARDS = adult respiratory distress syndrome; VD/VT = dead-space fraction; MVV = maximal voluntary ventilation; COPD = chronic obstructive pulmonary disease; VC = vital capacity; MIV = maximum inspiratory force; ID = inside diameter.
Source: Reproduced from DJ Pierson. Weaning from mechanical ventilation in acute respiratory failure: Concepts, indications and techniques. *Respir Care* 28:646, 1983.

collateral circulation via the ulnar artery. Prior to insertion, the status of this collateral circulation should be assessed with an Allen's test. With this test, both the ulnar and radial arteries are occluded by pressure at the wrist; after the hand becomes pale and cool, releasing only the ulnar artery occlusion should restore adequate circulation within 5 seconds. The femoral, dorsalis pedis, and brachial arteries may be cannulated also. Femoral arterial catheterization has not been associated with any increased risk of complication compared with that of the radial artery, providing that the catheters are inserted with sterile technique percutaneously [149].

COMPLICATIONS OF SYSTEMIC ARTERIAL CATHETERS

The major potential complications of peripheral arterial catheterization are infection and ischemia. Ischemia may occur secondary to either thrombosis with local occlusion or distal embolization. In one large prospective study, a 4 percent incidence of catheter-related septicemia and an 18 percent incidence of local infection (defined by semiquantitative culture of the catheter tip) were found [10]. The risk factors favoring infection include insertion by surgical cutdown rather than percutaneously, duration of cannulation exceeding 4 days, and inflammation at the catheter site [10]. Infection may originate in the transducer or fluid-delivery apparatus. One recent prospective study indicated that catheter-related infection can be decreased markedly if a continuous flush device is located immediately distal to the transducer apparatus rather than close to the insertion site [157]. This eliminates a long proximal static fluid column between the transducer and flush intake. With this design and careful sterile precautions at the blood-sampling stopcock, the incidence of catheter-related septicemia was reduced to less than 1 percent.

Clinically significant thrombosis or embolism is rare. In over 12,000 consecutive placements of arterial lines (including radial, brachial, and/or dorsalis pedis arteries), necrosis of fingers or toes occurred in only 15 (<0.2 percent) [154]. Similarly, in another study, only 3 (0.6 percent) of 531 patients required emergency thrombectomies for distal ischemia [59]. The clinical risk factors for acute distal ischemia include systemic hypotension, severe peripheral vascular disease, and the use of vasopressor drugs. Even though clinically important ischemia is rare, reversible subclinical arterial occlusion or reduced flow is common, with up to 24 percent of arteries still

occluded 1 week after catheter removal [15]. The risk factors for such occlusion include larger catheter size (18 versus 20 gauge), smaller wrist size (women and children), repeated attempts before successful cannulation, and duration of cannulation (risk increases after 3 to 4 days). Ulnar refill time determined by the Allen's test prior to insertion is also of some predictive value. As mentioned, a palmar blush due to filling via the ulnar artery should appear within 5 seconds. If 15 seconds is used as an acceptable upper limit, then distal ischemia is more frequent (approximately 10 percent) [14].

Once the catheter is placed, distal perfusion should be assessed at least daily by noting any changes in skin color, temperature, or capillary refill time. If the arterial pressure tracing becomes persistently dampened, or if blood drawing is difficult, thrombosis formation on the catheter tip is likely and the catheters should be removed, since the risk of occlusion is high [43].

Pulmonary Artery Catheterization

The availability of bedside pulmonary artery catheterization has had a major impact on the management of critically ill patients. In the last decade, for example, it was estimated that over 2 million pulmonary artery catheters were inserted into a wide variety of medical and surgical patients [96]. There are numerous clinical conditions for which pulmonary artery catheterization has been accepted as useful. These include shock associated with acute myocardial infarction, sepsis or major trauma, acute respiratory failure from cardiogenic or noncardiogenic pulmonary edema, and management of patients following cardiac or major vascular surgery. However, there has been increasing concern that clinicians need to be better informed regarding the risks and potential benefits of systemic and pulmonary artery catheterization [101,140,155,180]. The recent clinical literature contains numerous examples of how incorrect information may be conveyed from pulmonary arterial pressure measurements when physicians are not sufficiently skilled at interpreting pressure and waveform tracings [100, 133,180].

INSERTION TECHNIQUES

The pulmonary circulation can be monitored by percutaneous insertion of a balloon-tipped pulmonary artery catheter via the subclavian, internal jugular, external jugular, femoral, or antecubital vein. Catheterization can be done at the patient's bedside with only pressure waveform and amplitude and electrocardiographic monitoring. Fluoroscopy is not necessary, although the pressure waveform must be displayed on a bedside oscilloscope. The pulmonary artery catheter used most frequently has four lumina plus a small thermistor near the tip for thermodilution cardiac output measurements. One lumen is used to inflate the balloon on the tip of the catheter. After the catheter is advanced into the thorax, the balloon is inflated. The flow-directed catheter then usually passes easily from the right atrium across the tricuspid valve through the right ventricle and into the pulmonary artery (Fig. 46-7). If the catheter is advanced further with the balloon inflated, it will wedge in a pulmonary artery and occlude blood flow. The distal lumen, which opens at the tip of the catheter, will then record the downstream vascular pressure, the pulmonary arterial wedge pressure (see Fig. 46-7). When the balloon is deflated, the distal lumen records the phasic pulmonary arterial pressure. The proximal lumen, located 30 cm from the tip of the catheter, will then be positioned in the right atrium to measure central venous pressure when the tip of the catheter is in the pulmonary artery. This proximal lumen is also used to inject a bolus of indicator (10 ml of 5% dextrose) to determine cardiac output by thermodilution. The bolus is injected through the lumen in the right atrium so that the thermistor near the tip of the catheter in the pulmonary artery can sense the change in temperature as the bolus flows into the pulmonary artery. A small bedside computer then integrates the time-temperature curve and prints out the cardiac output. The fourth lumen, located 31 cm from the tip of the catheter, is used for infusion of intravenous solutions. An introducer sheath that has an additional lumen is also available for the intravenous infusion of fluids.

Fig. 46-7. Representative recording of pressures as a Swan-Ganz catheter is inserted through the internal jugular vein through the right side of the heart into the pulmonary artery. The first recorded waveform is a right atrial tracing with characteristic *a* and *v* waves. In the right ventricle, note that the end-diastolic pressure is zero. In the pulmonary artery, a normal pressure waveform is recorded. The catheter is then advanced to the wedge position with the balloon inflated. The wedge pressure tracing shows *a* and *v* waves transmitted from the left atrium. The wedge tracing is not always this clear, but it should not be overly dampened. The pressures shown here are normal. (Reproduced from MA Matthay. Invasive hemodynamic monitoring in critically ill patients. *Clin Chest Med* 4:234, 1983.)

OBTAINING RELIABLE PRESSURE MEASUREMENTS

Once the catheter is in place, the pressure is transmitted via the catheter through the fluid-filled tubing to the diaphragm of a transducer and then converted to an electronic signal. The signal is amplified, the pressure waveform is shown on an oscilloscope, and the pressure is shown on a digital display (see Fig. 46-7). Correct pressure measurements depend on accurately calibrated transducers, a fluid-filled catheter system without blood clots or air bubbles, and a monitor that displays the pressure tracing in an appropriate size to demonstrate the waveforms clearly. The

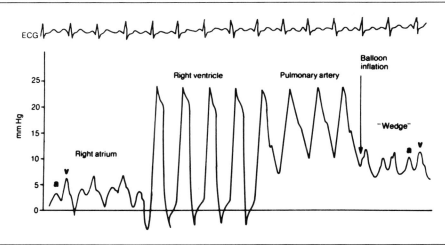

pulmonary arterial and wedge pressure tracing in Figure 46-7 fulfills these requirements. Note that there is a single major pulmonary arterial pressure wave for each spike on the electrocardiogram. Correct amplitude settings are needed to display the waveform correctly. In general, amplitudes in the range of 0 to 30 or 0 to 60 mmHg are appropriate for the pulmonary circulation. In addition to correct amplitude, the contour of the tracing is important. Figure 46-8 illustrates the dampening effect of a small air bubble in the catheter system. The dampening of the tracing also can be caused by a clot on the end of the catheter.

Calibration of the transducer should be done with a mercury manometer at the bedside. Because transducers may not be linear over a wide range, it is important that the transducer for the pulmonary artery catheter be calibrated for the lower pressures of the pulmonary circulation (0 to 40 mmHg) rather than for the higher pressure range of the systemic circulation [100,124]. Another common pitfall is improper location of the zero reference point, particularly because patients are moving from side to side or the head of the bed is raised or lowered. In general, the proper zero reference is the midchest position.

Perhaps the most common source of error in making intrathoracic pressure measurements is failure to take into account the effects of respiration on these pressure measurements [100, 124,180]. Pleural pressure becomes negative during spontaneous inspiration and positive during the inspiratory cycle of mechanical ventilation (IPPV). Consequently, the pressure readout and

the waveform on the oscilloscope will change, depending on the phase of respiration. In Figure 46-9, the recording of pulmonary arterial wedge pressure is interrupted by deep troughs in the tracing produced by the patient's spontaneous inspiratory efforts. During these troughs, the pressure reading was zero. The opposite pattern then occurs with positive-pressure ventilation, as the tracing shows a rise in the waveform as the ventilator is generating positive pressure during the inspiratory cycle. Thus, the problem is how to obtain a reliable transmural pressure measurement when the reference pressure (pleural pressure) is changing. To minimize the effects of changing pleural pressure, pulmonary arterial pressures should be measured at end-expiration when pleural pressures will be close to zero. In Figure 46-9, end-expiration can be clearly seen in both the pulmonary arterial pressure and the wedge pressure tracing. This approach enables the clinician to consider the measured pressure at end-expiration as a very close approximation of the true transmural pressure. This approach can be complicated if the patient is breathing so rapidly that the end-expiratory phase is very brief. In most circumstances, the best approach for obtaining a reliable pressure tracing is to obtain a

Fig. 46-8. Pulmonary artery tracing after introduction of 0.5 ml of air into the connecting tubing at *X*, with the electrocardiogram recorded below. The phasic contour of the pulmonary artery tracing is dampened out by the air bubble; the same pattern can be produced by clots in the catheter or on the catheter tip. (Reproduced from K Quinn, EJ Quebbeman. Pulmonary artery pressure monitoring in the surgical intensive care unit. *Arch Surg* 116:872, 1981.)

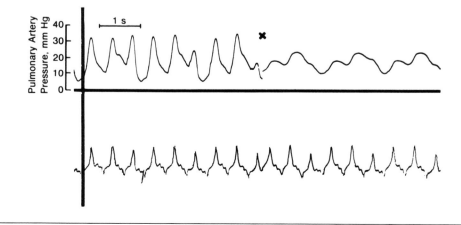

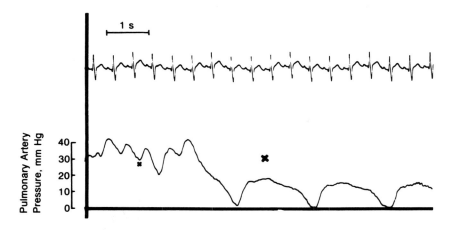

Fig. 46-9. Continuous monitoring of the electrocardiogram and the phasic pulmonary artery pressure, plus a segment of a pulmonary artery wedge tracing. Note that the troughs in the pulmonary artery and in the wedge tracings occur when the patient takes a spontaneous breath and pleural pressure becomes negative, thus causing a downward deflection in the tracing. The *X* marks indicate end-expiration in the respiratory cycle. At end-expiration, pleural pressure is zero; therefore, the measured intraluminal pressure should be close to the real transmural pressure. Wedge pressure is about 15 mmHg below the pulmonary artery end-diastolic pressure; the patient had pulmonary hypertension from acute pulmonary embolism, which accounts for the gradient between the end-diastolic and the wedge pressures. (Reproduced from K Quinn, EJ Quebbeman. Pulmonary artery pressure monitoring in the surgical intensive care unit. *Arch Surg* 116:872, 1981.)

printout of the actual pressure tracing, ideally on a strip-chart recorder, but alternatively on the oscilloscope electrocardiographic monitor paper. First, the calibration lines for the pressure range are recorded on the paper, then the actual pressure tracing is recorded, and then the end-expiratory period can be noted on the paper. The pressure at end-expiration can then be measured from the tracing on the paper. When the patient's respiratory rate is rapid, the digital readout will not be accurate because the frequency response of the electronic system is usually too slow to detect the brief period of end-expiration [124].

Accurate measurements of pulmonary arterial pressures can be particularly difficult in patients with acute, severe airways obstruction. In order to overcome the high airway resistance, patients generate very positive intrathoracic pressures throughout expiration, and this leads to an elevated pulmonary arterial pressure or an elevated wedge pressure. During inspiration, the patient's pleural pressure may be markedly negative and there will be a wide swing in the pulmonary arterial pressure tracing in the opposite direction. The problems posed by measuring pressures in patients on PEEP are considered in the next section after discussion of the relationship of wedge pressure to left atrial pressure.

RELATION OF WEDGE PRESSURE TO LEFT ATRIAL PRESSURE
The pulmonary arterial wedge pressure is used widely as an index of left atrial filling pressure. In general, most studies have demonstrated that the correlation between wedge pressure and left atrial pressure in patients is very good [124,180]. The correlation of left atrial pressure to left ventricular end-diastolic pressure likewise is good, provided there is no mitral valve disease. The pulmonary arterial end-diastolic pressure usually provides an accurate indication of the pulmonary arterial wedge pressure except when there is an increase in pulmonary vascular resistance, in which case the end-diastolic pressure will be higher than the wedge pressure.

EFFECT OF PEEP ON WEDGE PRESSURE MEASUREMENTS
Accurate transmural arterial and wedge pressure measurements may be more difficult to obtain in patients on PEEP in excess of 10 cmH$_2$O. PEEP may interfere with accurate measurements in two ways. First, it may result in an undetermined

increase in pleural pressure. Second, the airway pressure generated by PEEP may be transmitted to the pulmonary microcirculation [133]. Because PEEP prevents transpulmonary pressure from falling to zero at the end of expiration, this means the pleural pressure remains positive at the end of expiration; thus, the reference pressure for the pulmonary arterial pressure measurement is not zero. Hence, the recorded intraluminal pressure (central venous pressure, pulmonary arterial pressure, or wedge pressure) may be higher than the actual transmural pressure. One way to solve this problem is to measure esophageal pressure as an indicator of pleural pressure in order to obtain a more accurate reference pressure. However, reliable esophageal pressure measurements are difficult to obtain, especially in a supine patient in a critical care unit. The best working solution to the problem, in general, is to make an estimate of pleural pressure and subtract this value from the measured wedge pressure. In clinical studies in which pleural pressure was measured in patients with the adult respiratory distress syndrome (ARDS), pleural pressure does not usually become significantly positive with levels of PEEP below 10 cmH$_2$O [44,79]. With levels of PEEP above 10 cmH$_2$O, pleural pressure usually will be approximately 2 to 3 cmH$_2$O positive for every 5 cmH$_2$O increase in PEEP above 10 cmH$_2$O [44,79].

The other potential difficulty with levels of PEEP above 10 cmH$_2$O is that if alveolar pressure exceeds the pulmonary arterial pressure, the catheter tip may reflect airway pressure rather than vascular pressures. Theoretically, the wedge pressure will reflect left atrial pressure if the wedged catheter tip is located in a portion of the lung where pulmonary arterial and pulmonary venous pressures exceed the alveolar pressure (zone 3) [124,180]. If the catheter tip is in an area where alveolar pressure exceeds venous pressure when pulmonary arterial flow is occluded with balloon inflation, the recorded pressure will be airway pressure rather than pulmonary artery pressure. If the catheter is located in zone 3, the wedge catheter can look through the pulmonary vasculature to sense left atrial pressure. Thus, to have an accurate indication of left atrial pressure, the pulmonary artery catheter must be in a zone 3 area [124,180].

Usually, the flow-directed pulmonary artery catheter migrates to zone 3 and the wedge pressure accurately reflects left atrial pressure [180]. If PEEP is increased, it is possible that the zone

3 area, where the catheter was initially placed, may become a zone 2 area, where alveolar pressure exceeds venous pressure. Although this does not happen very often, it has been shown experimentally that if the tip of the pulmonary artery catheter is at or below the left atrium, the mean wedge pressure at end-expiration still reflects left atrial pressure, even with levels of PEEP up to 30 cmH$_2$O [170]. Therefore, it is reasonable to confirm the position of the catheter tip with an anteroposterior portable chest roentgenogram and, if necessary, a lateral chest radiograph [180]. When a question arises concerning the location of the catheter tip, there are a few maneuvers that can be done to verify zone 3 conditions [94] (Table 46-3). For wedge pressure tracings outside zone 3, the wedge contour appears unusually smooth and the pulmonary artery end-diastolic pressure tends to be lower than the balloon-occlusion pressure. In zones 1 and 2, changes in the wedge pressure tend to follow alveolar rather than left atrial pressure. Thus, the swings in the wedge pressure during ventilation with positive pressure are unusually wide because only half or less of the change in static airway pressure (peak greater than pressure) transmits to the pleural spaces, left atrium, and intrathoracic vessels. For the same reason, a trial of PEEP reduction causes a fall in the wedge pressure of unexpected magnitude (more than half the PEEP decrement) when the catheter tip is in zone 1 or 2 [94].

Table 46-3. Checklist for verifying position of pulmonary artery catheter

	Zone 3	Zone 1 or 2
Respiratory variation of PW	$\leq$ 1/2 ΔPalv	> 1/2 ΔPalv
PW contour	Cardiac ripple	Unnaturally smooth
Catheter tip location	LA level or below	Above LA level
$\downarrow$ PEEP trial	ΔPW $\leq$ 1/2 PEEP	ΔPW > 1/2 ΔPEEP
PPAD vs. PW	PPAD > PW	PPAD $\leq$ PW

PW = wedge pressure; Palv = static airway pressure; LA = left atrium; PEEP = positive end-expiratory pressure; PPAD = pulmonary artery diastolic pressure.
Source: Reproduced from JJ Marini. Obtaining meaningful data from the Swan-Ganz catheter. *Respir Care* 30:572, 1985.

CLINICAL INDICATIONS FOR PULMONARY ARTERY CATHETERIZATION

The most common clinical conditions for which pulmonary artery catheterization is used in intensive care units include acute pulmonary edema, shock, and management of patients after cardiac or major vascular surgery [161].

Acute Cardiogenic Pulmonary Edema. In general, acute cardiogenic pulmonary edema is accompanied by either systemic hypertension or hypotension. Indications for pulmonary artery catheterization depend mainly on the patient's systemic blood pressure. The diagnosis of cardiogenic pulmonary edema in the setting of systemic hypertension is nearly always accompanied by physical findings that point to left ventricular failure as the cause of the pulmonary edema [155]. Treatment of the heart failure almost always results in prompt improvement, making it unnecessary to insert a pulmonary artery catheter for diagnosis or management. In fact, the wedge pressure may return to the normal range even before the pulmonary artery catheter can be inserted [53]. Treatment of the acute pulmonary edema does not require pulmonary artery catheterization in these patients unless hemodynamic instability develops [155].

In contrast, patients with acute pulmonary edema in association with systemic hypotension secondary to an acute myocardial infarction present more difficult problems. A number of studies have documented that the hemodynamic profiles of patients within this group may vary considerably. Some patients will have markedly elevated left ventricular end-diastolic pressures in association with a very low cardiac output, while others may have a much more moderate elevation in the pulmonary arterial wedge pressure and better ventricular function [34,155]. Occasionally, patients thought to have left ventricular failure will be found to have noncardiogenic pulmonary edema. Rational decisions regarding the use of vasopressors, vasodilators, and volume replacement can best be made with knowledge of the left ventricular filling pressure and systemic vascular resistance [101,155].

Acute Noncardiogenic Pulmonary Edema. There are a number of reasons why pulmonary arterial catheterization may be indicated in most patients with suspected noncardiogenic pulmonary edema. First, differentiation of cardiogenic from noncardiogenic pulmonary edema can be difficult both radiographically [1] and clinically.

In one study, the clinical diagnosis of noncardiogenic pulmonary edema was substantiated on pulmonary artery catheterization in only 56 percent of patients [38]. In addition, patients who have primary lung injury also may have a mild elevation in the pulmonary arterial wedge pressure that contributes to the pulmonary edema [27,161]. Therefore, in most patients with pulmonary edema that appears to be of a noncardiac origin, it is reasonable to obtain pulmonary hemodynamic measurements to be certain that the diagnosis is correct.

The management of certain patients with noncardiogenic pulmonary edema is facilitated by hemodynamic measurements [27]. This is particularly true in patients with sepsis in whom hypotension and respiratory failure occur together. In this setting, the goals of management should be to produce optimal cardiac output and systemic perfusion with as little increase as possible in the pulmonary arterial wedge pressure. This balance can only be achieved with the use of invasive hemodynamic monitoring, although there is no definite proof that measurement of these physiologic variables ultimately results in an improved patient outcome [101].

Most patients with ARDS should have their pulmonary artery catheter removed within 3 to 4 days in order to reduce the risk of secondary infection and to convert the central line to a triple-lumen catheter that can be used for the administration of fluids, antibiotics, and hyperalimentation. There are some patients with ARDS who are very stable hemodynamically and in whom the oxygenation defect is not very severe. Some of these patients can be managed without pulmonary arterial catheterization [102,137].

Shock. One of the original justifications for pulmonary artery catheterization rests on the evidence that some patients with acute myocardial infarction may have a normal central venous pressure in the presence of an elevated pulmonary arterial wedge pressure [163]. Also, some patients with an acute myocardial infarction and shock are found to have low left ventricular filling pressures that can be best treated with volume expansion to increase preload. Thus, the argument has been that pulmonary arterial catheterization helps provide information that cannot be obtained by clinical examination alone. In fact, one study confirmed that clinical assessment of hemodynamic variables in patients with shock prior to insertion of a pulmonary artery catheter was poor [38]. In patients with pulmonary arterial wedge pressures greater than 18 mmHg, the wedge pressure was predicted correctly only 35 percent of the time. Similarly, in the same group of patients with a measured cardiac index of less than 2.2 liters/min/m^2, the cardiac index was predicted correctly only 55 percent of the time.

Management of Patients After Cardiac and Major Vascular Surgery. The indications for pulmonary artery catheterization in patients who have had cardiac surgery are controversial [101]. In some institutions, for example, clinicians insert pulmonary artery catheters in all patients who undergo cardiac surgery, whereas in other institutions, even cardiac transplant patients do not have routine pulmonary artery pressure monitoring. However, available data regarding risks versus benefits of pulmonary artery catheterization after cardiac surgery support a more selective approach, reserving pulmonary artery catheterization for patients with a reduced left ventricular ejection fraction [101]. Moreover, one study demonstrated that the pulmonary arterial wedge pressure was not a reliable indicator of left ventricular preload in the immediate period following coronary artery bypass surgery [68].

Patients who have undergone major vascular surgery often have coexistent cardiac and renal disease which places them at high risk for postoperative hemodynamic instability. In addition, it is common for these patients to have large collections of peritoneal fluid and a diffuse systemic capillary leak following cross-clamping of the aorta, so they have major fluid shifts postoperatively. Because these patients are at high risk of postoperative heart failure, volume overload respiratory failure, and renal failure, they may benefit from pulmonary artery catheterization, although the decision should be made on a case-by-case basis [101].

Respiratory Monitoring

A variety of direct and indirect methods have been used for monitoring respiratory status in both spontaneously breathing and mechanically ventilated patients. This section considers some of these methods, with an emphasis on both traditional and new methods for assessing respiratory failure.

RESPIRATORY RATE
The respiratory rate can be measured and recorded automatically in nonintubated, spontaneously ventilating patients with impedance devices to which alarms can be attached. In patients who are intubated and spontaneously breathing, respiratory rate and tidal volume can be monitored with a pneumotachygraph. Other approaches include the use of a respiratory inductance plethysmograph (RIP) to monitor lung volume by recording the inductance changes in wire coils applied to the abdomen and rib cage. RIP has been used to measure tidal volume in both normal subjects and those with respiratory disease [150]. This method may be useful for the early detection of respiratory failure in patients in critical care units, but further study of its sensitivity and clinical value is needed.

MUSCLE FATIGUE
Because respiratory muscle fatigue has been recognized as an important contributing factor in many patients with acute respiratory failure, attempts have been made to monitor respiratory muscle function [41,144]. In one study, investigators demonstrated that a fall in the ratio of high- to low-frequency power over the diaphragm often preceded clinical manifestations of impending respiratory failure in recently weaned patients [37]. The change in the power ratio preceded the development of tachypnea, altered breathing patterns (respiratory alternans and abdominal paradox), and the increase in PaCO$_2$ (Fig. 46-10). It is possible that monitoring respiratory muscle (electromyographic) signals may become clinically useful in following patients with early respiratory failure or in assessing patients during weaning with spontaneous breathing trials on a T-piece or CPAP.

NEUROMUSCULAR BLOCKADE
Recent studies have indicated that prolonged neuromuscular blockade occurs in critically ill patients who have been treated with L vecuronium or pancuronium to facilitate effective positive pressure ventilation [152]. The mechanisms for this effect may be related to multiple factors. These include persistent blockade of the neuromuscular junctions from drug accumulation, persistence of active metabolites, or a myopathy induced by the drug used to block the neuromuscular junction coupled with a possible additive or synergistic effect from the administration of corticosteroids [64]. Therefore, in patients being

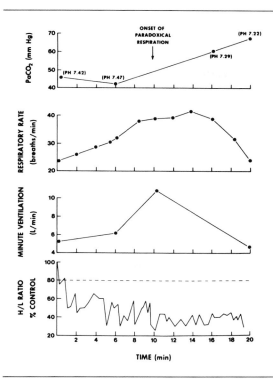

Fig. 46-10. Sequence of changes in a patient during a 20-minute attempt to discontinue mechanical ventilation. The initial change was a fall in the ratio of high- to low-frequency power of the respiratory muscles as detected by surface electromyography. After the change in high-low ratio (*H/L*), there was a progressive rise in respiratory rate and an initial respiratory alkalosis. After the onset of paradoxical respiration, minute ventilation progressively decreased and hypercapnia and respiratory acidosis developed. Thus, the fall in high-low ratio may be a useful predictor of diaphragmatic fatigue that precedes clinical evidence of impending respiratory failure. (Reproduced from CA Cohen et al. Clinical manifestations of inspiratory muscle fatigue. *Am J Med* 73:308, 1982.)

treated with neuromuscular blockade to facilitate mechanical ventilation, the effects of the drug on neuromuscular function should be monitored by use of nerve stimulation to assess the degree of response. In this way use of excessive amounts of the blocking agent can be avoided and prolonged paralysis prevented or at least diagnosed early. Although routine monitoring of neuromuscular blockade has not been used in intensive

care units it seems clear that it should be applied more frequently than it has been up to now.

AIRWAY PRESSURE
In patients who are mechanically ventilated, it is mandatory to monitor airway pressure. An acute decrease in airway pressure indicates a leak in the system or disconnection of the ventilator tubing from the endotracheal tube. Therefore, a low-pressure alarm system is essential. Acute increases in airway pressure may indicate simply the need for suctioning of the endotracheal tube or a change in chest-wall compliance because the patient is agitated or in pain. On the other hand, acute increases in airway pressure may herald a more serious problem, such as pneumothorax, lobar atelectasis, malposition of the endotracheal tube in the right mainstem bronchus, or acute bronchospasm. Some investigators recommend measurements of static and dynamic respiratory compliance to help determine the etiology of increases in airway pressure [21]. The equations for calculating respiratory compliance were described earlier (Eq. 46-14, 46-15). Patients with severe airways obstruction will have elevated peak airway pressure during gas flow but normal plateau pressures (measured by occluding outflow on the ventilator momentarily) during no flow. The effects of inhaled bronchodilator agents can be followed sequentially in patients with an increase in the peak-plateau pressure difference (>10 cmH_2O).

COMPLIANCE
In addition to the measurements of static and dynamic compliance described above, the interruptor technique has recently been adapted to determine the mechanical properties of the respiratory system in patients. Flow, volume, and tracheal pressure have been measured through a series of brief (1.5-second) interruptions of expiratory flow in patients to determine passive flow resistances as well as elastance of the total respiratory system. This method is yet another approach to assess respiratory compliance. The limitations of the method are that lung volume cannot be directly assessed and the chest wall needs to be relaxed [61].

WORK OF BREATHING
The work of breathing can be estimated by simultaneous recording of pressure changes and flow over time. Work (expressed in kilogram-

meters) is obtained by integration of power (pressure times flow in kilograms per meter per second) over time. Work can be analyzed as either total respiratory work (lung and chest wall) by using transthoracic pressure differences (airway opening minus atmosphere pressure) or only work done to move the lungs and produce airflow by using transpulmonary pressures (airway–esophageal balloon pressures). The inspiratory work of breathing during assisted mechanical ventilation has been measured, and evidence has been presented that even with the assist-control mode of ventilation, patients may expend considerable respiratory muscle work [96]. These measurements of the work of breathing are primarily useful for research studies in ventilated patients.

CARBON DIOXIDE PRODUCTION
Measurement of carbon dioxide production also can be useful in determining an etiology for persistent hypercapnic respiratory failure. For example, elevated carbon dioxide production has been associated with excessive calorie and carbohydrate nutritional therapy, thus making it difficult for the patient to be weaned from mechanical ventilation [131]. Hyperthermia, sepsis, and hyperthyroidism can also increase carbon dioxide production.

ARTERIAL BLOOD GASES
Monitoring of arterial oxygen and carbon dioxide tensions can be most accurately accomplished with direct arterial blood gas sampling. Indwelling catheter electrodes are now available for continuous intraarterial measurement of PaO_2, $PaCO_2$, and pH. They have some technical limitations, and their superiority over more conventional periodic blood sampling from an indwelling arterial line has not been proved. In addition, there is a fiberoptic pulmonary artery catheter for continuous measurement of oxyhemoglobin saturation in the mixed venous blood. The clinical value of this device remains to be established [23].

OTHER TECHNIQUES
The clinical value of a number of additional monitoring techniques is uncertain. Breath-by-breath measurements of respiratory system compliance and both volume-pressure and volume-flow relationships can be made. Also, mass spectrometer systems are available to measure FIO_2 and exhaled carbon dioxide and oxygen. These measurements of exhaled gases, especially the

$PeCO_2$, may provide an early indicator of changes in alveolar ventilation, but their utility in a critical care unit has not been clearly demonstrated.

In some patients with respiratory failure, however, measurement of mixed expired gas $PeCO_2$ concentration is useful for calculation of the dead-space fraction, as already described in the section, Calculations of Respiratory Variables (Eq. 46-4). Measurements of the dead-space fraction can be used to assess the physiologic basis of the respiratory failure. Physiologic dead space may be elevated in patients with pulmonary vascular disease, chronic obstructive lung disease, necrotizing pneumonitis, or ARDS. A dead-space fraction greater than 0.55 often correlates with major difficulty in weaning a patient from mechanical ventilation because the required minute ventilation and work of breathing are excessive.

Transcutaneous PO_2 and PCO_2 measurements are noninvasive methods that use heated skin electrodes and provide indirect reflections of PaO_2 and $PaCO_2$. They have been useful in infants but are not as clinically valuable in adults. A more useful noninvasive approach is pulse oximetry, which measures oxygen saturation in arterialized blood in a fingertip [51,151]. Pulse oximetry is an advance from the prior technique of using ear oximetry, which required preparation of the site and calibration. Pulse oximetry, unlike transcutaneous PO_2 and PCO_2 measurements, does not require skin preparation or rotation to a new site. Under conditions of poor perfusion from local vasoconstriction or a low cardiac output, both methods may become inaccurate [12]. The pulse oximeter can be very useful, particularly during weaning of patients from mechanical ventilation, evaluating oxygen saturation during sleep, and during procedures such as bronchoscopy and gastroscopy [151].

Pathophysiology of Respiratory Disorders for Which Critical Care May Be Necessary

Neuromuscular Etiologies of Respiratory Failure

There are numerous causes of acute respiratory failure from neuromuscular disorders. These include the Guillain-Barré syndrome, myasthenia gravis, botulism, poliomyelitis, heavy metal intoxication, organic phosphate poisoning, and rarely aminoglycoside antibiotics. Severe electrolyte disorders such as hypokalemia and hypophosphatemia also may be associated with muscle weakness sufficient to cause acute respiratory failure. There are, of course, a variety of congenital and acquired neuromuscular diseases that may be associated with progressive respiratory failure. Acute respiratory failure also may follow injury to the spinal cord, if the lesion is at a high enough level to affect function of the phrenic nerve [90].

Acute respiratory failure is the most life-threatening complication of the Guillain-Barré syndrome. In most large series, approximately 20 to 30 percent of patients with Guillain-Barré syndrome require mechanical ventilation [62,112]. The average duration of mechanical ventilation is 4 to 6 weeks, but the range is quite variable (7 to 93 days in one series) [62]. Characteristically, patients who require mechanical ventilation have a FVC less than 4 to 5 ml/kg of body weight, a progressive inability to handle oral secretions, and poor cough, and they develop hypoventilation. In addition, lobar atelectasis and pneumonia may occur [49]. The basic pathophysiology stems from a combination of inadequate neuromuscular strength leading to alveolar hypoventilation, low tidal volume breathing, and diffuse atelectasis. While this form of acute respiratory failure can be classified as primarily hypercapneic respiratory failure, it is frequently accompanied by a widened alveolar-arterial oxygen gradient secondary to atelectasis and pneumonia [78].

Patients who develop Guillain-Barré syndrome should be monitored closely with frequent measurements of VC and arterial blood gases and careful clinical evaluation of their ability to cough and protect their airway. Initial monitoring in a critical care unit is usually desirable so that immediate respiratory support can be provided if the patient's respiratory status deteriorates. Treatment for Guillain-Barré syndrome is mainly supportive, with mechanical ventilation, intravenous fluids, and nutritional support. In addition, the use of prophylactic subcutaneous heparin is recommended [62,112]. Careful attention to psychosocial issues is very important in managing Guillain-Barré patients in the intensive care unit [49,72].

In a prospective controlled study of 245 patients, it was reported that plasmapheresis was superior to conventional supportive therapy in hastening recovery of muscle strength [66]. If plasmapheresis was started before the patient required mechanical ventilation, the median time on the ventilator was 9 days, versus 23 days in the control group. There was no benefit of plasmapheresis in shortening the duration of mechanical ventilation if the patient already required ventilation (Table 46-4). Although the study was not blinded, the basic beneficial effects of plasmapheresis in this syndrome seem to have been well established [48]. Presumably, the process of plasmapheresis removes a circulating factor from the plasma that is important in the pathogenesis of acute paralysis.

A multicenter trial compared intravenous immunoglobulin therapy with plasmapheresis [172]. The intravenous immunoglobulin therapy was given by daily infusions of pooled gamma globulin (0.4 mg/kg/d) for the first 2 weeks of the treatment. The results showed that intravenous immunoglobulin therapy was as effective as plasmapheresis.

Myasthenia gravis may result in acute respiratory failure at any time during the clinical course of the disease. Some patients present with acute respiratory failure, others develop respiratory failure at some point during the course of their illness, and others may develop the need for mechanical ventilation following thymectomy. The muscle weakness caused by the disease results in a decrease in VC and consequent inadequate alveolar ventilation with the associated risks of atelectasis and secondary pneumonia. Frequent monitoring of the VC is useful, but it should not be seen as a substitute for clinical evaluation of the patient's degree of weakness, the ability to protect the airway, and the trend in arterial blood

Table 46-4. **Effect of ventilatory status in Guillain-Barré patients at time of randomization on duration of mechanical ventilation**

Group	Conventional treatment	Plasmapheresis treatment	p Value*
On ventilator before randomization	33*	27	NS
On ventilator after randomization	23	9	<0.05

*Results are given as median times in days.

gases. In trying to assess the need for postoperative mechanical ventilation in patients undergoing thymectomy, investigators in one study found that four risk factors were particularly helpful in predicting the need for mechanical ventilation: duration of myasthenia gravis, history of chronic respiratory disease, pyridostigmine dosage greater than 750 mg/day, and a preoperative VC of less than 2.9 liters [88]. Management of patients who require mechanical ventilation with myasthenia gravis is primarily supportive unless it is complicated by secondary pneumonia. Treatment with anticholinesterase agents is useful for improving muscle strength. Corticosteroids and plasmapheresis have been effective in treating acute exacerbations in many patients with myasthenia gravis [65].

The other causes of acute neuromuscular failure (Table 46-5) require supportive treatment similar to that described for Guillain-Barré syndrome and myasthenia gravis. Weaning patients from mechanical ventilation who have a neuromuscular cause for their acute respiratory failure must be done gradually. Therefore, relatively prolonged trials (12 to 24 hours) on a T-piece or CPAP ventilation are usually indicated to be certain that the patient can sustain sufficient respiratory effort to maintain adequate ventilation [131]. Measurements of the dead-space fraction, the frequency to tidal volume ratio, and the min-

ute ventilation during CPAP trials may be useful in deciding when the patient is ready for extubation and spontaneous ventilation.

Unilateral or bilateral impairment of diaphragm function also may lead to acute respiratory failure [108]. The diaphragm is the principal muscle of inspiration, being almost totally responsible for inspiration during quiet breathing. Weakness or paralysis of both hemidiaphragms is most likely to be associated with chronic neuromuscular disease, but it also may occur as an isolated abnormality and with spinal cord trauma. In addition, the phrenic nerves may be interrupted inadvertently during surgical procedures in the neck or thorax, such as during a coronary artery bypass operation [108]. Clinically, paradoxical or inward movement of the abdominal wall during spontaneous inspiration in the supine posture may be overlooked, and it is therefore necessary to use fluoroscopy or ultrasound to demonstrate paradoxical movement of the diaphragm with spontaneous inspiration. Additional evaluation with transdiaphragmatic pressure measurements and phrenic nerve conduction studies may be necessary [89]. Ventilatory support by pacing of the diaphragm has been developed and used in a number of patients with trauma or infarction of the cervical cord above C2 when it was certain that the lower motor neurons of the phrenic nerve were viable [60].

Table 46-5. **Clinical description of respiratory failure in derangements of the thorax**

Category	Incidence	Severity	Clinical course	Secretions, atelectasis, pneumonia
Mechanical				
Scoliosis	Common	+ + +	Slow	NL
Obesity-hypoventilation	Common	+ + +	Periodic	NL or ↑
Fibrothorax	Common	+ + +	Slow	NL
Thoracoplasty	Common	+ + +	Slow	NL or ↑
Ankylosing spondylitis	Rare	+	Slow	NL
Neuromuscular				
Postpoliomyelitis	Common	+ + +	Slow	↑
Amyotrophic lateral sclerosis	Common	+ + +	Fast	↑
Muscular dystrophies	Common	+	Slow	↑
Spinal cord injury	Common	+ +	Slow	↑
Multiple sclerosis	Uncommon	+	Slow	↑
Myasthenia gravis	Common	+ + +	Periodic	↑

+ = dyspnea on exertion; + + = dyspnea, mild hypoxemia, and hypercapnia only; + + + = severe hypoventilation; NL = normal lungs; ↑ = increased incidence.
Source: Reproduced from EH Bergofsky. Respiratory failure in disorders of the thoracic cage. *Am Rev Respir Dis* 119:643, 1979.

Drug Overdoses

There are a variety of sedative and hypnotic drugs that directly depress respiration and result in the need for mechanical ventilation. In particular, tricyclic depressant overdose is a common cause of acute respiratory failure. Cardiopulmonary complications of drug overdose occur commonly and may include hypotension, arrhythmias, and central nervous system dysfunction, including status epilepticus. This section focuses primarily on acute respiratory failure that may occur in drug-overdosed patients.

In general, the patient's history of specific drugs that have been ingested may not be reliable. Medication containers and samples of drugs or substances are helpful if they can be obtained in the emergency room. Gastric contents, urine, and blood also may be collected for toxicologic examination. Initial treatment of drug-overdosed patients in the emergency room includes attempts to remove any unabsorbed drug with emesis or gastric lavage. Activated charcoal can be used to bind and prevent absorption of some drugs that were not removed by emesis or lavage as well as helping to remove some drugs that undergo intrahepatic recirculation. Further discussion of these issues can be found in other texts [17,139].

Most patients who require intubation and mechanical ventilation from a drug overdose do not develop primary pulmonary complications. Their need for mechanical ventilation is usually related to a depression of the central ventilatory drive, and this recovers as the drug is removed from the circulation. The decision to intubate and ventilate patients with drug overdose is based on clinical evaluation of the patient, including mental status, hemodynamic stability, and ability of the patient to protect the airway. As a general rule, it is preferable to intubate patients with a known drug overdose who have a decrease in mental function, even if their arterial blood gas values remain acceptable.

Acute respiratory failure secondary to intrinsic lung disease, however, does occur in some patients following drug overdose and may become the primary clinical problem in the patient's management. For example, gastric aspiration can lead to diffuse and severe lung injury with secondary pulmonary and pleural space infections. In addition, there are some drugs that have been implicated in specifically causing acute lung injury even in the absence of gastric aspiration. In patients who have overdosed on these drugs, pulmonary edema may occur from an increase in lung vascular permeability, resulting in protein-rich edema fluid collecting in the interstitium and airspaces of the lung, even in the absence of elevated pulmonary microvascular pressures. For example, salicylate overdose has been associated with noncardiogenic pulmonary edema in a number of studies [71]. Other drugs that cause noncardiogenic pulmonary edema include heroin, other narcotics, and ethchlorvynol (Placidyl). Measurement of the alveolar-arterial oxygen difference [$P(A-a)O_2$] (Eq. 46-5) can be useful in determining if a patient with drug overdose has arterial hypoxemia secondary to an intrapulmonary process (like aspiration or pulmonary edema) or just from alveolar hypoventilation secondary to the depressant effect of the drug overdose on central ventilatory drive.

Management of patients with noncardiogenic pulmonary edema following drug overdose may be complicated by associated circulatory problems. In general, it is reasonable to place a pulmonary artery line to be certain that the cause of the pulmonary edema is not related to left ventricular failure, which may occur with cardiodepressant effects of the drug. If possible, it is best to maintain the pulmonary arterial wedge pressure in a normal or low-normal range, providing that the patient's cardiac output is adequate. If hypotension and low cardiac output accompany noncardiogenic pulmonary edema, then it is reasonable to try to improve the cardiac output with the use of low-dose vasoactive agents such as dobutamine or dopamine [27].

Chest-Wall Abnormalities as a Cause of Acute Respiratory Failure

Traumatic injury to the chest wall with subsequent rib fractures is a frequent cause of acute respiratory failure. Such an injury is usually associated with pain that prevents full lung inflation and results in atelectasis and occasionally alveolar hypoventilation. If multiple ribs are fractured in multiple locations, lung inflation may be limited because of loss of normal chest-wall rigidity and a subsequent paradoxical motion of the involved area (flail chest). Underlying injury to the lung will contribute to abnormalities of gas exchange. Some patients can be managed without intubation and mechanical ventilation depending on the severity of their injury and associated pulmonary dysfunction, as indicated by arterial blood gas tensions. The primary indications for placement of an endotracheal tube and mechanical ventilation are deteriorating gas exchange, particularly hypoxemia, and a requirement for large doses of narcotic agents to control pain [153].

Chronic deformities of the chest wall or marked pleural disease also may result in acute respiratory failure, although in these situations the pathophysiologic alterations are more complex than in acute injuries to the chest wall because they involve chronic parenchymal and pulmonary vascular abnormalities as well [18]. These abnormalities include ventilation-perfusion mismatching due to airway closure when lung volumes are reduced by a deformed thoracic cage, inability to cough, malfunction or an acquired defect of the respiratory center in conjunction with an increased work of breathing, and excessive blood volume and fluid retention that aggravates the work of breathing and ventilation-perfusion mismatch.

Table 46-5 includes a list of clinical conditions that can best be described as mechanical causes of respiratory failure. These include scoliosis, severe obesity, fibrothorax, thoracoplasty, and ankylosing spondylitis. The incidence of respiratory failure, its clinical course, and associated problems are also shown in Table 46-5 [18].

Many of the disorders that affect the chest wall are associated with chronic respiratory failure that may be accompanied by chronic alveolar hypoventilation and hypoxemia, which may in turn lead to chronic pulmonary hypertension. Thus, some patients who present with acute respiratory failure also may have associated cor pulmonale with signs and symptoms of right-sided heart failure in association with moderate to severe pulmonary hypertension. The pulmonary hypertension also may be related to mechanical compression of portions of the pulmonary circulation. There are some data suggesting that there is a relationship between pulmonary arterial pressures and the angle of spinal deformity in patients with scoliosis [18].

Treatment for acute respiratory failure in patients with chest-wall abnormalities must be directed toward reversing hypoxemia and improving alveolar ventilation. There is some evidence that hyperinflation with positive-pressure breathing devices or incentive spirometers may be useful in improving lung inflation and oxygenation. In many cases, acute respiratory failure occurs because of the development of an associated lung infection [18].

Endotracheal intubation and mechanical ventilation may be necessary to reverse acute deterioration of blood gases as well as to help clear pulmonary secretions. Mechanical ventilation also may be necessary in patients with the obesity-hypoventilation syndrome, in whom central respiratory drive is inadequate to maintain ventilation. Treatment of right-sided heart failure can best be accomplished by improving oxygenation. In general, digitalis has not been shown to be of major benefit in right-sided heart failure alone.

In some of the mechanical causes of respiratory failure, specific treatment may be helpful in reversing or preventing respiratory failure. For example, decortication of entrapped lungs or major weight loss in obese patients may help reverse the fundamental cause of respiratory failure. Orthopedic procedures have been useful in treating scoliosis and stabilizing the spine, but not after the development of alveolar hypoventilation with respiratory failure.

There are other mechanical causes of acute respiratory failure that should be remembered. These include tension pneumothorax, severe ascites, and metabolic disorders such as hypothyroidism. In addition, chest-wall or pleural abnormalities may contribute to respiratory failure in patients who have a primary pulmonary cause for their respiratory distress. For example, in patients with acute exacerbations of chronic obstructive lung disease, respiratory failure may be exacerbated by ascites, obesity, or an endocrine disorder such as hypothyroidism. Similarly, patients with primary chest-wall or pleural disease may develop secondary parenchymal abnormalities such as pneumonia or pulmonary edema that lead to acute respiratory failure. Thus, acute respiratory failure can often be attributed to multiple factors.

Upper Airway Obstruction

There are many possible causes of upper airway obstruction that may lead to acute respiratory failure and the need for emergency treatment. In children, croup and epiglottitis are the most common causes of upper airway obstruction. These also may occur in adults. Upper airway obstruction may be the result of obstructing tumors in the base of the tongue, the larynx, or the hypopharynx. Acute upper airway obstruction also may occur from aspirated liquid or food contents or any foreign object that becomes lodged in the airway. In some massively obese patients, obstruction of the upper airway may occur when the patient is supine.

Management of acute upper airway obstruction requires an understanding of the pathogenesis of the disorder. In patients who have severe carbon dioxide retention or apnea, emergency endotracheal intubation must be performed. If oral intubation is not possible, an emergency cricothyrotomy or tracheostomy must be done. In patients with progressive upper airway obstruction, as may occur in acute epiglottitis, a number of studies have shown that early intubation in a controlled setting by a skilled anesthesiologist is the treatment of choice. In some patients with tumors causing upper airway obstruction, temporizing measures such as treatment with helium-oxygen mixtures have been reported to preclude the need for intubation while the patient is receiving radiation therapy, chemotherapy, and corticosteroids to reduce the size of the tumor [40].

Pulmonary edema may complicate upper airway obstruction in both children and adults [166]. The mechanism for the relationship between upper airway obstruction and pulmonary edema has not been established.

Chronic Obstructive Airways Disease

PATHOGENESIS OF AIRWAYS OBSTRUCTION

The specific disorders causing chronic airways obstruction are chronic bronchitis and emphysema and, much less frequently, diffuse bronchiectasis. These processes are discussed in more detail in other chapters in this book. Although chronic bronchitis and emphysema are pathologically distinct processes, they usually occur together, producing a uniform pattern of respiratory failure. The physiologic hallmark of chronic airways obstruction is an increase in the resistance to airflow within the airways. In chronic bronchitis, the increased airflow resistance is related primarily to an increase in the size and number of tracheobronchial mucous glands with consequent hypersecretion of mucus [168]. The increase in mucous glands decreases the airway luminal area, which is further encroached upon by free mucus and mucous plugs. Metaplasia of goblet cells in the airways also may contribute to the obstruction [76]. Earlier in the course of chronic bronchitis, mucous gland abnormalities may be largely limited to more peripheral, smaller airways and not be associated with marked increases in the measured airways resistance [109]. Nevertheless, even with

so-called small airways disease, functional disturbances in gas exchange may be severe and occasionally result in respiratory failure. Much more commonly, however, these anatomic changes are present in more central as well as peripheral airways. Airway inflammation and edema also may play a role in causing airways narrowing.

Emphysema is probably more important in the pathogenesis of airways obstruction in chronic obstructive airways disease [118,119]. Because emphysema is a process in which there is destruction of lung parenchyma, the elastic forces that tether the airways and provide radial traction to maintain airway patency are reduced. At autopsy this leads to airway narrowing without any intrinsic disease of the airways necessarily being present. The severity of emphysema in autopsied lungs has been found to correlate positively both with anatomic findings of airways narrowing and distortion of bronchiolar dimensions and with premortem PaO_2 and measurements of airflow obstruction [119]. Correlations have been poor between anatomic findings and $PaCO_2$, which is consistent with the fact that control of this variable involves many factors other than the anatomic derangements within the lungs per se. Not surprisingly, the anatomic degree of emphysema has been found to correlate negatively with the degree of reversibility of airflow obstruction [119].

Inflammation and edema have been noted to have little correlation with the degree of airways obstruction, at least in stable chronic airways obstruction [109]. However, because infection with consequent inflammation is a common event that precipitates acute respiratory failure in patients with chronic airways obstruction, its role may be underestimated in autopsy studies.

As opposed to the finding in patients with asthma, an increase in airway smooth muscle tone is not a consistent feature in patients with chronic airways obstruction. In fact, recent studies have suggested that in the presence of emphysema, increased muscle in the airway may have a beneficial effect, perhaps tending to maintain airway dimensions [118]. The finding of increased airway smooth muscle has not been found, however, to correlate with reversibility of airflow obstruction.

Although morphologic findings cannot be relied on to guide therapy, the results of studies to date suggest that the abnormalities underlying chronic airways obstruction are not in themselves reversible. This underlines the importance of prevention of superimposed acute insults and of diligence in seeking out and treating processes that might be causing exacerbations of airflow obstruction leading to acute respiratory failure.

PATHOPHYSIOLOGY

As opposed to the disorders that primarily involve alveoli, respiratory failure in patients with chronic airways obstruction is characterized by an increase in $PaCO_2$ as well as a decrease in PaO_2. The pathogenesis of the hypoxemia is mainly dependent on mismatching of ventilation and perfusion [173]. This is a consequence of the anatomic abnormalities described previously. In addition, superimposed conditions such as pneumonia, atelectasis, and left ventricular failure cause hypoxemia from intrapulmonary right-to-left shunting of blood.

The mechanisms of impaired carbon dioxide elimination are more complex but also relate in part to mismatching of ventilation and perfusion [173]. Unless there is rather severe airways obstruction, reductions in ventilation to some alveoli can be offset by increased ventilation to other alveoli. However, with increasing airways obstruction, this compensatory mechanism is not sufficient to cope with the overall reduction in alveolar ventilation. At least three important factors also play a role in compounding the effects of airways obstruction. First, because of the increased work of breathing in the face of hypoxic conditions, the respiratory muscles may become fatigued and be unable to maintain the necessary level of minute ventilation [146]. Second, also related to the increased work of breathing, carbon dioxide production is increased [145]. Finally, there may be a decrease in central ventilatory drive, partly genetic [3,115] and partly acquired [28]. Also, the hypercapnia and hypoxemia or both may depress central respiratory drive, leading to further hypoventilation. In patients with acute decompensation, administration of oxygen leads to further hypercapnia. This may be due to a decrease in ventilatory drive from the loss of hypoxic stimulus, although some studies suggested that an increase in alveolar dead space associated with oxygen therapy may be responsible [7].

Chronic obstructive airways disease is generally regarded as an inexorably, albeit slowly, progressive disorder [31]. Patients may have symptoms of cough and sputum production for many years. As the airways obstruction progresses, however, patients become more vulnerable to what in persons with normal lungs would be minor insults. Although acute respiratory failure may be a consequence simply of severe progressive airways obstruction, first episodes are generally precipitated by some complicating disorder. Most commonly, the precipitating problem is a lower respiratory tract infection, either bronchitis or pneumonia [67]. The inflammation resulting from the infection, together with increased mucus production, causes further airways narrowing. If pneumonia is present, the alveolar filling causes shunting of blood and worsens lung mechanics. As a result, a cycle may be initiated in which the acute process superimposed on chronic airways disease results in further increases in airways resistance, worsening of gas exchange with both increases in $PaCO_2$ and decreases in PaO_2, and an increased work of breathing. As a consequence of increasing demands placed on respiratory muscles at a time when oxygen delivery is reduced, muscle fatigue ensues. The increased work of breathing also increases carbon dioxide production, as does fever if present, thereby presenting the lungs with an increased load of carbon dioxide that they are incapable of eliminating. This results in a progressively increasing $PaCO_2$ and decreasing PaO_2 unless the cycle is interrupted.

A number of other processes in addition to infection also may be involved, either alone or in combination, in producing acute respiratory failure. These include left ventricular failure, pneumothorax, pulmonary embolism, and worsening of the airways obstruction in response to inhaled irritants.

As the abnormalities of gas exchange become more severe, the function of other organs, especially the heart and central nervous system, may be affected. With regard to the heart, these effects may be manifested as arrhythmias, ischemia, heart failure, or actual myocardial infarction. Central nervous system effects include alterations in behavior, reduction in level of consciousness, coma, seizures, or myoclonus. Obviously, either cardiovascular or central nervous system effects could have a major adverse influence on the course of respiratory failure and themselves become a part of the progressive downward spiral.

ASSESSMENT OF SEVERITY

The symptoms associated with respiratory failure in patients with chronic airways obstruction usually represent an accentuation of the baseline symptoms. Most patients with airways obstruction have cough and sputum production. Acute lower respiratory tract infections generally increase these symptoms and are often associated with an increase in the volume of sputum and its being darker and thicker. It should be kept in mind, however, that as airways obstruction increases, the ability to clear mucus from the lungs may decrease. Thus, a report of a decrease in sputum production associated with other symptoms also may be indicative of worsening clinical status.

Increasing Dyspnea. Worsening gas exchange is nearly always associated with increasing dyspnea. In patients who have acclimated to their lung disease or who are very sedentary, dyspnea may not be reported as a prominent symptom. Nevertheless, a carefully taken history should always be structured to elicit indications of reduction in lung function.

In some patients, cardiovascular complaints may predominate. These include palpitations, orthopnea, paroxysmal nocturnal dyspnea, ankle swelling, and chest pain. Complaints related to central nervous system dysfunction also may be prominent. Headache, visual problems, sleep disturbances, memory loss, and behavioral alterations may be reported. In some patients, these may be of sufficient severity to obscure the respiratory symptoms.

Findings on physical examination may be quite helpful and provide an important context in which to evaluate the more objective measurements such as blood gas tensions. The general appearance of the patient is very important: A patient who looks reasonably well and is alert and able to cooperate with therapy obviously represents quite a different management problem than the patient who is confused, combative, stuporous, or comatose, even though both patients may have the same blood gas and pH values. Alterations in behavior or level of consciousness may not be caused by the abnormal blood gas tensions per se, but could be related to drugs or other factors; however, the implications for treatment are the same. In addition to providing information concerning the lung disease, the physical examination should be targeted to detect disorders that may have precipitated the acute deterioration (e.g., left ventricular failure). At least in the acute setting, the degree of pulsus paradoxus correlates with the severity of airways obstruction. Lung findings may or may not be helpful. Most patients with acute exacerbations of chronic airways obstruction have supraclavicular and intercostal space retractions. The chest usu-

ally is hyperinflated and tympanitic with very limited diaphragmatic excursion. Breath sounds commonly are markedly diminished. Wheezing may or may not be heard.

The chest film has considerable value in this setting, sometimes providing evidence of pneumonia, left ventricular failure, or pneumothorax that was not evident on physical examination. The electrocardiogram is less often helpful, but it is important if it shows right atrial or right ventricular enlargement, an arrhythmia, or evidence of left ventricular disease. Routine blood studies may provide evidence of other processes, but except for the hematocrit, they do not relate to lung disease. Patients who have been hypoxemic for long periods of time will, unless other factors supervene, have secondary polycythemia [116]. This finding gives some indication of the duration of the hypoxemia.

Assessment of Respiratory Function. Of all the assessments that can be made, measurements of arterial PO_2, PCO_2, and pH are the most important. Serial measurements of PaO_2, $PaCO_2$, and pH are much more helpful than a single determination and can indicate success or failure of initial therapy. Blood gas and pH values, taken together with the general status of the patient, often determine the necessary intensity of supportive measures, particularly whether or not endotracheal intubation and mechanical ventilation will be necessary. Many patients with chronic airways obstruction will have some degree of hypoxemia and some will have carbon dioxide retention when they are at their functional baseline. As noted earlier, chronicity of hypoxemia may be attested to by polycythemia and in addition by findings of pulmonary hypertension with or without right ventricular failure. A single measurement of $PaCO_2$ without a prior baseline value may be very difficult to interpret, hence, the importance of the clinical context. An elevated plasma bicarbonate concentration is an indication that an elevated $PaCO_2$ has been present for a sufficiently long period of time to allow metabolic compensation (see Fig. 46-3).

Direct measurements of airflow are often difficult to obtain in severely ill patients and may not be useful. Measurements of FEV_1 and FVC may be helpful, however, in evaluating the response to therapy.

MANAGEMENT

Effective management of acute respiratory failure in patients with chronic airways obstruction requires a critical care unit. The approach to treatment should always be directed toward providing supportive care while at the same time treating the specific processes such as lower respiratory tract infection that precipitated the acute deterioration.

General Principles. The major supportive intervention is provision of supplemental oxygen. Because the pathophysiologic mechanism by which hypoxemia develops is mismatching of ventilation and perfusion, increases in PaO_2 usually are easily achieved by administration of low concentrations of oxygen. Overadministration of oxygen causing an increase in $PaCO_2$ has been well described and is a potential problem in patients who have a chronically elevated $PaCO_2$ [7,32]. This concern, however, should not deter physicians from oxygen administration. The basic principle should be to administer the lowest amount of oxygen necessary to increase PaO_2 to approximately 60 mmHg. Frequently, this can be achieved using nasal prongs or a cannula with flows of 1 to 2 liters/min. Occasionally, higher flows are needed. The FiO_2 delivered by devices such as nasal prongs will vary considerably, depending on the patient's minute ventilation. Although this does not usually present a problem, more precise control of the FiO_2 can be provided by a mask with a Venturi device through which a high flow of oxygen is delivered that entrains sufficient room air to produce the desired FiO_2. The disadvantages of the Venturi delivery device are that the inspired gas is usually poorly humidified and that the mask interferes with talking and eating.

Regardless of the oxygen delivery system, arterial blood gas tension must be measured soon after oxygen therapy is begun. The goal, as cited above, is to increase the PaO_2 to 60 mmHg (i.e., 90 percent hemoglobin saturation) without undue effects on $PaCO_2$. Blood gas measurements should be made thereafter as frequently as the clinical circumstances dictate. Because of the concern with the interactions of PaO_2 and $PaCO_2$, noninvasive oximetric monitoring of oxyhemoglobin saturation alone is not sufficient. Because reductions in PaO_2 below the target value of 60 mmHg will cause reductions in saturation to less than 90 percent, monitoring of oxyhemoglobin saturation complements direct measurements of PaO_2 and $PaCO_2$.

For most patients, provision of supplemental oxygen will be the only supportive therapy needed. In some, however, endotracheal intubation and mechanical ventilation will be required. Precise criteria for intubation and mechanical ventilation are difficult to define and commonly involve subjective as well as objective assessments. Hypoxemia is usually not in itself an indication for intubation because of the relative ease with which PaO_2 can be increased with supplemental oxygen provided by external devices. The major indication for ventilatory assistance is poorly compensated respiratory acidosis. This may be apparent at the time of initial evaluation and dictate prompt application of mechanical ventilation. Commonly, however, the need for ventilatory assistance is indicated by the failure of the patient to improve or the patient's worsening with conservative management. This determination is made through careful monitoring of the response to oxygen administration as well as an assessment of such other variables as respiratory distress, fatigue, mental status, and ability to cooperate with conservative management.

In some patients, the need for mechanical ventilation may be avoided by the use of doxapram [114]. This agent increases carotid body sensitivity to hypoxemia; thus, less hypoxemia produces a larger response in minute ventilation. The drug also provides direct stimulation of the medullary respiratory centers. It can be given either by intermittent intravenous administration (approximately 2 mg/kg) or by continuous infusion (1 to 3 mg/min). Continuous infusion of doxapram has been shown in some patients to obviate endotracheal intubation while the causes of the acute deterioration are being treated. Although the drug is recommended only for a 2-hour period of infusion, patients have continued to receive the drug for 36 hours or more with continued stimulation of ventilation. The major adverse effects of the drug are on the central nervous system. It may cause hypertension, tachycardia, arrhythmias, tremulousness, restlessness, and seizures, all of which also may be caused by respiratory failure and by other agents, such as methylxanthines. Given the sorts of adverse reactions that may occur, the use of doxapram should not be undertaken lightly and should always be done in a critical care unit under continuous cardiac monitoring and close observation.

Another approach to avoiding mechanical ventilation is the use of positive airway pressure delivered by a tight-fitting face mask [29]. More studies of this therapy are needed.

When necessary, mechanical ventilation should be accomplished using a volume-cycled ventilator and IPPV or IMV with a low level of pressure support (5–10 cm H_2O). The primary initial goal of mechanical ventilation is to rest the respiratory muscles by providing mechanical assistance to achieve adequate oxygenation and alveolar ventilation. Respiratory muscle fatigue presumably plays a major role in the need for mechanical ventilation in this setting. Tidal volume should be set at approximately 7 to 10 ml/kg of body weight. When the patient is awake, he or she will determine the respiratory rate. Given the tachypnea that is common in such patients, sedation is often necessary to enable an optimal ventilatory pattern. Ideally, the rate should be relatively slow, providing sufficient time for full exhalation of the previous breath to avoid stacking breaths with a consequent further increase in functional residual capacity. A long inspiratory time also is desirable to improve the distribution of inspired gas. PEEP as a general rule should not be used. The effect of PEEP would be to further increase the already greatly enlarged functional residual capacity and cause further overdistension of the lungs. In patients with airways obstruction, an auto-PEEP effect may occur because of airway closure before full exhalation [127]. When the patient is being mechanically ventilated, there should be no concern with overadministration of oxygen, and the FIO_2 should be sufficient to maintain a PaO_2 of over 60 mmHg.

Within 10 minutes of beginning mechanical ventilation, arterial blood gases should be measured. Because many patients with acute respiratory failure and chronic airways obstruction have had carbon dioxide retention for days, months, or years, metabolic compensation has occurred. This compensation generally is insufficient in the setting of an acute deterioration but is appropriate for the baseline $PaCO_2$. When mechanical ventilation is applied, the $PaCO_2$ generally can be decreased very quickly, and if it is reduced well below the patient's baseline to a normal value of 40 mmHg, the patient will be left with an uncompensated, sometimes profound, metabolic alkalosis. Alkalosis has a number of potential adverse effects, including depression of cardiac output, increasing the risk of both supraventricular and ventricular arrhythmias, depressing the level of consciousness, and causing seizures [83]. Because of the concern with alkalosis, the adequacy of mechanical ventilation should be determined not by $PaCO_2$ but by pH. The $PaCO_2$ should be maintained at a level that keeps the pH no higher than 7.45 to 7.50, and preferably close to 7.40. Also, because of chronic increases in $PaCO_2$, patients commonly are deficient in potas-

sium and chloride. A reduction in plasma bicarbonate concentration will not occur until sufficient chloride, usually in the form of potassium chloride, has been given [80].

Weaning patients with chronic airways obstruction from mechanical ventilation can present a difficult problem. Implicit in the decision to intubate and ventilate is the assumption that a reversible factor contributes to the acute deterioration and that treatment will restore the patient to his or her baseline status. Thus, mechanical ventilation is simply supporting the patient until specific therapy has had its effect, although resting the muscles of respiration may be of value in itself. Given this assumption, weaning efforts should begin as soon as the reversible component has been improved. In the case of left ventricular failure, for example, this may occur quite rapidly in response to diuresis. On the other hand, if pneumonia caused the acute deterioration, improvement may be slow.

A number of criteria have been developed as predictors of ability to be weaned. Unfortunately, these criteria are rarely applicable to patients with chronic airways obstruction, who may not have been able to perform at the levels indicated by the criteria for many years. For this reason, assessment of ability to be weaned in this setting is more subjective [130]. Measurements such as VC and MIP can be made, but low values should not be assumed to predict failure. The patient should be alert and psychologically prepared for weaning. Serum electrolyte concentrations, especially potassium, phosphate, calcium, and magnesium, should be optimal, and the patient should be hemodynamically stable.

In general, prior to beginning the process of weaning, the PaO_2, $PaCO_2$, and pH should be maintained approximately at their baseline values, if known. Thus, patients may be mildly hypoxemic, hypercapneic, and acidemic. The technique of weaning is somewhat controversial, some clinicians preferring a trial of spontaneous breathing on a T-piece or a low level of CPAP (1 to 2 cmH_2O) while others favoring the use of IMV with progressively decreasing ventilatory rates, sometimes with the addition of low levels of pressure support [131]. A T-piece or CPAP trial offers the advantage of being able to determine fairly rapidly if a patient is ready to be extubated. If the patient ventilates adequately via a T-piece or a low level of CPAP for 1 or 2 hours without a deterioration in arterial blood gas tension and without a marked increase in respiratory rate, decrease in tidal volume, or other evidence of fatigue, then usually the endotracheal tube can be removed. Longer periods of spontaneous breathing, especially through a small endotracheal tube (<7 mm in diameter), may, because of the resistance of the tube, increase respiratory muscle fatigue [96,131].

In managing patients with acute respiratory failure and chronic airways obstruction, important and difficult ethical issues may be raised. As stated previously, in undertaking mechanical ventilatory support, it is assumed that the respiratory failure has a reversible component. This may not be the case. The respiratory failure may simply represent the end stage of a disease that is known to be inexorably progressive. Providing mechanical ventilation for a patient who has no reversible component usually means that the patient will not be able to be weaned successfully. Under ideal circumstances, the patient and his or her physician will have had the opportunity to discuss the outlook for the illness prior to acute deterioration, and the patient can make an informed decision regarding the use of mechanical ventilation. Such a patient may decide that ventilation should be undertaken on the chance that there is a reversible component. If facilities are available, the patient also may choose chronic ventilatory support. Given the multiplicity of clinical disorders commonly present in these sorts of patients, chronic mechanical ventilation is usually a very unattractive option even if available. Patients who are being ventilated mechanically also may elect to have this support discontinued. If mechanical ventilation is not undertaken or is discontinued, vigorous treatment can still be provided, but in addition, particular attention should be paid to the patient's comfort.

Hospital survival rates for acute respiratory failure in patients with chronic airways obstruction have been surprisingly similar in several studies, ranging from 58 to 79 percent. Not surprisingly, 24-month survival rates have been much lower, from 35 to 72 percent (Fig. 46-11) [98].

Specific Treatment. In addition to the general principles of care described in this section, treatment of the airways obstruction and of the precipitating disorder must be prompt and vigorous. Although there is controversy concerning the usefulness of bronchodilators in patients with chronic airways obstruction, it should always be assumed that there is a reversible component. Inhaled beta-adrenergic agonists such as albuterol, metaproterenol, and terbutaline should be used

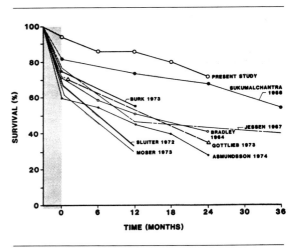

Fig. 46-11. A comparison of reported survival data for patients with chronic obstructive pulmonary disease after an episode of acute respiratory failure. The shaded area denotes the period of hospitalization. The "present study" refers to work presented by Martin [98]. (Reproduced from TR Martin et al. The prognosis of patients with chronic obstructive pulmonary disease after hospitalization for acute respiratory failure. *Chest* 82:310, 1982.)

at intervals of 2 to 4 hours at the beginning of treatment and decreased in frequency if adverse reactions are encountered. Also, inhaled ipratropium bromide, an anticholinergic compound, can be added to beta adrenergic agonist therapy in patients with marked bronchospasm [30]. They can be administered either directly via a nebulizer driven by a compressed-gas source or through a mechanical ventilator or as a metered dose inhaler through the ventilator. With either of these devices, the amount of drug actually delivered is difficult to quantify, and thus the dose given should be limited mainly by side effects. Intravenous theophylline also may be of benefit, albeit less than inhaled beta agonists. The loading dose of aminophylline in patients who have not been taking the drug is 5 to 6 mg/kg. Maintenance doses in patients with severe airways obstruction, some of whom may have heart failure, should be 0.3 to 0.5 mg/kg/min [177]. After 18 to 24 hours, a serum theophylline concentration should be measured and the infusion rate adjusted appropriately. The concentration should be maintained approximately 10 to 20 μg/ml, with 20 μg/ml being the usual threshold for toxicity. Theophylline has been shown to increase the strength of respiratory muscles, but it appears that to achieve this effect toxic concentrations are required [45].

Corticosteroids also may be of benefit [2], although response is not universal. The dose that should be given is not established, but a sufficient amount should be given to ensure an effect. Doses of 120 to 240 mg are commonly administered daily early in the course of treatment.

Antimicrobial drugs are given commonly and are of obvious value if there is a bacterial bronchitis or pneumonia [169]. The choice of agents should be guided initially by the results of sputum Gram stains. If Gram stains and cultures do not provide guidance, empiric therapy with ampicillin, trimethoprim-sulfamethoxazole, or tetracycline may be used.

Respiratory Failure in Asthma

PATHOGENESIS OF AIRWAYS OBSTRUCTION IN ASTHMA

Several factors contribute to the marked obstruction to airflow that is the hallmark of severe asthma. The initial event is contraction of bronchial smooth muscle as the result of an immunologically mediated process, direct stimulation of irritant receptors within the airways, or both. In patients who have had long-standing asthma, the amount of smooth muscle in the airways is increased [165]. This in itself may reduce the cross-sectional diameter of the airway and, in addition, may result in a greater response to a given stimulus than would be expected to occur in the absence of smooth-muscle hypertrophy [22].

The same stimuli that result in smooth-muscle contraction also influence the volume and composition of bronchial mucus. Gross and microscopic examinations of airways from patients who had fatal asthmatic attacks clearly show that mucociliary abnormalities play an important role in causing the airways obstruction. The mucous glands are hypertrophic and may encroach on the airway lumen, goblet cells are increased in numbers, and excessive secretions, often forming plugs, are present in the airways [47]. Loss of the ciliated epithelium of the airway contributes to the inability to clear the secretions. Moreover, the epithelial damage can lead to leakage of plasma proteins, including large-molecular-weight substances such as fibrinogen, that further impairs the removal of airway secretions and increases mucus viscosity. Inflammation also plays a role

by increasing vascular permeability and causing cellular infiltration and edema. In addition, mediators of inflammation may in themselves cause smooth-muscle contraction [77].

With time, there is a decrease in the relative contribution of smooth-muscle contraction to airways narrowing, while obstruction caused by mucous plugging and edema of the bronchial walls increases. Perhaps for this reason, the response to bronchodilating drugs in status asthmaticus is diminished. With the emergence of mucous plugging and airway edema as the major factors causing obstruction, a much longer period of intensive treatment is required.

PATHOPHYSIOLOGY

Acute airways obstruction in asthma results in increased resistance to airflow during both inspiration and especially expiration, and this leads to air trapping and overinflation of the lungs [183]. Because the airflow obstruction is not uniform, the distribution of inspired air is uneven, causing mismatching of ventilation and perfusion. This results in hypoxemia and an increase in wasted ventilation [148,174]. The hyperinflation serves to maintain airway patency, but as functional residual capacity increases and approaches the predicted normal total lung capacity (TLC), a greater change in transpulmonary pressure is required to produce an adequate tidal volume. This, together with the rise in airways resistance, markedly increases the work of breathing. Therefore, in severe airways obstruction there is an increased oxygen demand caused by the increased work of breathing at the same time that hypoxemia results from mismatching of ventilation and perfusion. Moreover, the increase in wasted ventilation and in carbon dioxide production requires a greater minute ventilation, which can be achieved only by imposing an additional work load on the respiratory muscles. Because of the hyperinflation, the intercostal, accessory, and diaphragmatic muscles are forced to work at a considerable mechanical disadvantage [97]. At some point, if the airways obstruction is not corrected, the system fails and carbon dioxide retention occurs. In addition, as the oxygen demands of the respiratory muscles exceed the supply of oxygen, anaerobic metabolism results with subsequent metabolic (lactic) acidosis. Because there is no possibility for respiratory compensation, the pH rapidly decreases. Metabolic acidosis in this setting must be dealt with promptly or rapid deterioration and death will occur.

ASSESSMENT OF SEVERITY

Assessment of the severity of an asthmatic episode is of obvious importance in determining the approach to management of the patient. Although the vast majority of asthmatic attacks are treated on an outpatient basis, it is essential that both the patient and the medical personnel be aware of when more intensive treatment is needed. Several groups of investigators have identified factors of importance in deciding which patients with asthma require hospital admission [11,56,81,135]. However, the utility and accuracy of numerical indices derived from such data have been questioned [33,142]. Thus, the severity of an asthmatic episode should be assessed both objectively and subjectively. Factors that should be taken into account in such evaluations are listed in Table 46-6.

Clinical and General Laboratory Evaluation.
The history is of major importance in assessing the severity of a given asthmatic episode and provides information that influences the interpretation of the more objective physiologic data. Persons with a history of severe attacks tend to continue to have severe attacks. Thus, information from the patient or from the medical record that he or she has previously required hospitalization increases the probability that the current episode will require hospitalization. The duration of the current attack is also important, since the mechanism of airways obstruction changes as

Table 46-6. Important factors in assessing severity of acute asthma

---

1. History of prior hospitalization for asthma
2. History of prior or current corticosteroid therapy
3. Patient's subjective sense of severity of attack
4. Failure to respond to usual treatment (i.e., persistent wheezing despite bronchodilator therapy)
5. Duration of attack
6. Patient too distressed to talk
7. Silent chest (i.e., minimal breath sounds)
8. Disturbances in mental status
9. Systemic hypertension, tachycardia > 110/min
10. Cardiac arrhythmias
11. Cyanosis
12. Prominent accessory muscle use
13. Pulsus paradoxus > 10 mmHg
14. Mediastinal emphysema, pneumothorax
15. FEV < 1.0 liter
16. Acute respiratory acidosis or arterial PaO_2 < 60 mmHg on room air

---

the attack persists. Early on in exacerbations of asthma the mechanism of obstruction is mainly smooth-muscle spasm, whereas later it is mucous plugging and edema. Spasm can resolve within minutes, but days may be required to improve obstruction that is caused by edema and plugging.

Patients with acute asthmatic episodes nearly always have tachypnea and tachycardia, neither of which correlates well with the degree of airways obstruction. The amount of pulsus paradoxus does, however, correlate with the degree of obstruction [134]. This finding can therefore be used both to indicate severity and to judge response to therapy. The intensity of wheezing cannot be used to infer the amount of airways obstruction, although prolongation of the expiratory phase varies roughly with obstruction. The absence of wheezing in a patient who, by all other indicators, has asthma is an ominous finding indicating that airflow is so reduced that there is not sufficient turbulence to cause wheezing. Unilateral absence of wheezing may be the result of a pneumothorax or a mucous plug in a large airway and likewise is indicative of a serious clinical problem.

Although not specific, abnormalities in mental status are important in patients with severe airways obstruction. Such findings may be the result of hypoxia or carbon dioxide retention or be unrelated to the asthma, but they influence management by interfering with patient cooperation.

Although an understanding of the alterations in pulmonary function is necessary to conceptualize the pathophysiology of asthma, in clinical practice the only measurements that are made routinely are the FEV_1, peak expiratory flow, and FVC. Of these, the peak expiratory flow is the most easily obtained because it does not require a full forced exhalation but rather a short forced puff similar to a cough after a full inhalation. Severe obstruction is indicated by a peak flow of less than 100 liters/min. This has been shown to correspond to an FEV_1 of less than 0.7 liter [122].

The FEV_1 is more difficult to measure because it requires a full inspiration followed by a full forced exhalation, maneuvers that a patient with severe asthma may not be able to perform because of dyspnea. In some patients, the forced expiration worsens the obstruction [117]. Nevertheless, the FEV_1 is the most direct measurement of airflow, and it correlates well with other variables and clinical outcomes. Nowak and associates [122] found that an FEV_1 of less than 1 liter or 20 percent of the predicted value was associated with a poor bronchodilator response, the need for hospitalization, and the likelihood of relapse. Similar findings were reported by Kelsen and coworkers [81]. Several investigators have related the FEV_1 to PaO_2 and $PaCO_2$ [136,164] and have demonstrated that in general, in acute asthma, carbon dioxide retention begins at an FEV_1 of approximately 750 ml or 25 percent of the predicted value. An increase in $PaCO_2$ is a direct consequence of worsening airways obstruction in patients with limited ventilatory capability in the face of increased carbon dioxide production. Because mild degrees of acute airways obstruction are usually associated with a lower than normal $PaCO_2$, the finding of a value in the range of 40 mmHg should be viewed with alarm.

Although there is a tendency for the PaO_2 to decrease with decreasing values of the FEV_1, the relationship is not as predictable as with $PaCO_2$ [52]. Nearly all patients with airways obstruction have some degree of arterial hypoxemia. Values of less than 50 mmHg are distinctly unusual, however, and suggest that factors in addition to airways obstruction are present.

Acute hypoventilation results in a reduction in arterial pH of about 0.008 pH unit for every millimeter of mercury increase in $PaCO_2$; thus, an increase in $PaCO_2$ from 40 to 60 mmHg would result in a pH of 7.24 (see Fig. 46-3). A reduction in pH that is in excess of the predicted change in $PaCO_2$ indicates the presence of a metabolic as well as respiratory acidosis. As discussed previously, metabolic acidosis in this setting is due to an imbalance between the supply and consumption of oxygen by the respiratory muscles plus a reduction in clearance of lactate from blood. The finding of metabolic acidosis in a patient with severe asthma is an ominous finding [5].

Chest radiographs should be obtained routinely in patients with severe asthma. The most common finding is overinflation of the lungs, but occasionally, pneumonia, pneumomediastinum, pneumothorax, or atelectasis from mucous plugging of larger airways may be found. Electrocardiograms also should be obtained, especially in older patients. The common abnormalities include P pulmonale, right ventricular strain, and right axis deviation, all of which may be reversible. Less commonly, changes indicative of ischemia or arrhythmias may be encountered.

MANAGEMENT

The treatment modalities employed in severe asthma are directed toward both support of the patient and reversal of the airways obstruction.

Supportive Care. Supplemental oxygen is an essential supportive measure that should be instituted in all patients with acute airways obstruction. Because there is no concern with depression of ventilatory drive by oxygen in patients with asthma, the choice of an oxygen delivery system should mainly be dictated by patient comfort. For example, face masks that fit tightly may not be tolerated, and humidification of the inspired gas mixture, although desirable, may stimulate more bronchoconstriction. Normal saline is less likely to produce this effect than distilled water. In addition, heated humidification is preferable.

Many patients who have had significant airways obstruction for days to weeks will have some degree of intravascular volume depletion, as indicated by an increased hematocrit and blood urea nitrogen level [162]. The goal of fluid therapy in this group is to restore normovolemia. Overly vigorous hydration does not improve mucus clearance and may be hazardous. Although electrolyte abnormalities are uncommon, patients with asthma who have been taking adrenal corticosteroids and/or diuretic agents may have hypokalemia and hypochloremia. These should be looked for and corrected when present.

It is difficult to determine when to institute mechanical ventilation in severe asthma. There are no uniformly applicable criteria that can guide the decision, and as with the general assessment, both subjective and objective criteria should be used. Generally, mechanical ventilation should not be undertaken before the patient has been given maximal bronchodilator therapy, even though marked abnormalities of gas exchange may be present. Exceptions to this generalization include the presence of significant mental status changes, life-threatening cardiac arrhythmias, electrocardiographic evidence of myocardial ischemia, or a history of previous severe asthmatic episodes requiring mechanical ventilation.

Patients who continue to deteriorate in the face of aggressive, in-hospital management generally require mechanical ventilation. This is indicated by increasing respiratory acidosis often accompanied by metabolic acidosis. Hypoxemia in itself, because it can be managed effectively with supplemental oxygen, is rarely an indication for mechanical ventilation.

Insertion of an endotracheal tube should be done semielectively rather than waiting until the patient is close to having a respiratory arrest. Nasotracheal intubation using adequate topical anesthesia may be performed after preoxygenation.

Because there are irritant receptors in the larynx and trachea, the process of endotracheal intubation may provoke increased bronchoconstriction. This response is mediated by the parasympathetic nervous system and may be reduced by premedication with atropine or topical lidocaine in the pharynx and larynx. In most patients, therefore, orotracheal intubation with sedation and paralysis is necessary.

Once control of the airway is achieved, sedation is generally necessary. Morphine sulfate, 3 to 5 mg given intravenously, is the agent of choice. Although some data indicate that morphine causes release of histamine and further bronchoconstriction, this has not been clinically significant.

Mechanical ventilation should be provided with a volume-cycled ventilator. The initial ventilatory mode should be IPPV rather than IMV. This will allow the respiratory muscles to rest completely. Tidal volume should be in the range of 6 to 10 ml/kg of body weight. Because the functional residual capacity is markedly increased, added PEEP, which will further increase the functional residual capacity, should not be used. In fact, in virtually all patients with sufficiently severe status asthmaticus that requires intubation and mechanical ventilation, auto-PEEP will be present [135].

Appropriate adjustment of the ratio of inspiration to expiration is the most difficult aspect of mechanical ventilation in the setting of severe airways obstruction. An interplay of four factors is involved: (1) marked slowing of the expiratory flow because of the airways obstruction, (2) dyspnea and tachypnea, (3) the need for a minute ventilation that will reduce the $PaCO_2$, and (4) the desirability of a slow inspiratory time to minimize peak airway pressures and enable optimal distribution of the inspired gas. Because of the reduction in expiratory flow, a relatively long expiratory time is needed. If expiratory time is too short, further air trapping will occur. To avoid this, either the inspiratory time can be shortened or the tidal volume reduced, neither of which is desirable. Thus, it is generally preferable to sedate the patient until apnea is produced so that a slow ventilatory rate can be used, thereby allowing both a slower inspiratory flow and a longer expiratory time. In addition to morphine or diazepam, muscle relaxants may be necessary. Pancuronium or vecuronium are the muscle relaxants of choice although, as described earlier, use of these agents can be associated with prolonged neuromuscular blockade or a myopathy [30,46, 64,152].

In one recent study, excellent results with controlled hypoventilation with hyperoxic mixtures in mechanically ventilated patients were reported [42]. In this study, the authors did not allow peak airway pressures to exceed 50 cmH$_2$O and thus allowed the patients to be hypercapnic but well oxygenated. Alveolar hypoventilation was maintained for hours or even up to 4 days until airway obstruction was relieved and the hypercapnia resolved. There were no deaths with this approach, in contrast with prior studies (Table 46-7).

During the course of mechanical ventilation, in addition to following PaO_2, $PaCO_2$, and pH, the peak airway pressure should be noted, since this provides a rough indication of the inspiratory flow resistance. With mechanical ventilation, PaO_2 and $PaCO_2$ generally can be brought into the normal range quite promptly; however, weaning cannot begin until the airways obstruction remits. This is indicated by a reduction in peak inspiratory pressure, a spontaneous maximum inspiratory force of at least -30 cmH$_2$O, and a VC of at least 15 ml/kg of body weight. If these are achieved, weaning can usually proceed using either conventional T-piece trials with spontaneous ventilation or IMV with a progressively decreasing frequency of mechanical breaths.

Specific Treatment. The principles for the use of bronchodilator agents apply equally in mild, moderate, and severe asthma. As discussed previously, however, one of the clinical features that serves to define severe asthma is a failure to respond promptly to the usual bronchodilators. In spite of the poor early response to bronchodilators in patients with severe asthma, these agents together with corticosteroids remain the keystone of treatment. In severe asthma, the general rule is to give both theophylline and beta-adrenergic agonists in maximal doses as determined by blood concentrations (theophylline) or toxicity (beta-adrenergic agents and theophylline). In at least two studies, this approach was substantiated as providing more bronchodilation than with either agent given alone in maximal doses, although in a third trial inhaled isoproterenol proved to have as much effect alone as when combined with aminophylline [143,182].

Beta-adrenergic agonists may be administered orally, by inhalation, subcutaneously, or intravenously. When given by inhalation, there is a much more favorable ratio between benefit and unto-

Table 46-7. **Prognosis in patients requiring mechanical ventilation in status asthmaticus**

Study	Year	Episodes (n)	Deaths	Mortality (%)
Riding and Ambiavagar	1967	26	4	15
Iisalo et al.	1969	29	4	14
Lissac et al.	1971	19	4	21
Sheehy et al.	1972	22	2	9
Scoggin et al.	1977	21	8	38
Cornil et al.	1977	58	6	10
Westerman et al.	1979	42	4	9.5
Webb et al.	1979	20	7	35
Picado et al.	1983	26	6	23
Darioli et al.	1983	34	0	0

Source: Reproduced from R Darioli, C Perret. Mechanically controlled hypoventilation in status asthmaticus. *Am Rev Respir Dis* 129:385, 1984.

ward effects [86,156,167]. Because of limitation of inspiratory flow, a metered-dose inhaler may not be adequate to deliver the aerosol. Placing a spacer or reservoir between the inhaler and the mouth may make the metered-dose inhaler more effective. Of the beta$_2$-selective agents, only metaproterenol, terbutaline, and albuterol are available in the United States. The usual dose for metaproterenol solution is 15 mg (0.3 ml of 5% solution) and for terbutaline, 1.5 to 2.5 mg. Normal saline is added to the drug to make a total volume of 2.5 to 3.0 ml. Using standard nebulizers, this volume should be completely aerosolized in 10 to 15 minutes. It should be realized that with most compressed gas–driven systems, nebulization is continuous, but only the portion of the nebulized drug that is inhaled constitutes an effective dose. Thus, the doses listed above are substantially in excess of the doses delivered.

When treating severe episodes of asthma, a beta$_2$-selective agent should be inhaled nearly continuously during the first hour unless toxicity develops, as indicated by cardiac arrhythmia or intolerable tremor. During the next several hours, inhalation can be given at hourly intervals with close monitoring for toxicity. As the airways obstruction improves, the dosing interval can be increased to 4 to 6 hours. Aerosolized agents have an onset of action within minutes, and the effect of a single dose peaks at 30 to 60 minutes. The duration of effect is 4 to 6 hours following a single dose. In patients with asthma who require mechanical ventilation, the drug can be delivered using an in-line nebulizer in the inspiratory limb of the ventilator circuit. Also, recent data suggests

that addition of inhaled ipratroprium bromide, an anticholinergic agent, may have additive bronchodilating properties in patients being treated for severe asthma with inhaled beta adrenergic agonists [30].

The use of theophylline was discussed in an earlier section and is not reviewed here. It should be noted, however, that the factors that tend to alter the pharmacokinetics of theophylline, such as pneumonia, heart failure, and severe airways obstruction, are more likely to be present in severe asthma than in milder forms. Because of the severity of the process and perhaps because of coexisting diseases, it is more difficult to determine if a given occurrence (cardiac arrhythmia, seizure) is due to theophylline. For these reasons, the use of theophylline in severe asthma must be monitored closely using measurements of serum concentration of the drug.

Treatment with corticosteroids is essential therapy in severe asthma. In patients who do not respond promptly to initial bronchodilator therapy, treatment with a systemic, generally intravenously administered, corticosteroid should be instituted [84]. This does not obligate the patient to a long course of corticosteroids nor cause him or her to become steroid-dependent. Because the peak effect occurs no sooner than 4 to 6 hours after intravenous administration, it is best to give the initial dose early in the course of treatment and reevaluate the need for continuation at a later time. There appears to be a dose-response relationship between increasing doses of methylprednisolone (15, 40, and 125 mg all given three times a day) and FEV$_1$ [69]. Given that the adverse effects of even high doses of corticosteroids are minimal if the duration of administration is short, it is better to err on the side of giving too much of the drug rather than too little. Based on the scant data available, a dose of methylprednisolone in the range of 60 to 120 mg given intravenously at 6- to 8-hour intervals for 48 to 72 hours represents a reasonable initial approach to corticosteroid administration in patients with severe asthma. Higher doses should be used in patients who have been taking corticosteroids before or who are taking other drugs, such as barbiturates, phenytoin, or rifampin, that accelerate the metabolism of corticosteroids [187]. In patients who respond promptly, the dose can be reduced rapidly to maintenance doses given orally or discontinued altogether. Aerosols of corticosteroids, although effective in maintenance therapy, have no role in management of the severe attack.

Because both airway smooth-muscle and mucociliary functions are modulated by the parasympathetic nervous system, with stimulation causing both bronchoconstriction and an increase in mucus production, it is logical to assume that antimuscarinic agents such as atropine might be of benefit in asthma. To date, however, there is no evidence that administration of atropine or related compounds results in more bronchodilation than that provided by maximal doses of beta-adrenergic agonists.

Antimicrobial agents are of questionable value in the routine management of acute asthmatic episodes [39]. However, antimicrobial therapy is clearly indicated in patients who have bacterial pneumonia as diagnosed by chest radiographs and the presence of bacteria and polymorphonuclear leukocytes in a Gram-stained sputum smear. Antimicrobial agents also should be used in patients with severe asthma and bacterial bronchitis.

In general, mucolytic agents are of little use in severe asthma. Although compounds such as N-acetyl-L-cysteine reduce mucus viscosity by breaking the disulfide bonds between strands of mucus, these compounds offer little benefit to the vast majority of patients with severe asthma. Occasionally, however, acetylcysteine may be helpful in patients in whom tenacious mucous plugs are suctioned from the tracheobronchial tree or in whom atelectasis caused by mucous plugging is noted on chest films. The drug should be administered via nebulizer (2 ml of 20% solution in 2 ml of normal saline) every 2 to 6 hours [188]. Since airway irritation with consequent

bronchospasm is the major side effect of the drug, it must be used with caution.

Occasionally, very large plugs of mucus may obstruct larger bronchi in patients with refractory asthma. Such plugs obviously interfere with the ability of the patient to breathe and may cause lobar or segmental atelectasis. Fiberoptic bronchoscopy can allow visualization of the plugs and facilitate their removal.

In a few instances when extensive mucous plugging of more peripheral airways prevents effective ventilation, bronchial lavage has been beneficial. This has been undertaken on a limited scale via a fiberoptic bronchoscope using various solutions that contain N-acetyl-L-cysteine [158]. More vigorous lavage using balloon-tipped catheters to isolate a portion of lung and then flooding that portion also has been employed with anecdotal reports of success.

General anesthesia with inhalational agents has been used in the treatment of refractory asthma for a number of years. Halothane, because it possesses inherent bronchodilating properties, is the current agent of choice [125]. The drug has been demonstrated to antagonize the effects on smooth muscle of acetylcholine and histamine as well as reducing antigen-induced bronchospasm in dogs. In addition to the pharmacologic effects of the anesthetic agent, general anesthesia may allow more effective mechanical ventilation, although this also could be achieved in the vast majority of instances by proper use of sedatives and muscle relaxants in patients already being ventilated mechanically.

The side effects of halothane must be considered in deciding to administer general anesthesia. These include myocardial depression and arrhythmias, both of which may be potentiated by hypoxia and acid-base disturbance and worsened hypoxemia caused by a loss of intrapulmonary regulation of blood flow.

Evaluation of Response to Therapy. The same measures used to evaluate the severity of the episode when the patient is first seen are also useful in determining the response to therapy. As the airways obstruction lessens, the abnormalities of gas exchange will become less severe. Metabolic acidosis should decrease initially, while a reduction of $PaCO_2$ may lag. However, once the FEV_1 increases above 750 to 1000 ml, the $PaCO_2$ should be normal. Hypoxemia may persist for considerably longer.

In general, patients who are recovering from a severe asthmatic episode should continue to receive vigorous treatment with bronchodilators and corticosteroids until a plateau in pulmonary function is reached. Premature discontinuation of corticosteroids may precipitate a recurrence of severe bronchospasm. Symptoms and physical findings are not good indicators of objective response [106]. Typically, when patients begin to respond to treatment, the physical examination reveals increased rales, rhonchi, and wheezing as inspissated sections are mobilized into larger airways.

DEATH FROM ASTHMA

Death from asthma is very uncommon. By and large, however, even these few deaths are preventable, as indicated by retrospective analyses of the circumstances of the deaths and of the features that characterize the high-risk patient [36,73,179]. Patients who died from asthma tended to have long-standing, poorly controlled or progressively worsening asthma. Also, patients with very labile airways obstruction and those who had on previous occasions required mechanical ventilation were at high risk of having subsequent severe or lethal attacks. Often, both patients and their physicians failed to recognize the severity of the illness, and objective evaluations, such as spirometry and arterial blood gas and pH measurements, were not obtained. Consequently, therapy was not optimal. Patients were admitted to general hospital wards rather than to critical care units. Corticosteroids were not given or were given only in low doses, and bronchodilator drugs were not given in maximal doses and their effects were not monitored. In many instances, sedating drugs were used to treat the anxiety associated with the attack. Also of note is that in at least one large series, mortality occurred primarily in the early morning hours [83]. Several studies have shown that there is a normal diurnal variation in airflow rates. Rates are highest in the evening (6 to 10 P.M.) and lowest in the early morning hours (4 to 6 A.M.) [35]. Exaggeration of the normal diurnal variation in airflow rates was found to be the only factor that distinguished patients who died during what by other criteria were mild attacks.

Parenchymal Causes of Acute Respiratory Failure

Clinical disorders of the lung parenchyma can be divided into those that primarily involve the pul-monary vascular bed, the lung interstitium, or the distal airspaces (alveoli) of the lung. The major effects of pulmonary vascular obstruction are usually circulatory rather than respiratory, although acute respiratory failure is characteristic of massive pulmonary embolism and severe pulmonary vasculitis [113]. Patients with acute respiratory failure due to pulmonary vascular obstruction may require intubation and mechanical ventilation while their hemodynamic status is being stabilized and attempts are being made to treat the primary vascular disorder [75,83]. Other sections in this text consider pulmonary vascular disease and pulmonary embolism in more detail.

Many interstitial lung diseases may progress to acute respiratory failure. Often the development of acute respiratory failure in the setting of chronic restrictive interstitial lung disease is a consequence of superimposed viral or bacterial lung infection. If the blood gas abnormalities are of sufficient severity, then mechanical ventilation may be needed. Appropriate antimicrobial therapy should be instituted. Occasionally, as in systemic lupus pneumonitis, an acute exacerbation may lead to acute respiratory failure and may be successfully treated with antiinflammatory agents.

The most common parenchymal causes of acute respiratory failure are diseases that result in accumulation of fluid, pus, or blood in the airspaces of the lungs. Acute respiratory failure may result from pulmonary edema (either cardiogenic or noncardiogenic), pneumonia, or aspiration syndromes that may be associated with widespread atelectasis as well as with increased permeability pulmonary edema.

CARDIOGENIC PULMONARY EDEMA

The pathogenesis of acute respiratory failure in patients with cardiogenic pulmonary edema may be complex. In addition to the edema in the lung, in some patients, particularly those with acute myocardial infarction, systemic hypotension contributes to inadequate tissue perfusion, metabolic acidosis, and decreased function of the respiratory muscles. In addition, the work of breathing may rise sufficiently to add significantly to the load on the ischemic myocardium. From a hemodynamic standpoint, the main goal of treating cardiogenic pulmonary edema is to reduce left ventricular filling pressures and thereby reduce myocardial oxygen consumption. This goal can usually be accomplished by bed rest, morphine, diuretics, and vasodilators. In addition, of course, supplemental oxygen should be given to maintain systemic arterial oxygen saturation above 95 percent.

In some patients with cardiogenic pulmonary edema, the acute respiratory failure is not satisfactorily relieved by the preceding treatments. In these patients, PaO_2 usually is less than 60 mmHg, the work of breathing is high, and the patients have metabolic acidosis. These patients will benefit from endotracheal intubation and positive-pressure ventilation, which treats both the cardiac and respiratory problems. First, mechanical ventilation reduces preload by decreasing venous return to the heart. Second, mechanical ventilation may decrease afterload on the left side of the heart by abolishing wide swings in pleural pressure produced by the dyspneic, spontaneously breathing patient. Also, mechanical ventilation improves arterial oxygenation because of better ventilation to lung units that were previously poorly ventilated. In addition, mechanical ventilation corrects respiratory acidosis and can provide appropriate respiratory compensation for a metabolic acidosis. Finally, positive-pressure ventilation takes over the work of breathing so that systemic and myocardial oxygen demand may be reduced. Ideally, endotracheal intubation can be accomplished by the nasotracheal route, thus avoiding the need for sedation or for paralyzing agents. In general, patients with cardiogenic pulmonary edema can be weaned from mechanical ventilation once their hemodynamic and gas-exchange status have improved so that they can reassume voluntary ventilation without developing myocardial ischemia or excessive work of breathing.

NONCARDIOGENIC PULMONARY EDEMA: ARDS
ARDS is a clinical constellation of symptoms that is the end result of a complex sequence of cellular and biochemical events following severe systemic or pulmonary injury [138,181]. The clinical syndrome is characterized by severe hypoxemia, diffuse infiltrates on chest radiograph, and decreased respiratory compliance (Fig. 46-12). A wide variety of clinical disorders have been associated with ARDS (Table 46-8).

Some patients develop milder forms of acute lung injury that do not reach the full-blown syndrome of severe pulmonary edema and respiratory failure [176]. It has been estimated that at least 150,000 patients develop ARDS annually in the United States, and mortality has remained high, in the range of 60 to 70 percent, which is similar to the mortality rate Petty and Asbaugh

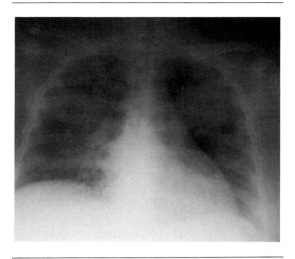

Fig. 46-12. Anteroposterior chest radiograph of a 42-year-old man with severe respiratory failure and adult respiratory distress syndrome from *E. coli* urosepsis. Note the bilateral infiltrates in both lung fields. A pulmonary artery line was inserted and revealed a pulmonary arterial wedge pressure of 5 mmHg. The patient required mechanical ventilation with an FiO_2 of 0.8 with a PaO_2 of 58 mmHg and PEEP of 10 cmH_2O.

Table 46-8. Clinical disorders associated with the adult respiratory distress syndrome

Sepsis	Shock of any etiology
Trauma	Hematologic disorders
Fat emboli	Thrombotic thrombocytopenic purpura
Lung contusion	Disseminated intravascular coagulation
Massive blood transfusions	
Liquid aspiration	Metabolic
Gastric contents	Acute pancreatitis
Fresh and salt water (drowning)	Miscellaneous
Hydrocarbon fluids	Lymphangiography
Drug-associated	Reexpansion pulmonary edema
Heroin	Neurogenic pulmonary edema
Ethchlorvynol	Postcardiopulmonary bypass
Aspirin	Eclampsia
Inhaled toxins	Air emboli
Smoke	Amniotic fluid embolism
Corrosive chemicals (NO_2, Cl_2, NH_3, phosgene)	Ascent to high altitude

reported when they first described the syndrome in 1967 [129]. It has been recognized subsequently that mortality in patients with ARDS can often be related to the clinical disorder (i.e., sepsis) that precipitated the lung injury or to associated multiorgan failure [54,111].

Epidemiology. Two large prospective studies have demonstrated that the most common clinical disorders placing patients at high risk for ARDS are sepsis and gastric aspiration. In one study from the University of Washington, 38 percent of the patients with the sepsis syndrome developed ARDS [126]. In another study from the University of Colorado, infection was associated with the development of ARDS in 44 percent of patients. This was broken down into bacteremia (10 percent), probable sepsis (10 percent), and pneumonia (11 percent) as single risk factors and infection as part of multiple risks (15 percent) [58]. Aspiration of gastric contents was the second most important cause of ARDS in these two studies. In both studies, patients were identified early, either at the time of admission to the hospital or very shortly after the development of one of the clinical disorders placing them at high risk. They were then followed closely for the devel-

opment of ARDS. There were some important differences between the two studies. First, the study by Pepe and colleagues included only patients who were intubated [126], thereby selecting a population at higher risk for developing ARDS. That study found an incidence of ARDS of 34 percent (46 of 134 patients). In contrast, the study by Fowler and associates included a broader group of patients, totaling 993 patients with a 7 percent incidence of ARDS [58]. Both studies found that the presence of more than one risk factor substantially increased the incidence of ARDS. In the study by Pepe and associates, the incidence of ARDS after a single risk factor was 18 percent, compared with 59 percent when there were multiple risk factors. Similarly, the study by Fowler and coworkers reported a 6 percent incidence of ARDS with a single risk factor, compared with a 25 percent incidence with multiple risk factors.

The results of the two studies are summarized in Table 46-9, with the specific incidence of ARDS for each clinical condition that placed patients at high risk. The estimated risk for the development of ARDS secondary to sepsis probably depends on whether investigators included evidence of systemic hypotension as part of the sepsis syndrome. For example, in the study by Fowler's

Table 46-9. Incidence of ARDS following clinical risks*

Clinical condition	Incidence of ARDS	
	Pepe et al. [126]	Fowler et al. [58]
Sepsis		
Bacteremia	—	9/239 (4%)
Sepsis syndrome	5/13 (38%)	—
Aspiration of gastric contents	7/23 (30%)	16/45 (36%)
Fractures	1/12 (8%)	2/38 (5%)
Multiple transfusions		
10 units/24 hours	—	9/197 (5%)
10 units/6 hours	4/17 (24%)	—
Cardiopulmonary bypass	—	4/237 (2%)
Burn	—	2/87 (2%)
Pneumonia in ICU	—	10/84 (12%)
Disseminated intravascular coagulation	—	2/9 (22%)
Pulmonary contusion	5/29 (17%)	—
Near-drowning	2/3	—
Pancreatitis	1/1	—
Prolonged hypotension	0/1	—

*These data refer to patients with only a single risk event. Not included are those with multiple risks.
Source: Reproduced from RJ Maunder. Clinical prediction of the adult respiratory distress syndrome. *Clin Chest Med* 6:413, 1985.

group, all patients with bacteremia were included regardless of whether they had systemic hypotension [58], and therefore the risk for developing ARDS from infection was lower. In the study from Pepe and coworkers, the risk for ARDS from bacteremia was higher because systemic hypotension was an entry criterion [126]. In addition, two studies from the University of California, San Francisco, reported that the risk of ARDS following sepsis is in the range of 30 to 40 percent when systemic hypotension is present [147,176].

Recently, Maunder reviewed various approaches for predicting the risk for ARDS using both the associated clinical disorder and hemodynamic and respiratory parameters [104]. Although it is impossible to predict with absolute certainty the development of ARDS, it is clear that a population of patients at very high risk for ARDS can be identified. In fact, this approach was successful enough for a prospective, randomized study of the possible prophylactic value of treatment with 8 cmH_2O PEEP in patients at high risk for developing ARDS. Although prophylactic PEEP did not decrease the incidence of ARDS, the study did demonstrate that a prospective evaluation of treatment for ARDS could be done on patients at high risk for developing ARDS.

One of the important discoveries from these clinical studies has been the evidence that patients may develop ARDS within 24 hours of the inciting clinical event [126]. In particular, the lag time between the development of sepsis and ARDS is short [176]. Therefore, the opportunity to begin treatment before the syndrome develops is limited. While the reported incidence of ARDS following sepsis ranges from 20 to 35 percent in retrospective and prospective studies [51,147, 176], some degree of lung injury in patients with sepsis syndrome occurs in 60 percent of patients [176]. Mortality from a combination of sepsis and ARDS approaches 90 percent, and the need for early intervention is therefore particularly important in this group of patients [147]. Further information regarding the clinical risk factors for ARDS is presented in the article by Pepe and coworkers [126].

Pathology. The morphologic alterations of the lung parenchyma in ARDS can be divided into those changes that occur in the acute phase of lung injury and those that occur in the subacute to chronic phase of ARDS. In general, the pathologic findings in ARDS are uniform and nonspe-

cific [8]. Occasionally, biopsy or postmortem specimens reveal a primary lung infection that was not previously suspected as a cause of the acute respiratory failure. The light microscopic findings in the acute phase of ARDS are characterized by diffuse alveolar damage where the alveolar spaces are inhomogeneously filled with a proteinaceous fluid that may be hemorrhagic [8]. This fluid contains abundant neutrophils and macrophages, a variety of cell fragments, and amorphous material that includes plasma proteins, fibrin strands, cell debris, and remnants of surfactant [8]. In addition, hyaline membranes are often present; these may represent the proteinaceous residue left by the protein exudate and the cell debris from the acute phase of lung injury (Fig. 46-13).

Ultrastructural studies of the lungs of patients dying in the acute phase of ARDS show that defects in the lung endothelium can be identified; however, epithelial lesions are seen more often [8]. Figure 46-14 is an electron micrograph of the lungs of a patient who died 4 days after fulminant septicemia from ARDS. This patient had both endothelial lesions and extensive epithelial injury. In summary, the morphologic findings in the acute stage of ARDS (about 2 to 5 days) are characterized by alveolar and interstitial edema with focal injury to the endothelial and epithelial barriers and an impressive increase in the number of both neutrophils and macrophages in the lung.

Some patients will have a gradual resolution of ARDS radiographically and clinically over a few days following the acute phase of lung injury, while other patients will have an acute phase of protein-rich pulmonary edema and then progress to a fibrosing alveolitis that is clinically manifested by worsening lung compliance, pulmonary hypertension, and persistent respiratory failure. It is not clear which biochemical and cellular factors control the transition from the acute to progressive fibrosis of the lungs in these ARDS patients. The light microscopic findings in patients with the subacute and chronic phases of ARDS show a marked decrease in the number of neutrophils and an increase in collagen and fibroblasts in the lungs. Ultrastructural studies have indicated that the type II alveolar epithelial cells proliferate to reepithelialize the alveolar barrier. The alveolar type II cells take on the appearance of what has been described as bulky cuboidal cells with poorly developed lamellar bodies. Generally, the type I epithelial cells that have been acutely injured cannot regenerate, and type II cells are therefore the primary reparative cells

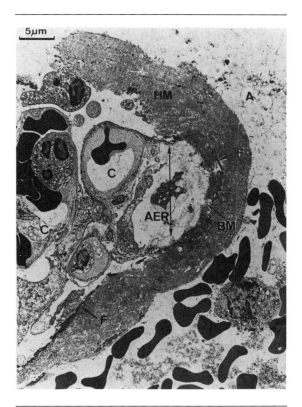

Fig. 46-13. Electron micrograph of a lung specimen from a 17-year-old woman who died of an acute fat embolism syndrome and the adult respiratory distress syndrome 3 days after a traffic accident. Alveolar entrance ring (*AER*) covered by a hyaline membrane (*HM*) composed of condensed plasma protein and fibrin strands (*F*). Close contact of hyaline membrane to the epithelial basement membrane (*BM*) is restricted to area of destroyed epithelial lamina. *A* = alveolar space; *C* = capillary. (Reproduced from M Bachofen, ER Weibel. Structural alterations of lung parenchyma in the adult respiratory distress syndrome. *Clin Chest Med* 3:35, 1982.)

that reconstitute the alveolar epithelial barrier. Plasma cells and lymphocytes are also present in the lungs at this phase [9]. In addition, there are often strands of fibrotic tissue that encompass both the airspaces and the interstitium of the lungs. The original architecture of the lungs can be completely lost. Histologic findings indicate compressed alveoli with fibrotic tissue plates surrounding the airspaces.

The total collagen content during this chronic phase was increased two- to threefold over baseline values [186]. In order to determine the con-

centration of collagen in the lungs correctly, a correction for the contribution of hemoglobin to the dry weight of lung tissue samples is necessary. It is likely that further correction is necessary, considering the protein left in the alveoli and the number of cells in the lung. Thus, the actual collagen content is probably even higher than what has been estimated.

Major changes in the vascular bed of the lungs occur in the subacute to chronic phase of ARDS. There is a partial or complete disruption and, in some cases, even disappearance of much of the pulmonary vascular bed [63]. These findings correlate with the progressive pulmonary hypertension as well as the marked decrease in single-breath carbon monoxide diffusing capacity that has been reported in some patients [50,185]. Many of these patients with the subacute to chronic phase of ARDS have thrombotic or embolic obstruction of much of the vascular bed of the lungs [63].

In the multihospital study of the extracorporeal membrane oxygenator as a treatment modality for ARDS, pathologic studies at autopsy in 59 patients showed rapid progression to fibrosis, particularly of the alveolar ducts and the distal alveolar spaces. Increased numbers of spindle-shaped fibroblastic cells in the lungs as well as some evidence of organized and active pneumonitis were also reported [74,132]. Other pathologic studies also have reported an increased frequency of secondary bacterial pneumonia in patients dying with ARDS [16].

In summary, the early pathologic changes indicate the acute phase of protein-rich pulmonary edema, associated with an influx of red blood cells, neutrophils, and a variable deposition of fibrin in both the interstitium and the airspaces of the lungs. After a few days, the acute inflammatory response usually resolves, and much of the edema fluid is removed. Hyaline membranes (precipitated protein) become prominent, and in some patients with persistent ARDS, variable degrees of fibrosis, loss of normal lung architecture, and obliteration of the normal vascular bed of the lungs occur. These changes are relatively nonspecific in terms of the etiology of acute lung injury.

Pathogenesis. The pathogenesis of the acute lung injury probably depends in part on the associated clinical disorder. For instance, most of the associated disorders can be divided into those in which the injury to the lung is delivered via the bloodstream (sepsis, fat emboli) or via the airways (gastric aspiration, inhaled toxic gases)

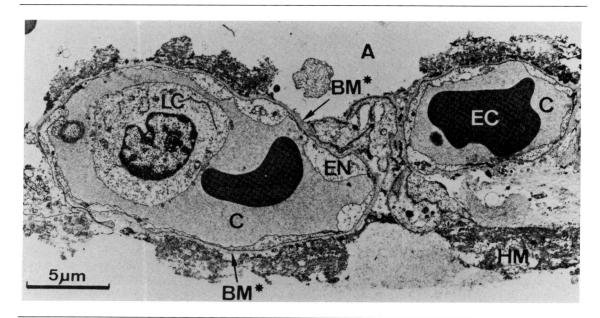

Fig. 46-14. Electron micrograph of the alveolar septum with extensive endothelial and epithelial destruction in a 19-year-old woman who died after 4 days of fulminant pulmonary edema from septicemia. Note the irregularly swollen but continuous endothelial cell layer. Also, there is some denuding of the epithelium. A = alveolar space; BM^* = denuded basement membrane; C = capillary; EC = intravascular erythrocyte; E = swollen endothelial cell; HM = hyaline membrane; LC = intravascular leukocyte. (Reproduced from M Bachofen, ER Weibel. Structural alterations of lung parenchyma in the adult respiratory distress syndrome. *Clin Chest Med* 3:35, 1982.)

[181]. Clinically, all the disorders lead to an increase in alveolar-capillary permeability and subsequent pulmonary edema and atelectasis, but the precise pathways for lung injury may be somewhat different.

A wide variety of mediators have been implicated in the pathogenesis of the lung injury, including complement, neutrophils, proteases, coagulation factors, platelets, prostaglandins, lymphokines, and tumor necrosis factor, a product of macrophages [181]. The specific role of these factors varies in different experimental models of lung injury, and no clinical studies have as yet identified one single common pathway. In fact, it appears that the pathogenesis of lung injury may vary depending on the associated clinical disorder. For example, activated neutrophils probably participate in increasing lung vascular permeability under some conditions, but ARDS has been well documented to occur in patients who are severely neutropenic [105]. Little information is available on the factors that influence the transformation of acute ARDS to the subacute to chronic phase, where fibrosis, pulmonary vascular destruction, and abnormalities of surfactant become important. As already mentioned, only about 20 percent of ARDS patients actually succumb to respiratory failure [111]. The majority die from recurrent sepsis or multiorgan dysfunction.

Pathophysiology. The severe hypoxemia in ARDS results primarily from right-to-left intrapulmonary shunts through fluid-filled and atelectatic alveoli (see Fig. 46-1). Lung volumes are decreased because of the edema fluid in the alveoli and microatelectasis [181]. There is a decrease in lung compliance due to the edema fluid in the alveoli and the interstitium and to increased surface tension resulting from intraalveolar protein exudate and inflammatory cells. The reduced compliance means that for any distending pressure the lung volume is smaller than normal. Therefore, higher pressures are required to ventilate these patients at tidal volumes of 12 to 15 ml/kg. Indeed, serial measurements of the static compliance of the chest wall and lung utilizing the end-inspiration plateau airway pressure and the expired tidal volume are useful in following the course of ARDS patients.

Some patients with noncardiogenic pulmonary edema or ARDS may have hemodynamic instability or frank cardiac dysfunction. Systemic hypotension and metabolic acidosis are characteristic of patients with sepsis syndrome and complicate management of patients with sepsis-induced ARDS [27]. Some patients have preexistent left ventricular disease that complicates the acute respiratory failure that develops in the presence of acute lung injury [171]. In addition, mild elevations of pulmonary arterial pressure are characteristic of the early phase of ARDS and may be associated with increased afterload on the right ventricle, particularly in the face of marked elevations of PEEP. Frank right-sided heart failure may develop later in the course of ARDS when patients have developed more severe pulmonary hypertension in association with diffuse parenchymal damage and obliteration of portions of the pulmonary vascular bed.

Management. Treatment of ARDS is primarily supportive, since there are as yet no pharmacologic agents that reverse the permeability defect and help to hasten the resolution of the pulmonary edema [181]. Treatment of the underlying disorder is critical. For example, if sepsis is the likely cause of acute lung injury, it is mandatory to treat with broad-spectrum antimicrobial agents and, if necessary, drain any collections of pus. It is also important to be certain that the diagnosis of ARDS does not obscure the possibility that a primary, treatable lung infection may be present, particularly if the patient is immunosuppressed.

The main goal of treatment is to guarantee adequate oxygenation and to achieve hemodynamic stability without worsening pulmonary function. Mechanical ventilation is required with high tidal volumes to reexpand atelectatic and partially fluid-filled alveoli that can then participate in gas exchange; PEEP should be delivered as a further means of increasing functional residual capacity and recruiting alveoli for ventilation; the FIO_2 can be controlled and, hopefully, reduced in the presence of optimal mechanical ventilation with high tidal volumes and PEEP; and mechanical ventilation allows the patient to rest and the work of breathing to be assumed by the mechanical ventilator.

One of the most common problems in managing patients with ARDS is to determine the optimal level of PEEP [27]. While PEEP improves oxygenation, it may decrease cardiac output and thus decrease tissue oxygen delivery. Higher levels of PEEP may be associated with an increased risk of barotrauma to the lungs. For these reasons, the risk-benefit ratio of PEEP must be weighed carefully. In most patients, a level of PEEP between 10 and 15 cmH_2O is satisfactory for achieving reasonable oxygenation without markedly impairing the cardiac output. PEEP does not reverse the course of acute lung injury but simply provides a means of improving oxygenation at a lower FIO_2 [128]. Also, all patients with ARDS have a marked increase in their dead-space or wasted ventilation fraction [see Eq. (46-4)], and PEEP does not alter this problem because the increase in wasted ventilation is related to loss of vascular perfusion to the lungs (see the section on the pathology of ARDS).

It is not clear at what oxygen concentrations or over what time period oxygen toxicity will complicate acute lung injury. Nevertheless, extrapolation from experimental data suggests that oxygen concentrations in the range of 50 to 60 percent are unlikely to contribute in a major way to progressive lung injury. Therefore, a reasonable goal is to adjust the level of PEEP to achieve an FIO_2 of approximately 0.5 to 0.6. This may not be possible in the first 24 to 48 hours of ARDS, particularly if the patient has septicemia.

Some investigators have recommended closely following the effects of different levels of PEEP on pulmonary and systemic hemodynamics with measurements of cardiac output, arterial-venous oxygen content differences, as well as end-organ indices of tissue perfusion such as urine output, pH, and mental status. It is useful in some patients to monitor the effects of different levels of PEEP on cardiac output and systemic oxygen transport [see Eqs. (46-7) and (46-8)]. However, there is no substitute for the clinical evidence of end-organ perfusion. For example, a patient may have a fall in cardiac output of 15 percent with an increase of PEEP from 10 to 15 cmH_2O; however, if urine flow, renal function, arterial pH, and mental status are not adversely affected, then there is no reason for concern. Measurement of arterial-venous oxygen content differences is not useful in patients with ARDS because the mixed venous oxygen tension does not reliably reflect the changes in cardiac output. There are some data, in fact, that suggest that mixed venous oxygen tension in patients with ARDS is more a function of changing oxygen consumption than of specific levels of oxygen transport or cardiac output [27].

Hemodynamic monitoring of pulmonary vascular filling pressures may be particularly useful in the early phase of ARDS. Measurement of the pulmonary arterial wedge pressure can help to confirm that the cause of the pulmonary edema is indeed noncardiogenic. It has been shown that some patients with primary acute lung injury have coexistent modest elevations in pulmonary arterial wedge pressure [171]. Treatment with diuretics may then lower the pulmonary venous pressures and in turn decrease the pulmonary edema. If the wedge pressure is in the normal range, then the monitoring of the filling pressure can be useful to guide fluid therapy, particularly in patients in whom there is associated systemic hypotension that requires treatment with intravenous fluids, packed red blood cells, or plasma expanders.

In general, if volume expansion is needed, the first choice should be packed red blood cells to maintain a hematocrit between 35 to 40 percent. If further volume expansion is required, then administration of crystalloid is preferable to colloid solutions because protein-containing solutions will simply extravasate from the circulation and worsen the pulmonary edema. In some patients, particularly those with mild to moderate systemic hypotension, it may be useful to administer a vasopressor agent to help maintain blood pressure and renal perfusion and to minimize the total volume of fluids administered in an attempt to maintain the pulmonary capillary wedge pressure as low as is compatible with a reasonable cardiac output.

Dopamine is particularly useful as an agent to increase renal blood flow, although it does usually result in a mild increase in pulmonary capillary wedge pressure [110]. For this reason, dobutamine is a preferred agent, although it does not increase renal blood flow and urine flow as well as dopamine [110]. In patients with frank left-sided heart failure, systemic vasodilators may be useful, although they may further impair oxygenation because of a direct inhibitory effect on hypoxic pulmonary vasoconstriction. In the last phases of ARDS with frank right-sided heart failure, vasodilating agents have been used with some success in increasing cardiac output, although no definitive effect on outcome has been demonstrated. Hydralazine is the vasodilator of choice for reducing right or left ventricular afterload because it has the least effect on compromising oxygenation.

Treatment with corticosteroids is not useful in patients with established ARDS [91,181]. In the future, replacement of surfactant may be shown to be a useful treatment to improve gas exchange and lung mechanics, permitting earlier extubation [99]. Monoclonal antibody therapy for sepsis may attenuate the acute lung injury and the associated multiorgan failure [13]. If tumor necrosis factor (TNF) is an important mediator of lung injury, then specific anti-TNF antibodies might be useful in treating ARDS early in the course.

Much more needs to be learned about the resolution of pulmonary edema and the process of recovery from lung injury. Experimental and clinical studies have shown that removal of alveolar edema across the alveolar epithelial barrier depends on active sodium transport, a process that can be stimulated with beta-adrenergic agonists [20]. The normality of function of the alveolar epithelial barrier after acute lung injury may be an imporant determinant of prognosis for recovery [103]. Type II epithelial cells probably play a role in the process of alveolar liquid clearance since they have been shown to transport Na^+ and form domes of fluid in in vitro studies. Also, type II cells synthesize and release surfactant, and they are responsible for restoring an epithelial barrier after type I epithelial cells are injured. More in vitro and in vivo physiology and cell biology studies are needed to provide insight into the pathogenesis and resolution of this syndrome. Efforts to prevent infection and sepsis are very important because it has been shown that sepsis is the leading cause of death in patients with ARDS [16,111].

The patients who survive ARDS will usually have some residual pulmonary function abnormalities, including a decrease in diffusing capacity, mild to moderate decrease in VC, and even mild obstructive lung disease in some individuals. However, these abnormalities usually improve gradually and are not usually severe [50,181].

Acknowledgments

This work was supported in part by Pulmonary Vascular SCOR grant HL 19155.

References

1. Aberle DR, et al. Hydrostatic versus increased permeability pulmonary edema: Diagnosis based on radiographic criteria in critically ill patients. *Radiology* 168:73, 1988.
2. Albert RK, Martin TR, Lewis SW. Controlled

clinical trial of methylprednisolone in patients with chronic bronchitis and acute respiratory insufficiency. *Ann Intern Med* 92:753, 1980.

3. Anthonisen NR, Cherniack RM. Ventilatory Control in Lung Disease. In C Roussos, PT Macklem (Eds), *The Thorax.* New York: Marcel Dekker, 1985. Pp 965–987.

4. Appel D, et al. Lactic acidosis in severe asthma. *Am J Med* 75:580, 1983.

5. Appel D, et al. Lactic acidosis in severe asthma. *Am J Med* 75:580, 1983.

6. Attose MD. Assessment and management of breathlessness. *Chest* 88(Suppl):779, 1985.

7. Aubier M, et al. Central respiratory drive in acute respiratory failure of patients with chronic obstructive lung disease. *Am Rev Respir Dis* 122:191, 1980.

8. Bachofen M, Weibel ER. Alterations of the gas exchange apparatus in adult respiratory insufficiency associated with septicemia. *Am Rev Respir Dis* 116:589, 1977.

9. Bachofen M, Weibel ER. Structural alterations of lung parenchyma in the adult respiratory distress syndrome. *Clin Chest Med* 3:35, 1982.

10. Band JD, Maki DG. Infections caused by arterial catheters used for hemodynamic monitoring. *Am J Med* 67:735, 1979.

11. Banner AS, Shah RS, Addington WW. Rapid prediction of need for hospitalization in acute asthma. *JAMA* 235:1337, 1976.

12. Barker SJ, Tremper KK, Gamel DM. A clinical comparison of transcutaneous PO_2 and pulse oximetry in the operating room. *Anesth Analg* 65:805, 1986.

13. Baumgartner JD, et al. Prevention of gram-negative shock and death in surgical patients by antibody to endotoxin core glycolipid. *Lancet* 2:59, 1985.

14. Bedford RF. Radial arterial function following percutaneous cannulation with 18- and 20-gauge catheters. *Anesthesiology* 47:37, 1977.

15. Bedford RF. Long-term radial artery cannulation: Effects on subsequent vessel function. *Crit Care Med* 6:64, 1978.

16. Bell RC, et al. Multiple organ system failure and infection in adult respiratory distress syndrome. *Ann Intern Med* 99:293, 1983.

17. Benowitz N, Rosenberg J, Becker CE. Cardiopulmonary Catastrophes in Drug-Overdosed Patients. In MM Scheinman (Ed), *Cardiac Emergencies.* Philadelphia: Saunders, 1984. Pp 316–348.

18. Bergofsky EH. Respiratory failure in disorders of the thoracic cage. *Am Rev Respir Dis* 119:643, 1979.

19. Bernhard WN, et al. Intracuff pressures in endotracheal and tracheostomy tubes. *Chest* 87:720, 1985.

20. Berthiaume Y, Staub NC, Matthay, MA. Beta-adrenergic agonists increase lung liquid clearance in anesthetized sheep. *J Clin Invest* 79:335, 1987.

21. Bone RC. Monitoring ventilatory mechanics in acute respiratory failure. *Respir Care* 28:597, 1983.

22. Boushey HA, et al. Bronchial hyperreactivity. *Am Rev Respir Dis* 121:389, 1980.

23. Boutros AR, Lee C. Value of continuous monitoring of mixed venous blood oxygen saturation in the management of critically ill patients. *Crit Care Med* 14:132, 1986.

24. Brackett NC Jr, Cohen JJ, Schwartz WB. Carbon dioxide titration curve of normal man: Effect of increasing degrees of acute hypercapnia on acid-base equilibrium. *N Engl J Med* 272:6, 1965.

25. Brackett NC Jr, et al. Acid-base response to chronic hypercapnia in man. *N Engl J Med* 280:124, 1969.

26. Branson RD, Hurst JM, DeHaven CB Jr. Mask CPAP: State of the art. *Respir Care* 30:846, 1985.

27. Broaddus VC, et al. Hemodynamic management of the adult respiratory distress syndrome. *J Intensive Care Med* 2:190, 1987.

28. Broadovsky D, McDonnell JA, Cherniack RM. The respiratory response to carbon dioxide in health and in emphysema. *J Clin Invest* 39:724, 1960.

29. Brochard L, et al. Reversal of acute exacerbations of chronic obstructive lung disease by inspiratory assistance with a face mask. *N Engl J Med* 323:1523, 1990.

30. Bryant DH, Rogers P. Effects of ipratropium bromide nebulizer solution with and without preservatives in the treatment of acute and stable asthma. *Chest* 102:742, 1992.

31. Burrows B, Earle RH. Course and prognosis of chronic obstructive pulmonary disease. *N Engl J Med* 280:397, 1969.

32. Campbell EJM. The management of acute respiratory failure in chronic bronchitis and emphysema. *Am Rev Respir Dis* 95:626, 1967.

33. Centor RM, Yarbrough B, Wood JP. Inability to predict relapse in bronchial asthma. *N Engl J Med* 310:577, 1984.

34. Chatterjee K, et al. Effects of vasodilator therapy for severe pump failure in acute myocardial infarction on short-term and late prognosis. *Circulation* 53:797, 1976.

35. Clark TJH, Hetzel MR. Diurnal variation of asthma. *Br J Dis Chest* 71:87, 1977.

36. Cochrane GM, Clark TJH. A survey of asthma mortality in patients between ages 35 and 64 in the greater London hospitals in 1971. *Thorax* 30:300, 1975.

37. Cohen CA, et al. Clinical manifestations of inspiratory muscle fatigue. *Am J Med* 73:308, 1982.

38. Connors AF Jr, McCaffree DR, Gray BA. Evaluation of right-heart catheterization in the criti-

cally ill patient without acute myocardial infarction. *N Engl J Med* 308:263, 1983.

39. Cook JL. Infection in asthma. *Semin Respir Med* 8:259, 1987.

40. Curtis JL, et al. Helium-oxygen gas therapy: Use and availability for the emergency treatment of inoperable airway obstruction. *Chest* 90:455, 1986.

41. Dantzker DR, Tobin MJ. Monitoring respiratory muscle function. *Respir Care* 30:422, 1985.

42. Darioli R, Perret C. Mechanical controlled hypoventilation in status asthmaticus. *Am Rev Respir Dis* 129:385, 1984.

43. Davis FM, Stewart JM. Radial artery cannulation. *Br J Anaesth* 52:41, 1980.

44. Dhainault JF, Devaux J, Monsallier J. Mechanisms of decreased left ventricular preload during continuous positive pressure ventilation in ARDS. *Chest* 90:74, 1986.

45. Dimarco A, et al. Comparative effect of aminophylline on diaphragm and cardiac contractility. *Am Rev Respir Dis* 132:800, 1985.

46. Douglass JA, et al. Myopathy in severe asthma. *Am Rev Respir Dis* 146:517, 1992.

47. Dunnhill MS. The pathology of asthma with special reference to changes in the bronchial mucosa. *J Clin Pathol* 13:27, 1960.

48. Dyck PJ, Kurtzke JF. Plasmapheresis in Guillain-Barré syndrome. *Neurology* 35:1105, 1985.

49. Eisendrath SJ, et al. Guillain-Barré syndrome: Psychosocial aspects of management. *Psychosomatics* 24:465, 1983.

50. Elliot CG, Morris AH, Cengiz M. Pulmonary function and exercise gas exchange in survivors of the adult respiratory distress syndrome. *Am Rev Respir Dis* 123:492, 1981.

51. Fanconi S, et al. Pulse oximetry in pediatric intensive care comparison with measured saturations and transcutaneous oxygen tension. *J Pediatr* 107:362, 1985.

52. Fanta CH, Rossing TH, McFadden ER Jr. Emergency room treatment of asthma. *Am J Med* 72:416, 1982.

53. Fein A, et al. Is pulmonary artery catheterization necessary for the diagnosis of pulmonary edema? *Am Rev Respir Dis* 129:1006, 1984.

54. Fein A, et al. The risk factors, incidence and prognosis of the adult respiratory distress syndrome following septicemia. *Chest* 83:40, 1983.

55. Fewell JE, et al. Mechanism of decreased right and left ventricular end-diastolic volumes during continuous positive-pressure ventilation in dogs. *Circ Res* 47:467, 1980.

56. Fischl MA, Pitchenik A, Gardner LB. An index predicting relapse and need for hospitalization in patients with acute bronchial asthma. *N Engl J Med* 305:783, 1981.

57. Fouts JB, Brashear RE. Intermittent positive-pressure breathing, a critical appraisal. *Postgrad Med* 59:103, 1976.

58. Fowler AA, et al. Adult respiratory distress syndrome: Prognosis after onset. *Am Rev Respir Dis* 132:472, 1985.

59. Gardner RM, et al. Percutaneous indwelling radial-artery catheters for monitoring cardiovascular function. *N Engl J Med* 290:1227, 1974.

60. Glenn WL, et al. Ventilatory support by pacing of the conditioned diaphragm in quadriplegia. *N Engl J Med* 310:1150, 1984.

61. Gottfried SB, et al. Interrupter technique for measurement of respiratory mechanics in anesthetized humans. *J Appl Physiol* 59:647, 1985.

62. Gracey D, et al. Respiratory failure in Guillain-Barré syndrome. *Mayo Clin Proc* 57:742, 1982.

63. Greene R, et al. Early bedside detectors of pulmonary vascular occlusion during acute respiratory failure. *Am Rev Respir Dis* 124:593, 1981.

64. Griffin D, et al. Acute myopathy during treatment of status asthmaticus with corticosteroids and steroidal muscle relaxants. *Chest* 102:510, 1992.

65. Grob D. Acute neuromuscular disorders. *Med Clin North Am* 65:189, 1981.

66. Guillain-Barré Syndrome Study Group. Plasmapheresis and acute Guillain-Barré syndrome. *Neurology* 35:1096, 1985.

67. Gump DW, et al. Role of infection in chronic bronchitis. *Am Rev Respir Dis* 113:465, 1976.

68. Hansen RM, et al. Poor correlation between pulmonary arterial wedge pressure and left ventricular end-diastolic volume after coronary artery bypass surgery. *Anesthesiology* 64:764, 1986.

69. Haskell RJ, Wong BM, Hansen JE. A double-blind, randomized clinical trial of methylprednisolone in status asthmaticus. *Arch Intern Med* 143:1324, 1983.

70. Heffner J, Miller KS, Sahn SA. Tracheostomy in the intensive care unit. *Chest* 90:269 (part I) and 430 (part II), 1986.

71. Heffner JE, Sahn SA. Salicylate-induced pulmonary edema. *Ann Intern Med* 95:405, 1981.

72. Henschel EO. The Guillain-Barré syndrome: A personal experience. *Anesthesiology* 47:228, 1977.

73. Hetzel MR, Clark TJH, Branthwaite MA. Asthma: Analysis of sudden deaths and ventilatory arrests in hospital. *Br Med J* 1:808, 1977.

74. Hill JD, et al. Pulmonary pathology in acute respiratory insufficiency: Lung biopsy as a diagnostic tool. *J Thorac Cardiovasc Surg* 71:64, 1976.

75. Hoagland PM. Massive Pulmonary Embolism. In SZ Goldhaber (Ed), *Pulmonary Embolism and Deep Venous Thrombosis*. Philadelphia: Saunders, 1985. Pp 179–208.

76. Hogg JC, Macklem PT, Thurlbeck WM. Site and nature of airways obstructive lung disease. *N Engl J Med* 278:1355, 1968.

77. Holtzman MJ, et al. Importance of airway inflammation for hyperresponsiveness induced by ozone. *Am Rev Respir Dis* 137:686, 1983.

78. Hund E, et al. Intensive management and treatment of severe Guillain-Barre syndrome. *Crit Care Med* 21:433, 1993.

79. Jardin F, et al. Influence of positive end-expiratory pressure on left ventricular performance. *N Engl J Med* 304:387, 1981.

80. Kassires JP, et al. The critical role of chloride in the correction of hypokalemic alkalosis in man. *Am J Med* 38:172, 1965.

81. Kelsen SG, et al. Emergency room assessment and treatment of patients with acute asthma. *Am J Med* 64:622, 1978.

82. Ketty SS, Schmidt CF. The effects of altered arterial tensions of carbon dioxide and oxygen on cerebral blood flow and cerebral oxygen consumption of normal young men. *J Clin Invest* 27:484, 1948.

83. Kilburn KH. Shock, seizures and coma with alkalosis during mechanical ventilation. *Ann Intern Med* 66:977, 1966.

84. King TE, Chang S-W. Corticosteroid therapy in the management of asthma. *Semin Respir Med* 8:387, 1987.

85. Lareau SC, Ryan KJ, Diener CF. The relationship between frequency of ventilator circuit changes and infectious hazard. *Am Rev Respir Dis* 118:493, 1978.

86. Larsson S, Svedmyr N. Bronchodilating effect and side effects of beta-adrenoceptor stimulants by different routes of administration (tablets, metered aerosol, and combinations thereof). *Am Rev Respir Dis* 116:861, 1977.

87. Leventhal JM. Clinical predictors of pneumonia as a guide to ordering chest roentgenograms. *Clin Pediatr* 21:730, 1982.

88. Leventhal SR, Orkin FK, Hirsh RA. Prediction of the need for postoperative mechanical ventilation in myasthenia gravis. *Anesthesiology* 53:26, 1980.

89. Loh L, Goldman M, Davis JN. The assessment of diaphragm function. *Medicine* 56:165, 1977.

90. Luce JM. Medical management of spinal cord injury. *Crit Care Med* 13:126, 1985.

91. Luce JM, et al. Ineffectiveness of high-dose methylprednisolone in preventing parenchymal lung injury and improving mortality in patients with septic shock. *Am Rev Respir Dis* 138:62, 1988.

92. Luce JM, Pierson DJ, Hudson LD. Intermittent mandatory ventilation. *Chest* 76:678, 1981.

93. MacIntyre NR. Respiratory function during pressure support ventilation. *Chest* 89:677, 1986.

94. Marini JJ. Obtaining meaningful data from the Swan-Ganz catheter. *Respir Care* 30:572, 1985.

95. Marini JJ. Weaning from mechanical ventilation. *N Engl J Med* 324:1496, 1991.

96. Marini JJ, Rodriguez RM, Lamb V. Bedside estimation of the inspiratory work of breathing during mechanical ventilation. *Chest* 89:56, 1986.

97. Martin J, et al. The role of respiratory muscles in the hyperinflation of bronchial asthma. *Am Rev Respir Dis* 121:441, 1980.

98. Martin TR, Lewis S, Albert RK. The prognosis of patients with chronic obstructive pulmonary disease after hospitalization for acute respiratory failure. *Chest* 82:310, 1982.

99. Mason RJ. Pulmonary alveolar type II epithelial cells and adult respiratory distress syndrome. *West J Med* 143:611, 1985.

100. Matthay MA. Invasive hemodynamic monitoring. *Clin Chest Med* 4:233, 1983.

101. Matthay MA, Chatterjee K. Bedside catheterization of the pulmonary artery: Risks compared with benefits. *Ann Intern Med* 109:826, 1988.

102. Matthay MA, Eschenbacher WL, Goetzl EJ. Elevated concentrations of leukotriene D_4 in pulmonary edema fluid of patients with the adult respiratory distress syndrome. *J Clin Immunol* 4:479, 1984.

103. Matthay MA, Wiener-Kronish JP. Intact epithelial barrier function is critical for the resolution of alveolar edema in humans. *Am Rev Respir Dis* 142:1250, 1990.

104. Maunder RJ. Clinical prediction of the adult respiratory distress syndrome. *Clin Chest Med* 6:413, 1985.

105. Maunder RJ, et al. Occurrence of the adult respiratory distress syndrome in neutropenic patients. *Am Rev Respir Dis* 133:313, 1986.

106. McFadden ER Jr, Kaiser R, DeGroot WJ. Acute bronchial asthma. *N Engl J Med* 288:221, 1973.

107. Mellemgaard K. The alveolar-arterial oxygen difference: Its size and components in normal man. *Acta Physiol Scand* 67:10, 1966.

108. Mickell JJ, et al. Clinical implications of postoperative unilateral phrenic nerve paralysis. *J Thorac Cardiovasc Surg* 75:297, 1978.

109. Mitchell RS, et al. The morphologic features of the bronchi, bronchioles and alveoli in chronic airway obstruction: A clinicopathologic study. *Am Rev Respir Dis* 114:137, 1976.

110. Molloy DW, et al. Hemodynamic management in clinical acute hypoxemia respiratory failure. *Chest* 89:636, 1986.

111. Montgomery AB, et al. Causes of mortality in patients with the adult respiratory distress syndrome. *Am Rev Respir Dis* 132:479, 1985.

112. Moore P, James O. Guillain-Barré syndrome: Incidence, management and outcome of major complications. *Crit Care Med* 9:549, 1981.

113. Moser KM. Pulmonary embolism. *Am Rev Respir Dis* 115:829, 1977.

114. Moser KM, et al. Respiratory stimulation with intravenous doxapram in respiratory failure. *N Engl J Med* 288:427, 1973.

115. Mountain R, Zwillich C, Weil JV. Hypoventilation in obstructive lung disease. *N Engl J Med* 10:521, 1978.

116. Murray JF. Classification of polycythemic disorders with comments on the diagnostic value of arterial blood oxygen analysis. *Ann Intern Med* 64:892, 1966.

117. Nadel JA, Tierney DF. Effect of a previous deep inspiration on airway resistance in man. *J Appl Physiol* 16:401, 1961.

118. Nagai A, et al. The National Institutes of Health Intermittent Positive Pressure Breathing Trial I: Interrelationship between morphologic lesions. *Am Rev Respir Dis* 132:937, 1985.

119. Nagai A, West WW, Thurlbeck WM. The National Institutes of Health Intermittent Positive Pressure Breathing Trial II: Correlation between morphologic findings, clinical findings and evidence of air-flow obstruction. *Am Rev Respir Dis* 132:946, 1985.

120. National Institutes of Health. Consensus-development conference on critical care medicine. *Crit Care Med* 11:466, 1983.

121. Newman JH, Neff TA, Zipporin P. Acute respiratory failure associated with hypophosphatemia. *N Engl J Med* 296:1101, 1977.

122. Nowak RM, et al. Comparison of peak expiratory flow and FEV$_1$ admission criteria for acute bronchial asthma. *Ann Emerg Med* 11:64, 1982.

123. O'Donohue WJ Jr, Baker JP. Controlled low-flow oxygen in the management of acute respiratory failure. *Chest* 63:818, 1973.

124. O'Quinn R, Marini JJ. Pulmonary artery occlusion pressure: Clinical physiology measurement, and interpretation. *Am Rev Respir Dis* 128:319, 1983.

125. O'Rourke PP, Crone RK. Halothane in status asthmaticus. *Crit Care Med* 10:341, 1982.

126. Pepe PE, et al. Clinical predictors of the adult respiratory distress syndrome. *Am J Surg* 144:124, 1982.

127. Pepe PE, Marini JJ. Occult positive end-expiratory pressure in mechanically ventilated patients with airflow obstruction: The auto-PEEP effect. *Am Rev Respir Dis* 126:166, 1982.

128. Pepe PE, Hudson CD, Carrico CJ. Early application of positive end-expiratory pressure in patients at risk for the adult respiratory distress syndrome. *N Engl J Med* 311:281, 1984.

129. Petty TL, Asbaugh DG. The adult respiratory distress syndrome: Clinical factors influencing prognosis and principles of management. *Chest* 60:233, 1971.

130. Petty TL. Acute Respiratory Failure in COPD. In TL Petty (Ed), *Chronic Obstructive Pulmonary Disease.* New York: Marcel Dekker, 1978. Pp 163–180.

131. Pierson DJ. Weaning from mechanical ventilation in acute respiratory failure: Concepts, indications, and techniques. *Respir Care* 28:646, 1983.

132. Pratt P, et al. Pulmonary morphology in a multihospital collaborative extracorporeal membrane oxygenation project: I. Light microscopy. *Am J Pathol* 85:210, 1976.

133. Quinn K, Quebbeman EJ. Pulmonary artery pressure monitoring in the surgical intensive care unit. *Arch Surg* 116:872, 1981.

134. Rebuck AS, Pengelly LD. Development of pulsus paradoxus in the presence of airways obstruction. *N Engl J Med* 288:66, 1973.

135. Rebuck AS, Read J. Assessment and management of severe asthma. *Am J Med* 51:788, 1971.

136. Rees HA, Millar JS, Wood KW. A study of the clinical course and arterial blood gas tensions of patients in status asthmaticus. *Q J Med* 148:541,1968.

137. Rinaldo JE. Indicators of risk, course, and prognosis in adult respiratory distress syndrome. *Annu Rev Respir Dis* 133:343, 1986.

138. Rinaldo JE, Rogers RM. Adult respiratory-distress syndrome. *N Engl J Med* 306:900, 1982.

139. Rippe JM, et al. *Intensive Care Medicine.* Boston: Little, Brown, 1985.

140. Robin ED. The cult of the Swan-Ganz catheter: Overuse and abuse of pulmonary flow catheters. *Ann Intern Med* 103:445, 1985.

141. Rochester DF, Martin LL. Respiratory Muscle Rest. In C Roussos, PT Macklem (Eds), *The Thorax* New York: Marcel Dekker, 1985. Pp 1303–1328.

142. Rose CC, Murphy JG, Schwartz JS. Performance of an index predicting the response of patients with acute bronchial asthma to intensive emergency department treatment. *N Engl J Med* 310:573, 1984.

143. Rossing TH, Fanta CH, McFadden ER Jr. Medical Housestaff of the Peter Bent Brigham Hospital: A controlled trial of single versus combined drug therapy in the treatment of acute episodes of asthma. *Am Rev Respir Dis* 123:190, 1981.

144. Roussos C, Macklem PT. Diaphragmatic fatigue in man. *J Appl Physiol* 43:189, 1977.

145. Roussos C. Ventilatory Failure and Respiratory Muscle. In C Roussos, PT Macklem (Eds), *The Thorax.* New York: Marcel Dekker, 1985. Pp 1253–1279.

146. Roussos C, Moxham J. Respiratory Muscle Fatigue. In C Roussos, PT Macklem (Eds), *The Thorax.* New York: Marcel Dekker, 1985. Pp 829–870.

147. Rubin D, et al. Elevated von Willebrand factor antigen is an early plasma predictor of acute lung injury in non-pulmonary sepsis syndrome. *J Clin Invest* 86:474, 1990.

148. Rubinfeld AR, Wagner PD, West JB. Gas ex-

change during acute experimental canine asthma. *Am Rev Respir Dis* 118:525, 1978.

149. Russell J, et al. Prospective evaluation of radial and femoral artery catheterization sites in critically ill patients. *Crit Care Med* 11:9, 1983.

150. Sackner JD, et al. Noninvasive measurement of ventilation during exercise using a respiratory inductive plethysmograph. *Am Rev Respir Dis* 122:867, 1981.

151. Schnapp LM, Cohen NH. Pulse oximetry: Uses and abuses. *Chest* 98:1244, 1990.

152. Segredo V, et al. Persistent paralysis in critically ill patients after long-term administration of vecuronium. *N Engl J Med* 327:524, 1992.

153. Shackford SR, Virgilio RW, Peters RM. Selective use of ventilator therapy in flail chest injury. *J Thorac Cardiovasc Surg* 81:194, 1981.

154. Shapiro BA. Monitoring gas exchange in acute respiratory failure. *Respir Care* 28:605, 1983.

155. Shaver JA. Hemodynamic monitoring in the critically ill patient (editorial). *N Engl J Med* 308:277, 1983.

156. Shim C, Williams MH Jr. Bronchial response to oral versus aerosol metaproterenol in asthma. *Ann Intern Med* 93:428, 1980.

157. Shinozaki T, et al. Bacterial contamination of arterial lines: A prospective study. *JAMA* 249:223, 1983.

158. Shridharani M, Reed TM. Pulmonary lavage in a patient in status asthmaticus receiving mechanical ventilation: A case report. *Ann Allergy* 49:156, 1982.

159. Sperelakis N. Pathophysiology of Skeletal Muscle and Effect of Some Hormones. In C Roussos, PT Macklem (Eds), *The Thorax*. New York: Marcel Dekker, 1985. Pp 115–140.

160. Stauffer JL, Silvestri RC. Complications of endotracheal intubation, tracheostomy and artificial airways. *Respir Care* 27:417, 1982.

161. Steingrub JS, et al. Therapeutic impact of pulmonary artery catheterization in a medical/surgical ICU. *Chest* 99:1451, 1991.

162. Straub PW, Buhlmann AA, Rossier PH. Hypovolemia in status asthmaticus. *Lancet* 1:923, 1969.

163. Swan HJ, et al. Catheterization of the heart in man with the use of a flow-directed balloon-tipped catheter. *N Engl J Med* 283:447, 1970.

164. Tai E, Read J. Blood gas tensions in bronchial asthma. *Lancet* 1:644, 1967.

165. Takizawa T, Thurlbeck WM. Muscle and mucous gland size in the major bronchi of patients with chronic bronchitis, asthma and asthmatic bronchitis. *Am Rev Respir Dis* 104:331, 1971.

166. Tami T, et al. Pulmonary edema and acute upper airway obstruction. *Laryngoscope* 96:506, 1986.

167. Thiringer G, Svedmyr N. Comparison of infused and inhaled terbutaline in patients with asthma. *Scand J Respir Dis* 57:17, 1976.

168. Thurlbeck WM. The Morphology of Chronic Bronchitis Asthma and Bronchiectasis. In JL Bennington (Ed), *Chronic Airflow Obstruction in Lung Disease*. Philadelphia: Saunders, 1976. Pp 31–95.

169. Toews GB. Use of antibiotics in patients with chronic obstructive pulmonary disease. *Semin Respir Med* 8:165, 1986.

170. Tooker J, Huseby J, Butler J. The effect of Swan-Ganz catheter height on the wedge pressure relationship in edema during positive pressure ventilation. *Am Rev Respir Dis* 117:721, 1978.

171. Unger KM, Shibel EM, Moser KM. Defection of left ventricular failure in patients with adult respiratory distress syndrome. *Chest* 67:8, 1975.

172. VanderMeche F, et al. A randomized trial comparing intravenous immune globulin and plasma exchange in Guillain-Barre syndrome. *N Engl J Med* 326:1123, 1992.

173. Wagner PD, et al. Ventilation-perfusion inequality in chronic obstructive pulmonary disease. *J Clin Invest* 59:203, 1977.

174. Wagner PD, et al. Ventilation-perfusion inequality in asymptomatic asthma. *Am Rev Respir Dis* 118:511, 1978.

175. Wasserman K. Exercise testing in the dyspneic patient: The chairman's postconference reflections. *Am Rev Respir Dis* 129 (Suppl):S1, 1984.

176. Weinberg P, et al. Biologically active products of complement and acute lung injury in patients with the sepsis syndrome. *Am Rev Respir Dis* 103:791, 1984.

177. Weinberger M, Hendeles L, Ahrens R. Pharmacologic management of reversible obstructive lung disease. *Med Clin North Am* 65:579, 1980.

178. Weisman IM, Rinaldo JE, Rogers RM. Positive end-expiratory pressure in adult respiratory failure. *N Engl J Med* 307:1381, 1982.

179. Westerman DE, et al. Identification of the high-risk asthmatic patient. *Am J Med* 66:565, 1979.

180. Wiedemann HP, Matthay MA, Matthay RA. Cardiovascular-pulmonary monitoring in the intensive care unit. *Chest* 85:537 (part I) and 656 (part II), 1984.

181. Wiedemann HP, Matthay MA, Matthay RA (Eds), *Acute Lung Injury*. Philadelphia: Saunders, 1986.

182. Wolfe JD, et al. Bronchodilator effects of terbutaline and aminophylline alone and in combination in asthmatic patients. *N Engl J Med* 298:363, 1978.

183. Woolcock AJ, Read J. Lung volume in exacerbations of asthma. *Am J Med* 41:259, 1966.

184. Yang KL, Tobin MJ. A prospective study of indexes predicting the outcome of trials of wean-

ing from mechanical ventilation. *N Engl J Med* 324:1445, 1991.

185. Zapol WM, Snider WT. Pulmonary hypertension in severe acute respiratory failure. *N Engl J Med* 296:476, 1977.

186. Zapol N, et al. Pulmonary fibrosis in severe acute respiratory failure. *Am Rev Respir Dis* 119:547, 1979.

187. Ziment I. Corticosteroids. In I Ziment (Ed), *Respiratory Pharmacology and Therapeutics.* Philadelphia: Saunders, 1978.

188. Ziment I. Mucokinetic Agents. In I Ziment (Ed), *Respiratory Pharmacology and Therapeutics.* Philadelphia: Saunders, 1978.

47

Pulmonary Rehabilitation

François Haas   Kenneth Axen
John Salazar-Schicchi   Albert Haas

The immediate roots of pulmonary rehabilitation can be traced to the era of sanatorium treatment for tubercular patients that emerged toward the end of the nineteenth century. Although absolute rest was the most widely used form of therapy in sanatoriums, the controversy between rest versus exercise therapy had never been fully resolved. Some experts of that era recognized that encouraging progressive exercise training within the limits of comfort could improve the quality of life of a large number of patients suffering from respiratory insufficiency.

Early in the twentieth century, for example, the physician Marcus S. Paterson in an article titled "Graduated labour in pulmonary tuberculosis" [108] stated that "Some consumptive persons ... under ideal conditions and with the work carefully graduated in accordance with their physical state, are able to undertake useful labour." He listed three advantages of such a program:

First, it would do much to meet the objection that members of the working class are liable to have their energy sapped, and to acquire lazy habits by ... (rest cures); secondly, it would make them more resistant to the disease, by improving their physical condition; and thirdly, would enable them by its effect upon their muscles to return to their work immediately after their discharge.

Data illustrating the positive aspects of work and exercise in treating tuberculosis continued to appear. A follow-up in the United States of 146 patients in the 1- to 2½-year interval after discharge showed that 92 percent were still at work, 6 percent were no longer working, and 1 percent had died. In a group discharged after only traditional rest therapy, 2 years later only 66 percent were well and working, 24 percent were invalids, and 10 percent had died [94].

Similar statistics obtained in England led to the following observations by Woodhead and Varrier-Jones [150]:

We have previously noted that it has been stated on the highest authority that the chances of recovery of a well-to-do person are three times as great as that of a working man, the only apparent difference between the two being that the rich man has an opportunity of gradually resuming his employment—employment of a suitable nature, whereas the poor man has to return to unsatisfactory work for unsatisfactorily long hours—*at once.*

It is agreed that according to the stages of the disease an ex-sanatorium patient can do only 30 to 60 per cent of the work done by the normal individual; and since this is an ascertained and undisputed fact it is foolish to ignore it. That we have ignored it in the past is only too evident and accounts for the story of failure which have followed most after-care efforts.

Just as the State recognizes that it must be responsible for the treatment and training of ex-soldiers who have been incapacitated by the war, so the State ought to shoulder the responsibility of these civilians who fall by the way, succumbing to tuberculosis. The stress of modern life, inadequate housing, and severe competition are responsible for the break-down of such men, and it seems that since the State has already shouldered so much of the responsibility it should go a step farther and *make sure that the opportunity be given to these men to do the work of which they are capable*, though it be but a percentage of a full day's work [italics represent authors' emphasis].

The combined impact of these alarming statistics and persuasive reasoning led to the birth of modern pulmonary rehabilitation, ushered in by the *sheltered workshop* in the United States and the *industrial colony* in Europe. On June 14,

1915, Altro Work Shops, a model garment factory, opened its doors in New York City to 22 former sanatorium patients. It was described as a "workshop [that] offers the post-sanatorium patient temporary sheltered factory employment through which he may condition himself, physically and psychologically, in preparation for his return to every-day life. Whenever necessary, the course at the workshop is followed by a period of vocational training" [123].

The English went even further. Papworth Colony near Cambridge housed not only patients, but their entire families as well. It comprised hospital and educational facilities in addition to numerous workshops. In their follow-up article, Varrier-Jones and Woodhead [144] elaborated on the Colony's philosophy:

As one intelligent patient [once] remarked: "We waste time; we wish to learn something, we have nothing to occupy our minds, we want to improve ourselves; you say that we cannot go back to our original trades, yet you do not attempt to provide us with a substitute; we cannot dig, to beg we are ashamed. If we cannot exert our bodies, can we educate our minds?"

As a temporary expedient, sanatorium treatment gives excellent results. By itself, as a means of permanently restoring the patient to health, it has proved to be a failure. It is a good thing in itself, but not by itself. Something more is needed, and that something is what is now known as after-care . . . a phrase as elastic as it is vague.

This statement transposes easily to the modern needs of pulmonary rehabilitation: *Medicine is a good thing in itself, but not by itself. Something more is needed, and that something is what we now call pulmonary rehabilitation.* . . . "a phrase as elastic as it is vague." Thus, by the end of World War I, the essential credo of pulmonary rehabilitation was already well understood [150]:

The gain to the community of a productive member in place of a useless consumer.

The education of patients in the "ritual" necessary *for their own "nutrition,"* maintenance in, or restoration to health and strength. . . .

The inculcation of a feeling of moral and physical self-respect involved in the knowledge that they are being cared for, not out of charity, but because their fellows—the State or community—recognize that they . . . still have a chance of making a success of their life and work.

The 1950s saw the second wave of pioneers in pulmonary rehabilitation establish the successful techniques that now allow patients with pulmonary impairment to resume useful, satisfying lives. Although the incidence of tuberculosis soon dropped precipitously, with the introduction of powerful antibiotics threatening to make these techniques obsolete, a new clientele for rehabilitation services was emerging—the patient with chronic obstructive pulmonary disease (COPD). Eventually, the relevance of pulmonary rehabilitation was extended beyond immediate pulmonary pathology to include respiratory problems due to neuromuscular diseases [123].

The aim of this chapter is to define the "elastic and vague" phrase *pulmonary rehabilitation*, outline its elements, with emphasis on often neglected areas such as nutrition, and review efficacy studies.

Definition

Broadly speaking, the two principal objectives of pulmonary rehabilitation are (1) to control and alleviate, as much as possible, the symptoms and pathophysiologic implications of the respiratory impairment, and (2) to teach the patient how to achieve his or her optimal capability for carrying out activities of daily living [65]. Although the basic principles of this field were well established by the end of World War I, it was not until 1974 that the American College of Chest Physicians developed a formal definition [109]:

Pulmonary rehabilitation may be defined as an *art* of medical practice wherein an *individually tailored, multidisciplinary* [italics represent authors' emphasis] program is formulated which through accurate diagnosis, therapy, emotional support, and education, stabilize or reverse both the physio- and psychopathology of pulmonary diseases and attempt to return the patient to the highest possible functional capacity allowed by his pulmonary handicap and overall life situation.

This definition was eventually accepted and endorsed by the American Thoracic Society in its position paper on pulmonary rehabilitation in 1981 [65].

The definition focuses on three critical features of effective rehabilitation: It is (1) an art, (2) individually tailored, and (3) multidisciplinary. Ironically, these same key features also make any "scientific" evaluation of its outcome extremely difficult. Defining pulmonary rehabilitation as an "art" carries the recognition that a certain degree of creative adaptation and skill is inherent in its practice. "Individually tailored" means that the criteria for success cannot be clear-cut or standard. The level of success achieved by any given patient depends on many factors, with severity of the underlying disease being only one. Outcome evaluation is further confounded by the multidisciplinary modalities (e.g., psychological and vocational counseling, physical therapy) involved. Not only is it difficult to assign treatment effects to a single therapy modality, but also improvement via one modality may initiate changes in other areas (Table 47-1). Improved exercise tolerance, for example, often improves psychological outlook.

Despite the difficulties inherent in demonstrating the value of pulmonary rehabilitation in general, and the individual modalities in particular, there is a growing body of scientific information available for guiding the health care personnel on the pulmonary rehabilitation team in working with the individual patient's particular symptoms and level of pulmonary impairment.

The Team

The complexity of the pulmonary patient's needs invariably calls for the services of a variety of specialists. Because this results in a rehabilitation team of specialists from many different fields, careful coordination and integration of their activities are required in order to arrive at realistic rehabilitation goals, and to ensure that maximum assistance is available to the patient in making the required readjustments in his or her life pattern.

Team makeup can vary depending on the available departmental and personnel resources in the specific health care environment. The responsibilities of individual team members often cross disciplines, sometimes to ensure that all of the patient's needs are met and sometimes because disciplines share overlapping areas (such as occupational therapists, some of whose work is traditionally regarded as part of physical therapy).

Table 47-1. **Benefits attributed to pulmonary rehabilitation**

Benefit	Major responsible program components	Possible contributing program components
Increased exercise capacity	Exercise training Inspiratory muscle training Oxygen administration	Psychological counseling Energy conservation Nutritional counseling
Improved ability to perform routine activities of daily living	Exercise training Oxygen therapy Inspiratory muscle training	Energy conservation Psychological counseling Nutritional counseling
Reduced mortality	Oxygen therapy	Outpatient medical care Education
Reduction in hospitalizations	Oxygen therapy Outpatient care	Education
Enhanced quality of life	Oxygen therapy Energy conservation Exercise training	Inspiratory muscle training Psychological counseling
Decreased respiratory symptoms	Exercise training Inspiratory muscle training Oxygen therapy	Psychological counseling Energy conservation Breathing retraining Nutritional counseling
Decreased anxiety and depression	Psychological counseling	Oxygen therapy Exercise training
Improved ability to be gainfully employed	Vocational training	Exercise training Oxygen therapy

Source: From BJ Make. Pulmonary rehabilitation: Myth or reality? *Clin Chest Med* 7:519, 1986.

Because of this, separating the responsibilities of individual team members must often be artificial and somewhat arbitrary. Whatever the makeup of the team, however, the appreciation by each specialist of the place and importance of the work of the others, and their cooperation in forming a coordinated and cohesive unit, are paramount if the program is to be successful. And irrespective of the makeup of a specific rehabilitation team, the keystone must be the patient.

The Patient

Pulmonary rehabilitation is for everyone with pulmonary disease, restrictive or obstructive, that has caused lung impairment sufficiently severe to limit the patient's normal life-style. Thus, pulmonary rehabilitation is not only for the patient with advanced COPD. Most patients with chronic lung disease will benefit, and the improvement will be obvious—if not necessarily quantifiable—in a variety of ways. Unfortunately, because most patients do not seek medical assistance until their disease is already well advanced, the majority entering rehabilitation programs are class IV or V on Moser's Disability Scale [66] (Table 47-2). Class III patients who for the most part

do not enter pulmonary rehabilitation programs could possibly derive even greater benefit than that experienced by patients with the most advanced disease [66].

The ideal patients are medically stable, recognize the physical limitations related to their disease, are willing and able to learn about their disease, and are motivated to devote the time and

Table 47-3. Possible reasons for failure of rehabilitation program

1. Cognitive deficits: Lack of understanding of:
   A. Illness
   B. Rehabilitation program
2. Emotional illness, depression, and anxiety
3. Secondary gain from illness (e.g., self-destructive needs due to masochism)
4. Mismatching of patient needs and rehabilitation services provided
5. Personal conflict between staff and the patient or family
6. Negative attitude toward rehabilitation on the part of patient and/or family and/or physician
7. Coexisting disease (e.g., cancer, arthritis, or psychiatric disease)

Table 47-2. Chronic obstructive pulmonary disease disability scale

Class I	No significant restriction of normal activities, but dyspnea on strenuous exercise
Class II	No dyspnea with essential activities of daily living; dyspnea on climbing stairs and in other climbs but not level walking; employability limited to sedentary occupations
Class III	Dyspnea with some activities of daily living (e.g., showering, dressing), but can perform all such activities without assistance; able to walk at own pace for a city block, but cannot keep up while walking with normal others of the same age
Class IV	Dependent on others in some activities of daily living; not dyspneic at rest, but dyspneic with minimal exertion
Class V	Dyspneic at rest; dependent on assistance from others for most activities of daily living

Source: From JE Hodgkin, EG Zorn, GL Connors (Eds), *Pulmonary Rehabilitation: Guidelines to Success.* Boston: Butterworth, 1984.

Table 47-4. Specific goals of pulmonary rehabilitation

1. An operative improvement in cardiopulmonary function
2. Prevention and treatment of complications associated with the particular nature of the pulmonary impairment
3. The recognition and treatment of disease-related anxiety and depression
4. Promotion of an active rather than passive life-style
5. Promotion of patient acceptance of and compliance with optimum medical care, wherein the patient assumes increasing responsibility for his or her own care and well-being
6. An increase in the understanding of the disease and the disease process
7. A reduction in numbers of exacerbations, emergency room visits, and hospitalization
8. A return to work and/or more active, productive, emotionally satisfying life
9. The provisions of tools with which the patient may regain independence and cope with the sense of loss, including loss of control of personal and social relationships, self-esteem, and self-worth
10. Improvement in the quality of life for both the patient and his or her family

effort necessary to benefit from a rehabilitation program. But many factors beyond the patient's characteristics affect the ultimate success of a rehabilitation program. Table 47-3 lists some of the reasons for a poor rehabilitation outcome. To minimize the chance of failure, it is essential to set realistic and specific short- and long-term goals (Table 47-4) that are mutually agreed on by the patient, his or her family, and the health professional team. Setting these goals requires a careful assessment of the patient prior to entrance into the program. This evaluation includes both a diagnostic medical workup and a psychosocial assessment.

Patient Evaluation

Medical Evaluation

An accurate diagnosis of the particular respiratory disease is essential. Despite the fact that respiratory conditions are generally divided into restrictive and obstructive pathologies, the specific diseases within these two broad categories can involve a very different clinical presentation, course, mode of treatment, prognosis, and final outcome. Evaluation involves not only careful review of the patient's medical history and pertinent laboratory data (including pulmonary function test results, arterial blood gases, chest radiographs, electrocardiogram, and blood chemistries). A nutritional assessment, which is often overlooked, should also be done.

Nutritional evaluation is essential in a comprehensive care program because the prognosis for critically ill patients is materially worsened by malnutrition. This generalization is highly relevant to patients with COPD, in whom low body weight or progressive weight loss is clearly associated with increased frequency of hospitalization and decreased life expectancy [20,63]. Prevalence of low body weight in this patient group is estimated to be as high as 70 percent [143], with undernutrition more prevalent among emphysema patients than among patients with chronic bronchitis [105]. Because low body weight and weight loss must be regarded as risk factors for progression of COPD, improving or preventing poor nutritional status requires serial monitoring and dietary intervention after the initial nutritional assessment.

Direct exercise testing is an important part of the evaluation process. Pulmonary function tests are a poor predictor of exercise capacity because the pulmonary patient's exercise tolerance depends considerably on his or her subjective perception of such symptoms as dyspnea and muscle fatigue [73,114]. Direct exercise testing not only permits assessment of the patient's current functional exercise tolerance and gas-exchange effectiveness (as reflected in the degree of hypoxemia or hypercapnia), but also provides a sound basis for prescribing subsequent rehabilitation training. This testing should use the same type of exercise that training will involve (e.g., treadmill testing for a walk-training program) [100].

Although blood gas sampling during exercise is important to assess the frequent occurrence of exercise-induced hypoxemia [120], it is an invasive technique that significantly complicates the procedure. Cutaneous oximetry, which is noninvasive, is useful for continuous monitoring of trends but cannot be relied on for accuracy. (The confidence limits for measurement of arterial oxygen saturation are ±4 to 5 percent saturation [119].)

Psychosocial Assessment

Because COPD patients develop a number of psychosocial problems as a consequence of their disease [1,117,127], successful pulmonary rehabilitation requires attention to these psychological and social sequelae. Psychological deterioration parallels the physical, so that these patients typically have become depressed, frightened, anxious, and dependent. COPD patients also show evidence of cognitive and neuropsychological dysfunction, possibly related to or exacerbated by the effects of hypoxemia on the central nervous system [54]. In order to cope with these problems, the patient's psychological status (i.e., cognitive capacity, depression, anxiety) and social status (i.e., family and social support, living arrangement, hobbies, and employment potential) must be evaluated.

Components of Pulmonary Rehabilitation

The components of a comprehensive program are outlined in Table 47-5, and described in subsequent sections of this chapter. It is important for the reader to remember that just as functionally delineating each team member's responsibilities must commonly be artificial and somewhat arbitrary, so must the division that is created in this chapter. Divisions are necessary in such a

Table 47-5. **Components of a comprehensive rehabilitation program**

EVALUATION	
Medical	*Psychosocial*
Pulmonary function testing	Cognitive assessment
Blood gas analysis	Psychological profile
Chest radiographs	Vocational profile
Nutritional assessment	Social profile
Exercise capacity testing	

PULMONARY REHABILITATION PROGRAM					
Medical	*Education*	*Physical therapy*	*Occupational therapy*	*Vocational counseling*	*Psychosocial counseling*
Pharmaceutical Oxygen Nutrition	Patient and family Smoking cessation Nutrition	Exercise retraining Relaxation techniques Breathing retraining Bronchial hygiene Assisted coughing	Energy conservation Training in activities of daily living	Vocational retraining	Psychological and social counseling

TEAM FOLLOW-UP

discussion, however, in order to present the rationale for incorporating each specific treatment modality into a pulmonary rehabilitation program.

Smoking Cessation

Discussion of any rehabilitation program for pulmonary insufficiency must begin with smoking cessation. *Smoking cessation is the most effective step in helping patients with chronic bronchitis and/or emphysema.* Motivation, though, is critical. Nothing, not the most effective program in the world, will help a patient become an ex-smoker if he or she does not really want to do it.

For the patient who sincerely wants to give up cigarettes, breaking the cycle of physical addiction is the first step. Complete physical withdrawal from nicotine normally varies from 2 days to more than 2 weeks [71]. Side effects of nicotine withdrawal include any of the following: light-headedness, headache, diarrhea, nervousness, and insomnia. In addition, the patient who stops smoking can expect to gain 3 to 6 kg in weight [21]. For smokers who cannot quit "cold turkey" or are afraid to try, various types of help exist: (1) drug therapy, (2) behavior modification, (3) hypnosis, and (4) acupuncture [129].

In surveying these various supports, the American College of Physicians' Health and Public Policy Committee concluded [140]:

A variety of methods and programs exist for the potential former smoker, and it is often best to combine a number of methods for an individualized program. Some of the most successful "programs" are those conducted largely by the individual, motivated to quit because of increasing awareness of the risks of smoking and the benefits of stopping. . . . The fact remains that despite the vast array of smoking cessation programs and methods, most people who have quit have done so largely on their own. [But] all persons who wish to quit, whether involved in a formal program or on their own, can benefit from some assistance, such as education presented in lay literature or as part of professional counseling, self-help guides, and more structured educational programs.

Medical Management

Failure to maintain patients in the best possible health via the proper medical regimen will undermine their confidence in the rehabilitation program, increase their anxiety and depression, and thus promote noncompliance in the program. As the pharmaceutical management of the pulmonary-impaired patient has been described elsewhere (see Chap. 39), this discussion of medical management focuses on nutritional management and the use of supplemental oxygen.

NUTRITIONAL MANAGEMENT

Undernutrition. *Undernutrition* includes deficient intake of nutrients that serve as energy sources (carbohydrate, fat, and protein), of substances that act as coenzymes or regulators of physiologic function, and/or of structural materials (primarily vitamins and minerals). In general, inadequate energy sources result in weight loss and a diversion of amino acids from their role as constituents of serum and tissue proteins to their use as substrates for energy extraction.

Undernutrition alone, uncomplicated by pulmonary or other disease, substantially stresses the respiratory system. There is a decrease in diaphragmatic and skeletal muscle mass [4,75], increased destruction of lung protein because of low antiprotease activity [147], increased surface tension forces because of reduced levels of surfactant [147], and reduced pulmonary and systemic immune function [122]. These changes are associated with respiratory muscle weakness [5,83], loss of connective tissue in the lung [147], and increased risk of respiratory infection [147,148]. Undernourished normal subjects also exhibit changes in ventilatory control; hypoxic drive, for example, has been reported to be depressed in acute semistarvation and to return to normal by refeeding [39].

These findings support the observed associations between declining prognosis and falling body weight in COPD patients [147], and between undernutrition and a detrimental effect on already compromised respiratory function [20,63, 83]. The association of weight loss or subnormal body weights in COPD with deteriorating respiratory function and increased mortality indicates the importance of nutritional care in this patient group.

If poor nutritional status is prognostic of ventilatory decline, then nutritional intervention should slow this decline. Studies of short-term (2 to 3 weeks) supplementation in COPD patients who were underweight (mean of 81 percent ideal body weight) [42] or experienced recent weight loss (at least 10 percent of body weight within the past year) [53] showed weight gain, increases in triceps skinfold thickness and midarm muscle circumference, increases in maximal inspiratory and expiratory mouth pressure and handgrip strength, improved endurance and walking distance, reduced dyspnea, and increased sense of well-being. These improvements were not accompanied by improved resting arterial blood gas levels when values were only marginally abnormal beforehand [53]. Although other studies of nutritional intervention in ambulatory COPD patients have failed to show improved respiratory function [81,84], equivocal results do not negate the value of more aggressive nutritional support of significantly underweight individuals [42,53] both to retard deterioration of respiratory function and to restore immune function, skeletal muscle strength, and a host of normal body functions. The potential vicious cycle of increased energy cost of breathing and consequent further weight loss and respiratory muscle wasting (Fig. 47-1) *must* be prevented or interrupted.

Intervention. Because the decision to initiate nutritional intervention must be based on documented nutritional need, not subjective assessment, evaluation should be done at initial contact and then periodically thereafter, especially following a change in therapy or diet. The total energy need of the patient may be estimated by calculation from a formula[1] or based on measurement of oxygen consumption. Adjustments to the normal calculated values are made to allow for the increased energy expenditure in COPD and for the extra calories needed to afford a gain in body weight. Provision of vitamins and minerals according to the recommended dietary allowance [102] guidelines set by the National

---

[1]For COPD, resting energy expenditure (in kcal/day) is estimated as 1.2 to 1.5 (the higher factor is used for emaciated patients) times the values calculated below [147]:

Men: 66 + 13.7 (weight in kg)
    + 5 (height in cm) − 6.8 (age in yr)

Women: 655 + 9.6 (weight in kg)
    + 1.7 (height in cm) − 4.7 (age in yr)

To this number is added the estimated caloric value of physical exercise if the individual is not confined to bed, and then the sum is multiplied by 1.06 so that the final product, total energy output, includes the thermic effect of food.

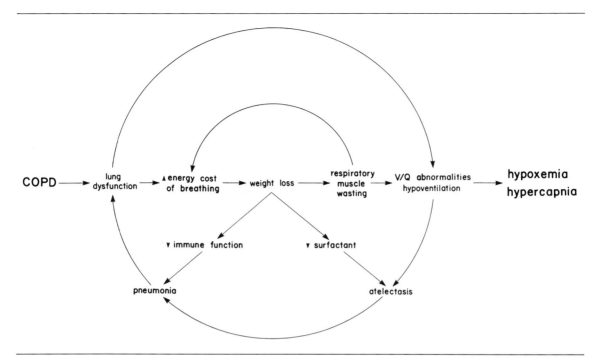

Fig. 47-1. Mechanisms whereby chronic obstructive pulmonary disease (*COPD*) ultimately leads to hypoxemia and hypercapnia. Irreversible lung destruction and partially reversible bronchial obstruction lead to ventilation-perfusion ($\dot{V}/\dot{Q}$) abnormalities and chronic hyperinflation of the lung. Hyperinflation shortens the inspiratory muscles, making them operate from a mechanically disadvantaged position, thereby increasing the energy cost of breathing and promoting alveolar hypoventilation. This increase in energy expenditure may lead to a vicious cycle of weight loss, respiratory muscle wasting, and exacerbation of lung dysfunction. (From K Axen. Nutrition in Chronic Obstructive Pulmonary Disease. In F Haas, K Axen (Eds), *Pulmonary Therapy and Rehabilitation: Principles and Practice* (2nd ed). Baltimore: Williams & Wilkins, 1991.)

Research Council is necessary, regardless of the type of diet.

The form of nutritional support is determined by the patient's ability to ingest, digest, and absorb food. These functions may be altered by concurrent disease (e.g., gastric ulcers, biliary disease). Patients with COPD may limit their food intake because of discomfort related to gastrointestinal distension or dyspnea. Eating small, frequent meals may obviate these problems because it reduces both the volume of the meal and the time dedicated to eating it. The latter issue is relevant to the oxygen desaturation observed during feeding in patients with severe COPD [17,22]. Low-fiber, low-water-content foods are calorically dense and can be used to advantage in promoting weight gain. Low-fiber foods also minimize abdominal bloating but then the problem of resultant constipation, which may diminish food intake, must be addressed.

Specialized, high-fat liquid meals for pulmonary patients are available for use as supplements. Care must be taken, however, to prevent their substitution for normal food intake because the net effect would be little or no increase in caloric intake. The same problem can occur with other specialized supplemental oral formula feedings that are often used to increase intake of energy sources, protein, vitamins, and minerals. Manipulation of the taste or timing of this supplemental feeding can minimize the problem of the patient who compensates by reducing his or her intake of regular food.

OXYGEN
A critical turning point in treating patients in chronic respiratory failure occurred with the availability of oxygen equipment for use outside

the hospital. First came the large oxygen containers with long tubes that enabled patients with advanced disease to move around their home while breathing supplemental oxygen. Then came portable units that opened up the outside world for them. Each advance in providing regular adequate oxygen has represented a major improvement in the health and life-style for these patients.

The use of oxygen in the treatment of chronic respiratory disease was initially suggested by Alvan Barach in 1936 [110]: "[O]xygen therapy in suitable cases relieves difficult breathing, restores strength and helps reduce the swelling of the patient's leg and back." He also often used it to relieve dyspnea [112]. Two studies, the Nocturnal Oxygen Therapy Trial (NOTT) [103] and the British Medical Research Council (MRC) study [117] established the positive effects of long-term continuous oxygen therapy on survival (Fig. 47-2). Increased survival is, in part, the result of improved hemodynamics as reflected in improved pulmonary vascular resistance (PVR), pulmonary artery pressure, and stroke volume index. The decrease in PVR is associated with improved cardiac function as reflected in increased baseline and exercise stroke volume index. Oxygen therapy also increases exercise tolerance [16,87] and generates neuropsychological improvements in COPD patients (Fig. 47-3).

Oxygen used at home for long periods is expensive whether paid for by the patient, a private insurer, or a government agency. But this cost must be weighed against the far greater economic impact from loss of employment, repeated hospitalizations, and eventual full-time health care at home or in an institution. (The large body of data documenting the benefits of supplemental oxygen coupled with the overwhelming acceptance of oxygen therapy make it highly unlikely, however, that large-scale studies such as the NOTT will be mounted to quantify the relative cost-effectiveness of oxygen versus no oxygen.)

Insurance payments have been complicated by legislation. Despite overwhelming acceptance of oxygen's benefits for patients with chronic hypoxemia, government regulations, in the form of Health Care Financing Administration requirements introduced in 1986, permit physicians little flexibility in prescribing oxygen therapy for patients who depend on insurance reimbursement. In brief, they allow home oxygen only for severe lung disease associated with these significant symptoms and signs of hypoxemia: pulmonary hypertension, congestive right-sided heart failure

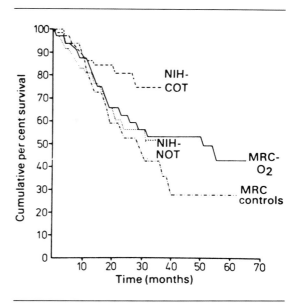

Fig. 47-2. Comparison of survival curves of the NIH Oxygen Therapy Trial (*NIH-NOT, NIH-COT*) and British Medical Research Council (*MRC*) studies. The worst survival was seen in the MRC controls who received no oxygen. The best survival occurred in patients using continuous oxygen (NIH-COT). Those receiving 12 hours and 15 hours (*NIH-NOT* and *MRC-O₂*, respectively) had significantly better survival than the group that received no oxygen. (From TL Petty. Ambulatory Oxygen Therapy in Chronic Respiratory Insufficiency. In F Haas, K Axen. (Eds), *Pulmonary Therapy and Rehabilitation: Principles and Practice* (2nd ed). Baltimore: Williams & Wilkins, 1991. Pp 160–176.)

from cor pulmonale, polycythemia, impaired neuropsychiatric function, nocturnal restlessness, and morning headaches.

The prescription must list the diagnosis, acceptable laboratory evidence of hypoxemia (the current criterion is a stable oxygen tension ≤ 55 mmHg or a blood saturation level ≤ 88 percent), required oxygen flow, and estimated frequency and duration of oxygen use calculated on a monthly basis. The patient who finds that his or her oxygen needs have increased must pay the difference until the physician writes a new prescription [110]. Prescriptions for portable oxygen must, in addition, be carefully worded. If it is not clearly stated that it is for the therapeutic purpose of promoting exercise and muscle conditioning, with concretely specified goals (e.g., to participate in a pulmonary rehabilitation pro-

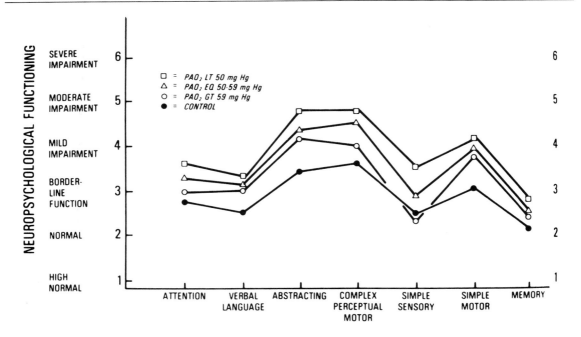

Fig. 47-3. Neuropsychiatric performance of patients with COPD at three levels of hypoxemia in comparison with the performance of age-matched control subjects. *LT* = <50 mmHg; *GT* = > 59 mmHgO_2; EQ = 50–59 mmHgO_2. (Reprinted from I Grant, RK Heaton. Neuropsychiatric Abnormalities in Advanced COPD. In TL Petty (Ed), *Chronic Obstructive Pulmonary Disease* (2nd ed). New York: Marcel Dekker, 1985, by courtesy of Marcel Dekker, Inc.)

gram, to increase activities of daily living), the cost of portable oxygen will not be reimbursed.

Physical Therapy

The meaning and exact role of *physical therapy* in the context of pulmonary rehabilitation tend to be poorly understood by most physicians. The physical therapy modalities appropriate for the treatment of patients with respiratory impairment are listed in Table 47-5. (A detailed review of physical therapy modalities can be found elsewhere [51].) The specific emphases in a given rehabilitation program are dictated by the needs of the individual. Treatments are often used in combination with each other for greater efficiency.

RELAXATION TECHNIQUES

Dyspneic patients become anxious and tense and may even panic because they fear suffocating. Unfortunately, their instinctive response—breathing faster—is maladaptive because they must then work harder to breathe. The substantial anxiety level of COPD patients is reflected in their greater skeletal muscle tension relative to that in a group of chronically anxious patients without lung disease [67]. There are a wide vari-

ety of muscle relaxation techniques that can be easily learned and performed at home. Methods such as progressive muscle relaxation, meditation, and listening to music work well in this population [130]. In addition, there has been growing interest in biofeedback as a relaxation modality.

Muscle Relaxation. Techniques selected to reduce muscle tension can significantly decrease anxiety [49]. Renfroe [116] used progressive muscle relaxation in a ten-patient study group and demonstrated reduced dyspnea and anxiety, compared to a control group that had been told to relax but had not been given specific instructions for doing it.

The Jacobson relaxation technique, the most widely used of the many relaxation methods, bears the name of the man who developed it in the early 1920s. Edmond Jacobson was a Chicago physician and physiologist who theorized that muscle relaxation and psychological stress cannot coexist. His technique is a prescribed sequence of quiet muscle exercises that alternately tense and relax all of the major muscle groups [70]. While one group is being focused on, all of the others are to remain as relaxed as possible.

Many relaxation techniques have their roots in Eastern religious traditions such as Zen or Yoga and Transcendental Meditation [130]. In a randomized clinical trial on 24 COPD patients comparing traditional physical therapy, including breathing retraining, and yoga, the yoga group had a significant increase in maximum work capacity, quicker recovery after exertion, and greater self-control over dyspnea [136]. Although yoga has not been used extensively, this study suggests its possible benefits.

Biofeedback. Biofeedback uses a learning situation to change the nature of a physiologic response (heart rate, for example). Electronic or mechanical equipment continuously measures and displays (for the eye and/or ear) this physiologic behavior, so that patients can see what happens when they attempt to change it. In this way they learn how to achieve the change at will. Biofeedback has been used primarily with asthmatics to help control their respiratory rate and dyspnea. It has been used successfully in a small group of COPD patients to decrease shortness of breath [67].

For relaxation training, the electrical activity of the muscles supplies the feedback that helps the patient do a more effective job of reducing the muscle tone. Electrical activity diminishes as the muscles relax. Any of several muscles may be monitored, but some consider facial muscle tone to be particularly important. Relaxing the forehead muscle automatically relaxes the scalp, neck, and upper part of the body. The mechanism behind this connection is presently a mystery, but the implications for relaxation training, particularly in COPD, are clear.

Music. The use of music to induce a state of relaxation was well known to the Greeks (Orpheus could calm the savage beasts with his song). Because the right kind of soft, slow music (e.g., Pachelbel's Kanon, Albinoni's Adagio) tends to produce a calming effect on physiologic responses, it can be used to elicit a relaxation response directly [38,88] or it can provide a soothing, helpful background for learning and practicing other relaxation exercises [106].

The earliest recorded scientific observation on the physiologic effects of music is attributed to the French musician A. E. M. Grétry (1741 to 1813). Grétry described this experiment in his "Essais sur la musique" [30]:

> I placed three fingers of my right hand on the artery of my left arm, or on any other artery in my whole body, and sang myself an air, the tempo of which was in accordance with the action of my pulse: some little time afterward, I sang with great ardor an air in a different tempo, when I distinctly felt my pulse quickening or slackening its action to accommodate itself by degrees to the tempo of the new air.

Guibaud's similar experiment on a number of subjects [56] identified reliable individual differences in respiratory response. Although different subjects responded differently to the same music, within the same individual the effects of a given stimulus were constant. Despite the overall variation in response, Guibaud did find that respiration generally became more regular with calm melodies and more irregular when rhythm or intensity were altered. He also observed that the rhythm of respiration tends to follow the music's rhythm, "especially when the latter grows slower." This finding was recently confirmed [60].

BREATHING RETRAINING

Breathing retraining seeks to gain better control of breathing by replacing rapid, shallow, less effective breathing patterns with slower, deeper, more effective breathing. The breathing retraining goals for COPD patients are listed in Table 47-6.

Pursed Lip Breathing. In COPD patients, pursed lip breathing has been reported to decrease respiratory rate significantly, increase tidal volume [99,141,142], and increase ventila-

Table 47-6. **Breathing retraining goals**

1. Controlling respiratory rate and breathing pattern to decrease air trapping
2. Improving the use of the diaphragm
3. Improving thoracic cage mobility
4. Improving ventilation without substantially increasing the energy cost of breathing
5. Teaching breathing patterns for handling dyspnea
6. Helping the patient to gain confidence in his or her ability to control breathing and promote relaxation

tion to poorly ventilated regions of the lung [141]. The change in rate may account for both the decreased resting $PaCO_2$ [99,141] and increased PaO_2 [141,142]. This association is supported by a similar improvement in arterial blood gases that was observed when patients with severe emphysema adopted a slower, deeper breathing pattern without the use of pursed lip breathing [98].

Several observations, however, suggest that the benefits from pursed lip breathing are based on more than improved blood gases. One is that the relief from dyspnea that this technique provides is too immediate [7] to be explained by alterations in blood gases. In addition, some subjects instinctively discover the benefits of pursed lip breathing on their own [69,141], while some never feel helped by it [99]. The most likely immediate mechanism is that pursed lip breathing creates an obstruction to exhalation at the mouth which slows the rate of exiting air and increases mouth pressure. It has been postulated that this pressure is reflected backward through the airways [141], thereby maintaining patency of collapsible airways during exhalation [128]. This in turn decreases airway resistance and air trapping [128]. Slowing the expiratory flow rates in these patients, therefore, helps to prevent airway closure and air trapping caused by high flow rates and the Bernoulli effect on collapsible airways [50]. Consequently, patients with increased airway compliance are most helped by pursed lip breathing [69,99,128].

Even though the mechanisms underlying the benefits of pursed lip breathing are not fully understood, the benefits themselves are so clearly demonstrable for many COPD patients that this technique will continue to be recommended to all patients with COPD for use before and during activities that may precipitate dyspnea.

Diaphragmatic Breathing. Because the diaphragm is the primary muscle of inspiration, instruction in diaphragmatic breathing is one of the mainstays of chest physical therapy. Miller [96] showed that such training is effective in increasing diaphragmatic excursion, which in turn increases tidal volumes and decreases respiratory rates. He also noted consequent improvement in blood gases. Comparing spontaneous breathing pattern to diaphragmatic breathing in COPD patients shows no alteration in the distribution of inspired air to the bases of the lung [15,124]. Because diaphragmatic breathing does not become

an automatic function, it is effective only as long as it is being performed [45]. However, in most studies on the effects of breathing exercises, at least some of the participants demonstrated physiologic improvements as well as subjective impressions of improved breathing [45].

Those patients with some diaphragmatic mobility may benefit the most from diaphragmatic breathing training [45]. In some patients with severe COPD and marked hyperinflation, the diaphragm may be so low and flattened that the technique is difficult to learn and may, as well, be ineffective in increasing lung volume [45]. These are probably the same patients noted clinically as being unable to perform diaphragmatic breathing. Until a method is found for identifying those patients who will respond to breathing retraining, however, the techniques should continue to be taught to everyone with COPD.

Paced Breathing. A second modality designed to reduce respiratory rate is paced breathing. Paced breathing attempts to improve lung emptying by having patients exhale for roughly twice the amount of time (in seconds) that they inhale (inspiratory to expiratory ratios of $2:4$, $3:6$, or $3:5$) [146]. A general introduction to this concept may be preferable to teaching a rigid counting pattern for use during breathing exercises and activities of daily living. Paced breathing is used in conjunction with pursed lip and/or diaphragmatic breathing.

Localized Lung Expansion Exercises. The three localized lung expansion exercises commonly used during chest physical therapy [52] are those for (1) apical expansion, (2) lateral costal expansion, and (3) posterior basal expansion. Their primary uses are either during postural drainage of a specific segment, or in achieving reexpansion of an atelectatic or collapsed segment or lobe. In addition, thoracic expansion exercises are often important in maintaining patency of these lobes.

Recovery from Shortness of Breath. An important part of breathing exercise instruction is teaching, and requiring practice in, the optimal positions and breathing patterns that help regain control of breathing once the dyspnea threshold has been exceeded. Most patients will discover on their own that sitting more upright, and especially bending forward at the waist, will help

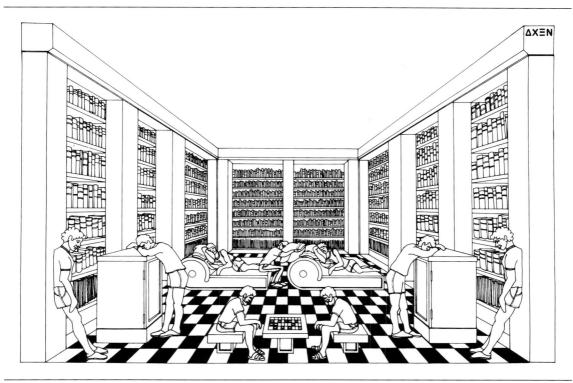

Fig. 47-4. Positions utilized for recovery from shortness of breath. (From F Haas, SS Haas. *The Chronic Bronchitis and Emphysema Handbook.* New York: Wiley, 1990.) Reprinted by permission of John Wiley & Sons, Inc. Copyright © 1990.

them to regain control. The same principles can be utilized while standing (Fig. 47-4).

This postural relief of dyspnea may result from a higher, and therefore improved, resting position of the diaphragm as the abdominal contents push it up with forward bending [131]. This improved resting position allows the diaphragm to contract from a more favorable segment of its length-tension relationship [131]. Relief from dyspnea might also be due to improving the length-tension inappropriateness of the inspiratory muscles, which Campbell and Howell [25] and Burki [24] suggest is partly responsible for the sensation of dyspnea.

MANAGEMENT OF SECRETIONS

Depending on diagnosis, clearance of secretions may be more or less of a priority. Patients with cystic fibrosis, bronchiectasis, or chronic bron-chitis and patients with critically located mucous plugs require an emphasis on management of secretions [28,32].

Postural Drainage. The 12 postural drainage positions (Fig. 47-5) utilize gravity to help drain secretions from a specific lobe or segment of the lung [52]. In addition to gravity drainage, manual techniques, such as percussion, vibration, and shaking, over a lung segment may be used in conjunction with the appropriate postural drainage position to speed the clearance of secretions from that area. (Table 47-7 indicates strategies that deal with thick and tenacious secretions prior to postural drainage [31].)

Studies using inhaled radioaerosol particles have shown that these techniques increase clearance from central, intermediate, and peripheral lung regions in COPD patients with excessive secretions [8,9] and also increase sputum production in patients with COPD and those with cystic fibrosis [8,9,89]. Some forced expiratory airflow parameters improve after postural drainage in cystic fibrosis patients [139], but not in patients with stable chronic bronchitis [91].

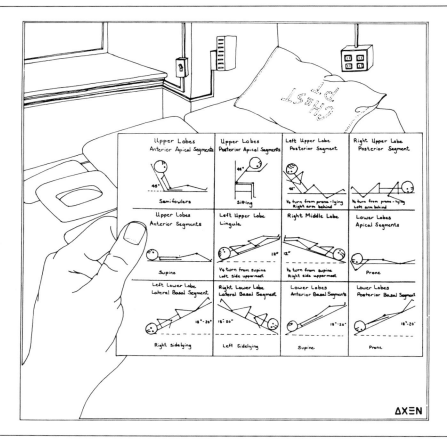

Fig. 47-5. Postural drainage positions for various lung segments. (From SL Garritan. Chest Physical Therapy Treatment of the Patient with Chronic Obstructive Pulmonary Disease. In F Haas, K Axen (Eds), *Pulmonary Therapy and Rehabilitation: Principles and Practice* (2nd ed). Baltimore: Williams & Wilkins, 1991.)

Table 47-7. **Methods for thinning secretions prior to postural drainage**

1. Increased fluid intake of 6–8 glasses of water daily (unless fluids need to be restricted due to the presence of other systemic diseases, such as cardiac or renal disorders)
2. Ultrasonic nebulizer or aerosol treatment
3. Hot, steamy shower
4. Drinking hot liquids, such as tea
5. Use of bronchodilators, administered by nebulizers or metered-dose inhalers, when bronchospasm is a component of the patient's disease

RESPIRATORY MUSCLE THERAPY

Respiratory Muscle Training. The findings that increased functional demands modify both the fiber and the oxidative composition of the diaphragm [76,86], and that diaphragmatic performance is related to its histologic characteristics [85], establish the fact that the diaphragm, like other skeletal muscles, can respond to training. It has also been shown in normal subjects that static contractions of the respiratory muscles increase muscle strength but not endurance [82], whereas deep-fast breathing exercises increase endurance [82,85] but not strength [82]. Thus, the observation in limb skeletal muscle that isometric and high-load isotonic exercises selectively build strength, while continuous submaximal exercises selectively build endurance, appears to apply to respiratory muscles.

In addition, exercises combining deep-fast breathing coupled with added resistance to muscle shortening have proved effective in increasing respiratory muscle strength and endurance in quadriplegic people [55] in whom the diaphragm is the only functionally significant respiratory muscle. These latter findings demonstrate that resistive exercises of sufficient intensity to induce diaphragmatic fatigue (as evidenced by alterations in the electromyogram [55]) can increase diaphragmatic strength and endurance at the same time.

In healthy people, respiratory muscle training effects require more rigorous protocols [55,82] than those producing training effects in limb skeletal muscle [95], probably because the respiratory muscles are normally in a comparatively higher state of training. In accordance with the overload principle, however, it may be that less strenuous programs could prove beneficial to sedentary patients, as their respiratory muscles are likely to be deconditioned in comparison to those of active healthy subjects.

Bearing this out, a number of respiratory muscle exercises using deep breathing against resistance have been shown to be effective in increasing lung volumes, and thus respiratory muscle shortening, in patients with muscular dystrophy [132] and COPD [3]. Breathing against added resistance also effectively improves respiratory muscle endurance in patients with COPD [3] and cystic fibrosis [77], as well as in the quadriplegic patients noted above. Isocapnic hyperventilation exercises without added resistance can also improve exercise tolerance in people with COPD [14]. Such improvements in respiratory muscle function are generally accompanied by increased exercise tolerance, decreased susceptibility to respiratory muscle fatigue, and improved ability to carry out activities of daily living.

Respiratory Muscle Fatigue. Respiratory muscle fatigue has been implicated in predisposing patients with advanced pulmonary disease to respiratory insufficiency [18,121]. In principle, fatigue can be defined as an inability to maintain the tension associated with a given neural drive. In practice, diaphragmatic fatigue can be inferred from the inability to maintain the same transdiaphragmatic pressure (Pdi) in the face of repeated presentations of an inspiratory resistive load [11].

Diaphragmatic fatigue can be promoted by increasing diaphragmatic pressure (i.e., the fraction of the maximum transdiaphragmatic pressure used during breathing, or *Pdi/Pdi$_{max}$*). In severe COPD, for example, hyperinflation of the lung reduces the maximum transdiaphragmatic pressure (Pdi$_{max}$), thereby amplifying Pdi/Pdi$_{max}$ and rendering the diaphragm more susceptible to fatigue.

Diaphragmatic fatigue can also be promoted by increasing duty cycle (T$_I$/T$_T$, an expression of that fraction of the breath associated with diaphragmatic contraction; the remaining fraction of the breath [T$_E$/T$_T$] is associated with diaphragmatic relaxation). Since increases in T$_I$/T$_T$ occur at the expense of decreases in T$_E$/T$_T$, breathing patterns that increase duty cycle render the diaphragm more susceptible to fatigue by not allotting sufficient time for the diaphragm to relax between successive contractions.[2] It has been proposed that diaphragmatic fatigue occurs when the tension time index—defined as the product of these two factors, (Pdi/Pdi$_{max}$) × (T$_I$/T$_T$)—exceeds a value of 0.15 [11].[3]

The failure of some patients to respond to respiratory muscle training has been attributed to chronic respiratory muscle fatigue [18,121]. In these patients, the use of mechanical ventilators to rest the respiratory muscles has been shown to improve arterial blood gases, inspiratory muscle strength, and 12-minute walking distance, and to reduce dyspnea [19,35,57]. Improvements in respiratory function were found with periods of mechanical ventilation ranging from as little as 8 hours once weekly to as much as 4 to 10 hours daily. These findings suggest that the degree and extent of respiratory muscle fatigue are probably important determinants of the appropriate rest period for any given individual.

Recommendations for Respiratory Muscle Therapy. In light of the above considerations, it would appear that the appropriate therapy for weak and/or deconditioned respiratory muscles is exercise to improve strength and endurance. However, because exercising a fatigued muscle can cause physical damage to the muscle fibers as well as degenerative changes within them [26,86,145], the appropriate therapy for chronically fatigued respiratory muscles would appear to be rest to restore strength and endurance. The judicious use of rest and/or respiratory muscle

---

[2]The sum of the inspiratory (T$_I$) and expiratory (T$_E$) durations determine the total respiratory duration (T$_T$); that is, T$_I$ + T$_E$ = T$_T$. Dividing by T$_T$, we find T$_I$/T$_T$ + T$_E$/T$_T$ = T$_T$/T$_T$ = 1. From this it follows that an increase in T$_I$/T$_T$ occurs at the expense of a decrease in T$_E$/T$_T$.

[3]As an example, a breathing pattern using 30 percent of the maximum pressure (Pdi/Pdi$_{max}$ = 0.30) for one-half of the respiratory cycle (T$_I$/T$_T$ = 0.50) and a breathing pattern using 60 percent of the maximum pressure (Pdi/Pdi$_{max}$ = 0.60) for one-fourth of the respiratory cycle (T$_I$/T$_T$ = 0.25) both yield the same critical tension time index of 0.15.

exercise therapies (tailored to each subject's specific needs) should be complemented by the appropriate pharmacologic, nutritional, and chest physical therapies.

Wind Instrument Playing. Among the claims put forth by the Renaissance composer William Byrd in *Reasons to purswade every one to learne to sing* was the following: "The exercise of singing is delightful to Nature & good to preserve the health of Man. It doth strengthen all the parts of the brest, & doth open the pipes...."

This principle has generally been ignored except for informal attempts earlier in this century, in Europe and somewhat in the United States, to have asthmatic children play the recorder or harmonica (personal communication, Albert Haas, 1992). It is interesting to note, however, two relevant developments over the last 10 years. One is that training the respiratory muscles has become a focus of experimental investigation. The other is the development of a large number of devices designed to train the respiratory system by making demands comparable to those of singing (encouraging large volumes) or playing a wind instrument (breathing against a resistance). One wonders if sticking to a long-term training program, which is especially difficult for children, might be far less of a problem if actual musical training, with its independent challenges and gradual sense of mastery, replaced boring plastic devices.

Recently Tateno and Suzuki [138] developed a new method of diaphragmatic respiratory training involving whistling and singing, which they termed *asthma music*. Although we could not find literature assessing this treatment's efficacy, we remain impressed by the authors' philosophy [138]:

Persistent asthma attacks tend to make us feel gloomy. We then desire to withdraw within ourselves. This would be an unfavorable reaction and delay the cure of the asthma. To enjoy singing on such an occasion would open the door to the heart, kindle hope, and invite sunshine into every corner. The experience of relieving an asthmatic attack without the use of drugs provides courage and confidence to fight against asthma. The mood of dependence on drugs and physicians will be transformed to a positive attitude in confronting this disease.... The enjoyment of singing a song will enable you to feel light at heart and overcome troubles that burden your mind. Singing songs is in itself nothing but breathing.

ENDURANCE EXERCISE AND THE EXERCISE PRESCRIPTION IN COPD

Ventilatory impairment drastically limits exercise capacity in people with severe COPD. This limitation is compounded in many patients by physical deconditioning due to the typical downward spiral caused by dyspnea (Fig. 47-6). Dyspnea causes anxiety and then abstention from an accustomed level of exertion, promoting deconditioning and eventually dyspnea at a lower level of exertion, then abstention from this degree of exertion, further deconditioning, and so on. As a result, these COPD patients ultimately become deconditioned out of proportion to their cardiopulmonary limitation.

Endurance exercise training can benefit these individuals by reversing this condition, permitting them to recondition themselves to the less restrictive limits set by their potential capacity to

Fig. 47-6. The dyspnea spiral. Exercise-induced dyspnea in COPD can ultimately cause physical deconditioning to the point where activities of daily living (*ADL*) are compromised out of proportion to the individual's potential capacity to exercise. (From F Haas, K Axen (Eds), *Pulmonary Therapy and Rehabilitation: Principles and Practice* (2nd ed). Baltimore: Williams & Wilkins, 1991.)

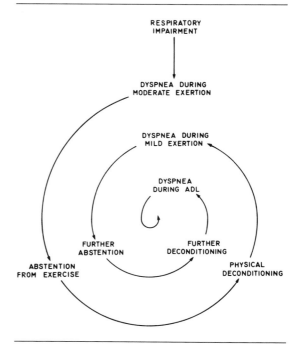

exercise. The exercise prescription aims to provide a safe, appropriate dose of exercise that is of sufficient intensity, duration, and frequency to achieve this training effect. Such an individualized training program takes the patient's initial exercise capacity as the starting point.

Training intensity, probably the most important factor in the exercise prescription, is moderated for healthy subjects and mildly impaired patients by exercise that requires a target heart rate that is some predetermined fraction (usually 75 to 85 percent) of the calculated maximum heart rate. Severely impaired patients, though, cannot exercise with the intensity needed to increase heart rate to the levels set by these guidelines. The lack of scientifically based criteria for choosing exercise intensity in severely impaired patients has led pulmonary rehabilitation centers to adopt their own empirical protocols.

In order to maintain adequate oxygenation of arterial blood during endurance training, supplemental oxygen (2 to 4 liters/min) should be provided for patients having (1) resting PaO_2 values less than 55 mmHg (obtained by blood gas analysis), (2) arterial blood saturations falling below 90 percent during exercise (obtained by oximetry), and (3) decreasing bicarbonate concentration ($[HCO_3^-]$) during exercise due to buffering of lactic acid (obtained by analysis of blood samples taken at rest and during exercise). Supplemental oxygen is effective in reducing the ventilation associated with a given level of external work [135], in improving PaO_2 during exercise [80], and in increasing endurance [16] in people with severe COPD. Since supplemental oxygen has also been shown to reduce dyspnea even in COPD patients who are not hypoxemic [149], it may be generally beneficial during the initial training period, especially with patients who experience anxiety.

Endurance exercise training programs (employing motorized treadmills and/or bicycle ergometers) consisting of three to five 20- to 30-minute sessions per week for several weeks can significantly increase physical work capacity and thereby significantly improve tolerance for activities of daily living in people with severe COPD. Although some studies have found that training also leads to some improvement in either cardiovascular [107] or pulmonary [101] function, most studies in this area report that such training does not improve the usual indices of cardiovascular or pulmonary function in people with severe COPD [12,13,23,29,113]. Such meager cardiopul-

monary responses to training, which are not shown at all by healthy [6,93,126] or mildly impaired people, support the view that patients with severe COPD cannot exercise with sufficient intensity to achieve appreciable cardiopulmonary training effects. *Since pulmonary function test parameters are poor predictors of one's exercise capacity [114], however, the failure of people with severe COPD to exhibit typical cardiopulmonary responses to training in no way negates their improved capacity to perform physical work* (Fig. 47-7) [12,13,23,29,101,107,113].

Fig. 47-7. Effect of a 5-week treadmill training program in 14 patients with severe COPD showing stress time (*upper-left panel*), oxygen consumption (*upper-right panel*), calculated total external work (*lower-left panel*), and derived efficiency (*lower-right panel*). Symbols denote the group's mean ± standard error before (*open circles, pre*) and after (*closed circles, post*) training. The significance level is indicated in the lower-right corner of each panel. *NS* = not significant. (From H Pineda, F Haas, K Axen. Treadmill exercise training in chronic obstructive pulmonary disease. *Arch Phys Med Rehabil* 67:155, 1986.)

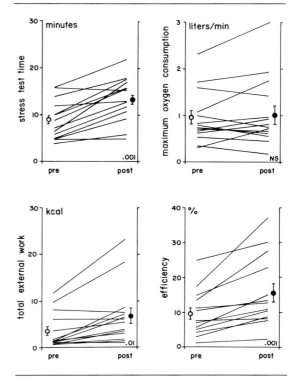

ACTIVITIES OF DAILY LIVING

With increasing disease severity, certain kinds of activities normally encountered in daily living (referred to as *activities of daily living* or *ADL*) can present special problems. This is particularly true with tasks involving the upper extremity. Something as basic as grooming or bathing can leave a severely involved patient breathless or fatigued [104]. Because many COPD patients report disabling dyspnea during simple daily tasks such as grooming, dressing, lifting, and carrying [27,34,137], upper-extremity exercise training is generally not a primary component of rehabilitation programs.

Celli and colleagues [27] suggested that unsupported arm work, in contrast with leg work, results in dyssynchronous breathing patterns that exacerbate dyspnea. Contrary to this concept, however, Keens and coworkers [77] reported improved ventilatory muscle function in cystic fibrosis children after a physical training program emphasizing upper-extremity activities. Similarly, Ellis and Ries [43] used upper-extremity training with COPD patients and demonstrated significantly increased upper-extremity endurance along with a lower level of fatigue and decreased dyspnea perception from arm work. These data strongly suggest that upper-extremity exercise may provide significant benefits for the COPD patient.

Until the value of upper-extremity training is more fully evaluated, however, patients can improve their capacity for activities of daily living by using three energy conservation approaches [104].

INCREASED AWARENESS OF PERFORMANCE

Breath-holding or uncoordinated shallow breathing during exertion, for example, is a common tendency of many COPD patients. Awareness of this problem along with an emphasis on using coordinating breathing patterns during movement can help alleviate it. In general, movements that compress the abdominal or thoracic regions should be coordinated with expiration. Movements that straighten or enlarge the thorax should be coordinated with inspiration.

Modification of Activity. Modification of activities of daily living involves performing a task in a way that eliminates unnecessary components, movements, and postures. Use of a shower commode, for example, eliminates the need for standing and so conserves energy. Bathing aides such as a long-handled back brush and soap on a rope,

which can conserve energy otherwise wasted in reaching movements, are other examples.

Compensation. When the preceding techniques alone are not sufficient to avoid dyspnea or fatigue during activities of daily living, the delegation of certain tasks to others may become necessary. This might involve hiring someone to provide cooking and cleaning services, or using a food-delivery service such as Meals on Wheels.

Vocational Counseling

The basic philosophy of rehabilitation is to attempt to return the patient to as self-sufficient and useful a role in society as feasible. This should include employability when possible. COPD patients who work are more gregarious and self-confident, and more likely to use denial to minimize the intrusive character of their physical problems. In contrast, those who do not work are found to be more anxious, self-doubting, and irritable [47]. The overall value of pulmonary rehabilitation for employability of COPD patients is controversial, however, because COPD usually appears in older patients who are more apt to be retired or less inclined to return to work. Although allied vocational rehabilitation efforts may be inappropriate for many older patients, it is clearly a valuable adjunct for the younger population with COPD.

Haas and Cardon [58] conducted a 5-year follow-up of patients under the age of 65 who had participated in a comprehensive rehabilitation program, finding 25 percent still employed full-time compared to only 3 percent of the patient group receiving only medical management. A study by Kass and colleagues 6 years later [74] found 21 percent of patients still employed full-time 31 months after completing a rehabilitation program.

In contrast, Petty and associates [111] found that patients were rarely able to return to work following a comprehensive rehabilitation program. These authors concluded that rehabilitation is more effective in helping patients to maintain their employability than is returning to work after a substantial hiatus. The working patients were significantly younger and had better exercise tolerance than the nonworking group, despite no significant differences in measurement of pulmonary function or blood gases.

Interestingly, although prospectively Kass and colleagues [74] found that the measurement of forced expiratory volume in 1 second (FEV$_1$) correlated with potential for vocational rehabilitation, in a retrospective analysis [36], with the vocational rehabilitation outcome already known, outcome appeared related primarily to IQ (IQ = 83 percent accuracy of prediction), with pulmonary lung function contributing relatively little to the overall prediction of success (IQ + FEV_1 = 90 percent accuracy of prediction). In general, those patients with both an IQ above 90 and an FEV_1 higher than 56 percent of predicted were more likely to remain employed. It was hypothesized that the direct relationship with IQ reflects the fact that jobs requiring more intelligence to perform also have lower energy demands.

It is apparent that—in addition to the level of pulmonary involvement—age, intelligence, motivation, education, capacity for retraining, physical demands of a particular job, and employer's support and understanding [7,36] determine the employability of an individual patient. It would appear, therefore, that patients who enter a pulmonary rehabilitation program while still employed, while relatively young, and with less severe airflow obstruction are better candidates for vocational rehabilitation, and that a specific vocational training program should be available for those patients in whom employment is a desired outcome [90].

Psychosocial Support

COPD patients often show typical psychosocial symptoms associated with chronic disease. They are often depressed, angry, isolated, anxious, and exhibit excessive body preoccupation [1]. These symptoms in turn contribute to an increasingly sedentary life-style, which further restricts their behavioral functioning and reinforces their negative self-perception. In addition, because of their fear of dyspnea, many patients repress any strong emotion (both anger and joy) because they fear these feelings will worsen their dyspnea. The inevitable result of this repression is further depression and isolation [40]. Combined, these psychological problems may make the patient unable to progress in the rehabilitation program [1,40].

The repression, irritability, and isolation inevitably precipitate withdrawal from one's spouse, and place often insurmountable stress on the one relationship that ideally should function as a primary source of support. Instead, the healthy partner, in turn, typically feels isolated and betrayed by his or her spouse's withdrawal and excessive irritability. Additionally, there is often anger if one's spouse becomes unable to work, limiting their life-style. Unless the healthy partner understands the disease, he or she may secretly feel that the patient is malingering [78].

These problems, however, are likely to improve with a comprehensive rehabilitation program [44]. The specific approach to these problems should depend on their nature and severity. Patients who have major psychopathology or whose depression or anxiety is so severe that they are unable to take even the first step need to be referred for psychiatric treatment [127].

Education. For the majority, improvement may be obtained through the immediate resources of the rehabilitation program. A thorough education is the necessary first step in getting emotions "out of the driver's seat." The essential prerequisites are a knowledgeable, caring, and available rehabilitation team. A sympathetic, supportive team can alleviate a great deal of the anxiety typically experienced by the average patient and the family by combining this nurturant character with a thorough, realistic educational program on COPD and how to live with it most effectively.

Although the exact role of the educational program as a single therapeutic modality has not been critically evaluated, a review of the effects of patient education in chronic diseases in general found improved patient compliance, especially in programs with a behavioral emphasis [92]. Psychological problems also tend to diminish as activity performance improves. Diminished depression and anxiety are also associated with improving exercise tolerance [2,44].

Sexual Adjustment. The long-term emotional impact of living with a chronic disease places a very real and very large burden on the patient's relationships, with the most intimate relationship one of the frequent casualties.

The capacity for the conscious exercise of sexual delight reflects the evolution-rooted dimension of human existence that distinguishes us from all other animals. While we continue to carry out the instinctive and reproductive aspects of sex, our level of cortical development allows us, as well, to take delight in its pleasures as an end in themselves. Because sex has become for us a multilayered source of deep pleasure and meaning, sexual activity and how one feels about it are basic components of one's identity and self-esteem. It follows that any sense of unhappiness with sexual performance and satisfactions has a deeply painful impact. Sexual dysfunction and loss of sexual pleasure are severely disturbing to the psychodynamics of both the individual and the marital relationship.

COPD patients are particularly harshly dealt with by their disease when it comes to their sexual rights. It is obvious that once pulmonary resources have substantially diminished, and especially if the patient has become significantly deconditioned, the breathlessness experienced is not love's intoxication, but intense dyspnea. Dyspnea in turn makes the patient highly anxious, and anxiety can substantially worsen the dyspnea. We know that the fear engendered by the experience of intense dyspnea causes most patients to renounce whatever activities provoke it. Sex is no exception.

Without education and support, patients usually become unable to manage their meager pulmonary resources in a way that permits satisfying sexual activity. Sex is very strenuous, and unless oxygen demands are minimized and pulmonary efficiency is maximized, the result can only be frightening dyspnea, powerful anxiety, withdrawal, anger, guilt, and self-loathing. These sequelae seriously compound the other stresses on the relationship precipitated by the impact of a severely limiting chronic disease.

Sexual dysfunctions fall into four categories: (1) inhibited sexual desire (i.e., decreased libido), (2) inhibited sexual arousal (e.g., lack of erection in men, decreased lubrication or vasocongestion in women), (3) inhibited orgasm, and (4) other problems (e.g., premature or retarded ejaculation, priapism, dyspareunia, vaginismus).

Although COPD obviously has a rich potential for devastating sex lives, there is a general paucity of data concerning sexual dysfunction as a consequence of chronic pulmonary disease. (Its effects on sexual dysfunction in women have been almost totally ignored. Until such data are obtained, we can only assume that the psychological and physiologic problems observed in men have their corollary in women.) Although the data on record are not consistent, the reported incidence of dysfunction in more recent investigations is relatively high. Of 128 men and women interviewed, 67 percent reported that their illness interfered with some physical aspect of their sexuality [62]. One smaller study noted a correlation between increasing sexual dysfunction and decreasing lung function, with 7 of 20 men reporting erectile dysfunction [48]. In another, 19 of 23 patients in a rehabilitation group reported both erectile dysfunction and decreased libido [1].

Whatever the cause, physical or psychological, change requires dealing with sexual problems on at least two levels. The psychological level involves feelings and attitudes. The technical level involves such aspects as the properly timed use of breathing-aiding medication, the use of energy-conserving techniques, and so on [125].

The first step is for the patient, the patient's partner, and their health professional to talk, really talk, about the disease. This discussion should include the couple's respective feelings about COPD and how it has affected their activities, including sex. Both partners must have an accurate understanding of what COPD is, and what their physical limitations really are and aren't.

For sexual problems that require more than facilitating the lines of communication between partners, the optimal next step is referring the couple to a support group. This is an ideal place to get them started on confronting and resolving their problems (sexual and otherwise!), and to help out if new problems appear, or old ones reappear. The support group offers the couple an excellent "education" and provides the crucial reassurance that comes from listening to other couples who have successfully worked through similar sexual and emotional difficulties.

Two Critical Emphases. Pulmonary rehabilitation programs engender substantial improvement in the quality of life for the overwhelming majority of patients. Although the consequent improvements, in general strength, flexibility and endurance, mental alertness, and self-esteem, all contribute to stronger sexual feelings, more is needed. *Given the importance of satisfying sexual intimacy to overall well-being, formal instruction regarding sex and sexuality should be an essential part of any comprehensive rehabilitation program for COPD patients. Unfortunately, it is often omitted.*

There are two essential concepts to communicate in this sex education course [125]. One is stressing the parallel between sex and strenuous exercise. Patients should be instructed to handle sex in the same way they would regular exercise. The second concept assumes critical importance for couples for whom COPD has progressed to the point at which orgasmic satisfaction, no matter how it is attempted, is often or permanently unattainable. When COPD makes orgasmic satisfaction difficult, it becomes particularly important to stress that not all stimulating interactions have to end in intercourse (or a manual/oral substitute) to be acceptable. COPD does not lessen the ability to hug, kiss, and caress. Each step along the way to intercourse—snuggling, hugging, taking a bath or shower together—can also be enjoyed as an end in itself. If these intermediary activities create a wonderful feeling of closeness and contentment, it is critical to discard any sense of pressure to go beyond them and consummate. Achieving intimacy and feeling loved is the ultimate point of it all.

Global Benefits

The above discussion emphasizes the many benefits that can be derived from the individual components of a comprehensive pulmonary rehabilitation program. In total, however, the overall benefits appear greater than the sum of its parts. Global benefits of a comprehensive rehabilitation program are reported as (1) decreased mortality, (2) reduced hospitalization, and (3) enhanced quality of life.

Decreased Mortality

Because there are no published prospective, randomly controlled studies of the effect of comprehensive pulmonary rehabilitation on survival rate, its role in reducing mortality remains equivocal. An analysis of existing data, however, strongly suggests that comprehensive rehabilitation *does* improve survival. In general, 78 [58] to

87 percent [10,134] of the COPD patients completing such a program were alive 5 years later, compared to only 50 percent of patients not undergoing rehabilitation [33,134].

Actual survival varied as a function of FEV_1. The 5-year survival rate for patients with an FEV_1 above 1.24 was 93 percent compared to 71 percent for patients with an FEV_1 less than 1.24. These data demonstrate that comprehensive rehabilitation can increase survival, and that its ability to do so is more effective if patients are enrolled earlier in the evolution of their disease [134].

Reduced Hospitalization

The effectiveness of pulmonary rehabilitation can also be measured in terms of its cost-effectiveness. A number of studies have shown a significant decrease in hospitalization, and therefore in medical costs, for these patients [37,41,68,72].

Table 47-8 illustrates a more recent cost-benefit analysis based on a 5-year follow-up of 150 patients who had been divided equally among (1) interviewed but not enrolled, (2) received only the education component, and (3) went through the complete program. The measurable effect of the complete program was a significant reduction in hospitalization and medical costs [134].

Table 47-8. **Cost savings analysis (N = 150)**

	Just interviewed (50 patients)	Educated (50 patients)	Complete program (50 patients)
Before being seen			
No. hospitalized	42	43	39
Total no. patient-days	1069	586	801
Average length of stay	25.5	13.6	20.5
Study period	5 y	5 y	5 y
Average cost per day at 1987 prices	$1193*	$1193*	$1193*
Total cost per patient at 1987 prices	$30,422	$16,225	$24,457
After being seen			
No. hospitalized	38	39	36
Total no. patient-days	1570	946	417
Average length of stay	41.3	24.3	11.6
Study period	5 y	5 y	5 y
Average cost per day at 1987 prices	$1193*	$1193*	$1193*
Total cost per patient at 1987 prices	$49,271	$28,990	$13,839

*Average cost including ventilators.
Source: From R Sneider, JA O'maley, M Kahn. Trends in pulmonary rehabilitation at Eisenhower Medical Center: An 11 years' experience (1976–1987). *J Cardiopulm Rehabil* 8:453, 1988.

Quality of Life

Many rehabilitation programs have documented an improvement in patient symptoms [1,2,44, 46,59,62,64,79,97]. In addition, a majority of patients who have undergone comprehensive pulmonary rehabilitation report improvement in a variety of subjective variables including dyspnea, increased ability to go outside, reduced number of episodes of breathing difficulty, increased self-assurance, and improved quality of life (assessed by a variety of quality-of-life questionnaires) [90,118]. For patients, then, the major benefits of pulmonary rehabilitation are related to improved quality of life, reduction in debilitating respiratory symptoms, increased exercise tolerance and level of physical activity, more independence and ability to perform activities of daily living, and improved psychological function (less anxiety and depression, increased feelings of hope, control, and self-esteem). Evaluating the effectiveness of any given rehabilitation program, therefore, must incorporate measurements that reflect quality of life as well as variables reflecting pulmonary function and oxygen use.

One Person's Experience

When all the numbers are collected, however, the impact of rehabilitation is a very personal experience. Given that, we decided to include one patient's own experience in his words [61]. Leon Lewis, now in his mid-70s, participated in our outpatient comprehensive pulmonary rehabilitation program 10 years ago. His pulmonary function test results from then are given in Table 47-9.

I started smoking cigarettes when I was 8 or 9. I don't remember why, but I guess smoking was an important part of the image I was holding up for people to see. Most candy stores and soda fountains sold them for a penny each. I bought them when I had the money, and begged them from friends and strangers when I didn't. That was par for kids who moved in my circle.

When I reached the point where I could support my habit, I was smoking a pack every 2 days, then every day. Then I became a radio disc jockey in Albany, New York. Something happened, and I found myself smoking the better part of two packs a day. Then as sales manager at an Albany radio and TV station, I was dipping into three packs a day. And by the time I got to New York City doing a telephone talk show from midnight until 6 A.M., I was well into four packs a day.

Working at night, I had a good part of the day to myself. The jogging craze was setting in, and I wanted to jog, but I couldn't. So I began a walking program. I was soon walking a couple of miles a day, and for the first time I began to experience the "high" that exercise produces. I soon found that smoking was interfering with my walking, and so I did the impossible, the thing I'd had no urge or inclination to do for years. I stopped smoking. I just woke up one morning and didn't light a cigarette. But, oddly enough, my problems began after I stopped smoking.

I pushed myself hard because I still had this dream about jogging. I thought when I got in shape, I would be able to do it. I don't remember exactly when it was that I developed a cough. The doctor said I had chronic bronchitis. He gave me some antibiotics and a cough syrup, and it went away. In time I learned that when the stuff I coughed up was yellow or green, I had an infection, which meant antibiotics and cough syrup.

Table 47-9. Pulmonary function tests

Parameter	Units	Predicted	Actual	% Predicted
Forced vital capacity (FVC)	Liters	3.65	1.30	36
FEV_1	Liters	2.41	0.66	27
FEV_1/FVC	%	68	51	
Peak expiratory flow (PEF)	Liter/s	7.14	3.09	43
V_{max50}	Liter/s	2.24	0.27	12
Residual volume (RV)	Liters	2.35	2.70	115
Total lung capacity (TLC)	Liters	5.48	4.29	78
RV/TLC	%	42	63	
Carbon dioxide diffusing capacity (DLCO)	ml/min/mmHg	16.7	8.8	53

$PO_2 = 55$ mmHg, $PCO_2 = 50.2$, pH = 7.362.

The treatment always relieved the condition, but the condition itself remained.

However, my walking program continued. On my bad days when I couldn't walk up the hill, I took the bus up and walked down.

I left my job in radio for the Community Film Workshop, helping train women and minority group people for entry-level jobs in TV news. It was fascinating and successful work (many of our students found jobs in TV stations all over the country, several with the networks right here in New York), but the old building we had converted into a newsroom, studios, and classrooms was the last place on earth I should have been. It was dusty, drafty, and often cold. And the hours were such that I virtually abandoned my exercise program.

In a little over a year, I left for a job with a public relations firm. It was part-time, but I never got back to my exercise program. At that point it was an effort for me to walk up the stairs from the subway. The cough and the infections began to plague me again.

In my search for more competent medical care, I came up with a Park Avenue doctor I thought was the answer to my prayers. He introduced me to anti-flu shots, anti-pneumonia shots, and a monthly intake of antibiotics he called a "flush." The last time I saw him, he listened to my chest and said I seemed a little congested. He sent me home. I didn't feel too well, but I didn't make too much of it until I went to lie down that night. I found I couldn't. I couldn't breathe. I thought I was living the last hours of my life.

The most comfortable position I could find was standing up and leaning on our grand piano. I was still there when my wife discovered me in the morning. I told her I was dying. She suggested I call a nearby university hospital to see if they could help me. The answer was "Yes, but you have to get here." Breathing was a real struggle, but my wife and I got a cab, and we made it. I was in the emergency room roughly 5 hours before I began to think I might live.

I never went back to my Park Avenue doctor. I began seeing an internist in private practice at the local university hospital. She put me on Theo-Dur [theophylline] and the Proventil inhaler [albuterol]. I thought I was out of the woods. But one evening after dinner at a friend's house, I had an attack and ended up back in the emergency room. I was not so frightened this time, because I knew what they could do.

They also got in touch with my doctor, who wanted me admitted. While I was waiting, I met another man who had already survived one such attack and was also waiting to be admitted. In 1 hour I learned more about my disease from him than I had learned from all the doctors I had seen. Maybe that isn't quite right. Let's say I learned more about how to take care of myself than anyone else had taught me till then. And he told me that the hospital had a chest clinic and a chest physiotherapy department. I learned about percussion and vibration, the way they thump the chest to loosen up mucus.

Shortly after I left the hospital, a friend saw a news story about an experimental rehabilitation program for pulmonary patients at New York University's Rusk Institute. They needed volunteers. I applied. I was eventually accepted. It was the turning point of my life.

I was put on the program, and I began to feel like a human being again. This program set me free. I no longer had to plan ahead to make a trip to the bank or keep a business appointment. I no longer had to avoid hills, stairs, and any unnecessary exertion.

Then, wonder of wonders, I was offered a job opportunity on the island of Jamaica. It was both exciting and frightening. I was afraid to be that far away from the NYU program, but I was intrigued with the idea of living in Jamaica. For years I had dreamed of living in another country, learning another culture and language.

I talked it over with the people directing my program at Rusk. They didn't foresee any problems as long as I took my medicine on schedule and continued my exercise program. I wasn't so sure, but I closed my eyes and jumped. I lived nearly 5 years in Jamaica with, as predicted, regular medicine and exercise and no problems.

Three days a week I got up at 5:30 A.M. and drove up to the Mona Reservoir in Kingston. It was a popular place to be that early in the morning. Jamaica's Prime Minister was often there, joining many of the city's professional and business people. The walk around the reservoir is 1.7 miles. Normally, I made it around in just under 30 minutes. I wasn't trying to set any records. I simply needed 30 minutes of aerobic exercise. And at that hour, just before dawn, with the moonlight shining on the water and the stars burning brightly in the sky, it was almost a spiritual experience.

When I returned to New York, I went back to NYU's program immediately. I credit it with saving my life. I have learned a great deal about my problem, and a great deal about how to take care of myself.

Not all patients benefit maximally from pulmonary rehabilitation. Patients with strong psychosocial assets are more likely to benefit [40]. In our informal but extensive observation, one of the biggest differences between patients who experience successful rehabilitation and those who do not is that the former have held on to their sense of humor. They take their disease seriously, but not too seriously. Those who make it have not forgotten how to laugh.

Conclusion

Careful analysis of the achievements of large numbers of programs unequivocally confirms the benefits of a comprehensive pulmonary rehabilitation program, that is, reduced hospital and emergency room visits, increased exercise capacity, reduced dyspnea, improved ability to perform activities (work and leisure), decreased anxiety and depression, and even decreased mortality. Although it may not always be possible to determine which modality is responsible for what kind of improvement, the documented improvements strongly indicate that implementation of a comprehensive rehabilitation program is the most effective means available for the treatment of COPD patients.

Despite this evidence, however, the medical establishment has treated pulmonary rehabilitation with benign neglect at best and outright hostility at worst. It branded it a waste of time and money to rehabilitate patients with a disease that can only get worse. In 1918, 2 weeks after the Varrier-Jones and Woodhead article on Papworth Colony appeared, for example, the *Lancet* printed this response [115]:

Very few early cases of pulmonary tuberculosis require more than three months in a sanatorium, and those that require more would seldom be better for being made to work.... Whether the expense involved in treating cases of this kind for prolonged periods is justified is more than open to doubt....

Seventy-two years later, a pulmonary physician was overheard complaining to another specialist about a COPD patient in common: "His problem is all the reconditioning exercises he does." Sadly, this is not an isolated instance. In fact, only the minority of pulmonary physicians regularly refer patients for rehabilitation.

The explanation for this hostility is not clear. One aspect of the problem is the underlying mindset that nothing can be done to arrest the disease. In this regard, there is a widespread tendency to confuse the total irreversibility of airway obstruction with the potential reversibility of the life-style impairment that derives from it. This notion is reinforced because improvements due to a comprehensive rehabilitation program have far greater value than can be measured objectively.

This nihilistic approach to COPD patients (i.e., that nothing more can be done for them) is further complicated by economic pressures that will make pulmonary rehabilitation inaccessible to all but the rich. One source of pressure is the enormous increase in people 65 and older in the United States. There were only 3 million at the turn of the century (4 percent of the 76 million US inhabitants), but at least 26 million now (over 11 percent of the roughly 235 million people living here in the 1980s). Older people inevitably place a disproportionate stress on the medical delivery system, and COPD patients fall primarily in this group.

The second source of pressure is that both private and governmental insurers are reluctant to pay for preventive medical care, even though, as far as the COPD patient is concerned, prevention of exacerbation is the most effective form of therapy. Approximately 25 percent of the Medicare patients interviewed in 1991 for pulmonary rehabilitation at the Rusk Institute were arbitrarily turned down by Medicare on advice of Medicare's consulting physician (personal communication, Horacio Pineda, 1991). As the United States becomes poorer and must rely more and more on "lifeboat ethics"—saving only those who can benefit society or who do not tax remaining resources—rehabilitation will be reserved primarily for patients young enough to repay society with many productive years of work. So older patients, whose remaining years of economic productivity would be few or nil, and whose annual medical costs would be more substantial, would be unlikely to get high priority.

Two things, however, give us some cause for optimism. One is that there are a growing number of professionals around the country who are working to develop the field, and a growing number of medical organizations, if not individual physicians, that are realizing its importance (e.g., the American Thoracic Society). The other source of optimism is a change in patient attitude from one of compliance to one of insistence on retaining involvement in one's treatment. This means that patients are now becoming more educated about their disease, and so are taking the lead in demanding rehabilitation.

References

1. Agle DP, Baum GL. Psychological aspects of chronic obstructive pulmonary disease *Med Clin North Am* 61:749, 1977.
2. Agle DP, et al. Multidiscipline treatment of chronic pulmonary insufficiency. 1. Psychological aspects of rehabilitation. *Psychosom Med* 35:41, 1981.
3. Anderson JB, et al. Resistive breathing training in severe chronic obstructive pulmonary disease patients. *Scand J Respir Dis* 60:151, 1979.
4. Arora NS, Rochester DF. Effect of body weight and muscularity on human diaphragm muscle mass, thickness, and area. *J Appl Physiol* 52:64, 1982.
5. Arora NS, Rochester DF. Respiratory muscle strength and maximal ventilation in undernourished patients. *Am Rev Respir Dis* 126:5, 1982.
6. Astrand P-O, Rodahl K. *Textbook of Work Physiology: Physiological Bases of Exercise* (3rd ed). New York: McGraw-Hill, 1986.
7. Barach AL. Physiological advantages of grunting, groaning, and pursed-lip breathing: Adaptive symptoms related to the development of continuous positive pressure breathing. *NY Acad Med Bull* 49:666, 1973.
8. Bateman JR, et al. Regional clearance of excessive bronchial secretions during chest physiotherapy. *Lancet* 1:294, 1979.
9. Bateman JR, et al. Is cough as effective as chest physiotherapy in the removal of excessive tracheobronchial secretions? *Thorax* 36:683, 1981.
10. Bebout DE, et al. Clinical and physiological outcomes of a university-hospital pulmonary rehabilitation program. *Respir Care* 28:1468, 1983.
11. Bellemare F, Grassino A. Effect of pressure and timing of contraction on human diaphragm fatigue. *J Appl Physiol* 53:1190, 1982.
12. Belman MJ, Kendregan BA. Exercise training fails to increase skeletal muscle enzymes in patients with chronic obstructive pulmonary disease. *Am Rev Respir Dis* 118:239, 1978.
13. Belman BJ, Kendregan BA. Physical training fails to improve ventilatory muscle endurance in patients with chronic obstructive pulmonary disease. *Chest* 81:440, 1982.
14. Belman BJ, Mittman C. Ventilatory muscle training improves exercise capacity in chronic obstructive pulmonary disease patients. *Am Rev Respir Dis* 121:273, 1980.
15. Brach BB, et al. Xenon washout patterns during diaphragmatic breathing. *Chest* 71:735, 1977.
16. Bradley BL, et al. Oxygen-assisted exercise in chronic obstructive lung disease: Effect on exercise capacity and arterial blood gas tensions. *Am Rev Respir Dis* 118:239, 1978.
17. Brandstetter RD, et al. Effect of nasogastric feedings on arterial oxygen tension in patients with symptomatic chronic obstructive pulmonary disease. *Heart Lung* 17:170, 1988.
18. Braun NMT, et al. When should respiratory muscles be exercised? *Chest* 84:76, 1983.
19. Braun NMT, Marino WD. Effect of daily intermittent rest of respiratory muscles in patients with severe chronic airflow limitation (CAL) (abstract). *Chest* 85S:59S, 1984.
20. Braun SR, et al. Predictive clinical value of nutritional assessment factors in COPD. *Chest* 85:853, 1984.
21. British Thoracic Society report. Smoking withdrawal in hospital patients: Factors associated with outcome. *Thorax* 39:651, 1984.
22. Brown E, Casciari RJ, Light RW. Arterial saturation during meals in patients with severe chronic obstructive pulmonary disease. *South Med J* 76:194, 1983.
23. Brundin A. Physical training in severe chronic obstructive lung disease. I. Clinical course, physical working capacity and ventilation. *Scand J Respir Dis* 55:25, 1974.
24. Burki NK. Dyspnea in chronic airways obstruction. *Chest* 77(Suppl):298, 1980.
25. Campbell EJM, Howell JBL. The sensation of breathlessness. *Br Med Bull* 19:36, 1963.
26. Campbell JA, et al. Alterations in intercostal muscle morphology and biochemistry in patients with obstructive lung disease. *Am Rev Respir Dis* 122:679, 1980.
27. Celli BR, Rassulo J, Make BJ. Dyssynchronous breathing during arm but not leg exercise in patients with chronic airflow obstruction. *N Engl J Med* 314:1485, 1986.
28. Cherniack RM, Lertzman MM. Management of patients with chronic airflow obstruction. *Med Clin North Am* 61:1219, 1977.
29. Chester EH, et al. Multidisciplinary treatment of chronic pulmonary insufficiency: 3. Effect of physical training on cardiopulmonary performance in patients with chronic obstructive pulmonary disease. *Chest* 72:695, 1977.
30. Chomet H. *The Influence of Music on Health and Life* (LA Flin, transl). New York: Putnam, 1875.
31. Chopra SK, et al. Effects of hydration and physical therapy on tracheal transport velocity. *Am Rev Respir Dis* 115:1009, 1977.
32. Cochrane GM, Webber BA, Clarke SW. Effects of sputum on pulmonary function. *Br Med J* 2:1181, 1977.
33. Commission on Professional and Hospital Activities (CPHA). *Risk Adjusted Mortality Norms.* 1986 Workbook. Ann Arbor, MI: CPHA Publications, 1987. P 62.
34. Criner GJ, Celli BR. Effect of unsupported arm exercise on ventilatory muscle recruitment in patients with severe chronic airflow obstruction. *Am Rev Respir Dis* 138:856, 1988.
35. Cropp A, DiMarco AF. Effects of intermittent

negative pressure ventilation on respiratory muscle function in patients with severe chronic obstructive pulmonary diseases. *Am Rev Respir Dis* 135:1056, 1987.

36. Daughton DM, et al. Physiological-intellectual components of rehabilitation success in patients with chronic obstructive pulmonary diseases. *J Chronic Dis* 32:405, 1979.

37. DeFlorio GP, et al. A prospective study of morbidity and cost/benefit outcomes for in-hospital pulmonary rehabilitation of patients with chronic obstructive lung disease. *Am Rev Respir Dis* 121:127, 1980.

38. DiMotto JW. Relaxation. *Am J Nurs* 84:757, 1984.

39. Doekel RC Jr, et al. Clinical semistarvation: Depression of hypoxic ventilatory response. *N Engl J Med* 295:358, 1976.

40. Dudley DL, et al. Psychosocial concomitants to rehabilitation in chronic obstructive pulmonary disease. *Chest* 77:413, 544, 677, 1980.

41. Dunham JL, et al. Cost Effectiveness of Pulmonary Rehabilitation Programs. In JE Hodgkin, EG Zorn, GL Connors (Eds), *Pulmonary Rehabilitation: Guidelines to Success.* Boston: Butterworth, 1984.

42. Efthimiou J, et al. The effect of supplementary oral nutrition in poorly nourished patients with chronic obstructive pulmonary disease. *Am Rev Respir Dis* 137:1075, 1988.

43. Ellis B, Ries AL. Upper extremity exercise training in pulmonary rehabilitation. *J Cardiopulm Rehabil* 11:227, 1991.

44. Emery CF, et al. Psychological outcomes of a pulmonary rehabilitation program. *Chest* 100:613, 1991.

45. Faling LJ. Pulmonary rehabilitation-physical modalities. *Clin Chest Med* 7:599, 1986.

46. Fishman DG, Petty TL. Physical, symptomatic and psychological improvement in patients receiving comprehensive care for chronic airway obstruction. *J Chronic Dis* 24:755, 1971.

47. Fix AJ, et al. Personality traits affecting vocational rehabilitation success in patients with chronic obstructive pulmonary disease. *Psychol Rep* 43:939, 1978.

48. Fletcher EC, Martin RJ. Sexual dysfunction and erectile impotence in chronic obstructive pulmonary disease. *Chest* 81:413, 1982.

49. Freedberg PD, et al. Effects of progressive muscle relaxation on the objective symptoms and subjective responses associated with asthma. *Heart Lung* 16:27, 1987.

50. Fry DL, Hyatt RE. Pulmonary mechanics: A unified analysis of the relationship between pressure, volume, and gas flow in lungs of normal and diseased human subjects. *Am J Med* 29:672, 1960.

51. Garritan SL. Chest Physical Therapy Treatment of the Patient with Chronic Obstructive Pul-

monary Disease. In F Haas, K Axen (Eds), *Pulmonary Therapy and Rehabilitation: Principles and Practice* (2nd ed). Baltimore: Williams & Wilkins, 1991.

52. Gaskell DV, Webber BA. Breathing Exercises and Postural Drainage. In *The Brompton Hospital Guide to Chest Physiotherapy* (2nd ed). Oxford: Blackwell Scientific, 1973. Pp 5–15.

53. Goldstein SA, et al. Nitrogen and energy relationships in malnourished patients with emphysema. *Am Rev Respir Dis* 138:636, 1988.

54. Grant I, Heaton RK. Neuropsychological Findings in Advanced COPD. In TL Petty (Ed), *Chronic Obstructive Pulmonary Disease* (2nd ed). New York: Marcel Dekker, 1985.

55. Gross D, et al. The effect of training on strength and endurance of the diaphragm in quadriplegia. *Am J Med* 68:27, 1980.

56. Guibaud M. Contribution a l'etude experimentale de l'influence de la musique sur la circulation et la respiration. *Annee Physiol* 5:645, 1898.

57. Gutierrez M, et al. Weekly cuirass ventilation improves blood gases and inspiratory muscle strength in patients with chronic air-flow limitations and hypercarbia. *Am Rev Respir Dis* 138:617, 1988.

58. Haas A, Cardon H. Rehabilitation in chronic obstructive pulmonary disease: A 5 year study of 252 male patients. *Med Clin North Am* 53:593, 1969.

59. Haas F, Axen K (Eds), *Pulmonary Therapy and Rehabilitation: Principles and Practice* (2nd ed). Baltimore, Williams & Wilkins, 1991.

60. Haas F, Distenfeld S, Axen K. The effects of perceived musical rhythm on respiratory pattern. *J Appl Physiol* 61:1185, 1986.

61. Haas F, Haas SS. *The Chronic Bronchitis and Emphysema Handbook.* New York: Wiley, 1990.

62. Hanson EI. Effect of chronic lung disease on life in general and on sexuality: Perception of adult patients. *Heart Lung* 11:435, 1982.

63. Hoch D, et al. Nutritional status as an index of morbidity in chronic airflow limitation. *Chest* 85(Suppl):66, 1984.

64. Hodgkin JE, et al. Benefits and Limitations and the Future of Pulmonary Rehabilitation. In JE Hodgkin, EG Zorn, GL Connors (Eds), *Pulmonary Rehabilitation: Guidelines to Success.* Boston: Butterworth, 1984.

65. Hodgkin JE, et al. Pulmonary rehabilitation. *Am Rev Respir Dis* 124:663, 1981.

66. Hodgkin JE, Zorn EG, Connors GL. *Pulmonary Rehabilitation: Guidelines to Success.* Boston: Butterworth, 1984.

67. Holliday JE. Biofeedback. In JA O'Ryan, DG Burns (Eds), *Pulmonary Rehabilitation from Hospital to Home.* Chicago: Year Book Medical, 1984.

68. Hudson LD, Tyler MD, Petty TL. Hospitalization needs during an outpatient rehabilitation pro-

gram for severe chronic airway obstruction. *Chest* 70:606, 1976.

69. Ingram RH, Schilder DP. Effect of pursed lips expiration on the pulmonary pressure-flow relationship in obstructive lung disease. *Am Rev Respir Dis* 96:381, 1967.

70. Jacobson E. *Progressive Relaxation.* Chicago: University of Chicago Press, 1938. Pp 40–80.

71. Jaffe ME. Drug Addiction and Drug Abuse. In AG Gillman et al (Eds), *Goodman and Gillman's The Pharmacological Basis of Therapeutics* (7th ed). New York: Macmillan, 1985.

72. Johnson NR, DeFlorio GP, Einstein H. Cost/benefit outcomes of pulmonary disease. *Am Rev Respir Dis* 127:111, 1983.

73. Jones NL. *Clinical Exercise Testing* (3rd ed). Philadelphia: Saunders, 1988.

74. Kass I, et al. Correlation of psychophysiological variables with vocational rehabilitation outcome in patients with chronic obstructive pulmonary disease. *Chest* 67:433, 1975.

75. Kelsen SG, Ferrence M, Kapoor S. Effects of prolonged undernutrition on structure and function of the diaphragm. *J Appl Physiol* 58:1354, 1985.

76. Keens TG, et al. Cellular adaptations of the ventilatory muscles to a chronic increased respiratory load. *J Appl Physiol* 44:905, 1978.

77. Keens TG, et al. Ventilatory muscle endurance training in normal subjects and patients with cystic fibrosis. *Am Rev Respir Dis* 116:853, 1977.

78. Kierna J, Pleatt N. No end to love. *Am Lung Assoc Bull* 2, 1981.

79. Kimbel P, et al. An in hospital program for rehabilitation of patients with chronic obstructive pulmonary disease. *Chest* 60(Suppl):6S, 1971.

80. King AJ, et al. Effects of 30% oxygen on respiratory response to treadmill exercise in chronic respiratory failure. *Clin Sci* 44:151, 1973.

81. Knowles JB, et al. Dietary supplementation and respiratory muscle performance in patients with COPD. *Chest* 93:977, 1988.

82. Leith DL, Bradley M. Ventilatory muscle strength and endurance training. *J Appl Physiol* 41:508, 1976.

83. Lewis MI, Belman MJ. Nutrition and the respiratory muscles. *Clin Chest Med* 9:337, 1988.

84. Lewis MI, Belman MJ, Dorr-Uyemura L. Nutritional supplementation in ambulatory patients with chronic obstructive pulmonary disease. *Am Rev Respir Dis* 135:1062, 1987.

85. Lieberman DA, et al. Performance and histochemical composition of guinea pig and human diaphragm. *J Appl Physiol* 34:233, 1973.

86. Lieberman DA, Maxwell LC, Faulkner JA. Adaptation of guinea pig diaphragm muscle to aging and endurance training. *Am J Physiol* 222:556, 1972.

87. Lilker ES, Karnick A, Lerner L. Portable oxygen in chronic obstructive lung diseases with hypoxemia and cor pulmonale: A controlled double-blind cross over study. *Chest* 68:236, 1975.

88. Look JD. Music as an intervention in the oncology setting. *Cancer Nurs* 9:23, 1986.

89. Lorin MI, Denning CR. Evaluation of postural drainage by measurement of sputum volume and consistency. *Am J Phys Med* 50:215, 1971.

90. Make BJ. Pulmonary rehabilitation: Myth or reality? *Clin Chest Med* 7:519, 1986.

91. May DB, Munt PW. Physiologic effects of chest percussion and postural drainage in patients with stable chronic bronchitis. *Chest* 75:29, 1979.

92. Mazzuca SA. Does patient education in chronic disease have a therapeutic value? *J Chronic Dis* 35:521, 1982.

93. McArdle WD, Katch FI, Katch VI. *Exercise Physiology. Energy, Nutrition, and Human Performance* (2nd ed). Philadelphia: Lea & Febiger, 1985.

94. Meek WO. The value and limitations of sanatorium treatment as regards the working classes. *Lancet* 2:785, 1917.

95. Merrick J, Axen K. Inspiratory muscle function following abdominal weight exercises in healthy subjects. *Phys Ther* 61:651, 1981.

96. Miller WF. A physiologic evaluation of the effects of diaphragmatic breathing training in patients with chronic pulmonary emphysema. *Am J Med* 17:471, 1954.

97. Miller WF. Rehabilitation of patients with chronic obstructive lung disease. *Med Clin North Am* 51:349, 1967.

98. Motley HL. The effects of slow deep breathing on the blood gas exchange in emphysema. *Am Rev Respir Dis* 88:485, 1963.

99. Mueller RE, Petty TL, Filley GF. Ventilation and arterial blood gas changes induced by pursed lips breathing. *J Appl Physiol* 28:784, 1970.

100. Mungall IPF, Hainsworth R. Assessment of respiratory function in patients with chronic obstructive airways disease. *Thorax* 34:784, 1979.

101. Mungall IPF, Hainsworth R. Objective assessment of value of exercise training to patients with chronic obstructive airways disease. *Q J Med* 49:77, 1980.

102. National Research Council. *Recommended Dietary Allowances* (10th ed). Washington, DC: National Academy Press, 1989.

103. Nocturnal Oxygen Therapy Trial Group. Continuous or nocturnal oxygen therapy in hypoxemic chronic obstructive lung disease: A clinical trial. *Ann Intern Med* 93:391, 1980.

104. Ogden LM, deRenne C (Eds), *Chronic Obstructive Pulmonary Disease: Program Guidelines for Occupational Therapists and Other Health Professionals.* Laurel, MD: RAMSCO, 1985.

105. Openbrier D, et al. Nutritional status and lung

function in patients with emphysema and chronic bronchitis. *Chest* 83:17, 1983.

106. Ostrander S, Schroeder L, Ostrander N. *Superlearning.* New York: Delacorte, 1979. P 74.

107. Paez PN, et al. Physiologic basis of training patients with emphysema. *Am Rev Respir Dis* 95:944, 1967.

108. Paterson MS. Graduated labour in pulmonary tuberculosis. *Lancet* 1:216, 1908.

109. Petty TL. Pulmonary rehabilitation. *Basics RD* 4:1, 1975.

110. Petty TL. Ambulatory Oxygen Therapy in Chronic Respiratory Insufficiency. In F Haas, K Axen (Eds), *Pulmonary Therapy and Rehabilitation: Principles and Practice* (2nd ed). Baltimore: Williams & Wilkins, 1991. Pp 160–176.

111. Petty TL, et al. Chronic airway obstruction, respiratory insufficiency, and gainful employment. *Arch Environ Health* 21:71, 1970.

112. Petty TL, Nett LM. The history of long-term oxygen therapy. *Respir Care* 28:859, 1983.

113. Pineda H, Haas F, Axen K. Treadmill exercise training in chronic obstructive pulmonary disease. *Arch Phys Med Rehabil* 67:155, 1986.

114. Pineda H, et al. Accuracy of pulmonary function tests in predicting exercise tolerance in chronic obstructive pulmonary disease. *Chest* 86:564, 1984.

115. Prest EE. Colonies in the treatment of pulmonary tuberculosis (letter). *Lancet* 2:220, 1918.

116. Renfroe KL. Effect of progressive relaxation on dyspnea and state anxiety in patients with chronic obstructive pulmonary disease. *Heart Lung* 17:408, 1988.

117. Report of the Medical Research Council Working Party: Long term domiciliary oxygen therapy in chronic hypoxic cor pulmonale complicating chronic bronchitis and emphysema. *Lancet* 1:681, 1981.

118. Ries AL. Position paper of the American Association of Cardiovascular and Pulmonary Rehabilitation: Scientific basis of pulmonary rehabilitation. *J Cardiopulm Rehabil* 10:418, 1990.

119. Ries AL, Farrow JT, Clausen JL. Accuracy of two ear oximeters at rest and during exercise in pulmonary patients. *Am Rev Respir Dis* 132:685, 1985.

120. Ries AL, Farrow JT, Clausen JL. Pulmonary function tests cannot predict exercise-induced hypoxemia in chronic obstructive pulmonary disease. *Chest* 93:454, 1988.

121. Rochester DF. Does respiratory muscle rest relieve fatigue or incipient fatigue? *Am Rev Respir Dis* 138:516, 1988.

122. Rothkopf MM, Askenazi J. Nutrition and respiration. *World Rev Nutr Diet* 56:43, 1988.

123. Rusk HA. *Rehabilitation Medicine* (3rd ed). St. Louis: Mosby, 1971. Pp 501–568.

124. Sackner MA, et al. Distribution of ventilation

125. Salazar-Constain J, Haas SS, Salazar-Schicchi J. Sexual Aspects of the Pulmonary-Impaired Person. In F Haas, K Axen (Eds), *Pulmonary Rehabilitation: Principles and Practice (2nd ed).* Baltimore: Williams & Wilkins, 1992. Pp 315–326.

126. Saltin B, et al. Response to exercise after bed rest and aftertraining: Longitudinal study of adaptive changes in oxygen transport and body composition. *Circulation* 38(Suppl 7):1, 1968.

127. Sandhu HS. Psychosocial issues in chronic obstructive pulmonary disease. *Clin Chest Med* 7:629, 1986.

128. Schmidt RW, Wasserman K, Lillington GA. The effect of air flow and oral pressure on the mechanics of breathing in patients with asthma and emphysema. *Am Rev Respir Dis* 90:564, 164.

129. Schwartz JL, Rider G. *Review and Evaluation of Smoking Control Methods: United States and Canada, 1969–1977.* DHEW Publication no (CDC) 79-8369. Washington, DC: Department of Health, Education and Welfare, 1978.

130. Sexton DL, Neureuter A. Relaxation Techniques and Biofeedback. In F Haas, K Axen (Eds), *Pulmonary Therapy and Rehabilitation: Principles and Practice* (2nd ed). Baltimore: Williams & Wilkins, 1991. Pp 277–288.

131. Sharp JT, et al. Postural relief of dyspnea in severe chronic obstructive pulmonary disease. *Am Rev Respir Dis* 122:201, 1980.

132. Siegel IM. Pulmonary problems in Duchenne muscular dystrophy: Diagnosis, prophylaxis, and treatment. *Phys Ther* 55:160, 1975.

133. Siltzbach LE. Medical aspects of the rehabilitation of the tuberculous. *Am Rev Tuberc* 45:489, 1942.

134. Sneider R, O'maley JA, Kahn M. Trends in pulmonary rehabilitation at Eisenhower Medical Center: An 11 years' experience (1976–1987). *J Cardiopulm Rehabil* 8:453, 1988.

135. Stein DA, Bradley BL, Miller WC. Mechanisms of oxygen effects on exercise in patients with chronic obstructive pulmonary disease. *Chest* 81:6, 1982.

136. Tandon MK. Adjunct treatment with yoga in chronic severe airways obstruction. *Thorax* 33:514, 1978.

137. Tangri S, Woolf CR. The breathing pattern in chronic obstructive lung disease during the performance of some common daily activities. *Chest* 63:126, 1873.

138. Tateno K, Suzuki I. Asthma music. *Br J Music Ther* 13:2, 1982.

139. Tecklin JS, Holsclaw DS. Evaluation of bronchial drainage in patients with cystic fibrosis. *Phys Ther* 55:1081, 1975.

140. The Health and Public Policy Committee of the

American College of Physicians (position paper). Methods for stopping cigarette smoking. *Ann Intern Med* 105:281, 1986.

141. Thoman RL, Stoker GL, Ross JC. The efficacy of pursed-lips breathing in patients with chronic obstructive pulmonary disease. *Am Rev Respir Dis* 93:100, 1966.

142. Tiep BL, et al. Pursed lips breathing training using ear oximetry. *Chest* 90:218, 1986.

143. Vandenburg F, Van De Woestigne K, Gyselen A. Weight changes in the terminal stages of chronic obstructive lung disease. *Am Rev Respir Dis* 96:565, 1967.

144. Varrier-Jones PC, Woodhead GS. Further experiences. Colony treatment and after-care. *Lancet* 2:133, 1918.

145. Vihko V, Rantamaki J, Salimen A. Exhaustive physical exercise and acid hydrolase activity in mouse skeletal muscle. *Histochemistry* 45:237, 1978.

146. Willeput R, et al. Thoracoabdominal motion during chest physiotherapy in patients affected by chronic obstructive lung disease. *Respiration* 44:204, 1983.

147. Wilson DO, Rogers RM, Hoffman RM. Nutrition and chronic lung disease. *Am Rev Respir Dis* 132:1347, 1985.

148. Winick M (Ed), *Hunger Disease: Studies by the Jewish Physicians in the Warsaw Ghetto.* New York: Wiley, 1979.

149. Woodcock AA, Gross ER, Geddes DM. Oxygen relieves breathlessness in "pink puffers." *Lancet* 1:907, 1981.

150. Woodhead GS, Varrier-Jones PC. Experiences in colony treatment and after-care. *Lancet* 2:779, 1917.

48

Lung Transplantation

Neil A. Ettinger   Joel D. Cooper

Following the initial unsuccessful attempt by Hardy and colleagues in 1963 [20], approximately 40 lung transplantations were attempted during the next two decades. One patient survived to hospital discharge but died shortly thereafter. The majority of patients died of primary graft failure, sepsis, or rejection and many patients experienced fatal disruption of the bronchial anastomosis [3].

The clinical success of lung transplantation was delayed until those factors responsible for its failure were identified. The adverse effect of prednisone on bronchial healing [31] and the recognition that bronchial omentopexy could provide mechanical support and promote revascularization of the anastomoses [32] were major advances. However, the introduction of cyclosporine proved revolutionary, permitting highly effective immunosuppression without interfering with airway healing [18].

The first successful lung transplantation was performed at the University of Toronto in 1983 in a patient with idiopathic pulmonary fibrosis [47]. Since that time, both the surgical technique of lung transplantation and the medical management of lung transplant recipients have undergone substantial evolution. Through August 1992, 1536 isolated lung transplant procedures have been reported to the St. Louis International Lung Transplant Registry. Although lung transplantation is still in its early phase, 1- and 2-year survival rates now approach those observed in liver, kidney, and heart transplant recipients [52]. Moreover, the indications for isolated lung transplantation have expanded as the indications for heart-lung transplantation (HLT) have decreased.

This chapter discusses the indications for lung transplantation, recipient selection, management of complications, and overall outcome.

Preoperative Considerations

Indications and Choice of Procedure

The diseases for which lung transplantation has been utilized are listed in Table 48-1. Although interstitial lung disease was the primary indication for transplantation during the early part of the last decade, chronic obstructive pulmonary disease (COPD) is now the most common indication for lung transplantation, reflecting primarily the success of single-lung transplantation (SLT). The choice of procedure requires consideration of a number of factors, including age, physiology, and the presence or absence of chronic infection in the native lungs.

SINGLE-LUNG TRANSPLANTATION

SLT was first performed in patients with idiopathic pulmonary fibrosis because the distribution of ventilation and perfusion following transplantation was expected to be favorable. In such patients, the low compliance and high pulmonary vascular resistance of the native lung preferentially direct both ventilation and perfusion to the allograft. Gas exchange improves dramatically following transplantation, and excellent, long-term functional results have been attained [19]. In the last several years, the indications for SLT have been expanded to include patients with a variety of other interstitial lung diseases as well as primary and secondary pulmonary hypertension (see Table 48-1).

Because of early unfavorable results, SLT was viewed as physiologically inappropriate for patients with COPD [43]. Preferential ventilation of the highly compliant native lung was observed to cause hyperinflation, resulting in compression of the allograft. The relative increase in perfusion to the allograft in conjunction with the increase in ventilation to the native lung also caused signifi-

Table 48-1. Diseases for which lung transplantation has been utilized

Chronic obstructive pulmonary disease	27.3%
Idiopathic pulmonary fibrosis	20.1%
Antitrypsin deficiency emphysema	14.8%
Cystic fibrosis	14.7%
Primary pulmonary hypertension	9.7%
Other	13.4%

    Secondary pulmonary hypertension
    Secondary pulmonary fibrosis
    Eosinophilic granuloma
    Lymphangioleiomyomatosis
    Sarcoidosis
    Hypersensitivity pneumonitis
    Eosinophilic pneumonia
    Lymphoid interstitial pneumonitis
    Alveolar microlithiasis
    Alveolar proteinosis
    Bronchiectasis
    Allergic bronchopulmonary aspergillosis
    Bronchiolitis obliterans
    Silicosis
    Asbestosis
    Berylliosis
    Chronic pulmonary embolism
    Fat embolism
    ARDS
    Scleroderma
    Systemic lupus erythematosus
    Ciliary disorders
    Pulmonary arteriovenous malformations
    Paraquat poisoning
    Bronchoalveolar cell carcinoma

Source: Based on data obtained from the St. Louis International Lung Transplant Registry through August 1992.

cant ventilation-perfusion ($\dot{V}/\dot{Q}$) mismatching. In retrospect, the problems encountered during the initial attempts at SLT for COPD reflected complications occurring in the allograft and were not an inevitable consequence. In the last 3 years, SLT has been performed in numerous patients with COPD and the results have been excellent [34,50].

The most recent advance in lung transplantation has been the performance of SLT in patients with primary pulmonary hypertension and selected patients with Eisenmenger's syndrome [30,49]. Traditionally, HLT has been the procedure of choice for these disorders. However, recent experience indicates that insertion of a single-lung allograft can normalize pulmonary artery pressure and relieve right ventricular afterload, allowing recovery of right ventricular function [38]. A

threshold value of right ventricular function below which the right ventricle cannot recover has not been identified. Surgical correction of atrial and ventricular septal defects can also be performed during SLT [35]. Although SLT can be applied to most patients with pulmonary hypertension, those with irreparable cardiac defects, inoperable coronary artery disease, or severe left ventricular dysfunction require HLT.

DOUBLE-LUNG AND BILATERAL SINGLE-LUNG TRANSPLANTATION
Double-lung transplantation (DLT) was initially applied to younger patients with COPD [4]. Using tracheal anastomoses and cardiopulmonary bypass, many centers experienced unfavorable results [39]. Recently, the surgical approach was altered to one using a transverse, bilateral thoracosternotomy with sequential replacement of both lungs (bilateral single-lung transplantation [BLT]). This approach, which incorporates bilateral bronchial anastomoses, is now widely utilized and permits better surgical exposure, improved control of bleeding, and avoidance of cardiopulmonary bypass in most patients [37].

BLT is the procedure of choice for patients with any pulmonary disorder complicated by chronic airway infection, such as bronchiectasis, cystic fibrosis, and chronic bronchitis. The possibility of spillover of infection from the native lung to the allograft precludes SLT in such patients. Whether to use BLT or SLT for patients with COPD is controversial. The choice of procedure is often based on individual considerations such as age, the presence of intraoperative risk factors such as cardiac function, malnutrition, and overall degree of debilitation, as well as the availability of donor lungs.

HEART-LUNG TRANSPLANTATION
The indications for HLT have decreased as the indications for isolated lung transplantation have expanded. As a result, the numbers of patients waiting for HLT have decreased while the number waiting for isolated lung transplants have grown [27]. The shift to isolated lung transplantation has permitted a more efficient distribution of donor organs and eliminated the unnecessary risk of complications that affect the transplanted heart, such as accelerated coronary atherosclerosis and chronic rejection. HLT should be reserved for patients with pulmonary hypertension associated with either a congestive cardiomyopathy or irreparable cardiac defects.

Recipient Selection

Guidelines for selecting recipients of lung transplants vary slightly from center to center and generally reflect a particular program's experience with the procedure. Some standard guidelines are detailed in Table 48-2. In general, the optimal patient must have severe underlying disease with a poor short-term prognosis. The patient should be stable enough to survive the waiting period, should be well enough to tolerate the operation, and should have the potential for full recovery. Among the primary factors considered are the patient's age; typical criteria are ages less than 50 years for HLT, less than 50 to 55 years for DLT, and less than 65 years for SLT. Although these guidelines are arbitrary, they reflect the prevalent philosophy of offering the limited number of donor organs to the youngest patients and to those most likely to withstand the procedure.

Table 48-2. **Recipient selection guidelines**

Severe and progressive obstructive or restrictive defect or pulmonary hypertension

No alternative, effective, medical, or surgical therapy

Limited life expectancy

Adequate left ventricular function without significant coronary artery disease

Ambulatory with potential for rehabilitation

Acceptable nutritional status

Satisfactory psychosocial profile with well-defined emotional support system

Table 48-3. **Contraindications to lung transplantation**

Absolute
　Systemic disease with nonpulmonary vital-organ involvement
　Active or uncontrolled pulmonary or extrapulmonary infection
　Significant liver or kidney disease of any cause
　Significant left ventricular dysfunction or coronary artery disease
　Recent or active cigarette smoking
　Significant psychosocial disturbances or recent history of substance abuse
　History of medical noncompliance
Relative
　Current systemic steroid therapy
　Prior cardiothoracic surgery or pleurodesis

The contraindications to lung transplantation are outlined in Table 48-3. Several contraindications have been modified or deleted as experience with the procedure has grown, and others have become the focus of considerable controversy. For example, the need for mechanical ventilatory support is no longer a contraindication for lung transplantation as success in such patients has been demonstrated [33]. Prior cardiothoracic surgery, although increasing the technical difficulty and risk of the operation, is no longer considered a contraindication in most patients since improvements in technique have maximized surgical exposure and minimized intraoperative bleeding.

Early published reports included the prior use of corticosteroids as an absolute contraindication to lung transplantation [10]. This recommendation was based primarily on experimental evidence of impaired airway healing in animals [31] and on adverse experience with airway dehiscence during the pre-cyclosporine era. This issue is now controversial. Recent, relatively small studies found no adverse effect of the use of low doses (up to 20 mg/day) of corticosteroids before transplantation [42]. Moreover, while steroid therapy may have no obvious benefits, its withdrawal is often associated with symptomatic and physiologic deterioration. In light of the current controversy, the optimal approach appears to be the use of the lowest tolerated dose of corticosteroids if attempted withdrawal is unsuccessful.

Timing of Transplantation

The timing of referral for lung transplantation and the decision of when to perform the procedure is purely a matter of clinical judgment and is therefore highly individualized. Factors that must be considered include the natural history of the underlying disease, the patient's present clinical condition, and the rate of deterioration. Included in this assessment is the average waiting time to obtain a donor organ, which may approach 1 year in some centers [27].

Guidelines for the referral of patients for transplantation are listed by disease in Table 48-4. These guidelines are arbitrary and reflect the experience at the Washington University Lung Transplant Program. Although a variety of survival indices or scoring systems have been devised for different disease states, none have been studied in the context of identifying the optimum time for transplantation.

Table 48-4. Guidelines for timing of referral for lung transplantation

Chronic obstructive pulmonary disease
    Postbronchodilator FEV_1 < 30% predicted
    Resting hypoxemia (PaO_2 < 55 mmHg) or hyper-
        capnia ($PaCO_2$ > 50 mmHg)
    Secondary pulmonary hypertension
    Accelerating rate of deterioration, frequent
        hospitalizations
Idiopathic pulmonary fibrosis
    Total lung capacity or vital capacity < 60%
        predicted
    Resting hypoxemia
    Secondary pulmonary hypertension
    Worsening clinical status despite medical
        therapy
    Accelerating rate of deterioration
Cystic fibrosis
    Postbronchodilator FEV_1 < 30% predicted
    Resting hypoxemia (PaO_2 < 55 mmHg) or hyper-
        capnia ($PaCO_2$ > 50 mmHg)
    Secondary pulmonary hypertension
    Increasing frequency of hospitalizations
    Accelerating weight loss
Primary or secondary pulmonary hypertension
    New York Heart Association functional class III
        or IV
    Mean right atrial pressure > 10 mmHg
    Mean pulmonary artery pressure > 50 mmHg
    Cardiac index < 2.5 liters/min/m^2
    Increasing frequency of syncope or hemoptysis

Postoperative Considerations

Airway Complications

Approximately 25 percent of isolated lung transplant recipients develop an airway abnormality following transplantation [39], but only a minority (15 percent) develop bronchial disruption or stenosis [11]. The most common abnormality is superficial necrosis involving the mucosa at or distal to the bronchial anastomoses. This type of lesion is typically of minor significance and usually resolves spontaneously within a few weeks.

Dehiscence of the bronchial anastomosis may cause obstruction of the mainstem bronchus with or without associated atelectasis. In such cases, placement of a Silastic stent may be required to maintain airway patency (Fig. 48-1). The development of an anastomotic stricture typically follows early problems with airway healing. Treatment of airway stricture includes balloon dilatation [24] and/or endoscopic stent placement.

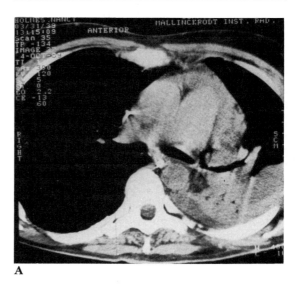

A

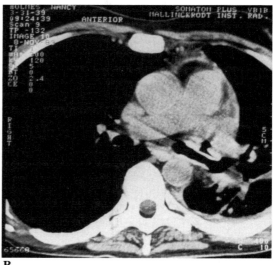

B

Fig. 48-1. A 50-year-old woman with lymphangioleiomyomatosis who underwent left-lung transplantation. A. Computed tomography (CT) scan obtained on posttransplantation day 14 following the onset of increasing dyspnea reveals dehiscence of the left bronchial anastomoses with significant luminal obstruction. B. Repeat CT scan following endoscopic placement of a Silastic stent. (Reproduced from NA Ettinger. Single Lung Transplantation: Early and Late Results. In *Current Topics in Thoracic Surgery.* Amsterdam: Elsevier, 1993.)

Surgical repair of airway complications is rarely required and is considered a procedure of last resort [25].

Acute Lung Injury

The development of severe gas-exchange abnormalities and progressive pulmonary infiltrates early following lung transplantation can have many causes, including transient edema due to reimplantation, pulmonary edema due to hypervolemia, acute allograft rejection, and pneumonia. Failure to respond to empiric diuresis, antibiotics, or corticosteroids suggests the presence of acute lung injury.

The development of acute lung injury following lung transplantation is unpredictable. Estimates of incidence vary, ranging from 8 to 20 percent [11,21]. The histologic findings include diffuse alveolar damage with hyaline membrane formation and/or organizing alveolitis. A variety of causes have been identified and include sepsis syndrome, pneumonia, and mechanical obstruction of the pulmonary venous anastomoses to the left atrium. Other postulated causes include poor allograft preservation, prolonged allograft ischemia, reperfusion injury, and unrecognized aspiration pneumonitis in the donor lung [21].

Histologic documentation should be obtained in all cases to exclude rejection. Infection also should be excluded by bronchoscopy. Treatment of acute lung injury following lung transplantation is usually supportive. Prolonged mechanical ventilation is often required and in extreme cases where oxygenation cannot be maintained, extracorporeal membrane oxygenation may be useful until retransplantation can be performed or spontaneous improvement occurs (Fig. 48-2). Recovery from early acute lung injury may occur with no long-term impairment in pulmonary function or exercise capacity [21]; therefore, an aggressive approach to treatment is warranted.

Acute Rejection

Acute allograft rejection occurs in the vast majority of lung transplant recipients during the first few weeks following transplantation, with a peak incidence occurring during the second week [28]. The clinical manifestations of acute rejection are listed in Table 48-5. Acute rejection may also occur late following transplantation but its clinical presentation is typically more subtle.

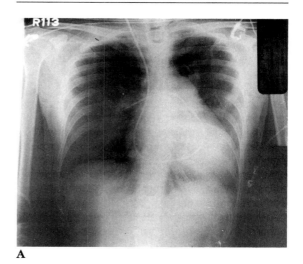

A

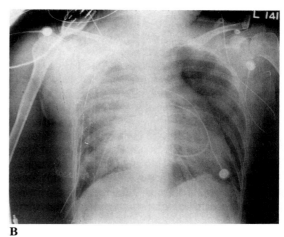

B

Fig. 48-2. A 32-year-old woman with primary pulmonary hypertension who underwent single-lung transplantation. A. Baseline chest radiograph obtained immediately prior to the procedure, demonstrating normal lung fields. B. Chest radiograph obtained 8 hours following the transplantation, demonstrating opacification of the allograft. The patient developed stenosis of the pulmonary venous anastomoses, which caused severe pulmonary congestion at the time of reperfusion. Extracorporeal membrane oxygenation was required for 72 hours prior to stabilization. The patient ultimately made an uneventful recovery. (Reproduced from NA Ettinger. Single Lung Transplantation: Early and Late Results. In *Current Topics in Thoracic Surgery.* Amsterdam: Elsevier, 1993.)

Table 48-5. Clinical manifestations of lung rejection

Acute

Temperature: Rise of > 0.5°C above usual baseline

Oxygenation: Fall of > 10 mmHg below baseline PaO_2

Chest radiograph: New pulmonary infiltrates or no change

Spirometry: Decline in FEV_1 of > 10% below baseline value

Symptoms: Dyspnea, malaise, chest tightness, myalgias

Improvement in the above with high-dose methylprednisolone

Infection excluded

Chronic

Temperature: None or slight increase above baseline

Oxygenation: Early—normal, late—hypoxemia

Chest radiograph: No change from baseline or hyperinflation

Spirometry: Progressive decline in FEV_1, FVC, $FEF_{25-75\%}$

Lung volumes: Progressive decline

Symptoms: Cough, nasal congestion, chest tightness, dyspnea

Transient improvement with high-dose methylprednisolone

Chronic airway infection is commonly present

At the present time, the diagnosis of acute rejection requires histologic documentation, as less invasive diagnostic methods such as bronchoalveolar lavage (BAL) and blood-based assays do not yet permit reliable differentiation of infection from rejection. The detection of donor-specific alloreactivity in BAL-derived lymphocytes has been demonstrated to correlate with acute rejection; however, it may also be detected during episodes of infection and the assay is time-consuming and cumbersome to perform [40]. In a recent study, large increases in serum levels of soluble interleukin-2 (IL-2) receptor correlated with episodes of acute rejection. However, smaller increases also occurred during episodes of infection and the number of patients studied was small [29].

The characteristic histologic findings of acute rejection include perivascular mononuclear infiltrates (Fig. 48-3). Other, less commonly observed patterns include interstitial and/or alveolar edema or hemorrhage, alveolar type II cell hyperplasia, and interstitial fibrosis [28]. A histo-

logic grading system was recently introduced [54] in an effort to standardize the histologic description of rejection and airway inflammation (Table 48-6).

Standard treatment of acute allograft rejection typically consists of bolus doses of intravenous methylprednisolone (500 mg to 1 gm) given over 3 consecutive days. Clinical and radiographic improvement is often observed following the first dose. Such improvement may be itself diagnostic of acute rejection although cytomegalovirus (CMV) pneumonitis may also demonstrate transient improvement in response to corticosteroids. In general, if a rapid and sustained improvement is not observed following empiric steroid therapy, the diagnosis should be confirmed or excluded by transbronchial lung biopsy (see Diagnostic Procedures). Refractory episodes of acute rejection may require treatment with antilymphocyte agents such as antithymocyte globulin or OKT3 [5].

Chronic Rejection

The experience at Washington University indicates that approximately one-third of lung transplant recipients develop chronic allograft rejection. Longer follow-up may reveal an even higher incidence, considering the 50 percent long-term incidence observed in heart-lung transplant recipients [17]. With improvements in both surgical technique and the treatment and prevention of infection, chronic rejection has emerged as the single most limiting factor to the long-term success of lung transplantation.

Chronic rejection may develop within months of transplantation or it may appear years after the procedure. Its clinical onset is usually heralded by a fall in spirometric indices (forced expiratory volume [FEV_1], forced vital capacity [FVC], and forced expiratory flow in midexpiratory phase [$FEF_{25-75\%}$]) that is often refractory to repeated courses of corticosteroids (Fig. 48-4). Exertional dyspnea, decreased exercise tolerance, fatigue, and cough are common symptoms that may precede or accompany the objective changes in pulmonary function (see Table 48-5). The chest radiograph usually remains unchanged or may demonstrate hyperinflation. Many patients in the later stages of chronic rejection develop chronic airway infection with gram-negative organisms such as *Pseudomonas aeruginosa* [46].

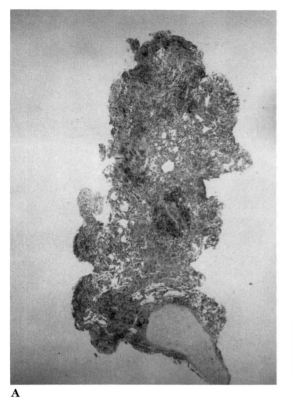

A

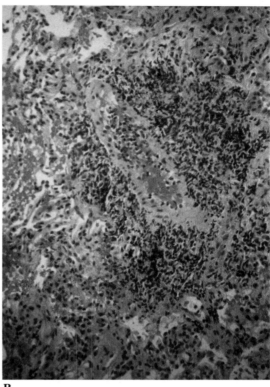

B

Fig. 48-3. Transbronchial lung biopsy specimen obtained from a 60-year-old woman following single-lung transplantation for COPD. A. Low-magnification view demonstrates multiple foci of perivascular inflammation consistent with acute allograft rejection. B. Higher magnification of the same specimen demonstrates extension of the inflammatory infiltrate into surrounding parenchyma, consistent with grade 3 (moderate) rejection.

The diagnosis of chronic rejection may be made by transbronchial lung biopsy, although the yield is lower than with acute rejection [56]. Open lung biopsy may be required for histologic confirmation. The histologic findings are usually those of bronchiolitis obliterans and are characterized by dense submucosal and peribronchiolar fibrosis with obliteration of small airways by concentric fibrous plugs [55]. Vascular-directed obliteration and fibrosis may also accompany the airway lesions. Although histologic confirmation of chronic rejection is desirable, the clinical and spi-rometric presentation is highly characteristic and is usually sufficient to make the diagnosis in most patients, after infection is excluded.

The etiology of chronic rejection is unclear, although several mechanisms have been proposed. The common denominator appears to be the up-regulation of class II major histocompatibility antigen (MHC-II) expression in the bronchial epithelium, resulting in lymphocyte activation and a predominately airway-directed rejection process. A variety of stimuli are associated with such MHC-II upregulation, including both viral (CMV) and bacterial infections as well as exposure to other environmental antigens [1]. The precise role of these infectious and environmental stimuli in the development of the rejection process remains to be defined.

Treatment of chronic rejection usually consists of antilymphocyte agents such as antithymocyte globulin or OKT3. Corticosteroids are also utilized but are often ineffective when used alone.

Table 48-6. **Classification and grading of acute pulmonary rejection**

Grade 0—No rejection
  Normal pulmonary parenchyma

Grade 1—Minimal acute rejection
  Scattered, infrequent perivascular mononuclear infiltrates not overtly obvious at low magnification; vessels cuffed by a ring of transformed lymphocytes 2–3 cells thick

Grade 2—Mild acute rejection
  Frequent perivascular mononuclear infiltrates surrounding venules and arterioles that are easily observed at low magnification; subendothelial infiltration and expansion of perivascular interstitium by inflammatory cells

Grade 3—Moderate acute rejection
  Cuffing of venules and arterioles by dense perivascular mononuclear infiltrate; subendothelial infiltration and degeneration usually present; the inflammatory cell infiltrate extends into the perivascular and peribronchiolar alveolar septa and airspaces

Grade 4—Severe acute rejection
  Diffuse perivascular, interstitial, and alveolar mononuclear infiltration; type I pneumocyte damage with hyaline membrane formation, neutrophilic infiltration, and necrotic cellular debris; associated parenchymal necrosis, infarction, or vasculitis may be present

Source: From SA Yousem et al. A working formulation for the standardization of nomenclature in the diagnosis of heart and lung rejection: Lung Rejection Study Group. *J Heart Lung Transplant* 9:593, 1990.

Treatment may result in improvement or stabilization of lung function, but many patients sustain a permanent and substantial loss of pulmonary function. Although a small proportion of patients progress to respiratory failure, the majority of deaths in patients with chronic rejection are due to infection, arising as a result of the intensive augmentation of immunosuppression. More novel approaches to the treatment of chronic rejection, such as the use of agents that interfere with cell adhesion [6], have not yet been studied in lung transplant recipients.

Infection

BACTERIAL
Approximately one-third of lung transplant recipients develop bacterial pneumonia during the first 2 weeks following transplantation [7,22]. These early pneumonias usually arise as a result of donor lung infection [7]. The majority of lung transplant donors have sustained head injuries or other trauma and have been intubated for over

Fig. 48-4. Longitudinal plot of FEV_1 obtained from a 34-year-old woman who had bilateral lung transplantation for alpha$_1$-antitrypsin deficiency. The patient experienced multiple episodes of acute allograft rejection, treated with corticosteroids. Lung function continued to deteriorate despite treatment. Histologic confirmation of bronchiolitis obliterans was obtained by open lung biopsy. Closed arrows indicate treatment with high-dose methylprednisolone. Open arrows indicate treatment with antilymphocyte agents.

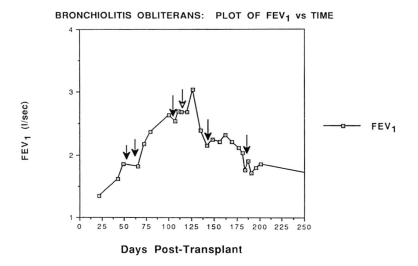

24 hours. Aspiration and pulmonary contusion are relatively common among lung donors and may go unrecognized. Accordingly, organisms cultured from the donor airway are usually the cause of early bacterial pneumonia in the recipient. Gram-negative pathogens and *Staphylococcus aureus* are the most common etiologic agents, although prevailing hospital pathogens may cause nosocomial pneumonia at any time during the initial hospitalization. Patients with cystic fibrosis are typically colonized with *Pseudomonas* species which are a common cause of early bacterial pneumonias among these patients.

The late development of bacterial pneumonia may represent a sporadic, community-acquired infection. Gram-negative or gram-positive pathogens, including *Legionella* species, may be causative (Fig. 48-5). More commonly, late bacterial pneumonias arise in patients with chronic allograft rejection. Bacterial colonization of the airways is common in such patients and the necessary massive immunosuppressive treatment further predisposes the patient to develop pneumonia.

The immediate postoperative use of broad-spectrum antibiotics has proved effective at minimizing the risk of early pneumonia [7]. Empiric antibiotic coverage based on donor sputum Gram stains may be further narrowed when culture results are available. Diagnosis of late bacterial pneumonias should include a bronchoscopic evaluation to exclude the presence of opportunistic pathogens and *Legionella*.

FUNGAL

The majority of lung transplant recipients demonstrate airway colonization with *Candida* species at some point following transplantation [7]. True, invasive *Candida* pneumonia is rare, however. The most common, clinically important fungal pneumonia is caused by *Aspergillus* species, the incidence of which is directly related to the intensity of environmental contamination [13].

Aspergillus infection in lung transplant recipients may present with limited tracheobronchial involvement [26], with localized pulmonary infiltration, or as a rapidly progressive, invasive pneumonia. Airway colonization with *Aspergillus* species represents a significant problem, particularly in patients treated for chronic rejection (Fig. 48-6). The treatment of choice for established aspergillus infections is amphotericin B, although itraconazole may prove useful for patients with limited, slowly progressive infections [26] or

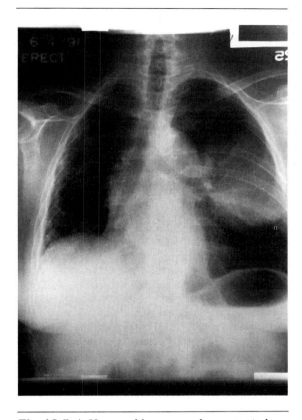

Fig. 48-5. A 60-year-old woman who presented with dyspnea, fever, hypoxemia, and pleuritic chest pain 8 months following lung transplantation. The chest radiograph demonstrates dense left-upper-lobe consolidation. Bronchoalveolar lavage fluid cultures and stains revealed *Legionella pneumophila*. The patient required both erythromycin and rifampin to achieve a lasting clinical response. (Reproduced from NA Ettinger. Immunocompromised Patient: Transplant, Solid Organ, Bone Marrow. In Niederman, Sarosi, Glassroth (Eds), *Respiratory Infections*. Philadelphia: Saunders [in press].)

for those who develop excessive amphotericin-related toxicity.

VIRAL

CMV infection is the most common infectious complication following lung transplantation (Fig. 48-7). Over 90 percent of lung transplant recipients at risk for either a primary or reactivation CMV infection will shed the virus in the blood or the lung during the first year following lung transplantation, and over 70 percent of these patients will have histologic confirmation of CMV pneu-

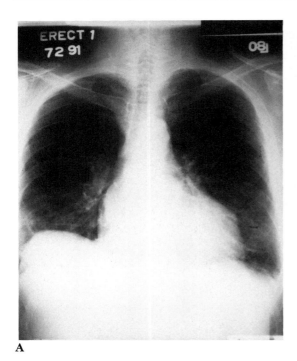

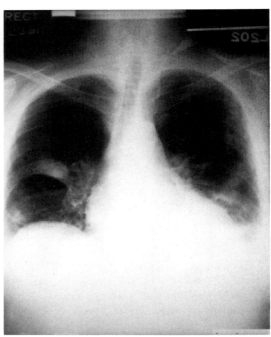

A   B

Fig. 48-6. A 55-year-old man who developed chronic rejection 6 months following bilateral lung transplantation for COPD. A. Baseline chest radiograph obtained at the time of initial treatment with antilymphocyte globulin. Sputum cultures at the time of treatment were positive for *Aspergillus fumigatus.* B. Chest radiograph obtained 3 weeks later, revealing progressive bilateral pulmonary infiltrates. Transbronchial lung biopsy confirmed invasive aspergillus pneumonitis. The patient subsequently died of overwhelming aspergillus infection despite treatment with amphotericin.

monitis if aggressive histologic surveillance is utilized [12].

The clinical presentation of CMV infection in lung transplant recipients is often mistaken for rejection. Fever and malaise are frequently present, but are nonspecific. Radiographic infiltrates rarely accompany milder episodes of CMV infection or pneumonitis [12], but may be present during more severe episodes. The diagnosis of CMV pneumonia is usually made histologically and is often found unexpectedly following routine surveillance lung biopsies (see Diagnostic Procedures). The detection of CMV in BAL fluid is associated with histologic evidence of underlying pneumonitis in only one-third of cases and is therefore not predictive of CMV pneumonitis on biopsy.

Patients at risk for primary CMV infection tend to develop more frequent and more severe episodes of CMV pneumonitis than patients in other donor-recipient serologic risk groups, and most life-threatening episodes occur during the course of a primary infection. CMV infection has been associated with a negative impact on long-term pulmonary function, an increase in the incidence of chronic rejection and lower overall survival

[9]. These findings are controversial, however, and will require larger, multicenter studies for confirmation [12].

Ganciclovir is effective therapy for most cases of CMV pneumonia in lung transplant recipients although foscarnet may be successfully used for patients with severe ganciclovir toxicity or those with ganciclovir-resistant strains of CMV. The issue of ganciclovir prophylaxis for patients at risk for primary CMV infection is controversial. Many centers provide such prophylaxis, although the effectiveness of this approach and the optimal duration of treatment have not yet been determined in large-scale studies.

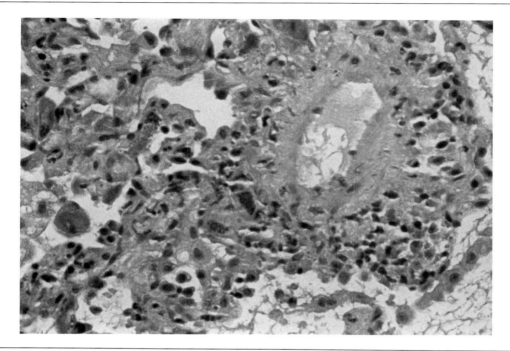

Fig. 48-7. Photomicrograph of transbronchial lung biopsy specimen obtained from a 55-year-old man with COPD who underwent single-lung transplantation. The biopsy confirmed the presence of cytomegalovirus (CMV) pneumonitis. Characteristic cytomegalic cells are seen in association with a perivascular mononuclear infiltrate. This specimen points out the difficulty in diagnosing rejection in the presence of CMV pneumonitis, as both processes may cause perivascular inflammation.

Diagnostic Procedures

Invasive diagnostic procedures are frequently required in lung and heart-lung transplant recipients, particularly since the clinical features of acute allograft rejection and CMV pneumonitis are often indistinguishable. Transbronchial lung biopsy has proved extremely useful in heart-lung [23] and lung transplant recipients [51] and is used extensively in the management of these patients.

In a recent analysis of 203 procedures performed on 55 lung transplant recipients, the sensitivities of transbronchial biopsy for the diagnosis of acute rejection and CMV pneumonitis were 72 and 91 percent, respectively [51]. On average, 10 biopsy specimens were obtained during each procedure. When biopsies were performed for clinical indications, a specific, treatable diagnosis was obtained in 69 percent of cases. Likewise, when a procedure was performed routinely in asymptomatic patients as part of a surveillance program, a specific, unexpected diagnosis, usually CMV pneumonia or acute rejection, was found in 57 percent of cases.

The high positivity rate during routine transbronchial biopsy surveillance suggests that this surveillance is useful and should be employed. However, the high positivity rate also suggests that lung biopsy is not the optimal method of surveillance as it is performed relatively infrequently, is time-consuming, and is not without risk. A less invasive method of surveillance that can be performed frequently and that can distinguish infection from rejection is not presently available but remains an important objective.

As in other immunocompromised hosts [44], BAL is useful for the diagnosis of opportunistic infection in lung transplant recipients. However, its utility for the diagnosis of rejection has not been proved. Differential analysis of BAL-derived cell populations does not appear to be able to reliably distinguish rejection from infection [14]. As previously mentioned, functional studies of BAL-derived lymphocytes have proved useful in the identification of acute allograft rejection in some centers [40]. However, these assays are time-consuming and require donor splenocytes, which are often not available.

Although the majority of pathologic processes affecting the allograft may be identified by trans-bronchial biopsy, open lung biopsy is occasionally required. Chronic allograft rejection, adult respiratory distress syndrome (ARDS), posttransplantation lymphoproliferative disorder, and opportunistic fungal infections are some examples of pulmonary processes in lung transplant recipients that commonly require histologic confirmation by open lung biopsy.

Results

The outcome of lung transplantation can be measured in terms of improvement in lung function, hemodynamics, exercise capacity, and survival. These results may vary according to the type of underlying disease and according to the type of transplantation performed.

Pulmonary Function Testing

Steady improvements in spirometric measurements and lung volumes typically occur for the first 2 months following lung transplantation, followed by more gradual improvement or plateau [11]. As expected, the degree of improvement is greater in bilateral or double-lung transplant recipients when compared to single-lung transplant recipients (Fig. 48-8). The development of early complications in the allograft can delay the usual pace of improvement.

Gas exchange recovers at a more variable pace following lung transplantation. In patients with preoperative carbon dioxide retention, hypercapnia often persists for 2 to 3 weeks following the transplant procedure. In such patients, carbon dioxide rebreathing studies have demonstrated a blunting of the ventilatory response to carbon dioxide that returns toward normal levels at the same time the hypercapnia resolves (G. Trachiotis, personal communication, 1992). This delay in recovery of central chemoreceptivity does not usually impair withdrawal of mechanical ventilation during the immediate perioperative period. Other centers have noted similar or conflicting findings related to hypercapneic chemosensitivity in lung transplant recipients [8,15,41]. However, significant differences in methodology exist between the studies.

Hemodynamics

SLT for primary or secondary pulmonary hypertension results in dramatic improvement of all hemodynamic indices in the majority of patients who receive a successful transplant (Fig. 48-9). Mean pulmonary artery pressures fall and cardiac output increases immediately following the procedure [38].

The early perioperative course is unusually labile following SLT for pulmonary hypertension. Nearly all pulmonary blood flow is directed to the allograft, with ventilation shared nearly equally between the two lungs. Although normal gas exchange is usually maintained despite such $\dot{V}/\dot{Q}$ mismatch, the allograft remains unusually sensitive to insults [30]. Significant levels of hypoxemia can develop with relatively minor episodes of rejection or infection or even during routine bronchoscopy. Recurrence of pulmonary hypertension following lung transplantation has not been documented.

Exercise Capacity

Cardiopulmonary exercise testing has consistently demonstrated significant exercise limitation in terms of maximum oxygen consumption at peak exercise in both heart-lung and isolated lung transplant recipients [16,36,45,53]. Maximum oxygen consumption typically ranges from 45 to 50 percent of predicted and no significant differences are found between single-lung and bilateral lung transplant recipients. Circulatory factors and deconditioning appear to be limiting in most patients.

As measured by 6-minute walking distance, exercise capacity improves dramatically following lung transplantation. Although the results appear to be better among bilateral lung transplant recipients when compared to single-lung transplant re-

Fig. 48-8. Pulmonary function testing obtained from single-lung (*squares*) ($n = 18$) and bilateral lung (*black diamonds*) ($n = 17$) transplant recipients during the first year after transplantation. A. FEV_1. B. Total lung capacity (*TLC*). C. $DLCO/Va$. D. PaO_2. The asterisk indicates $P < 0.05$ using analysis of variance. SD = standard deviation. (Reproduced from NA Ettinger. Single Lung Transplantation: Early and Late Results. In GA Patterson, L Couraud (Eds), *Current Topics in General Thoracic Surgery.* Amsterdam: Elsevier, 1993.)

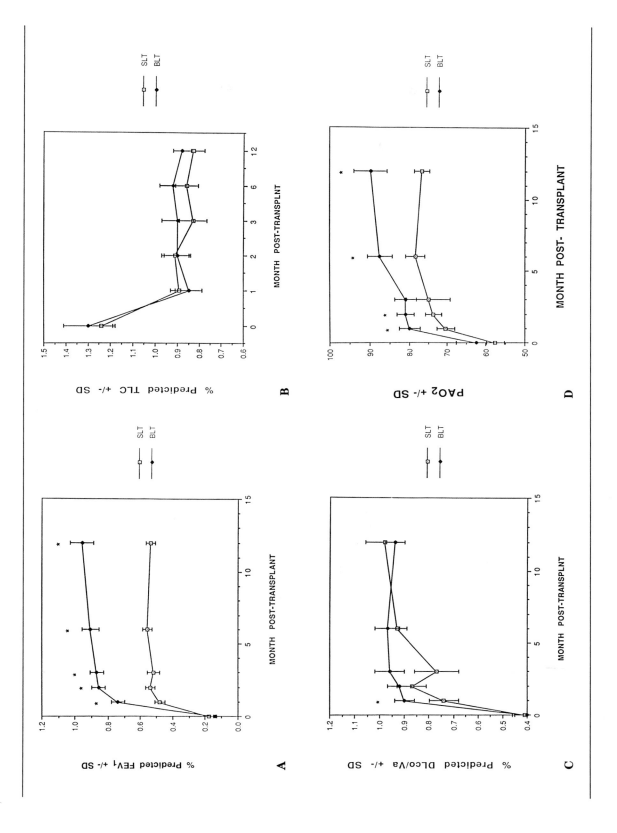

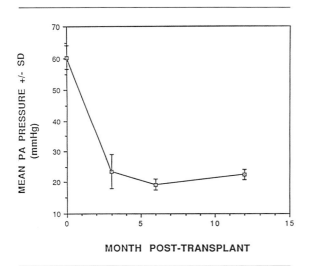

MONTH POST-TRANSPLANT

Fig. 48-9. Longitudinal plot of mean pulmonary artery (*PA*) pressure obtained from eight patients who underwent single-lung transplantation for primary or secondary pulmonary hypertension. Measurements are obtained at baseline and 3, 6, and 12 months following transplantation. *SD* = standard deviation.

cipients, these differences do not appear to translate into perceptible inequalities between these groups in terms of activities of daily living or lifestyle. However, further comparisons using quality-of-life indices are needed to detect such differences.

Survival

Information obtained from the St. Louis International Lung Transplant Registry through August 1992 reveals 1- and 2-year actuarial survival figures of 68 and 60 percent, respectively (n = 1362). Results at individual centers [2,48] exceed these figures obtained from over 81 centers worldwide.

Significant survival differences between single-lung and bilateral lung transplant recipients are not observed (Fig. 48-10*A*). Survival appears to

Fig. 48-10. St. Louis International Lung Transplant Registry 2-year actuarial survival curves by (A) type of transplantation and (B) underlying diagnosis. *PH* = pulmonary hypertension; *CF* = cystic fibrosis; *EMP* = emphysema; *PF* = pulmonary fibrosis; *S* = single; *B* = bilateral; *E* = en bloc double.

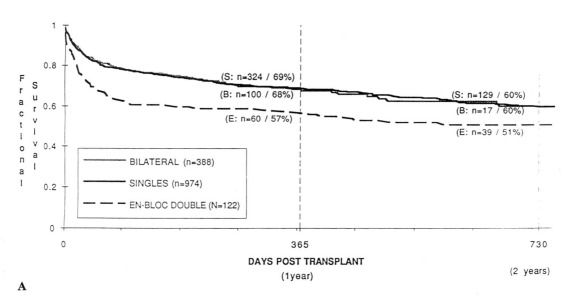
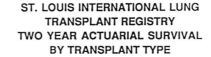

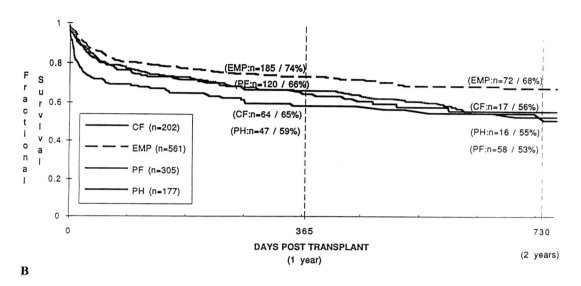

ST. LOUIS INTERNATIONAL LUNG
TRANSPLANT REGISTRY
TWO YEAR ACTUARIAL SURVIVAL
BY DIAGNOSIS

B

Fig. 48-10. (continued)

be best among patients undergoing transplantation for emphysema and worst for patients undergoing transplantation for pulmonary hypertension (Fig. 48-10*B*).

Causes of death following lung transplantation vary by time following the procedure. During the early perioperative period, the most common causes of death are mechanical complications related to the airway and cardiac complications occurring intraoperatively or immediately postoperatively. ARDS is an increasingly recognized early cause of death. Late deaths are primarily related to chronic rejection and its treatment. Infection commonly supervenes during periods of intensive augmentation of immunosuppression and is the most common cause of death in patients with chronic rejection.

The Future

Although lung transplantation can no longer be considered experimental, it is by no means a routine procedure. Many advances will be required before lung transplantation can be provided to those who need it and long-term survival can be regularly expected. Improvements in lung preservation are needed to improve early graft function and to increase the availability of donor organs. Risk factors for the development of chronic rejection must be identified and better methods of prevention and treatment must be developed. In addition, the performance of lung transplantation in patients who have systemic diseases with limited pulmonary involvement, such as scleroderma, systemic lupus erythematosus, and rheumatoid arthritis, warrants further study. Finally, the possibility of utilizing lung xenografts may ultimately provide an answer to the problem of limited organ availability.

References

1. Burke CM, et al. Lung immunogenicity, rejection, and obliterative bronchiolitis. *Chest* 92:547, 1987.
2. Calhoon JH, et al. Single lung transplantation: Alternative indications and techniques. *J Thorac Cardiovasc Surg* 101:816, 1991.
3. Cooper JD. The evolution of techniques and indications for lung transplantation. *Ann Surg* 212:249, 1990.
4. Cooper JD, et al. Double lung transplantation for advanced chronic obstructive lung disease. *Am Rev Respir Dis* 139:303, 1989.
5. Cosimi AB. The clinical usefulness of anti-

lymphocyte antibodies. *Transplant Proc* 15:583, 1983.

6. Cosimi AB, et al. In vivo effects of monoclonal antibody to ICAM-1 in nonhuman primates with renal allografts. *J Immunol* 144:4604, 1990.

7. Dauber JH, Paradis IL, Dummer JS. Infectious complications in pulmonary allograft recipients. *Clin Chest Med* 11:291, 1990.

8. Duncan SR, et al. Hypercarbic ventilatory responses of human heart-lung transplant recipients. *Am Rev Respir Dis* 144:126, 1991.

9. Duncan SR, et al. Sequelae of cytomegalovirus pulmonary infections in lung allograft recipients. *Am Rev Respir Dis* 146:1419, 1992.

10. Egan TM, et al. Analysis of referrals for lung transplantation. *Chest* 99:867, 1991.

11. Ettinger NA. Single Lung Transplantation: Results—Early and Late. In GA Patterson (Ed), *Current Topics in Thoracic Surgery.* Amsterdam: Elsevier, 1993.

12. Ettinger NA, et al. Cytomegalovirus pneumonitis: Impact following isolated lung transplantation. *Am Rev Respir Dis* (in press).

13. Ettinger NA, Trulock EP. Pulmonary considerations of organ transplantation. *Am Rev Respir Dis* Part 1, 143:1386; Parts 2 and 3, 144:213, 433, 1991.

14. Ettinger NA, et al. The use of bronchoalveolar lavage to distinguish rejection from infection in single and double lung transplant recipients. *Am Rev Respir Dis* 143:A600, 1991.

15. Frost AE, et al. Hypercapneic ventilatory response in recipients of double-lung transplants. *Am Rev Respir Dis* 146:1610, 1992.

16. Gibbons WJ, et al. Cardiopulmonary exercise responses after single lung transplantation for severe obstructive lung disease. *Chest* 100:106, 1991.

17. Glanville AR, et al. Obliterative bronchiolitis after heart-lung transplantation: Apparent arrest by augmented immunosuppression. *Ann Intern Med* 107:300, 1987.

18. Goldberg M, Limo O, Morgan E. A comparison between cyclosporine A and methylprednisolone plus azathioprine on bronchial healing following canine lung autotransplantation. *J Thorac Cardiovasc Surg* 85:821, 1983.

19. Grossman RF, et al. Results of single-lung transplantation for bilateral pulmonary fibrosis. *N Engl J Med* 322:727, 1990.

20. Hardy JD, Webb WR, Dalton ML. Lung homotransplantation in man. *JAMA* 186:1065, 1963.

21. Haydock DA, et al. Management of dysfunction in the transplanted lung: Experience with 7 clinical cases. *Ann Thorac Surg* 53:635, 1992.

22. Haydock DA, et al. Lung transplantation: Analysis of thirty six consecutive procedures performed over a twelve month period. *J Thorac Cardiovasc Surg* 103:329, 1992.

23. Higenbottam T, et al. Transbronchial lung biopsy for the diagnosis of rejection in heart-lung transplant patients. *Transplantation* 46:532, 1988.

24. Keller C, Frost A. Fiberoptic bronchoplasty: Description of a simple technique for the management of bronchial stenosis following lung transplantation. *Chest* 102:995, 1992.

25. Kirk AJB, et al. Successful surgical management of bronchial dehiscence after single-lung transplantation. *Ann Thorac Surg* 49:147, 1990.

26. Kramer MR, et al. Ulcerative tracheobronchitis after lung transplantation. *Am Rev Respir Dis* 144:552, 1991.

27. Kriett JM, Kaye MP. The registry of the International Society for Heart and Lung Transplantation: Eighth official report—1991. *J Heart Lung Transplant* 10:491, 1991.

28. Lawrence EC. Diagnosis and Management of Lung Allograft Rejection. In RF Grossman, JR Maurer (Ed), *Pulmonary Considerations in Transplantation.* Philadelphia: Saunders, 1990. Pp 269–278.

29. Lawrence EC, Holland V, Young JB. Dynamic changes in soluble interleukin-2 receptor levels following lung or heart-lung transplantation. *Am Rev Respir Dis* 140:789, 1989.

30. Levine SM, et al. Single lung transplantation for primary pulmonary hypertension. *Chest* 98:1107, 1990.

31. Lima O, et al. Effects of methylprednisolone and azathioprine on bronchial healing following lung transplantation. *J Thorac Cardiovasc Surg* 82:211, 1981.

32. Lima O, Goldberg M, Peters WJ. Bronchial omentopexy in canine lung allotransplantation. *J Thorac Cardiovasc Surg* 83:418, 1982.

33. Low DE, et al. Lung transplantation of ventilator dependent patients. *Chest* 101:8, 1992.

34. Mal H, et al. Unilateral lung transplantation in end stage pulmonary emphysema. *Am Rev Respir Dis* 140:797, 1989.

35. McCarthy PM, et al. Single-lung transplantation with atrial septal defect repair for Eisenmenger's syndrome. *Ann Thorac Surg* 52:300, 1991.

36. Miyoshi S, et al. Cardiopulmonary exercise testing after single and double lung transplantation. *Chest* 97:1130, 1990.

37. Pasque MK, et al. Improved technique for bilateral lung transplantation: Rationale and initial clinical experience. *Ann Thorac Surg* 49:785, 1990.

38. Pasque MK, et al. Single-lung transplantation for pulmonary hypertension: Three-month hemodynamic follow-up. *Circulation* 84:2275, 1991.

39. Patterson GA, Todd TR, Cooper JD. Airway complications after double lung transplantation. *J Thorac Cardiovasc Surg* 99:14, 1990.

40. Rabinowich H, et al. Proliferative responses of bronchoalveolar lavage lymphocytes from heart-

lung transplant patients. *Transplantation* 49:115, 1990.

41. Sanders MH, et al. Ventilation and breathing pattern during progressive hypercapnea and hypoxia after human heart-lung transplantation. *Am Rev Respir Dis* 140:38, 1989.

42. Schafers HJ, et al. Preoperative corticosteroids: A contraindication to lung transplantation? *Chest* 102:1522, 1992.

43. Stevens PM, et al. Regional ventilation and perfusion after lung transplantation in patients with emphysema. *N Engl J Med* 282:245, 1970.

44. Stover DE, et al. Bronchoalveolar lavage in the diagnosis of diffuse pulmonary infiltrates in the immunosuppressed host. *Ann Intern Med* 101:1, 1984.

45. Theodore J, et al. Cardiopulmonary function at maximum tolerable work rate exercise following human heart-lung transplantation. *Chest* 92:433, 1987.

46. Theodore J, Starnes VA, Lewiston NJ. Obliterative bronchiolitis. *Clin Chest Med* 11:309, 1990.

47. Toronto Lung Transplant Group. Experience with single-lung transplantation for pulmonary fibrosis. *JAMA* 259:2258, 1988.

48. Trulock EP, et al. The Washington University-Barnes Hospital experience with lung transplantation. *JAMA* 266:1943, 1991.

49. Trulock EP, et al. Unilateral lung transplantation for pulmonary hypertension. *Am Rev Respir Dis* 143:A467, 1991.

50. Trulock EP, et al. Single lung transplantation for severe chronic obstructive pulmonary disease. *Chest* 96:738, 1989.

51. Trulock EP, et al. The role of transbronchial lung biopsy in the treatment of lung transplant recipients. *Chest* 102:1049, 1992.

52. UNOS. *Transplantation Statistics—1990.* Press release. Richmond, VA: United Network for Organ Sharing (UNOS), 1991.

53. Williams TJ, et al. Maximal exercise testing in single and double lung transplant recipients. *Am Rev Respir Dis* 145:101, 1992.

54. Yousem SA, et al. A working formulation for the standardization of nomenclature in the diagnosis of heart and lung rejection: Lung Rejection Study Group. *J Heart Lung Transplant* 9:593, 1990.

55. Yousem SA, Burke CM, Billingham ME, Pathologic pulmonary alterations in long-term human heart-lung transplantation. *Hum Pathol* 16:911, 1985.

56. Yousem SA, et al. Efficacy of transbronchial lung biopsy in the diagnosis of bronchiolitis obliterans in heart-lung transplant recipients. *Transplantation* 47:893, 1989.

VII

Pulmonary Vascular Diseases

49

The Normal Adult Pulmonary Circulation

Steven M. Scharf   Harly E. Greenberg

The survey of the adult pulmonary circulation that follows in the next few chapters emphasizes the interplay between structure and function in determining the behavior of the normal and abnormal pulmonary vascular bed. We especially emphasize the clinical course of patients with pulmonary hypertension and cor pulmonale (right ventricular failure on the basis of lung disease). There are four chapters in this section. The Normal Adult Pulmonary Circulation is devoted to a description of the anatomy, physiology, and biochemistry of the pulmonary vascular bed. In this chapter, we also consider newer aspects of the physiology of lung extravascular water homeostasis and the physiologic-anatomic basis for pulmonary edema. In addition, we consider the normal function of the bronchial circulation. Pulmonary Hypertension: Pathophysiology and Clinical Disorders discusses the mechanisms by which disease causes pulmonary hypertension and the natural history and prognosis of this disorder. Consideration is given to treatment modalities of primary pulmonary hypertension. Pulmonary Embolism describes the pathogenesis, natural history, diagnosis, and management of deep vein thrombosis and pulmonary thromboembolism. Finally, in Pulmonary Heart Disease, we describe the response of the right ventricle to acute and chronic elevations in pulmonary vascular resistance and abnormal right ventricular loading conditions, and we consider the natural history of cor pulmonale and its treatment.

Pulmonary Vascular Anatomy

General Considerations

The principal function of the lungs is to transport the respiratory gases, O_2 and CO_2, into and out of the bloodstream. In the mammalian lung, this is done by a remarkable system of air- and blood-containing vessels, folded together in an elastic structure in such a way that the air- and blood-containing vessels are in intimate contact yet their contents do not physically mix. The normal adult man requires the transfer of 200 to 250 ml/min of O_2 into the body at rest. However, the transport of O_2 can increase to 3000 to 4000 ml/min at maximum exercise [46]. In diseased lungs, O_2 transport capacity can be limited, which in turn limits the transport of O_2 into peripheral tissues, the ultimate target.

To accomplish its task, the pulmonary vasculature affords a capillary surface area (i.e., blood vessels exposed to air-containing compartments) measuring 50 to 80 m^2 and being some 300 nm thin [97–99]. In normal lungs, which receive all the output from the right ventricle (approximately 5 liters/min), there is 290 ± 50 ml/m^2 volume in the pulmonary circulation. Of this pulmonary blood volume, approximately 50 ml/m^2 is found in the gas-exchanging vessels, the capillaries. Any given red cell normally spends approximately 0.75 seconds in air-exchanging vessels, which affords ample time for gas exchange across the wall of the vessel by the process of diffusion.

Several differences between systemic and pulmonary circulations should be emphasized [27]. First, the major site of flow resistance in the pulmonary circulation is in alveolar capillaries, as opposed to precapillary vessels in the systemic circulation. Second, pulmonary microvascular pressures are extremely variable within the lung depending on the anatomic location of the vessel (dependent versus independent regions), the site of the vessel within the parenchyma (intraalveolar versus extraalveolar), and the state of lung inflation. Third, the systemic vessels within the lung (bronchial circulation and pleural vessels) drain into the same venous bed as the pulmonary vessels by a network of anastomoses that constitute potential shunts from one bed to another.

Careful morphometric analysis of the pulmonary vascular tree reveals that there are more arteries than airways [37,84,85,96,98,99]. After a few generations, pulmonary arteries lose their muscular media and the most peripheral branches consist only of endothelium and internal elastic membrane. This flimsy structure is very susceptible to direct mechanical interactions, either compression or tethering open, by surrounding lung parenchyma. Extension of muscular coats from arterial generations that normally have them (diameter 100 to 500 μm) into peripheral arteries that normally do not is one of the prime histologic manifestations of pulmonary hypertension. The muscular coat in pulmonary arterioles is relatively smaller (3 to 4 percent of cross sectional diameter) than that in systemic arterioles (40 to 50 percent of cross sectional diameter) [94]. Sympathetic and parasympathetic innervation to pulmonary vessels is sparser than to systemic vessels [41,104]. The pulmonary circulation has no valves. Pulmonary veins are also relatively more thin-walled than systemic veins of the same diameter. These factors mean that the pulmonary circulation normally has an enormous capacity to accommodate increased blood flow by either distension or recruitment of pulmonary vessels (see next section), with little increase in pressure.

Pulmonary Capillaries

The pulmonary capillary network is different from that in the systemic circulation. Systemic arterioles give rise to successive generations of capillaries as a spreading brush, which reunite on the venous side. One can trace the connection between systemic arterioles and the capillaries to which they give rise. The situation is different in the pulmonary system. Weibel [98] characterized pulmonary capillaries in the alveolar walls as forming a dense hexagonal network of cylindric tubes into and out of which conducting vessels were connected. Other, more complicated models have been proposed to account for biologic irregularity and to make mathematic analysis feasible [27]. Fung and Sobin [23] have modeled the alveolar microvascular network as a sheet perforated by holes and have idealized pulmonary alveolar flow as occurring between two membranes held apart by evenly spaced posts, much like the geometry of an underground parking garage. Both the tube flow model [99] and the sheet flow model [23] are probably oversimplifications of the real situation. There are advantages to each model. However, Fung and Sobin [23] have pointed out that Poiseuille type flow would not pertain to either model.

It is useful to distinguish between three types of vessels in the pulmonary microvasculature: intraalveolar, alveolar corner, and extraalveolar vessels. *Intraalveolar* microvessels are contained within and virtually fill the walls between separate adjacent alveoli. They are subject to changes in intraalveolar pressure, being compressed when alveolar pressure increases relative to pleural pressure (lung inflation) and vice versa. They are also subject to the effects of alveolar surface tension. Thus, capillary morphology depends on lung volume, vascular pressures, and alveolar surface forces [28].

Corner vessels are found at the junction of three alveoli. They are contained within folds of the endothelium, or pleats, beneath sharp curvatures of the alveolar surfactant film [28]. In this way, corner vessels are contained within a space surrounded by smooth curved tissue surfaces, which protect them from perturbations of alveolar pressure. Hence, when intraalveolar pressure is increased, thus shutting off flow through alveolar walls, flow can continue from arterial to venous channels, even when there are swings in alveolar pressure [27].

Extraalveolar vessels are small vessels not exposed to alveolar pressure and are surrounded by a connective tissue sheath. They are exposed to interstitial pressure, which decreases as the lungs inflate (i.e., as intraalveolar pressure increases relative to pleural pressure). Hence, lung inflation tends to open extraalveolar vessels while closing intraalveolar vessels. The differing behavior of intraalveolar and extraalveolar vessels accounts for lung volume–dependent changes in pulmonary vascular volume and resistance, as discussed later.

Pulmonary Vascular Pressures

The pulmonary vascular bed is a low-pressure, low-resistance bed that accommodates all the cardiac output. Normally, pulmonary vascular pressures are measured relative to atmospheric pressure and are zero-referenced to a level 5 cm below the angle of Louis in the supine patient (approximate level of the right atrium). When comparing data between different laboratories, it is important to keep in mind possible differences in zero reference points. Normal limits for pressure values in the pulmonary circulation are given in Table 49-1. Pulmonary arterial pressure contours resemble those seen at the aortic root, with a dicrotic notch (Fig. 49-1). However, pulmonary arterial pressures recorded from bedside balloon-tipped catheter systems may not resemble those recorded under ideal conditions. Under ideal conditions, the frequency response of the catheter transducer system used to record pulmonary arterial pressure should be flat to approximately 80 Hz [57]. The presence of bubbles in the line or, as is common in long indwelling catheters used in critical care units, fibrin clots at the catheter tip can severely dampen this response such that high-frequency components of the signal are damped and the signal can resemble a mean. Other causes of damped recording include tubing kinks, an excessive number of stopcocks, and cracked fittings. On the other hand, pulmonary artery catheters may demonstrate excessive high-frequency components, sometimes due to vibration or knocking of the catheter, which may make interpretation difficult. Finally, pulmonary arterial pressure is subject to transmitted changes in intrathoracic pressure. With normal quiet breathing (i.e., under catheterization laboratory conditions), these are small. However, in the presence of abnormal ventilatory patterns (e.g., airway obstruction or positive-pressure ventilation), these may be considerable. In such cases, referencing pulmonary vascular pressures to atmosphere may be confusing at best and misleading at worst.

Pulmonary venous pressure is equal to left atrial (LA) pressure. Both left and right atrial (RA) pressures exhibit three waveforms per beat, the *a*, *c*, and *v* waves (see Fig. 49-1). The *a* wave

coincides with atrial contraction and peaks approximately 80 ms after the P wave on the surface electrocardiogram (ECG). The *v* wave is due to atrial filling during ventricular systole, aided by descent of the atrioventricular (AV) valve ring. The origin of the *c* wave, a minor deflection, is not as well established but may be due to bulging of the AV valves into the atria at the onset of ventricular systole. The pressure descent following the *a* wave is called the *x* descent, that following the *c* wave is the *x'* descent, and the *y* descent follows the *v* wave. The right ventricular (RV) waveform (see Fig. 49-1) is characterized by a gradual upsloping curve during diastole (ventricular filling) with a rapid steep upstroke at the onset of ventricular systole. RV end-diastolic pressure is normally equal to mean RA pressure since there is no flow across the open tricuspid valve.

During diastole, there is normally no flow across the pulmonary bed. Hence, there is no pressure gradient from pulmonary artery to vein, and so pulmonary artery end-diastolic pressure is normally equal to pulmonary venous and left atrial pressure. Because mean LA pressure is normally equal to left ventricular (LV) end-diastolic pressure, pulmonary artery end-diastolic pressure becomes a measure of LV filling pressure. Of course, if pulmonary vascular resistance is elevated (see below), then flow continues throughout diastole, and pulmonary artery end-diastolic pressure is greater than pulmonary venous pressure. If a catheter is wedged into a small pulmonary vessel such that flow ceases through the vessel, then there is no longer a pressure drop from catheter tip to pulmonary vein and the pressure recorded from the wedged catheter is equal to LA and LV end-diastolic pressure, provided the catheter is wedged in a so-called zone 3 portion of the lung (defined below). A similar recording

Table 49-1. **Approximate normal pulmonary hemodynamic values**

Pulmonary arterial pressure	
Systolic	22–30 mmHg
Diastolic	6–12 mmHg
Mean	10–12 mmHg
Left ventricular end-diastolic pressure (= left atrial mean)	6–12 mmHg
Right ventricular end-diastolic pressure (= right atrial mean)	0–6 mmHg
Cardiac index	2.7–3.5 liters/min/m^2
Pulmonary vascular volume	290 ml/m^2
Capillary blood volume	80–120 ml
Pulmonary vascular resistance	150–200 dynes/cm^2

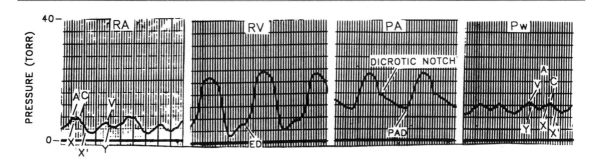

Fig. 49-1. Normal pulmonary and right heart pressures. These were measured using a standard saline-filled balloon-tipped catheter and are of particularly excellent quality for this type of system. Note mean right atrial (*RA*) pressure is equal to right ventricular (*RV*) end-diastolic (*ED*) pressure. Pulmonary arterial diastolic (*PAD*) pressure is equal to mean pulmonary wedge pressure (*Pw*) which, under most circumstances, is equal to left ventricular end-diastolic pressure. (Courtesy of Dr. Gary Friedman.)

can be made by using a balloon-tipped catheter in a small branch of the pulmonary artery to stop flow [89]. The pressure recorded often is called the *capillary wedge pressure*, although it has very little to do with pulmonary capillary pressure when blood is flowing.

Pulmonary Capillary Pressures

Pulmonary capillaries are interposed between arterioles and veins. As will be discussed in detail later, it is the capillary hydrostatic pressure that provides the gradient for filtration of fluid into the interstitium and alveoli (pulmonary edema). Thus, one would ideally want to measure this in clinical situations where pulmonary edema is a consideration. For any given arterial to venous channel, capillary pressure depends on the longitudinal distribution of resistance along the channel as well as flow. Capillary pressure (Pc) is related to blood flow through the channel ($\dot{Q}c$), venous resistance (Rv), and pulmonary venous pressure (Ppv) by the laminar flow equation:

$$Pc = Ppv + \dot{Q}cRv$$

Since flow is related to inflow pressure (Ppa) and arterial resistance (Ra) for each channel, Pc can be shown to be related to Ppa and the ratio of venous to arterial resistance (Rv/Ra):

$$Pc = \frac{(Rv/Ra)\ Ppa\ +\ Ppv}{1\ +\ Rv/Ra}$$

This is easily derived from laminar flow relationships. Thus, pulmonary capillary pressure is, in part, a function of the ratio of venous to arterial resistance (Rv/Ra), downstream pressure (Ppv), and arterial pressure (Ppa). The longitudinal dis-

tribution of the pulmonary vasculature has been reviewed extensively [18,19].

A number of techniques have been devised to measure capillary pressure, with varying degrees of agreement between them [66]. One such technique, the arterial occlusion technique, has been proposed as clinically useful [12,13,19]. The technique is based on the assumption that most pulmonary vascular compliance between a catheter tip in a branch of the pulmonary artery and venous outflow is located in pulmonary capillaries. When arterial flow in the branch is stopped by wedging the catheter tip distally or inflating a balloon just proximal to the catheter tip, pressure immediately falls to the level in the pulmonary capillaries (no flow = no pressure gradient). Then as the capillary reservoir empties, pressure falls exponentially to that of the pulmonary veins. Thus two phases can be distinguished in the wedged catheter: first an initial fall to the level of pulmonary capillary pressure and then a slower fall leading to equilibration with the pulmonary venous pressure and with the usually measured wedge pressure (Fig. 49-2) [36]. Knowing capillary pressure, one could calculate the longitudinal distributions of resistances. However, a number of theoretic and practical problems remain before this technique can be recommended as a routine clinical measure [36,66].

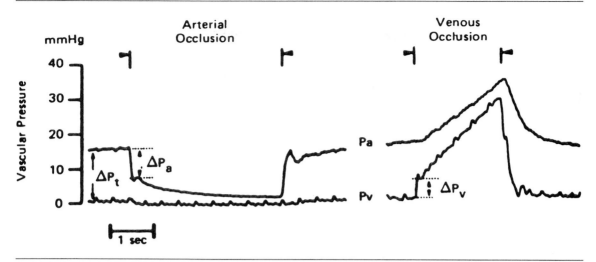

Fig. 49-2. Time course of separate pulmonary arterial and venous occlusions. With arterial occlusion, pulmonary arterial pressure (Pa) suddenly falls to a level equal to true capillary pressure (Pt), not to be confused with so-called capillary wedge pressure. There is then a slower fall as Pa equilibrates with pulmonary venous pressure (Pv), which is the usual "wedge" pressure measured clinically. (Reprinted with permission from TS Hakim, RP Michel, HK Chang, Partitioning of pulmonary vascular resistance by arterial and venous occlusion. *J Appl Physiol* 52:710, 1982.)

Pulmonary Blood Flow

Although the pulmonary circulation receives all the cardiac output, the distribution of blood flow within the lung is far from uniform. Physiologists frequently speak about *upstream* and *downstream* loci in a vascular bed. These terms are relative and connote an orientation more toward the arterial (upstream) or more toward the venous (downstream) side of the circulation. In the upright human, there is a hydrostatic gradient down the lung due to gravitational effects on the column of blood (approximately 30 cmH$_2$O, the approximate height of the adult human lung). West and coworkers [101,102] conceived of the distribution of blood flow within lung according to the relation between pulmonary arterial (PPA), alveolar (PALV), and venous (PPV) pressures. Pulmonary hydrostatic pressures increase from apex to base of the upright lung due to the gravitational acceleration and are equal to pgh, where p is fluid density (1.05 gm/cm^3 for blood), g the

gravitational acceleration constant (980 cm/s^2 on the planet earth at sea level), and h the vertical distance down the lung. Since p and g remain constant, vascular pressure increases approximately 1 cmH$_2$O for each centimeter down the lung.

With a mean PPA of 20 cmH$_2$O, PPA falls to zero 20 cm from the bottom of the lung. With a mean PPV of 10 cmH$_2$O, PPV falls to zero 10 cm from the bottom of the lung. With the lung at rest and the glottis open, alveolar pressure (PALV) is constant throughout the lung (PALV = 0) [32]. This distribution of pressures results in three zones of flow within the lung (Fig. 49-3). In zone 1 (more than 20 cm from the bottom of the lung), both PPA and PPV are less than zero (= PALV). Pulmonary vessels are collapsed and flow is zero. In zone 2 (in our example, 10 to 20 cm from the bottom of the lung), PPA exceeds PALV which exceeds PPV. Flow is thus determined by the gradient between PPA and PALV, *not* the gradient between PPA and PPV. In zone 3 (less than 20 cm from the lung base in our example), PPA is less than PPV which is less than PALV. Here, flow is determined by the gradient between PPA and PPV, as in standard ohmic resistances. According to this scheme, the distribution of blood flow is explained by a series of simple Starling resistors (collapsible tubes with a pressure surrounding the collapsible segment). In fact, the theory predicts that when PPA is greater than PALV which, in turn, is greater than PPV (zone 2), raising and lowering PPV would have little effect on pulmonary blood flow since the ef-

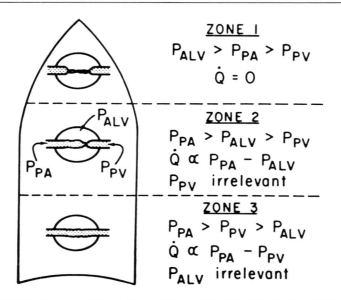

$$\text{ZONE 1}$$
$$P_{ALV} > P_{PA} > P_{PV}$$
$$\dot{Q} = 0$$

$$\text{ZONE 2}$$
$$P_{PA} > P_{ALV} > P_{PV}$$
$$\dot{Q} \propto P_{PA} - P_{ALV}$$
$$P_{PV} \text{ irrelevant}$$

$$\text{ZONE 3}$$
$$P_{PA} > P_{PV} > P_{ALV}$$
$$\dot{Q} \propto P_{PA} - P_{PV}$$
$$P_{ALV} \text{ irrelevant}$$

Fig. 49-3. Schematic drawing of the three zones according to the model of West and coworkers [101, 102]. P_{PA} = pulmonary arterial pressure; P_{ALV} = alveolar pressure; P_{PV} = pulmonary venous pressure; $\dot{Q}$ = regional blood flow. (Reprinted with permission from JF Green, The Pulmonary Circulation, in R Zelis [Ed], *The Peripheral Circulation.* New York: Grune & Stratton, 1975.)

fective back pressure to flow is P_{ALV}, not P_{PV}. Only as P_{PV} is raised above P_{ALV} does P_{PV} become the effective back pressure to flow. These concepts were the basis for the now classic studies of Permutt and colleagues [70–72], which confirmed these predictions.

As with most models, the simple Starling resistor model does not explain all experimental results, as illustrated in Figure 49-4. As expected, in zone 1 there is no blood flow. Flow in zone 2 increases down the lung because the gradient ($P_{PA} - P_{ALV}$) increases one to one with decreasing height. Further increases in flow are not expected in zone 3 because both P_{PA} and P_{PV} increase one to one down the lung and the gradient for flow ($P_{PA} - P_{PV}$) thus remains constant. However, as shown in Figure 49-4, actual flow does increase in zone 3, although at a slower rate than in zone 2. Further, a new zone, zone 4, is found—especially at low lung volumes—in which flow actually decreases toward the base. Flow may increase down the lung in zone 3 because pulmonary vascular resistance decreases, due to either distension of vessels or recruitment of closed vessels [29,56,102]. The explanation for zone 4 may be that with increased capillary pressure, there is an increased hydrostatic gradient for transudation of fluid into the interstitium, possibly decreasing the diameter of microvessels in the interstitium [39]. On the other hand, at low lung volume, the tendency for extraalveolar ves-

sels to be held open is less, which would result in increased pulmonary vascular resistance toward the lung base since transpulmonary pressure decreases toward the lung base as well [63].

During normal spontaneous ventilation, most lung is in zone 3, with little of the lung in zone 1. In supine patients, there is practically no lung in zone 1 conditions. With hypovolemia, pulmonary vascular pressures fall, which leads to an increased proportion of the lung in zone 1, manifest as an increase in measured anatomic dead space [55]. With positive-pressure mechanical ventilation, alveolar pressures can increase relative to vascular pressures, especially at high levels of positive end-expiratory pressure (PEEP). This leads to an increased proportion of the lung in zones 1 and 2 and increased numbers of lung units with high ventilation-perfusion ratios [16]. Conversely, when pulmonary vascular pressures increase, as in congestive heart failure or pulmonary hypertension, the proportion of the lung in zone 3 increases, thus making blood flow more uniform within the lung [4]. Of course, as blood flow increases in the apex, zone 1 diminishes. Be-

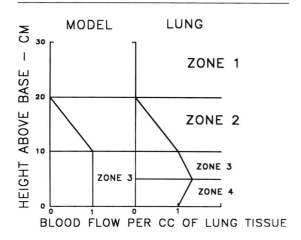

Fig. 49-4. Theoretical distribution of blood flow within the lung according to the model in Figure 49-3 (*Model*) and as measured in actual lungs (*Lung*). See text for explanation.

cause the apices receive relatively poor ventilation, units with decreasing ventilation-perfusion relationships could be created, thus contributing to hypoxemia in congestive heart failure. As previously indicated, there is normally a large reserve in the pulmonary vascular bed. A significant portion of the bed is underperfused (zone 1), thus allowing substantial reserve for recruitment of new vessels. In addition, there may be a significant reserve for distension of already perfused vessels. For these reasons, PPA normally does not rise substantially with pneumonectomy [14]. With exercise, pulmonary blood flow (cardiac output) can increase considerably with only small increases in PPA. This is because, due to passive dilation of the pulmonary vascular bed, the resistance to blood flow through the pulmonary vascular bed decreases passively. We will consider next the factors that actively regulate pulmonary vascular resistance.

Pulmonary Vascular Resistance

The pulmonary bed often is modeled as a straightforward Poiseuille type of system where flow ($\dot{Q}$) is laminar and is determined by the gradient between mean PPA and left atrial pressure (PLA), and a resistance term called *pulmonary vascular resistance* (PVR):

$$\dot{Q} = \frac{1}{\text{PVR}} (\text{PPA} - \text{PLA})$$

If pulmonary blood flow were truly laminar and the pulmonary vascular bed were a simple ohmic resistance, then plotting the pressure drop across the bed as a function of flow would yield a straight line. As shown in Figure 49-5, PPA − PLA rises in a roughly hyperbolic manner, with $\dot{Q}$ illustrating that PVR *decreases* with increasing flow [51]. As we have seen, the gradient (PPA − PLA) is the driving pressure only for zone 3 lung. Thus measurements of PVR by the usual equation or plot of PPA − PLA against $\dot{Q}$ may fail to differentiate between changes in cross sectional area due to recruitment or distension and critical closing pressure (usually equal to alveolar pressure).

As noted earlier, the presence of a gradient that develops between pulmonary arterial end-diastolic and pulmonary venous pressure (i.e., wedge pressure) is indicative of flow at end-diastole. The magnitude of this gradient increases with increased pulmonary vascular resistance, compliance, and blood flow.

A number of workers have performed studies plotting PPA against $\dot{Q}$. When these plots are extrapolated to zero flow, the critical closing pressure of the vascular bed may be measured as the

Fig. 49-5. An averaged curve of pressure drop across the pulmonary bed (pulmonary arterial to left atrial pressure gradient [$P_a - P_{la}$]) versus flow in isolated cat lungs. The shape is hyperbolic (i.e., flow resistance decreases at higher flows). (Reprinted with permission from A Krishnan et al, Cat lung hemodynamics: Comparison of experimental results and model predictions. *J Appl Physiol* 61:2023, 1986.)

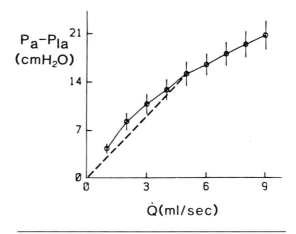

pressure at zero flow. The slope of the line is the true laminar flow resistance such that:

$$\dot{Q} = \frac{1}{PVR} (P_{PA} - P_C)$$

where P_C = the critical closing pressure of the bed when P_C exceeds P_{LA} (zone 2). Although alveolar pressure can function as the critical closing pressure (when P_{ALV} exceeds P_{LA}), any pressure surrounding the pulmonary vessels can act similarly, whether due to vasomotor tone [72] or even increased interstitial pressure, as might occur in pulmonary edema. These plots sometimes lead to surprising conclusions. For example, Figure 49-6 shows pulmonary pressure–flow curves obtained in dogs by Prewitt and Ducas [77]. With oleic acid–induced pulmonary edema, a model of adult respiratory distress syndrome, there was an increase in the critical downstream pressure compared to a time-dependent control, which suggests that an increase in critical closing pressure of the pulmonary vascular bed is an important contributor to increased P_{PA} in this form of edema.

Hydralazine and pulmonary emboli also lead to changes in critical closing pressure [76]. Differentiating between effects on critical closing pressure and resistance of the pulmonary vascular bed has implications for the interaction between cardiac and pulmonary causes of pulmonary hypertension. For example, if pulmonary hypertension is produced by increased critical closing pressure, changes in P_{LA} would have little effect on upstream pressure or flow. On the other hand, vasodilators such as hydralazine, which lower critical closing pressure, could make upstream pressures or flow *more* sensitive to fluctuations in P_{LA}. Thus it must be obvious that calculating the ratio $(P_{PA} - P_{LA})/\dot{Q}$ may not give adequate information to infer the caliber of pulmonary resistance vessels or the state of vasomotor tone. This is because of the effects of passive dilation of the pulmonary bed (recruitment or distension), the intrapulmonary distribution of blood flow (percent flow in any given lung zone), and the differential effects of resistance versus critical closing (or alveolar) pressure. Finally, Mitzner and Huang [60] have shown that when vasoconstriction or dilation produce changes in the compliance as well as resistance of a vessel, a parallel shift in the curve can result. The distensible vessel model of vascular pressure–flow relations may be an alternative to the Starling resistor–ohmic resistor model we have presented here.

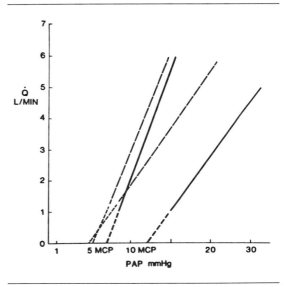

Fig. 49-6. Mean pressure-flow curves before and during oleic acid–induced pulmonary edema. *Dashed lines* represent controls at time zero and at 5 hours. *Solid lines* represent before and 5 hours after oleic acid infusion. With time alone, there is a decrease in the slope (conductance) of the dashed lines but no change in the zero intercept, which represents the critical closing pressure of the pulmonary bed. With pulmonary edema, a similar decrease occurs in conductance (*solid lines*). However, note that the zero intercept pressures also increase, suggesting an increase in the critical closing pressure of the vascular bed. $\dot{Q}$ = volume of regular blood flow; *PAP* = pulmonary artery pressure; *MCP* = mean circulatory pressure. (Reprinted with permission from RM Prewitt, J Ducas, Hemodynamic Management of Acute Respiratory Failure, in SM Scharf, SS Cassidy [Eds], *Heart-Lung Interactions in Health and Disease.* New York: Marcel Dekker, 1989.)

Pulmonary Vascular Impedance

The usual laminar flow approximations governing pulmonary resistance calculations assume that pulmonary vessels have rigid walls and flow is nonpulsatile ($\dot{Q}$ = mean flow). We have already noted that the vessels are markedly distensible and flow is pulsatile, being zero at end-diastole. Thus calculations of PVR based on laminar flow profiles may be misleading, even taking into consideration the factors previously discussed.

It has been suggested that the calculation of input impedance (z) at the pulmonary arterial root is a better way of assessing the state of the pulmonary vascular bed [57,59,90]. Input imped-ance is the ratio of instantaneous pressure to in-stantaneous flow at a given frequency. Pressure and flow signals are analyzed, usually by Fourier transformation, and broken down into their re-spective harmonic series, each harmonic being a sine wave characterized by a frequency, a multi-ple of heart rate, the dominant frequency, ampli-tude (called the *modulus*), and phase angle. The pressure modulus is divided by the flow modulus to calculate impedance magnitude, and the phase angles are subtracted to yield the impedance phase. One advantage for using impedance anal-ysis is that it takes into account two major deter-minants hindering RV ejection (i.e., two major determinants of RV afterload). These are the flow-resistive and capacitative behavior of the pulmonary bed [26], and they explain data not otherwise understandable from mean data. For example, for the same increase in Ppa, constriction of the proximal pulmonary artery produces a greater dynamic RV afterload than distal pulmo-nary arterial occlusion by microembolization [10]. With proximal occlusion, the compliance of the proximal pulmonary artery is severely de-creased, causing a decrease in capacitance. This increases the relative importance of the capaci-tative component of impedance more than for distal occlusion. The development of electromag-netic catheter-tipped measurements of instanta-neous flow velocity has enabled impedance mea-surements to be made in humans [64].

Effects of Lung Volume on Pulmonary Vascular Resistance and Blood Volume

In their pioneering work, Permutt and coworkers [38,71] demonstrated that the responses of in-traalveolar and extraalveolar vessels to lung inflation are different. With increased transpul-monary pressure, intraalveolar vessels are com-pressed whereas extraalveolar vessels are ex-posed to expanding forces. The net effect on pulmonary vasculature is biphasic, such that vas-cular capacitance is maximal at lung volumes close to functional residual capacity (FRC). As lung volume decreases below FRC, vascular ca-pacity diminishes due to compression of extraal-veolar vessels. As lung volume increases above FRC (as with ventilation with PEEP or in ob-structive airways disease), vascular capacity di-minishes due to compression of intraalveolar ves-sels. As lung volume increases, the tendency for pulmonary edema to form around intraalveolar vessels diminishes due to increased interstitial

pressure, whereas the tendency for edema for-mation increases around extraalveolar vessels due to decreased interstitial pressure. The bal-ance of these tendencies may lead to increased rate of edema formation as lung volume in-creases in noncardiogenic pulmonary edema [31]. Biphasic compressive effects on the pulmonary circulation lead to biphasic effects of lung infla-tion on calculated PVR. As lung volume de-creases below FRC, PVR rises, and as lung vol-ume increases above FRC, PVR also rises [103]. At high lung volumes, increased PVR due to in-traalveolar compression can lead to substantial increase in RV afterload, especially in the pres-ence of pulmonary edema [22].

Pulmonary Vasomotion

The normal pulmonary vascular bed has very little resting vasomotor tone, PVR is low, and infusion of potent vasodilators rarely leads to decreases in baseline resistance. Whether the normally low PVR is the baseline natural state or is due to the continued chronic production of va-sodilator substances is a matter of controversy [96]. Nevertheless, it is clear that there are many influences capable of regulating pulmonary va-somotor tone. These include endogenously pro-duced vasoconstrictors and vasodilators (Table 49-2) [3,5–7,9,42,45,47,50,79,88,93,105], changes in autonomic tone mediated by central nervous sys-tem reflexes, a variety of pharmacologic agents, and changes in arterial blood gases, such as hy-poxia, hypercapnia, and changes in pH. Changes in pulmonary vasomotor tone should be viewed on three levels: (1) global effects, or changes in overall PVR; (2) regional effects, or changes in the distribution of blood between various parallel channels (a good example is pulmonary hypoxic vasoconstriction); and (3) changes in longitudi-nal distribution of resistance, which could affect microcirculatory pressure gradients responsible for edema formation.

The state of initial vasomotor tone is important in determining the action of a given vasoactive agent. An example is histamine, which acts as a constrictor on dilated vessels and a dilator on constricted vessels [3,88]. In addition, many en-dogenously produced mediator substances act not directly on smooth muscle but via other me-diators. An example is the vasodilating action of acetylcholine, which acts only on precontracted smooth muscle in the presence of endothelium to produce vasodilation [24], working via an endo-thelial-derived relaxing factor (EDRF). This fac-

Table 49-2. Vasoactive mediators in the pulmonary circulation

Vasoconstrictors
Alpha-adrenergic agonists: norepinephrine,
    phenylephrine
Angiotensin II
Thromboxane A_2 [5]
Serotonin [6]
Histamine (relaxed bed) [3]
Prostaglandins $F_{2\alpha}$ and E_2 [45,47]
Leukotrienes C_4 and D_4 [93]
Interleukin-2 [7]
Tumor necrosis factor [105]
Prostaglandin D_2 [9]
Endothelin [50]

Vasodilators
Histamine (preconstricted bed) [88]
Prostacyclin (PGI_2) [42]
Beta agonists: isoproterenol
Bradykinin
Prostaglandins E_1 and E_2 (neonates)
Platelet-activating factor (preconstricted bed) [79]
Endothelium-derived relaxing factor (nitric oxide)
Acetylcholine
Adenosine

tor, now known to be nitric oxide [68], in turn acts by stimulating soluble guanylate cyclase, leading to increased levels of cyclic guanosine 3′5′ monophosphate, which is the agent bearing a direct effect on smooth muscle cells [44]. While a thorough review of all that is known about the regulation of pulmonary vasomotor tone is beyond the scope of this chapter, some mention of the factors involved is important because of the importance of pulmonary vasomotor tone both physiologically and clinically.

Pulmonary Vasomotor Mediators

Vasoactive mediator substances (Table 49-2) are produced by many cell types within the lung, including interstitial mast cells and neutrophils, interstitial monocytes, alveolar macrophages, marginated neutrophils, and pulmonary endothelium. Many mediator substances are hypothesized to be released in response to acute lung injury [7] and pulmonary embolism, which are responsible for changes in vasomotor tone (usually vasoconstriction) and vascular permeability [7,52,54]. Among the most potent vasoactive substances are the eicosanoids, derived from arachidonic acid. Arachidonic acid is a 20-carbon polyunsaturated fatty acid released from tissue by the dea-

cylation of cellular phospholipids. It may be metabolized by one of two pathways: The *cyclooxygenase* pathway leads to the production of the prostenoids—prostacyclin (PGI_2), thromboxane A_2, prostaglandin D_2 (PGD_2), PGE_2, and $PGF_{2\alpha}$—and it is inhibited by a variety of pharmacologic agents including nonsteroidal antiinflammatory agents (e.g., aspirin and indomethacin). The *lipoxygenase* pathway leads to the production of the leukotrienes. Whereas the prostenoids have been recognized as powerful vasoactive agents, the leukotrienes are also vasoactive agents. This allows for cross-talk between endothelium-derived factors such as PGE_2 and neutrophil-derived factors such as leukotriene D_4 in the regulation of vasomotor tone and permeability [7]. A number of pharmacologic uses have been found for naturally occurring mediators. Prostacyclin, a powerful vasodilator, has been used in the treatment of primary pulmonary hypertension [81], and infusion of PGE_2 or PGE_1 can maintain patency of the ductus arteriosus of newborns.

Finally, the pulmonary endothelium processes a number of vasoactive substances which, when released into the systemic circulation, can play an important role in the regulation of systemic vasomotor tone. Prostacyclin and PGE_2 are produced by pulmonary endothelial cells. Serotonin is extracted by pulmonary capillary cells [62]. Angiotensin I is converted into the powerful vasoconstrictor angiotensin II by the enzyme angiotensin-converting enzyme (ACE) found in pulmonary endothelium [82]. The same enzyme metabolizes bradykinin [75], a potent vasodilator. Thus inhibition of ACE would decrease angiotensin II levels and increase bradykinin levels, leading to decreased systemic pressure and vice versa. The pulmonary circulation is thus an important regulator of the systemic circulation.

Autonomic Vascular Reflexes

The role of autonomic reflexes in controlling pulmonary vascular tone is less well understood than that for the systemic circulation [41]. One should bear in mind that interspecies differences occur that may partially account for varying results in the literature. Relatively little is known about these responses in humans. In a number of species, both adrenergic and cholinergic nerve endings can be demonstrated in the pulmonary arterial bed in the adventitia of large and small intrapulmonary arteries. Further, alpha- and beta-adrenergic responses can be demonstrated after administration of exogenous selective alpha- or beta-adrenergic agonists. Blocking of these responses by specific blockers can be demonstrated as well. Electric stimulation of pulmonary sympathetic nerves (e.g., by stimulating the stellate ganglion) causes pulmonary vasoconstriction [35], which has been variously manifest as an increase in pulmonary resistance [47] or decreased pulmonary vascular compliance, primarily of large pulmonary arteries. Stimulation of the vagus nerve is more complex since it contains both sympathetic and parasympathetic fibers. In one model, vagal stimulation under baseline conditions causes modest vasoconstriction, which is blocked by alpha-adrenergic blockade. However, when baseline vascular resistance is elevated, vagal stimulation causes pulmonary vasodilation [40]. One interpretation is that sympathetic effects predominate with low baseline tone and cholinergic effects predominate with high baseline tone. We have already alluded to the mediating role of nitric oxide in cholinergic vasodilation.

A number of efferent brain-pulmonary vascular connections exist. For example, stimulation of discrete areas of the forebrain causes a two-phase response. The early phase consists of two subphases, initial constriction followed by dilation. The late phase consists of vasodilation. The early phase may be mediated by neural mechanisms, the late phase by release of epinephrine from the adrenal medulla [41]. A number of other such brain pulmonary connections are identified that may be responsible for the sympathetic component of the response to elevated cerebrospinal fluid pressure (Cushing's reflex) [53]. The ultimate change in PVR depends on the interaction of sympathetic-mediated pulmonary vasoconstriction, cholinergic vasodilation, resting tone, and concomitant changes in venous return and cardiac output, which lead to passive dilation of the bed. The role of neural control in maintaining oxygenation by matching ventilation and perfusion is not well-known; nor are the mechanisms understood by which pathologic central nervous system stimulation may lead to abnormal water exchange, as in neurogenic pulmonary edema.

Finally, there are a number of afferent reflexes from pulmonary vasculature that lead to changes in ventilatory pattern. The existence of CO_2-sensitive receptors that can regulate ventilation has been the subject of considerable controversy ever since originally postulated by Pisuner and Bellido in 1919 [74] (reviewed by Adams and colleagues [1]). These receptors have been postulated to contribute to the hyperpnea of exercise. Indeed, when the pulmonary circulation is separated from the systemic circulation, CO_2 loading or unloading of pulmonary arterial blood leads to concomitant changes in ventilation [84]. The mixed venous CO_2 receptor may be identical to slowly adapting stretch receptors in the lung. However, a role for vagally carried bronchopulmonary C fibers has been postulated as well [91].

There is a large body of literature reporting that pulmonary vascular congestion can reflexively evoke systemic hypotension, bradycardia, and tachypnea [20,48]. Paintal [67] first hypothesized unmyelinated C-fiber innervated receptors in the interstitium of the lung stimulated by congestion of pulmonary microcirculation. Called *J receptors* (for "juxtacapillary"), the role of the vagally carried fibers in mediating the tachypnea accompanying many pulmonary disorders such as pulmonary edema, pulmonary embolus, and fibrosis remains controversial, with evidence on each side of the argument [1]. Whether these fibers are stimulated directly by vascular congestion or by release of a mediator substance such as serotonin [2] is not known.

A number of chemical substances lead to the triad of bradycardia, hypotension, and apnea. This pulmonary chemoreflex [17] can occur with the injection of certain naturally occurring mediators such as prostaglandins I_2 and E_2 and opiate peptides [2]. Numerous other substances when injected into the pulmonary artery through balloon-tipped catheters, including iced saline, are capable of causing this reflex.

The Pulmonary Endothelium

Because the pulmonary circulation receives the entire cardiac output, it is in an ideal location for performing a number of biologic operations on the entire blood supply. We have alluded earlier to the clearance or production of vasomediators. The reader is referred elsewhere for review articles [75,83,100]. Table 49-3 summarizes some of the known metabolic functions of the pulmonary endothelium. Endothelial cells bear receptors for a host of substances that lead to release of many biologically active mediators. Signal transduction leading to prostacyclin and EDRF release is not completely understood but may involve stimulation of intracellular calcium [83]. The same anatomic location that makes endothelium conducive to vasomotor biochemistry also makes endothelial cells subject to vascular injury from a number of distant organ sources. As shown in Table 49-3, endothelial cells possess a number of binding sites for biologically active bloodborne substances, including those involved in hemostasis and inflammation as well as complex interactions with cellular elements of the blood. Thus the lung is a frequent site of injury in distant processes, such as infections, leading to associated diffuse lung injury.

The endothelium also interacts with surrounding vascular smooth muscle. We have already discussed the role of endothelial-derived vasoactive mediators (such as nitric oxide) and prostacyclin in regulating smooth-muscle tone. However, PVR also is a function of the histologic structure of the vascular tree. Endothelial cells secrete several growth factors that can lead to smooth-muscle proliferation, including a platelet-derived growth factor–like substance, fibroblast growth factors, and a growth inhibitory factor [80]. Endothelial injury denudes the vessel, removes growth-inhibiting factors, and exposes the vessel media to interactions with bloodborne elements that could interact with smooth muscle. Thus the balance between mitogens and growth-inhibiting factors

Table 49-3. Pulmonary metabolic functions associated with vascular endothelium

Enzymes	Binding sites
Angiotensin-converting enzyme	Thrombin
Carboxypeptidase N	Insulin
5' Nucleotidase	Atrial natriuretic factor
Adenosine triphosphatase	Muscarinic-receptor
Lipoprotein lipase	Alpha and beta receptors; adenosine, adenosine triphosphate; histamine; Fc portion of IgG; C3b, C1q; growth factors
Transport Processes	*Biosynthesis*
5-Hydroxytryptamine	Eicosanoids (prostacyclin, PGE$_2$)
Norepinephrine	Adenosine
Prostaglandins E and F series	Endothelial-derived relaxing factor (nitric oxide)
	Endothelin

Source: Adapted from BR Pitt, G Lister, GN Gillis. Metabolic functions of the lung and cardiopulmonary physiology. In SM Scharf and SS Cassidy (Eds), Heart-Lung Interactions in Health and Disease. NY: Dekker, 1989. Pp. 331–406.

in vascular endothelium might be responsible for preserving or altering normal pulmonary architecture.

Effects of Altered Gas Exchange on Pulmonary Circulation

It would be in the interest of preserving pulmonary ventilation-perfusion relationships if there were a mechanism allowing for local vascular control by regional gas tensions such that areas of poor ventilation receive less blood flow. Hypoxic, hypercapnic, or acidotic lung regions would thereby undergo local vasoconstriction, shunting blood away from diseased areas. Both severe hypercapnia and acidosis are capable of causing vasoconstriction. However, the mechanism most studied is that of hypoxic vasoconstriction, and it is this that we review briefly. It should be noted that interspecies differences regarding the strength of, and possibly the mechanisms involved in, hypoxic vasoconstriction exist and should lead to caution in extrapolating between studies in different species. Failure of hypoxic vasoconstriction is often postulated to be the cause of hypoxemia seemingly out of proportion to the estimated size of pulmonary lesion, such as pneumonia and atelectasis.

Figure 49-7 shows a pressure-flow curve for an isolated lung before and during perfusion by hypoxic blood. Note that P$_{PA}$ is higher at any given flow. In this pressure-flow curve [61], the hypoxic curve appears parallel shifted relative to normal, suggesting a change in critical closing pressure rather than vessel diameter (see above). Normally, precapillary vascular smooth muscle dilates on exposure to hypoxia. This mechanism normally serves to increase blood oxygen supply to end organs when the oxygen content of blood decreases. Pulmonary smooth muscle, when stripped of surrounding adventitia, behaves in the same way. Thus hypoxic vasoconstriction appears to be the result of secondary mediation produced by interactions between interstitium, endothelium, and pulmonary smooth muscle rather than an intrinsic property of pulmonary vascular smooth muscle.

A number of substances have been proposed as the mediator of hypoxic vasoconstriction. Much recent attention has been focused on endothelial-derived factors, previously proposed mediators such as vasoactive intestinal peptide, histamine, potassium, angiotensin, and substance P no longer being considered viable candidates. In some species, inhibition of the cyclooxygenase

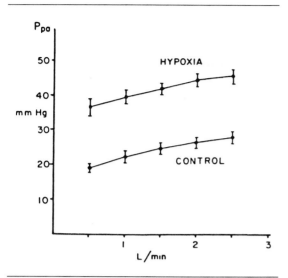

Fig. 49-7. The effect of hypoxic vasoconstriction on pressure-flow curves of isolated pig lungs. The slope of the line does not change; only the critical closing pressure of the vascular bed changes. Therefore, pulmonary vascular resistance which, strictly speaking, is represented by the slope of the pressure-flow curve, does not change in this model. Hypoxic vasoconstriction manifests itself as an increase in the critical closing pressure of the pulmonary vascular bed such that the curve has shifted parallel to itself. Thus, at any given flow, pulmonary arterial pressure is increased. (Reprinted with permission from W Mitzner, JT Sylvester, Hypoxic vasoconstriction and fluid filtration in pig lungs. *J Appl Physiol* 57:1065, 1981.)

pathway of arachidonic acid metabolism inhibits hypoxic vasoconstriction, whereas in others inhibition of the lipoxygenase pathway has the same effect [100]. The endothelium-derived vasoconstrictor endothelin may also play a role in hypoxic vasoconstriction [50].

Finally, the effect of local hypoxia on regional blood flow is the end result of a number of factors besides regional gas tensions. These effects include local compression or malformation of vessels as well as the systemic effects of hypoxemia. Thus systemic adrenergic stimulation could add to the local mechanisms involved in hypoxic vasoconstriction.

Chronic hypoxemia, as occurs in high-altitude dwellers, is associated with structural changes in the pulmonary vascular bed in addition to the vasospasm of acute hypoxia. We have already alluded to the cross-talk between pulmonary endothelial-derived growth factors and smooth muscle, which may be responsible for architectural remodeling, including hyperplasia and hypertrophy of pulmonary arterial and arteriolar walls (e.g., smooth muscle and medial layers). In chronic high-altitude dwellers who move to sea level, pulmonary arterial pressures remain elevated and dilatory reserve remains limited for an extended period of time, due to structural changes in pulmonary vasculature [95].

Pulmonary Edema Formation and Prevention in the Lung

Exchange of nutrients and fluids occurs at the capillaries, arterioles, and small veins, vessels that may be lumped under the term *microvasculature*. Fluid exchange at the microvascular level occurs by filtration, diffusion, and micropinocytosis. Filtration and diffusion are passive processes in which substances flow down a potential energy gradient.

THE STARLING EQUATION

In 1896, Starling [86] described the balance of forces that regulate the flow of fluid (filtration) across microvasculature into and out of the interstitium. The force driving fluid *out* of microvasculature is the gradient between hydrostatic pressure across the vessel, and that driving fluid *into* the microvessels is the colloid oncotic (or osmotic) pressure gradient across the vessel. The classic relationship may be written:

$$\dot{Q}_f = K_f [(P_m - P_{is}) - k(\pi_m - \pi_{is})]$$

where $\dot{Q}_f$ is fluid flow across the microvessel, P_m is microvasculature hydrostatic pressure, P_{is} is interstitial hydrostatic pressure, π_m is microvascular plasma oncotic pressure, and π_{is} is interstitial oncotic pressure. The constant k is the reflection coefficient, which represents the degree to which proteins can move across the vessel wall. If $k = 0$, then protein moves freely and there can be no oncotic gradient driving fluid back into the microvasculature. If $k = 1$, then the vessel wall is impermeable to protein. Constant k is usually close to 1 [49]. K_f is the filtration coefficient, which is made of terms representing the filtration constant of the microvascular membrane, membrane surface area, filtrate viscosity, and the distance across the vessel wall, and thus represents the conductance for fluid flux across the membrane. It can be seen that with a large K_f, even a small balance of forces in favor of fluid movement results in a large-volume flow of fluid [65].

Plasma and interstitial fluid each contain approximately 280 mmol of crystalloid, which is freely interchangeable between the two compartments. Thus the osmotic forces governing transvessel fluid exchange are dominated by the protein concentration gradient, approximately 7 gm/100 ml, giving a plasma osmotic (oncotic) pressure of 28 mmHg. Pulmonary interstitial protein content is not known for certain and is often assumed to be close to zero. Thus the edemagenic potential of the lung depends on the balance of forces, which is not necessarily constant but is related to regional variations in vascular and interstitial compartments. In addition, the lung is richly endowed with a lymphatic system, which can drain the interstitium (Fig. 49-8).

We have already considered most of the factors that govern microvascular filtration pressure. It should be noted that both extraalveolar and intraalveolar vessels contribute to edema formation [43], and the gradients across the walls of these vessels may be very different depending on the state of lung inflation. In general, microvascular filtration pressure increases from less to more dependent lung regions and, for any given arterial pressure, microvascular filtration is greater as the ratio of arterial to venous resistance decreases. Thus it is difficult to consider *the* capillary filtration pressure within the lung as if it were a unique entity, although various techniques have been used to estimate the overall mean filtration pressure for any given set of conditions (see Oppenheimer and Goldberg [66]).

It is important for preservation of normal gas exchange that the pulmonary interstitium, particularly in the intraalveolar compartment, remain dry—that is, without free fluid. Pulmonary interstitium, far from being a space, is composed of cellular elements, elastin, collagen, glycosamines, and proteoglycans [73], and probably has a consistency similar to gelatin. Like microvascular pressure, interstitial pressure varies locally between extraalveolar and intraalveolar compartments, with lung inflation, along hydrostatic gradients and from hilum to parenchyma. In general, interstitial pressure is *less* than pleural pressure, is more negative in the extraalveolar than in the intraalveolar compartments, and is more negative in hilar than in peripheral lung regions. This leads to different transmicrovascular fluid pressure gradients within the lung such that the edemagenic potential varies within the lung, leading to a sequence of edema formation [87]. Edema

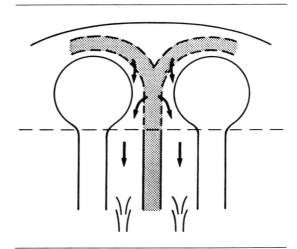

Fig. 49-8. Representation of the lung as three concentric compartments: airway, vascular, and interstitial. *Arrows* indicate the net filtration volume. Lymphatics drain the interstitium. (Reprinted with permission from L Oppenheimer, HS Goldberg, Pulmonary Circulation and Edema Formation, in SM Scharf, SS Cassidy [Eds], *Heart-Lung Interactions in Health and Disease.* New York: Marcel Dekker, 1989.)

forms initially in the connective tissue of the alveolar septa. Following pressure gradients, it then accumulates around arterioles and bronchioles as cuffs of fluid and travels to the interstitium around larger arteries, veins, and airways. This leads to the perivascular and peribronchial cuffing sign seen on chest roentgenograms. Ultimately, fluid may penetrate into the alveolar space to cause alveolar flooding.

The pulmonary interstitium has a number of defense mechanisms to prevent alveolar flooding. First, pressure gradients tend to encourage flow toward extraalveolar regions, around large vessels, and ultimately to the hilum. Second, to maintain a pressure gradient for flow through the interstitium, there must be a significant resistance to fluid flow [34,66]. Tissue resistance decreases as interstitial hydration increases [92], which is protective: As vessels leak fluid, tissue resistance decreases, thus allowing easier redistribution of fluid away from the local area of fluid accumulation. We have alluded to the matrix quality of the interstitium. The matrix normally excludes macromolecules such as albumin. However, as free fluid accumulates, the matrix becomes looser and more albumin penetrates into the interstitium. As this occurs, the volume into which albumin equilibrates increases which, in turn, decreases the oncotic pressure exerted by interstitial albumin. Hence, with interstitial hydration, changes in the interstitial matrix act to buffer the tendency for fluid accumulation [69].

INTERSTITIAL COMPLIANCE

Like other interstitial areas, the pulmonary interstitium has a biphasic pressure-volume curve [30,33]. At low levels of hydration (low free fluid volume), large changes in fluid pressure produce small changes in volume. This stiff portion of the pressure-volume curve is found when interstitial pressure is negative and protects against edema formation because large pressure gradients, such as might be produced by lung inflation, are tolerated with little change in fluid volume. As water accumulates and the matrix opens up, the pressure-volume curve becomes more compliant, such that relatively small changes in pressure produce large volume changes. This allows the interstitium to soak up considerable amounts of fluid, thereby buffering against alveolar flooding.

Finally, pulmonary lymphatics, which drain into the systemic venous system, act as sump drains, removing excess interstitial fluid. Lymphatics flow increases with either increased microvascular pressure or increased microvascular permeability [25,106]. With high microvascular pressures resulting in transudation of fluid, lymph is essentially an ultrafiltrate of plasma and has a low protein content. With increased vascular permeability, macromolecules usually leak through and the protein content of lung lymph is high. Injection of substances that damage pulmonary microvessels often demonstrate two phased alterations of lung lymph. In stage 1, lymph protein content is low, although lung lymph flow is increased. This is consistent with elevation of pulmonary microvascular filtration pressure with little change in vascular permeability. In phase 2, lung lymph flow is also increased, but protein content is high, consistent with permeability or leaky capillary type pulmonary edema (Fig. 49-9) [8].

Although the overall Starling balance for the lung is difficult to ascertain, estimates of microvascular fluid filtration pressure usually hover around 15 mmHg, albeit with considerable variation (see Oppenheimer and Goldberg [66]). Interstitial hydrostatic pressure is subatmospheric, approximately −8 mmHg. This gives a 23-mmHg (15 to −8 mmHg) gradient for outward fluid movement, which is more than counterbalanced by the inward-acting oncotic pressure gradient

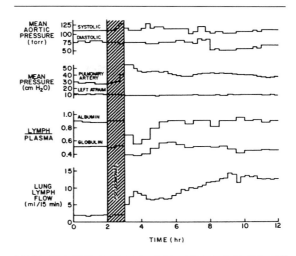

Fig. 49-9. Effect of intravenous infusion of *Pseudomonas aeruginosa* on vascular pressures, lymph plasma-protein concentration (L/P) ratio, and lung lymph flow in an unanesthetized sheep. Note there are two phases. Initially, L/P ratio falls, lymph flow increases, and pulmonary arterial pressure increases. This is consistent with the hemodynamic or hydrostatic phase in which the microvascular pressure increase is responsible for edema formation. After 4 hours, the L/P ratio increases, vascular pressure begins to decrease, and lung lymph flow increases even more. This late phase is consistent with the increased permeability or leaky capillary phase of edema formation in this model. (Reprinted with permission from KL Brigham et al, Increased sheep lung vascular permeability caused by *Pseudomonas* bacteremia. *J Clin Invest* 54:792, 1974.)

of 28 mmHg. Therefore, the overall balance of forces is approximately 5 mmHg in favor of movement of fluid out of the interstitium into the microvasculature. This does not leave much room for increases in microvascular filtration pressure as might well occur with physiologic maneuvers (e.g., exercise). Thus the other mechanisms discussed that keep the interstitium fluid-free assume a particular importance.

THE BRONCHIAL CIRCULATION

The bronchial circulation is the systemic vascular supply to the airways, arising from the bronchial arteries, intercostal arteries, and aorta. The bronchial circulation constitutes the major nutritive blood supply to the bronchi down to the level of the respiratory bronchioles. Below this level, the pulmonary circulation performs this function. There is considerable anatomic variation in the origin of the bronchial arteries, which has practical importance in clinical situations where embolization of the bronchial circulation is used to treat massive hemoptysis [15]. The bronchial circulation also sends branches to mediastinal and other extrapulmonary structures, including hilar lymph nodes and pleura (Fig. 49-10). The extrapulmonary bronchial circulation drains via the azygos and hemiazygos veins, whereas the intrapulmonary bronchial circulation drains via the pulmonary veins. There is evidence for anastomoses or potential anastomoses between bronchial and pulmonary circulations at every level of the vasculature, including arteries, capillaries, and veins [11,78]. To supply airways to the level of the terminal bronchioles, the bronchial circulation forms two plexuses, one inside the airways in the submucosa and one outside the airway in the peribronchial tissue.

The bronchial circulation normally constitutes only 1 to 2 percent of the cardiac output [15,21]. However, this belies its potential importance. Because of its location and extensive networking,

total bronchial blood volume is considerable; hence bronchial blood velocity is slow. Thus the bronchial circulation is well situated to participate in fluid and even gas exchange in the lung [21]. When there is pulmonary vascular obstruction, bronchial blood flow via anastomoses to the pulmonary circulation helps maintain inflow from surrounding pulmonary networks and acts to prevent infarction. Of particular importance may be the role of the bronchial circulation in airway inflammation, when bronchial blood flow increases considerably.

Clearly, the bronchial circulation is important when considering the edema, bronchospasm, and inflammatory changes found in airways in a variety of disorders. In addition, the bronchial circulation acts to condition air in the bronchial tree

Fig. 49-10. Schematic depiction of the bronchial circulation. The numbers indicate possible sites of absorption of edema fluid. Note the many intrapulmonary and extrapulmonary sites supplied by the bronchial circulation. (Reprinted with permission from ME Deffeback, J Butler, The Bronchial Circulation and Lung Edema, in SM Scharf, SS Cassidy [Eds], *Heart-Lung Interactions in Health and Disease.* New York: Marcel Dekker, 1989.)

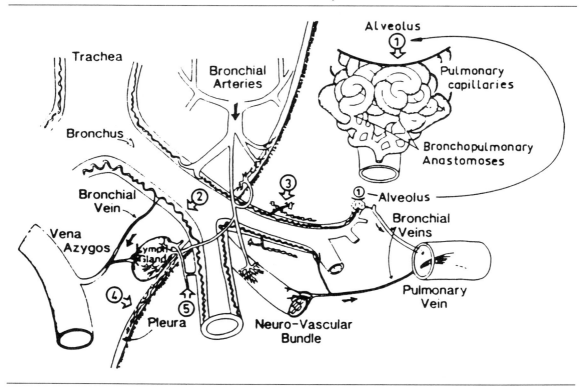

that is not conditioned in the upper airways. The blood vessels of the airways may act to minimize heat loss during hyperventilation such as that induced by exercise. McFadden [58] suggested that airway mucosal surfaces were cooled during inspiration. Thus, during exhalation, heat and water would be given back to the air, cooling the airway surface but minimizing heat loss to the outside. Similarly, the bronchial circulation plays an important role in regulating airway water, which can influence the rheology of mucus and thus affect the clearance of particulate matter from the lung as well as change the osmolality of the mucous lining layer. The latter is believed to affect airway smooth-muscle tone, especially in asthmatic patients. Finally, in pathologic situations—most notably bronchiectasis, tumor, and lung abscess—local bronchial circulation increases considerably, in part because of opening of previously closed bronchial-pulmonary anastomoses [15,21]. The hypertrophied bronchial circulation is responsible for hemoptysis in these situations, which may be life-threatening. Conditions associated with bronchial arterial hypertrophy and proliferation may be associated with right-to-left extracardiac shunting, hypoxemia, and increased cardiovascular load. Left-to-left shunts have been demonstrated but only when the expansion of the bronchial circulation is large. Interestingly, these conditions are often associated with the clinical sign of digital clubbing.

References

1. Adams L, Schertel ER, Green JF. Reflexes Elicited from the Pulmonary Vasculature in the Control of Breathing. In SM Scharf, SS Cassidy (Eds), *Heart-Lung Interactions in Health and Disease*. New York: Marcel Dekker, 1989. Pp 365–389.
2. Armstrong DJ, Miller SA. Lung irritant and C-fiber responses in thrombocytopenic rabbits. *J Physiol (Lond)* 303:41P, 1980.
3. Aviado DM. *The Lung Circulation* (vol 1). London: Pergamon Press, 1965.
4. Bencowitz HZ, LeWinter MM, Wagner PD. Effect of sodium nitroprusside on ventilation perfusion matching in heart failure. *Am J Cardiol* 4:918, 1984.
5. Bowers R, et al. Effects of prostaglandin cyclic endoperoxides on the lung circulation of sheep. *J Clin Invest* 63:131, 1979.
6. Braun K, Stern S. Pulmonary and systemic blood pressure responses to serotonin. Role of chemoreceptors. *Am J Physiol* 201:369, 1961.
7. Brigham KL. Mediators in the Pulmonary Circulation. In AP Fishman (Ed), *The Pulmonary Circulation: Normal and Abnormal*. Philadelphia: University of Pennsylvania Press, 1990. Pp 91–107.
8. Brigham KL, et al. Increased sheep lung vascular permeability caused by *Pseudomonas* bacteremia. *J Clin Invest* 54:792, 1974.
9. Brigham KL, Ogletree ML. Effects of prostaglandins and related compounds on lung vascular permeability. *Bull Eur Physiopath Respir* 17:703, 1981.
10. Calvin JE, Baer RW, Glantz SA. Pulmonary artery constriction produces a greater right ventricular dynamic afterload than lung microvascular injury in the open chest dog. *Circ Res* 56:40, 1985.
11. Charan NB, Turk GM, Dhand R. Gross and subgross anatomy of the bronchial circulation in sheep. *J Appl Physiol* 57:658, 1984.
12. Collee GG, et al. Bedside measurements of pulmonary capillary pressure in patients with acute respiratory failure. *Anesthesiology* 66:614, 1987.
13. Cope DK, et al. Measurements of effective pulmonary capillary pressure using the profile after pulmonary artery occlusion. *Crit Care Med* 14:16, 1986.
14. Cournand A, et al. Pulmonary circulation and alveolar ventilation-perfusion relationships after pneumonectomy. *J Thorac Surg* 19:80, 1950.
15. Cudkowitz L. Bronchial Arterial Circulation in Man: Normal Anatomy and Responses to Disease. In K Moser (Ed), *Pulmonary Vascular Diseases*. New York: Marcel Dekker, 1979. Pp 111–232.
16. Dantzker DR, et al. Gas exchange in adult respiratory distress syndrome and the effects of positive end-expiratory pressure. *Am Rev Respir Dis* 120:1039, 1979.
17. Dawes GS, Comroe JH, Chemoreflexes from the heart and lungs. *Physiol Rev* 34:167, 1954.
18. Dawson CA. Role of pulmonary vasomotion in physiology of the lung. *Physiol Rev* 64:544, 1989.
19. Dawson CA, et al. On the estimation of pulmonary capillary pressure from arterial occlusion. *Am Rev Respir Dis* 140:1228, 1989.
20. DeBurgh Daly M. Interactions between Respiration and Circulation. In AP Fishman, N Cherniack (Eds), *Handbook of Physiology* (Sec 3, vol 2, part 2). Baltimore: Williams & Wilkins, 1986.
21. Deffeback ME, Butler J. The Bronchial Circulation and Lung Edema. In SM Scharf, SS Cassidy (Eds), *Heart-Lung Interactions in Health and Disease*. New York: Marcel Dekker, 1989. Pp 131–154.
22. Dhainaut JF, Aoute P, Brunet F. Circulatory Effects of Positive End-Expiratory Pressure in Patients with Acute Lung Injury. In SM Scharf, SS

Cassidy (Eds), *Heart-Lung Interactions in Health and Disease.* New York: Marcel Dekker, 1989. Pp 809–838.

23. Fung Y-C, Sobin SS. Pulmonary Alveolar Blood Flow. In JB West (Ed), *Bioengineering Aspects of the Lungs.* New York: Marcel Dekker, 1977. Pp 267–359.

24. Furchgott RF, Zawdzki JV. The obligatory role of endothelial cells in the relaxation of arterial smooth muscle by acetylcholine. *Nature* 288:373, 1980.

25. Gee MH, Havill AM. The relationship between perivascular cuff fluid and lung lymph flow in dogs with edema. *Microvasc Res* 19:209, 1979.

26. Gessner U. Vascular Input Impedance. In DH Bergel (Ed), *Cardiovascular Fluid Dynamics.* New York: Academic Press, 1972. Chapter 10.

27. Gil J. The Normal Pulmonary Microcirculation. In AP Fishman (Ed), *The Pulmonary Circulation: Normal and Abnormal* Philadelphia: University of Pennsylvania Press, 1990. Pp 3–16.

28. Gil J, et al. Alveolar to surface area relationships in air and saline filled lungs fixed by vascular perfusion. *J Appl Physiol* 47:990, 1979.

29. Glazier JB, et al. Measurement of capillary dimensions and blood volume in rapidly frozen lungs. *J Appl Physiol* 26:65, 1969.

30. Goldberg HS. Pulmonary interstitial compliance and microvascular filtration coefficient. *Am J Physiol* 239:H189, 1980.

31. Goldberg HS, Mitzner W, Batra G. Effect of transpulmonary and vascular pressures on the rate of edema formation. *J Appl Physiol* 43:14, 1977.

32. Green JF. The Pulmonary Circulation. In R Zelis (Ed), *The Peripheral Circulation.* New York: Grune & Stratton, 1975. Pp 193–209.

33. Guyton AC. Interstitial fluid pressure II. Pressure-volume curves of interstitial space. *Circ Res* 16:452, 1965.

34. Guyton AC, Scheel K, Murphee D. Interstitial fluid pressure III. Its effect on resistance to tissue fluid mobility. *Circ Res* 19:412, 1966.

35. Hakim TS, Dawson CA. Sympathetic nerve stimulation and vascular resistance in pump-perfused dog lung lobe. *Proc Soc Exp Med* 160:38, 1979.

36. Hakim TS, Michel RP, Chang HK. Partitioning of pulmonary vascular resistance by arterial and venous occlusion. *J Appl Physiol* 52:710, 1982.

37. Horsfield K. Morphometry of the small pulmonary arteries in man. *Circ Res* 42:593, 1978.

38. Howell JBL, et al. Effect of inflation of the lung on different parts of the pulmonary bed. *J Appl Physiol* 16:71, 1961.

39. Hughes JMB, et al. Factors determining the distribution of pulmonary blood flow in patients with raised venous pressure. *Clin Sci* 37:847, 1969.

40. Hyman AL. The Dickenson W. Richards Memorial Lecture. Neural control of the pulmonary vascular bed. *Circulation* 74(II):IID, 1986.

41. Hyman AL, et al. Autonomic Control of the Pulmonary Arterial Circulation. In EK Weir, JT Reeves (Eds), *Pulmonary Vascular Physiology and Pathophysiology.* New York: Marcel Dekker, 1989. Pp 291–324.

42. Hyman AL, Kadowitz PJ. Pulmonary vasodilator activity of prostacyclin (PGI_2) in the cat. *Circ Res* 45:404, 1979.

43. Iliff LD. Extra-alveolar vessels and edema development in excised dog lungs. *Circ Res* 28:524, 1971.

44. Ingarro LJ, et al. Activation of purified soluble guanylate cyclase by endothelium-derived relaxing factor from intrapulmonary artery and vein. Stimulation by acetylcholine, bradykinin and arachidonic acid. *J Pharmacol Exp Ther* 237:893, 1987.

45. Joiner PD, et al. Actions of prostaglandins E_1 and E_{2a} on isolated intrapulmonary vascular smooth muscle. *Proc Soc Exp Biol Med* 150:414, 1975.

46. Jones EL, Campbell EM. *Clinical Exercise Testing.* Philadelphia: Saunders, 1982.

47. Kadowitz PJ, Joiner PD, Hyman AL. Effect of prostaglandin E_2 on pulmonary vascular resistance in intact dog, swine and lamb. *Eur J Pharmacol* 31:72, 1975.

48. Kauffman MP, Cassidy SS. Reflex Effects of Lung Inflation on the Heart and Circulation. In SM Scharf, SS Cassidy (Eds), *Heart-Lung Interactions in Health and Disease.* New York: Marcel Dekker, 1989. Pp 339–364.

49. Kinasewitz GT, et al. Effect of hypoxia on permeability of pulmonary endothelium of canine visceral pleura. *J Appl Physiol* 61:554, 1986.

50. Kotlikoff MI, Fishman AP. Endothelin: Mediator of Hypoxic Vasoconstriction? In AP Fishman (Ed), *The Pulmonary Circulation: Normal and Abnormal.* Philadelphia: University of Pennsylvania, 1990. Pp 85–89.

51. Krishnan A, et al. Cat lung hemodynamics: Comparison of experimental results and model predictions. *J Appl Physiol* 61:2023, 1986.

52. Kuhl PG, et al. Thromboxane receptor mediated bronchial and hemodynamic responses in ovine endotoxemia. *Am J Physiol* 254:R310, 1988.

53. Long WA, Brown DL. Central Neural Regulation of the Pulmonary Circulation. In AP Fishman (Ed), *The Pulmonary Circulation: Normal and Abnormal.* Philadelphia: University of Pennsylvania Press, 1990. Pp 131–149.

54. Malik AB, Johnson A. Role of Humoral Mediators in the Pulmonary Vascular Response to Pulmonary Embolism. In EK Weir, JT Reeves (Eds), *Pulmonary Vascular Physiology and Pathophysiology.* New York: Marcel Dekker, 1988. Pp 445–468.

55. Malik AB, Newell JC. Pulmonary perfusion and

gas exchange in hemorrhagic shock. *J Appl Physiol* 42:279, 1977.

56. Maseri A, et al. Determinants of vascular volume: Recruitment vs. distensibility. *Circ Res* 31:218, 1972.

57. McDonald DA. *Blood Flow in Arteries.* Baltimore: Williams & Wilkins, 1974.

58. McFadden ER. Respiratory heat and water exchange: Physiologic and clinical implications. *J Appl Physiol* 54:331, 1983.

59. Milnor WR. Pulsatile blood flow. *N Engl J Med* 287:27, 1972.

60. Mitzner W, Huang I. Interpretation of Pressure-Flow Curves in the Pulmonary Vascular Bed. In JA Will, et al. (Eds), *The Pulmonary Circulation in Health and Disease.* Orlando, FL: Academic Press, 1987. Pp 215–230.

61. Mitzner W, Sylvester JT. Hypoxic vasoconstriction and fluid filtration in pig lungs. *J Appl Physiol* 57:1065, 1981.

62. Morel DR, et al. Pulmonary extraction of serotonin and propranolol in patients with adult respiratory distress syndrome. *Am Rev Respir Dis* 132:479, 1985.

63. Muir A, et al. Distribution of blood flow in the lungs in acute pulmonary edema in dogs. *J Appl Physiol* 33:763, 1972.

64. Murgo JP, Westerhof N. Input impedance of the pulmonary arterial system in normal man. *Circ Res* 54:666, 1984.

65. Oppenheimer L, et al. Transvascular fluid flux measured from intravascular water concentration changes. *J Appl Physiol* 54:64, 1983.

66. Oppenheimer L, Goldberg HS. Pulmonary Circulation and Edema Formation. In SM Scharf, SS Cassidy (Eds), *Heart-Lung Interactions in Health and Disease.* New York: Marcel Dekker, 1989. Pp 93–130.

67. Paintal AS. Mechanism of stimulation of type J pulmonary receptors. *J Physiol (Lond)* 203:511, 1969.

68. Palmer RMJ, Ferrige AG, Moncada S. Nitric oxide release accounts for the biological activity of endothelium derived relaxing factor. *Nature* 327:524, 1987.

69. Parker JC, et al. The effect of increased vascular pressure on albumin excluded volume and lung lymph flow in the dog lung. *Circ Res* 47:866, 1980.

70. Permutt S, Bromberger-Barnea B, Bane HN. Alveolar pressure, pulmonary venous pressure and the vascular waterfall. *Med Thorac* 19:239, 1962.

71. Permutt S, et al. Effects of lung inflation on static pressure-volume characteristics of pulmonary vessels. *J Appl Physiol* 16:64, 1961.

72. Permutt S, Riley RL. Hemodynamics of collapsible vessels with tone: the vascular waterfall. *J Appl Physiol* 18:924, 1963.

73. Pickerel JA. *Lung Connective Tissue: Location,* *Metabolism, and Response to Injury.* Boca Raton, FL: CRC Press. Pp 5–100, 1973.

74. Pisuner A, Bellido JM. Segona nota sobre la sensibilitat guimica del neumogastric pulmonar. *Treballs Soc Biol Barc* 4:311, 1919.

75. Pitt BR, Lister G, Gillis CN. Metabolic Functions of the Lung and Cardiopulmonary Physiology. In SM Scharf, SS Cassidy (Eds), *Heart-Lung Interactions in Health and Disease.* New York: Marcel Dekker, 1989. Pp 391–406.

76. Prewitt RM. Pathophysiology and treatment of pulmonary hypertension in acute respiratory failure. *J Crit Care* 2:206, 1987.

77. Prewitt RM, Ducas J. Hemodynamic Management of Acute Respiratory Failure. In SM Scharf, SS Cassidy (Eds), *Heart-Lung Interactions in Health and Disease.* New York: Marcel Dekker, 1989. Pp 879–914.

78. Pump KK. The bronchial arteries and their anastomoses in the human lung. *Dis Chest* 43:245, 1963.

79. Reeves JT, McMurty IF, Voelkel NF. Possible role of membrane lipids in the function of the normal and abnormal pulmonary circulation. *Am Rev Respir Dis* 136:196, 1987.

80. Reidy MA. A reassessment of endothelial injury and arterial lesion formation. *Lab Invest* 53:513, 1985.

81. Rubin LJ, et al. Treatment of primary pulmonary hypertension with continuous intravenous prostacyclin (epoprosterol): Results of a randomized trial. *Ann Intern Med* 112:485, 1990.

82. Ryan JW. Processing of endogenous polypeptides by the lung. *Annu Rev Physiol* 44:241, 1982.

83. Ryan US. Endothelial Processing of Biologically Active Materials. In AP Fishman (Ed), *The Pulmonary Circulation: Normal and Abnormal.* Philadelphia: University of Pennsylvania Press, 1990. Pp 69–84.

84. Sheldon MI, Green JF. Evidence for pulmonary CO_2 chemosensitivity: Effects on ventilation. *J Appl Physiol* 52:1192, 1982.

85. Singal S, et al. Morphometry of the human arterial tree. *Circ Res* 33:190, 1973.

86. Starling EH. On absorption of fluid from connective tissue spaces. *J Physiol (Lond)* 19:312, 1896.

87. Staub NC, Nagano H, Pearce ML. Pulmonary edema in dogs, especially the sequence of fluid accumulation in the lungs. *J Appl Physiol* 22:227, 1967.

88. Stecenko AA, et al. Vasodilatory effect of aerosol histamine during pulmonary vasoconstriction in the unanesthetized sheep. *Pediatr Pulmonol* 3:94, 1987.

89. Swan HJC, et al. Catheterization of the heart in man with use of a flow directed balloon-tipped catheter. *N Engl J Med* 283:447, 1970.

90. Taylor MG. The input impedance of an assem-

bly of randomly branching elastic tubes. *Biophys J* 6:29, 1966.

91. Trenchard D, Russell NJW, Reybould H. Non-myelinated vagal lung receptors and their reflex effects on respiration in rabbits. *Respir Physiol* 55:63, 1984.

92. Unruh HW, Goldberg HS, Oppenheimer L. Pulmonary interstitial compartments and tissue resistance to fluid flux. *J Appl Physiol* 57:1512, 1984.

93. Voelkel NF, et al. Actions of lipoxygenase metabolites in isolated rat lungs. *J Appl Physiol* 57:860, 1984.

94. Wagenvoort CA. Vasoconstriction and medial hypertrophy in pulmonary hypertension. *Circulation* 22:535, 1960.

95. Wagner PD. Hypobaric Effects on the Pulmonary Circulation and High Altitude Pulmonary Edema. In EK Weir, JT Reeves (Eds), *Pulmonary Vascular Physiology and Pathophysiology.* New York: Marcel Dekker, 1989. Pp 173–198.

96. Walker BR, Voelkel NF, Reeves JT. Pulmonary pressor response following prostaglandin synthesis inhibition in conscious dogs. *J Appl Physiol* 52:705, 1982.

97. Weibel ER. Morphologic basis of alveolar-capillary gas exchange. *Physiol Rev* 53:419, 1973.

98. Weibel ER. *Morphometry of the Human Lung.* New York: Academic Press, 1963.

99. Weibel ER, Gomez EM. Architecture of the human lung. *Science* 137:577, 1962.

100. Weir EK, Reeves JT. *Pulmonary Vascular Physiology and Pathophysiology.* New York: Marcel Dekker, 1989. P 762.

101. West JB, Dollery CT. Distribution of blood flow and the pressure-flow relations in the whole lung. *J Appl Physiol* 20:175, 1965.

102. West JB, Dollery CT, Naimark A. Distribution of blood flow in isolated lung relative to vascular and alveolar pressures. *J Appl Physiol* 19:713, 1964.

103. Whittenberger JL, et al. Influence of state of inflation of the lung on pulmonary vascular resistance. *J Appl Physiol* 15:878, 1960.

104. Widdicombe JG, Sterling GM. The autonomic nervous system and breathing. *Arch Intern Med* 126:311, 1970.

105. Yanagisawai M, et al. A novel potent vasoconstrictor peptide produced by vascular endothelial cells. *Nature* 332:411, 1988.

106. Zumsteg TA, Havill AM, Gee MH. Relationships among lung extravascular fluid compartments with alveolar flooding. *J Appl Physiol* 53:267, 1982.

50

Pulmonary Hypertension: Pathophysiology and Clinical Disorders

Harly E. Greenberg   Steven M. Scharf

The pulmonary circulation accommodates the entire cardiac output, but because of its low resistance characteristics, it normally does so at systolic and diastolic pressures that are vastly lower than in the systemic circulation [59]. As emphasized in the preceding chapter, primary factors responsible for the lower resistance of the pulmonary compared to systemic vasculature are that pulmonary precapillary arterioles are compliant with thinner media and less smooth muscle than corresponding systemic arterioles. In addition, the cross sectional area of the pulmonary vascular bed is large and highly distensible, with recruitable vessels available to accommodate increases in flow such as occurs with exercise.

Diseases have a variable effect on pulmonary hemodynamics. A framework for assessing the nature of pulmonary hypertension is presented in Figure 50-1. Under normal circumstances and in the presence of left heart dysfunction, pulmonary arterial and left ventricular blood pressures are equal at end-diastole. With acute elevations in left heart pressures, pulmonary venous pressure is increased passively, leading to elevation of pulmonary arterial pressure (PAP). When these changes occur acutely, the walls of the pulmonary vessels remain thin and distensible, and pulmonary vascular resistance may actually decrease due to vascular recruitment. As a result, an end-diastolic pressure gradient is not generated across the pulmonary vascular bed. This form of pulmonary hypertension is sometimes classified as *passive*, implying that the elevation in PAP is a consequence of elevated left-sided pressures.

Alternatively, structural or functional abnormalities of the pulmonary vessels themselves, or pulmonary parenchymal processes that destroy the vasculature or expose it to stimuli which cause vasoconstriction, curtail its cross sectional area and increase pulmonary vascular resistance (PVR) [72]. This form of pulmonary hypertension is sometimes called *active* pulmonary hypertension, implying that pulmonary hypertension develops consequent to direct changes in the pulmonary vessels. In these disorders, pulmonary arterial diastolic pressure exceeds left ventricular end-diastolic pressure. This pressure gradient reflects the level of PVR [42] and can be measured clinically by pulmonary artery catheterization.

In diseases causing chronic and severe elevation of pulmonary venous pressure, such as mitral stenosis and pulmonary veno-occlusive disease, PAP may be disproportionately elevated in relation to pulmonary venous pressure. This form of pulmonary hypertension has been termed *reactive* pulmonary hypertension, implying that the pulmonary vasculature has reacted to chronic elevation in pulmonary downstream pressure. The additional increase in PAP above and beyond what is expected on the basis of elevated pulmonary downstream pressure is due to structural alteration and vasoconstriction of precapillary pulmonary arterioles and may be reversible with normalization of pulmonary venous pressure. Table 50-1 lists the major causes of pulmonary hypertension in these categories.

The natural history of pulmonary hypertension, and its response to treatment, depends on the mechanisms responsible for its initiation. When a reversible stimulus such as hypoxia or increased pulmonary blood flow secondary to left-to-right intracardiac shunting is present, pulmonary hypertension can be ameliorated by appropriate timely therapy. In disorders in which

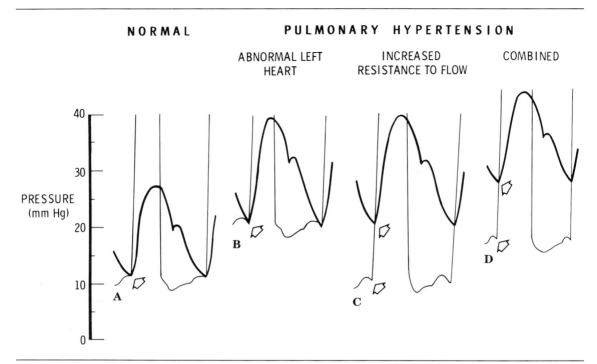

Fig. 50-1. The relation between left ventricular (*thin line*) and pulmonary arterial (*thick line*) end-diastolic pressures may be used to characterize the nature of pulmonary hypertension. Under normal circumstances (*A*) end-diastolic pressures at these sites are identical (*arrow*). When abnormal left heart function elevates left ventricular end-diastolic pressure above normal levels (*B*), pulmonary arterial pressure rises passively to the same extent. Resistance to pulmonary blood flow does not change. When pulmonary hypertension stems from abnormal structure or function of the pulmonary vessels (*C*), pressure in the pulmonary artery exceeds that in the left ventricle at end-diastole (*arrows*). The vertical distance between the arrows reflects the level of pulmonary vascular resistance. Passive pulmonary hypertension and increased resistance to blood flow may also occur simultaneously (*D*).

the inciting stimulus is irreversible or unknown, the disease tends to run an inexorably progressive course, leading to permanent anatomic changes of the vasculature with severely decreased cross sectional area and increased resistance. Eventually, cor pulmonale develops. Unfortunately, as described later, attempts at vasodilation to reverse this process are often disappointing, and management is limited to supportive measures. Recently, however, single-lung transplantation has been demonstrated to be effective in improving cardiac output, gas exchange, and exercise tolerance in selected cases.

Pulmonary Vascular Remodeling

Increased pulmonary artery pressure or flow due to various inciting conditions eventually leads to structural alterations of the pulmonary vasculature characteristic of long-standing pulmonary hypertension. The progressive nature of these histologic changes was recognized by Heath and Edwards [44] in 1958 in a study of pulmonary hypertension in congenital heart disease. They proposed a classification of these progressive vascular alterations ranging from mild and possibly reversible, grades I and II, to severe and irreversible, grades IV through VI (Table 50-2). The pathologic process leading to these changes in the pulmonary vasculature has been termed *vascular remodeling.*

Normal pulmonary arterioles are thin-walled vessels in which the intima is only one cell layer thick and the media occupies less than 7 percent of vessel thickness. The major feature of remodeled vessels is an increase in smooth muscle in already muscularized arteries and an extension of smooth muscle into vessels that are normally

Table 50-1. Causes of pulmonary hypertension

I. Elevated transmural pulmonary venous pressure
  A. Abnormal left heart function
    1. Left ventricle: failure, hypertrophy, aneurysm
    2. Pericardium: tamponade, restriction
    3. Mitral valve obstruction: stenosis, myxoma, thrombus
  B. Pulmonary venous obstruction
    1. Extrapulmonic: massive mediastinal fibrosis
    2. Intrapulmonic: veno-occlusive disease
  C. Hypervolemia: massive obesity, polycythemia vera
II. Normal transmural pulmonary venous pressure
  A. Abnormal gas exchange with vasoconstriction
    1. Ventilation-perfusion disturbance: chronic bronchitis, cystic fibrosis, acute bronchiolitis, bronchial asthma
    2. General hypoventilation: thoracic cage deformities, neuromuscular disorders, obesity hypoventilation, sleep apnea syndromes, upper airway obstruction, central depression
  B. Anatomic restriction of the bed
    1. Extravascular: diffuse, chronic interstitial lung diseases
    2. Intravascular: pulmonary arteritides, schistosomiasis, filariasis, tumor emboli, sickle cell disease
  C. Anatomic restriction and vasoconstriction
    1. Extravascular: emphysema, diffuse healed tuberculosis, anthracosilicosis
    2. Intravascular: pulmonary thromboemboli
  D. Overperfusion of the bed: congenital and acquired left-to-right shunts
  E. High alveolar pressure: positive end-expiratory pressure ventilation
  F. Unknown cause: "primary" pulmonary hypertension

Table 50-2. Heath and Edwards' classification of progressive pulmonary vascular changes in pulmonary hypertension [44]

Grade	Pathologic features
I	Medial hypertrophy
II	Cellular intimal proliferation
III	Luminal occlusion due to intimal hyperplasia ("onion-skinning")
IV	Plexiform lesions with dilatation and bypass channels around occluded vessels
V	Angiomatoid formation
VI	Fibrinoid necrosis

thin and nonmuscular. Other changes observed in various animal models include damage to the intimal endothelium with intimal hyperplasia and fibrosis. After a more prolonged course, proliferation of fibrous tissue in periadventitial regions may be seen as well. Eventually, the vasculature is obliterated by thrombus formation and fibrosis. Precursor cells, which after appropriate stimulation proliferate into mature smooth muscle and contribute to remodeling, are found in nonmuscular vessels where they are termed *pericytes*. Intermediate cells are also smooth-muscle precursors that more closely resemble mature smooth-muscle cells and are located in more muscular vessels [55,76].

A major stimulus to remodeling is hypoxia, which has been well studied in various animal models. Pulmonary hypertension following chronic hypoxia thus serves as a useful model for detailed consideration. On exposure to hypoxic conditions, acute increases in PAP occur; further elevation is observed with continued exposure. The early increase in PVR is predominantly due to hypoxia-mediated vasoconstriction, although some early cell proliferation in vessel walls has been observed. Subsequent pressure increases are predominantly due to vascular remodeling as well as to secondary polycythemia, which alters the rheologic properties of blood and, hence, pulmonary vascular pressure gradients. Within several days of exposure to hypoxia, pericytes and intermediate cells in precapillary arterioles proliferate and differentiate into smooth muscle, thereby decreasing vascular cross sectional area. Elastin and collagen synthesis and deposition in the vessel wall also occur [66,78]. Because of increased vascular resistance, pressure is increased in more proximal arteries, which may lead to remodeling in these vessels as well. Smooth-muscle proliferation is seen in the media of these larger vessels, and fibroblast proliferation is observed in perivascular regions. These changes contribute to further increases in PVR and pulmonary hypertension. In addition, vasomotor function may be altered in these remodeled vessels, with impairment of both vasodilatory and vasoconstrictive properties.

Remodeling has been demonstrated in several other experimental conditions, including inflammation secondary to sepsis or endotoxin and exposure to monocrotaline, a substance that produces pulmonary hypertension in animal models. Similar changes have been observed in humans with the adult respiratory distress syndrome (ARDS) [87]. A common feature of these processes is endothelial cell injury with subsequent progressive vascular remodeling. Remodeling is also observed when pulmonary blood flow is increased, as in congenital heart disease with intracardiac shunt leading to development of the Eisenmenger reaction. It has been postulated that the inflammatory process and increased blood flow lead to vascular remodeling by damaging endothelial cells, which then secrete factors that initiate smooth-muscle proliferation. Alternatively, damaged endothelial cells may fail to produce inhibitory factors, possibly heparin-like substances [39], which decrease smooth-muscle proliferation. Other data suggest a role for platelet-derived growth factors, which may stimulate proliferation of smooth muscle and fibroblasts. Increased pressure and mechanical shear forces also may stimulate remodeling directly. These mechanical factors apparently act via the endothelium as they require intact endothelium to induce collagen synthesis in the vessel wall [93].

Traditionally, once histologic remodeling occurred, the process was considered to be irreversible. Recent studies in rats have demonstrated that removal of the inciting stimulus can lead to reversal of structural changes. Increased pulmonary arterial proteolytic activity occurs after return of chronically hypoxic rats to normal conditions. This proteolysis may lead to resolution of vascular structural changes that have occurred as a result of remodeling. The decrease in wall tension resulting from release of hypoxic vasoconstriction may be one factor responsible for initiating proteolysis [94].

Clinical Disorders Causing Pulmonary Hypertension

Abnormal Left Heart Function

End-diastolic pressure in the left ventricle is the major determinant of blood volume and pressure in the pulmonary circulation under normal circumstances. Disease may increase pressure in the left ventricle as a consequence of myocardial failure, myocardial hypertrophy, or pericardial restriction or tamponade. In each instance, pulmonary blood volume and pressure rise in a fashion analogous to the behavior of the normal pulmonary vascular bed during blood volume expansion. Alternatively, disorders of the left venoatrial system, such as veno-occlusive disease, or mitral stenosis also elevate pulmonary venous pressure, although left ventricular end-diastolic pressure remains normal (see Table 50-1).

The vascular response to increased left ventricular pressure consists of a sequence of events that can be grouped into three phases depending on severity of the cardiac disturbance. During the initial phase, as pulmonary blood volume increases, the pulmonary vascular bed becomes fully recruited, with equalization of the normal pattern of apical and basal perfusion [45]. At this point, the patient may have relatively few symptoms, and no major abnormalities are demonstrable on physical examination. Upright roentgenographic examination of the chest may identify the abnormal distribution of perfusion.

With further increases in intravascular pressure, the second phase develops, in which fluid shifts from the vascular compartment to the adjacent interstitial space to produce interstitial edema. Roentgenographic examination reveals the presence of interstitial edema with reversal of the normal pattern of basal and apical perfusion [21]. The reversal stems from several mechanisms. Luminal dimensions are decreased and resistance to basal blood flow is increased as vessels are compressed by the accumulation of interstitial fluid. Local vasoconstriction, evoked by hypoxia in the basal regions, also contributes to this diversion of blood flow. Physical examination may reveal tachypnea as well as inspiratory crackles or expiratory wheezing. The latter finding is due to compromise of luminal dimensions of conducting airways by the surrounding cuff of interstitial edema [20]. If the process is sustained as occurs in mitral stenosis [43] or, rarely, in advanced protracted left ventricular failure [86], structural changes are generated in the vessel walls and remodeling occurs. This may lead to the development of reactive pulmonary hypertension, which is due to a combination of passive and active mechanisms with PAPs rising out of proportion to left ventricular end-diastolic pressure.

As described in Chapter 49, a balance of hydrostatic and colloid osmotic forces determines the extent of extravasation of fluid into the extravascular compartment. The third phase, with development of alveolar edema, is therefore a late manifestation of pulmonary congestion. Pulmonary function abnormalities may reflect these pathologic changes. Lung compliance is diminished, vital capacity falls, closing volume increases, and ventilation-perfusion abnormalities and shunt develop, giving rise to hypoxemia [40]. In the vast majority of instances, pulmonary hypertension due to abnormal left ventricular function is reversible with improvement of the underlying cardiac abnormality.

Pulmonary Parenchymal Disease as a Cause of Pulmonary Hypertension

Pulmonary parenchymal diseases produce pulmonary hypertension by one of two mechanisms: hypoxia (as described earlier) and obliteration of pulmonary vasculature. Hypoxia may be caused by hypoventilation, ventilation-perfusion imbalances and, in some cases, right-to-left shunting of blood.

OBSTRUCTIVE AIRWAYS DISEASE

A strict distinction between chronic bronchitis and emphysema is artificial because most patients with chronic obstructive pulmonary disease (COPD) exhibit pathophysiologic features common to both disorders. It is nevertheless useful to separate these disorders to emphasize the different pathophysiologic mechanisms responsible for development of pulmonary hypertension.

In chronic bronchitis, airway narrowing reduces alveolar ventilation in a large portion of the lung, with consequent development of alveolar hypoxia, which then contributes to pulmonary vasoconstriction [27,31]. The vasoconstrictive response to alveolar hypoxia is enhanced by acidosis, which may occur as a result of hypercapnia. Of note, hypercapnia itself does not lead to increased PAP; it only induces pulmonary vasoconstriction when accompanied by acidosis.

As the extent of alveolar hypoxia or acidosis increases, PVR increases (Fig. 50-2). The dominant site of hypoxic vasoconstriction is in vessels smaller than 200 μm [35,48]. Acidosis may also cause vasoconstriction in this as well as other segments of the pulmonary vasculature [27]. The mechanism responsible for hypoxic vasoconstriction is not well understood, and several mediators may be involved. Pulmonary hypertension associated with chronic hypoxia due to chronic bronchitis is, theoretically, at least partially reversible with correction of hypoxia and acidosis [30]. This reversibility is limited if structural changes in the vasculature have occurred secondary to remodeling. Similarly, pulmonary hypertension may occur in other disorders such as cystic fibrosis and asthma, which perturb ventilation-perfusion relationships.

In patients with emphysema, the characteristics of pulmonary hypertension have recently been investigated. Elevation of PAP is not common at rest unless pulmonary dysfunction is advanced [84]. It is more commonly increased, however, with exercise. In Oswald-Mommosser and colleagues' study [61], the degree of pulmonary

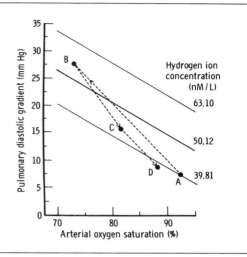

Fig. 50-2. Effect of alveolar oxygen tension (reflected by arterial blood oxyhemoglobin saturation) and blood hydrogen ion concentration on pulmonary vascular resistance in chronic bronchitis [42]. Left ventricular end-diastolic pressure is fixed at 10 mmHg in this consideration. Hypoxia and acidemia interact to increase resistance to blood flow by evoking vasoconstriction. This effect is reversed by corrected respiratory gas exchange. The fluctuating course of pulmonary hypertension is indicated by the sequence of arrows from the interval state (*A*) to hospitalization with acute respiratory failure (*B*), to an improved condition after 24 hours in the intensive care unit (*C*) and at the time of discharge from hospital (*D*).

hypertension correlated with the 1-second forced expiratory volume (FEV_1), diffusion capacity, and PO_2 during exercise but not with resting PO_2 and PCO_2. This suggests that pulmonary hypertension in emphysema is related to airways obstruction and extent of obliteration of the pulmonary vascular bed due to destruction of lung parenchyma in addition to hypoxic vasoconstriction. Nevertheless, the relationship between emphysema and cor pulmonale has been difficult to establish, particularly since many patients with severe emphysema do not demonstrate right ventricular hypertrophy. Thurlbeck [91] has suggested that the incidence of cor pulmonale increases with increasing severity of emphysema, ranging from 5 percent in mild to 40 percent in severe emphysema. This is supported by histologic studies demonstrating the presence of vascular remodeling in muscular pulmonary arteries of emphysema patients, with severity of vascular alterations correlating with extent of emphysema [52].

As mentioned previously, most patients with COPD have an admixture of emphysema and chronic bronchitis, and pulmonary hypertension in these patients often has features of both diseases. The chronic bronchitic component contributes to development of pulmonary hypertension by producing hypoxic vasoconstriction, whereas the emphysematous component increases PVR by decreasing the available pulmonary vascular bed.

Although obliteration of the vasculature and hypoxic vasoconstriction are major factors responsible for pulmonary hypertension in COPD, other mechanisms may contribute to development and maintenance of pulmonary hypertension. In a recent study of COPD patients, platelet aggregation and beta-thromboglobulin levels were found to be increased in blood samples taken from the pulmonary circulation of those with pulmonary hypertension in comparison to those with peripheral blood [79]. This difference was not observed in COPD patients with normal PAP, and the degree of platelet aggregation was found to correlate with mean PAP [79]. This find-

ing suggests the possibility that the coagulation cascade and platelet aggregation are involved in the pathogenesis of pulmonary hypertension in this disorder.

OBLITERATION OR COMPRESSION OF THE PULMONARY VASCULATURE IN DIFFUSE INTERSTITIAL LUNG DISEASES

Chronic interstitial lung diseases such as idiopathic pulmonary fibrosis, pneumoconioses, and asbestosis are believed to be initiated by alveolitis but may ultimately progress to fibrosis with decreased pulmonary compliance and reduced

Fig. 50-3. Relationship between lung volume, pulmonary blood volume (*PBV*), and pulmonary vascular resistance in chronic diffuse interstitial lung diseases [28]. PBV is expressed as a percentage of the total circulating blood volume (*TBV*) to permit comparison of subjects of different sizes. As interstitial inflammation and fibrosis act to diminish vital capacity, they also encroach on the small pulmonary vessels, and PBV falls linearly (*A*). Pulmonary vascular resistance rises hyperbolically as PBV falls (*B*).

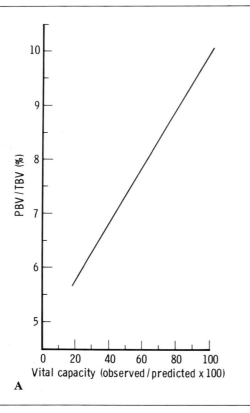

A

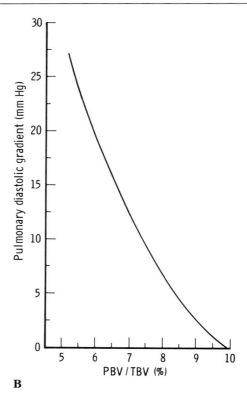

B

lung volumes [8]. This process eventually leads to compression and obliteration of the pulmonary vasculature by the inflammatory process itself, thrombosis [4], and fibrosis. The consequences of encroachment by the fibrotic process on the pulmonary vascular bed are illustrated in Figure 50-3 for idiopathic pulmonary fibrosis. When vital capacity is normal, so is the pulmonary blood volume. As pulmonary fibrosis encroaches on alveolar spaces and causes vital capacity to decrease, it also impinges on the small pulmonary vessels, and pulmonary blood volume falls linearly. PVR increases hyperbolically as pulmonary blood volume falls. Compression and obliteration of the vasculature by interstitial disease therefore leads to increased PVR [26]. When vital capacity is reduced to between 50 and 80 percent of predicted, pulmonary hypertension is generally demonstrable only during exercise, despite some elevation of PVR [26,96]. This finding is in keeping with loss of vascular reserve available for recruitment during exercise. As vital capacity is further reduced, pulmonary hypertension appears at rest. Since carbon monoxide diffusion capacity (DLCO) reflects pulmonary capillary blood volume, this measure also decreases with obliteration of pulmonary vessels as the fibrotic process progresses. In contrast, in sarcoidosis, limitation of DLCO but not vital capacity correlates with the degree of pulmonary hypertension [26]. This suggests that in sarcoidosis, the pathogenesis of pulmonary hypertension may differ from that in idiopathic pulmonary fibrosis, with the disease process directly affecting the pulmonary vasculature and resulting in decreased capillary blood volume, with reduced DLCO despite variable reduction of vital capacity.

Gas exchange is affected in a manner paralleling the progression of pathologic changes, with near-normal resting PO_2 early in the disorder and hypoxemia evident only during exercise. As the disease progresses, hypoxemia worsens with the evolution of pulmonary hypertension and eventual cor pulmonale. Early in the course of these disorders, if the pulmonary parenchymal inflammatory process is reversed, pulmonary hypertension may be averted. As fibrosis and vascular obliteration become a more prominent component of the disease process, little improvement can be expected with therapy. However, progression to significant pulmonary arterial hypertension and cor pulmonale is not ubiquitous. In some cases, cor pulmonale does not occur, probably due to development of numerous dilated vessels that serve as anastomotic channels between the pulmonary and systemic circulations that bypass occluded pulmonary vessels [96].

PULMONARY HYPERTENSION IN COLLAGEN-VASCULAR DISORDERS

Pulmonary hypertension is often observed in connective tissue diseases involving the lungs. The primary process may be vascular (i.e., vasculitis) or parenchymal (i.e., fibrosis). The disease process may directly injure the vascular endothelium or it may induce hypoxic vasoconstriction as a result of accompanying pulmonary parenchymal disease. Serum from patients with systemic lupus erythematosus (SLE) and progressive systemic sclerosis has been demonstrated to be cytotoxic to pulmonary endothelial cells and may be one factor initiating vascular remodeling in these disorders [46,63]. Alternatively, diffuse arteritis occurring as a consequence of collagen-vascular disease as well as other vasculitides may obstruct blood flow sufficiently to cause pulmonary hypertension.

Elevation of PAP is particularly common in progressive systemic sclerosis, with 33 to 67 percent of patients affected [81,106]. Similarly, evidence of pulmonary hypertension has been demonstrated in up to 40 percent of patients with SLE [29]. In many of these cases, minimal or no interstitial fibrosis or other pulmonary parenchymal disease is evident, suggesting that the primary lesion is in the pulmonary vasculature [81,83]. Histologic abnormalities of pulmonary vessels in these diseases include intimal proliferation with luminal narrowing, medial hypertrophy, and fibrosis indicative of vascular remodeling. Necrotizing arteritis, however, has also been observed. In addition, hypoxic vasoconstriction may contribute to pulmonary hypertension in these disorders as PVR can be reduced by administration of high inspired oxygen tension [58]. Hypercoagulability and intravascular thrombosis may also contribute to vascular obliteration, particularly since antiphospholipid antibodies have been demonstrated in SLE patients with pulmonary hypertension [3].

Those patients with collagen-vascular diseases who develop pulmonary hypertension are most frequently young women with a history of Raynaud's phenomenon and exertional dyspnea [31,67]. The major pulmonary function abnormality is a marked reduction of DLCO, which has been demonstrated to be a sensitive noninvasive indicator of pulmonary vascular disease and pulmonary hypertension in collagen-vascular disorders [67,89,97]. The DLCO may be reduced even in the absence of roentgenographic abnormalities. Among patients with collagen-vascular diseases, those with limited scleroderma or the variant known as CREST syndrome are at greatest risk for developing severe progressive pulmonary hypertension. As vasodilator therapy has been largely unsuccessful, structural changes in the vasculature rather than vasospasm is likely the predominant factor responsible for this progressive elevation of PVR [1,44,105,107].

Pulmonary Hypertension in Sleep-Disordered Breathing and Primary Alveolar Hypoventilation

Pulmonary hypertension has been noted in patients with obstructive sleep apnea (OSA). Whereas chronic awake pulmonary hypertension is relatively uncommon, affecting 12 to 20 percent of OSA patients [2,64], acute elevations of PAP during apneic episodes may be more frequent. Hypoxic vasoconstriction resulting from apnea-related hypoxemia may play an important role in the cyclic oscillations of PAP observed during sleep in OSA [92]. Hemodynamic factors may also be important in the pathogenesis of elevated PAP during apneic episodes. Because of continued respiratory efforts occurring against an obstructed upper airway, large negative swings in intrathoracic pressure occur during apneas. This results in augmented venous return during inspiration, which increases right ventricular output and may lead to acute increases in PAP during apnea. Furthermore, because of ventricular interdependence, any apnea-associated increase in right ventricular volume may decrease left ventricular compliance and contribute to increased PAP [65].

Although acute oscillations of PAP may commonly occur during individual obstructive apneas, most patients do not demonstrate prolonged nocturnal elevations. Such sustained elevations of PAP are probably due to extended periods of hypoxia and hypercapnia resulting from prolonged nocturnal alveolar hypoventilation, which may be due to concomitant pulmonary disease or abnormalities of ventilatory control.

As mentioned earlier, chronic awake pulmonary hypertension can be a serious sequela of OSA, although it is relatively uncommon. Interestingly, the development of pulmonary hypertension does not correlate with the severity or frequency of apneic events but rather depends on the presence of daytime hypoxemia, pulmonary

dysfunction, and obesity. Abnormalities in ventilatory control are also associated with chronic pulmonary hypertension in OSA because chronic hypercapnia and reduced ventilatory sensitivity to CO_2 are more common in OSA patients with pulmonary hypertension [9].

Whereas resting pulmonary hypertension is relatively infrequent in this disorder, elevated PAP during exercise may be more common [64,104]. In many of these individuals, concomitant elevations of pulmonary wedge pressure occur during exercise, suggesting that left ventricular dysfunction often contributes to pulmonary congestion and elevation of PAP [104].

Primary alveolar hypoventilation while awake may accompany sleep-disordered breathing in a small subset of patients with the pickwickian syndrome and OSA [70], or it may be a result of an isolated defect of ventilatory control without associated sleep-disordered breathing. These patients with obesity hypoventilation demonstrate a complex interaction of abnormalities that ultimately are responsible for the development of pulmonary hypertension. Decreased chest wall compliance due to obesity and decreased pulmonary compliance due to concomitant pulmonary congestion or other lung disease increase the work of breathing [60,85]. However, these mechanical abnormalities usually are not sufficiently severe to diminish alveolar ventilation to the extent observed, implicating an accompanying abnormality of ventilatory control. Once established, the resultant alveolar hypoxia and acidosis cause pulmonary vasoconstriction and pulmonary hypertension. Correction of respiratory gas exchange abnormalities can return PAP to near-normal levels [34,98].

Patients with respiratory muscle dysfunction due to neuromuscular disorders such as myasthenia gravis, multiple sclerosis, and amyotrophic lateral sclerosis or those with chest wall abnormalities such as kyphoscoliosis can also develop similar degrees of hypoxia and acidosis and develop pulmonary hypertension by similar pathogenetic mechanisms.

Overperfusion of the Pulmonary Vascular Bed

Congenital abnormalities that produce communications between the systemic and pulmonary circulations are often associated with pulmonary hypertension. Atrial septal defect is the most common of these disorders in the adult population, affecting between 0.2 and 0.7/1000 individuals [49]. Though these congenital heart disorders are characterized by elevated pulmonary blood flow due to left-to-right shunting, the observed changes in the pulmonary vasculature cannot be explained solely on the basis of increased flow. In certain forms of congenital heart disease, PAP is disproportionately elevated in comparison with the increase in pulmonary blood flow, suggesting that structural alterations or vasoconstriction contributes to elevation of PAP in these cases.

Factors that may be responsible for the development of pulmonary hypertension in these disorders become evident from data which demonstrate that the degree of pulmonary hypertension is dependent on the site of communication between the pulmonary and systemic circulations. Pulmonary hypertension develops only after many years in pretricuspid shunts such as atrial septal defect, whereas it develops much more rapidly when the site of communication is distal to the tricuspid valve as in ventricular septal defect. In fact, some patients have been reported to survive with atrial septal defect for 80 or more years, although the average survival is 50 years [49]. The greater pressures, velocity, and shearing forces transmitted through the shunt in communications distal to the tricuspid valve may be responsible for the more rapid development of pulmonary hypertension in these cases [68]. The size of the septal defect also influences the development of pulmonary hypertension, with defects greater than 1.5 cm in diameter more likely to be associated with pulmonary vascular abnormalities [6].

Increased perfusion of the pulmonary vascular bed at high kinetic energy has been demonstrated to delay or prevent maturation of the thick-walled fetal vessels, which is normally complete by the second month of life. Hence, the pulmonary hypertension of fetal life persists throughout the neonatal period in these congenital disorders and is perpetuated by the development of reactive lesions in small pulmonary arteries [6]. Current hypotheses concerning the pathogenesis of delayed maturation of pulmonary vessels and of reactive lesions suggest that high pulse pressures and shearing forces resulting from left-to-right shunting damage pulmonary vascular endothelial cells both structurally and functionally. Electron-microscopic studies have demonstrated coarsening of the endothelial surface in these hypertensive pulmonary arteries [68,69]. This endothelial injury may increase platelet adherence, aggregation, and activation with the liberation of growth factors that may, in part, be responsible for remodeling of the vasculature and development of reactive lesions. Other endothelium-derived factors released in response to injury may also be responsible for initiating and maintaining the remodeling process, which is similar to that which occurs in response to many other inciting stimuli [68]. Vasoconstriction, as evidenced by decreased PAP in response to acetylcholine and oxygen administration [41], is often present early in the course of pulmonary hypertension. Its role in the genesis of this disturbance remains unclear.

After surgical correction of the shunt, pulmonary hypertension and vascular remodeling may be reversible if histologic changes are limited to medial hypertrophy and intimal cellular proliferation (Heath and Edwards' classification grades I and II; see Table 50-2) [99,100]. Progression to intimal fibrosis and higher-grade abnormalities is unlikely to be reversible even after surgical correction of the shunt [107]. When PAP reaches systemic levels and right ventricular end-diastolic pressure exceeds that in the left ventricle, right-to-left shunting develops [10] and severe hypoxemia occurs.

Pulmonary Thromboembolic Disorders

Under experimental conditions, approximately one-half to two-thirds of the pulmonary vascular bed must be obliterated before pulmonary hypertension develops (Fig. 50-4). Mechanical obstruction of the pulmonary vasculature approximating these conditions can occur in various clinical diseases such as acute and chronic thromboembolism; vascular occlusion secondary to sickle cell crises; and schistosomal, fat, tumor, and amniotic fluid embolization, among other disorders in which particulate emboli lodge in the pulmonary vasculature. Once pulmonary hypertension is established, it may run a progressive course leading to cor pulmonale. Pulmonary thromboembolic disorders are discussed in full elsewhere; the following discussion is limited to the effects of thromboembolism on the pulmonary vessels and development of pulmonary hypertension.

The hemodynamic consequences of thromboembolism include increased pulmonary vascular resistance and pulmonary hypertension, with right ventricular dysfunction occurring if impedance to right ventricular outflow rises significantly. In patients with no prior history of cardiopulmonary disease, the maximum mean PAP observed with acute pulmonary embolism is less

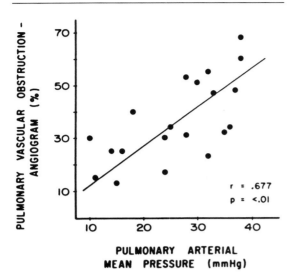

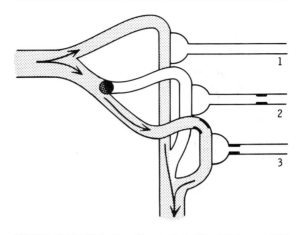

Fig. 50-4. The effect of thromboembolism on pulmonary arterial pressure in previously normal individuals. Pressure increases linearly with increasing extent of obstruction of the pulmonary vascular bed, as documented angiographically. The mean pulmonary arterial pressure does not exceed 30 mmHg until more than 50 percent of the vascular bed is occluded. (Reproduced with permission from McIntyre KM, Sassahara AS. The hemodynamic response to pulmonary embolism in patients without prior cardiopulmonary disease. *Am J Cardiol* 28:288, 1971.)

Fig. 50-5. Effect of thromboembolism on pulmonary vessels and associated airways. Clot is shown at a vascular bifurcation completely obstructing one branch and only partially occluding the other. Fibrin and platelets aggregate on the free surface of the clot (*crosshatched area*), which is bathed by blood. Vasoactive substances liberated by platelet degranulation are carried to precapillary vessels downstream of the clot. Three populations of airways can be characterized: (*1*) those ventilating normal areas of the bed; (*2*) those ventilating totally occluded vessels, which constrict and increase airway resistance; and (*3*) other more distal airways that constrict and cause compliance to fall. (Reproduced with permission from Y Enson, Pulmonary heart disease: Relation of pulmonary hypertension to abnormal lung structure and function. *Bull NY Acad Med* 53:551, 1977.)

than 40 mmHg and peak systolic pressure is less than 60 mmHg [53]. This upper limit of pressure is related to the maximal pressure-generating capacity of the nonhypertrophied right ventricle, which functions essentially as a capacitance chamber. Further increases in PVR result in right ventricular dilatation and failure, with elevation of right atrial pressure. Hemodynamic collapse with syncope or shock can occur [14]. PAPs above this level indicate prior cardiopulmonary disease with right ventricular hypertrophy. As shown in Figure 50-4, in previously normal individuals, as the degree of mechanical obstruction increases, resistance to blood flow rises linearly. Substantial pulmonary hypertension occurs only with massive embolization. However, in patients with prior cardiopulmonary disease, the increase in PAP in response to pulmonary embolism is accentuated. Obstruction of even 30 percent of the pulmonary vasculature can result in significant elevations of PAP, suggesting that pressure flow characteristics are altered in this setting [16,54].

The vascular consequences of thromboembolism are indicated in Figure 50-5. Emboli usually lodge at vascular bifurcations where narrowing occurs. One branch vessel may be totally obstructed while the other is only partially occluded. Both mechanical obstruction of the vessels and vasoconstriction appear to contribute to increased PVR. Hypoxia in remaining perfused lung zones may be one factor responsible for vasoconstriction. Hypoxemia in pulmonary thromboembolism results, in part, from a decline in ventilation-perfusion ratios in nonembolized regions as they now accommodate flow previously directed to obstructed vessels, resulting in overperfusion relative to ventilation. In addition, decreased cardiac output can lead to lower mixed venous oxygen tension, which may contribute to hypoxic vasoconstriction. Other vasoconstrictive

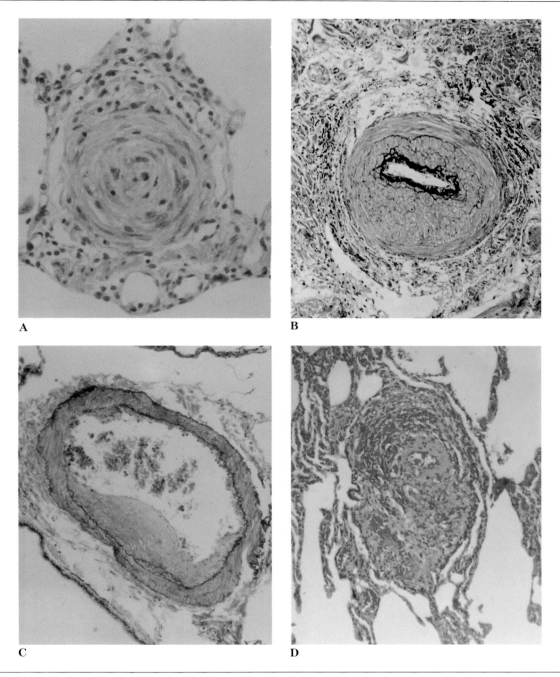

Plate 50-1. (A) Small muscular pulmonary artery showing almost complete occlusion by myointimal hyperplasia and fibrosis. This is also termed *concentric laminar intimal fibrosis* or an *onion-skin lesion* (H&E). (Courtesy of Dr G Pietra.) (B) Muscular pulmonary artery demonstrating eccentric intimal fibrosis, which is suggestive of remote thromboembolism (H&E). (Courtesy of Dr G Pietra.) (C) Medium-size pulmonary artery showing medial muscular hypertrophy between the external muscular coat and the internal elastic lamina (elastic stain). (Courtesy of Dr D Dantzker.) (D) Plexiform lesion.

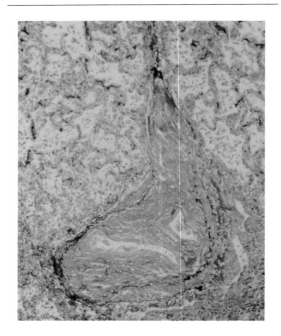

Plate 50-2. Medium-size pulmonary vein in a case of veno-occlusive disease demonstrating intraluminal fibrosis and variably sized intravascular channels, suggesting recanalization of prior thrombosis. (Courtesy of Dr D Dantzker.)

influences may contribute to increased PVR. Fibrin and platelets aggregate on the free surface of the clot. These platelets interact with thrombin in blood bathing this surface, degranulate, and release vasoactive substances [103]. Downstream, precapillary vessels respond by vasoconstriction, augmenting the increase in PAP caused by the mechanical obstruction. However, the duration of this vasoconstrictive response may be brief and limited to the immediate postembolic period. The precise nature of these vasoactive substances has not been characterized in humans, although serotonin, histamine, and vasoconstrictive prostaglandins ($PGF_{2\alpha}$) are possible candidates.

Chronic pulmonary hypertension is not a common sequela of acute pulmonary embolism; angiographic evidence of clot retraction and fibrinolysis is apparent by 10 to 14 days, and resolution is almost complete by 21 days, by which time pulmonary hypertension and hypoxemia have been substantially corrected in previously normal individuals. Fewer than 2 percent of patients continue to have repeated showers of thromboemboli or fail to lyse the emboli and pass into a chronic phase of sustained pulmonary hypertension [13]. These patients frequently do not present with acute episodes of pulmonary emboli but rather complain of the insidious onset of dyspnea and, occasionally, syncope due to developing chronic pulmonary hypertension. Lung perfusion scans are often helpful diagnostically in distinguishing unresolved pulmonary emboli in large vessels from other causes of pulmonary hypertension. The degree of elevation of PVR may be out of proportion to the extent of vascular obstruction documented angiographically in patients with chronic recurrent emboli or chronic unresolved thromboembolic disease. This may relate to vascular remodeling of nonobstructed arteries exposed to increased pressures [73] as well as vasoconstriction secondary to hypoxia or other inciting factors, including abnormal neural tone [5,17].

Pulmonary Hypertension in ARDS

ARDS arises from a heterogeneous group of disorders causing injury to the lung parenchyma that results in increased microvascular permeability. Regardless of the origin, the clinical manifestations of ARDS are uniform. Edema and atelectasis cause the lungs to become stiff, interfere with oxygenation of mixed venous blood, and result in progressively severe hypoxemia.

Although PAP often is normal in ARDS, pulmonary hypertension has been demonstrated in this syndrome [107] and is the result of an increase in PVR that is not entirely due to pulmonary congestion and decreased functional residual capacity. Factors initially responsible for lung injury, such as endotoxin, or products of the ensuing inflammatory process may damage the pulmonary endothelium and contribute to vasoconstriction, thus initiating and perpetuating the process of pulmonary vascular remodeling. Thromboxane A_2, released from platelets and neutrophils in response to endotoxin administration, may be one such factor as it has been found to produce a transient increase in PAP [19]. In addition, the pulmonary endothelial cell may be rendered more thrombogenic by procoagulant effects present in ARDS [56]. This may contribute to the pulmonary intravascular coagulation and fibrin deposition noted during gram-negative sepsis [82]. Hypoxia resulting from alveolar flooding and ventilation-perfusion inequality also contributes to pulmonary vasoconstriction in ARDS. Initially, PVR can be reduced by vasodilatory agents such as prostaglandin E_1 (PGE_1), although this has not been demonstrated to improve survival [7]. Later in the course of ARDS, thrombotic and fibrotic occlusion of pulmonary vessels predominates, and pulmonary hypertension is unresponsive to vasodilators [28].

Pulmonary Hypertension of Unknown Cause

In a subset of patients with pulmonary hypertension, no underlying etiologic factor can be found. In 1951, Dresdale and associates [22] described 39 cases of unexplained pulmonary hypertension and coined the term *primary pulmonary hypertension* (PPH). Subsequently, in 1973, the World Health Organization categorized PPH into three subtypes based on histopathologic findings: plexogenic pulmonary hypertension, thrombotic pulmonary arteriopathy, and pulmonary veno-occlusive disease (Table 50-3). However, the demonstration that pathologic features of both plexogenic and thrombotic forms of pulmonary hypertension coexist in individuals with familial PPH [50] brings into question the validity of separating PPH into these categories. Therefore, the following discussion will consider two clinically distinct diseases, PPH and pulmonary veno-occlusive disease. This would seem justifiable as patients with PPH can exhibit primary plexo-

Table 50-3. **Pathologic subtypes of pulmonary hypertension of unknown cause**

Subtype	Pathologic features
Plexogenic pulmonary hypertension	Concentric intimal fibrosis and plexiform lesions
Thrombotic pulmonary arteriopathy	Eccentric fibrotic lesions and organized microthrombi
Pulmonary veno-occlusive disease	Intimal proliferation with fibrosis and thrombosis of pulmonary venules

genic or thrombotic lesions or a mixture of these findings, whereas patients with pulmonary veno-occlusive disease rarely demonstrate pulmonary arterial lesions.

PRIMARY PULMONARY HYPERTENSION

PPH is most prevalent in women in the third and fourth decades of life, with a female-male ratio of 1.7 : 1 [15]. Cases have been documented in persons older than 60 years. The syndrome carries a grim prognosis, with a median survival of approximately 3 years from the time of diagnosis in those patients presenting with New York Heart Association functional class III status. Those presenting with class IV function have a median survival of only 6 months [15]. Other poor prognostic features include elevated right atrial pressure indicating right ventricular failure, decreased cardiac index, decreased diffusion capacity (DLCO), and the presence of Raynaud's phenomenon.

Since the initial description of PPH, interest has focused on mechanisms responsible for injury to the pulmonary arteries, which then give rise to the characteristic pathologic findings (Plate 50-1). The pathologic features seen in PPH can be observed also in pulmonary hypertension secondary to known cause and therefore represent the histologic consequence of injury to the pulmonary vasculature. Affected vessels demonstrate concentric intimal fibroelastosis, with complex plexiform lesions associated with vascular dilatations, and fibrinoid necrosis of muscular pulmonary artery walls. Pathologic features

may progress from initial smooth-muscle proliferation in the media to intimal hyperplasia and fibrosis with eventual luminal occlusion. Vessels are said to demonstrate a characteristic onion-skin pattern. Some vessels, seen in a subset of patients, demonstrate eccentric intimal fibrosis, with asymmetric rather than concentric fibrosis. This lesion may be associated with thrombosis and subsequent recanalization of the affected pulmonary artery, although this etiologic association has been questioned [24]. This histopathologic finding is the predominant feature in thrombotic pulmonary arteriopathy and may portend a somewhat better prognosis, as mentioned earlier, but many patients demonstrate an admixture of pathologic findings.

Many diverse inciting factors have been implicated in PPH, suggesting that multiple agents are capable of injuring the pulmonary vasculature and causing the pathologic and clinical features of PPH. Some substances associated with PPH are the appetite suppressant aminorex, oral contraceptives, and elevated catecholamine levels [38]. An interesting association between PPH and hepatic cirrhosis with portal hypertension has emerged, suggesting that pulmonary vascular damage may occur as a result of exposure to toxic substances that enter the circulation due to hepatic dysfunction [23,77]. In addition, in 5 to 10 percent of cases, an increased incidence of PPH has been observed within families, suggesting genetic susceptibility to this disorder [51].

Abnormal pulmonary vasoconstriction was initially hypothesized by Wood [108] to be an important factor in the pathogenesis of PPH. Once initiated, vasoconstriction could then lead to self-perpetuating damage to pulmonary vessels due to chronically elevated PAP. Eventually, obliteration of the vascular bed would occur. The pathologic lesions observed suggest that damage to the pulmonary endothelium may be an integral factor in this disorder, leading to intimal proliferation, fibrosis, and vascular remodeling. The search for vasoconstrictive factors or substances responsible for damaging the endothelium and initiating smooth-muscle and fibrous tissue proliferation has largely been unrewarding for many years. Investigations have focused on the role of factors produced by the endothelium, circulating platelets, and immune cells in the regulation of vasoconstriction and vascular remodeling. Recent identification of a peptide, endothelin-1, with vasoconstrictive properties and the concomitant ability to induce proliferation of vascular smooth muscle has suggested a role for this agent in the pathogenesis of PPH. Levels of endothelin-1 have been shown to be elevated in PPH, with higher concentrations in systemic arterial compared to systemic venous blood, suggesting that the peptide is produced in the pulmonary system [88]. Whether endothelin-1 has a direct role in the pathogenesis of PPH or is merely a marker of endothelial damage remains to be determined.

Platelet- and macrophage-derived growth factors have also been implicated in remodeling of the pulmonary vasculature in PPH [78]. Alternatively, damage to the endothelium may render it unable to produce protective vasodilatory or antiproliferative factors. Possible protective factors include prostacyclin and endothelium-derived relaxing factor, both products of the endothelial cell, which have been demonstrated to produce pulmonary vasodilation and to decrease platelet aggregability and adherence to endothelial surfaces [32,36,57].

Other evidence suggests that microthromboembolic disease is important in PPH. Thrombosis probably occurs in situ as no identifiable source of recurrent emboli can be demonstrated in most cases [62]. In support of this theory, elevated levels of fibrinopeptide A have been demonstrated in PPH, which is suggestive of an ongoing thrombotic process, possibly induced by damaged endothelium [25].

Immunologic factors also may contribute to PPH, as serologic abnormalities such as a positive antinuclear antibody and Raynaud's phenomenon are seen in 29 percent and 11 percent of cases, respectively [15]. Thus PPH has many features of connective tissue–autoimmune disorders, which may explain the overlap between identifiable collagen-vascular disease and pulmonary vasculopathy. In addition, abnormalities in neural activity regulating pulmonary vessels have been postulated in the pathogenesis of PPH. Whatever the inciting factor, narrowing of the vascular lumen due to intimal proliferation, plexiform lesions, and fibrosis as well as in situ thrombosis increases PVR and PAP. The resultant increase in shear stress and wall tension may further perpetuate damage to the endothelium and lead to additional remodeling and obliteration of vessels.

The earliest clinical manifestations of PPH are easy fatigability and exertional dyspnea with vague precordial chest pain, which may be secondary to right ventricular strain. These vague and nonspecific symptoms are often overlooked. A long asymptomatic period probably occurs prior to diagnosis, with most patients presenting late in the course of the disease when structural damage to the pulmonary vasculature is widespread [15,101]. Syncope during exercise is another manifestation, and sudden death has been reported to be increased in this disorder.

Pulmonary Veno-occlusive Disease

Pulmonary veno-occlusive disease is a rare form of idiopathic pulmonary hypertension, accounting for fewer than 10 percent of cases, and it is rapidly fatal, with death usually occurring within 2 years of diagnosis. It affects children and young adults, but large studies of its demographics are not available. Pulmonary hypertension in this condition stems from lesions that predominantly involve the pulmonary venules and veins rather than pulmonary capillaries and arterioles. Both children and adults are affected, with a slight male predominance. Although the diagnosis can be made on clinical, radiologic, and morphologic grounds, other entities capable of producing postcapillary pulmonary hypertension such as mitral stenosis, fibrosing mediastinitis, and congenital venous atresia or stenosis must be excluded. Biopsy specimens reveal obliteration of the intima of pulmonary veins and venules with fibrosis (Plate 50-2). Although the inciting factors for this disease process are unknown, speculation has centered on in situ thrombosis with recanalization as well as proliferative changes secondary to chronically elevated intravascular pressures.

Because the pulmonary venous system is obstructed in this disorder, pulmonary congestion may occur, manifested by orthopnea and paroxysmal nocturnal dyspnea with Kerley B lines present on chest roentgenography despite normal left atrial pressure. Measurement of pulmonary wedge pressure is of little use in this disease because observed values can reflect pressure in veins in which flow has ceased owing to obstruction rather than true left atrial pressure. According to principles outlined in Chapter 49, left atrial pressure can be accurately assessed only if the catheter is wedged in a region drained by patent and communicating veins. In the majority of cases of veno-occlusive disease in which it is measured, the pulmonary capillary wedge pressure is found to be normal [90].

The onset of this disorder is usually insidious, but progression is inexorable, and most patients die within 2 years of becoming symptomatic. Exertional dyspnea is the first symptom, which progresses to dyspnea at rest. Signs and symptoms of pulmonary congestion and exertional syncope follow. When the clinical picture is fully developed, physical examination indicates the presence of pulmonary hypertension, right ventricular enlargement, and elevated central venous pressure. Tricuspid regurgitation may appear.

When manifestations of pulmonary congestion are absent and the pulmonary capillary wedge pressure is normal, it is not possible to distinguish pulmonary veno-occlusive disease from plexogenic pulmonary hypertension on clinical grounds. Open-lung biopsy can demonstrate the characteristic pathology. No meaningful therapeutic measures are available, although various modalities have been employed, as described below.

CLINICAL AND LABORATORY FEATURES

The major goal in evaluating patients who present with signs and symptoms suggestive of pulmonary hypertension is to identify treatable causes of secondary pulmonary hypertension and to assess the severity of pulmonary hypertension and right ventricular dysfunction. In secondary pulmonary hypertension, clinical features are those of the underlying disorder. In PPH, the onset may be insidious, without specific historical features.

Findings present on physical examination depend on the severity and chronicity of the disorder. Frequently, narrow splitting of the second heart sound is evident, with an accentuated pulmonic component and ejection murmur. Signs of right ventricular hypertrophy such as a right parasternal heave may be present, along with murmurs of tricuspid regurgitation. Right ventricular failure is heralded by jugular venous distension and a prominent A wave. At the end stage, peripheral edema and hepatic congestion may appear.

Enlargement of the main pulmonary arteries and its branches with "pruning" of peripheral vessels may be seen on chest roentgenography, along with signs of right ventricular enlargement (Fig. 50-6). Lung fields are usually clear. However, in veno-occlusive disease, increased interstitial markings by Kerley B lines may be present, and the chest roentgenogram may be reminiscent of congestive heart failure. Pulmonary function tests may demonstrate a restrictive ventilatory defect with reduced diffusion capacity (DLCO). The latter is a common but relatively nonspecific marker of PPH [15]. Mild to moderate hypoxemia is frequently observed and is due to a low mixed venous oxygen tension resulting from low car-

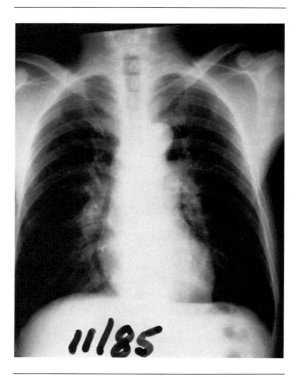

Fig. 50-6. Chest roentgenogram in pulmonary hypertension, demonstrating enlargement of the main pulmonary arteries with pruning of peripheral vessels. (Courtesy of Dr D Dantzker.)

diac output with increased peripheral O_2 extraction combined with mild ventilation-perfusion inequality. A mild chronic respiratory alkalosis may also be present [15]. The electrocardiogram may demonstrate evidence of right ventricular strain or hypertrophy and right atrial enlargement. Other laboratory abnormalities include abnormal liver function tests secondary to hepatic congestion and positive antinuclear antibodies.

Perfusion lung scans are an important part of the evaluation to rule out chronic large-vessel thromboembolic disease. In plexogenic PPH, these scans are normal or demonstrate nonspecific defects, whereas a patchy distribution may indicate microthrombi or veno-occlusive disease [75]. Perfusion lung scanning may theoretically be hazardous in severe cases because of further obstruction of the pulmonary vascular bed by macroaggregates used for scanning. However, no adverse consequences of perfusion scanning were observed in the National Institutes of Health (NIH) National Registry of PPH [15].

The need to rule out occult chronic proximal pulmonary artery thromboemboli and to clarify results of ventilation-perfusion lung scanning that may suggest thromboembolic disease necessitates pulmonary angiography in many cases. Although a potential for increased risk of this procedure exists in severe pulmonary hypertension, the NIH National Registry did not demonstrate significant adverse consequences of angiography in this population [15].

Echocardiography may be a useful noninvasive adjunct in the evaluation of PPH. It can identify anatomic abnormalities due to congenital or other causes and can estimate severity of pulmonary hypertension. M-mode evaluation can demonstrate paradoxic septal motion and partial systolic closure of the pulmonic valve in up to 60 percent of cases [15]. Doppler ultrasonography may also be useful to assess the severity of pulmonary hypertension. Features such as tricuspid velocity, pulmonary velocity acceleration time, and right ventricular relaxation time have been used to estimate PAP noninvasively [12].

Cardiac catheterization is essential to confirm the diagnosis and to assess severity. It is also essential to rule out unsuspected congenital heart disease with Eisenmenger's reaction. The details of pressure measurements and assessment of PVR are fully described in Chapter 49.

The role of open-lung biopsy in the evaluation of pulmonary hypertension is controversial. This procedure may identify an unsuspected cause of pulmonary hypertension such as vasculitis or interstitial fibrosis. However, in practice it is rare to demonstrate histologic findings other than those of PPH in patients whose clinical presentation is characteristic and who have undergone an extensive evaluation. In addition, qualitative analysis of histologic features fails to predict response to therapy [62]. Therefore, when the morbidity of this procedure is considered, it usually is advocated only for those cases in which the possibility of secondary pulmonary hypertension still exists after noninvasive evaluation.

TREATMENT OF PRIMARY PULMONARY HYPERTENSION

Treatment directed at pulmonary hypertension of unknown cause should be considered only after secondary pulmonary hypertension has been meticulously excluded. Therapeutic modalities currently available include anticoagulant therapy, vasodilators, and lung transplantation.

Because thrombosis of muscular pulmonary arteries and arterioles in various stages of orga-

nization has been demonstrated in pulmonary hypertension of unknown cause, there is a rationale for anticoagulant therapy. Thrombi probably arise in situ as a result of a procoagulant state induced by injured vascular endothelium. A distant source of emboli cannot be identified in most cases, despite extensive evaluation. A retrospective study of PPH has demonstrated a survival benefit of chronic anticoagulation in all histologic subtypes [33]. However, such therapy confers additional risk, and prospective studies are needed to assess its utility better.

In addition to structural changes of the pulmonary vasculature, endothelial injury may lead to vasoconstriction, which may contribute to increased PVR in some cases. As a result, many investigations have focused on the therapeutic role of vasodilators in PPH. One of the problems in assessing efficacy of vasodilators is that current clinical measurements of PVR are influenced by cardiac output, as described in Chapter 49. An increase in cardiac output without lowering PAP can result in a calculated fall in PVR. Such a calculated response is probably without significant clinical benefit, as right ventricular overload is unaffected and abnormal pressure and shear forces on the pulmonary vessels persist.

A meaningful response to vasodilators should include a rise in cardiac output, associated with reductions of PVR and PAP, and improved exercise tolerance. Different criteria have been proposed to define the degree of improvement necessary to indicate a favorable vasodilator response. However, the significant short-term and long-term variability observed in these hemodynamic parameters at baseline as well as long-term variability of response to treatment confounds the selection of a specific degree of improvement necessary to indicate vasodilator responsiveness [18]. Criteria developed by Rich and colleagues [74] for defining a positive response to high-dose calcium channel blocker therapy include a 50 percent reduction in PVR accompanied by a 33 percent fall in PAP. In another vasodilator trial, Weir and coworkers [102] utilized a 10 percent increase in cardiac output accompanied by a 5-mmHg decrease in mean PAP, a 20 percent reduction of PVR, and a decrease in the ratio of pulmonary to systemic vascular resistance to define vasodilator responsiveness.

Further complicating this issue is the significance of a positive response to vasodilators. Although improved long-term survival is predicted by vasodilator responsiveness, this may reflect less extensive obliteration of the pulmonary vasculature in responsive cases rather than a survival benefit of drug therapy. It must also be recognized that these drugs may cause significant adverse effects, particularly in those patients in whom the predominant cause of elevated PVR is structural change in the vasculature rather than vasoconstriction. In such cases, accompanying systemic vasodilation may produce severe hypotension and fatal hemodynamic collapse because the failing right ventricle cannot augment cardiac output in the presence of fixed pulmonary vascular obstruction.

Predominance of medial muscular hypertrophy on histopathologic examination would be expected to predict responsiveness to vasodilators whereas predominant intimal hyperplasia, thrombosis, and fibrosis should suggest lack of efficacy, but accurate prediction of vasodilator response is not possible by qualitative assessment of pathologic features [62]. Quantitative morphometric analysis of lung biopsy specimens does, however, predict unresponsiveness to vasodilators when obliteration of the vasculature is extensive. Baseline hemodynamic parameters also do not predict acute vasodilator response [62]. Because of the inability to predict therapeutic response to vasodilators on clinical or histologic grounds, and because of the possibility of adverse effects, short-term vasodilator trials under close hemodynamic monitoring are necessary before instituting this mode of treatment. A significant decrease in PVR during a short-term vasodilator trial has been demonstrated to be useful in predicting long-term efficacy [71].

Several vasodilators have been evaluated, including calcium channel blockers, hydralazine, acetylcholine and, more recently, prostacyclin and its analogues, PGE_1, adenosine, and other agents. Prostacyclin is particularly useful for vasodilator trials because of its short half-life. A beneficial response to prostacyclin during short-term trials has been demonstrated to predict response to other vasodilator agents such as hydralazine and nifedipine [37]. In addition to vasodilation, prostacyclin inhibits platelet aggregation, which may be induced by injured endothelium. Continuous long-term administration of prostacyclin via intravenous infusion pump has resulted in sustained hemodynamic improvement [80].

Recent studies have evaluated another approach using high-dose calcium channel blocker therapy titrated under close hemodynamic monitoring (right heart catheterization). In this protocol, described by Rich and colleagues [74], nifedipine or diltiazem is administered in an initial test dose of 20 or 60 mg, respectively. Hemodynamic measurements are made after 1 hour. Further oral doses of calcium channel blocker are administered hourly until a favorable hemodynamic response is observed, marked by a 33 percent fall in PAP and a 50 percent fall in PVR, or until adverse effects force discontinuation. Adverse consequences that may preclude continuation include a decrease in systemic systolic blood pressure below 90 mmHg or gastrointestinal distress. In those patients in whom a favorable hemodynamic response is achieved, the cumulative effective dose is then administered every 6 to 8 hours and continued on a chronic basis. A sustained reduction in PAP and PVR with regression of right ventricular hypertrophy was noted after 1 year in 4 of 5 patients who initially responded to this protocol, although a survival benefit has not been clearly demonstrated [74]. Further placebo-controlled prospective trials are necessary to document clear physiologic and survival benefit because calcium channel blockers have the potential to induce severe adverse effects.

Heart-lung transplantation has been employed in treating patients with severe pulmonary hypertension. One-year survival has ranged from 64 to 76 percent [95]. However, limited availability of heart-lung donors has decreased the applicability of this procedure. Single-lung transplantation has been demonstrated to be a reasonable alternative in selected cases with reversible cardiac dysfunction [11,95] and is rapidly replacing heart-lung transplantation in this disorder. Remarkably, despite performing this procedure on patients with severe right ventricular dysfunction (mean right ventricular ejection fraction [RVEF], 22 ± 15 percent), Trulock and associates [95] demonstrated regression of right ventricular hypertrophy with functional recovery (mean posttransplantation RVEF 51 ± 11 percent) with return of PAP and cardiac index to normal. Eleven of 12 patients in this study have survived up to 22 months. All patients demonstrated significant improvement in New York Heart Association functional class. This mode of therapy merits serious consideration in selected cases of pulmonary hypertension with severe functional impairment.

Right ventricular failure is the primary determinant of prognosis in PPH [47]. The importance of improving right ventricular function by various therapeutic modalities is emphasized by the fact that neither PVR nor PAP are, by themselves, predictive of clinical outcome. Methods of assessing right ventricular function and its response to therapy is the subject of the next chapter.

References

1. Al-Sabbagh MD, et al. Pulmonary arterial morphometry in systemic sclerosis: A case control autopsy study. *Arthritis Rheum* 29:552, 1986.
2. Apprill M, et al. Frequency and mechanism of daytime pulmonary hypertension in patients with obstructive sleep apnea syndrome. *Cor Vasa* 33:42, 1991.
3. Asherson RA, Mackworth-Young CG, Boey MC. Pulmonary hypertension in systemic lupus erythematosus. *Br Med J* 287:1024, 1983.
4. Bignon J, Hem B, Molinier B. Morphometric and angiographic studies in diffuse interstitial pulmonary fibrosis. *Prog Respir Dis* 8:141, 1975.
5. Bjornsson J, Edwards MD. Primary pulmonary hypertension: A histopathologic study of 80 cases. *Mayo Clin Proc* 60:16, 1985.
6. Bloomfield DK. The natural history of ventricular septal defect in patients surviving infancy. *Circulation* 29:914, 1964.
7. Bone RC, et al. Randomized double blind multicenter study of prostaglandin E1 in patients with the adult respiratory distress syndrome. *Chest* 96:154, 1989.
8. Boushy SP, North LB. Pulmonary function in infiltrative lung disease. *Chest* 64:448, 1973.
9. Bradley D, et al. Role of daytime hypoxemia in the pathogenesis of right heart failure in the obstructive sleep apnea syndrome. *Am Rev Respir Dis* 137:835, 1985.
10. Brammell HL, et al. The Eisenmenger syndrome. *Am J Cardiol* 28:679, 1971.
11. Calhoun JH, et al. Single lung transplantation alternative indications and technique. *J Thorac Cardiovasc Surg* 101:816, 1991.
12. Chan K, et al. Comparison of three Doppler ultrasound methods in the prediction of pulmonary artery pressure. *J Am Coll Cardiol* 59:662, 1987.
13. Dalen JE, Alpert JS. Natural history of pulmonary embolism. *Prog Cardiovasc Dis* 17:259, 1975.
14. Dalen JE, Dexter L, Ockene IS. Precapillary pulmonary hypertension: Its relationship to pulmonary venous hypertension. *Trans Am Clin Climatol Assoc* 86:207, 1974.
15. D'Alonzo GE, et al. Survival in patients with primary pulmonary hypertension: Results from a national prospective registry. *Ann Intern Med* 115:343, 1991.
16. Dantzker DR. Pulmonary Embolism. In RG Crystal, GB West (Eds), *The Lung: Scientific Foundations*. New York: Raven Press, 1991. Pp 1198–1207.
17. Dantzker DR, Bower JS. Partial reversibility of chronic pulmonary hypertension caused by pulmonary thromboembolic disease. *Am Rev Respir Dis* 124:129. 1981.
18. Dantzker DR, D'Alonzo GE, Gianotti L. Vasodilators and primary pulmonary hypertension: Variability of long term response. *Chest* 95:1185, 1989.
19. Demling RH. Role of prostaglandins in acute microvascular injury. *Ann NY Acad Sci* 384:517, 1982.
20. Detroyer A, Yernault J, Englert M. Mechanisms of breathing in patients with atrial septal defect. *Am Rev Respir Dis* 115:413, 1977.
21. Dollery CT, West JB. Regional uptake of radioactive oxygen, carbon monoxide and carbon dioxide in the lungs of patients with mitral stenosis. *Circ Res* 8:765, 1960.
22. Dresdale DT, Schultz M, Michtom RJ. Primary pulmonary hypertension: I. Clinical and hemodynamic study. *Am J Med* 11:686, 1951.
23. Edwards BS, et al. Coexistent pulmonary and portal hypertension: Morphologic and clinical features. *J Am Coll Cardiol* 10:1233, 1987.
24. Edwards WD, Edwards JE. Clinical primary pulmonary hypertension: Three pathologic types. *Circulation* 56:884, 1977.
25. Eisenberg PR, Lucore C, Kaufman L. Fibrinopeptide-A levels indicative of pulmonary vascular thrombosis in patients with primary pulmonary hypertension. *Circulation* 82:841, 1990.
26. Emirgil C, et al. The lesser circulation in pulmonary fibrosis secondary to sarcoidosis and its relationship to respiratory function. *Chest* 60:371, 1971.
27. Enson Y, et al. The influence of hydrogen ion concentration and hypoxia on the pulmonary circulation. *J Clin Invest* 43:1146, 1964.
28. Enson Y, Thomas HM, Bosken CH. Pulmonary hypertension in interstitial lung disease. *Trans Assoc Am Physicians* 88:248, 1975.
29. Fayemi AO. Pulmonary vascular disease in systemic lupus erythematosus. *Am J Clin Pathol* 65:284, 1976.
30. Ferrer MI, et al. Some effects of digoxin upon the heart and circulation in man: Digoxin in cor pulmonale. *Circulation* 1:161, 1950.
31. Fishman AP, et al. Effects of acute hypoxia on the circulation and respiration in patients with chronic pulmonary disease studied during the steady state. *J Clin Invest* 31:770, 1952.
32. Funchgott RM, Vanhoutte PM. Endothelium derived relaxing and contracting factors. *FASEB J* 3:2007, 1989.
33. Fuster V, Steele PM, Edwards WD. Primary pulmonary hypertension: Natural history and importance of thrombosis. *Circulation* 70:580, 1984.

34. Gillam PMS, Mymin D. Hypoventilation and heart disease. *Lancet* 2:853, 1961.

35. Glazier JB, Murray JF. Sites of pulmonary vasomotor reactivity in the dog during alveolar hypoxia and serotonin and histamine infusion. *J Clin Invest* 50:2250, 1971.

36. Griffith TM, et al. Endothelium derived relaxing factor. *J Am Coll Cardiol* 12:797, 1988.

37. Groves BM, et al. Comparison of the acute hemodynamic effects of prostacyclin and hydralazine in PPH. *Am Heart J* 110:1200, 1985.

38. Guazzi MD, et al. Hypersensitivity of lung vessels to catecholamines in systemic hypertension. *Br Med J* 293:291, 1986.

39. Hales CA, et al. Impairment of hypoxic pulmonary artery remodeling by heparin in mice. *Am Rev Respir Dis* 128:747, 1983.

40. Hales CA, Kazemi H. Pulmonary function after uncomplicated myocardial infarction. *Chest* 72:350, 1977.

41. Harris P. Influence of acetylcholine in the pulmonary arterial pressure. *Br Heart J* 19:272, 1957.

42. Harvey RM, Enson Y, Ferrer MI. A reconsideration of the origins of pulmonary hypertension. *Chest* 59:82, 1971.

43. Heath D, Whitaker W. The pulmonary vessels in mitral stenosis. *J Pathol Bacteriol* 70:291, 1955.

44. Heath DA, Edwards JE. The pathology of hypertensive pulmonary vascular disease. *Circulation* 18:533, 1958.

45. Hogg JC, et al. Distribution of airway resistance with developing pulmonary edema in dogs. *J Appl Physiol* 32:20, 1972.

46. Kahaleh MB, Sherer GK, LeRoy EC. Endothelial injury in scleroderma. *J Exp Med* 149:1326, 1979.

47. Kanemoto N, Sasamoto H. Pulmonary hemodynamics in primary pulmonary hypertension. *Jpn Heart J* 20:395, 1979.

48. Kato M, Staub NC. Response of the small pulmonary arteries to unilobar hypoxia and hypercapnia. *Circ Res* 19:426, 1966.

49. Konstananides S, et al. The natural history of atrial septal defect in adults—a still unsettled issue. *Klin Wochenschr* 69:506, 1991.

50. Loyd JE, et al. Heterogeneity of pathologic lesions in familial PPH. *Am Rev Respir Dis* 138:952, 1988.

51. Loyd LE, Primm RK, Newman JH. Familial primary pulmonary hypertension: Clinical patterns 1,2. *Am Rev Respir Dis* 129:1947, 1984.

52. Magee F, et al. Pulmonary vascular structure and function in chronic obstructive pulmonary disease. *Thorax* 43:183, 1988.

53. McIntyre KM, Sasahara AA. The hemodynamic response to pulmonary embolism in patients without prior cardiopulmonary disease. *Am J Cardiol* 28:288, 1971.

54. McIntyre KM, Sasahara AA, Sharma GVRK. Pulmonary thromboembolism: Current concepts. *Ann Intern Med* 18:192, 1972.

55. Meyrick B, Reid L. The effect of continued hypoxia on rat pulmonary arterial circulation: An ultrastructural study. *Lab Invest* 38:188, 1978.

56. Moalli R, et al. Fibrinolysis in critically ill patients. *Am Rev Respir Dis* 140:287, 1989.

57. Moncada S, Vane JR. Pharmacology and endogenous roles of prostaglandin endoperoxides, thromboxane A2 and prostacyclin. *Pharmacol Rev* 30:293, 1979.

58. Morgan JM, et al. Hypoxic pulmonary vasoconstriction in systemic sclerosis and primary pulmonary hypertension. *Chest* 99:551, 1991.

59. Murray JF. *The Normal Lung.* Philadelphia: Saunders, 1976. Pp 113–150.

60. Naimark A, Cherniack RM. Compliance of the respiratory system in health and obesity. *J Appl Physiol* 15:377, 1960.

61. Oswald-Mommosser M, et al. Pulmonary hemodynamics in chronic obstructive pulmonary disease of the emphysematous type. *Respiration* 58:304, 1991.

62. Palevsky H, et al. Primary pulmonary hypertension: Vascular structure, morphometry and responsiveness to vasodilator agents. *Circulation* 80:1207, 1989.

63. Penning CA, et al. Antibody-dependent cellular cytotoxicity of human vascular endothelium in systemic lupus erythematosus. *J Clin Lab Immunol* 17:125, 1985.

64. Podszus T, Bauer W, Mayer J. Sleep apnea and pulmonary hypertension. *Klin Wochenschr* 64:131, 1986.

65. Podzus T, Greenberg H, Scharf S. The Influence of Sleep State and Sleep-Disordered Breathing on Cardiovascular Function. In N Saunders, C Sullivan (Eds), *Sleep and Breathing,* (Vol 2). New York: Marcel Dekker, (in press).

66. Poiani GJ, Toggi CA, Yohn SE. Collagen and elastin metabolism in hypertensive pulmonary arteries in rats. *Circ Res* 66:968, 1990.

67. Pronk LL, Swaak AJ. Pulmonary hypertension in connective tissue disease. Report of three cases and review of the literature. *Rheumatol Int* 11:83, 1991.

68. Rabinovitch M. Mechanisms of Pulmonary Hypertension in Chronic High Flow States. In EK Weir, JT Reeves (Eds), *Pulmonary Vascular Physiology and Pathophysiology.* New York: Marcel Dekker, 1989. Pp 469–511.

69. Rabinovitch M, et al. Pulmonary artery endothelial abnormalities in patients with congenital heart defects and pulmonary hypertension: A correlation of light with scanning electron microscopy and transmission electron microscopy. *Lab Invest* 55:632, 1986.

70. Rapoport DM, et al. Hypercapnea in the ob-

structive sleep apnea syndrome: A reevaluation of the pickwickian syndrome. *Chest* 89:627, 1986.

71. Reeves JT, Govesm BM, Turkevich D. The case for treatment of selected patients with primary pulmonary hypertension. *Am Rev Respir Dis* 134:342, 1986.

72. Reid L. Structural and Functional Reappraisal of the Pulmonary Artery System. In *The Scientific Basis of Medicine* (ann rev). London: Atholone Press, 1968. Pp 289–307.

73. Reid L. Structure and function in pulmonary hypertension. *Chest* 89:279, 1986.

74. Rich S, Brundage BH. High dose calcium channel blocking therapy for primary pulmonary hypertension: Evidence for long term reduction in pulmonary artery pressure and regression of right ventricular hypertrophy. *Circulation* 76:135, 1987.

75. Rich S, et al. Primary pulmonary hypertension: Radiographic and scintigraphic patterns of histologic subtypes. *Ann Intern Med* 105:233, 1986.

76. Riley DJ. Vascular Remodeling. In RG Crystal, GB West (Eds), *The Lung: Scientific Foundations*, New York: Raven Press, 1991.

77. Robalino BD, Moodie DS. Association between primary pulmonary hypertension and portal hypertension: Analysis of its pathophysiology and clinical laboratory and hemodynamic manifestations. *J Am Coll Cardiol* 17:492, 1991.

78. Ross R. The Pathogenesis of Atherosclerosis. In E Braunwald (Ed), *Heart Disease: A Textbook of Cardiovascular Medicine.* Philadelphia: Saunders, 1988. P 1135.

79. Rostagno L, et al. Evidence for local platelet activation in pulmonary vessels in patients with pulmonary hypertension secondary to chronic obstructive pulmonary disease. *Eur Respir J* 4:147, 1991.

80. Rubin LJ, et al. Treatment of primary pulmonary hypertension with continuous intravenous prostacyclin (Epoprostenol): Results of a randomized trial. *Ann Intern Med* 112:485, 1990.

81. Sackner MA, et al. Pathophysiology of scleroderma involving the heart and respiratory system. *Ann Intern Med* 60:611, 1964.

82. Saldeen T. Fibrin-derived peptides and pulmonary injury. *Ann NY Acad Sci* 483:310, 1982.

83. Salerni R, et al. Pulmonary hypertension in the CREST syndrome variant of progressive systemic sclerosis (scleroderma). *Ann Intern Med* 86:394, 1977.

84. Schulman L, et al. Pulmonary vascular resistance in emphysema. *Am Rev Respir Dis* 133:223A, 1986.

85. Sharp JT, et al. Total respiratory inertiance and its gas and tissue components in normal and obese men. *J Clin Invest* 48:503, 1964.

86. Smith RC, Burchell HB, Edwards JE. Pathology of the pulmonary vascular tree: IV. Structural changes in the pulmonary vessels in chronic left ventricular failure. *Circulation* 10:801, 1954.

87. Snow RL, et al. Pulmonary vascular remodeling in the adult respiratory distress syndrome. *Am Rev Respir Dis* 126:887, 1982.

88. Steward DJ, et al. Increased plasma endothelin-1 in pulmonary hypertension: Marker or mediator of disease. *Ann Intern Med* 114:464, 1991.

89. Stupi AM, et al. Pulmonary hypertension in the CREST syndrome variant of systemic sclerosis. *Arthritis Rheum* 29:515, 1986.

90. Thadani U, et al. Pulmonary veno-occlusive disease. *QJ Med* 44:133, 1975.

91. Thurlbeck WM. Chronic Airflow Obstruction: Correlation of Structure and Function. In TL Petty (Ed), *Chronic Obstructive Pulmonary Disease* (2nd ed). New York: Marcel Dekker, 1985. Pp 129–204.

92. Tilkian AG, et al. Hemodynamics in sleep induced apnea. *Ann Intern Med* 85:714, 1976.

93. Tozzi CA, et al. Pressure induced connective tissue synthesis in pulmonary artery segments is dependent on intact endothelium. *J Clin Invest* 84:1005, 1989.

94. Tozzi CA, et al. Vascular connective tissue is rapidly degraded during early regression of pulmonary hypertension. *Chest* 99(3 Suppl):418, 1991.

95. Trulock EP, et al. The Washington University–Barnes Hospital experience with lung transplantation. Washington University Lung Transplantation Group. *JAMA* 266:1943, 1991.

96. Turner-Warwick M. Pre-capillary systemic pulmonary anastomoses. *Thorax* 18:225, 1963.

97. Ungerer RG, Tashkin DP, Furst D. Prevalence and clinical correlation of pulmonary arterial hypertension in progressive systemic sclerosis. *Am J Med* 75:65, 1983.

98. Vogel J, Blount G. The role of the hydrogen ion concentration in the regulation of pulmonary artery pressure: Observations in a patient with hypoventilation and obesity. *Circulation* 32:788, 1965.

99. Wagenvoort C, Wagenvoort N, Draulans Y. Reversibility of plexogenic pulmonary arteriopathy following banding of the pulmonary artery. *J Thorac Cardioavasc Surg* 87:876, 1984.

100. Wagenvoort CA, Heath DA, Edwards JE. *The Pathology of the Human Vasculature.* Springfield, IL: Thomas, 1964.

101. Wagenvoort CA, Wagenvoort N. Primary pulmonary hypertension: A pathologic study of the lung vessels in 156 clinically diagnosed cases. *Circulation* 42:1163, 1970.

102. Weir EK, Rubin LJ, Hyers JM. The acute administration of vasodilators in PPH. *Am Rev Respir Dis* 140:1623, 1989.

103. Weiss HJ. Platelet physiology and abnormalities of platelet function. *N Engl J Med* 293:531, 1975.

104. Weitzenblum E, et al. Daytime pulmonary hypertension in patients with obstructive sleep apnea. *Am Rev Respir Dis* 138:345, 1988.

105. Young D, Mark H. Fate of the patient with the Eisenmenger syndrome. *Am J Cardiol* 28:658, 1971.

106. Young RH, Mark GJ. Pulmonary vascular changes in scleroderma. *Am J Med* 64:998, 1978.

107. Zapol WM, Snider MJ. Pulmonary hypertension in severe acute respiratory failure. *N Engl J Med* 296:476, 1976.

108. Wood P. Pulmonary hypertension with special reference to the vasoconstrictive factor. *Br. Heart J.* 20:557, 1958

51

Pulmonary Embolism

Kenneth M. Moser

Over the last two decades, there have been major advances in our understanding of venous thromboembolism. These advances have included new insights into pathogenesis, improved diagnostic techniques, and new therapeutic approaches. However, perhaps the most important advances have been conceptual—that is, recognition of a series of basic concepts that compose a structural framework to guide a logical sequence of decision making.

Perhaps the most important concept that has emerged is that venous thromboembolism is one disorder, and pulmonary embolism is simply a complication of venous thrombosis [25,33,85]. This powerful basic concept has multiple management ramifications. For example, when coupled with the recognition that venous thrombosis is a largely preventable entity, this concept emphasizes that a campaign aimed at prevention of venous thrombosis is the most vital action that can be taken to reduce the morbidity and mortality due to acute pulmonary embolism [80].

Unfortunately, the incidence of venous thrombosis, and therefore pulmonary embolism, does not appear to be decreasing. It is estimated that 5 million patients on the North American continent develop deep venous thrombosis each year, of whom 500,000 (10 percent) suffer pulmonary embolism, 50,000 of which prove fatal. There are probably a number of factors responsible for maintaining this incidence despite the many improvements that have been realized. As technologic advances have occurred, more patients are salvaged from previously lethal disorders or have invasive procedures performed. For example, hip and knee replacements have become common, cardiac surgery is widely performed, and larger numbers of patients survive acute myocardial infarction and severe trauma. Thus, as our knowledge of venous thromboembolism has expanded, so has the population at risk.

However, the major "missing link" in achieving a reduction in venous thromboembolism is a failure to modify physician behavior. Specifically, there has been a gap between what is known and its application in daily medical practice. Certain important investigative goals remain to be achieved. But application of existing information about pathogenesis, natural history, diagnosis, prevention, and management of venous thromboembolism is the major clinical deficit requiring remedy.

Pathogenesis

It has long been recognized that three factors promote venous thrombosis and, therefore, the potential for thrombus detachment in the form of pulmonary embolism: stasis, injury to the venous intima, and alteration in the coagulation-fibrinolytic system. This triad, enunciated by Virchow in the last century, remains intact. In recent years, this triad has been translated into a clinically usable form; that is, the specific risk factors associated with the development of venous thrombosis have been identified and, to a large degree, quantified. These data have been generated by studies in which objective tests have been employed to detect the presence of deep venous thrombosis or pulmonary embolism in well-characterized patient populations [2,8,9,24,26,52,53,74]. Such data were not available during the long era in which these diagnoses were based on clinical judgment. As we now know, clinical diagnosis is subject to a completely unacceptable rate of both false-positive and false-negative diagnoses [6,39,40,52,68]. Thus, valid data began to be accumulated only after objective tests—namely, contrast venography, ^{125}I-fibrinogen leg scanning [52], and impedance plethysmography [39] in the case of deep vein thrombosis (DVT), and lung scanning [44,61] and pulmonary angiography [14] in the case of pulmonary embolism—became available and were employed.

Employing such methods, it has been possible to identify the risk factors associated with venous thromboembolism (Table 51-1). Furthermore, it has become evident that these risk factors are cumulative (i.e., the more risk factors present, the more likely is the development of venous thromboembolism). For example, the risk of venous thrombosis in uncomplicated myocardial infarction is rather low (10 to 15 percent) [96]. However, if an infarction is associated with prolonged immobility, congestive heart failure, obesity, and advanced age, the risk becomes substantially higher. Conversely, it is clear that venous thromboembolism rarely occurs among individuals with no identifiable risk factor(s). Venous thromboembolism is almost exclusively a disorder of otherwise ill, hospitalized, or recently hospitalized (or operated) patients [24,33].

Another important feature of venous thromboembolism now recognized is that embolism arises almost exclusively from DVT of the lower-extremity veins. Necropsy observations and other investigations have disclosed that approximately 95 percent of all pulmonary emboli arise from the deep veins of the lower extremities [25,33,85]. Occasionally, venous thrombosis at other sites can be incriminated. For example, mural thrombi in the right atrium or right ventricle and vegetations on the tricuspid or pulmonary valves can embolize. Patients with unusual sites of embolic origin usually are not difficult to identify; they are chiefly individuals with myocardial infarction, chronic right ventricular failure, and septic endocarditis. Even among these patients, however, the legs are a frequent embolic source. Rarely, renal or hepatic vein thrombosis proves to be the site from which emboli rise.

Table 51-1. Risk factors predisposing to venous thromboembolism

Major surgery (general anesthesia lasting more than 1 hour)

Trauma or surgery of pelvis and lower extremities

Prior deep venous thrombosis

Lower-extremity stasis, any cause

Prolonged immobility

Pregnancy, postpartum state

Other: Age > 60 years, use of estrogen-containing compounds, cancer, obesity, specific coagulopathies

In the past, upper-extremity veins were rarely an embolic source. However, this has changed somewhat in recent years because of the increasing use of indwelling devices in the major veins [63]. Ventriculoatrial shunts, indwelling catheters for hyperalimentation or drug delivery, and intraventricular pacing wires are particularly common embolic sources because of their size, long residence, and the materials delivered through them. Upper-extremity thrombosis (most often of the subclavian vein related to vigorous upper-extremity exercise) is another potential, though uncommon, source. Finally, intravenous drug users can induce bland venous thrombosis (as well as septic phlebitis) by trauma to upper- and lower-extremity venous injection sites. Beyond these patients with special circumstances leading to venous thrombosis in unusual locations, however, embolism connotes that there has been thrombosis in the deep veins of the lower extremities.

We know that thrombi that remain limited to the calf veins do not pose an embolic threat of clinical significance, whereas those in the popliteal veins or higher pose substantial embolic risk [37,45,71]. The most likely explanation for this disparity relates to thrombus size. Calf thrombi are usually small and, if they do embolize, are not likely to give rise to symptoms (or be detected by lung scan or pulmonary angiography). Thus, while such veins may be a thromboembolic source, emboli arising from them rarely are clinically significant. On the other hand, above-knee venous thrombosis is associated with a 40 to 50 percent incidence of emboli that induce symptoms and can be detected by scan or angiogram (Fig. 51-1).

Periprostatic and uterine veins are often invoked as sources of embolism when no other source is clinically apparent, but such attribution rarely is correct. These veins are small and, like calf veins, it is improbable that they will deliver emboli of a size that induces symptoms. Thus, unless such veins have become markedly enlarged, they should not be incriminated as the source of emboli that occlude segmental or larger pulmonary arteries.

Natural History

The natural history of venous thrombosis of the lower extremities is now reasonably well characterized. Patients at risk develop a platelet nidus in the region of a venous valve, most commonly in a calf vein [84]. (Thrombosis originating in

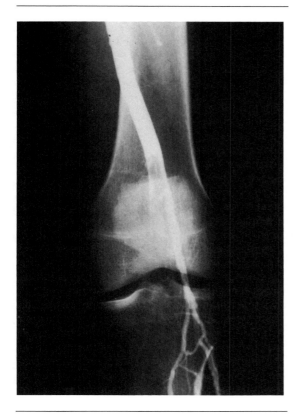

Fig. 51-1. Contrast venogram demonstrating acute venous thrombus in the femoral vein.

above-knee veins is substantially less common, although it does occur after trauma or surgery involving the femur or pelvis.) The platelet nidus then initiates the coagulation cascade and, fairly rapidly, a red fibrin thrombus appears. The thrombus does inflame the valve and venous wall, but early in its career it has rather fragile attachments. If it is not swept away—and in the face of stasis or venous wall injury, it may not be—the thrombus grows. Such growth occurs by layering of fibrin and platelets supplied by the flowing blood. The growth may be rapid (minutes), and it continues until the thrombus is swept away (embolism), stasis is relieved, the vessel becomes totally occluded, or therapy is initiated. As thrombosis is initiated, the intrinsic fibrinolytic system is activated and promotes lysis of the thrombus even as other factors seek to extend it. How activation of the fibrinolytic system is achieved is not yet understood. Clearly, this stage of thrombosis is a highly dynamic event

subject to multiple outcomes. These early events are subclinical.

If the thrombus becomes sizable and remains attached, the inflammation of the venous wall (thrombophlebitis) continues. However, clinically detectable expression of this inflammation (local heat, redness, tenderness) often does not occur. The next step is organization of the thrombus, during which the fibrin clot is converted into an organized venous wall plaque or scar or, if it is totally occlusive, a plug. Recanalization of the plug may then occur, or collateral veins may develop to relieve the obstruction.

If there are venous valves along the course of the thrombus, these are incorporated into the organizing mass and may be rendered permanently incompetent. This process—from nidus formation to dissolution or organization—takes place over approximately 7 days. Of course, it may be over in minutes or hours if the thrombus is swept away or lysed. Alternatively, with renewed thrombus growth, the period to resolution may be longer.

At any time during this sequence, and until organization occurs, embolism is a threat. Obviously, the threat to the patient is the greatest when large thrombi have been formed whose attachment to the venous wall is insecure. Thus, embolic risk is greatest soon after thrombus formation and diminishes with time.

The prognosis for the patient, in terms of recurrent DVT, obviously depends on the outcome of this initial episode. If the patient restores venous integrity, the risk of future episodes returns to baseline. However, if significant residual obstruction, or valvular incompetence, persists, the patient remains at increased risk of recurrent DVT (and, therefore, pulmonary embolism).

The natural history of acute pulmonary embolism also has been fairly well defined. Sudden obstruction of pulmonary arteries may induce several pulmonary consequences, including hyperventilation, creation of an alveolar dead space, hypoxemia, pneumoconstriction, and surfactant depletion.

The pathogenesis of the hyperventilation is obscure, although tachypnea is one of the most constant consequences of embolism both in animal investigations and in patients. Stimulation of various intrapulmonary receptors has been invoked, but whether this is operative in humans is unknown.

The creation of an alveolar dead space is an obvious consequence of total occlusion (Fig. 51-2). A zone of nonperfused but ventilated lung is cre-

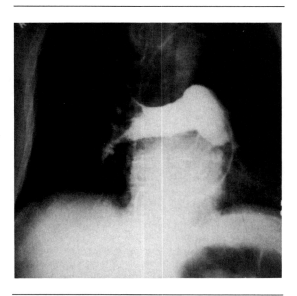

Fig. 51-2. Massive acute pulmonary embolism. Angiogram demonstrates multiple filling defects in distal portion of right main pulmonary artery and its branches. Subsequent injection of left main pulmonary artery (not shown) disclosed several segmental artery obstructions. Both lungs remained well ventilated with no evidence of volume loss. The patient complained only of moderate tachypnea; tachycardia (110 beats/min) was present.

ated. However, most emboli are not totally occlusive; thus, a high $\dot{V}/\dot{Q}$ zone tends to result. Other events may further reduce the extent of this dead space. One such event is pneumoconstriction. It has been demonstrated in animals that the marked alveolar hypocapnia that occurs beyond the point of pulmonary artery obstruction induces contraction of the alveolar spaces [83]. How often this occurs in humans is not clear. However, patients are free to rebreathe their dead-space air (which contains CO_2); also, they rather promptly open bronchial arterial channels (which provide CO_2 at systemic levels) and, because emboli are rarely totally occlusive, hypocapnia will not occur. Furthermore, hyperinflation reduces (experimental) pneumoconstriction. All these factors limit the extent to which pneumoconstriction may occur in patients.

Arterial hypoxemia as a consequence of embolism has attracted substantial investigative attention, but its basis has escaped full explanation, probably because the mechanism varies from patient to patient and over time in a fashion not replicated by animal models [58]. Perhaps the most important clinical points are that hypoxemia does *not* occur in all patients with embolism but that the more extensive the embolic occlusion, the more likely and severe is arterial hypoxemia. In extensive embolism, a fall in cardiac output leads to a widened arteriovenous oxygen difference, which is reflected in arterial hypoxemia. In an animal model, it has been shown that major embolism does not induce hypoxemia as long as cardiac output is maintained [7]. Other mechanisms for hypoxemia include the induction of ventilation-perfusion disturbances—perhaps the most common basis of hypoxemia—and right-to-left shunting through a patent foramen ovale. The key clinical point is that absence of hypoxemia does *not* exclude the diagnosis of pulmonary embolism [67].

Surfactant depletion, the last pulmonary consequence of acute embolism, occurs, if at all, later than the others. Available animal data and such clinical experience as is available indicate that complete arterial obstruction is needed to interrupt surfactant production and allow time for surfactant depletion [20]. If complete occlusion persists, atelectasis and transudation of plasma and formed elements occur in the affected zones. The resultant lesion has been called *congestive atelectasis*. The clinical expression is the radiographic appearance of lesions that combine volume loss and alveolar filling (Fig. 51-3). These radiographic shadows are often called *infarcts*, implying that tissue death has occurred. In fact, animal and human investigations have demonstrated that, given time and restoration of pulmonary arterial circulation or development of bronchial arterial collateral flow, surfactant production is restored, the debris is cleared, and the architectural integrity of the affected zones is restored [20]. Thus, true pulmonary infarction (tissue death with scarring) is an uncommon consequence of embolism. The lung parenchyma is especially equipped to avoid infarction because it has three sources of oxygen supply, via the pulmonary arteries, the bronchial arteries, and the tracheobronchial tree, with nutrient supply available from the first two. In the experimental animal, it is extremely difficult to induce infarction unless there is embolism plus compromise of at least one of the other two (and usually both) nutrient oxygen pathways. The same appears true in humans. Except in patients with coexisting left ventricular failure or lung disease, infarction is rare.

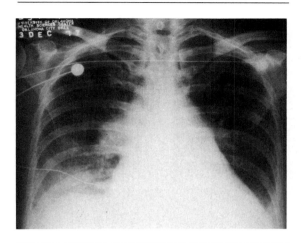

Fig. 51-3. Chest roentgenogram 36 hours after angiographically proved acute embolic obstruction of descending branch of right pulmonary artery. Artery is markedly distended by embolus. Congestive atelectasis has developed in right lower lobe. This cleared slowly without scarring.

The acute *hemodynamic* consequence of embolism is an increase in pulmonary vascular resistance (PVR), which is almost always accompanied by tachycardia. The severity of the increase in PVR is conditioned by several factors, one of which is undisputed whereas the others are controversial. The undisputed determinant is the extent of embolic obstruction: The greater the extent, the greater is the increase in resistance [17,60]. Disputed are mechanisms that may induce pulmonary arterial constriction, thereby exaggerating the degree-of-resistance increment. Various reflexes promoting such constriction have been suggested [99] and a variety of mediators of vasoconstriction also have been postulated, particularly serotonin and thromboxane released from the platelets known to coat emboli [31,91]. None of these mechanisms has been proved to operate in patients, but clinical observations do suggest that one or more of them may exaggerate, early on, the PVR increase that follows embolism.

The clinical consequences of this increase in PVR depend on two major factors: the extent of the increase and the prior cardiopulmonary status of the patient. The right ventricle, thin-walled as it normally is, is poorly equipped to deal with an acute major increase in afterload. Available data indicate that the right ventricle cannot tol-

erate acute elevations in mean pulmonary arterial pressure above the range of 40 to 50 mmHg [60]. In this range and higher, right ventricular ischemia and failure ensue, perhaps abruptly, with death of the patient.

Clearly, patients with diminished cardiopulmonary reserve may show substantial clinical deterioration after embolization of rather modest degree [60]. Preexisting severe lung disease may exaggerate the extent of hypoxemia and acutely increase an already elevated PVR. Coronary artery disease may express itself as right or left ventricular ischemia, acute ischemic dysfunction, or an arrhythmia. On the other hand, previously normal individuals often tolerate major emboli with no expression of acute hemodynamic impairment other than perhaps tachycardia.

Another important consideration concerning acute embolism is the timing of mortality following a major embolic event. Fatal episodes of pulmonary emboli leave little time for diagnosis and treatment because the vast majority of fatalities occur within a few hours [1]. Those few deaths (perhaps 10 percent) that occur later probably are due to recurrences of emboli.

If the patient survives the acute embolic event, the natural history of embolism parallels that of DVT. Most emboli tend to resolve, within days to weeks, by a combination of lysis and organization (Fig. 51-4) [14]. Within 6 weeks, most of the embolic obstructions have resolved in the majority of treated patients, though modest residuals often persist [93,94]. However, there are uncommon exceptions to this rule in which patients permanently maintain substantial chronic obstruction. Most of these chronic obstructions have escaped diagnosis and have not received treatment. In a small number of such patients, despite apparent adequate treatment, major emboli fail to resolve for reasons that remain obscure [64].

Diagnosis

The diagnostic approaches to DVT and pulmonary embolism derive directly from our understanding of the natural history and pathophysiology of these related phenomena.

Deep Venous Thrombosis

In the case of DVT, we have learned that venous thrombi do three things that may be used to assist us diagnostically: They (1) inflame veins, (2) obstruct veins, and (3) grow by platelet-fibrinogen accretion. If inflammation is severe, local

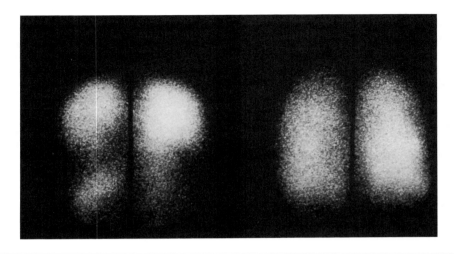

heat, redness, or tenderness may be detectable clinically. If obstruction is marked, edema may appear. Unfortunately, in substantial numbers of patients with DVT, neither inflammation nor edema is detectable and, in many patients with such findings, DVT is not the cause. Thus, it is not surprising that multiple studies have shown that the clinical diagnosis of DVT is unreliable [2,33,39,40,52,53,70]. Objective tests must be done to confirm or deny the diagnosis. Perhaps the most important clinical point, then, is that most venous thrombi are asymptomatic and will not be detected clinically. Conversely, many patients clinically suspected of having venous thrombosis (due to leg pain, swelling, heat) do not have it.

Among the available diagnostic tests, the gold standard is contrast venography (see Fig. 51-1). However, this procedure is not without hazard and discomfort, and it is not easy to perform correctly or to interpret. Further, the procedure must be performed in the radiology suite, making it necessary to move the patient. Therefore, in recent years, much attention has focused on the validation of other techniques that do not share certain of these disadvantages. From among the many already studied or being investigated, two have achieved adequate validation: impedance plethysmography (IPG) and radiofibrinogen leg scanning. A third, duplex scanning, holds promise.

IPG is based on the detection of venous outflow obstruction from the lower extremities (Fig. 51-5). Careful guidelines for test performance and

Fig. 51-4. Posterior perfusion scans in patient with angiographically proved pulmonary emboli. At left is admission scan showing extensive defects. At right is scan 4 weeks later demonstrating excellent resolution on therapy with anticoagulant drugs.

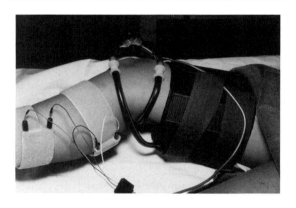

Fig. 51-5. Impedance plethysmography. A standardized sequence of cuff occlusion is employed as measurements of impedance are made by the electrodes.

interpretation have been developed, and the results have been validated against contrast venography [39–41,45]. These investigations have disclosed that IPG will detect approximately 95 percent of thrombi in above-knee veins that have been present for 5 days or less. Because the degree of venous outflow obstruction induced by thrombi in veins below the popliteal vein is often modest, the test detects 30 percent or fewer of such thrombi. Further, collateral channels may develop rapidly around persistent above-knee occlusions, so that test reliability falls off beyond the fifth day. Nevertheless, IPG is an invaluable addition to our diagnostic arsenal. It detects the very thrombi that are most likely to embolize—recent above-knee thrombi. False-negative IPG results are uncommon, whereas the frequency of false-positive tests depends on the population being studied. Any cause of venous obstruction, including tumor obstruction in the pelvic area, will result in a positive test. False-positive results also are encountered in patients with severe right ventricular failure (whose venous outflow is impeded by a high right atrial pressure), in patients on mechanical ventilation with positive end-expiratory pressure, and in patients with a low cardiac output.

In addition to its high sensitivity and specificity, IPG is noninvasive, can be done quickly at the bedside, and can be repeated frequently if needed. It has become, at our institution as at others, a centerpiece of our diagnostic and management approach [39,41]. Recent reports, however, suggest that IPG may lack sensitivity in one high-risk population, namely, those undergoing hip replacement [48], possibly because these thrombi generally arise high in the femoroiliac system and often are only partially occlusive.

The second well-validated diagnostic test was ^{125}I-fibrinogen leg scanning [52]. The agent is no longer available for clinical use owing to complexities in its production by the pharmaceutical industry. However, this test is worthy of review here because of its great contributions to our understanding of DVT and because it serves as the prototype for other agents now being developed. The success of ^{125}I-fibrinogen leg scanning depends on a fundamental characteristic of thrombi—namely, growth. If ^{125}I-fibrinogen is injected and a thrombus subsequently forms or actively grows, the thrombus incorporates fibrinogen and can be detected by counting radioactivity over the legs with an appropriately collimated, hand-held gamma-detecting probe. Extensive evaluation has clarified both the advantages and the disadvantages associated with this test [40,52,53,68]. On the positive side were its safety and simplicity. Further, it was shown that the test was highly sensitive to detecting thrombi located from the ankle to midthigh. The frequency of false-positive tests was low, and those false-positive results encountered were due to such events as hemorrhage and Baker's cysts.

Cellulitis, unless very severe, was not a source of false-positive results.

The negative features of the test included the fact that reliable diagnosis was not available until 24 hours after injection, a period required to allow development of an adequate target (thrombus)–to–background (circulating fibrinogen) ratio. Even at that time, thrombi located in midthigh or higher could not be reliably detected because of radioactivity circulating in the large pelvic blood pool. In addition, the method detected only active thrombi (i.e., those that were forming or grew after ^{125}I-fibrinogen injection). Thus, thrombi more than 5 days old rarely were detected and, if effective heparin therapy had been applied, the test was not reliable.

Although ^{125}I-fibrinogen is no longer available, its application led to significant advances in our understanding of the diagnosis, natural history, and treatment of venous thromboembolism. Furthermore, the concept of this diagnostic modality—incorporation of a radionuclide into a formed or growing thrombus—is currently being applied in a number of variations of the original test. These include the use of ^{111}In-labeled platelets (Fig. 51-6) [66,69] and radiolabeled monoclonal antibodies or Fc fragments directed against specific components of fibrin or platelet membranes [32,57,77]. The ultimate value of these tests is not yet clear.

Other methods have been studied or are under investigation. The most widely used of these has been Doppler ultrasonography [11,52,98]. This technique uses both ultrasound visualization and Doppler estimates of flow to assess the presence of venous thrombi, thus leading to use of the term *duplex* for the approach. Some have suggested that this approach can replace other tests, but problems remain in objective assessment of its role in the diagnosis of DVT. First, criteria for establishing a test as positive or negative vary from study to study and institution to institution. At present, only visualization of the femoral and popliteal veins plus demonstration of noncompressibility have been established as reliable criteria [98]. Also, technical performance of the test varies widely. An experienced operator who has validated his or her diagnoses against venography may provide accurate interpretations. However, if such validation has not occurred, the reliability of the test is uncertain. Finally, like IPG, duplex scanning is insensitive to the detection of calf thrombi. As these issues are clarified, the true value of this technique will be defined.

Another modality that had achieved wide pop-

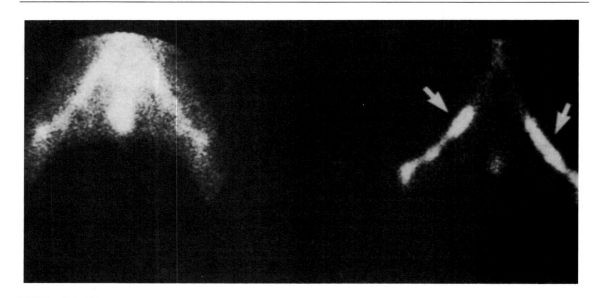

Fig. 51-6. Animal (dog) study in which bilateral femoral vein thrombi were induced, and homologous platelets labeled with indium 111 were injected after thrombus formation. At left, gamma-camera image 30 minutes after injection. At right, image 3 hours later demonstrates extensive thrombi bilaterally (*arrows*).

ularity, but failed ultimately to be validated, was radiovenography, in which a radionuclide—usually ^{99m}Tc-labeled macroaggregated albumin (or albumin microspheres)—is injected into a pedal vein and the progress of the radionuclide through the venous system of the legs and pelvis is followed by gamma-camera imaging [29]. It had been suggested that the technique could suggest the diagnosis of DVT in two ways: (1) by disclosing obstruction or diversion of the radionuclide flow in the venous system and (2) by deposition of the radionuclide on thrombi, resulting in residual "hot spots" in the venous system. Unfortunately, radiovenography proved unreliable in both regards and has been largely abandoned.

Hence, at this time, IPG remains the most reliable noninvasive approach for detecting above-knee DVT. No available modality except contrast venography is reliable in detecting calf-limited thrombi.

Pulmonary Embolism

As is the case with DVT, the clinical diagnosis of pulmonary embolism is unreliable, and objective tests are required. The inaccuracy of clinical diagnosis derives from the fact that the symptoms and signs of embolism (e.g., tachypnea, tachycardia, chest pain, hemoptysis) are nonspecific and occur with variable frequency among patients with acute embolism [4,90]. Nevertheless, the clinical context and findings provoke the practitioner to take the next steps toward the diagnosis of embolism and are worthy of review.

Perhaps the most important consideration in stimulating a suspicion of embolism is the clinical context of the patient; that is, does the patient have any of those risk factors, described previously, that promote the embolic forerunner, DVT? Such contexts are obvious among inpatients who have suffered trauma, recently have undergone operation, or have been immobilized by medical illness. Less obviously at risk are patients recently discharged from the hospital (who probably developed DVT in-hospital, but suddenly suffer an embolic event some days later) and patients with a prior history of DVT. Less commonly, patients without obvious risk factors may develop DVT and embolism after immobility during prolonged air travel.

Almost universal as a symptom of embolism is sudden onset of dyspnea. A feeling of impending doom is often reported. Occasionally, syncope is the presenting complaint. Less frequently, because infarction is uncommon, pleuritic chest pain or hemoptysis occurs, usually some hours after the onset of dyspnea. Among patients with cardiac disease, abrupt onset of an irregular heart rhythm (most frequently atrial fibrillation) may mark the embolic episode.

The most common signs of embolism include tachypnea and tachycardia. Low-grade fever (to 101°F) may occur. Examination is otherwise not suggestive unless massive embolism has occurred, in which case cardiac examination may disclose an augmented pulmonary closure sound, a fixed splitting of S2, or a right ventricular S3. The lower extremities may reveal signs of DVT, but the absence of such signs does not rule out this associated diagnosis.

Unfortunately, none of these signs or symptoms is either sensitive or specific. Furthermore, it has been shown in several studies that among patients with DVT, asymptomatic pulmonary embolism occurs in some 40 percent [18,38,62]. Thus, all patients with venous thrombosis are automatically suspects for embolism. Whether the suspicion of embolism is initiated by context or onset of compatible signs and symptoms, the suspicion must be confirmed (or denied) by objective tests.

The spectrum of differential diagnosis is a wide one, ranging from myocardial infarction, pneumonia, pneumothorax, and left ventricular failure through neurologic disease (with a syncopal presentation) to psychiatric diagnoses (such as hyperventilation) when the patient complains of dyspnea and a feeling of impending doom. Unfortunately, standard laboratory tests are not helpful because the findings are nonspecific. For example, the hematocrit and white blood cell count are usually normal, although mild leukocytosis ($<15,000/mm^3$) may occur. The chest roentgenogram may be normal, although it often shows some reduction in lung volume and, after 24 hours, may show infiltrates due to congestive atelectasis (see Fig. 51-3) or, rarely, infarction with pleural effusion. Occasionally, other radiographic clues are present (Fig. 51-7). The electrocardiogram may disclose right axis deviation, an S1, Q3 pattern, and right ventricular ischemia, but most often only sinus tachycardia is present [89]. Arterial blood gas analysis often shows hypoxemia, but it may be normal. Nevertheless, these standard laboratory tests should be performed, chiefly to rule out competing diagnoses.

Having excluded competing diagnoses to the extent possible, the next procedures that should be performed are an IPG study of the legs and a perfusion lung scan. A positive IPG does not con-

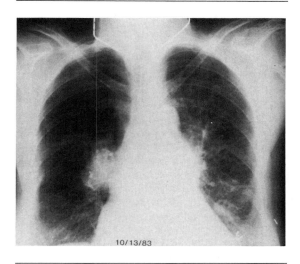

10/13/83

Fig. 51-7. Striking chest roentgenogram in patient with total embolic occlusion of the right pulmonary artery, which is large (distended by impacted embolus) and lacks visible branches. Right lung is oligemic; left lung is hyperperfused.

firm the diagnosis of embolism nor does a negative test exclude it. Nonetheless, results of this test are very useful in developing a therapeutic and, to a degree, diagnostic strategy in patients suspected of embolism. The results of the perfusion scan are invaluable. A perfusion scan should be obtained in all embolism-suspected patients regardless of concern about false-positive results.

One major reason for obtaining a perfusion ($\dot{Q}$) scan in all embolism suspects is that a negative (normal) scan rules out the diagnosis of embolism as the basis for the patient's acute cardiopulmonary symptoms. A normal scan has the same diagnostic power as a normal pulmonary angiogram in such patients [47,56,75]. This does not mean that either test rules out very small peripheral emboli, as both angiography and scanning may miss such small emboli. It *does* mean that with a negative scan and angiogram, therapy is not necessary. Thus, a normal scan is a powerful decision maker. The frequency of normal scans at a given institution will depend on the patient mix seen at the institution in terms of age and coexisting cardiopulmonary disease. At the UCSD Medical Center, approximately 40 percent of all perfusion scans in embolism suspects are normal.

If the perfusion scan is positive (i.e., shows zones of absent or reduced perfusion), a logical approach to the assessment of the abnormal perfusion scan has been devised based on information provided by clinical investigations [44,61,79]. This approach is based on three considerations: the size of the perfusion defect(s), the findings on chest roentgenography, and the results of the ventilation scan. It should be noted that we do not perform ventilation scans in all embolism suspects and that when they are performed, they are done immediately *after* the perfusion scan. Many patients do not benefit from a ventilation scan and so are saved this expense and the radiation exposure. In addition, the perfusion scan indicates the best ventilation scan view. We use ^{133}Xe gas for ventilation scans because we regard the washout phase as very useful, and this phase is not available when particulate inhalation scans are employed. There is no difficulty in interpreting ^{133}Xe ventilation scans done immediately after perfusion scans [55].

In assessing abnormal perfusion scans, we first determine where and how large are the perfusion defects. If all perfusion defects occur in areas abnormal by chest roentgenogram (infiltrates, effusions, bullae), ventilation scanning is not useful. Thus, only in patients with defects in areas normal by chest roentgenogram is ventilation scanning done. Likewise, if all defects are subsegmental (or smaller) in size, we have not found ventilation scanning useful.

After such an analytic sequence, we are left with a subgroup who have segmental or larger perfusion defects in areas normal by chest roentgenogram. In these, a ventilation scan is done. If the ventilation scan is normal, these patients are extremely likely to have an embolism (>90 percent), and we regard such a result as diagnostic (Fig. 51-8). However, if ventilation of the zones of the perfusion defects is abnormal, the study is regarded as nondiagnostic.

In summary, then, I regard only one pattern as sufficiently reliable to be characterized as diagnostic: segmental or larger defects in lung zones clear by roentgenography that are ventilated normally on ^{133}Xe study. All other scan findings are *nondiagnostic* (a term I prefer to *low probability*).

This relatively simple approach to scan interpretation appears preferable [49] to the rather complex multiple-subcategory classifications suggested by other investigators [79]. In reaching clinical decisions concerning pulmonary embolism, a diagnostic versus nondiagnostic approach to lung scan findings seems most useful. Furthermore, in those patients with nondiagnostic scans, there should be no hesitancy in proceeding to the next step: pulmonary angiography. If essential appropriate procedures are employed, a scan-guided angiography in embolic suspects is a safe procedure. First, catheter insertion should be via neck or upper-extremity veins, *not* via the femoral vein, unless an antecedent IPG or venogram is available and indicates that the femoral vein

Fig. 51-8. Anterior-view perfusion scan (*A*) in patient suspected of embolism. Chest roentgenogram showed no parenchymal abnormalities. Multiple perfusion defects are evident. In anterior view, ^{133}Xe ventilation scans were normal during washin (*B*), at equilibrium (*C*), and washout (not shown). Findings are diagnostic of pulmonary embolism at the 90 percent and greater level (see text).

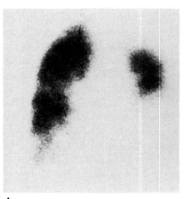
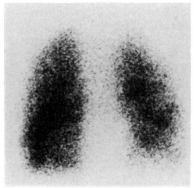
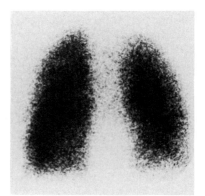

A   **B**   **C**

route is thrombus-free. Second, appropriate therapy should be maintained throughout the procedure. Specifically, if oxygen is needed to maintain an adequate PaO_2, if pressor agents are required, and if anticoagulant therapy is considered indicated, these should not be interrupted. Third, adequate hemodynamic measurements must be made as part of the procedure (right atrial, right ventricular, pulmonary arterial, and pulmonary capillary wedge pressures, and cardiac output). Fourth, if pulmonary hypertension exists, nonionic contrast media should be used. Finally, and most vital, *the objective of the angiogram should be clearly stipulated.* The usual objective is to determine whether embolism explains the patient's symptoms and scan findings. Thus, all that usually is necessary is one contrast injection of 20 to 30 ml, guided by the lung scan, into the right or left main pulmonary artery (Fig. 51-9). With appropriate positioning, such an injection should provide adequate visualization of the main, lobar, and segmental arteries. If a thrombus is visual-

Fig. 51-9. Pulmonary angiogram in embolic suspect whose scan disclosed left lower-lobe perfusion defect and slight decrease in ventilation. Single injection of contrast into left pulmonary artery disclosed large filling defect with "tracks" of contrast material around it (*arrows*). No further injections were required.

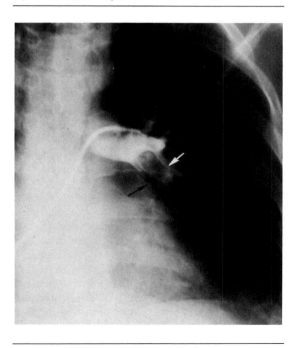

ized, the procedure has done its job and can be terminated. If such vessels have no abnormalities, it is rarely necessary to proceed to magnification or other studies because tiny defects in very distal vessels are probably irrelevant in explaining the patient's symptoms or scan findings.

After one side is injected, the films should be developed and reviewed before further catheter manipulations or contrast injections are undertaken, because often they are not required. I prefer large, cut-film studies rather than cineangiograms or digital subtraction angiograms because the latter approaches usually do not provide the clear, detailed images available with large, sequential films. Following such guidelines, the angiographic studies are usually accomplished quickly and with minimal difficulty.

Question often arises as to how long after symptom onset an angiogram can be obtained without the possibility of a false-negative result. This question really asks how rapidly an embolus can completely resolve. Absolute answers are not available, but reasonable guidelines are. The most rapid resolution ever reported was 54 hours, and this case appears exceptional [51]. In the large urokinase-streptokinase study (as well as in my own experience), residual scan defects were the rule 1 week after initiation of therapy [94]. The scan normalizes when the involved artery or arteries regain 20 percent luminal patency. At this time, the angiogram would still show an abnormality. Therefore, angiography will remain diagnostic for at least a week or more in the vast majority of patients. Nonetheless, the procedure should be performed as early as possible so that appropriate therapeutic decisions can be made promptly.

Other diagnostic procedures are currently being evaluated. For example, radiolabeled monoclonal antibodies or Fc fragments targeted against specific sites on fibrin or platelets may prove useful [32,57,77]. Chest computed tomography scans with contrast may identify emboli in the *main* pulmonary arteries, as may magnetic resonance imaging. Standard or transesophageal ultrasound examination may allow detection of main pulmonary artery emboli, especially those in the right main artery. However, the ability of any of those methods to detect emboli reliably in more distal sites remains to be established. Another promising technique for the direct visualization of emboli is the fiberoptic pulmonary angioscope, which has proved successful in visualizing acute emboli in the dog [87] and in identifying chronic thromboemboli in patients [88]. As the equipment improves, it is likely that scan-guided angioscopy will prove to be a rapid means for diagnosing acute embolism in patients or for ruling out such a diagnosis.

Management

Deep Venous Thrombosis

The management of DVT and pulmonary embolism flows logically from knowledge of the natural history of venous thromboembolism and the judicious application of diagnostic tests. As emphasized earlier, venous thromboembolism is one disease. Any patient with DVT may have, or is at risk for, pulmonary embolism; and in any patient with pulmonary embolism, DVT was, or is, likely to be present. Hence, it is my policy to perform a lung scan to rule out embolism in any patient with proved DVT and to rule out DVT in any patient with embolism. The high incidence of asymptomatic embolism in patients with DVT has been discussed previously; the same is true about the presence of asymptomatic DVT in patients with embolism.

Management of the patient with suspected DVT begins with proving the diagnosis with an objective test. My choice is to use IPG. If this is negative, above-knee thrombosis has been effectively ruled out and therapy can be safely withheld, even though thrombosis limited to the calf veins may be present [37,43]. In other centers, in which duplex evaluation of the above-knee veins has been validated and performed with close physician supervision, the same approach may be followed. However, since 15 to 20 percent of initially calf-limited thrombi may extend into the popliteal vein and higher, these noninvasive tests should be repeated every other day for 10 to 14 days if a no-treatment policy is adopted. If such follow-up is not feasible, then either the DVT suspect should be treated or a contrast venogram should be performed.

Any patient with a positive IPG or duplex scan, either initially or during the follow-up period, is admitted and treated. In such patients, a perfusion lung scan also is obtained as a baseline and to detect asymptomatic emboli. The treatment regimen in most patients consists of heparin administration as a 5000-unit bolus, followed by a continuous intravenous infusion of approximately 1000 units/hour. There is no convincing evidence that administration of heparin by either intermittent intravenous bolus (e.g., 5000 units every 4 hours) or subcutaneously (e.g., 10,000

units every 8 hours or 15,000 units every 12 hours) is any less effective or any more hazardous. Indeed, studies indicating equal efficacy and safety for each of these regimens are available [5,27,72]. Most authorities, however, favor continuous intravenous administration [3,46,82].

Uncertainty surrounds the most appropriate means for monitoring heparin dosing or, indeed, whether monitoring of coagulation tests is even necessary. Hemorrhagic risk does not appear to relate to heparin dose but rather to the clinical status of the patient [73]. As to efficacy, animal investigations in our laboratory have indicated that constant maintenance of the activated partial thromboplastin time (APTT) at one and a half times control values does prevent deposition of fibrinogen and platelets on existing thrombi (i.e., it prevents thrombus growth) [19]. Because this is the only role of heparin, such animal data indicate that maintenance of APTT at such a level is appropriate. The consensus from human investigations endorses the same policy [35]. However, despite suggested nomograms [13], such stable maintenance of the APTT is not easy; substantial diurnal variation in the APTT occurs [16,21].

To ensure that the control value is normal and that antithrombin III deficiency is not present, I obtain a control APTT and another APTT 1 hour after the initial heparin bolus to ascertain whether the APTT at that time is substantially prolonged (i.e., >1.5 times control). Thereafter, I infuse heparin at 1000 units/hour and monitor the APTT once daily. Others recommend more frequent monitoring, with periodic adjustments of the heparin dose [42]. Perhaps the growing availability of bedside finger-stick measurement of APTT will make such monitoring more feasible. Regardless of the monitoring approach employed, it is particularly important to avoid lowering the daily dose of heparin below 1000 units/hour based on a single APTT. I would maintain a tested dose unless repeat values the same day show marked APTT prolongations (e.g., >2.5 times control).

These considerations of heparin dose and monitoring are likely to undergo substantial revision in the years ahead as low-molecular-weight heparins gain regulatory approval and are introduced into clinical use. As these heparins replace the complex mixtures that constitute standard current heparins, available data suggest major alterations in approach. First, it appears likely that the subcutaneous route of administration will become standard, perhaps with a single dose per day being given [35]. Second, it appears that no monitoring will be recommended because the APTT does not reflect the activity of these heparins, and the more sophisticated assays that may reflect the in vivo activity of these heparins will not be available in most clinical laboratories. Physicians will need to familiarize themselves with these significant differences as the new heparins become available.

After implementing the initial heparin regimen, the practitioner must decide how long anticoagulant protection should be maintained. Again, no absolute guidelines are available, although opinions abound. My own approach is to base the decision about duration on three factors: (1) the presence of continuing clinical risk factors, (2) the results of sequential IPG studies, and (3) the findings on perfusion lung scan. If there are no persistent clinical risk factors, the IPG becomes negative, and the lung scan shows no defects, the minimum duration of anticoagulant protection should be 7 to 10 days, a period that allows for adequate resolution of the venous thrombi.

However, few patients will meet these three criteria for early cessation. Therefore, the majority of patients merit long-term protection. Such protection should be maintained until all three criteria for cessation are met. With respect to the IPG, it has been shown that 65 percent of patients with an abnormal IPG test revert to normal at 3 months and 90 percent at 12 months.

The decision about long-term protection should be made as early as possible so that prolonged hospitalization is avoided. Several strategies are available to accomplish this. They relate to the choice of agent for long-term prophylaxis: heparin or warfarin sodium (Coumadin) [42]. If Coumadin is to be used, it can be initiated early in the patient's course (e.g., day 2 or 3 of heparin therapy). However, it is important to recognize that initiation of Coumadin does not protect the patient. The prothrombin time must be in the therapeutic range (1.3 to 1.8 times control) for at least 3 days before protection is achieved [97]. Heparin should therefore be continued until that goal is achieved. The IPG can be repeated prior to contemplated discharge of the patient and, if it is negative, risk factors are absent, and the lung scan normal, the Coumadin can be discontinued.

Alternatively, subcutaneous heparin in a dose of 7500 to 10,000 units subcutaneously every 12 hours can be chosen for long-term protection. The patient (or significant others) can be taught the procedure, and the transition from continuous intravenous to subcutaneous heparin can be made smoothly. A third alternative also exists; discharge on subcutaneous heparin and implementation of Coumadin therapy as an outpatient.

As to other aspects of acute management, I allow patients bathroom (or bedside commode) privileges very early; struggling with a bedpan is a greater risk. I also encourage them to ambulate as soon as pain has abated.

Pulmonary Embolism

The management of pulmonary embolism is, in most regards, identical to that of acute above-knee DVT. Indeed, the impedance test is, in my view, as much a key to long-term decisions as are the lung scan and angiographic results. The differences in management are as follows.

Data indicate that, in animals, a large dose of heparin is needed to prevent further platelet aggregation and release of potential vasoconstrictive agents [91]. Therefore, I use a larger initial heparin dose (15,000 to 20,000 units). Beyond this first dose, I follow the same regimens as described for DVT. The same bases for deciding about long-term therapy also are invoked. As noted previously, a predischarge lung scan is valuable. In my view, the persistence of one or more segmental or larger defects warrants continued anticoagulant therapy, as anticoagulation may prevent in situ thrombus extension. With stability of the lung scan for 6 months, a normal IPG, and no clinical risk factors, therapy may be discontinued.

In the acute phase of embolism, normal supportive measures are provided to the patient. These include oxygen, if hypoxemia is present, and the use of pressor agents if required. Isoproterenol is often a particularly useful agent in this context because it may induce pulmonary vasodilatation and may increase cardiac output [59,86]. However, selection of vasoactive agents is guided by the specific hemodynamic measurements obtained.

The regimen described is successful in managing the great majority of patients with acute pulmonary embolism. However, there are patient subgroups in whom special management approaches are warranted. One such subgroup consists of those patients in whom embolism is of such magnitude as to induce cardiopulmonary compromise (i.e., marked hypoxemia or right ventricular failure resulting in persistent systemic hypotension). In such patients, I require both angiography (for diagnostic confirmation) and hemodynamic assessment (pulmonary arterial pressure, wedge pressure, and cardiac output). There are then three options that can be exercised: (1) inferior venacaval (IVC) protection to prevent recurrence, (2) surgical embolectomy, and (3) thrombolytic therapy.

If DVT is present (i.e., the embolic source is the leg veins), I prefer IVC protection. The rationale behind this choice is twofold: (1) Death due to embolism rarely occurs unless there is embolic recurrence, even in the compromised patient and (2) in such patients, caval protection is associated with less risk of morbidity and mortality than the other alternatives. My choice of IVC protection is insertion of a Greenfield filter [30,54]. The device can be placed via the femoroiliac route (if venography demonstrates no thrombi in the insertion pathway) or via a neck vein. Migration of the filter is rare. Perhaps most important is the excellent long-term patency rate demonstrated for this device; in our experience, approximately 95 percent remain patent during more than 5 years of follow-up. Other devices are available and may have advantages (e.g., smaller size at insertion, ability to filter cavae of large diameter), but data regarding the long-term patency rates of these devices are limited. We no longer use caval interruptive procedures that require surgery (e.g., clips, fenestration procedures, ligation).

There is, of course, a group of patients—those in whom anticoagulant treatment is contraindicated due to hemorrhagic risk—in whom IVC protection is indicated as primary therapy. In such patients, caval protection to prevent embolic recurrence is the only alternative.

Acute surgical embolectomy is an attractive option in theory. Unfortunately, it is a major undertaking in already compromised patients and has consistently been associated with a 50 percent mortality [12], which is a higher mortality than that associated with anticoagulant therapy alone. Embolectomy must be combined with caval protection if the patient has DVT; otherwise the patient is not protected against recurrence in the postoperative period.

Role of Thrombolytic Agents

The proper role of thrombolytic agents in the treatment of venous thromboembolism remains unsettled. With respect to the treatment of DVT, the use of the three thrombolytic agents available—streptokinase, urokinase, and tissue plasminogen activator—like anticoagulant therapy, need be considered only in patients with thrombosis of the popliteal and higher veins. Throm-

bolytic agents have conceptual appeal because their use promises rapid restoration of luminal patency (and valvular rescue), whereas heparin alone simply halts further thrombosis. However, practical realization of this conceptual promise has not occurred for several reasons. First, the major objectives of DVT therapy are to alleviate patient symptoms, limit the likelihood of acute embolism (if it has not already occurred), reduce the frequency of subsequent recurrences of venous thrombosis (and embolism), and reduce the frequency of long-term postphlebitic symptoms. Given these goals, the outcomes of patients treated with anticoagulants have been satisfactory. In contrast, available reports have not, in my view, demonstrated that thrombolytic therapy has significantly improved these short- or long-term results [28,92]. Furthermore, thrombolytic therapy does not *replace* heparin or Coumadin therapy. Indeed, it is essential that thrombolysis be followed by anticoagulant therapy to prevent rethrombosis. Also, many patients with DVT (often a postoperative problem) have contraindications to the use of thrombolytic agents. Finally, even in the absence of contraindications, hemorrhagic risk exists.

Given these considerations, my current opinion is to limit the use of thrombolytic therapy to that group of patients with DVT of iliofemoral origin. The long-term outlook for such patients is poor with heparin therapy, with many exhibiting marked postphlebitic problems [76]. It should be noted that even in this group, there are no data indicating that thrombolytic agents improve outcome. Nonetheless, I believe that the poor results with heparin alone justify the use of thrombolytic drugs, providing there are no major contraindications to their use.

In embolism, essentially the same considerations have prompted me to use thrombolytic agents only rarely. In most patients, the emboli resolve nicely under heparin therapy (see Fig. 51-4). Despite large-scale studies, there are no data which document that thrombolytic therapy alters short- or long-term morbidity or mortality [15,93–95]. Therefore, I reserve the use of thrombolytic agents for patients with marked hemodynamic compromise in whom hypotension persists for an hour or more despite heparin and good supportive therapy. Although in most such patients heparin, support, and caval protection are my first choices, a trial of thrombolytic therapy is justified [15] because the mortality in this small subgroup of patients with persistent hypotension is 30 to 35 percent. No data are yet available, however, which demonstrate that such therapy improves these figures. It should be noted that thrombolytic agents do enhance, at 24 to 48 hours, the extent of embolus resolution. Nonetheless, until it is demonstrated that such enhancement translates into reduced short-term or long-term morbidity or mortality, such observations cannot be used to support more widespread application of thrombolytic agents. Patient outcome, not enhanced early embolus resolution, is the only rational basis for application of thrombolytic or other therapies.

Prophylaxis

Although the treatment of venous thromboembolism excites substantial interest and controversy, it has been abundantly clear for some years that improvements in therapy will have little impact on the morbidity and mortality of this disorder [1]. Many episodes of DVT escape clinical detection and, therefore, laboratory confirmation and therapy. Further, most deaths due to pulmonary embolism occur unexpectedly and so suddenly (within hours) that neither diagnosis nor therapy can be established [65].

Consequently, the only effective means for reducing the frequency of DVT and its major complication, pulmonary embolism, is by establishing prophylactic regimens for DVT. To achieve prophylaxis, two elements are needed: (1) a reliable means for identifying patients at risk for DVT and (2) adequate prophylactic treatment. Both these requirements have been well met in recent years. Therefore, prophylaxis should be widely used.

Clinically determined risk factors, discussed previously, identify those patients most likely to develop DVT (e.g., patients with pelvic or lower-extremity injury or surgery, patients undergoing major surgery, patients facing prolonged immobility). Examination of trials of prophylactic regimens has provided useful insights into the proper selection of regimens [58,80]. Aspirin and other antiplatelet agents (e.g., sulfinpyrazone) have not been shown to be effective prophylactic agents in DVT and should not be recommended for this purpose. Low-molecular-weight dextran has a variable record as a prophylactic agent. It probably is effective but is not widely used due to potential toxicity (fluid overload, allergic reactions) and patient inconvenience (repetitive intravenous infusions are necessary), as well as uncertainty as to efficacy compared to other alternatives.

Prothrombinopenic drugs (e.g., Coumadin) ac-

tually have the longest history of efficacy as well as a highly acceptable safety record, even among patients with trauma and burns. Despite such documentation, substantial resistance to its prophylactic use remains. Coumadin is a viable alternative nonetheless, in patients at risk [36]. Its use is slowly gaining acceptance, particularly in patients undergoing orthopedic surgery in whom low-dose regimens have proved effective and safe [23].

So-called low-dose heparin also has been established as an effective and safe modality for prophylaxis in most patient groups at high risk for DVT. The standard regimens are 5000 units given subcutaneously every 8 or 12 hours. These regimens have been shown to be effective in prophylaxis in many high-risk patient groups [8] but not as effective in patients with hip replacement or prostatic surgery [10].

Most recently, devices that provide intermittent lower-extremity compression have been added to the prophylactic armamentarium (Fig. 51-10). All such devices provide intermittent compression by a simple pump delivered to an inflatable cuff [9,34,81]. The cuffs vary in design, some compressing calf only, some calf and thigh, and some providing a sequence of calf-thigh compression. All seem of equal efficacy, so that cost, reliability, availability, and patient acceptance are the major selection criteria. These devices are a major advance because they can be applied to patients in whom anticoagulant prophylaxis is contraindicated (e.g., neurosurgical patients) or in whom, for a variety of reasons, the physicians involved

Fig. 51-10. One of several types of systems that provide periodic mechanical compression of the lower extremities.

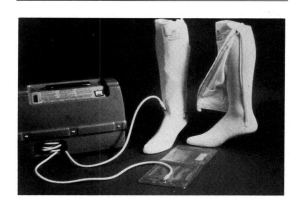

do not wish to apply anticoagulant prophylaxis. The antistasis and, therefore, antithrombotic effect of these devices is substantially different from the marginal value of elastic stockings. Only stockings designed to apply a reliable calf-to-thigh pressure gradient appear to be of value [50], and these may be difficult to obtain and fit.

Although none of the three major prophylactic options is perfect, clearly there is no longer any medical reason that each patient at risk is not provided at least one preventive option. Furthermore, as risk escalates, the prophylactic regimen can be increased. In the lowest-risk population (e.g., postpartum), mechanical compression can be applied, whereas in high-risk patients (e.g., hip replacement), such devices plus Coumadin or heparin would appear warranted.

The key to effective prophylaxis is physician and institutional attention to its need and delivery. At the UCSD Medical Center, hospital policy mandates consideration of prophylaxis, and a service has been established to implement this policy. Such efforts are not only medically sound but also cost-effective.

Chronic Thrombotic Obstruction of Major Pulmonary Arteries

As already noted, most patients in whom pulmonary embolism is diagnosed and treated demonstrate excellent resolution of their emboli. Chronic pulmonary hypertension in particular is a rare postembolic event [78]. However, in recent years it has become apparent that there is a small group of patients in whom emboli fail to resolve and who present, months to years after their acute event, with pulmonary hypertension due to chronic organized thrombi in the major (main, lobar, segmental) pulmonary arteries [64]. Increased attention has been directed toward this entity because of the demonstration that it is remediable by surgical thromboendarterectomy. As is often the case, the availability of such treatment has led to sharply increased recognition. More than 500 patients with this condition now have been recognized in the United States. Our own estimates of its frequency suggest that in 0.1 percent of patients major emboli fail to resolve adequately, giving a rate for this condition in the United States of approximately 450 patients per year.

It is now clear that, in the majority of these patients, the initial episode of pulmonary embolism was either undiagnosed or misdiagnosed. As these patients progress in symptoms, alternative diagnoses have been assigned for periods of months to years. Such diagnoses have included myocardial infarction, pneumonia, asthma (particularly exercise-induced asthma), interstitial fibrosis, and psychogenic hyperventilation.

The dominant symptoms suggesting the diagnosis are nonspecific: dyspnea on exertion and easy fatigue. Effort syncope or near-syncope, anginal pain (due to right ventricular ischemia) and, ultimately, evidence of right ventricular failure (hepatomegaly, ascites, edema) may develop. Chest roentgenography, electrocardiography, and spirometric studies often are normal, but they may provide some clues to the diagnosis. For example, the chest roentgenogram may disclose asymmetry in pulmonary arterial size and blood flow distribution; the electrocardiogram may reveal right axis deviation; and spirometry, by being normal, may suggest an alternative (vascular) basis for the patient's dyspnea. Arterial blood gases commonly disclose hypoxemia at rest or during exercise, with normocapnia or hypocapnia.

The test that most commonly suggests the diagnosis is the perfusion lung scan, which uniformly discloses segmental or larger bilateral perfusion defects that, on ventilation scan, are normally ventilated [22]. Such a pattern also may be seen in fibrosing mediastinitis, pulmonary artery agenesis, or coarctation, as well as with arterial obstruction due to tumor. Nonetheless, this pattern should lead to right heart catheterization and pulmonary angiography. Catheterization is required to confirm the presence (and severity) of pulmonary hypertension and to rule out competing diagnoses. Angiography also is needed to rule out other lesions and to define the location of chronic thrombi.

The angiogram often is definitive. However, unlike the situation in acute embolism, the angiogram in chronic thrombotic obstruction may be difficult to interpret (Figs. 51-11, 51-12). Such difficulties relate to the odd patterns of partial resolution and recanalization that occur. Therefore, in some patients, direct visualization of the pulmonary arterial system through a balloon-tipped fiberoptic angioscope may be very helpful (Fig. 51-13) [88].

In patients in whom the diagnosis is confirmed and no contraindication to surgical intervention exists, pulmonary thromboendarterectomy should be considered. This open heart procedure is a true thromboendarterectomy, not an embolectomy (Fig. 51-14). It is a difficult, complex pro-

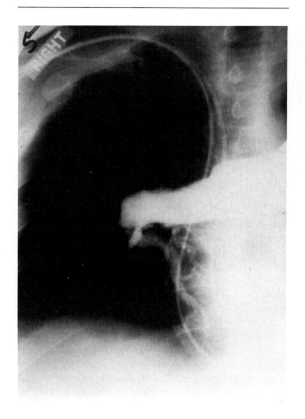

Fig. 51-11. Pulmonary angiogram (right lung) in a patient with severe chronic thromboembolic pulmonary hypertension. Proximal "bump" is obstructed in right upper-lobe branch. Ragged appearance of right pulmonary artery is due to chronic thrombus.

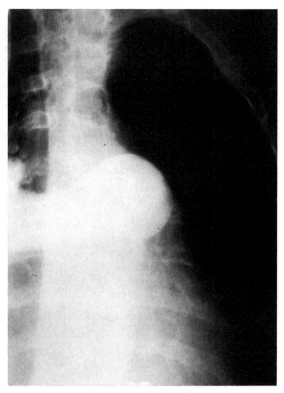

Fig. 51-12. Smooth termination of left pulmonary artery, which mimics agenesis. Chronic thrombus obstructing this artery was removed.

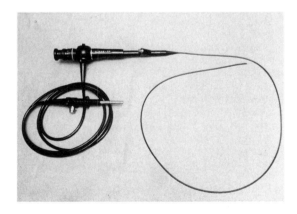

Fig. 51-13. Fiberoptic angioscope (120-cm device) inserted transvenously. Balloon on distal tip is inflated to allow visualization of pulmonary artery walls.

cedure that, for optimal outcome, should be carried out only by those experienced with it. When properly performed, the short- and long-term outcomes are rewarding, even among patients with prolonged right ventricular failure.

Unfortunately, the frequency of this entity is not likely to decline in the near future, because in most of these patients acute embolism has not been diagnosed, and therefore the patients have not been appropriately treated. It is hoped that further investigations of these patients will provide insight into the issue of why their emboli fail to resolve.

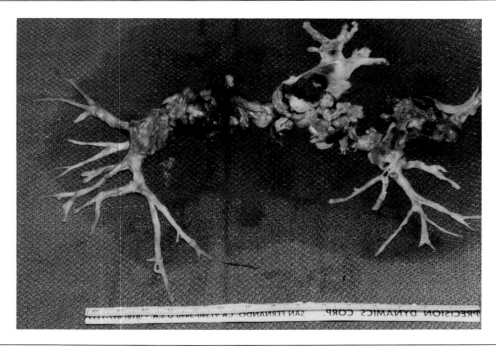

Fig. 51-14. Organized thrombotic material removed from a patient with chronic major vessel thromboembolic pulmonary hypertension. Virtually the entire pulmonary arterial system was obstructed. (Scale below is 15 cm.)

References

1. Alpert JS, et al. Mortality in patients treated for pulmonary embolism. *JAMA* 236:1477, 1976.
2. Anderson FA Jr, et al. A population-based perspective of the hospital incidence and case fatality rates of deep vein thrombosis and pulmonary embolism. The Worcester DVT Study. *Arch Intern Med* 151:933, 1991.
3. Basu D, et al. A prospective study of the value of monitoring heparin treatment with the activated partial thromboplastin time. *N Engl J Med* 287:324, 1972.
4. Bell WR, Simon TL, DeMets DL. The clinical features of submassive and massive pulmonary emboli. *Am J Med* 62:355, 1977.
5. Bentley PG, et al. An objective study of alternative methods of heparin administration. *Thromb Res* 18:177, 1980.
6. Buller HR, et al. Deep vein thrombosis: New non-invasive diagnostic tests. *Thromb Haemost* 66:133, 1991.
7. Channick RN, et al. Central pulmonary vascular obstruction does not lead to hypoxemia in canine acute pulmonary embolism. *Am Rev Respir Dis* 141:A740, 1990.
8. Clark-Pearson DL, et al. Venous thromboembolism prophylaxis in gynecologic oncology: A prospective, controlled trial of low-dose heparin. *Am J Obstet Gynecol* 145:606, 1983.
9. Coe NP, et al. Prevention of deep venous thrombosis in urologic patients: A controlled, randomized trial of low-dose heparin and external pneumatic compression boots. *Surgery* 83:230, 1978.
10. Collins R, et al. Reduction of fatal embolism and venous thrombosis by perioperative administration of subcutaneous heparin: Overview of results of randomized trials in general, orthopedic and urologic surgery. *N Engl J Med* 318:1162, 1988.
11. Cronan JJ, et al. Deep venous thrombosis: US assessment using vein compression. *Radiology* 162:191, 1987.
12. Cross FS, Mowlem A. A survey of current status of pulmonary embolectomy for massive pulmonary embolism. *Circulation* 35(Suppl 1):86, 1967.
13. Cruickshank MK, et al. A standard heparin nomogram for the management of heparin therapy. *Arch Intern Med* 151:333, 1991.
14. Dalen JE, et al. Pulmonary angiography in acute pulmonary embolism: Indications, techniques and results in 367 patients. *Am Heart J* 81:175, 1971.

15. Dalen JE. Controversy: The case against fibrinolytic therapy. *J Cardiovasc Med* 5:799, 1980.
16. Decousus HA, et al. Circadian changes in anticoagulant effect of heparin infused at a constant rate. *Br Med J* 290:341, 1985.
17. Dexter L, Smith GT. Quantitative studies of pulmonary embolism. *Am J Med Sci* 247:644, 1964.
18. Dorfman GS, et al. Occult pulmonary embolism: A common occurrence in deep venous thrombosis. *Am J Radiol* 148:263, 1987.
19. Fedullo PF, et al. Indium-111-labeled platelet: Effect of heparin on uptake by venous thrombi and relationship to the activated partial thromboplastin time. *Circulation* 66:632, 1982.
20. Finley TH, et al. Changes in mechanical properties, appearance and surface activity of extracts of one lung following occlusion of its pulmonary artery in the dog. *Physiologist* 3:56, 1960.
21. Fishmann AJ, Moser KM, Fedullo PF. Sequential hourly activated partial thromboplastin time monitoring during heparin therapy in venous thromboembolism. *Chest* 84:329, 1983.
22. Fishmann AJ, Moser KM, Fedullo PF. Perfusion lung scans vs. pulmonary angiography in evaluation of suspected primary pulmonary hypertension. *Chest* 84:679, 1983.
23. Francis CW, et al. Two-step warfarin therapy. *JAMA* 249:374, 1983.
24. Frantantoni J, Wessler S. *Risk Factors and the Epidemiology of Venous Thromboembolism* (NIH publication no. 76-866). Washington, DC: US Government Printing Office, 1976, Pp 18–27.
25. Freiman DG, Suyemoto J, Wessler S. Frequency of pulmonary thromboembolism in man. *N Engl J Med* 272:1278, 1965.
26. Gillum RF. Pulmonary embolism in the United States. *Am Heart J* 114:1262, 1987.
27. Glazier RL, Crowell EB. Randomized prospective trial of continuous versus intermittent heparin therapy. *JAMA* 236:1365, 1976.
28. Goldhaber SZ, et al. Pooled analysis of randomized trials of streptokinase and heparin in phlebographically documented deep venous thrombosis. *Am J Med* 76:393, 1984.
29. Gomez A, Webber MM, Buffkin D. Contrast venography vs. radionuclide venography: A study of discrepancies of their possible significance. *Radiology* 142:719, 1982.
30. Greenfield LJ, et al. Greenfield vena cava filter experience: Late results in 150 patients. *Arch Surg* 116:1451, 1981.
31. Gurewich V, Cohen JL, Thomas DP. Humoral factors in massive pulmonary embolism. *Am Heart J* 76:784, 1968.
32. Hashimoto Y, et al. Fragment of an anti-human fibrin monoclonal antibody in a rabbit model. *Radiology* 171:223, 1989.
33. Havig O. Deep venous thrombosis and pulmonary embolism. *Acta Chir Scand* 478:1, 1978.
34. Hirsh J. Choosing the best of old and new ways

to prevent venous thrombosis. *J Cardiovasc Med* 6:691, 1981.
35. Hirsh J. Heparin. *N Engl J Med* 324:156, 1991.
36. Hirsh J. Oral anticoagulant drugs. *N Engl J Med* 324:1865, 1991.
37. Huisman MV, et al. Serial impedance plethysmography for suspected deep venous thrombosis in outpatients. *N Engl J Med* 314:823, 1986.
38. Huisman AV, et al. Unexpected high prevalence of silent pulmonary embolism in patients with deep venous thrombosis. *Chest* 95:498, 1989.
39. Hull RD, et al. Impedance plethysmography using the cuff technic in the diagnosis of venous thrombosis. *Circulation* 53:696, 1976.
40. Hull RD, et al. The combined use of leg scanning and impedance plethysmography in suspected venous thrombosis: An alternative to venography. *N Engl J Med* 296:1497, 1977.
41. Hull RD, et al. Impedance plethysmography: The relationship between venous filling and sensitivity and specificity for proximal vein thrombosis. *Circulation* 58:898, 1978.
42. Hull RD, et al. Adjusted subcutaneous heparin versus warfarin sodium in the long-term treatment of venous thrombosis. *N Engl J Med* 306:189, 1982.
43. Hull RD, et al. The diagnosis of acute, recurrent deep vein thrombosis: A diagnostic challenge. *Circulation* 67:901, 1983.
44. Hull RD, et al. Pulmonary angiography, ventilation lung scanning and venography for clinically suspected pulmonary embolism with abnormal perfusion lung scan. *Ann Intern Med* 98:891, 1983.
45. Hull RD, et al. Diagnostic efficacy of impedance plethysmography for clinically suspected deep-vein thrombosis: A randomized trial. *Ann Intern Med* 102:21, 1985.
46. Hull RD, et al. Continuous intravenous heparin compared with intermittent subcutaneous heparin in the initial treatment of proximal vein thrombosis. *N Engl J Med* 315:1109, 1986.
47. Hull RD, et al. Clinical validity of a normal perfusion lung scan in patients with suspected pulmonary embolism. *Chest* 97:23, 1990.
48. Hull RD, et al. Effectiveness of intermittent pneumatic leg compression for preventing deep vein thrombosis after total hip replacement. *JAMA* 263:2313, 1990.
49. Hull RD, Raskob GE. Low-probability lung scan findings: A need for change. *Ann Intern Med* 114:142, 1991.
50. Ishak MA, Morley KD. Deep venous thrombosis after total hip arthroplasty: A prospective controlled study to determine the prophylactic effect of graded pressure stockings. *Br J Surg* 68:429, 1981.
51. James WS, Moser KM. Rapid resolution of a pulmonary embolus in man. *West J Med* 129:60, 1978.

52. Kakkar VV. The diagnosis of deep vein thrombosis using the ^{125}I-fibrinogen test. *Arch Surg* 104:152, 1972.

53. Kakkar VV. International multicentre trial: Prevention of fatal postoperative embolism by low doses of heparin. *Lancet* 2:145, 1975.

54. Kanter B, Moser KM. The Greenfield vena caval filter. *Chest* 93:170, 1988.

55. Kipper MS, Alazraki N. The feasibility of performing ^{133}Xe ventilation imaging following the perfusion study. *Radiology* 82:411, 1982.

56. Kipper MS, et al. Long-term follow-up of patients with suspected pulmonary embolism and a normal lung scan. *Chest* 82:411, 1982.

57. Kudryk B, et al. Specificity of a monoclonal antibody for the NH-2-terminal region of fibrin. *Mol Immunol* 21:89, 1984.

58. Levy SE, Simmons IH. Mechanism of arterial hypoxemia following pulmonary thromboembolism in dogs. *Circ Res* 42:92, 1978.

59. McDonald IG, et al. Isoproterenol in massive pulmonary embolism: Hemodynamic and clinical effects. *Med J Aust* 2:201, 1968.

60. McIntyre KM, Sasahara AA. The hemodynamic response to pulmonary embolism in patients without prior cardiopulmonary disease. *Am J Cardiol* 28:288, 1971.

61. Mercandetti AJ, Kipper MS, Moser KM. Influence of perfusion and ventilation scans on therapeutic decision making and outcome in cases of possible embolism. *West J Med* 142:208, 1985.

62. Monreal H, et al. Asymptomatic pulmonary embolism in patients with deep vein thrombosis. *J Cardiovasc Surg* 30:104, 1989.

63. Monreal M, et al. Upper-extremity deep venous thrombosis and pulmonary embolism. *Chest* 99:280, 1991.

64. Moser KM, Auger WR, Fedullo PF. Chronic major-vessel thromboembolic pulmonary hypertension. *Circulation* 81:1735, 1990.

65. Moser KM. Pulmonary embolism: Where the problem is not. *JAMA* 236:1500, 1976.

66. Moser KM. Indium-111 Platelets in Thromboembolism: Can Labeled Platelets Be Used to Evaluate Antithrombotic Therapy? In ML Thaker (Ed), *Radiolabeled Cellular Blood Elements*. New York: Plenum, 1985, Pp 155–176.

67. Moser KM. Venous thromboembolism. State of the art. *Am Rev Respir Dis* 141:235, 1990.

68. Moser KM, Brach BB, Dolan GT. Clinically suspected deep venous thrombosis of the lower extremities. *JAMA* 237:2195, 1971.

69. Moser KM, et al. Study of factors that may condition scintigraphic detection of venous thrombi and pulmonary emboli with In-111-platelets. *J Nucl Med* 21:1051, 1980.

70. Moser KM, Fedullo PF. Venous thromboembolism: Three simple decisions. *Chest* 83:117, 1983.

71. Moser KM, LeMoine JR. Is embolic risk conditioned by location of deep venous thrombosis? *Ann Intern Med* 94:439, 1981.

72. Nelson JE, Bynum LJ, Parkey RW. Heparin therapy in venous thromboembolism. *Am J Med* 70:808, 1981.

73. Nelson PH, et al. Risk of complications during intravenous heparin therapy. *West J Med* 136:189, 1982.

74. Nicolaides AN, Field ES, Kakkar VV. Prostatectomy and deep vein thrombosis. *Br J Surg* 50:487, 1972.

75. Novelline RA, et al. The clinical course of patients with suspected embolism and a negative pulmonary angiogram. *Radiology* 126:561, 1978.

76. O'Donnell TE, et al. The socioeconomic effects of an iliofemoral thrombosis. *J Surg Res* 22:481, 1977.

77. Oster SN, et al. Thrombus radioimmunoscintigraphy: An approach using monoclonal antiplatelet antibody. *Proc Natl Acad Sci* 82:3465, 1985.

78. Paraskos JA, Adelstein SL. Late prognosis of acute pulmonary embolism. *N Engl J Med* 289:55, 1973.

79. The PIOPED Investigators. Value of the ventilation/perfusion scan in acute pulmonary embolism. Results of the prospective investigation of pulmonary embolism diagnosis (PIOPED). *JAMA* 263:2753, 1990.

80. Prevention of venous thrombosis and pulmonary embolism. NIH Consensus Development. *JAMA* 256:744, 1986.

81. Roberts VC, Colton LT. Failure of low-dose heparin to improve efficacy of perioperative intermittent calf compression in preventing postoperative deep vein thrombosis. *Br Med J* 3:458, 1975.

82. Salzman EW, et al. Management of heparin therapy: Controlled prospective trial. *N Engl J Med* 292:1046, 1975.

83. Severinghaus JW, et al. Unilateral hypoventilation produced by occlusion of one pulmonary artery. *J Appl Physiol* 16:53, 1961.

84. Sevitt S. The structure and growth of valve pocket thrombi in femoral veins. *J Clin Pathol* 27:517, 1974.

85. Sevitt S, Gallagher NG. Venous thrombosis and pulmonary embolism: A clinical pathologic study in injured and burned patients. *Br J Surg* 48:475, 1961.

86. Shepard JW, et al. Effects of isoproterenol on distribution of perfusion in embolized dog lungs. *Mich Med* 20:950, 1979.

87. Shure D, et al. Identification of pulmonary emboli in the dog: Comparison of angioscopy and perfusion scanning. *Circulation* 64:618, 1981.

88. Shure D, Gregoratos G, Moser KM. Fiberoptic angioscopy: Role in the diagnosis of chronic pulmonary arterial obstruction. *Ann Intern Med* 103:844, 1985.

89. Stein PD, et al. The electrocardiogram in acute pulmonary embolism. *Prog Cardiovasc Dis* 17:247, 1975.

90. Stein PD, Willis PW III, DeMets DL. History and physical examination in acute pulmonary embolism without preexisting cardiac or pulmonary disease. *Am J Cardiol* 47:218, 1981.

91. Thomas DP, Gurewich J, Ashford TP. Platelet adherence to thromboemboli in relation to the pathogenesis and treatment of pulmonary embolism. *N Engl J Med* 274:953, 1966.

92. Tsapogas MJ, Peabody RA, Wu KT. Controlled study of thrombolytic therapy in deep venous thrombosis. *Surgery* 74:973, 1973.

93. Urokinase Pulmonary Embolism Trial. Phase 1 results. *JAMA* 214:2163, 1970.

94. Urokinase-Streptokinase Embolism Trial. Phase 2 results. *JAMA* 229:1606, 1974.

95. Verstrate M, Miller GAH, Bounnameaux H. Recombinant tissue-type plasminogen activator in the treatment of acute massive embolism. *Circulation* 77:353, 1988.

96. Warlow C, et al. A double-blind trial of low doses of subcutaneous heparin in the prevention of deep venous thrombosis after myocardial infarction. *Lancet* 2:934, 1973.

97. Wessler S, Ballon JD, Katz JH. Studies in intravascular coagulation: V. A distinction between the anticoagulant and antithrombotic effects of dicumarol. *N Engl J Med* 256:1223, 1957.

98. White RH, et al. Diagnosis of deep-vein thrombosis using duplex ultrasound. *Ann Intern Med* 111:297, 1989.

99. Widdicombe JG. Reflex Mechanisms in Pulmonary Thromboembolism. In KM Moser, M Stein (Eds), *Pulmonary Thromboembolism*. Chicago: Year Book, 1973.

52

Pulmonary Heart Disease

Marissa Llanera   Harly E. Greenberg
Steven M. Scharf

The right ventricle (RV) develops embryologically from two separate components of the primitive cardiac tube. The bulbus cordis is incorporated into the conus (outflow tract), and the sinus venosus is incorporated into the sinus (inflow) portion of the RV [45]. Analysis of the functional characteristics of RV contraction reveals that RV systole occurs by sequential contraction, beginning at the inflow tract and extending into the outflow tract [2,70]. That these two regions of the ventricle retain their separate nature is illustrated by the fact that under sympathoadrenal stimulation, a pressure gradient can develop within the ventricular cavity [63]. Thus RV contraction can be thought of as peristaltic in nature. The RV is therefore ideally suited to be a low-pressure, high-volume pump.

Dysfunction of the left ventricle (LV) has been clearly recognized as a threat to life. Normally, the RV appears to play little role in regulating blood flow. For example, the entire RV free wall may be ablated or removed with little change in cardiac output at rest, suggesting that the RV functions as a passive conduit. However, when pulmonary arterial pressures are increased or cardiac output demand is elevated, the RV is necessary for maintaining normal homeostasis. Dysfunction of the RV in clinical circumstances such as sepsis, adult respiratory distress syndrome, increased lung volume, RV infarction, or even exercise can severely disturb cardiac output homeostasis. Thus, under many clinical circumstances, RV malfunction can be life-threatening, and overt RV failure can lead to circulatory collapse.

In this chapter, we describe the characteristics of normal RV function, the etiologies of RV disease caused by increased pulmonary vascular resistance (pulmonary heart disease or cor pulmonale), diagnosis, and therapeutic options under differing circumstances. Because of controversial findings in some areas, we have chosen to present some representative individual studies pertinent to certain topics. We could not hope to review in detail all the excellent work in this field and have chosen some particular studies for their representational qualities. For a more detailed review, the reader is referred to the references cited throughout the chapter.

Normal RV

Because the normal RV is crescent-shaped, accurate determination of RV volume from the limited number of dimensions that can be assessed using imaging techniques is more difficult than corresponding measurements made from the LV. The difficulty is further compounded during RV dilation when the configuration becomes more ellipsoidal. Therefore, RV volume measurements are not easily obtained. The interaction between RV and low pulmonary vascular impedance results in RV and pulmonary arterial pressures of less than one-fourth of the corresponding LV pressures. Thus the work capacity of the RV is considerably smaller than that of the LV. Similarly, the ability of the RV to maintain stroke volume in the face of increased afterload is less than that of the LV for the same increase in systolic pressure (Fig. 52-1). Data such as those shown in Figure 52-1 [54] are often said to demonstrate that the RV is a volume pump, whereas the LV is a pressure pump. However, the principles of determination of ventricular function are the same for the two ventricles [52]. This can be illustrated, using the data shown in Figure 52-1, by plotting on the abscissa not absolute pressures but rather pressure expressed as a percent of baseline (normalized); the lines expressing de-

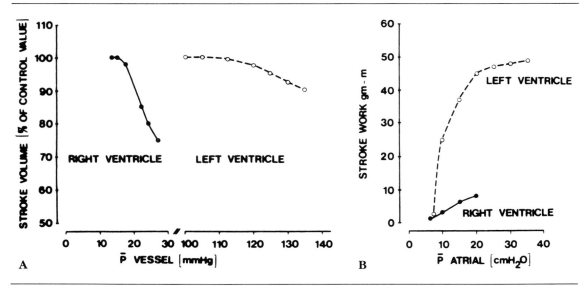

Fig. 52-1. Effects of increasing afterload (*A*) and preload (*B*) on right and left ventricular function. The data in the left panel were obtained by constriction of the main pulmonary artery or aorta in dogs. Note that with stroke volume falls more rapidly in the right ventricle. $\bar{P}$ = change in pressure. (Reprinted with permission from ER McFadden, E Braunwald, Cor pulmonale; in E Braunwald [Ed], *Heart Disease—A Textbook of Cardiovascular Medicine.* Philadelphia: Saunders, 1992.)

crease in stroke volume would be practically superimposable (Fig. 52-2).

The pressure-flow relationships of the pulmonary vasculature and mechanisms by which the normal pulmonary vasculature can accommodate large increases in flow with little change in pressure (RV afterload) have been discussed already in Chapter 49. However, acute and chronic derangements in the pulmonary vasculature (see Chapter 50) that result in elevated pulmonary arterial pressures will cause cor pulmonale and even RV failure.

Cor Pulmonale

McGinn and White [55] first used the term *acute cor pulmonale* to describe right heart strain resulting from massive pulmonary embolism. This contrasts with *chronic cor pulmonale*, which is defined as "an alteration in structure and function of the RV resulting from disease affecting the structure and function of the lung except when this alteration results from disease of the left side of the heart or congenital heart disease" [34].

Acute Cor Pulmonale

Although massive pulmonary embolism is the best-known cause of acute cor pulmonale, the same syndrome can be seen in any patient in whom pulmonary vascular resistance acutely and

severely increases. For example, acute cor pulmonale is being recognized with increasing frequency in patients with pulmonary hypertension who are ventilated at high lung volumes [20], which increase pulmonary vascular resistance as a result of compression of pulmonary vessels from overdistended alveoli (see Chapter 49).

PATHOPHYSIOLOGIC FEATURES
Numerous studies have confirmed that a previously normal RV can tolerate an acute rise in systolic pressure produced by pulmonary vascular occlusion up to approximately 55 to 60 mmHg (mean pressure of 40) without engendering circulatory failure [70]. Figure 52-3 depicts the results of animal experiments in which the main pulmonary artery was gradually constricted to the point of circulatory collapse. At the point just before overt circulatory failure (the highest load tolerable in Fig. 52-3), arterial pressure and cardiac output were subnormal but stable. If, however, systemic arterial systolic pressure is al-

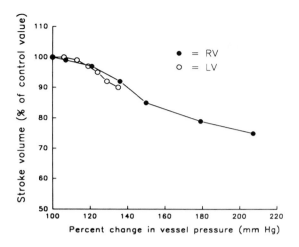

Fig. 52-2. Data from Figure 52-1 (increased afterload) replotted as a function of the percent change in afterload rather than as absolute change. Note that for the same percent increase in afterload, the right ventricle (*RV*) responds equivalently to the left ventricle (*LV*). In fact, RV afterload was increased percentage-wise to a greater extent than was LV afterload.

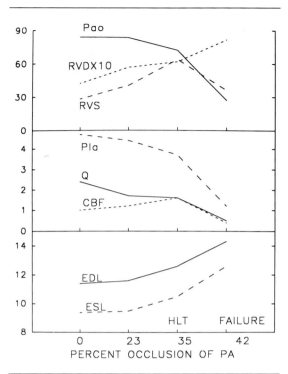

Fig. 52-3. Summary of experiments conducted by Scharf and coworkers [70] illustrating the effects of main stem pulmonary arterial (*PA*) constriction in dogs on right ventricular (*RV*) function. PA diameter could be reduced by 35 percent to produce the highest load tolerable (*HLT*). Further constriction produced circulatory collapse. *Pao* = mean aortic pressure (mmHg); *RVD* = RV end-diastolic pressure (mmHg); *RVS* = RV end-systolic pressure (mmHg); *Pla* = mean left atrial pressure (mmHg); $\dot{Q}$ = cardiac output (liters/min); *CBF* = right coronary arterial flow normalized to baseline; *EDL* = end-diastolic myocardial segment length in the outflow tract (mm); *ESL* = end-systolic myocardial segment length in the outflow tract (mm). (Reprinted with permission from SM Scharf, *Cardiopulmonary Physiology for Critical Care.* New York: Marcel Dekker, 1992.)

lowed to decrease below 60 mmHg, circulatory collapse ensues even though the degree of pulmonary artery constriction is unchanged [31]. Conversely, if systemic arterial pressure is increased by occlusion of the descending aorta or infusion of pressors, the degree to which RV systolic pressure can be increased without producing circulatory collapse is greater. That is, the tolerance of the RV to augmented afterload increases [18,24,77]. These phenomena illustrate the importance of the interaction between systemic and pulmonary factors in determining the response to increased RV afterload.

The mechanisms involved in acute RV failure are still a matter of controversy, but an imbalance between RV myocardial O_2 demand and supply is almost certainly involved [78]. With increased RV work, RV O_2 demand increases. Though this is partially met by increased coronary blood flow to the RV (see Fig. 52-3), according to some authors, a point is reached when RV O_2 demand outstrips supply. This is because the gradient for RV coronary perfusion is aortic – RV end-diastolic pressure. As RV afterload increases, aortic pressure decreases because of reduced cardiac output (see Fig. 52-3). Furthermore, as RV end-diastolic cavitary pressure increases, the back pressure to

coronary perfusion increases, further decreasing the gradient for coronary perfusion. Thus, at the same time RV O_2 demand increases, the gradient for blood flow to the RV myocardium decreases.

Some investigators believe that RV myocardium actually becomes ischemic during RV failure [77,78], whereas others believe that ischemia is not a necessary precondition for failure [70]. At some point, RV coronary blood flow does not increase proportionally to O_2 demand, and cardiac output falls. This in turn leads to decreased coronary perfusion pressure and worsening RV function. Thus a vicious cycle ensues, leading to circulatory collapse. These comments have a number of consequences as regards therapy for acute cor pulmonale. At the point of highest load tolerable, the administration of agents that increase cardiac contractility could be ineffective or even dangerous because they increase RV myocardial O_2 demand [57]. Similarly, massive fluid infusion, beyond the point of adequate RV filling, could have the same effect [27]. At less than maximal RV afterload, fluid infusion could, however, be useful. The presence of concomitant right coronary artery disease could further decrease the ability of the RV to tolerate increased afterload. This has been shown experimentally for partial pulmonary arterial occlusion [10] and high levels of positive end-expiratory pressure [72].

The manner in which pulmonary arterial pressure is increased can also influence the degree to which the RV can tolerate an increase in loading conditions. For example, for the same increase in RV systolic pressure, proximal pulmonary artery constriction leads to a greater dynamic RV afterload than distal pulmonary artery constriction [14]. This may be because pulmonary arterial input impedance (see Chapter 49) is increased more with proximal occlusion, due to decreased proximal pulmonary arterial compliance that leads to an increase in the capacitative component of pulmonary input impedance.

CLINICAL FEATURES

The clinical manifestations of acute cor pulmonale are nonspecific and include dyspnea, orthopnea, and cough. Physical examination may reveal distended neck veins with prominent a and v waves, pulsus paradoxus, and peripheral cyanosis. Inspection of the precordium may demonstrate a right ventricular lift, whereas palpation of the cardiac impulse may reveal a parasternal or subxyphoid heave. On cardiac auscultation, an S3 gallop and a loud pulmonic second sound are usually present. A holosystolic murmur, accentuated during inspiration, along the left parasternal border is suggestive of tricuspid regurgitation. Auscultation of the lung fields may be normal or may reveal crackles bilaterally. Although the patient's history and a carefully performed physical examination may be suggestive of acute cor pulmonale, additional diagnostic studies (discussed later) may be necessary to confirm the diagnosis.

Chronic Cor Pulmonale

Chronic cor pulmonale (CCP) develops when pulmonary disease is bilateral, diffuse, and chronic. Causes of pulmonary hypertension are discussed in the preceding chapters, and Table 52-1 lists many of the known causes of CCP. Chronic airways obstruction (CAO) or chronic obstructive lung disease (COPD) is the most common etiology of CCP. Although the true incidence of cor pulmonale is unknown, 10 to 30 percent of the hospital admissions in the United States for congestive heart failure are attributed to pulmonary heart disease [34]. As discussed in the previous chapters, both hypoxia and vascular remodeling can cause chronically elevated pulmonary arterial pressures. Considerable controversy exists vis-à-vis the relative importance of hypoxemia versus vascular remodeling. However, hypoxemia remains the most directly correctable pathophysiologic entity.

RIGHT VENTRICLE IN CCP

CCP leads to uniform hypertrophy of the RV. The cross-sectional area through the ventricular wall increases, as does myocardial fiber thickness [9,42,84]. Baseline coronary blood flow increases proportionally to muscle mass [84]. RV end-diastolic pressure increases only in the later stages of pulmonary hypertension and RV hypertrophy. Because of increased muscle mass and RV chamber size (dilatation), RV myocardial O_2 demand is increased, thus possibly rendering the RV more susceptible to demand and supply imbalance, as discussed earlier.

In contrast to acute cor pulmonale, RV systolic pressure in CCP can be very high, approaching or even equaling systemic pressures. Thus RV systolic pressures of this range signify a chronic problem in which hypertrophy has been an adaptive change.

Cardiac output at rest is usually normal or elevated in patients with CCP [39]. Patients with poor prognosis demonstrate progressively decreasing cardiac output over time. This suggests that maintaining peripheral blood flow is an important adaptive response to chronic tissue hypoxia. Polycythemia develops in many patients with CCP, and this may augment peripheral O_2 delivery in the setting of decreased cardiac output. However, polycythemia increases blood viscosity, thereby increasing pulmonary vascular resistance according to the laminar flow equation. The development of polycythemia may therefore be maladaptive as it may contribute to further decreases in cardiac output [78].

Table 52-1. Classification of cor pulmonale according to a causative factor

Diseases affecting air passages of the lung and alveoli

Chronic obstructive pulmonary disease
Cystic fibrosis
Congenital developmental defects
Infiltrative or granulomatous defects
    Idiopathic pulmonary fibrosis
    Sarcoidosis
    Pneumoconiosis
    Scleroderma
    Mixed connective tissue disease
    Systemic lupus erythematosus
    Rheumatoid arthritis
    Polymyositis
    Eosinophilic granuloma
    Malignant infiltration
    Radiation
Upper airways obstruction
Pulmonary resection
High-altitude disease

Diseases affecting thoracic cage movement

Kyphoscoliosis
Thoracotomy
Neuromuscular diseases
Sleep apnea syndrome
Idiopathic hypoventilation

Diseases affecting the pulmonary vasculature

Primary diseases of the arterial wall
    Primary pulmonary hypertension
    Pulmonary arteritis
    Toxin-induced pulmonary hypertension
        Aminorex fumarate
        Intravenous drug abuse
    Chronic liver disease
    Peripheral pulmonary stenosis
Thrombotic disorders
    Sickle cell disease
    Pulmonary microthrombi
Embolic disorders
    Thromboembolism
    Tumor embolism
    Other embolisms (amniotic fluid, air)
    Schistosomiasis and other parasites

Pressures on pulmonary arteries by mediastinal tumors, aneurysms, granulomas, or fibrosis

Source: Reproduced with permission from IJ Rubin (Ed), *Pulmonary Heart Disease*. Boston: Martinus Nijhoff, 1984. P 4.

Patients with CCP frequently experience syncope during exercise. The cause is multifactorial. Increased venous return during exercise could lead to increased RV pressure and volume, thus increasing O_2 demand. This could produce RV myocardial O_2 supply-demand imbalance. In addition, during exercise, systemic vascular resistance normally falls. However, systemic blood pressure increases because cardiac output increases even more than systemic vascular resistance decreases. In patients with CCP, cardiac output may increase minimally or not at all during exercise. In this case, arterial pressure may fall because of the peripheral vasodilation.

PATHOPHYSIOLOGIC FEATURES

The pulmonary hemodynamics of patients with COPD have been investigated by several authors. Weitzenblum and colleagues [81] evaluated 93 patients with severe COPD, 74 of whom were bronchitic and 19 of whom were emphysematous. None of these patients was receiving domiciliary oxygen or vasodilator therapy during the study. Each patient underwent both initial and follow-up right cardiac catheterization approximately 5 years later. Patients were divided into two groups: Group I had a mean pulmonary arterial pressure (mPAP) of 20 mmHg or less and group II had a mPAP exceeding 20 mmHg. The changes in mPAP over the study period were small—0.65 mmHg/yr and 0.39 mmHg/yr, for groups I and II, respectively. Pulmonary wedge pressure, RV end-diastolic pressure, and cardiac output remained unchanged. Hemodynamic deterioration, defined as an increase in mPAP of 5 mmHg or more, was observed in 27 patients. Because these patients demonstrated progressive hypoxemia, the authors suggested that worsening hypoxemia was responsible for the progression of pulmonary arterial hypertension.

Boushy and coworkers [7] reported similar findings in a larger patient population of 136 patients. The hemodynamic changes consisted of a 6 percent decrease in cardiac index and an increase of 7 percent in mPAP. As hypoxemia worsened, pulmonary arterial pressures at rest and during exercise became increasingly elevated.

Mahler and coworkers [44] also reported similar findings in patients with severe COPD during exercise. In this study, both pulmonary vascular resistance and mPAP increased during exercise, thus increasing RV afterload and leading to RV dilatation at end-systole and end-diastole. These results suggest that exercise performance may be limited by RV dysfunction in addition to ventilatory impairment in some patients with COPD.

Schrijen and associates [71] evaluated 35 patients with chronic bronchitis. The patients were divided into two groups, group I having an mPAP of less than 20 mmHg and group II an mPAP of 20 mmHg or more. There were no significant changes in mPAP when measured 3 years later. The mPAP increased from 15.8 mmHg at rest to 25.2 mmHg during exercise in group I, whereas the mPAP increased from 27.0 mmHg to 44.1 mmHg during exercise in group II. In this study, it was noted that there was a decrease in systemic arterial pressure over time in the patients with pulmonary hypertension (group II). The authors postulated that this decrease in LV afterload could be partly responsible for the fact that mPAP did not rise in these patients. Decreased systemic arterial pressure may have been due to the peripheral vasodilating effect of hypoxia and hypercapnia. There had been earlier reports that patients with severe emphysema have lower cardiac output compared to those with milder disease [12]. Other studies, however, demonstrated no correlation between cardiac output and severity of chronic obstructive airway disease [69,80,81].

In summary, except for mPAP, other hemodynamic parameters do not change significantly after several years of follow-up in patients with cor pulmonale. The mPAP and arterial oxygen tension are inversely correlated, suggesting that hypoxic vasoconstriction and subsequent remodeling of the pulmonary vascular bed play an important role in the pathogenesis of cor pulmonale [40].

LEFT VENTRICLE IN CCP

With acute dilatation of the RV, ventricular interdependence acts to impede LV filling [35]. Ventricular interdependence acts both by leftward shift of the septum and the fact that both ventricles are located within a common pericardial sac. In experimental animals, chronic banding of the pulmonary artery can lead to LV as well as RV hypertrophy [42], supporting the whole-heart concept of cor pulmonale. The clinical implications of these findings are, however, less well understood. In patients with no identifiable cause of LV disease in whom RV dysfunction is apparent, anatomic changes in the LV are rarely found, systolic function is normal, and LV failure is not common [13,23,37,74,79]. However, some patients with CCP do demonstrate overt LV failure in the absence of an identifiable cause [67]. Krayenbuehl and colleagues [41] found elevated LV filling pressure and decreased LV compliance in pa-

tients with CCP due to COPD, in keeping with postulated interdependence effects due to RV dilation [8].

Patients with airflow obstruction may generate large negative swings in intrathoracic pressure during inspiration. This increases venous return, acting to decrease LV compliance further due to increased RV volume during inspiration, as demonstrated in experimental animals [69] and humans [36]. COPD can lead to pulmonary hyperinflation. By direct mechanical heart-lung interaction, increased lung volume, especially of the lower lobes, acts to impede LV filling [36,69]. Finally, hypoxemia can impair active diastolic ventricular relaxation [29].

It is apparent that the effects of cor pulmonale on LV function depend on many factors. However, most evidence points to diastolic rather than systolic dysfunction. In addition, patients with COPD frequently exhibit concomitant coronary artery disease, which can affect LV systolic function, leading to LV failure.

Diagnosis

Both the clinical history and physical examination are critical in the diagnosis of cor pulmonale. There are several noninvasive methods that can aid in the assessment of secondary pulmonary hypertension and its cardiac complications.

ELECTROCARDIOGRAM

The electrocardiographic (ECG) abnormalities in cor pulmonale depend on its etiology. Patients with COPD have a characteristic ECG pattern due to major structural changes of the thorax and its contents [59,60,65]. The resulting ECG patterns, such as shift of the P wave and QRS axis, will then be superimposed on the changes due to cor pulmonale [33]. The ECG criteria for cor pulmonale listed in Table 52-2 illustrate the common patterns associated with COPD as well as other parenchymal lung diseases. A combination of these criteria are suggestive of, but not specific for, pulmonary heart disease.

In addition, many rhythm disturbances may be present in CCP. These range from premature atrial contractions to supraventricular tachycardias of all types, including paroxysmal atrial tachycardia, multifocal atrial tachycardia, atrial fibrillation, atrial flutter, and junctional tachycardias. These dysrhythmias often are present in patients with so-called acute exacerbations of COPD and frequently are related to secondary causes associated with the disease process, such

Table 52-2. **Electrocardiographic changes in cor pulmonale**

ECG criteria for cor pulmonale without obstructive disease of the airways

1. Right-axis deviation with a mean QRS axis to the right of + 110 degrees
2. R/S amplitude ratio in V1 >1
3. R/S amplitude ratio in V6 <1
4. Clockwise rotation of the electric axis
5. P-pulmonale pattern
6. S1,Q3 or S1,S2,S3 pattern
7. Normal voltage QRS

ECG changes in chronic cor pulmonale with obstructive disease of the airways

1. Isoelectric P waves in lead I or right-axis deviation of the P vector
2. P-pulmonale pattern (an increase in P-wave amplitude in II, III, AVF)
3. Tendency for right-axis deviation of the QRS
4. R/S amplitude ratio in V6 <1
5. Low-voltage QRS
6. S1,Q3 or S1,S2,S3 pattern
7. Incomplete (and rarely complete) right bundle-branch block
8. R/S amplitude ratio in V1 >1
9. Marked clockwise rotation of the electric axis
10. Occasional large Q wave or QS in the inferior or midprecordial leads, suggesting healed myocardial infarction

as RV overload, hypoxemia, acidosis, electrolyte disturbance, and therapy with beta agonists, methylxanthines, and digoxin. Reported incidences of supraventricular arrhythmias range from 20 to 71 percent [58]. The incidence of ventricular tachydysrhythmias is reported to be somewhat lower (7 to 24%) [58,73] and, in patients with primary pulmonary hypertension, ventricular tachycardia and atrioventricular junctional block are probably unusual [38].

CHEST ROENTGENOGRAM

Routine chest radiography demonstrating a right descending pulmonary artery greater than 16 mm in diameter or a left artery greater than 18 mm in diameter indicates pulmonary hypertension [58]. RV enlargement on the posteroanterior view results in displacement and increased transverse diameter of the heart shadow to the right. In the lateral view, RV enlargement leads to filling of the retrosternal airspace.

ECHOCARDIOGRAPHY

The diagnostic application of M-mode echocardiography in evaluating the RV is limited. Be-

cause the right-sided cardiac structures are anatomically situated posterior to the echo-dense sternum, accurate assessment is technically difficult. Pulmonary hyperinflation and excessive chest motion in patients with COPD also impose a limitation to this technique [51].

Two-dimensional (2-D) echocardiography provides multiple cross-sectional views of the heart, improves visualization of right-sided cardiac structures, and is useful in assessing RV hypertrophy in patients with COPD [22,61]. In addition, the use of multiple cross-sectional views can be used to obtain relatively accurate estimations of RV volume using the Simpson's rule approximation technique. Bommer and coworkers [6] performed 2-D echocardiograms on 8 human right-heart casts obtained at autopsy and on 50 patients who underwent complete left and right heart catheterization. Measurements of individual dimensions of the long and short axis correlated with the volume of these structures as determined by water displacement and with actual cast dimensions. Measurements of the right atrial and ventricular size by 2-D echocardiography distinguished normal patients from those with RV volume overload and correlated with the data obtained from catheterization.

Doppler echocardiography has been used by several investigators to estimate pulmonary arterial pressure. The combination of Doppler technique and echocardiography can estimate mPAP in patients with COPD by measuring the velocity of blood flow in the main pulmonary artery or in a regurgitant jet from the tricuspid valve. The time to peak velocity, defined as the time interval between the onset of RV ejection and peak flow velocity, is inversely correlated with mPAP [40]. Doppler echocardiography appears to be the most useful noninvasive technique for assessing pulmonary arterial pressure. When used with either 2-D or M-mode echocardiography, it is helpful in detecting mPAP in cor pulmonale in a semiquantitative fashion.

Chronic overload leads to RV dilation. This effect may be exaggerated during inspiration owing to venous return effects. Such changes can result in a configurational distortion of the interventricular septum, which may impair LV diastolic filling, as discussed previously [51,61]. These effects have echocardiographic manifestations. Normally, the interventricular septum is concave toward the LV, resulting in a relatively circular shape of the LV in the axial plane during diastole. During systole, there is symmetric inward motion of the ventricular walls, which results in constriction of the LV while maintaining its circular shape in the axial plane. Thus, during systole, the interventricular septum functions as part of the LV.

With RV volume overload, in diastole, septal abnormalities may range from slight flattening of the normal curvature to complete reversal of the direction of curvature such that the septum becomes concave toward the RV and convex toward the LV [83]. In extreme cases, the septum may actually bulge into the LV cavity during diastole.

With increased RV afterload, during systole the septum may demonstrate so-called paradoxical motion. This is defined as motion away from the LV posterolateral wall during systole and toward the RV free wall. That is, the septum becomes functionally part of the RV. Paradoxical septal motion was first reported by Popp and associates [66] and was later confirmed by Diamond and coworkers [21]. Using echocardiographic studies, Weyman and colleagues [83] were able to demonstrate paradoxical septal motion in 19 patients with RV volume overload. Figure 52-4 illustrates a normal M-mode echocardiogram of the left ventricle. During systole, the interventricular septum moves posteriorly toward the LV free wall. The

line diagram demonstrates the concentric inward motion of the LV endocardium during systole and that its geometric center is moved anteriorly. Figure 52-5 is an echocardiographic recording of a patient with RV overload due to pulmonary insufficiency. The accompanying diagram illus-

Fig. 52-4. A normal M-mode echocardiogram of the left ventricle (LV). During ventricular systole, the septum moves posteriorly toward the posterior LV wall. Corresponding anterior motion of the posterior ventricular wall results in shortening of the anteroposterior minor axis during ejection. The corresponding line drawing shows the shape of the LV cavity at five points during the cardiac cycle from end-diastole (*1*) to end-systole (*5*). Note the symmetrical concentric inward contraction of the LV endocardium during systole. The geometrical center of the LV moves anteriorly as the LV moves in space during contraction. The cross-sectional diagram is drawn as if one were looking from the apex up toward the mitral valve. *CW* = chest wall; *RV* = right ventricular cavity; *RS* = RV aspect of the septum; *LS* = LV aspect of the septum; *AML* = anterior mitral valve leaflet; *LV* = LV cavity; *EN* = LV posterior wall endocardium; *EP* = LV posterior epicardium. (Reprinted with permission from AE Weyman et al, Mechanism of abnormal septal motion in patients with right ventricular volume overload. *Circulation* 54:179, 1976.)

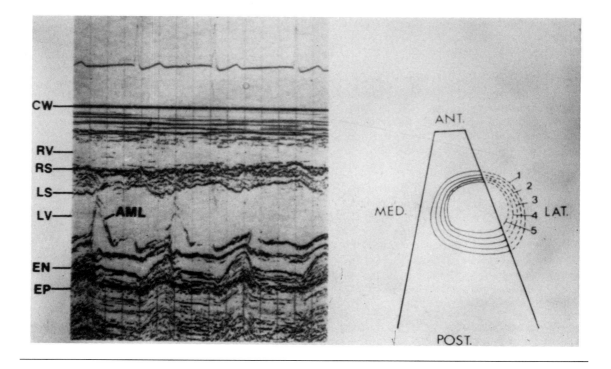

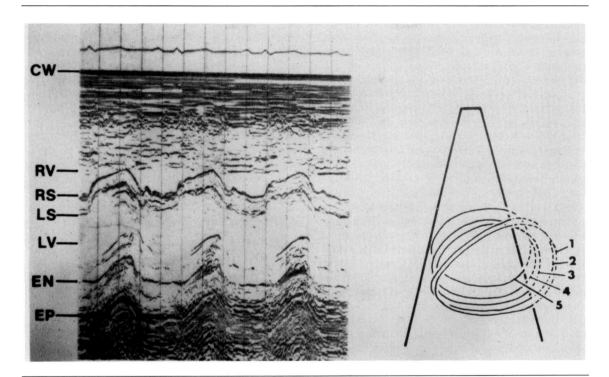

Fig. 52-5. M-mode echocardiogram from a patient with chronic respiratory insufficiency. The line drawing shows the cross-section during the contraction sequence from end-diastole (*1*) to end-systole (*5*). Note that during systole the septum moves anteriorly rather than posteriorly. *CW* = chest wall; *RV* = right ventricular cavity; *RS* = RV aspect of the septum; *LS* = LV aspect of the septum; *LV* = left ventricular cavity; *EN* = LV posterior wall endocardium; *EP* = LV posterior epicardium. (Reprinted with permission from AE Weyman et al, Mechanism of abnormal septal motion in patients with right ventricular volume overload. *Circulation* 54:179, 1976.)

trates the paradoxical motion of the interventricular septum during systole. The LV reassumes its normal circular configuration during diastole. With sufficient compromise of LV end-diastolic volume owing to septal bulging, it is possible that cardiac output could be compromised [83].

RADIONUCLIDE TECHNIQUES
The equilibrium-gated blood pool imaging technique allows continuous monitoring of RV performance by tagging erythrocytes with technetium 99m. Ejection fraction is calculated by comparing counts at end-systole with those at end-diastole over approximately 10 minutes [51]. Although equilibrium-gated blood pool imaging allows continuous monitoring of RV performance and provides reliable measurements of RV ejection fraction (RVEF), RV dimensions are difficult to evaluate because the ventricular borders are obscured by the presence of background counts in other cardiac chambers and the lungs [40]. The "first-pass" technique also involves labeling with technetium 99m but is based on principles of indicator dilution theory, whereby counting is done sequentially over each cardiac chamber as a function of time [51,61]. The advantage of the first-pass technique is that data are gathered over only a few heartbeats. Further, the high number of counts relative to background allows for definition of the RV border and estimates of diastolic and systolic size. Both first-pass and equilibrium-gated techniques can be used to evaluate ventricular function at rest and during exercise. The first-pass technique allows the patients to be studied in the supine or upright position, which is a major advantage. The 30-degree right anterior oblique position is optimal for assessing the RV [61]. It should be noted that while radionuclide

studies can detect severely elevated pulmonary arterial pressure, they cannot accurately assess mild pulmonary hypertension. The prediction of the actual level of mPAP from radionuclide measurements is also difficult.

RV function in COPD depends on the cause, duration, and severity of cor pulmonale. Biernacki and colleagues [4] performed radionuclide ventriculography in 100 patients with COPD. There was no significant correlation between RVEF and pulmonary arterial pressure. However, there was a weak correlation between pulmonary vascular resistance and RVEF. Despite the presence of pulmonary hypertension, RV wall motion remained normal. Matthay and coworkers [49], by contrast, observed an abnormal RVEF in 8 of 30 patients at rest with COPD, whereas 23 of the 30 patients demonstrated an abnormal RVEF during submaximal exercise.

Thallium 201 imaging is another technique used to evaluate RV function in patients with pulmonary hypertension [61]. Several investigators reported that the RV cannot be well visualized at rest in normals, but others have shown that visualization of RV at rest is common in patients with RV hypertrophy secondary to volume and pressure overload [48]. Weitzenblum and coworkers [82] evaluated 73 patients with lung disease, COPD being the most common etiology. The authors noted that the thallium imaging technique was more sensitive in detecting RV hypertrophy or RV pressure overloading when the mPAP exceeded 30 mmHg.

In summary, with the availability of noninvasive studies, invasive procedures often are not indicated for diagnosing cor pulmonale. However, if unexplained RV dysfunction presents in a patient without previously diagnosed pulmonary disease, other diagnoses such as primary pulmonary vascular disease, pulmonary embolism, or left heart failure should be considered. Right heart catheterization and pulmonary angiography may be indicated in such cases.

Therapy

ACUTE COR PULMONALE

There are few data on the optimal care of patients with acute RV failure as might be caused by massive pulmonary thromboembolism. In patients with acute cor pulmonale, hypotension or shock on the basis of RV failure frequently is observed, especially if prior cardiopulmonary disease is present. Recommendations for cardiopulmonary support have included fluid loading and

isoproterenol. However, as noted earlier, animal studies suggest this may be contraindicated. In these studies, which used the infusion of autologous clots to produce RV failure, administration of the vasoconstrictor norepinephrine was superior to either volume infusion or isoproterenol in improving RV function, increasing cardiac output, and decreasing mortality [27,57]. It would seem reasonable to reserve volume infusion for those patients with dehydration or low central venous pressure. Of course, the primary problem should be corrected if possible. For example, with massive pulmonary embolism, administration of thrombolytic agents or surgical embolectomy should be considered emergently, especially if circulatory support is a major problem.

OXYGEN THERAPY IN COPD

Short-Term Effects. The short-term effects of O_2 therapy in 35 patients with acute decompensation of COPD were studied by Degaute and coworkers [19]. Arterial blood gas and O_2 delivery were recorded while the patients were breathing room air and 28% O_2. Two patterns of hemodynamic response to 28% O_2 were noted. One group of patients (N = 15) was severely hypoxemic (PaO_2 = 40 mmHg) and demonstrated increased O_2 content but no change in cardiac output with O_2 administration. The other group was moderately hypoxemic (N = 20; PaO_2 = 49 mmHg) and also demonstrated an increase in O_2 content but a decrease in cardiac output. The latter effect may have been due to withdrawal of hypoxia-induced sympathoadrenal stimulation with O_2 administration. In these patients, O_2 delivery did not change with O_2 administration. The authors also noted that mPAP remained elevated despite O_2 therapy, suggesting that hypoxic vasoconstriction was not the sole cause of pulmonary hypertension.

MacNee and colleagues [43] investigated the effects of controlled O_2 therapy on ventricular function in patients with stable and decompensated cor pulmonale. Pulmonary hemodynamics, cardiac output, and RVEF were measured simultaneously to assess RV function in 14 patients with pulmonary hypertension due to COPD. Eight patients were clinically stable without edema, whereas 6 patients presented with gross peripheral edema indicating decompensated cor pulmonale. Measurements were made while the patients were breathing room air and O_2 (1 to 3 liters/min). The mPAPs for stable and for unstable patients were 30 ± 8 mmHg and 33 ± 6 mmHg, respectively. Although the mPAPs were similar, RVEF was lower in edematous (0.23 ± 0.11) as compared to nonedematous patients (0.47 ± 0.04). Cardiac output was normal in all patients. Oxygen therapy did not change right or left ventricular ejection fraction or the ventricular end-systolic pressure-volume relationship. These data indicate that ventricular function was normal in patients with COPD without edema and was reduced in decompensated patients with COPD. However, in the latter, reduced RV function was not the result of increased RV afterload insofar as RV afterload was estimated from mPAP. When given acutely, O_2 did not improve ventricular contractility.

In summary, based on these studies, O_2 administration primarily increases O_2 delivery by increasing O_2 content in severely hypoxemic patients. However, in moderately hypoxemic patients, O_2 therapy may not increase O_2 delivery because decreased cardiac output may counteract the effects of improved blood oxygen content. Although definitive improvement in RV function has not been shown when O_2 is given acutely, O_2 therapy still plays an important role in managing patients with cor pulmonale. The beneficial effects of O_2 probably stem from its peripheral circulatory effects (e.g., reducing sympatho-adrenal-related increases in myocardial O_2 demand, alleviating renal artery vasospasm, improving mental functioning, and relieving dyspnea).

Long-Term O_2 Therapy in CCP. Most of the studies demonstrating beneficial effects of long-term O_2 therapy have been carried out in patients with COPD. However, only two controlled trials have demonstrated improved survival rate. The British trial [75] consisted of 87 patients with severe COPD (with severe hypoxemia and hypercapnia) who were randomized to O_2 therapy (treated group) and no O_2 (control group). Forty-two patients received O_2 at 2 liters/min or greater, to achieve a PaO_2 in excess of 60 mmHg for at least 15 hr/day. The two groups were matched clinically in terms of lung function and other laboratory findings. Patients were followed for up to 5 years. Figure 52-6 demonstrates that the mortality rate in treated men was lower (11.9% per year) compared to the control group (29.4% per year). Figure 52-7 demonstrates that the mortality rate for treated women was dramatically lower (5.7% per year) than in the untreated control group (36.5% per year). The authors were unable to explain the marked difference in mortality between male and female patients since there was

no evidence of greater severity of lung disease in the women. The mPAP remained unchanged in the O_2-treated group but increased in the untreated patients. In addition, long-term O_2 therapy prevented the progressive decline in room air PaO_2 seen in untreated patients without significantly increasing arterial PCO_2.

The American trial [1,17,76] included six centers where patients with hypoxemic COPD were randomly assigned to either 12-hour nocturnal O_2 or continuous O_2 (17.7 hr/day) therapy for at least 12 months (mean, 19.3 months). The overall mortality in the nocturnal O_2 therapy group was approximately twice that in the continuous O_2 therapy group [17]. Pulmonary vascular resistance increased by 6.5 percent in patients who were given nocturnal O_2, whereas those who received continuous O_2 therapy demonstrated an 11 percent decrease. The mPAP fell from 28.0 mmHg to 26.4 mmHg in 6 months in both groups. Exercise tolerance did not improve in either group. Hematocrit decreased significantly for patients who received nocturnal O_2.

The effects of long-term O_2 therapy on RV function reported in the literature are inconsistent. Olvey and associates [62] reported that 4 of 10 patients with COPD who were given O_2 therapy during exercise demonstrated a normal RV response, defined as more than a 5 percent increase in RVEF. Other authors, however, reported that although there were improvements in RV function, as measured by RV end-diastolic pressure or RV stroke work index, the measured changes were not statistically significant [76,82].

In summary, because there is an inverse correlation between arterial hypoxemia and survival rate in patients with cor pulmonale, some O_2 is better than none, but continuous O_2 therapy is optimal [25]. Because most of the studies regarding the beneficial effects of O_2 therapy were conducted in patients with COPD, conclusions drawn may not be directly applicable to other forms of pulmonary heart disease.

Recommendations for Oxygen Therapy. The benefits of long-term domiciliary O_2 therapy for selected patients with chronic respiratory disease have been established [1]. However, because of continued inconsistencies and lack of uniformity of guidelines, a second O_2-prescribing consensus conference was convened [26]. The committee agreed that long-term O_2 therapy is known to prolong survival and improve both hemodynamic and neuropsychological function. The committee also reaffirmed that O_2 given during

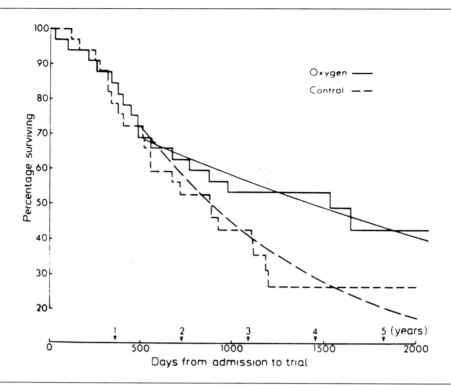

Fig. 52-6. Mortality in male patients receiving chronic O_2 therapy versus controls. Smooth curves indicate expected percentage of patients surviving from 500 days at a constant risk of 11.9 percent per year for O_2 therapy versus 29.4 percent per year for controls (received no oxygen). (Reprinted with permission from C Stuart-Harris et al, British Medical Research Council Working Party: Long-term domiciliary oxygen therapy in chronic hypoxic cor pulmonale complicating bronchitis and emphysema. *Lancet* 1:681, 1981.)

ambulation increases endurance and reduces disabling dyspnea. The committee recommended that O_2 be prescribed only when resting PaO_2 is 55 mmHg or less or when PaO_2 is 56 to 59 mmHg with cor pulmonale, polycythemia, or dependent edema. Oximetry is an acceptable method for demonstrating hypoxemia during activity and sleep. It is also an acceptable tool for follow-up evaluation and for monitoring the efficacy of long-term O_2 therapy. The need for continued O_2 therapy should be verified annually by the physician.

VASODILATOR THERAPY
The treatment of both primary and secondary pulmonary hypertension with vasodilators is discussed in Chapter 51. The reader is referred there.

ALMITRINE
Almitrine bismesylate is a triazine derivative that increases the sensitivity of peripheral arterial chemoreceptors to hypoxia. Bell and colleagues [3] studied the effects of almitrine in 67 patients with hypoxemia due to COPD in a placebo-

controlled, double-blinded study. The group that received 100 mg twice daily demonstrated an 11.2-mmHg increase in PaO_2 and a decrease of 3.8 mmHg in $PaCO_2$. In the group that received 50 mg twice daily, PaO_2 increased by 6.0 mmHg, whereas $PaCO_2$ remained unchanged. Thus a dose-response relationship could be demonstrated.

Connaughton and coworkers [16] studied the effects of almitrine in patients with chronic bronchitis and emphysema who were hypoxic while awake and asleep. Patients who received 50 mg almitrine twice daily for 14 days demonstrated a rise of 8 mmHg in PaO_2 and a decrease of 4 mmHg in $PaCO_2$ while awake. Almitrine also im-

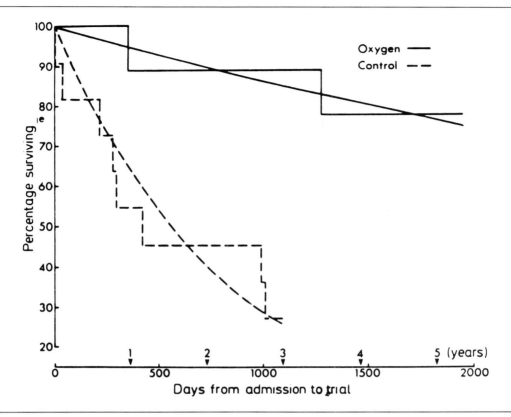

Fig. 52-7. Mortality in female patients receiving chronic O_2 therapy versus controls. Smooth curves indicate expected percentage of patients surviving at constant risk of 5.7 percent per year for O_2 therapy versus 36.5 percent per year for controls. (Reprinted with permission from C Stuart-Harris et al, British Medical Research Council Working Party: Long-term domiciliary oxygen therapy in chronic hypoxic cor pulmonale complicating bronchitis and emphysema. *Lancet* 1:681, 1981.)

proved nocturnal oxygenation, although the quality of sleep did not improve.

Because almitrine improves oxygenation in hypoxemic patients with COPD, many authors advocate the use of almitrine as an alternative to O_2 therapy. One possible mechanism for the observed improvement in arterial blood gas measurements is the reduction in ventilation-perfusion mismatching [56]. However, elevations in mPAP and pulmonary vascular resistance have been reported [3,43], and it has been suggested that increasing pulmonary vasomotor tone with almitrine could worsen cor pulmonale in patients with COPD. The other major adverse reaction

was unexplained worsening dyspnea, which occurred in some patients, perhaps related to increased sensitivity to hypoxia.

CARDIAC GLYCOSIDES
The efficacy of cardiac glycosides as therapy for cor pulmonale is controversial. In a clinical trial by Mathur and associates [46] in patients with severe COPD, RVEF improved only when left ventricular ejection fraction also was initially abnormal. Brown and colleagues [11] found no improvement in RVEF, either at rest or during exercise, in stable patients with severe COPD and no LV failure.

The utility of cardiac glycosides is demonstrable only in the presence of coexisting left ventricular dysfunction. The possibility that digoxin may have favorable effects when used as adjunctive therapy with other medications such as oxygen, vasodilators, beta$_2$-adrenergic agents, and theophylline has not been excluded [70]. Patients with chronic respiratory disease are at increased risk of developing digitalis toxicity, which may be mediated in part by acute hypoxia and its neuroexcitatory and adrenal effects [30].

PHLEBOTOMY

Reduction in intravascular volume may improve the patient's functional status. Diuretics should be used cautiously, and care should be taken to prevent hypokalemia and metabolic alkalosis, which may blunt respiratory drive.

Chronic hypoxemia may result in polycythemia in some patients. This augments blood viscosity and, to the extent that flow is laminar, increases pulmonary vascular resistance, thereby elevating mPAP. Phlebotomy should be considered when the hematocrit meets or exceeds 55 percent [15,40]. Chetty and coworkers [15] studied the effects of therapeutic phlebotomy on exercise tolerance of polycythemic patients with COPD. Maximum exercise tolerance improved, and this was associated with increased cardiac output and stroke volume. The authors hypothesized that increased stroke volume was due to higher RVEF secondary to decreased pulmonary arterial pressure [15].

THEOPHYLLINE

Although theophylline often is routinely prescribed as a bronchodilator agent in patients with COPD, its efficacy remains controversial. Matthay [47] reported that intravenous aminophylline acutely reduces both the pulmonary vascular resistance and pulmonary arterial pressures. Oral theophylline was also noted to improve right and left ventricular ejection fraction after 72 hours of therapy [50]. A combination of decreased afterload and inotropy was postulated to account for the beneficial effects of aminophylline. However, in an animal model, Gomez and colleagues [28] found that under hypoxic conditions, aminophylline did not actually have a positive inotropic effect. These authors observed that aminophylline caused a decrease in LV end-diastolic dimensions by augmenting hypoxia-induced increases in myocardial resting tension.

DECIDING AMONG THE THERAPEUTIC ALTERNATIVES

The specific therapeutic options to apply in any given patient depend on the cause of cor pulmonale. Correcting hypoxemia is the primary goal, to prevent progression of pulmonary hypertension. Long-term oxygen is the only therapy that has been shown to improve survival in patients with cor pulmonale due to severe COPD. Methylxan-thine derivatives and inhaled beta agonists for bronchodilation are commonly used in COPD patients. Vasodilators such as hydralazine and calcium channel blockers may improve pulmonary hemodynamics in some patients with primary pulmonary hypertension, but sustained benefits have not been demonstrated in such patients. Cardiac glycosides may improve RV function if LV dysfunction coexists. Finally, although almitrine may improve oxygenation in patients with COPD, its long-term effects on patients with pulmonary heart disease are unknown.

Treatment by Lung Transplantation

Lung transplantation was originally introduced to treat end-stage restrictive lung disease. However, the indications for transplantation have continued to evolve, and it has been successfully applied to patients with obstructive disease and pulmonary vascular diseases (see Chapter 48). Initially, patients with end-stage pulmonary hypertension were limited to en bloc heart-lung transplantation (HLT) [68]. Because of the scarcity of donor organs, single lung transplantation (SLT) has become more popular.

Bolman and coworkers [5] described their experience with HLT and SLT in 23 and 21 patients, respectively. In HLT patients, the preoperative mPAP was 70 ± 17 mmHg, whereas the postoperative mPAP was 18 ± 9 mmHg. The SLT recipients also demonstrated a reduction in mPAP, from 57 ± 21 mmHg to 25 ± 5 mmHg. Pasque and associates [64] noted that pulmonary arterial systolic pressure decreased from 92 ± 7 mmHg to 29 ± 6 mmHg in 7 patients who underwent SLT. In these patients, radionuclide ventriculography before and 17 weeks after transplantation demonstrated an increase in RVEF from 22 ± 15 percent to 51 ± 11 percent. Bolman's group [5] also observed a marked improvement in ventilatory function as shown by an increase in the mean 1-second forced expiratory volume (FEV_1) in both groups postoperatively, from 0.60 ± 0.25 liters to 2.03 ± 0.70 liters in the HLT patients and from 0.69 ± 0.29 liters to 1.73 ± 0.67 liters, in the SLT patients. Patients who underwent HLT have a survival of 85 and 74 percent at 1 and 2 years, respectively, compared with 80 percent at 1 and 2 years for recipients of SLT [5]. Hutter and colleagues [32] reported similar survival rates in 31 patients with HLT: 78 and 70 percent at 1 and 2 years, respectively. The recently reported excellent survival rates are no doubt attributable to improvement in immunosuppressive regimens [53].

The indications for lung transplantation are end-stage pulmonary disease of various etiologies such as primary pulmonary hypertension, cystic fibrosis, idiopathic pulmonary fibrosis, obliterative bronchiolitis, alpha$_1$-antitrypsin deficiency, and emphysema. Strict selection criteria for lung transplant recipients must be met because of the limited availability of organ donors. With the developments in organ preservation, as well as better patient management, the survival rate continues to improve. Because there were no significant differences in the survival rates between HLT and SLT recipients, SLT would seem to be the better alternative, especially when faced with limited resources. Finally, lung transplantation appears to reverse many of the features of pulmonary heart disease caused by chronically elevated pulmonary arterial pressures and so can lead to improved RV function. The mechanisms by which long-standing changes in RV function are alleviated remain to be elucidated.

References

1. Anthonisen NR. Long-term oxygen therapy. *Ann Intern Med* 99:519, 1983.
2. Armour JA, Pace JB, Randall WC. Interrelationships of architecture and function of the right ventricle. *Am J Physiol* 218:174, 1970.
3. Bell RC, et al. The effect of almitrine bismesylate on hypoxemia in COPD. *Ann Intern Med* 105:342, 1986.
4. Biernacki W, et al. Pulmonary hypertension and right ventricular function in patients with C.O.P.D. *Chest* 94:1169, 1988.
5. Bolman RM, et al. Lung and heart-lung transplantation. Evolution and new applications. *Ann Surg* 214(4):456, 1991.
6. Bommer W, et al. Determination of right atrial and right ventricular size by two-dimensional echocardiography. *Circulation* 60:91, 1979.
7. Boushy SF, North LB. Hemodynamic changes in chronic obstructive pulmonary disease. *Chest* 72:565, 1977.
8. Bove AA, Santamore WP. Ventricular interdependence. *Prog Cardiovasc Dis* 23:365, 1981.
9. Brenner O. Pathology of the vessels of the pulmonary circulation. *Arch Intern Med* 56:211, 1935.
10. Brooks H, et al. Performance of the right ventricle under stress: Relation to right coronary flow. *J Clin Invest* 50:2176, 1971.
11. Brown SE, et al. Effects of digoxin on exercise capacity and right ventricular function during exercise in chronic airflow obstruction. *Chest* 85:187, 1984.
12. Burrows B, et al. Patterns of cardiovascular dysfunction in chronic obstructive lung disease. *N Engl J Med* 286:912, 1972.
13. Caldwell EN. The Left Ventricle in Chronic Obstructive Lung Diseases. In LJ Rubin (Ed), *Pulmonary Heart Disease.* The Hague: Martinus Nijhoff, 1984. Pp 247–272.
14. Calvin JE, Baer RW, Glantz SA. Pulmonary artery constriction produces a greater right ventricular dynamic afterload than lung microvascular injury in the open chest dog. *Circ Res* 56:40, 1985.
15. Chetty KG, Brown SE, Light RW. Improved exercise tolerance of the polycythemic lung patient following phlebotomy. *Am J Med* 74:415, 1983.
16. Connaughton JJ, et al. Almitrine improves oxygenation when both awake and asleep in patients with hypoxia and carbon dioxide retention caused by chronic bronchitis and emphysema. *Am Rev Respir Dis* 132:206, 1985.
17. Continuous or nocturnal oxygen therapy in hypoxemic chronic obstructive lung disease. A clinical trial. *Ann Intern Med* 93:391, 1980.
18. Cooper N, Brazier J, Buckley G. Effects of systemic-pulmonary shunts on regional blood flow in experimental pulmonary stenosis. *J Thorac Cardiovasc Surg* 70:166, 1975.
19. Degaute JP, et al. Oxygen delivery in acute exacerbation of chronic obstructive pulmonary disease. *Am Rev Respir Dis* 124:26, 1981.
20. Dhainaut JF, Aoute P, Brunet FB. Circulatory Effects of Positive End-Expiratory Pressure in Patients with Acute Lung Injury. In SM Scharf, SS Cassidy (Eds), *Heart-Lung Interactions in Health and Disease.* New York: Marcel Dekker, 1989. Pp 809–838.
21. Diamond MA, et al. Echocardiographic features of atrial septal defect. *Circulation* 43:129, 1971.
22. Feigenbaum H. *Echocardiography* (4th ed). Philadelphia: Lea & Febiger, 1986. Pp 157–167.
23. Fishman AP. The left ventricle in chronic bronchitis and emphysema (edit). *N Engl J Med* 285:402, 1971.
24. Fixler DE, et al. Effects of acute right ventricular systolic hypertension on regional myocardial blood flow in anesthetized dogs. *Am Heart J* 85:491, 1973.
25. Flenley DC. Long-term home oxygen therapy. *Chest* 87:99, 1985.
26. Further recommendations for presenting and supplying long-term oxygen therapy. Conference report. *Am Rev Respir Dis* 138:745, 1988.
27. Ghignone M, Girling L, Prewitt RM. Volume expansion vs. noradrenaline in treatment of a low cardiac output complicating an acute increase in right ventricular afterload in dogs. *Anesthesiology* 60:48, 1984.
28. Gomez A, Eng J, Mink SN. Aminophyllin has little positive inotropic effect and a slightly negative diastolic effect on the left ventricle during hypoxic conditions. *Am Rev Respir Dis* 137:1246, 1988.

29. Gomez A, Mink S. Increased left ventricular stiffness impairs filling in dogs with pulmonary emphysema in respiratory failure. *J Clin Invest* 78:228, 1986.

30. Green LH, Smith TW. The use of digitalis in patients with pulmonary disease. *Ann Intern Med* 87:459, 1977.

31. Guyton AC, Adkins LH. Quantitative aspects of the collapse factor in relation to venous return. *Am J Physiol* 177:523, 1954.

32. Hutter JA, et al. Heart-lung transplantation: Better use of resources. *Am J Med* 85:4, 1988.

33. Ikeda K, et al. P-wave changes in obstructive and restrictive lung diseases. *J Electrocardiol* 18:233, 1985.

34. Inter-Society Commission for Heart Disease Resources. Primary prevention of pulmonary heart disease. *Circulation* 41:A17, 1970.

35. Janicki JS, Weber KT. The pericardium and ventricular interaction, distensibility and function. *Am J Physiol* 238:H494, 1980.

36. Jardin F, et al. Mechanism of paradoxic pulse in bronchial asthma. *Circulation* 66:887, 1982.

37. Kachel RG. Left ventricular function in chronic obstructive pulmonary disease. *Chest* 74:266, 1978.

38. Kanemoto N, Sasamoto H. Arrhythmias in primary pulmonary hypertension. *Jpn Heart J* 20:765, 1979.

39. Kawakami Y, et al. Relations of oxygen delivery, mixed venous oxygenation and pulmonary hemodynamics to prognosis in chronic obstructive pulmonary disease. *N Engl J Med* 308:1045, 1983.

40. Klinger JR, Hill NS. Right ventricular dysfunction in chronic obstructive pulmonary disease. *Chest* 99:715, 1991.

41. Krayenbuehl HP, Turina J, Hess O. Left ventricular function in chronic pulmonary hypertension. *Am J Cardiol* 41:1150, 1978.

42. Laks MM, Morady F, Swan HJC. Canine right and left ventricular sarcomere lengths after banding of the pulmonary artery. *Circ Res* 24:705, 1969.

43. MacNee W, et al. The effects of controlled oxygen therapy on ventricular function in patients with stable and decompensated cor pulmonale. *Am Rev Respir Dis* 137:1289, 1988.

44. Mahler DA, et al. Right ventricular performance and central circulatory hemodynamics during upright exercise in patients with chronic obstructive pulmonary disease. *Am Rev Respir Dis* 130:722, 1984.

45. March HW, Ross JK, Lower RR. Observations on the behavior of the right ventricular outflow tract, with reference to its developmental origins. *Am J Med* 32:835, 1962.

46. Mathur PN, et al. Effect of digoxin on right ventricular function in severe chronic airflow obstruction. *Ann Intern Med* 95:283, 1981.

47. Matthay RA. Effects of theophyllin on cardiovascular performance in chronic obstructive pulmonary disease. *Chest* 88:1125, 1985.

48. Matthay RA, Berger HJ. Cardiovascular function in cor pulmonale. *Clin Chest Med* 4:269, 1983.

49. Matthay RA, et al. Right and left ventricular exercise performance in chronic obstructive pulmonary disease: radionuclide assessment. *Ann Intern Med* 93:234, 1980.

50. Matthay RA, et al. Improvement in cardiac performance by oral long-acting theophyllin in chronic obstructive pulmonary disease. *Am Heart J* 104:1022, 1982.

51. Matthay RA, Niederman MS, Weidemann HP. Cardiovascular-pulmonary interaction in chronic obstructive pulmonary disease with special reference to the pathogenesis and management of cor pulmonale. *Med Clin North Am* 74:571, 1990.

52. Maughan WL, Oikawa RY. Right Ventricular Function. In SM Scharf, SS Cassidy (Eds), *Heart-Lung Interactions in Health and Disease*. New York: Marcel Dekker, 1989. Pp 179–220.

53. McCarthy PM, et al. Improved survival after heart-lung transplantation. *J Thorac Cardiovasc Surg* 99:54, 1990.

54. McFadden ER, Braunwald E. Cor Pulmonale. In E Braunwald (Ed), *Heart Disease—A Textbook of Cardiovascular Medicine*. Philadelphia: Saunders, 1992. Pp 1581–1601.

55. McGinn S, White PD. Acute cor pulmonale resulting from pulmonary embolism. *JAMA* 104:1473, 1935.

56. Melot C, et al. Improvement in ventilation-perfusion matching by almitrine in COPD. *Chest* 83:528, 1983.

57. Molloy WD, et al. Treatment of shock in a canine model of pulmonary embolism. *Am Rev Respir Dis* 130:870, 1984.

58. Murphy ML, Dinh H, Nichelson D. Chronic cor pulmonale. *Dis Mon* 35(10):653, 1989.

59. Nicholas WJ, Liebson PR. ECG changes in COPD: What do they mean? Part I: Atrial and ventricular abnormalities. *J Respir Dis* 8:13, 1987.

60. Nicholas WJ, Liebson PR. ECG changes in COPD: What do they mean? Part II: Right ventricular and biventricular hypertrophy and low voltage. *J Respir Dis* 8:103, 1987.

61. Niederman MS, Matthay RA. Cardiovascular function in secondary pulmonary hypertension. *Heart Lung* 15:341, 1986.

62. Olvey SK, et al. First-pass radionuclide assessment of right and left ventricular ejection fraction in chronic pulmonary disease: Effect of oxygen upon exercise response. *Chest* 78:4, 1980.

63. Pace JB, et al. Influence of sympathetic nerve stimulation on right ventricular outflow tract pressures in anesthetized dogs. *Circ Res* 24:397, 1969.

64. Pasque MK, et al. Single-lung transplantation for

pulmonary hypertension. Three-month hemodynamic follow-up. *Circulation* 84:2275, 1991.

65. Phillips RW. The electrocardiogram in cor pulmonale secondary to pulmonary emphysema: A study of 18 cases proved by autopsy. *Am Heart J* 56:352, 1958.

66. Popp RL, et al. Estimation of right and left ventricular size by ultrasound. A study of echos from the interventricular septum. *Am J Cardiol* 24:523, 1969.

67. Rao BS, et al. Left ventricular failure secondary to chronic pulmonary disease. *Am J Med* 45:229, 1968.

68. Reitz BA, et al. Heart-lung transplantation: Successful therapy for patients with pulmonary vascular disease. *N Engl J Med* 306:557, 1982.

69. Scharf SM. Cardiovascular effects of airways obstruction. *Lung* 169:1, 1991.

70. Scharf SM, et al. Load tolerance of the right ventricle: Effect of increased aortic pressure. *J Crit Care* 1:163, 1986.

71. Schrijen F, et al. Pulmonary and systemic hemodynamic evolution in chronic bronchitis. *Am Rev Respir Dis* 117:25, 1978.

72. Schulman DS, et al. Coronary flow limits right ventricular performance during positive end-expiratory pressure. *Am Rev Respir Dis* 141:1531, 1990.

73. Shih HT, Webb CR, Conway WA. Frequency and significance of cardiac arrhythmias in chronic obstructive lung disease. *Chest* 94:44, 1988.

74. Steele P, et al. Left ventricular ejection fraction in severe chronic obstructive airways disease. *Am J Med* 59:21, 1975.

75. Stuart-Harris C, Flenley DC, Bishop JH. British Medical Research Council Working Party: Long-term domiciliary oxygen therapy in chronic hyp-

oxic cor pulmonale complicating bronchitis and emphysema. *Lancet* 1:681, 1981.

76. Timms RM, et al. Hemodynamic response to oxygen therapy in chronic obstructive pulmonary disease. *Ann Intern Med* 102:29, 1985.

77. Vlahakes GJ, Turley K, Hoffman JIE. The pathophysiology of failure in acute right ventricular hypertension: Hemodynamic and biochemical correlations. *Circulation* 63:87, 1981.

78. Weideman HP, Matthay RA. The Management of Cor Pulmonale. In SM Scharf, SS Cassidy (Eds), *Heart-Lung Interactions in Health and Disease*. New York: Marcel Dekker, 1989. Pp 915–981.

79. Weisse AB. Contralateral effects of cardiac disease affecting either the left or right chambers of the heart. *Am Heart J* 87:654, 1974.

80. Weitzenblum E, et al. Course of pulmonary hemodynamics in patients with chronic obstructive pulmonary disease. *Chest* 75:656, 1979.

81. Weitzenblum E, et al. Long-term course of pulmonary arterial pressure in chronic obstructive pulmonary disease. *Am Rev Respir Dis* 130:993, 1984.

82. Weitzenblum E, et al. Long-term oxygen therapy can reverse the progression of pulmonary hypertension in patients with chronic obstructive pulmonary disease. *Am Rev Respir Dis* 131:493, 1985.

83. Weyman AE, et al. Mechanism of abnormal septal motion in patients with right ventricular volume overload. *Circulation* 54:179, 1976.

84. Wyse RKH, et al. Cardiac performance and myocardial blood flow in pigs with compensated right ventricular hypertrophy. *Cardiovasc Res* 18:733, 1985.

VIII

Neoplastic Diseases

53

Bronchogenic Carcinoma

Israel Bruderman

Lung cancer is the most common cancer in humans in the Western world, and in recent years, a most alarming increase in the incidence has been recognized in women. This increase in morbidity and mortality from lung cancer is in spite of the advances in diagnostic procedures and management of this disease. The results of treatment of pulmonary neoplasms are discouraging, since the 5-year survival rate is still very low, and this in spite of the advances in surgical techniques and postoperative care. The increase in smoking habits among women in recent years resulted in an "epidemic" of lung cancer, and it is now the leading cause of female cancer death in the United States [178]. The association of cigarette smoking with lung cancer has been known for more than 50 years [41]. It is most depressing, therefore, that the great efforts and expense connected with the medical and surgical treatment of lung cancer are still unsuccessful in a disease which in a majority of the cases is preventable.

Incidence and Etiology

Cancer of the lung has been the leading cause of cancer death among men in the United States since the 1950s. Mortality rates for this disease have increased from 4.9 per 100,000 in 1930 to 71.6 per 100,000 in 1980 for men, and there has been a tenfold increase among women for the same period of time (Fig. 53-1). Mortality rates for lung cancer were higher among whites than among nonwhites in the 1960s, whereas in the 1970s and 1980s mortality rates for nonwhite males surpassed those of white males. The average female rates were similar in whites and nonwhites [216].

In recent years, the rate of increase in age-adjusted lung cancer among American men has been leveling off, and under the age of 50 it has shown an actual decline. On the other hand, in women, age-adjusted rates have continued to show a dramatic increase, especially at age 45 and above. Accordingly, the age-adjusted lung cancer mortality rates for American women increased 337 percent over the years 1950–1980.

Smoking and Lung Cancer

The association of smoking and lung cancer is well known from many retrospective and prospective studies in humans [163,194,196,197,198]. These studies also showed the increased relative risks for this disease in smokers versus nonsmokers, and it is agreed that among men, the overall risk of lung cancer in smokers is about 10 times that of nonsmokers [195]. In the United States, it is estimated that 85 to 90 percent of lung cancer cases among men and 70 percent [44] among women are attributable to cigarette smoking. The epidemiologic data on smoking and lung cancer fulfill the criteria for causal association, and these are consistency of results in various studies, the time sequence between exposure and disease, the specificity, and a dose-response relationship.

The smoking prevalence for men was somewhat higher than 50 percent from the 1930s to the 1950s, while about a third of women were regular smokers during the same period. In men, smoking prevalence since that time decreased markedly to 36.9 percent in 1979, while among women, the decrease was relatively slight from 33.3 to 28.2 percent [196]. However, smoking prevalence is not a sufficient indicator of smoking patterns. The age of initiation, the number and type of cigarettes smoked, the tar and nicotine content of the cigarettes, the use of filtered or nonfiltered cigarettes, and inhalation practices are all important risk factors. These may well explain the possible differences between men and women vis-à-vis the relationship between smoking and lung

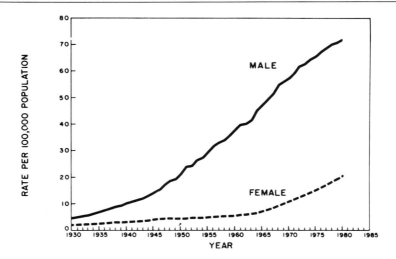

cancer. Although there is a decreasing tendency of smoking prevalence in recent years, the total lifetime exposure to cigarette smoking has increased, especially for later-born cohorts of women, the estimated age of onset being now at 15 to 16 years for cohorts of women born between 1950 and 1960, as opposed to 35 years for those born in 1900 [196]. This also may explain the time lag in the lung cancer explosion among women in recent years, as indicated by the time sequence between exposure and disease. Allowing for a time lag of 20 years, lung cancer rates followed and paralleled smoking prevalence first in men and later in women (Fig. 53-2). Accord-

Fig. 53-1. Age-adjusted lung cancer mortality rates, 1930 to 1980, United States, males and females. Standardized for age on the 1970 population of the United States. (Reproduced with permission from the Department of Epidemiology and Statistics, American Cancer Society.)

Fig. 53-2. Trends in smoking prevalence and lung cancer, British males and females. The data for this chart are for England and Wales. In men, smoking (○) began to increase at the beginning of the twentieth century, but the corresponding trend in deaths from lung cancer (●) did not begin until after 1920. In women, smoking (□) began later, and the increase in lung cancer deaths in women (■) has only appeared recently. (Reprinted with permission from LA Loeb et al. Smoking and lung cancer: An overview. *Cancer Res* 44:5940, 1984.)

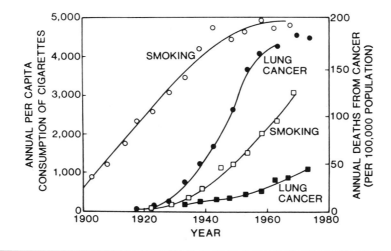

ingly, the lung cancer mortality rates today among women are slightly lower than those of men 25 years ago, reflecting again the lag of smoking patterns by women and suggesting similar risks in both sexes [196].

In the last 20 years, an increase in the proportion of heavy smokers has been noted, while the decreasing trend in smoking prevalence continues (Fig. 53-3). For example, only 13 percent of women smoked 25 or more cigarettes daily in 1965; this number almost doubled by 1979. During the same time period, the consumption of filter-tipped and low-tar cigarettes increased markedly, particularly among women. This may to some extent explain the average increase in the number of cigarettes smoked daily as a compensation for the low tar and nicotine content of cigarettes.

The smoking behaviors among teenage boys and girls are of great concern, since surveys indicated a steady increase in smoking since the 1960s. National survey data from 1979 showed a higher smoking rate among girls in the subgroup ages 17 to 18 years—26.2 versus 19.3 percent for boys of the same age group [196]. This relatively high smoking rate among teenagers is a most disturbing phenomenon, since early initiation is associated with heavier smoking, the attempts to stop smoking are very difficult, and the exposure time at the age of 30 to 40 is 15 to 20 years. This long exposure to cigarette smoking will no doubt have an influence on lung cancer mortality at the end of this century. It is reassuring, however, that in 1985 the smoking rate among high school seniors decreased significantly.

The association between passive smoking and impaired or decreased pulmonary function among children exposed to their parents' cigarette smoke or of nonsmoking adults of either sex exposed to cigarette smoke of spouses is well known [107,185,198,207]. Several studies reported on a possible association of lung cancer with exposure to passive (involuntary, sidestream) smoking [32,36,66,192]. The most impressive is the large prospective study of Hirayama [91,92], indicating elevated rates of lung cancer in nonsmoking wives of husbands who smoked when compared to nonsmoking wives of nonsmoking husbands. All these studies are very suggestive of a positive association between lung cancer and passive smoking, but they are not conclusive. They do raise a concern, however, about a possible serious public health problem [195].

Early Lung Cancer Detection

The great difficulties encountered in the management of lung cancer, the very low "curability" rate, and the poor prognosis of this disease are due to the fact that in the vast majority of patients the disease has already spread at the time the patient seeks medical help. Therefore, it is logical to assume that early detection screening might improve the grim outlook of this disease. In the past, early screening studies by chest roentgenography were ineffective in lowering mortality from this disease [3,122,206]. In the 1970s, a prospective study of 31,360 male heavy smokers aged 45 and over was initiated at Johns Hopkins [63], Memorial Sloan-Kettering [60], and the Mayo Clinic [61] in order to determine the effectiveness of chest x-ray and sputum cytology screening techniques in the early detection of lung cancer and whether these types of screening procedures can reduce significantly lung cancer mortality. The addition of sputum cytology to chest x-ray screening tests did not provide a better early detection of cancer of the lung.

There were 223 pathologically confirmed lung cancers detected among the 31,360 participants at the three institutions. Of these confirmed lung

Fig. 53-3. Trends in smoking prevalence, 1930s to present, United States, males and females. ————, prevalence of regular cigarette smoking among United States adults; -------, estimated percentage of adult regular smokers who smoked brands with less than 15 mg of "tar"; ⋯⋯⋯, estimated percentage of adult smokers who smoked 25 cigarettes or more daily. (*Source:* United States Surgeon General [196].)

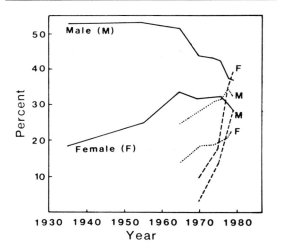

cancers, 160 were discovered by the dual screening technique, 123 cancers (77 percent) were detected roentgenographically, and 37 (23 percent) were detected by cytologic testing alone. Sputum cytology was highly specific in the detection of squamous cell cancers (35 of 37), especially those involving the subsegmental and larger, centrally located bronchi. In the dual-screen group, nearly twice as many lung cancer cases were detected by x-ray as by cytology and the chest roentgenogram was the better test for detection of adenocarcinomas located peripherally. Stage I cancers, which are potentially curable, are effectively detected by either the chest x-ray or the sputum cytology screening tests, while stage III cancers are mostly detected by chest films (Table 53-1). The percentages of patients with stage I or stage III cancer detected by both dual and x-ray screening methods are almost the same—47 percent for stage I and 45 percent for stage III lung cancers. This relatively high percentage of stage III patients proves again that chest x-ray and sputum cytology tests are still inadequate to detect the majority of patients in stage I when the disease might be curable.

On the other hand, the survival figures for the dual-screen and x-ray only are most impressive (33 to 35 percent) (Fig. 53-4) when compared to cancer survival data derived from the general population (15 percent) using a similar method of analysis [11,60,61,63,143]. However, this comparison cannot be interpreted as indicating that screening has an impact on mortality from lung cancer for the following reasons: First, a prevalence screen examines a population with slow-growing cancers, while rapidly growing tumors progress very quickly from initial diagnosis/

symptoms to death; thus they are undetected in a prevalence population. This explains the small number of small-cell carcinomas found in prevalence screening. Second, early asymptomatic cases picked up by screening have the lead time to appearance of symptoms added to their observed survival. Third, it is probable that some of the patients whose lung cancers were detected

Fig. 53-4. Survival from the time of lung cancer diagnosis by study group. The Kaplan-Meier method is used. Deaths caused by second primary lung cancers are indicated by X, deaths from other causes are indicated by diamonds, and survival times of patients who are still alive are represented by vertical bars. The number of cases appears in parentheses.

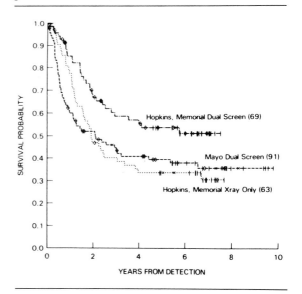

Table 53-1. Confirmed lung cancer cases classified by screening group, method of detection, and stage

Method of detection	Stage I (n)	Stage I (%)	Stage II (n)	Stage II (%)	Stage III (n)	Stage III (%)	Total (n)	Total (%)
Dual screen group*								
X-ray only	44	47	8	9	41	44	93	100
Cytology only	30	81	2	6	5	14	37	100
X-ray and cytology	7	23	2	7	21	70	30	100
Total	81	51	12	8	67	42	160	100
X-ray-only group[†]	24	38	5	8	34	54	63	100
Total	105	47	17	8	101	45	223	100

*Includes cases from Hopkins, Memorial and Mayo.
[†]Includes only cases from Hopkins and Memorial.
Source: From MR Melamed et al., Early lung cancer detection: Summary and conclusions. *Am Rev Respir Dis* 130:565, 1984.

by screening who are still alive today after successful resection would have died of their disease had they not been screened. Therefore, only these patients would have a positive impact on lung cancer mortality.

The survival of the 223 prevalence cases by means of detection showed a very high (85 percent) 5-year survival rate for those detected by sputum cytology only as compared to a 33 percent survival rate for those detected by x-ray (Fig. 53-5). This proves again that most tumors when detected radiologically are already disseminated. Figures 53-6 and 53-7 demonstrate clearly the importance of the stage and cell type of the lung tumor on the survival rate. While stage I lung tumors treated by surgical resection have an 80 percent 5-year survival rate, less than 10 percent of the patients will survive for 5 years with stage III lung cancer. Similarly, patients with squamous cell carcinoma have an estimated 5-year survival rate of almost 70 percent, while only 25 percent with large-cell carcinoma or adenocarcinoma survive 5 years. None of the patients with small-

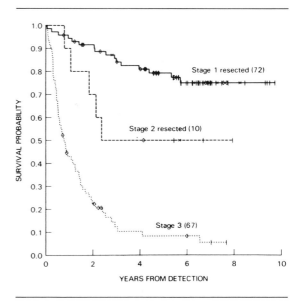

Fig. 53-6. Survival from the time of lung cancer diagnosis by AJCC stage. Cases from the dual-screen group at the three institutions are combined. Symbols are as in Fig. 53-4. (*Source:* See Fig. 53-5.)

Fig. 53-5. Survival from time of lung cancer diagnosis by means of detection. Results from the three institutions are combined. Symbols are as in Fig. 53-4. (Reprinted from JL Young et al. *Surveillance, Epidemiology, and End Results: Incidence and Mortality Data 1973–1977* [National Cancer Institute Monograph 57]. Bethesda, Md: US Dept of Health and Human Services, 1981.)

Fig. 53-7. Survival from the time of lung cancer diagnosis by cell type. Cases from the dual-screen group at the three institutions are combined. Symbols are as in Fig. 53-4. (*Source:* See Fig. 53-5.)

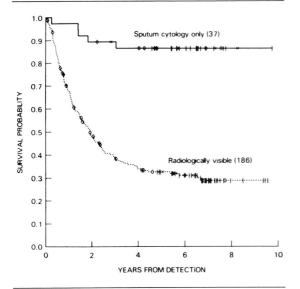

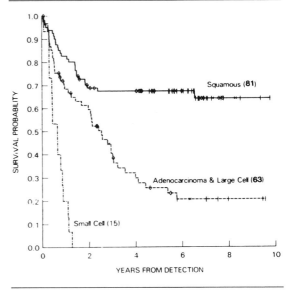

cell carcinoma survived as long as 2 years (Fig. 53-7).

Pathology and Classification

The correct choice of treatment and the assessment of prognosis of carcinoma of the lung are related to tumor size, the extent of tumor spread, its histologic cell type, and the anatomic location of the growth, that is, central or peripheral. Most malignant tumors of the lung have an infiltrative pattern of growth. At the beginning, the tumor spreads along the bronchus within the mucosa. At this time, the tumor may be visualized during bronchoscopy as a mucosal plaque, as an irregular, warty pattern, or as a focal luminal narrowing. At this stage, only a biopsy specimen will determine whether the mucosal irregularity is a carcinoma in situ or a malignant tumor invading the bronchial wall, adjacent lymphoid tissue, and alveolar parenchyma.

The classification of epithelial tumors of the lung is difficult, and none of the present classifications [29,129] is ideal. From all the recent classifications (based on the 1967 WHO classification, Table 53-2), the most satisfactory for the pathologist and the clinician is the Edinburgh 1982 (Table 53-3) classification for the following

Table 53-2. **Histologic typing of lung tumors WHO 1967**

I. Epidermoid carcinomas
II. Small cell anaplastic carcinomas
  1. Fusiform cell type
  2. Polygonal cell type
  3. Lymphocyte-like ('oat-cell') type
  4. Others
III. Adenocarcinomas
  1. Bronchogenic
    a. acinar   ⎰ with or without
    b. papillary   ⎱ mucin formation
IV. Large cell carcinomas
  1. Solid tumours with mucin-like content
  2. Solid tumours without mucin-like content
  3. Giant cell carcinomas
  4. 'Clear' cell carcinomas
V. Combined epidermoid and adenocarcinomas
VI. Carcinoid tumours
VII. Bronchial gland tumours
  1. Cylindromas
  2. Mucoepidermoid tumours
  3. Others

Source: D Lamb, The Pathology and Classification of Lung Cancer. In JF Smith (Ed), *The Management of Lung Cancer.* London: Edward Arnold, 1984.

reasons: First, it improves the compatibility between pathologists by describing criteria and rules for attribution of the different cell types. Accordingly, it enables the pathologist to differentiate between large-cell undifferentiated carcinoma (4/1 in Table 53-3) and the least differentiated squamous cell or adenocarcinoma (1/4 and 3/4 in Table 53-3), as well as between small-cell carcinoma (2/2 and 4/1 in Table 53-3) and large-cell undifferentiated carcinoma (Figs. 53-8 and 53-9). The differentiation between those two types of lung carcinoma is particularly important in view of the distinctive treatment of small-cell carcinoma. Second, the subdivision of squamous cell carcinomas and adenocarcinomas into well, moderate, and poorly differentiated enables the clinician to make an intelligent decision vis-à-vis the appropriate type of treatment and in many instances to avoid unnecessary surgery and radical chemotherapy. However, not even the Edinburgh 1982 classification of lung tumors is perfect, since like all the other classifications, it is based on limited parameters at the light-microscope level and the classification is based solely on the presence or absence of squamous and glandular differentiation and cell size.

In recent years, some progress has been made in ultrastructural and immunocytochemical studies of lung tumors, especially in separation of neuroendocrine oat cell carcinomas from the small variety of squamous cell carcinoma and in relating subtypes of adenocarcinomas to tumor behavior. Also, ultrastructural criteria were developed to diagnose mesothelioma versus primary lung carcinoma and to identify so-called metastatic neoplasms, primarily adenocarcinomas, as being primary carcinomas of the lung [89].

The ultrastructural and immunocytochemical studies in animal and human lungs have shown that cell populations in the normal bronchial mucosa can undergo various phenotypic changes and even a single cell type can apparently show a range of phenotypic expression from a predominantly mucous cell with a few tonofilaments to a keratinizing cell that still retains markers of its original mucin production [81]. Multiple phenotypes appear to be expressed not only in normal but also in the preneoplastic bronchial epithelium. Accordingly, current evidence supports the thesis that many lung carcinomas at the ultrastructural level contain both squamous and mucous features, expressing the mixed phenotypic patterns [22]. This can explain the difficulties encountered when using only the light microscope

Table 53-3. **Edinburgh classification of epithelial tumors of the lung (June 1982)**

Cell type 10 Squamous carcinoma

1/1 well differentiated—much keratinization (evident in up to 50 percent of islands of tissue)

1/2 moderately differentiated—less obvious keratinization but more than 1/3

1/3 poorly differentiated—very occasional squamous pearl of single cell keratinization, or cells with dense margins and obvious prickles. (Allocation of borderline cases: if pattern is consistent throughout—give higher group, but if patchy, e.g., an area of 1/2 other areas 1/3, bias case down to 1/3)

1/4 'undifferentiated' (squamoid)—shows stratification and resembles 1/3 but does not show prickles or keratinizing cells. (This group may be found under the heading undifferentiated large cell carcinoma in some classifications)

Cell type 20 Small cell carcinoma

2/1 oat cell carcinoma showing classical oat or lymphocyte-like pattern

2/2 intermediate type—a tumour composed of cells having nuclei similar to type 2/1 but with more abundant cytoplasm. The cells may be polygonal or fusiform and less regular in appearance, but the cell size may not be small and may show ribboning or rosettes

2/3 combined oat cell carcinoma—a tumour in which there is obvious oat cell carcinoma with focal squamous and/or adenocarcinomatous areas

Cell type 30 Adenocarcinoma

3/1 well differentiated—predominantly formed by obvious acinar formation, some of which may be cribriform

3/2 moderately differentiated—less marked glandular formation, includes cribriform pattern, gland formations in less than 50 percent of HP fields—but more than in 3/3

3/3 poorly differentiated—scanty glandular spaces less than 1 per 10 HP field—needs searching for!

3/4 undifferentiated adenocarcinoma showing no glandular differentiation but the presence of intracellular mucin production. (This group may be found under heading large cell carcinoma with mucin production in some alternative classifications)

3/5 broncho-alveolar

Cell type 40 Undifferentiated large cell carcinoma

4/1 large cell undifferentiated carcinoma (not showing stratification, mucin production, or any glandular differentiation). Cells, large, rounded with round to oval nuclei and often prominent nucleoli

Cell type 50 Tumours showing mixed differentiation

5/1 Adeno-squamous—tumours showing squamous and glandular differentiation in the same tumour, or squames and mucin without glands

5/2 other, including possible collision tumours, e.g., oat and squame, or oat and adeno

Cell type 60 Carcinoid tumours

6/1 classical carcinoid tumours

6/2 atypical ('malignant') carcinoid tumours showing features of carcinoid tumours but with cellular pleomorphism, necrosis, increased mitotic rate but not showing features of small cell carcinoma

Cell type 70 Bronchial gland carcinomas

7/1 adenoid cystic carcinoma

7/2 muco-epidermoid carcinoma

7/3 other

Cell type 80 Miscellaneous epithelial tumours

8/1 giant cell carcinoma

8/2 clear cell carcinoma

8/3 carcinosarcoma

8/4 spindle cell variant of squamous carcinoma

Cell type 90 Undiagnosable patterns (not conforming to the above types)

includes those in which difficulty is found in attribution to any of the groups

Comment: Subgroups 1/1 to 1/3 may be amalgamated, as may subgroups 3/1 to 3/3. Groups 1/4 and 3/4 must be kept separate to aid comparison with other classifications. Subgroups 6/1 and 6/2 must also be kept separate

Source: See Table 53-2.

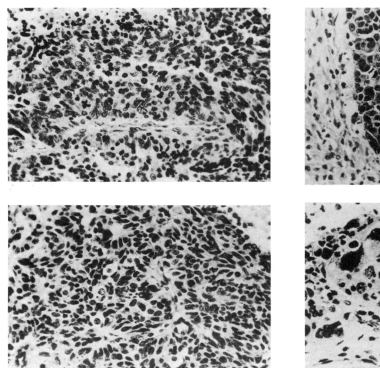

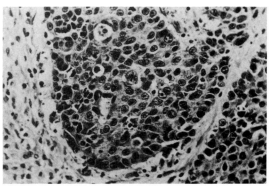

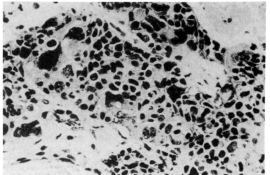

Fig. 53-8. Both show small-cell carcinoma of intermediate cell type, subgroup 2B in the WHO (1981) classification or 2/2 in the Edinburgh classification. The cells show more cytoplasm and a more irregular pattern, and may be significantly larger than in the classic types (hematoxylin and eosin; × 320). (Reprinted with permission from JF Smith. *The Management of Lung Cancer.* London: Edward Arnold, 1984.)

Fig. 53-9. (*Top*) A large-cell carcinoma not showing any mucin production or stratification, an example of group 4 in the WHO (1981) classification of undifferentiated large-cell carcinoma, group 4/1 in the Edinburgh classification. (*Bottom*) A tumor with large, pleomorphic cells. This is another area from the tumor illustrated as an example of a small-cell carcinoma of intermediate type. Such large-celled areas do not prohibit the diagnosis of small-cell carcinoma but may pose problems for diagnosis based on small biopsy specimens (hematoxylin and eosin; × 320). (Reprinted with permission from JF Smith. *The Management of Lung Cancer.* London: Edward Arnold, 1984.)

in classifying the small-cell anaplastic, large-cell anaplastic, and poorly differentiated squamous carcinomas and adenocarcinomas (Figs. 53-10 and 53-11).

Current evidence supports the thesis that most large-cell carcinomas, when studied ultrastructurally, are poorly differentiated adenocarcinomas [89]. In the case of small-cell anaplastic and carcinoid tumors containing neurosecretory granules and producing peptide hormones, the assessment of histogenesis is difficult, since the normal Kulchitzky cells are present in small number as preneoplastic lesions in human bronchial mucosa. Recent observations, however, suggest

that goblet cells containing neurosecretory granules can express this phenotype, and thus the potential cells of origin for peptide hormone–associated tumors are the same as for all other lung tumors. It seems, therefore, that at the present time the ultrastructural analysis of lung tumors supports the statement that Willis [211] made more than 40 years ago: "There is only one entity, *carcinoma of the lung.*" Thus future classifica-

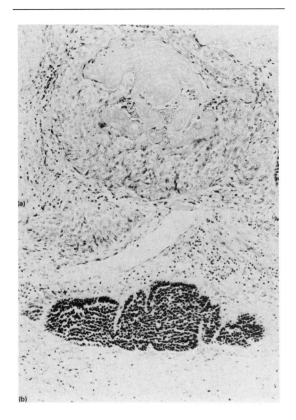

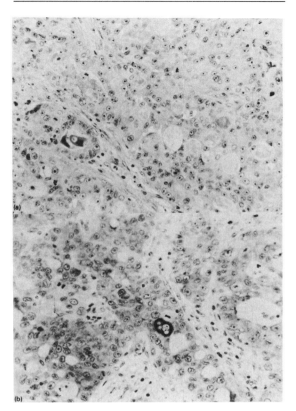

Fig. 53-10. This tumor consisted predominantly of intermediate-sized anaplastic cells arranged in a trabecular pattern with areas of keratin formation (*A*). Within this tumor there was a carcinoid-like focus with smaller cells arranged in definite trabeculae (*B*). On leveling, this region merged through cytologically intermediate areas to form a morphologic continuum with the larger anaplastic cells seen in the top left hand corner (hematoxylin and eosin; × 150). (Reprinted with permission from RL Carter. *Precancerous States.* New York: Oxford University Press, 1984.)

Fig. 53-11. Photomicrographs of a large-celled anaplastic carcinoma with mucin production. The majority of the mucin was cytoplasmic or in pools as shown by periodic acid–Schiff staining after diastase digestion (*A*). No clear ductal structures or acini were formed. (*B*) The same tumor stained immunocytochemically for keratin. The majority of cells contained keratin-like immunoreactive material and occasional mononuclear and multinucleate cells were strongly positive (× 250). (Reprinted with permission from RL Carter. *Precancerous States.* New York: Oxford University Press, 1984.)

tions of lung tumors will be based on the development of new markers of biologic significance that will rationalize the predicted response to treatment, as well as identify early precancerous states.

Structural Characterization of Lung Tumors

The classification of lung tumors is a complex one (see Table 53-3); however, 90 to 95 percent of all the pulmonary neoplasms fall into the four major types of epidermoid or squamous carcinoma, adenocarcinoma, small-cell carcinoma, and undifferentiated large-cell carcinoma. The relative frequency of these types varies at different centers. According to the National Cancer Institute Cooperative Early Lung Cancer Detection Program [60,61,63], the prevalence of squamous cell carcinoma is 39 to 45 percent, of adenocarcinoma 28 to 30 percent, and about 30 percent of tumors are small-cell and undifferentiated large-cell carcinomas. The type of treatment (surgical, chemotherapy, radiotherapy) and the prognosis depend very much on the differentiation of various cell types of which the tumor is composed [57]. Therefore, in the poorly differentiated lung carcinomas, the parameters available at the light microscope level are limited. In order to prevent unnecessary, and in some cases life-endangering, surgical interventions or "drastic" chemotherapy, ultrastructural characterization by electron microscopy in these cases is indicated. These four main types of pulmonary neoplasms are discussed here.

SQUAMOUS CELL CARCINOMA

These tumors occur mainly in the segmental, lobar, or mainstem bronchi and make up the majority of so-called central tumors. Occurring almost entirely in cigarette smokers, they are appreciably more common in men than in women. Compared with other malignant neoplasms of the lung, they are relatively slow growing and late to metastasize. By the time squamous cell tumors are discovered, they are generally large, bulky, and white with tiny yellow, necrotic, or larger, soft, central foci of yellow necrosis. Most are moderately desmoplastic and are firm or hard in consistency, but in as many as 10 percent there is central cavitation [27,128] (Fig. 53-12). Their growth pattern is that of spread along the bronchial wall with direct invasion of peribronchial lymph nodes and replacement of adjacent pulmonary parenchyma. They may obstruct the venae cavae by their invasive growth into the mediastinum or by sizable mediastinal node metastases, although the latter is a more common complication of oat cell carcinomas. Peripheral squamous carcinomas commonly invade the chest wall, and when situated near the apex, the brachial plexus and sympathetic chain may be involved, producing the syndrome described by Pancoast [148]. Microscopically, the spectrum of differentiation may be broad, even in the same tumor. Well-differentiated squamous carcinomas usually produce keratin, epithelial pearls, and a clearly squamous pattern (Fig. 53-13), while poorly differentiated squamous tumors have less obvious keratinization or cells with dense margins and obvious prickles.

Arising as they do as a consequence of the local irritating and carcinogenic effects of cigarette smoke, these tumors are preceded by focal squamous metaplasia, atypical proliferation, desmoplasia, carcinoma in situ, and microinvasion in

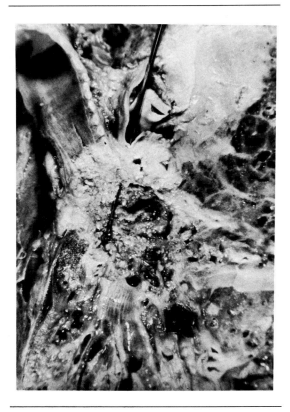

Fig. 53-12. Central cavitated squamous cell carcinoma of left lung. This tumor eroded into the adjacent pulmonary artery (*probe*), leading to fatal hemorrhage. (Reprinted with permission from WKC Morgan and MR Hales. Bronchogenic Carcinoma. In GL Baum and E Wolinsky (Eds), *Textbook of Pulmonary Diseases* (3rd ed). Boston: Little, Brown, 1983.)

that order [128]. Careful microscopic study of the lungs of cigarette smokers with squamous cell carcinoma may reveal all these changes focally in other bronchi [6]. In spite of this, grossly evident multiple squamous cell carcinomas are uncommon.

Metastases of squamous cell carcinomas are initially to hilar and mediastinal lymph nodes and then to the liver, adrenals, bones, and brain. Occasionally, a large tumor with extensive mediastinal lymph node metastases will still be free of demonstrable distant metastases at the time of the patient's death.

Electron microscopic examination reveals that squamous cell carcinomas are characterized by electron-lucent cytoplasm rich in organelles and

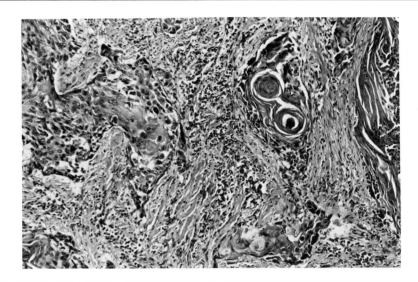

Fig. 53-13. Well-differentiated squamous cell carcinoma with two keratinized epithelial pearls. There are numerous lymphocytes and plasma cells in the desmoplastic stroma. (*Source:* See Fig. 53-12.)

by variable numbers of tonofilament bundles (Fig. 53-14). With less differentiated tumors, the number of tonofilament bundles decreases and the cytoplasmic appearance is more electron dense due to increased numbers of polyribosomes. Keratin immunocytostaining is positive in these squamous cell carcinomas; however, such positivity also may be present in adenosquamous carcinomas, other epithelial tumors, and epithelial mesotheliomas. Ultrastructural analysis is particularly useful in diagnosing the spindle cell variant of squamous cell carcinoma and in differentiating this type of carcinoma from pulmonary sarcoma or spindle cell carcinoid. Some neoplasms diagnosed by light microscopy as large-cell carcinomas or undifferentiated pulmonary carcinomas are diagnosed ultrastructurally as squamous cell carcinomas. On the other hand, squamous differentiation can be identified in otherwise typical pulmonary adenocarcinomas [22]. Therefore, the ultrastructural finding has to be correlated with the light microscopic findings before the final diagnosis of squamous cell carcinoma is made, since the squamous cell component may represent focal squamous differentiation in another type of neoplasm.

SMALL-CELL CARCINOMA (OAT CELL CARCINOMA)

Approximately one-fifth of all primary lung tumors are small-cell carcinomas. The majority of these tumors originate in the major bronchi at or near the hilum (Fig. 53-15). The most striking difference between small-cell carcinoma and other forms of malignant lung neoplasms is the aggressiveness of this tumor, resulting in a more rapid growth and early local and distant metastasis via the lymphatic and blood vessels. This behavior of the small-cell carcinoma renders surgical treatment inappropriate. On the other hand, this tumor is sensitive to chemotherapy and radiotherapy. This sensitivity has led to new treatment programs which have resulted in a significant change in the prognosis of these patients during the last 10 years.

Macroscopically, the small-cell carcinomas and their metastases are homogeneous and soft in consistency and have shiny gray cut surfaces. Microscopically, the malignant cells have scanty cytoplasm and hyperchromatic nuclei and several nucleoli. The cells are round, ovoid, or spindle-shaped, and accordingly, several subtypes are known. The classic small-cell carcinoma is the oat cell carcinoma consisting of lymphocyte-like cells growing in sheets or nests in a sparse connective-tissue stroma. The intermediate type is composed of polygonal or fusiform cells, quite large in size, which may show rosettes. The cytoplasm is more abundant, and the nuclei are

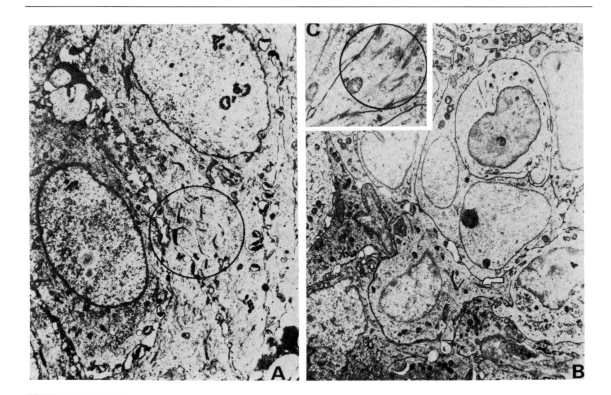

Fig. 53-14. Squamous cell carcinoma. *A, B.* Note the overall low-power ultrastructural appearance of this squamous cell carcinoma. Note prominent nucleoli and evenly dispersed nuclear chromatin. *A.* Note (within the circle) the well-formed desmosomes joining apposing outpouchings of adjacent cells and clusters of tonofilaments in the neighborhood of the intercellular junctions, as well as in paranuclear location. *B.* Note that only a few scattered bundles of tonofilaments are identifiable. *C.* Note the well-formed desmosomes joining apposing cellular membranes and nearby clusters of tonofilaments ($A \times$ 10,000; $B \times$ 7500; $C \times$ 22,000). (Reprinted with permission from Herrera et al. Ultrastructural characterization of pulmonary neoplasms. *Surv Synth Pathol Respir* 3:520, 1984.)

similar to those seen in oat cell carcinoma. The various subtypes of small-cell carcinoma often represent a major problem to the pathologist in differentiating them from large-cell undifferentiated carcinoma, squamous cell carcinomas with small cells, and carcinoid tumors. Since the treatment and prognosis of small-cell carcinoma differ significantly from the non–small-cell carcinomas, a precise diagnosis is most desirable.

Electron microscopy is of great help in differentiating the various neoplasms. In the typical oat cell carcinoma, the cells have evenly dispersed chromatin, small nucleoli, slight amounts of cytoplasm with well-defined cytoplasmic processes (Fig. 53-16), and few membrane-bound neuroendocrine granules [69]. On the other hand, the small variety of squamous cell carcinoma usually shows prominent heterochromatin aggregates and nucleoli. There are no membrane-bound neurosecretory granules, and tonofilament bundles are present in the cytoplasm.

Differentiation of small-cell neuroendocrine carcinomas from atypical malignant carcinoid tumors poses another problem, because of overlap [70,105,

106,204]. The typical carcinoid tumor is characterized ultrastructurally by numerous granules diffusely distributed throughout the cytoplasmic matrix, generally uniformly ovoid to round, and larger than in small-cell carcinoma (Fig. 53-17). Desmosomes are not uncommon in carcinoid tumor, and prominent nucleoli are seen as compared to few desmosomes and rare nucleoli in small-cell carcinoma. Regarding the origin of the neuro-

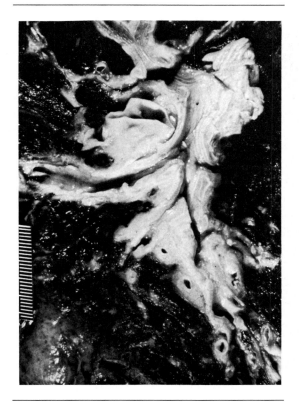

Fig. 53-15. Small-cell anaplastic carcinoma arising in the distal portion of the right intermediate bronchus and extending both proximally and distally along the bronchovascular rays. Although small in mass, this tumor was responsible for widespread metastases, inappropriate ACTH secretion, adrenal cortical hyperplasia, and death from severe intractable hypokalemia. (*Source:* See Fig. 53-12.)

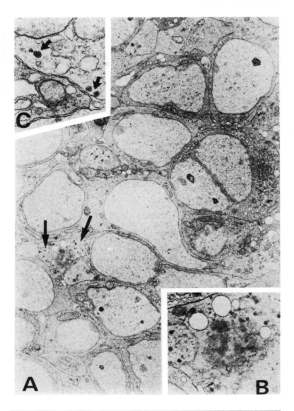

Fig. 53-16. Small- (oat) cell neuroendocrine carcinoma. *A.* Note the overall low-power ultrastructural appearance of this neuroendocrine (small-cell) carcinoma with cells showing evenly dispersed nuclear chromatin, small or absent nucleoli, and interdigitating cytoplasmic processes with aggregates of membrane-bound granules varying in size from 60 to 240 nm. *B, C.* Note the details of the aggregates of membrane-bound granules within the cytoplasmic processes. *A.* These processes are marked with arrows, and the granules (*C*) are also marked with arrows (*A* × 7500; *B* × 17,500; *C* × 22,000). (*Source:* See Fig. 53-14.)

endocrine small-cell carcinomas and carcinoid tumors, it is assumed that they arise from the Kulchitsky-type cells existing among the exocrine cells of the bronchial submucosal glands and among the cells lining bronchi and bronchioles [9,10,15]. Lamy and colleagues [116] suggested, however, because of the presence of several cell types within the same tumors, that small-cell carcinomas, squamous carcinomas, and adenocarcinomas may have a common origin, a multipotential epithelial stem cell. This concept contradicts the suggestion that neuroendocrine tumors derive from Kulchitsky-type cells [28,71, 116,166,167,213].

ADENOCARCINOMA

About one-third of all malignant lung neoplasms are adenocarcinomas, and their relative incidence appears to be increasing, especially among women, in whom this tumor represents about 40 percent of the total [82,201]. In contrast to squamous cell and small-cell carcinomas, adenocarcinomas arise mostly in the periphery of lung parenchyma, often in relation to focal scars, or in

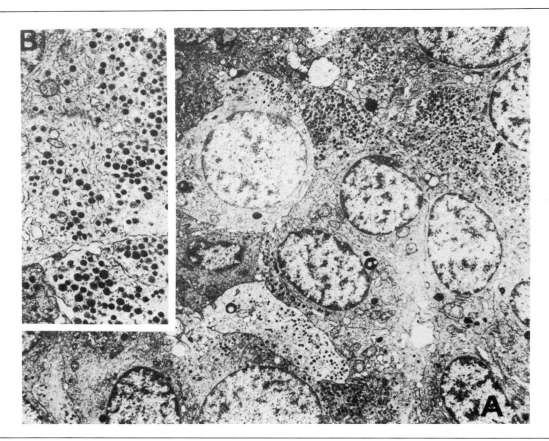

Fig. 53-17. Typical carcinoid tumor. *A.* Note the overall ultrastructural appearance of this typical carcinoid tumor. A monotonous cellular proliferation with regular ovoid to round nuclei without evidence of nuclear atypicality is observed. Also note the diffuse granularity within the cells. *B.* Note the homogeneous round and uniform membrane-bound granules (*A* × 7600; *B* × 10,000). (*Source:* See Fig. 53-14.)

regions of interstitial fibrosis [131]. Tumors with abundant mucus and little stroma are relatively soft and gelatinous in consistency and appearance, while desmoplastic tumors with little mucus production are gray, dense, and firm and resemble the usual squamous cell carcinoma. In general, the less differentiated the tumor, the more cellular and desmoplastic are the stroma [128]. Although adenocarcinomas are usually slow-growing tumors, they invade lymphatics and blood vessels early and thus produce early metastases. The invasive behavior of this tumor is the cause for the lower 5-year survival rate as compared to squamous cell carcinoma.

Microscopically, the well-differentiated tumors are characterized by predominantly acinar formation, some of which may be cribriform. In the less differentiated adenocarcinomas, glandular formation is less marked, while the undifferentiated adenocarcinoma shows no glandular differentiation. However, using the appropriate

stain, intracellular mucin production can be demonstrated (see Table 53-3).

The prognostic value of the current light microscopic classification has been challenged by the new information provided by electron microscopic studies of lung neoplasms. This is especially true with regard to the ultrastructural classification of adenocarcinomas, which in most cases can aid in the differentiation of primary versus metastatic pulmonary adenocarcinoma.

Ultrastructurally, these main cell–derived types of adenocarcinomas have been identified: *mu-*

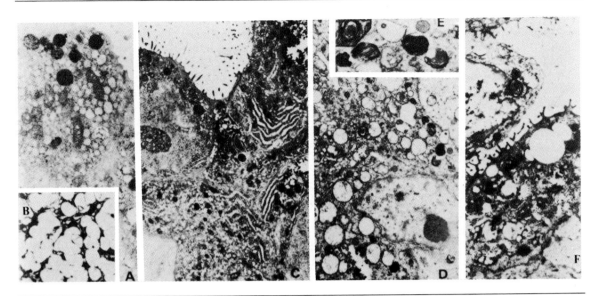

Fig. 53-18. Adenocarcinomas. *A.* Note the poorly formed surface microvillous border and the collections of coalescent mucin vacuoles. Coalescent mucin vacuoles are better illustrated in *B. C.* Note the dark, electron-dense granules, typical of clara cell adenocarcinomas. Also note the better developed microvillous border. *D.* Note the collections of typical lamellar bodies, indicative of pneumocyte type II differentiation. *E.* Note the details of the lamellar bodies. *F.* Note a combination of coalescent mucin vacuoles and clara cell granules within the same cell, indicative of a mixed adenocarcinoma (*A* × 13,000; *B* × 22,000; *C* × 10,000; *D* × 7500; *E* × 28,000; *F* × 13,000). (*Source:* See Fig. 53-14.)

cus, clara, and alveolar cell and the combination of these cells [14,113,133,159,160,176]. The *mucus cell*–derived group consists of cells with numerous mucus-secreting granules with a rough endoplasmic reticulum system and poorly developed microvilli (Fig. 53-18A and B). The *clara cell*–derived neoplasms contain electron-dense granules located in the apical portions of the cells. The microvillous borders are well developed, and the microvilli line the glandular spaces (Fig. 53-18C). The *alveolar cell*–derived adenocarcinomas are characterized by numerous lamellar bodies, while electron-dense and mucin granules are absent in this group (Fig. 53-18D and E). The microvillous borders are well developed and resemble those of the clara cell group. According to this ultrastructural classification of pulmonary adenocarcinomas, the clara and alveolar cell neoplasms have a better prognosis than the mucus cell neoplasms or mixed neoplasms with a mucus cell component (Fig. 53-18F) [88]. Therefore, the identification of a mucus cell component in a pulmonary adenocarcinoma represents a poor prognostic sign.

The separate classification of bronchoalveolar carcinoma is probably not warranted today [16,39, 43,78,88,99,114,141], since a variety of proliferating cell types is recognized in these tumors when analyzed ultrastructurally, and their behavior depends on the specific cell type that characterizes the tumor [42]. Immunohistologic analysis of surfactant apoprotein in bronchoalveolar carcinoma supports the concept that a certain percentage of these tumors are derived from the type II pneumocytes [39].

UNDIFFERENTIATED LARGE-CELL CARCINOMA
The large-cell undifferentiated carcinoma group is heterogeneous, defined mainly in a negative way, that is, not showing squamous or glandular differentiation and not being of small-cell type. Accordingly, the large-cell carcinoma group includes different subgroups in different classifications. The 1967 WHO classification (see Table 53-2) included, under the heading large-cell carcinoma, solid tumors with and without mucin-like content, giant-cell carcinomas, and clear-cell

carcinomas, whereas the 1981 WHO classification (Table 53-4) includes only two variants of large-cell carcinoma, namely, the giant-cell and clear-cell carcinomas; the solid tumors with mucin-like content are now included in the group of adenocarcinoma–solid carcinoma with mucus production. According to Herrera and associates [89], most large-cell carcinomas, when studied ultrastructurally, are poorly differentiated adenocarcinomas, while the minority are poorly differentiated squamous cell carcinomas and very rarely neuroendocrine carcinomas.

The large-cell undifferentiated carcinomas are similar to small-cell (oat cell) carcinomas in their rapid growth and early metastases. In a study of 26 patients with the diagnosis of large-cell carcinoma, an attempt was made to correlate the ultrastructure of these tumors with patient survival [96]. Ultrastructurally, four types of large-cell carcinomas were defined: squamous cell carcinoma, adenosquamous carcinoma, adenocarcinoma, and giant-cell carcinoma. The squamous type had a better prognosis than the adenosquamous and adenocarcinoma types. On the other hand, neoplasms with light microscopic features of giant-cell carcinoma usually represent ultrastructurally a highly malignant, anaplastic form of poorly differentiated adenocarcinoma of mucus cell type. A minority of giant-cell carcinomas have no recognizable differentiation even when studied by electron microscope. Thus the ultrastructural analysis of the so-called large-cell carcinomas eliminates the subgroup classification and makes this group of pulmonary neoplasms less heterogeneous.

Metastases

Lung cancer is highly malignant, and because of its tendency to invade pulmonary lymphatic channels and blood vessels, it metastasizes early. This applies to all of the major histologic types, although well-differentiated squamous cell carcinoma is notably slower to involve mediastinal lymph nodes and extrathoracic tissue than the others, and oat cell carcinoma is somewhat faster. Nohl [144] reported that in surgically excised specimens 100 percent of oat cell cancers and 86 percent of squamous cell growths had spread to the hilar lymph nodes. Overall, hematogenous or lymphatic spread has already taken place in one-third to one-half of subjects with lung cancer by the time they are first seen.

There is some variation among the different reported series collected and summarized by Engelman and McNamara [53] and by Spencer [181], but in general there is a clear predilection for malignant growths arising in the lung to spread centrifugally from lymph node group to lymph node group and to spread distally to liver, adrenals, brain, bones, and kidneys in that order of preference. Galluzzi and Payne [65] found brain metastases in over 25 percent of their subjects, and it may be that anastomoses between pulmonary and vertebral veins are in part responsible for these rather selective intracranial metastases.

Carcinoma of the lung, incidentally, is the most common cause of secondary tumor of the heart. Invasion of pulmonary arteries followed by direct or retrograde tumor embolization is the probable mechanism for spread of tumor to the remaining lung or to the other lung; contralateral pulmonary metastases occur in about 10 to 14 percent of subjects seen postmortem. Although it had not been documented by thorough statistical study, it is the impression of many pathologists that radiation and chemotherapy are altering the pattern of metastases as well as their frequency.

Table 53-4. **Histologic classification of lung tumours WHO 1981**

Group C Malignant epithelial tumors
1. Squamous cell carcinoma (epidermoid carcinoma)
   Variant:
   a. Spindle cell (squamous) carcinoma
2. Small cell carcinoma
   a. Oat cell carcinoma
   b. Intermediate cell type
   c. Combined oat cell carcinoma
3. Adenocarcinoma
   a. Acinar adenocarcinoma
   b. Papillary adenocarcinoma
   c. Bronchiolo-alveolar carcinoma
   d. Solid carcinoma with mucus formation
4. Large cell carcinoma
   Variants:
   a. Giant cell carcinoma
   b. Clear cell carcinoma
5. Adenosquamous carcinoma
6. Carcinoid tumor
7. Bronchial gland carcinoma
   a. Adenoid cystic carcinoma
   b. Mucoepidermoid carcinoma
   c. Others
8. Others

Source: See Table 53-2.

Genetic Factors

In malignant disease, the contribution of environmental factors seems to be greater than that from genetic factors, although both factors usually interact in causing the disease. From the great variety of environmental factors, smoking and asbestos are the most important ones in increasing the risks of lung cancer.

In 1973, Kellerman and coworkers [108,109] indicated possible genetically determined differences in susceptibility to lung cancer. This increased susceptibility is based on the readiness with which aryl hydrocarbon hydroxylation (AHH, an enzyme whose levels in the body are genetically determined) activity is inducible in cultures of lymphocytes. Since AHH converts some substances contained in cigarette smoke, such as 3,4-benzo(a)pyrene, to carcinogenic epoxides, a high AHH inducibility would serve as a genetic marker to increased lung cancer susceptibility. Accordingly, Emery and colleagues [52] found a significantly higher proportion of high inducers among patients with lung cancer than in patients with cancers at other sites (colon, rectum, pancreas) and control subjects matched by age, sex, and smoking habits. Increased AHH inducibility also was reported in mouth, larynx, and skin cancers [118], diseases thought to be due to exposure of polycyclic aromatic hydrocarbons (PAHs) [190,191].

However, the fundamental weakness of all these studies is that the measurement of inducibility was made after the cancers had developed. Therefore, AHH susceptibility may be more relevant to the effects of cancers than to their causation or the patient's susceptibility to cancer development. Thus at the present time there are no reliable means of distinguishing between individuals more likely or less likely to develop lung cancer in response to tobacco smoke or other environmental factors.

Mechanisms of Carcinogenesis

The association between lung cancer and cigarette smoking is epidemiologically and statistically firmly established [197]. However, which substances in cigarette smoke are carcinogenic and how they transform normal cells into malignant cells are two unanswered questions.

The process of carcinogenesis involves an alteration in the DNA of a cell by *mutation* (sometimes referred to as *tumor initiation*). This process involves a wide variety of mechanisms known as second-stage carcinogenesis, or *tumor promoter activity*, and includes hormone effects, various forms of chemical irritation, and immunosuppression.

Chemical analysis of tobacco smoke has identified more than 3000 chemicals obtained from smoke machines under uniform conditions [195]. The question remains as to which of these many chemicals are responsible for the development of human cancer. Two methods are currently used to answer this question: (1) chemical separation of the various constituents of tobacco smoke, and (2) biologic assays for carcinogenicity.

Chemical Constituents of Tobacco Smoke

Tobacco smoke is collected in two phases: the gaseous or volatile phase and the particulate phase. The particulate phase, using high-pressure liquid and gas chromatography, is fractionated into *acidic, neutral, and basic* components [94]. There is also an insoluble residue which contains metal carcinogens such as nickel and cadmium [184].

The *neutral fraction* contains a variety of PAHs which exhibit most of the tumorigenic activity of cigarette smoke. The best-known carcinogens in this fraction are benzo(a)pyrene and dibenz(a)anthracene (Table 53-5). It is commonly believed that these chemicals bind covalently with DNA, resulting in the primary initiating event in carcinogenesis. The damage caused to cellular DNA by these chemicals is of a random nature; thus the cells with malignant characteristics arise by accident, and therefore, the damage sometimes is reparable.

Contrary to this random chemical damage, in the case of viral oncogenesis, highly specific genetic information is introduced into the cell which in a way changes the cell's structure, behavior, and relationship with surrounding cells and usually is a one-stage process. Thus injection of the Rous sarcoma virus into rats or the polyoma virus into mice will result in development of macroscopically visible tumors within days or weeks, and the process will not be hastened by further injections of these viruses.

In the case of cancerous growth caused by the chemicals of tobacco smoke, there is always a long latent interval between exposure and the first visible sign of cancer. Moreover, following a single application of a potent carcinogen to the dorsal skin of a mouse, several different tumors

Table 53-5. **Major mutagens and carcinogens and related substances in tobacco smoke**

	Amount in smoke from one cigarette
I. Particulate phase	
A. Neutral fraction	
Benzo(a)pyrene	10–50 ng
Dibenz(a)anthracene	40 ng
5-Methylchrysene	0.6 ng
Benzofluoranthenes	90 ng
B. Basic fraction	
Nicotine	0.06–2 mg
N-Nitroeonornicotine	0.2–3.7 μg
C. Acidic fraction	
Catechol	40–280 μg
Unidentified tumor promoters	
D. Residue	
Nickel	0–3 μg
Cadmium	80 ng
^{210}Po	0.03–1.0 pCl
II. Vapor phase	
Hydrazine	32 μg
Vinyl chloride	1–16 ng
Urethan	10–35 μg
Formaldehyde	20–90 μg
Nitrogen oxides	16–600 μg
Nitrosodiethylamine	0.1–28 ng

Source: United States Public Health Service. *The Health Consequences of Smoking—Cancer: A Report of the Surgeon General.* Rockville, MD: United States Department of Health and Human Services, Office on Smoking and Health, 1980.

may arise at different sites on the body surface with different rates of growth.

Finally, repeated exposures to chemical carcinogens shorten to some extent the latent interval between first exposure and tumor appearance, a situation not observed with oncogenic virus exposure.

The *acidic fraction* contains compounds that have tumor-promoting activity as well as a number of potent mitogens. Tumor promoters are reversible potentiators of carcinogenesis, but by themselves they are not carcinogenic. The decline in lung cancer incidence with cessation of smoking suggests that the association between smoking and lung cancer is reversible owing to tumor-promoting activity. The tumor-promotion activity of some of the ingredients in cigarette smoke is substantiated also by epidemiologic studies. The mortality from lung cancer in uranium miners who are smokers is 440 times greater than in nonsmoking, nonexposed control individuals, whereas in nonsmoking uranium miners it is only 5 times greater [195]. Similar increased mortality rates from lung cancer exist also among asbestos workers who smoke cigarettes.

The *insoluble residue* of cigarette smoke contains nickel, cadmium, polonium, and other metals. Despite the fact that the lung concentration of ^{210}Po in smokers is 2.5 to 3.0 times greater than that in nonsmokers [85], it seems that the trace amount of polonium in cigarette smoke is not an important factor in causing lung cancer, as can be seen from the low lung cancer incidence in uranium miners who do not smoke and are exposed to higher concentrations of radioactivity.

The volatile phase of cigarette smoke contains nickel carbonyl, hydrazine, formaldehyde, and trace amounts of nitrosamines [195]. Nickel is a potent carcinogen, as shown by a marked increase in lung and nose cancer incidence in nickel refinery workers. The nitrosamines are very potent carcinogens, especially the N'-nitrosonornicotine and 4-(methylnitrosamino)-1-(3-pyridyl)-1-butanone. The installation of small amounts of these tobacco-specific nitrosamines into the trachea of Syrian golden hamsters results in the development of lung cancer [93]. Although constituents of tobacco smoke have been shown to be carcinogenic when applied directly to multiple tissues in animals, the results of inhalation studies in animals are rather disappointing. This may be due to the fact that animals are reluctant to inhale cigarette smoke and demonstrate shallow breathing.

Biological Assays for Carcinogenicity

The Ames bacterial assay is largely used for analyzing mutagenicity of tobacco constituents on histidine-dependent bacteria. Noted is their ability to grow in the absence of histidine [110]. The assay is very sensitive, and it permits the detection of mutagenicity of a quantity of cigarette smoke that is produced by the equivalent of 1/100 of a cigarette. On the basis of enhanced mutagenesis in bacteria, these substances can be classified as carcinogens.

ABSORPTION AND METABOLISM

The carcinogens in tobacco smoke are not only absorbed by the large epithelial surface which lines the airways and alveoli, but they are also metabolized, as evidenced by the presence of mutagens in the urine of smokers. The mutagenicity of cigarette smoke in humans has been established by chromosomal analysis of lymphocytes from smokers and nonsmokers [200].

Symptoms, Diagnosis, and Staging

Symptoms and Signs

A wide variation of symptoms is present in bronchogenic carcinoma, and in most cases, these symptoms are a manifestation of an advanced stage of the disease, since the tumor is present in the body many years before symptoms develop [56]. According to the doubling time of the various histologic types of lung cancer, the small-cell (oat cell) carcinoma starts to develop 2 to 3 years before symptomatology, while adenocarcinomas grow very slowly and are present in the lung 15 to 17 years before symptoms develop.

The symptoms and signs of lung cancer can be divided into (1) *local manifestations*, (2) *metastatic manifestations*, and (3) *nonmetastatic systemic manifestations*, also known as *paraneoplastic syndromes*. The diagnosis of bronchogenic carcinoma may be made on a routine chest x-ray while the patient is asymptomatic. In such a case, especially if the tumor is of squamous type, the prognosis is most favorable.

LOCAL MANIFESTATIONS

Cough and Sputum. In most cases, cough and sputum are nonspecific symptoms, since the majority of these patients suffer from chronic bronchitis and emphysema due to cigarette smoking. However, a change in the character of an established cough, that is, sudden onset of paroxysms of dry, hacking cough, or a change in the quality and quantity of sputum should raise the suspicion of a lung tumor.

Cough is caused by erosion and ulceration of the bronchial mucosa and by obstruction of a central airway. In the latter case, the airway obstruction results in an impairment of mucus clearance and thus causes infection and obstructive pneumonia.

Dyspnea. As in the case of cough and sputum, the symptom of dyspnea may be nonspecific, since most of these patients also suffer from chronic bronchitis and emphysema. It is sometimes difficult to determine whether the shortness of breath is due to the tumor or to chronic

bronchitis. However, sudden development of shortness of breath is usually associated with the obstruction of a main bronchus, most commonly caused by the squamous or small-cell (oat) variety of lung cancer. The airway obstruction causes an increase in airway resistance, and thus the dyspnea is severe.

Hemoptysis. Hemoptysis is caused in most cases by ulceration of the bronchial mucosa, and therefore, the amount of blood in sputum is minimal. In rare cases, when there is erosion of a bronchial artery by the tumor, massive and sometimes fatal bleeding occurs. This symptom, as opposed to cough and dyspnea, brings the patient to the physician immediately, and in the case of a heavy smoker, even a single episode of hemoptysis should be investigated by chest x-ray and bronchoscopy.

Wheezing. Unilateral, localized wheezing that does not disappear after cough in a smoker is pathognomonic of bronchogenic carcinoma and is caused by a narrowing of a central airway. In case the tumor is localized in the trachea, severe dyspnea is present. The performance of an expiratory and inspiratory flow-volume curve may localize the tumor in the extrathoracic or intrathoracic part of the trachea.

Chest Pain. The pain is usually dull and intermittent, localized in the midline or on the side of the tumor. This type of pain is constant and debilitating and is usually due to erosion of the first or second rib. Tumor invasion of the cervical sympathetic plexus results in Horner's syndrome.

METASTATIC MANIFESTATIONS

In 70 percent of the patients with lung cancer, the presenting symptoms are due to either *local intrathoracic* or *distant extrathoracic metastases* [137]. The percentage of metastatic lesions is especially high in small-cell (oat) carcinoma.

Local Intrathoracic Manifestations. In the majority of cases, *pleural effusion* is caused by direct extension of the tumor to the pleural surface. The sharp pleuritic pain is due to invasion of the pain receptors in the parietal pleura by the tumor. With accumulation of pleural fluid, the pain frequently disappears. Pleural effusion may be caused also by obstruction of the draining lymphatics. The pleural fluid may be clear and straw-colored, but usually it is bloodstained.

Superior vena cava syndrome is caused either by compression or direct invasion of the great veins of the thoracic outlet by paratracheal lymph nodes or the tumor itself. Patients usually complain of dyspnea, severe headaches, and swellings around the eyes or of the face. On physical examination, periorbital, facial, neck, and upper trunk edema is present with well-developed collateral circulation across the upper thorax and neck. The superior vena cava syndrome in most cases is life-threatening, and therefore, immediate treatment is mandatory.

Brachial neuritis is caused by a superior sulcus tumor invading the brachial plexus. Involvement of the cervical and first thoracic segments of the sympathetic nerve trunk results in enophthalmos, ptosis, myosis, and lack of sweating on that half of the face—*Horner's syndrome.*

Prolonged hoarseness after a common cold or hoarseness without a common cold is most suspicious of *left recurrent laryngeal palsy* due to lymph node pressure on the nerve as it encircles the aortic arch or to direct invasion of the nerve by the tumor.

Pericardial effusion is a serious complication that is usually due to direct extension of the tumor to the pericardium and epicardium. It causes retrosternal pain, neck vein distension, cardiac arrhythmias, and even cardiac tamponade.

Distant Extrathoracic Manifestations. The most commonly involved organs by metastases are bones, liver, brain, adrenals, and skin.

Lung cancer may metastasize to any *bones* in the body; however, the most frequent ones are the ribs and vertebrae. Bone metastases cause severe, dull pain that is aggravated by respiration if the ribs are involved. The bone lesions are usually osteolytic. At the beginning of symptomatology, radiologic examination of the bones and bone scans may be negative. On the other hand, a positive bone scan of the vertebrae with negative x-rays is usually indicative of degenerative rather than metastatic changes of the vertebrae.

Weakness and weight loss are usually characteristic of *hepatic* metastases and in the majority of cases indicate a poor prognosis. The intrahepatic metastases are small and not palpable, rarely affect liver function test results, and usually are not detected by a liver scan.

Hemiplegia, personality changes, epileptic seizures, confusion, and headaches are manifestations of *brain* metastases. Bronchogenic carcinoma accounts for 10 to 15 percent of intracranial metastases, and thus it is one of the most common brain tumors in neurosurgical units. Brain metastases may be single or multiple and are best identified on computed tomography (CT) scan.

Metastatic spread to *lymph nodes* leads usually to specific symptoms: vocal cord palsy, Horner's syndrome, superior vena cava syndrome, and others.

NONMETASTATIC SYSTEMIC MANIFESTATIONS
The paraneoplastic syndromes are not caused directly either by the tumor itself or by its metastases. The following are the main syndromes: metabolic (weight loss), thrombophlebitis migrans, endocrine-related syndromes (inappropriate antidiuretic hormone secretion, Cushing's syndrome, hypercalcemia), polyneuritis, and neuromuscular disorders. The cause for these syndromes is unknown, and their possible mechanism and treatment are discussed in Chapter 56.

Diagnosis

The symptoms and signs of bronchogenic carcinoma are nonspecific. However, they may suggest the presence of a lung tumor, especially in a man over 40 years old who has been a cigarette smoker for many years. The aim of the diagnostic procedures are twofold: (1) to confirm the clinical diagnosis by cytology or histology, and (2) to establish the extent of dissemination of the disease in order to determine the most suitable treatment, that is, surgical or irradiation and chemotherapy. In deciding on surgical treatment, the histologic type of the tumor has to be taken into account, since small-cell (oat) carcinoma and poorly differentiated squamous cell carcinoma and adenocarcinoma are also contraindications for surgery, even if no demonstrable dissemination of the disease is present.

RADIOLOGY
In most cases of lung cancer, the chest x-ray is abnormal when the patient is symptomatic. Moreover, in a prospective study it has been shown that the chest x-ray in the early detection of lung cancer is superior to cytology, especially in peripherally located lung tumors and stage III cancers [60,61,63].

Most frequently, a central (squamous cell carcinoma) or a peripheral mass (adenocarcinoma) is present on chest x-ray. The size of the mass is usually 2 to 4 cm in diameter with irregular borders (see Fig. 53-12). Later in the disease, hilar enlargement occurs (Fig. 53-19). However, in poorly differentiated tumors and in small-cell carcinoma, an enlarged hilum and hilar mass may occur simultaneously. Large squamous cell carcinomas may develop central necrosis and sub-

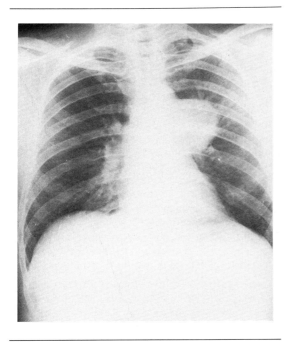

Fig. 53-19. A large hilar mass due to carcinoma of the lung. (*Source:* See Fig. 53-12.)

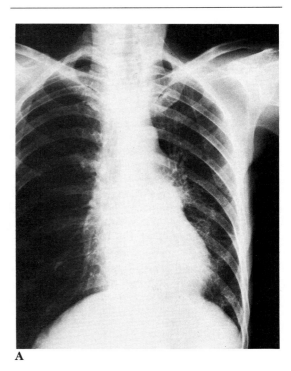

A

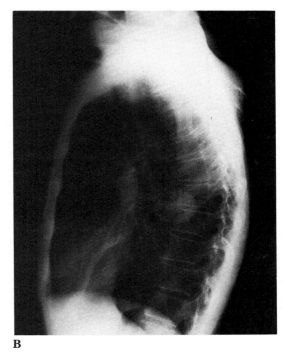

B

sequently lung abscess. Tumors located in the apical segment of the lower lobes may be present as hilar shadows. A lateral view or linear tomography will differentiate this parenchymal shadow from hilar lymph node enlargement. Lateral-view x-rays are most important also in localizing masses behind the cardiac shadow (Fig. 53-20).

Obstruction of a main or segmental bronchus may be associated with the following radiologic abnormalities: atelectasis or lobar emphysema, caused by partial obstruction of the airway and best seen on a maximal expiratory chest film, where in addition to air trapping, shift of the mediastinum to the healthy side occurs. Sometimes partial obstruction of the bronchus results in a slowly resolving pneumonia. In such cases, linear tomography of the area may reveal a nodular appearance in addition to the infiltrative lesion.

Intrathoracic metastatic spread can be seen as an enlarged upper and middle mediastinum due to increased paratracheal and hilar lymph nodes, an elevated diaphragm due to secondary phrenic nerve involvement, and pleural effusion. Careful examination of the thoracic bone structures may detect metastatic lesions visible as rib erosion or collapsed thoracic vertebra.

A solitary nodule on chest x-ray poses a diagnostic problem, since it may be a primary lung

Fig. 53-20. *A.* Carcinoma of the lung hidden behind the cardiac silhouette on posteroanterior roentgenogram. *B.* Lateral view of the chest reveals the carcinoma. (*Source:* See Fig. 53-12.)

cancer, a benign tumor, a secondary metastasis, or a granuloma. In most cases, such a nodule is either a primary bronchogenic carcinoma or a secondary lung tumor, and therefore, in such cases a thoracotomy is imperative, even if a benign tumor or granuloma is suspected.

COMPUTED TOMOGRAPHY AND MAGNETIC RESONANCE IMAGING

CT has revolutionized radiology and has become indispensable in the diagnosis, staging, and management of lung cancer. It is most useful in localizing and evaluating solitary or multiple nodules in the lung parenchyma, in assessing mediastinal and hilar lymphadenopathy, and in determining the extent of spread to mediastinal structures and distant sites such as the liver and adrenals [171].

Evaluation of Pulmonary Solitary Nodules. A solitary pulmonary nodule of less than 3 cm in diameter may be a primary lung carcinoma or a metastasis from a distant organ, or it may be a granuloma.

In 1980 Siegelman and colleagues [177] showed that nodules with a density greater than 175 Hounsfield units (HU) were benign. However, other observers were unable to confirm Siegelman's results. Some years later it had become apparent that many factors influence the Hounsfield number (kilovoltage, filtration, reconstruction algorithm), and that these factors differ from one manufacturer's unit to another.

To overcome this obstacle, Zerhouni and coworkers [219] developed a phantom (rods constructed of material with a density of 164 HU) that allows nodule density determinations to be made on units of any manufacturer. With this method in a cooperative study of 300 nodules reported from 10 institutions, only one false-negative diagnosis occurred [218].

However, a solitary noncalcified lesion greater than 3 cm in diameter seen on a plain chest film should be approached surgically without density determination by CT, due to the high likelihood of its being a carcinoma.

Assessment of Hilar and Mediastinal Lymphadenopathy. The accuracy of CT in diagnosing hilar abnormalities is controversial [121], especially in determining whether the hilar enlargement is due to direct extension from a peripheral lung carcinoma or whether it is due to enlargement of hilar lymph nodes secondary to lymphatic spread from a peripheral carcinoma. In spite of these diagnostic difficulties, CT is supe-

rior to conventional tomography in assessing hilar lymphadenopathy.

Hilar abnormalities caused by primary carcinoma in the main bronchi or in the central portions of the lobar bronchi can be clearly shown on standard CT examinations made with images at 1-cm intervals.

CT is a more sensitive modality to distinguish malignant from benign mediastinal lymph node enlargement, based on node size rather than on density criteria [86]. At the present, lymph nodes in the paratracheal, paraesophageal, and subcarinal regions that are smaller than 1 cm in diameter are considered normal, nodes 1 cm to 1.5 cm are considered suspicious, and those larger than 1.5 cm are abnormal with a high probability of being malignant. Some lymph nodes of this size may prove to be reactive, especially in cases of infection behind an obstructed bronchus.

Determination of the Extent of Disease. CT is most useful in demonstrating direct spread of tumor into the chest wall, pleura, vertebrae, or sternum, as well as in locating distant metastases to liver and adrenals by including scans of the upper abdomen [171]. However it should be emphasized that adrenal masses may be due to benign lesions as well.

Magnetic resonance imaging (MRI) is able to distinguish vessels with blood flow from solid tissue such as hilar lymph nodes but offers no other advantage, except the absence of any radiation exposure, over CT scans. Thus at the present time there are no indications for performing MRI rather than CT scans of the thorax.

CYTOLOGY

The study of desquamated individual cells in the diagnosis of malignant disease was introduced by Papanicolaou in the early 1930s. The usefulness and limitations of this technique in the diagnosis of bronchogenic carcinoma have become better appreciated during the ensuing years. Fresh sputum and bronchial washings are rapidly fixed and stained. The preparation is then carefully examined for malignant cells. The sensitivity of the test (relationship of number of positive test results to the number of proved cases) is 70 to 80 percent and probably cannot be increased without lowering its reliability.

There are two inherent limitations of the test that refinements of technique cannot completely eliminate. First, the presence or absence of tumor cells in any particular sputum sample is dependent on random sloughing of cells from the tumor. This can be partially circumvented by obtaining a significant number of sputum specimens for examinations: Evaluating five different samples increases the yield of proved cancer to 90 percent versus 40 percent from a single specimen [54]. The second limitation concerns the patency of the bronchus containing the tumor. If the bronchial lumen proximal to the tumor is occluded by inflammation or mucous plugs, tumor cells will not be found in the sputum. A similar situation exists in certain peripheral tumors with no large bronchial communication.

In one large series there was a diagnosis of cell type in 84 percent of patients in whom it was possible to establish a cytologic diagnosis of lung cancer. Yield from cytology is higher in central tumors (90 percent) than it is in peripheral tumors (50 percent).

If high degrees of sensitivity and reliability are to be obtained, careful attention must be paid to all phases of technique in performing the test. Careful sputum collection is the first prerequisite. The patient should first rinse his or her mouth so that all food particles and debris are removed. As soon as possible thereafter, he or she should cough up material for examination, and the specimen should be fixed as soon as it is obtained.

Care must be taken to ensure that the specimen is actually sputum and not saliva or nasal secretions. What is often not realized is that cytologic specimens taken at the time of bronchoscopy are far less likely to be positive than those taken in the following 24 to 36 hours. The persistent coughing that follows this procedure seems to produce an increase in the shedding of malignant cells. At least three or four sputum specimens should be obtained in the immediate 36 hours following endoscopy. In instances where the patient is having difficulty coughing up sputum, the use of heated aerosol of saline will often yield a positive examination. Occasionally, positive smears are found in the absence of a demonstrable lung lesion. A persistently positive cytologic smear in the absence of an obvious lung tumor demands an intensive search for tumors elsewhere in the upper respiratory tract or esophagus.

The interpretation of the stained smears requires considerable experience if the test is to attain a high degree of accuracy. The diagnosis of malignancy is based on morphologic changes in the nuclei of individual cells. Three changes are usually found in the malignant cell. The nucleus is increased in size with a consequent increase in the nuclear-cytoplasmic ratio. Hyperchromatism of the nucleus occurs, and the chromatin particles are irregularly placed with a thickened rim at the edge of the nucleus. Finally, large nucleoli are usually seen (Fig. 53-21). In any one specimen

Fig. 53-21. Photomicrograph of bronchial washings stained by the Papanicolaou technique showing malignant cells. Note the hyperchromatic nuclei with irregularly placed chromatin particles (× 900). (*Source:* See Fig. 53-12.)

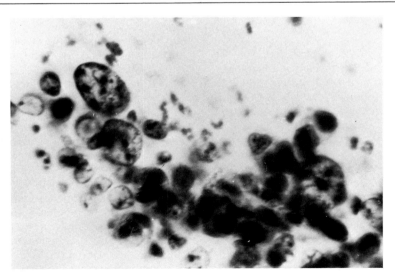

these changes may be subtle and difficult to interpret.

Other diseases of the lung and bronchi may induce changes in cells from the bronchial mucosa that resemble malignant changes. Bronchial metaplasia, as seen in chronic bronchitis, may be difficult to distinguish. Sputum from patients with asthma frequently contains clumps of cells that resemble adenocarcinoma, but the nuclei of these cells are normal. Lipoid pneumonia and pulmonary infarction also may lead to cellular changes that may be confused with malignancy. Farber and colleagues [55] believed that cellular changes associated with these diseases can be distinguished from those caused by malignancy if reliance is placed on the appearance of individual nuclei instead of on the appearance of clumps of cells. Tumors of the respiratory tract other than lung cancer can occasionally be diagnosed by the experienced cytologist.

Unfortunately, cytologic studies are least helpful in the same type of patient for whom bronchoscopy offers the least aid, that is, patients with peripheral lesions or solitary nodules. Sputum cytology is equally disappointing in early screening studies. In the 1970 prospective study, twice as many lung cancer cases were detected by x-ray than by cytology in the dual-screen group, and the chest roentgenogram was a better test to detect peripherally located tumors [143].

Cytologic examination of sputum specimens compared well with histologic diagnosis by bronchial biopsy, surgically resected specimens, or autopsy material [146,154]. Concordance is approximately 90 percent for squamous cell carcinoma and somewhat lower for small-cell (oat) carcinoma.

BRONCHOSCOPY

The flexible fiberoptic bronchoscope has added a new dimension to invasive diagnosis of lung tumors [168] for the following reasons: It is easy to use under local anesthesia, it causes less discomfort for the patient, and it has increased the range of visualization of the bronchial tree, and thus all the lobar and segmental bronchi can easily be examined and tumors located in these airways can be biopsied. Under fluoroscopic control, transbronchial biopsies, brushing [217] of lesions not visible in the airways, and bronchial washings for cytologic diagnosis can be obtained. In addition, the extent and operability of lung cancer are assessed by the site of the tumor, abnormal rigidity of the airway wall, tumor infiltration, narrowing of the airway, and widening of the carina due to external pressure of subcarinal, mediastinal, or hilar lymph nodes.

Complications related directly to fiberoptic bronchoscopy are rare. In a major study [38], serious complications or mortality were encountered in 0.08 and 0.01 percent of patients, respectively. Cardiac arrhythmias are common, especially in elderly patients, as a result of hypoxemia, while cardiac arrest is very rare. Complications related to transbronchial biopsies are low as well. Pneumothorax occurs in about 5 percent of patients, while hemorrhage of more than 50 ml occurs only in 1 to 2 percent.

PERCUTANEOUS TRANSTHORACIC NEEDLE ASPIRATION BIOPSY

The use of fine-needle aspiration biopsy (FNA) for cytologic examination is most suitable for peripheral lung tumors. The FNA is performed under biplane fluoroscopy using an image intensifier, and thus tumors of 2 cm in diameter or larger can easily be aspirated. Since the needle is a fine-bore spinal needle, tumors as far as 10 to 12 cm deep can be reached by this method. Nodules less than 2 cm in diameter are best visualized under CT scan [59]. The incidence of pneumothorax is somewhat higher than in transbronchial biopsies; however, it seldom requires drainage.

The FNA method yields a very high rate (80 to 90 percent) of cytologic diagnoses in lung cancer patients [43], yet conventional cytologic examination is often handicapped by the absence of well-defined histologic and morphologic features [158]. Moreover, Johnston and Frable [103] showed that in 80 percent of cytologically diagnosed squamous cell carcinomas from FNA, the diagnosis was not confirmed by subsequent tissue biopsies. It is thus apparent that cytologic examinations should be corroborated by complementary tests that might provide more specific and definitive cell typing, thus increasing the reliability of the FNA technique.

Based on the immunocytologic labeling of FNA samples with a variety of monoclonal antibodies reacting with intermediate filaments, Bruderman and coworkers [22] demonstrated that the majority of tumors cytologically identified as squamous cell carcinoma turned out to be adenocarcinomas or mixed adenosquamous carcinomas. Thus immunocytochemical labeling for FNA samples provides a complementary test for the differential diagnosis of squamous cell carcinoma and adenocarcinoma. Such diagnosis is of fundamental importance for arriving at the correct prognosis and selection of optimal therapy.

MEDIASTINOSCOPY AND MEDIASTINOTOMY

In approximately half of lung cancer patients, mediastinal lymph nodes are already involved with tumor when the patients first come to diagnosis. Some, but not all, surgeons believe that mediastinal node involvement is an absolute contraindication to resection. Because this information is critical, various approaches have been developed to accomplish exploration of the mediastinum. Carlens introduced anterior cervical mediastinoscopy in 1959. It has been quite generally accepted worldwide, but some controversy persists regarding its exact place in the workup of a patient with suspected lung cancer.

If mediastinoscopy is carried out routinely in lung cancer patients, tumor tissue will be obtained in 30 to 40 percent of cases [5,157]. After introduction of mediastinoscopy, the fraction of exploratory thoracotomies without resection decreased from approximately 50 to 10 to 20 percent [147,149,157]. Many surgeons perform a mediastinoscopy on all patients preoperatively. Others have attempted to establish criteria for selecting only certain patients for mediastinoscopy.

There is also debate regarding the exact approach to exploring the mediastinum. The anterior cervical approach is most frequently used, but it affords limited access to the mediastinum. In approximately 10 percent of explorations, the nodes will be too small to be detected, and in a similar fraction, they will be inaccessible [115,157]. Parasternal mediastinotomy has been advocated to overcome these problems and to permit better control of bleeding or other complications [104,183]. Some surgeons use this approach routinely; others select it for left-sided lesions or when there is suspicion that nodes below the aortic arch are involved. Here, and with the question of who should have mediastinoscopy, no blanket recommendation is possible. The prior experiences of each surgeon and the features unique to each patient will determine whether the mediastinum should be explored and which approach should be used.

The major controversy surrounding this topic is the issue of what to do with patients found to have tumor involvement of mediastinal nodes. Because these patients have such a poor prognosis, many surgeons consider that involvement of any mediastinal node is an absolute sign of unresectability. Some have argued otherwise. In epidermoid carcinoma confined to the superior mediastinum, the claim has been made that resection and radiation therapy can still effect a 20 to 25 percent 5-year survival rate [111,157].

Carlens [26] reviewed this debate and may have identified the factor responsible for the differing results reported by various groups. Tumor confined within the capsule of nodes seems to carry a more favorable prognosis than tumors with metastases extending out from the nodes [117,130,151].

At present, it is not possible to make a definite recommendation regarding the resectability of epidermoid carcinomas with mediastinal node involvement. If such tumors are resected, it should be carefully determined whether the metastases are intranodal or perinodal.

Staging

Surgical resection of lung cancer is still the best treatment available at the present time. Since it is well known that bronchogenic carcinoma disseminates very early (Table 53-6), clinical-diagnostic staging of lung cancer is imperative in order to select the right treatment and avoid unnecessary thoracotomy [182]. The staging based on the tumor-node-metastasis (TNM) system adopted in 1974 by the American Joint Committee for Cancer Staging [136] permits definition of the extent and stage of the disease (Table 53-7). The letter T represents the primary tumor and the numerical suffixes (T1 to T4), the increasing size and involvement or both. The letter N refers to the regional lymph node involvement, and the suffixes (N1 to N3) describe the levels of metastatic disease (hilar, mediastinal, subcarinal, contralateral). The letter M represents distant metastases. Thus the TNM system makes it possible to choose the appropriate treatment and predict the survival rate.

Table 53-6. Distribution of lung cancer at postmortem in patients dying within 1 month of "curative" resection: Death unrelated to lung cancer

Type	No.	No. with persistent disease	Distant metastasis
Squamous	131	44 (33%)	22 (37%)
Small cell	19	13 (70%)	12 (63%)
Adeno	30	12 (40%)	12 (40%)
Large cell	22	3 (16%)	3 (16%)

Source: MJ Matthews et al. Frequency of residual and metastatic tumor in patients undergoing curative resection for lung cancer. *Cancer Chemother Rep* 4:63, 1973.

However, the TNM staging system groups findings in broad categories, and therefore, it is too coarse. For example, T1, N0, M0 and T1, N1, M0 lesions are classified as stage I disease in spite of the fact that the prognosis is very different in these two cases, and the outcome for patients with T1, N1, M0 tumors closely resembles the survival pattern of patients with stage II lung cancer. Stage III represents another broad category, since it includes patients amenable to surgical resection (T1 to T3, N0 to N2, M0) as well as patients with contralateral lymph node involvement (N3) and distant metastases (M1).

To resolve these problems, a revision of the TNM system was developed, based on end-result studies in the United States and the proposals made by the international TNM study committees of the Union Internationale Contre le Cancer (UICC), Japan, and Germany [135,215]. Thus the new staging system for lung cancer shown in Table 53-8 is an international one. According to the new TNM system, patients with T1, N1 and T2, N1 subsets are classified as stage II disease. Stage III disease is subdivided into stage IIIa (T1 to T3, N1, N2, M0) and IIIb (T1 to T4, N1 to N3, M0) disease, while patients with distant metastases (M1) are classified as stage IV. Figure 53-22 shows the end results applied to a large contemporary data base [134] derived from clinical estimates of disease extent, based on the new TNM system's definitions and stage groupings. Patients with non–small-cell lung cancer and clinical stage I, II, or IIIa are candidates for surgical treatment, while those with stage IIIb or IV disease are candidates for radiotherapy, chemotherapy, or combined treatment.

Table 53-7. **Definitions for staging bronchogenic carcinoma**

T0:	No evidence of primary tumor.
TX:	Tumor proved by the presence of malignant cells in bronchopulmonary secretions but not visualized roentgenographically or bronchoscopically, or any tumor that cannot be assessed.
TIS:	Carcinoma in situ.
T1:	A tumor that is 3.0 cm or less in greatest diameter, surrounded by lung or visceral pleura, and without evidence of invasion proximal to a lobar bronchus at bronchoscopy.
T2:	A tumor more than 3.0 cm in greatest diameter, or a tumor of any size that either invades the visceral pleura or which has associated atelectasis or obstructive pneumonitis extending to the hilar region. At bronchoscopy, the proximal extent of demonstrable tumor must be within a lobar bronchus at least 2.0 cm distal to the carina. Any associated atelectasis or obstructive pneumonitis must involve less than an entire lung, and there must be no pleural effusion.
T3:	A tumor of any size with direct extension into an adjacent structure such as the parietal pleura, the chest wall, the diaphragm, or the mediastinum and its contents; or a tumor demonstrable bronchoscopically to involve a main bronchus less than 2.0 cm distal to the carina; or any tumor associated with atelectasis or obstructive pneumonitis of an entire lung or pleural effusion.
N0:	No demonstrable metastasis to regional lymph nodes.
N1:	Metastasis to lymph nodes in the peribronchial or the ipsilateral hilar region, or both, including direct extension.
N2:	Metastasis to lymph nodes in the mediastinum.
M0:	No distant metastasis.
M1:	Distant metastasis such as in scalene, cervical, or contralateral hilar lymph nodes, brain, bones, liver, or contralateral lung.

Occult carcinoma	Stage 1	Stage 2	Stage 3
TX N0 M0	TIS N0 M0	T2 N1 M0	T3 any N or M
	T1 N0 M0		N2 any T or M
	T1 N1 M0		M1 any T or N
	T2 N0 M0		

Source: SG Spiro. The Diagnosis and Staging of Lung Cancer. In JF Smith (Ed), *The Management of Lung Cancer.* London: Edward Arnold, 1984.

Table 53-8. **Staging of lung cancer: 1986 American Joint Committee on Cancer**

Primary tumor (T)

TX   • Tumor proved by the presence of malignant cells in bronchopulmonary secretions but not visualized roentgenographically or bronchoscopically, or any tumor that cannot be assessed as in a retreatment staging.

T0   • No evidence of primary tumor.

TIS   • Carcinoma in situ.

T1   • A tumor that is 3.0 cm or less in greatest dimension, surrounded by lung or visceral pleura, and without evidence of invasion proximal to a lobar bronchus at bronchoscopy.*

T2   • A tumor more than 3.0 cm in greatest dimension; or a tumor of any size that either invades the visceral pleura or has associated atelectasis or obstructive pneumonitis extending to the hilar region. At bronchoscopy, the proximal extent of demonstrable tumor must be within a lobar bronchus or at least 2.0 cm distal to the carina. Any associated atelectasis or obstructive pneumonitis must involve less than an entire lung.

T3   • A tumor of any size with direct extension into the chest wall (including superior sulcus tumors), diaphragm, or the mediastinal pleura or pericardium without involving the heart, great vessels, trachea, esophagus, or vertebral bodies; or a tumor in the main bronchus within 2 cm of the carina without involving the carina.

T4   • A tumor of any size with invasion of the mediastinum or involving heart, great vessels, trachea, esophagus, vertebral bodies or carina; or with the presence of malignant pleural effusion.†

Nodal involvement (N)

N0   • No demonstrable metastasis to regional lymph nodes.

N1   • Metastasis to lymph nodes in the peribronchial or the ipsilateral hilar region, or both, including direct extension.

N2   • Metastasis to ipsilateral mediastinal lymph nodes and subcarinal lymph nodes.

N3   • Metastasis to contralateral mediastinal lymph nodes, contralateral hilar lymph nodes, ipsilateral or contralateral scalene or supraclavicular lymph nodes.

Distant metastasis (M)

M0   • No (known) distant metastasis

M1   • Distant metastasis present; specify site(s)

Stage grouping			
Occult carcinoma	TX	N0	M0
Stage 0	TIS	Carcinoma in situ	
Stage I	T1	N0	M0
	T2	N0	M0
Stage II	T1	N1	M0
	T2	N1	M0
Stage IIIa	T3	N0	M0
	T3	N1	M0
	T1–3	N2	M0
Stage IIIb	Any T	N3	M0
	T4	Any N	M0
Stage IV	Any T	Any N	M1

T1*The uncommon superficial tumor of any size with its invasive component limited to the bronchial wall, which may extend proximal to the main bronchus, is classified as T1.

T4†Most pleural effusions associated with lung cancer are due to tumor. There are, however, some few patients in whom cytopathologic examination of pleural fluid (on more than one specimen) is negative for tumor, and the fluid is not bloody and is not an exudate. In such cases where these elements and clinical judgment dictate that the effusion is not related to the tumor, the patients should be staged T1, T2, or T3, excluding effusion as a staging element.

Source: Modified from CF Mountain. A new international staging system for lung cancer. *Chest* 89:225S, 1986.

The survival rate of a patient with lung cancer depends not only on the extent of the disease, but also on the histologic type of the tumor. As can be seen, the 2-year survival rate in stage I is good for all histologic types except small-cell (oat) carcinoma; the rates for stages II and III are uniformly poor, except stage II squamous cell carcinoma [136] (Table 53-9).

Fig. 53-22. Cumulative proportion of patients surviving 5 years by clinical stage of disease. (Reproduced from CF Mountain. A new international staging system for lung cancer. *Chest* 89:225S, 1986. With permission.)

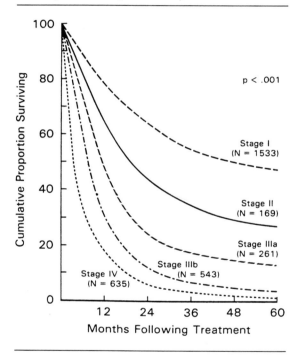

In addition to the type and extent of lung tumor, the clinical performance status of the individual patient has to be taken into account for the survival rate and for selection of the right treatment. For example, in two patients with localized squamous cell carcinoma of similar size, the prognosis will depend on their clinical status; that is, the asymptomatic patient's prognosis will be much better than the patient who has hemoptysis, weight loss, and/or other systemic manifestations. The most widely used scale to assess the clinical status is the Karnofsky Performance Scale (Table 53-10).

Diagnostic Procedures for Metastases

The extent of spread of the tumor at the time of diagnosis is critical in making both prognostic and therapeutic decisions. Unfortunately, the TNM staging system is still very crude and so are the procedures for diagnosing metastases. This is well documented in a study of 202 lung cancer patients dying 1 month following a "curative" resection, the cause of death being unrelated to the lung tumor (see Table 53-6). Persistence of tumor was noted in 33 percent of patients with squamous cell carcinoma, and half these patients also had distant metastasis. In small-cell (oat) carcinoma persistence of tumor was seen in 70 percent, with distant metastasis in almost every case.

The pattern of spread of lung cancer is best demonstrated from autopsy studies in advanced disease [123]. The most common organs involved are liver, adrenals, bone, and brain, and again, the highest percentages of metastases are present in small-cell (oat) carcinoma. Liver metastases are found in 74 percent of patients with small-cell (oat) carcinomas, in about half the cases of adenocarcinomas and large-cell carcinomas, and

Table 53-9. Two-year survival experience for 1975 patients with carcinoma of the lung, shown as fraction of patients surviving 2 years or more after diagnosis and total number of patients in each group

| Histologic type | Stage | | | | | |
| | I | | II | | III | |
	(%)	(no.)	(%)	(no.)	(%)	(no.)
Epidermoid	47	331	40	66	12	524
Small cell anaplastic	6	38	5	20	4	302
Adenocarcinoma	46	151	14	28	8	334
Large cell	43	61	13	17	13	103

Source: C Mittman, I Bruderman. Lung cancer: To operate or not? *Am Rev Respir Dis* 116:477, 1977.

Table 53-10. **The Karnofsky Performance Scale**

Definition	%	Criteria
Able to carry on normal activity and to work; no special care is needed.	100	Normal; no complaints; no evidence of disease.
	90	Able to carry on normal activity; minor signs or symptoms of disease.
	80	Normal activity with effort; some signs or symptoms of disease.
Unable to work; able to live at home, care for most personal needs; a varying amount of assistance is needed.	70	Cares for self; unable to carry on normal activity or to do active work.
	60	Requires occasional assistance but is able to care for most of his needs.
	50	Requires considerable assistance and frequent medical care.
Unable to care for self; requires equivalent of institutional or hospital care; disease may be progressing rapidly.	40	Disabled; requires special care and assistance.
	30	Severely disabled; hospitalization is indicated, although death may not be imminent.
	20	Very sick; hospitalization necessary; active supportive treatment necessary.
	10	Moribund; fatal processes progressing rapidly.

only in 25 percent of patients with squamous cell carcinomas. Brain metastases are found in approximately 15 percent of patients with squamous cell carcinomas and are twice as common in small- and large-cell carcinomas. Metastases to the adrenals are present in about 25 percent of patients with squamous cell carcinomas, while in patients with the other cell types it ranges from 50 to 59 percent. Bone metastases are found in one-fifth of patients with squamous cell carcinomas and in one-third of patients with other cell types. Only 4 percent of cases of small-cell (oat) carcinoma are limited to the thorax at autopsy, as opposed to 46 percent in squamous cell carcinoma.

The procedures to diagnose the presence of metastases are radioisotope scans and CT. As published, however, the liver and brain scans were negative in asymptomatic patients, while bone scans were positive in less than 4 percent of these cases [95]. Also, the interpretation of increased uptake on a bone scan may be difficult in the presence of degenerative bone disease, old fractures, hyperparathyroidism, and other metabolic bone disease. Therefore, radioisotope scans of liver, brain, and bones in asymptomatic patients are indicated only in small-cell carcinoma.

Therapy

The treatment of pulmonary neoplasms is most discouraging in spite of the advances made in the last 20 years in diagnostic procedures, surgical techniques, and postoperative care. The poor prognosis and the low "curability" rate of this disease are due to the fact that in the majority of patients the disease has already spread at the time the diagnosis is made. The grim outlook of this disease did not change even when early detection screening was used in a prospective study [11,60,61,63,143]. Thus the choice of treatment and the survival rate are influenced by the histologic cell type of the tumor and the stage of the disease. The highest 5-year survival rate (60 to 70 percent) is observed in patients with squamous cell carcinoma and stage I disease, as compared to less than 10 percent [161] in all lung cancer patients taken as a group.

Surgical Treatment

Radical surgical resection of a lung tumor is still the best available therapy for bronchogenic carcinoma in stage I and II disease. It is indicated but is less effective in stage IIIa cancer.

Preoperative evaluation of the patient's general condition is most important, since more than 70 percent of postoperative morbidity and mortality is due to cardiopulmonary complications [68, 139]. The postoperative mortality is almost 5 times higher in patients with cardiopulmonary disease (8.3 versus 1.7 percent) [150].

However, the most immediate postoperative threat is not cardiac but pulmonary. Therefore, in these patients a thorough preoperative pulmonary function evaluation is imperative. In patients with hypoxia and/or moderate impairment of ventilatory function, the expected postoperative 1-second forced expiratory volume (FEV_1) has to be calculated using equations based on ventilation-perfusion scans [2,140].

Patients with a slight to moderate decrease in mechanical function, normal arterial blood gases, and an expected postoperative FEV_1 of greater than 50 percent have a low probability of postoperative respiratory insufficiency, while patients with moderate exercise dyspnea, reduced mechanical function, hypoxia with normal arterial carbon dioxide pressure ($PaCO_2$), and an expected preoperative FEV_1 between 25 and 50 percent of predicted value should undergo ventilation-perfusion scans and an exercise tolerance test. Surgical treatment is contraindicated in patients with significant dyspnea, hypoxia and hypercapnia, and an expected postoperative FEV_1 of less than 25 percent of predicted value [140].

It is well known that the spread of primary lung tumor to regional lymph nodes (N1, N2 disease) decreases significantly the 5-year survival rate in surgically managed patients. There is also a controversy among surgeons regarding operability in these cases. Therefore, many surgeons recommend preoperative mediastinoscopy in most stage IIIa patients and in stage II patients with abnormal mediastinal lymph nodes on CT scan (nodes 1.5 cm in diameter or larger). Although mediastinoscopy is an invasive procedure, in patients with positive nodes it gives a precise histologic diagnosis, site, extent, and degree of invasiveness of the cancer [149]. Thus patients with contralateral node involvement (N3 disease) of small-cell carcinoma and extranodal extension of cancer are excluded from surgical treatment [155]. In patients with tumors of the left upper lobe or left hilum, an anterior mediastinotomy may be indicated.

Contraindications to Surgical Therapy

It is much simpler to define those patients who will not benefit from an operation than to predict those who will. Contraindications to operative therapy in patients with, or suspected of having, carcinoma of the lung are summarized as follows:

ABSOLUTE SIGNS OF INOPERABILITY:
1. Distant metastases to brain, bone, abdominal organs, skin, or contralateral lung
2. Mediastinal involvement (lymphatic metastases or direct extension of tumor):
   a. Vocal cord paralysis
   b. Vena caval obstruction
   c. Esophageal involvement
   d. Involvement of carina or trachea
   e. Pleural effusion with malignant cells
   f. Paralysis of diaphragm

Relative contraindications:

1. Diminished pulmonary function
2. Serious cardiac, renal, hepatic, or cerebral disease

Evidence of metastasis to a distant organ contraindicates operative therapy. Approximately 15 percent of patients with lung cancer will present with central nervous system signs and symptoms as the first manifestation of the disease. Even though about a third of these patients have a solitary metastasis, a combined approach of removing both the cerebral and pulmonary lesions is seldom worthwhile. Such a procedure usually does not prolong the patient's life and offers little palliation.

The vertebral bodies and rib cage are the most frequent sites of osseous metastases. Severe, localized, knifelike pain with occasional radiation along known nerve pathways is the most frequent symptom of this complication. Tenderness over the suspected area with no other obvious explanation contraindicates operation on the pulmonary lesion, and bone scans are usually positive under such conditions. Radiation therapy may offer some relief of the pain.

Abdominal organs are frequent sites of spread of this tumor. An enlarged, nodular liver may be present, but more commonly there is only slight hepatomegaly or the liver feels entirely normal. An elevated alkaline phosphatase level with other results of liver function tests within normal limits usually indicates hepatic metastasis. Adrenal involvement is frequent, but signs of overt adrenal insufficiency are rare.

Lymphatic spread via the peribronchial nodes to the mediastinum occurs frequently in cancer of the lung. Occasionally, it is possible to resect involved mediastinal nodes, although this procedure will rarely prolong life [175]. Extension of the tumor into the mediastinum directly or via metastases so that operation is contraindicated can be predicted when certain findings are present. Hoarseness secondary to vocal cord paralysis indicates involvement of the recurrent laryngeal nerve. Because of its deeper location under the arch of the aorta, the left nerve is more frequently involved. Bilateral swelling and venous engorgement of the neck, shoulders, and upper chest indicate obstruction of the superior vena cava. Dysphagia may indicate spread of the tumor into the posterior mediastinum with invasion of the esophagus. Roentgenographic studies with a barium swallow will usually confirm the presence or absence of esophageal involvement.

Bronchoscopic observation of the tumor may reveal evidence of inoperability. Any visible evidence of tumor at the carina or in the trachea is a sign of inoperability. There must be a large enough segment of normal bronchus to allow adequate closure of the bronchial stump after resection. Fixation of a major bronchus and widening or distortion of the carina occur with mediastinal extension of the tumor and contraindicate operation. A biopsy of the distorted area may reveal tumor even though the mucosa appears normal.

Extension of tumor outside the lung to pleura or chest wall usually contraindicates operation. In this group of patients, intrapleural chemotherapy offers better palliation of the symptoms resulting from excessive fluid accumulation.

Paralysis of the diaphragm on the involved side indicates invasion of the phrenic nerve. This is not an absolute contraindication to operation, since with lower lobe lesions it may occasionally be possible to resect the tumor and the involved portion of the nerve and pericardium.

The frequent association of emphysema and bronchogenic carcinoma necessitates a careful evaluation of pulmonary reserve prior to thoracotomy. If the patient already has severe respiratory impairment, this may represent an absolute contraindication to operation. The patient must have sufficient pulmonary reserve to survive both thoracotomy and the effects of loss of functioning pulmonary tissue following lobectomy or pneumonectomy.

The decision as to whether to operate on a patient with lung cancer plus airway obstruction and emphysema is often difficult. Since the results of surgery are so poor, it is unwise to recommend surgery with enthusiasm in subjects whose pulmonary function is borderline.

Many techniques have been used to assess whether a subject can stand a pneumonectomy.

These include differential bronchospirometry, ventilation-perfusion scans [18], and temporary occlusion of the pulmonary artery with a balloon. All are useful in individual cases but cannot be recommended for routine use. Significant pulmonary hypertension at rest is a contraindication, as is the development of pulmonary hypertension following occlusion of the pulmonary artery of the affected lung. Nonetheless, most such subjects have clinical evidence of severe lung impairment with grossly abnormal spirometry or significant arterial oxygen desaturation occurring with or without carbon dioxide retention.

Associated cardiac, hepatic, or renal disease also may be an absolute contraindication if it is of sufficient severity to make unlikely the chance of the patient surviving the operation. Surgery also should be avoided in a patient who has had a myocardial infarction within the past 3 months.

Pneumonectomy and Lobectomy

In the early 1930s, pneumonectomy was thought to be the only proper surgical treatment of bronchogenic carcinoma, and in the years 1930 to 1940, 75 percent of all pulmonary resections for lung cancer were pneumonectomies [209]. However, in the last 30 years, with the improvement of techniques in thoracic surgery, the tendency is to perform lesser resections rather than routine pneumonectomy, and today the choice of surgical treatment in lung cancer is lobectomy. As a result, pneumonectomy is performed only if the location of the tumor is such that a lesser resection is technically impossible. Contrary to simple pneumonectomy, radical pneumonectomy increases only operative mortality and morbidity without any increase in survival rate [120].

Bronchoplastic Resection and Segmentectomy

In a smaller percentage of patients, in whom the tumor is located proximally in a mainstem bronchus, bronchoplastic (sleeve) resection with lobectomy is possible. This conservative procedure enables resection of the tumor and at the same time conservation of lung tissue. Bronchoplastic resections account for 5 to 10 percent of all resections [8,100,138,142,153]. Another surgical procedure to conserve lung tissue is segmentectomy. This procedure is indicated only in very special circumstances, that is, a small peripheral tumor in an aged patient with limited respiratory and cardiovascular reserve [7,101].

Palliative Resection

Palliative resection is indicated only in patients in whom obstructive pneumonia has led to abscess formation or in whom the tumor causes severe, repeated pulmonary hemorrhages, or to relieve the symptoms of pulmonary hypertrophic osteoarthropathy.

Postoperative Mortality and Morbidity

The postoperative complications and death in lung cancer patients are relatively low. The Lung Cancer Study Group found an overall 30-day mortality of 3.7 percent in 2200 patients [68]. Small resections (less than lobectomy) carried a 1.4 percent mortality; lobectomy, 2.9 percent; and pneumonectomy, 6.2 percent. Age is an important factor in predicting operative mortality [134,140]. The mortality rate is 1.3 percent in patients under 60 years old, 4.1 percent in those between 60 and 69 years old, and 7.1 percent in those over 70 years old. The most common causes for early postoperative death are pulmonary embolism, pneumonia with respiratory failure, and bronchopleural fistulas with empyema.

Survival

Survival of patients with bronchogenic carcinoma is directly related to the patient's general condition, histologic cell type of the tumor, and the stage of the disease.

Patients with stage I disease (T1, T2, N0, M0) following surgical resection of the primary tumor have an expected 70 percent 5-year survival rate, independent of the histologic cell type (Fig. 53-23).

For patients with clinical stage II disease (T1, T2, N1, M0) the expected 5-year survival rate decreases to 50 percent (Fig. 53-24) and the prognosis is much less favorable for those with adenocarcinoma and large-cell carcinoma [175,186]. Moreover, at the time of thoracotomy the disease may be found to be more extensive than what was clinically diagnosed, and the postsurgical pathologic staging may change to stage IIIa, IIIb or even IV disease.

Patients with clinical stage IIIa disease (T1 to T3, N1, N2, M0) the expected 5-year survival rate is less than 20 percent and only a minority of these patients are candidates for surgical resection. The prognosis is even worse in patients with N2 disease. Pearson and associates [156] reviewed 141 patients with mediastinal lymph nodes in whom curative resection was deemed possible. In 79 patients with positive findings on

Fig. 53-23. Probability of survival of 488 patients with postsurgical stage I non–small-cell lung cancer, according to cell type; only deaths from lung cancer are considered. Seven patients with mixed and multiple cell types were excluded from the analysis. *Asterisks* indicate that 20 or fewer patients were alive at the beginning of that interval. Zero time on the *abscissa* represents 30 days after operation. (Reproduced from DE Williams et al. Survival of patients surgically treated for stage I lung cancer. *J Thorac Cardiovasc Surg* 82:70, 1981. With permission.)

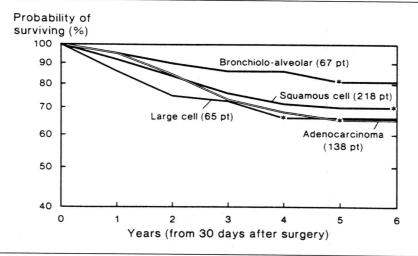

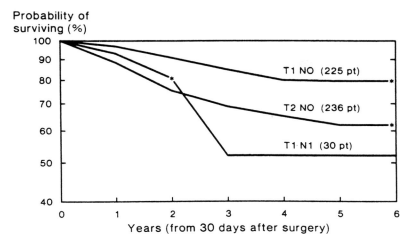

Fig. 53-24. Probability of survival of 491 patients with postsurgical stage I non–small-cell lung cancer, according to TN classification; only deaths from lung cancer are considered. Four patients with in situ squamous carcinoma were excluded from the analysis. *Asterisks* indicate that 20 or fewer patients were alive at the beginning of that interval. Zero time on the *abscissa* represents 30 days after operation. (Reproduced from DE Williams et al. Survival of patients surgically treated for stage I lung cancer. *J Thorac Cardiovasc Surg* 82:70, 1981. With permission.)

preoperative mediastinoscopy, the 5-year survival rate for all patients was 9 percent, versus 24 percent in 62 patients with negative results on preoperative mediastinoscopy. Curative resections almost doubled the 5-year survival rate from 9 to 18 percent in the first group, and from 24 to 41 percent in the second group.

Regarding the histologic cell type in stage IIIa disease, with subcarinal lymph nodes (N2), there is some controversy about surgical treatment of adenocarcinoma because of the very low survival rate. However, there is agreement that in those patients surgical resection alone is inadequate and adjuvant therapy (radiotherapy, combined chemotherapy) is recommended [187].

Patients with clinical stage IIIb or IV disease are not candidates for surgical treatment.

Second Primary Tumors

Second primary tumors occur in about 3 percent of patients postoperatively. In selected cases, the second primary tumor may also be resectable. However, only about 30 percent of these patients with resection survive 5 years, and the operative mortality is high, 10 to 20 percent [64,102]. The median survival time for patients with stage I disease is 26 months, while for stage II and stage IIIa disease it is less than 1 year.

Surgical Treatment for Small-Cell Lung Cancer

Until recently, it was generally accepted that surgical treatment was contraindicated in patients with small-cell carcinoma. However, over the past years, there has been experience that suggests that surgical resection of local disease combined with vigorous chemotherapy may enhance survival of patients with small-cell carcinoma [132].

Medical Therapy

Since fewer than half the patients with bronchogenic carcinoma are candidates for resection and only a small percentage of these are cured, most patients with this disease require some form of palliation. In caring for the group with nonresectable lesions, the physician is concerned not only with prolonging the patient's life, but also with making his or her last months as comfortable and productive as possible. Therapy should include efforts to slow the growth of the tumor and to treat complications as they arise, but above all, symptoms should be relieved.

Palliation implies the use of therapeutic measures that relieve symptoms and discomfort without necessarily changing the basic course of the disease. Inherent in this concept is the idea that the physician should not prescribe medication that will make the patient's symptoms worse. Agents or procedures that offer little or no hope of cure and whose use is associated with a significant incidence of unpleasant side effects should be avoided.

Pain and cough are the specific symptoms most frequently requiring therapy. Opiates offer the best relief, but because of the side effects and the problem of addiction associated with their use, it is better to avoid these drugs if less potent agents will suffice. When either cough or pain can be relieved only by opiates, they should be given only in doses sufficient to afford relief. Many physicians have an unreasoning reluctance to prescribe morphine and its derivatives even to patients with inoperable carcinoma. This is a serious omission, for the prime function of the medical attendant under such circumstances should be to render the last weeks of the patient's life as comfortable as possible.

Granting the preceding circumstances, heroic measures to prolong life by a few hours or days can only be classified as misplaced enthusiasm. Addiction often has to be accepted as the price of allowing a patient to die without undue suffering. For many years, the Brompton Hospital in London has relieved the pain and cough of inoperable lung cancer with a mixture known as the Brompton cocktail, the essential ingredients of which are morphine, cocaine, and gin. If opium alone is given, the patient tends to become withdrawn and difficult to nurse. The addition of cocaine counteracts this effect of opium, and the patient becomes extroverted and more easily managed. Alcohol is used as a vehicle for the narcotics, and it makes the cocktail more palatable; furthermore, it is a potent pain reliever itself. The concentrations of the constituents are adjusted according to the needs. Chlorpromazine and related drugs are sometimes helpful in that they decrease the dosage of narcotics needed for effect.

Steroids and irradiation therapy for the syndrome of superior vena caval obstruction are indicated as soon as the syndrome is recognized. Although irradiation, as discussed below, may have more lasting benefit, steroid therapy works quickly and offers the patient prompt relief from a terrible situation.

The problem usually arises as to how much to tell the patient about his or her disease. Some members of the patient's family must always be informed of the nature of the illness and prognosis. Relatives usually have definite ideas as to how much the patient should be told. If their wishes are contrary to the physician's ideas of what should be done, every attempt should be made to resolve these differences before there is any discussion of the problem with the patient.

Radiation Therapy

The basic indication for radiation therapy is inoperability [79]. This form of therapy can modify the natural course of the disease, relieve distressing symptoms, and produce an apparent cure in an occasional patient. It is imperative to distinguish between irradiation given for palliation and that given in the hope of producing a cure. Palliative irradiation usually involves a lesser dose given over a shorter time to a limited area, while curative radiation therapy is given over a longer period, a higher dose is used, and the area irradiated is not confined to the lesion itself but includes the regional lymph nodes, hilum, and mediastinum. Enthusiasm for radiation therapy is low, probably because of improper selection of patients and a lack of expertise among those who practiced this type of therapy in the past.

In general, radiation therapy should not be used without histologic proof of the presence of a tumor. Accurate histologic examination is the only method that ensures a correct diagnosis of cancer and avoids mismanagement of other lesions that may simulate a pulmonary malignancy, that is, tuberculosis.

The response to x-ray therapy depends primarily on the cell type of the tumor and the presence of blood vessel invasion. Squamous cell carcinomas and adenocarcinomas in general are less affected by irradiation, and the tumor seldom shrinks much with this mode of therapy. In contrast, undifferentiated carcinomas, in particular the oat cell type, have an excellent initial response to therapy and rapidly melt away. However, recurrence with decreased sensitivity to radiation is usual within a few weeks or months.

Palliative Radiation Therapy

This form of therapy is often helpful in relieving the distressing symptoms of cough and hemoptysis in patients with a large hilar growth. Symptoms secondary to mediastinal invasion and superior vena caval obstruction, as well as compression of the trachea or paralysis of recurrent laryngeal nerves, may be relieved temporarily. Nonetheless, it is important to remember that one cannot palliate an asymptomatic patient, and radiation is seldom indicated in the absence of symptoms. Occasionally, the dyspnea and facial edema seen in patients with the superior vena caval syndrome may become worse after the first two or three treatments owing to tissue destruction and inflammation produced by the irradiation. Prior treatment with steroids may prevent this complication, especially if the patient has an anaplastic carcinoma.

Metastatic lesions outside the lung are usually best managed by chemotherapy; the outstanding exception is bone metastases, for which usually a simple course of low-dose irradiation gives marked relief of pain.

Large, localized peripheral tumors may lead to recurrent pleural effusion and dyspnea. X-ray and cobalt radiation may decrease the size of the tumor; however, appreciable pleural fluid is a contraindication to radiation therapy. Recurrent pleural effusion associated with diffuse or hilar tumors is best managed by intrapleural injection of agents designed to obliterate the pleural space [119].

Radiation treatment of brain metastases from lung cancer is also often worthwhile since the brain is the only site of secondary deposits in about 25 percent of subjects. The use of high-dose dexamethasone further increases symptomatic relief by decreasing raised intracranial pressure and tissue edema. The 1-year survival rate of these patients is about 14 percent while 4 percent survived 3 years [40].

Contraindications to radiation must be considered in terms of the type of irradiation to be given. Severe anemia, cardiac failure, azotemia, and visceral metastases are the only contraindications to small doses given over a limited area to relieve symptoms.

Preoperative Irradiation

Because of the high rate of nonresectability and the poor results from surgery alone in stage IIIa lung cancer, various workers in the field have suggested that preoperative irradiation might possibly improve the results of therapy [12,13,21]. The most vigorous proponents of this mode of therapy have been Bloedorn and associates [12,13]. Initially, it was suggested that preoperative x-ray therapy might render resectable some tumors that would otherwise be inoperable due to direct spread and fixation to vital structures. It

also was thought that lymph node metastases might be sterilized and that systemic and local dissemination at the time of operation would be less likely. The main objections to preoperative irradiation relate to the fact that healing is delayed and there is a greater incidence of bronchopleural fistula and wound breakdown. The experience of most workers suggests that when a curative dose of radiation (5000 to 6000 rads) is given preoperatively, there is an appreciable increase in surgical morbidity and mortality. If the preoperative irradiation is reduced to about 4000 rads, serious postoperative sequelae are less frequent. Improved survival in apical lung tumors was reported by Paulson [152] and Mallams and coauthors [127] with preoperative radiotherapy compared with irradiation alone. Hilaris and coworkers [90] showed that preoperative irradiation of apical lung tumors greatly increased resectability but did not change survival.

Two randomized trials conducted by the National Cancer Institute and the Veterans Administration [202] showed no survival advantage even if moderate doses of preoperative irradiation were used. Thus the few nonresectable tumors that become operable as a consequence of preoperative irradiation are more than counterbalanced by the increase in surgical mortality.

Postoperative Irradiation

The effectiveness of postoperative irradiation in patients with locally advanced disease, tumor sites inaccessible to the surgeon, or possible nodal micrometastases is most doubtful. A large number of prospective studies have shown no benefit from postoperative radiotherapy in patients after pneumonectomy and in patients without lymph node metastases [33,187,199]; in patients with stage IIIa disease (T3, N1, N2, M0) a significant 5-year survival rate was seen [34,77] in patients given this treatment.

Complications of Radiation Therapy

Radiation reactions during the treatment are anorexia, nausea, and vomiting. Dysphagia due to radiation esophagitis often appears after 3 to 4 weeks of therapy and may be most distressing; it usually clears spontaneously in 1 to 2 months. A persistent, dry cough may appear at about the same time as the esophagitis, but this often lasts for 6 to 12 months. Presumably, the bronchial mucous glands and goblet cells are affected by the radiation.

Radiation pneumonitis and fibrosis may occur as early as 6 months after radical x-ray therapy for lung cancer (Fig. 53-25). They are usually, but by no means always, limited to the area irradiated and consequently in lung cancer are most often seen in paramediastinal regions (Fig. 53-26). The initial reaction is that of a pneumonitis, but with time there is a gradual transition to fibrosis [31,80,164]. Eventually the patient may become short of breath, and the pulmonary function demonstrates several abnormalities from an interrelationship of preexisting lung disease, the tumor, and postradiation fibrosis [67].

Following irradiation of the lungs, the early findings are pulmonary congestion, edema, lymphangiectasis, and hyaline membrane formation. The production of surfactant is reduced, and the alveolar cells desquamate. There is necrosis of bronchial and bronchiolar epithelium, and endarteritis of the small vessels of the lung may occur [203]. Later, fibrosis becomes more evident, and the pleura, capillary membranes, and small vessels all may be involved. Retraction of the lung to the affected side occurs. Cor pulmonale is a rare complication (see Chap. 52).

Steroids have been used to treat the symptoms of radiation pneumonitis. Symptomatically, they seem to be very effective, dyspnea and cough often being relatively rapidly relieved. Despite the symptomatic relief afforded by steroids, the

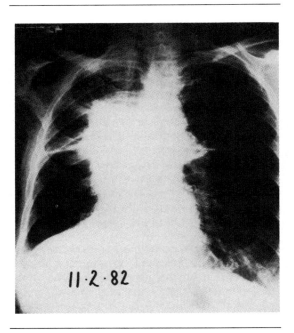

Fig. 53-26. Postirradiation pulmonary fibrosis in right hilar region. (*Source:* See Fig. 53-9.)

Fig. 53-25. Computed tomographic (CT) evidence of pulmonary fibrosis 6 months following radical irradiation (5500 cGy in 25 fractions) for squamous cell carcinoma of right upper lobe bronchus. Plain chest radiograph at the time was unremarkable, and there was no clinically evident respiratory embarrassment. (*Source:* See Fig. 53-9.)

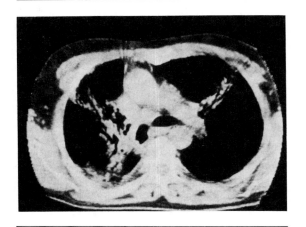

routine administration of these agents concomitantly with radiation therapy has been shown to avert neither radiation pneumonitis nor fibrosis. Furthermore, the decrease in pulmonary function that may occur as a result of this mode of therapy is apparently not affected by concomitant administration of steroids.

Aside from the effects of radiation on the lungs and esophagus, the bony thorax, skin, heart, and spinal cord may be affected. An excellent review of the possible complications is that of Whitfield, Bond, and Arnott [208]. The use of supervoltage and cobalt therapy has done much to reduce the side effects of irradiation; nevertheless, in certain patients there will be some side effects no matter what technique is used.

Measures to Potentiate Radiotherapy

Since the irradiation treatment of bronchogenic carcinoma is most disappointing, various measures to potentiate radiotherapy have been tried. It is known that high oxygen tension increases radiosensitivity of the tumor [76,188], just as hyperthermia increases the tumoricidal effect of ionizing radiation [58]. However, radiotherapy in hyperbaric oxygen, as well as in hyperthermia, is technically most difficult, with no advantage in remission, duration, or survival. Therefore, use of these modalities has not been generally accepted.

Chemotherapy

NON–SMALL-CELL CARCINOMA OF THE BRONCHUS

Lung cancer patients with advanced, unresectable lesions (stage IIIb or IV disease) have a very poor prognosis, since 70 percent die within 1 year and 85 to 90 percent die within 2 years. With mediastinal node involvement, the prognosis is even worse, regardless of histologic type.

At the present time, the only treatment modality offered to these patients with advanced disease is chemotherapy. Unfortunately, the response rates to single-agent or combined-drug chemotherapy are low, and contrary to small-cell carcinoma, it is not clear whether combined chemotherapy improves survival in these patients. In addition, chemotherapy is often associated with toxic effects that may shorten and make miserable the life of these patients. Therefore, a careful selection of patients with advanced disease is mandatory in order to avoid more distress and suffering as a result of chemotherapy.

SINGLE-AGENT CHEMOTHERAPY

The response rates to single-agent chemotherapy are low, and in general, there has been little change even with new agents tested in recent years [172] (see Table 53-11).

Alkylating Agents. In earlier reports, the effectiveness of nitrogen mustard in the treatment of squamous cell carcinoma was overoptimistic [25], since Edmonson and coauthors [50,51] reported less than 10 percent partial responses in patients with squamous cell and large-cell carcinoma using large intermittent doses of nitrogen mustard (see Table 53-11). Because of the low partial response, high toxicity, and side effects, the use of this drug in the treatment of lung cancer has been discontinued. The introduction of cyclophosphamide increased slightly the response in adenocarcinoma, but this drug is practically ineffective in squamous cell carcinoma [50] (see Table 53-11).

Methotrexate. Contrary to cyclophosphamide, methotrexate is partially effective in the treatment of squamous cell carcinoma, while its effectiveness is very small or none in adenocarcinoma and large-cell carcinoma [173,179].

Antitumor Antibiotics. As with other single agents, the response rates in non–small-cell carcinoma to doxorubicin (Adriamycin) and bleomycin are low, while in combination with other agents the partial response rate increases [17,112, 145].

Nitrosoureas. The various forms of nitrosourea are used in a wide variety of combination regimens. The addition of CCNU (chloroethyl-cyclohexyl-nitrosourea) or BCNU (bis-chloroethyl-nitrosourea) to cyclophosphamide and methotrexate increased the partial response rate as well as survival [84]. Since the use of nitrosourea as a single agent in the treatment of lung cancer is very disappointing, the encouraging results of this drug in combination with other agents may be due to synergism between these drugs.

Vinca Alkaloids and New Agents. Use of the vinca alkaloids vincristine and vinblastine causes some partial response in adenocarcinoma [25], while the newer alkaloid vindesine has shown some activity in all types of non–small-cell lung cancer [75]. From the newer agents (mitomycin C, cis-platinum, vindesine) tried in the last few years, the results of the Eastern Cooperative Oncology Group are summarized in Table 53-12. The results are rather disappointing, since the response rates to these drugs in adenocarcinoma and squamous cell carcinoma are low.

COMBINATION CHEMOTHERAPY

Since the results of single-agent chemotherapy for non–small-cell lung cancer are most discouraging, combination chemotherapy using two to five different agents [48,72,124,162,169] was introduced in the hope to achieve better results. Unfortunately, the results of combination chemotherapy so far are highly variable, owing to too small a number of patients in each investigation, and the response rates are not much higher than with single agents. However, there is a tendency for higher partial regression with combination chemotherapy in squamous cell carcinoma and adenocarcinoma than with single agents (Table 53-13). Since the results of chemotherapy in terms of survival are very low and the toxicity with any combination very high, none of the reported drugs or drug combinations should be used routinely.

COMBINED CHEMOTHERAPY AND RADIOTHERAPY

Radiotherapy of limited, nonresectable lung cancer (stages IIIb and IV) is associated with a high

Table 53-11. **Studies on established single agents**

Drug	Tumor type*	No.	CR[†]	PR	NR[‡]	Reference
Actinomycin D	SCC	47	0	3	40	165
Adriamycin 1	UC	10	0	3	7	145
	AC	17	0	1	16	
	SCC	13	0	0	13	
Adriamycin 2	SCC	58	1	3	54	112
	AC	45	0	2	43	
	LCC	37	0	2	35	
Cyclophosphamide	AC	79	1	9	69	50
Nitrogen mustard	SCC	70	0	6	64	50
	LCC	39	0	3	36	51
Methyl CCNU	SCC	46				
	AC	32				212
	LCC	35				
BCNU	SCC	35	No details of response rate			
	AC	16	given, but no group showed			
	LCC	10	improved survival			
CCNU	SCC	77	compared with control			
	AC	41				
	LCC	32				
Methotrexate						
0.6 mg/kg twice	SCC	23	0	8	15	173
weekly	AC	3	0	0	3	
0.2 mg/kg twice	SCC	11	0	1	10	
weekly	AC	4	0	0	4	
400 mg/ml/24	SCC	27	0	7	20	179
hrs with						
rescue						
800 mg/24 hrs	SCC	13	0	1	12	189
with rescue						
Vincristine	SCC	10	0	1	9	25
	LCC	10	0	0	10	
	AC	15	0	5	10	

*AC = adenocarcinoma; SCC = squamous cell carcinoma; LCC = large-cell carcinoma; UC = undifferentiated carcinoma.
[†]CR = complete response; PR = partial response; NR = no response.
[‡]Stable disease scored as no response.
Source: RL Souhami. The Management of Advanced Non-Small Cell Carcinoma of the Bronchus. In JF Smith (Ed), *The Management of Lung Cancer.* London: Edward Arnold, 1984.

rate of regression (75 to 90 percent), but a low 5-year survival rate (5 to 10 percent) mainly due to local relapses and distant metastases [174]. These results suggest that the tumor is often microscopically disseminated at the time of diagnosis. Thus the combination of chemotherapy and radiotherapy seems to be the most promising approach to the treatment of patients with stage IIIb or IV disease. Table 53-14 summarizes the various combined-modality therapies [1,4,83,87,126,193,214]. The response rate was 60 to 80 percent; however,

the median survival time was low, 5 to 18 months. The only 5-year survival rate was achieved with radiotherapy followed by combined chemotherapy with cyclophosphamide, doxorubicin, methotrexate, and procarbazine.

Most of the currently available combined regimens result in additive toxicity to the heart, lung, esophagus, and bone marrow. The low survival rate and the high toxicity of combined-modality therapy are disappointing in a similar way to the single or combined chemotherapy, in the treat-

Table 53-12. **New single agents**

Drug	Tumor*	No.	CR	PR	NR†	Reference
ACNU	SCC	10	0	0	10	62
	AC	13	0	0	13	
Adriamycin/DNA complex	SCC	7	0	0	7	112
	AC	1	0	0	1	
Dianhydrogalacticol 1	SCC	26	0	4	22	
	AC	16	0	0	16	62
	LCC	13	0	2	13	
Dianhydrogalacticol 2	SCC	26	0	0	22	165
Ftorafur	AC	33	0	1	32	165
	LCC	3	0	0	3	
ICRF 159	SCC	15	0	1	14	45
	AC	20	0	2	18	
	LCC	8	0	0	8	
Ifosfamide	SCC	28	2	9	17	37
	AC	4	0	0	4	
	LCC	6	0	3	3	
L-Asparaginase (2 different schedules)	SCC LCC AC	Numbers unclear, response rate not given. Survival shortened in high dose group				19
Maytansine	SCC	12	0	1	11	46
	AC	17	0	2	15	
	LCC	13	0	1	12	
Mitomycin C1	AC	20	1	4	15	170
	LCC	15	0	2	13	
Mitomycin C2	SCC	27	0	5	22	165
Piperazinedione	AC	27	0	2	25	165
	LCC	3	0	0	3	
Platinum 1	AC	22	0	2	20	20
Platinum 2	AC	9	0	0	9	30
	SCC	6	0	1	5	
	LCC	3	0	0	3	
Pyrazofurin	SCC	14	0	0	14	73
	AC	10	0	0	10	
Quelamycin	SCC	11	0	0	11	23
	LCC	7	0	3	4	
	AC	1	0	0	1	
Rubidazone	SCC	16	0	0	16	62
Vindesine	SCC	14	0	3	11	74
	AC	29	0	6	23	
	LCC	3	0	1	2	
VP-16-213	SCC	20	0	5	15	47
	AC	24	0	3	21	

*See Table 53-11 for abbreviations.
†Stable disease scored as no response.
Source: See Table 53-11.

Table 53-13. **Mean response rate (percent, with range) in chemotherapy studies on 10 or more patients**

No. of drugs	SCC		AC		LCC	
	No. of studies	Percent response	No. of studies	Percent response	No. of studies	Percent response
1	18	11.1 (0–39)	14	9.6 (0–33)	6	8.2 (0–15.2)
2	5	10.1 (3–20)		14.3 (5.8–33)	3 (72*)	11.5 (7.1–16.6)
3	7	22.4 (0–37.5)	9	26.2 (0–42.8)	3 (63*)	14.6 (0–32)
4 or more	11	29.4 (8.9–87)	9	32.5 (6.3–64)	4 (56*)	14.8 (0–35)

*Combined total of all patients in these studies.
Source: See Table 53-11.

ment of nonresectable, non–small-cell lung carcinoma.

CHEMOTHERAPY FOR SMALL-CELL LUNG CANCER

The abysmal results of surgery in the treatment of oat cell carcinoma have prompted a search for other therapeutic approaches. The most promising to date has been chemotherapy, with or without radiation. Since small-cell carcinoma of the lung grows rapidly, the TNM system has little relevance to the management of small-cell carcinoma of the lung. Therefore, the Veterans Administration Lung Cancer Study Group divided these patients into two groups: those with limited and those with extensive disease. Localization of the disease to one hemithorax and ipsilateral lymph nodes is defined as limited, while dissemination beyond this is termed extensive. Today, when chemotherapy is the choice of treatment of small-cell lung cancer, this simple division into two stages is important in assessing the outcome of different treatment modalities [35,125].

Since experience has shown that other rapidly growing tumors such as Burkitt's lymphoma and acute lymphatic leukemia tend to respond well to chemotherapy, it seemed logical to try various therapeutic regimens in oat cell cancer in the hope that this condition might be similarly responsive. All the drugs mentioned in the previous paragraphs have some chemotherapeutic effect by themselves, but it has become abundantly clear that multiple-drug regimens are more effective than is a single drug. Thus various combinations of cyclophosphamide with vincristine, methotrexate, doxorubicin, CCNU, and other agents have been tried, and virtually all have been

shown to extend the life of persons with oat cell carcinoma [205]. For the most part, at least three drugs and sometimes four are given. A good review of the treatment of small-cell carcinoma was written by Sorensen [180].

Prophylactic brain irradiation also has been tried because chemotherapeutic agents do not traverse the blood-brain area and it is known that secondaries from oat cell carcinoma are present in 40 percent of subjects with the condition when they are first seen. Prophylactic irradiation appears to reduce the likelihood of the development of brain metastases. Immunotherapy with BCG also has been tried, but the benefits of this treatment appear to be negligible [49].

While it is true that multiple-drug regimens have definitely prolonged the life of persons afflicted with the dreadful condition so that 2- and 3-year remissions are occurring in a significant number of cases, it is far too early to say whether cure ever occurs. Moreover, the side effects of multiple-drug regimens are by no means negligible; too often, although the tumor shrinks, so also does the quality of life. For this reason, while continued therapeutic trial of various agents is entirely justified, the haphazard administration of combinations of these toxic agents *faute de mieux* is to be avoided at all costs.

Immunotherapy

It is known that immunologic responsiveness is suppressed in lung cancer patients and that those showing less immune suppression have a better prognosis [24,97]. Moreover, immune responsiveness is suppressed in lung cancer patients by radiation and chemotherapy. Therefore, immuno-

Table 53-14. **Combined chemotherapy and radiotherapy phase II studies for non–small-cell lung cancer***

Reference	No. of evaluable patients	Stage	Thoracic irradiation dose	Type of chemotherapy	Timing of chemotherapy[†]	Objective response rate, %	Median survival (months)
83	27	LD	5,000	CPA + MTX + DACT + VCR	1 + 3	60	13
87	26	LD, DD	4,000 (split)	CPA + ADR	1 + 2 + 3	15[‡]	—
1	22	III	5,000	VCR + ADR + CPA	3	—	5
193	69	LD	4,500	CPA + ADR + MTX + PCZ	3	62	13
126	101	III, Mo	3–4,200	CPA + ADR + MTX + PCZ	3	63	8.8[§]
4	31	DD	4,800‖	CPA + ADR + MTX	2 + 3	68	6
214	20	LD	5–7,000	CPA + ADR + CDDP	1 + 3	80	18

*LD = limited disease; DD = disseminated disease; CPA = cyclophosphamide; MTX = methotrexate; DACT = actinomycin D; VCR = vincristine; ADR = Adriamycin; PCZ = procarbazine; CDDP = cis-platin.
[†]Pre = 1; concomitant = 2; post = 3 radiotherapy.
[‡]Response to chemotherapy only.
[§]5-year survival = 10%.
‖Multiple fractions daily.
Source: Modified from J Klastersky, JP Soulier. Nonsurgical combined modalities in non-small cell lung cancer. *Chest* 89:291S, 1986.

therapy seemed a logical approach to treat this dreadful disease. Unfortunately, the use of non-specific immune stimulants—*Corynebacterium parvum* and BCG [98]—did not fulfill these hopes, and therefore, immunotherapy has no justified use in the treatment of lung cancer.

Laser Therapy

Use of the YAG laser through a bronchoscope to vaporize inoperable tumors that are choking the patient or causing uncontrollable hemoptysis appears justified as humane palliation.

References

1. Aakbiyik N, et al. Comparison of survival in patients with non-oat cell carcinoma of the lung using various types of treatment modalities. *Int J Radiat Oncol Biol Phys* 8:1597, 1982.
2. Ali MK, et al. Regional and overall pulmonary function changes in lung cancer. *J Thorac Cardiovasc Surg* 86:1, 1983.
3. American Joint Committee on Cancer. *Manual for Staging of Cancer*. Philadelphia: Lippincott, 1983. Pp 99–105.
4. Arcangeli G, et al. Pilot study of multi-fraction daily radiotherapy alternating with chemotherapy in patients with stage IV non-oat cell lung cancer. *Cancer Treat Rep* 69:25, 1985.
5. Ashbaugh DG. Mediastinoscopy. *Arch Surg* 100:568, 1970.
6. Auerbach O, et al. Carcinoma in situ and early invasive carcinoma occurring in the tracheobronchial tree in cases of bronchial carcinoma. *J Thorac Surg* 34:298, 1957.
7. Bennett WF, Abbey Smith R. Segmental resection for bronchogenic carcinoma: A surgical alternative for the compromised patient. *Ann Thorac Surg* 27:169, 1979.
8. Bennett WF, Abbey Smith R. A twenty-year analysis of the results of sleeve resection for primary bronchogenic carcinoma. *J Thorac Cardiovasc Surg* 76:840, 1978.
9. Bensch KG, et al. Oat-cell carcinoma of the lung: Its origin and relationship to bronchial carcinoid. *Cancer* 22:1163, 1968.
10. Bensch KG, Gordon GB, Miller LR. Electron microscopic and biochemical studies on the bronchial carcinoid tumor. *Cancer* 18:592, 1965.
11. Berlin NI, et al. The National Cancer Institute Cooperative Early Lung Cancer Detection Program: Results of the initial screen (prevalence): Introduction. *Am Rev Respir Dis* 130:545, 1984.
12. Bloedorn FG, Wizenberg MJ. Preoperative irradiation. *Radiol Clin North Am* 33:287, 1964.
13. Bloedorn FG, et al. Preoperative irradiation in bronchogenic carcinoma. *AJR* 92:77, 1964.
14. Bolen JW, Thorning D. Histogenetic classification of pulmonary carcinomas: Peripheral adenocarcinomas studied by light microscopy, histochemistry, and electron microscopy. *Pathol Annu* 17:77, 1982.
15. Bonikos DS, Archibald R, Bensch KG. On the origin of the so-called tumorlets of the lung. *Human Pathol* 7:461, 1976.
16. Bonikos DS, Hendrickson M, Bensch, KG. Pulmonary alveolar cell carcinoma: Fine structural and in vitro study of a case and critical review of this entity. *Am J Surg Pathol* 1:93, 1977.
17. Bosly A, et al. Adriamycin and adriamycin-DNA in inoperable bronchogenic carcinoma: A randomized study with cyclophosphamide vinblastine. *Eur J Cancer* 14:639, 1978.
18. Boysen PG, et al. Prospective evaluation for pneumonectomy using the ^{99m} technetium quantitative lung scan. *Chest* 72:422, 1977.
19. Brindley CO, et al. An analysis of comparative trials of L-asparaginase (NSC-109929), cyclophosphamide and placebo in patients with inoperable bronchogenic carcinoma using corrected survival estimates. *Oncology* 35:33, 1978.
20. Britell JC, et al. *cis*-Dichlorodiammineplatinum (II) alone followed by adriamycin plus cyclophosphamide at progression versus *cis*-dichlorodiammineplatinum (II), adriamycin, and cyclophosphamide in combination for adenocarcinoma of the lung. *Cancer Treat Rep* 62(8):1207, 1978.
21. Bromley LL, Szur L. Combined radiotherapy and resection for carcinoma of the bronchus: Experience with 66 patients. *Lancet* 2:937, 1955.
22. Bruderman I, et al. Immunocytochemical characterization of lung tumors in fine needle aspiration: The use of cytokeratin monoclonal antibodies for the differential diagnosis of squamous cell carcinoma and adenocarcinoma. *Cancer* 68:1817, 1990.
23. Brugarolas A, et al. Phase I clinical study of quelamycin. *Cancer Treat Rep* 62(10):1527, 1978.
24. Brugarolas A, Takita H. Immunologic status in lung cancer. *Chest* 64:427, 1973.
25. Brugarolas D, et al. Vincristine (NSC 67574) in non-small-cell bronchogenic carcinoma: Results of a phase II clinical study. *Eur J Cancer* 14:501, 1978.
26. Carlens E. Appraisal of choice and results of treatment of bronchogenic carcinoma. *Chest* 65:442, 1974.
27. Carlisle JC, McDonald JR, Harrington SW. Bronchogenic squamous cell carcinoma. *J Thorac Surg* 22:74, 1951.
28. Carney DN, et al. Demonstration of the stem cell nature of clonogenic tumor cells from lung cancer patients. *Stem Cells* 1:149, 1981.
29. Carter D, Eggleston JCE. Tumors of the Lower Respiratory Tract. In *Atlas of Tumor Pathology* (Second Series Fascicle 17). Washington: Armed Forces Institute of Pathology, 1980.

30. Casper ES, et al. Phase II study of high-dose *cis*-dichlorodiammineplatinum (II) in the treatment of non-small-cell lung cancer. *Cancer Treat Rep* 63(11):2107, 1979.

31. Castellino RA, et al. Latent radiation injury of lungs or heart activated by steroid withdrawal. *Ann Intern Med* 80:593, 1974.

32. Chan WC, Fung SC. Lung Cancer in Nonsmokers in Hong Kong. In E. Grundman (Ed), *Cancer Campaign*, Vol 6. New York: Verlag, 1982. Pp 199–202.

33. Choi NC. Role of Postoperative Radiation Therapy in Lung Cancer with Either Metastases to Regional Lymph Nodes (N1 or Unforeseen N2) or Direct Invasion Beyond Visceral Pleura (T3). In NC Choi, HC Grileo (Eds), *Thoracic Oncology*. New York: Raven, 1983. Pp 129–146.

34. Choi NCH, et al. Basis for new strategies in postoperative radiotherapy of bronchogenic carcinoma. *Int J Radiat Oncol Biol Phys* 6:31, 1980.

35. Cohen MH, et al. Cyclic alternating combination chemotherapy for small-cell bronchogenic carcinoma. *Cancer Treat Rep* 63:163, 1979.

36. Correa P, et al. Passive smoking and lung cancer. *Lancet* 2:595, 1983.

37. Costanzi JJ, et al. Ifosfamide in the treatment of recurrent or disseminated lung cancer. *Am Cancer Soc* 41:1715, 1978.

38. Credle WF, Smiddy JF, Elliot RC. Complications of fiberoptic bronchoscopy. *Am Rev Respir Dis* 109:67, 1974.

39. Dairaku M, et al. Immunohistochemical analysis of surfactant-apoprotein in the bronchiolo-alveolar carcinoma. *Virchows Arch [Pathol Anat]* 400:223, 1983.

40. Deeley TJ, Rice-Edwards JM. Radiotherapy in the management of cerebral secondaries from bronchial carcinoma. *Lancet* 1:1209, 1968.

41. Department of Health, Education and Welfare. *Smoking and Health: A Report of the Surgeon General.* (DHEW Publication No. PHS 79-50066). Washington: Department of Health, Education and Welfare, 1979.

42. Dermer GB. Origin of bronchioloalveolar carcinoma and peripheral bronchial adenocarcinoma. *Cancer* 49:881, 1982.

43. Dick R, Heard BE, Hinson KFW. Aspiration needle biopsy of thoracic lesions: An assessment of 227 biopsies. *Br J Dis Chest* 68:86, 1974.

44. Doll R, Peto R. The causes of cancer: Quantitative estimates of avoidable risks of cancer in the United States today. *J Natl Cancer Inst* 66:1191, 1981.

45. Eagan RT, et al. ICRF-159 versus polychemotherapy in non-small-cell lung cancer. *Cancer Treat Rep* 60(7):947, 1976.

46. Eagan RT, et al. Phase II evaluation of maytansine in patients with metastatic lung cancer. *Cancer Treat Rep* 62(10):1577, 1978.

47. Eagan RT, et al. VP-16-213 chemotherapy for advanced squamous cell carcinoma and adenocarcinoma of the lung. *Cancer Treat Rep* 62(5):843, 1978.

48. Eagan RT, et al. Platinum-based polychemotherapy versus dianhydrogalactitol in advanced non-small-cell lung cancer. *Cancer Treat Rep* 61(7):1339, 1977.

49. Editorial. Adjuvant therapy for lung cancer. *Br Med J* 1:187, 1977.

50. Edmonson JH, et al. Cyclophosphamide and CCNU in the treatment of inoperable small-cell carcinoma and adenocarcinoma of the lung. *Cancer Treat Rep* 60(7):925, 1976.

51. Edmonson JH, et al. Mechlorethamine (NSC-762) plus CCNU (NSC-79037) in the treatment of inoperable squamous and large-cell carcinoma of the lung. *Cancer Treat Rep* 60(5):625, 1976.

52. Emery AEH, et al. Aryl-hydrocarbon-hydroxylase inducibility in patients with cancer. *Lancet* 1:469, 1978.

53. Engelman RF, McNamara WL. Bronchogenic carcinoma: Statistical review of 234 autopsies. *J Thorac Surg* 27:227, 1954.

54. Farber SM, et al. *Cytologic Diagnosis of Lung Cancer.* Springfield, Ill.: Thomas, 1950.

55. Farber SM, et al. Significant cytologic findings in nonmalignant pulmonary disease. *Dis Chest* 31:1, 1957.

56. Feinstein AR. Symptomatic patterns, biologic behavior, and prognosis in cancer of the lung. *Ann Intern Med* 61:27, 1964.

57. Feinstein AR, Gelfman NA, Yesner R. The diverse effects of histopathology on manifestations and outcome of lung cancer. *Chest* 66:225, 1974.

58. Field SB, Bleehan NM. Hyperthermia in the treatment of cancer. *Cancer Treat Rep* 6(2):63, 1979.

59. Fink I, Gamsu G, Harter LP. CT guided aspiration biopsy of the thorax. *J Comput Assist Tomogr* 6:958, 1982.

60. Flehinger BJ, et al. Early lung cancer detection: Results of the initial (prevalence) radiologic and cytologic screening in the Memorial Sloan-Kettering study. *Am Rev Respir Dis* 130:555, 1984.

61. Fontana RS, et al. Early lung cancer detection: Results of the initial (prevalence) radiologic and cytologic screening in the Mayo Clinic study. *Am Rev Respir Dis* 130:561, 1984.

62. Fraile RJ, et al. Clinical trial of rubidazone in advanced squamous cell carcinoma of the lung and adenocarcinoma of the large intestine. *Cancer Treat Rep* 62(10):1599, 1978.

63. Frost JK, et al. Early lung cancer detection: Results of the initial (prevalence) radiologic and cytologic screening in the Johns Hopkins study. *Am Rev Respir Dis* 130:549, 1984.

64. Gale MH, et al. Prognostic factors in patients

with resected stage I non-small cell cancer. *Cancer* 54:1802, 1984.

65. Galluzzi S, Payne PM. Bronchial carcinoma: A statistical study of 741 necropsies with special reference to the distribution of blood-borne metastases. *Br J Cancer* 9:511, 1955.

66. Garfinkel L. Time trends in lung cancer mortality among nonsmokers and a note on passive smoking. *J Natl Cancer Inst* 66:1061, 1981.

67. Germon PA, Brady LW. Physiologic changes before and after radiation treatment for carcinoma of the lung. *JAMA* 206:809, 1968.

68. Ginsberg RG, et al. Modern thirty-day operative mortality for surgical resections in lung cancer. *J Thorac Cardiovasc Surg* 86:654, 1983.

69. Gould VE, Chejfee, G. Ultrastructural and biochemical analysis of "undifferentiated" pulmonary carcinomas. *Human Pathol* 9:377, 1978.

70. Gould VE, et al. Neuroendocrine cells and neuroendocrine neoplasms of the lung. *Pathol Annu* 18:287, 1983.

71. Gould VE, Memoli VA, Dardi LE. Multidirectional differentiation in human epithelial cancers. *J Submicroscopic Cytol* 13:97, 1981.

72. Gralla RJ, et al. Cisplatin and vindesine combination chemotherapy for advanced carcinoma of the lung: A randomized trial investigating two dosage schedules. *Ann Intern Med* 95:414, 1981.

73. Gralla RJ, et al. Phase II evaluation of pyrazofurin in patients with carcinoma of the lung. *Cancer Treat Rep* 62(3):451, 1978.

74. Gralla RJ, Cvitkovic E, Golbey RB. *cis*-Dichlorodiammineplatinum (II) in non-small-cell carcinoma of the lung. *Cancer Treat Rep* 63(9):1585, 1979.

75. Gralla RJ, et al. Phase II evaluation of vindesine in patients with non-small-cell carcinoma of the lung. *Cancer Treat Rep* 63(8):1343, 1979.

76. Gray LH, et al. The concentration of oxygen dissolved in tissues at the time of irradiation as a factor in radiotherapy. *Br J Radiol* 26:638, 1953.

77. Green N. Lung Cancer Post-resection Irradiation. In RB Livingston, (Ed), *Lung Cancer,* The Hague: Martinus Nijhoff, 1981. Pp 75–111.

78. Greenberg SD. Histology and Ultrastructure of Bronchiolo-Alveolar Carcinoma. In *Morphogenesis of Lung Cancer,* Vol 1. Boca Raton, Fla: CRC Press, 1982. Pp 121–145.

79. Gregor A. Radiotherapy for Inoperable Non-Small-Cell Carcinoma of the Bronchus. In JF Smith (Ed), *The Management of Lung Cancer.* London: Edward Arnold, 1984.

80. Gross NJ. Pulmonary effects of radiation therapy. *Ann Intern Med* 86:81, 1977.

81. Gusterson BA. Preneoplasia in the Lungs and the Potential of Cells to Have Modulated Phenotypes. In RL Carter (Ed), *Precancerous States.* New York: Oxford University Press, 1984. Pp 161–184.

82. Hammond EC. Smoking in relation to mortality and morbidity: Findings in first thirty-four months of follow-up in a prospective study started in 1959. *J Natl Cancer Inst* 32:1161, 1964.

83. Hansen HH, et al. Intensive combined chemotherapy and radiotherapy in patients with nonresectable bronchogenic carcinoma. *Cancer* 30:315, 1972.

84. Hansen HH, et al. Combination chemotherapy of advanced lung cancer: A randomized trial. *Cancer* 38:2201, 1976.

85. Harley NH, Cohen BS, Tso TC. Polonium-210: A Questionable Risk Factor in Smoking-Related Carcinogenesis. In GB Gori and FG Bock (Eds), *Banbury Report 3-A Safe Cigarette?* Cold Spring Harbor, NY: Cold Spring Harbor Laboratory, 1980. Pp 93–104.

86. Heitzman ER. The role of computed tomography in the diagnosis and management of lung cancer. *Chest* 89:237S, 1986.

87. Herman TS, et al. Combination chemotherapy with Adriamycin and cyclophosphamide (with or without radiation therapy) for cancer of the lung. *Cancer Treat Rep* 61:875, 1977.

88. Herrera GA, Alexander CB, DeMoraes HP. Ultrastructural subtypes of pulmonary adenocarcinoma: A correlation with patient survival. *Chest* 84:581, 1983.

89. Herrera GA, Alexander CB, Jones JM. Ultrastructural characterization of pulmonary neoplasms. *Surv Synth Pathol Respir* 3:520, 1984.

90. Hilaris BS, et al. The value of preoperative radiation therapy in apical cancer of the lung. *Surg Clin North Am* 54(4):831, 1974.

91. Hirayama T. Nonsmoking wives of heavy smokers have a higher risk of lung cancer: A study from Japan. *Br Med J* 282:183, 1981.

92. Hirayama T. Passive smoking and lung cancer: Consistency of association. *Lancet* 2:1425, 1983.

93. Hoffmann D, et al. Tobacco Carcinogenesis: Metabolic Studies in Humans. In H Autrup (Ed), *Human Carcinogenesis.* New York: Academic Press, 1983. Pp 809–832.

94. Hoffmann D, Wynder EL. A study of tobacco carcinogenesis: XI. Tumor initiators, tumor accelerators, and tumor promoting activity of condensate fractions. *Cancer* 27:848, 1971.

95. Hooper RG, Beechler GR, Johnston MC. Radioisotope scanning in the initial staging of bronchogenic carcinoma. *Am Rev Respir Dis* 118:279, 1978.

96. Horie A, Ohta M. Ultrastructural features of large-cell carcinoma of the lung with reference to the prognosis of patients. *Human Pathol* 12:423, 1981.

97. Israel L. Cell-mediated immunity in lung cancer patients: data, problems, and propositions. *Cancer Chemother Rep* 4:279, 1973.

98. Israel L. Nonspecific Immune Stimulation with

Corynebacteria in Lung Cancer. In L Israel, AP Chahinian (Eds), *Lung Cancer: Natural History, Prognosis and Therapy.* New York: Academic Press, 1976. Pp 107–140.

99. Jacques J, Currie W. Bronchiolo-alveolar carcinoma: A clara cell tumor? *Cancer* 40:2171, 1977.

100. Jensik RJ, et al. Sleeve lobectomy for carcinoma: A ten-year experience. *J Thorac Cardiovasc Surg* 64:400, 1972.

101. Jensik KJ, et al. Segmental resection for lung cancer: A fifteen-year experience. *J Thorac Cardiovasc Surg* 66:563, 1973.

102. Jensik RJ, et al. Survival following resection for second primary bronchogenic carcinoma. *J Thorac Cardiovasc Surg* 82:658, 1981.

103. Johnston WW, Frable WJ. Cytopathology of the respiratory tract: A review. *Am J Pathol* 84:372, 1976.

104. Jolly PC, et al. Parasternal mediastinotomy and mediastinoscopy: Adjuncts in the diagnosis of chest disease. *J Thorac Cardiovasc Surg* 66: 549, 1973.

105. Kameya T, Kodama T, Shimosato Y. Morphology of Lung Cancer in Relation to Its Function. In *Morphogenesis of Lung Cancer,* Vol 2. Boca Raton, Fla: CRC Press, 1982. Pp 107–129.

106. Kameya T, Kodama T, Shimosato Y. Ultrastructure of Small-Cell Carcinoma of the Lung (Oat and Intermediate Cell Types) in Relation to Histogenesis and to Carcinoid Tumor. In *Morphogenesis of Lung Cancer,* Vol 2. Boca Raton, Fla: CRC Press, 1982. Pp 16–43.

107. Kauffman F, Tessier JF, Oriol P. Adult passive smoking in the home environment: A risk factor for chronic airflow limitation. *Am J Epidemiol* 117:269, 1983.

108. Kellermann G, Luyten-Kellermann M, Shaw CR. Aryl hydroxylase inducibility and bronchogenic cancer. *N Engl J Med* 289:934, 1973.

109. Kellermann G, Luyten-Kellermann M, Shaw CR. Genetic variations of aryl hydroxylase hydrocarbon in human lymphocytes. *Am J Hum Genet* 25:325, 1973.

110. Kier LD, Yamasaki E, Ames BN. Detection of mutagenic activity in cigarette smoke condensates. *Proc Natl Acad Sci USA* 71:4159, 1974.

111. Kirsh MM, et al. Carcinoma of the lung: Results of treatment over ten years. *Ann Thorac Surg* 21:371, 1976.

112. Knight EW, et al. Adriamycin in the treatment of far-advanced lung cancer. *Cancer Treat Rep* 60(7):939, 1976.

113. Kodama T, et al. Ultrastructural Study of 50 Cases of Well-Differentiated Adenocarcinoma of the Lung (Abstract). In *Proceedings of the 2nd World Conference on Lung Cancer.* Copenhagen: International Association for the Study of Lung Cancer, 1980.

114. Kreyberg L, Liebow AA, Vehlinger EA. *Histological Typing of Lung Tumors* Geneva: World Health Organization, 1967.

115. Labeau F, Vanderhoeft P. Analysis of 500 mediastinoscopies. *Acta Chir Belg* 69:365, 1970.

116. Lamy P, et al. Pulmonary small cell carcinoma: New concept of its histologic origin-ultrastructural study in 18 cases (Abstract). *Eur J Respir Dis* 63(Suppl 125):29, 1982.

117. Larsson S. Pretreatment classification and staging of bronchogenic carcinoma. *Scand Thorac Cardiovasc Surg* 7(Suppl. 10):1, 1973.

118. Leading Article. Aryl hydrocarbon hydroxylase inducibility and lung cancer. *Lancet* 1:910, 1974.

119. Leff A, Hopewell PC, Costello J. Pleural effusion from malignancy. *Ann Intern Med* 88:532, 1978.

120. Le Roux BT. The Surgical Management of Bronchial Carcinoma. In JF Smith (Ed), *The Management of Lung Cancer.* London: Edward Arnold, 1984.

121. Lewis JW Jr, et al. The value of radiographic and computed tomography in the staging of lung carcinoma. *Ann Thorac Surg* 34:553, 1982.

122. Lilienfeld AP, et al. An evaluation of radiologic and cytologic screening for the early detection of lung cancer: A cooperative pilot study of the American Cancer Society and the Veterans Administration. *Cancer Res* 26:2083, 1966.

123. Line DH, Deeley TJ. The necropsy finding in carcinoma of the bronchus. *Br J Dis Chest* 65:238, 1971.

124. Livingston RB. Combination chemotherapy of bronchogenic carcinoma: I. Non-oat-cell. *Cancer Treat Rep* 4:153, 1977.

125. Livingston RB, et al. Small-cell carcinoma of the lung: Combined chemotherapy and radiation. *Ann Intern Med* 88:194, 1978.

126. Madej PJ, et al. Combined modality therapy for stage III, M0, non-small cell lung cancer: A five year experience. *Cancer* 54:5, 1984.

127. Mallams J, et al. Presurgical irradiation in bronchogenic carcinoma, superior sulcus type. *Radiology* 82:1050, 1964.

128. Matthews MJ. Morphology of lung cancer. *Semin Oncol* 1:175, 1974.

129. Matthews MJ. Problems in Morphology and Behavior of Bronchopulmonary Malignant Disease. In L Israel, AP Chahinian (Eds), *Lung Cancer: Natural History, Prognosis and Therapy.* New York: Academic Press, 1976. Pp 23–63.

130. Matthews MJ, et al. Frequency of residual and metastatic tumor in patients undergoing curative surgical resection for lung cancer. *Cancer Chemother Rep* 4:63, 1973.

131. Meyer CE, Liebov· AA. Relationship of interstitial pneumonia, honeycombing and atypical epithelial proliferation to cancer of the lung. *Cancer* 18:322, 1965.

132. Meyer JA, et al. The prospect of disease control

by surgery combined with chemotherapy in stage I–II small cell cancer. *Ann Thorac Surg* 36:37, 1983.

133. Montes M, et al. Clara cell adenocarcinoma: Light and electron microscope studies. *Am J Surg Pathol* 1:245, 1977.

134. Mountain CF. The biologic operability of stage III non-small cell lung cancer. *Ann Thorac Surg* 40:60, 1985.

135. Mountain CF. A new international staging system for lung cancer. *Chest* 89:225S, 1986.

136. Mountain CF, Carr DT, Anderson WAD. A system for the clinical staging of lung cancer. *AJR* 120:130, 1974.

137. Muggia FM, Krezoski SK, Hanson HH. Cell kinetic studies in patients with small-cell carcinoma of the lung. *Cancer* 34:1683, 1974.

138. Naef AP, de Gruneck J. Right pneumonectomy or sleeve lobectomy in the treatment of bronchogenic carcinoma. *Ann Thorac Surg* 17:168, 1974.

139. Nagasaki F, Flehinger BG, Martini N. Complications of surgery in the treatment of carcinoma of the lung. *Chest* 82:25, 1982.

140. Nakahara K, et al. A method for predicting postoperative lung function and its relation to postoperative complications in patients with lung cancer. *Ann Thorac Surg* 39:260, 1985.

141. Nakamura M, et al. A case of bronchioloalveolar carcinoma: Ultrastructural and lipid-biochemical studies. *Cancer* 52:861, 1983.

142. Naruke T, et al. Bronchoplastic procedures for lung cancer. *J Thorac Cardiovasc Surg* 73:927, 1977.

143. The National Cancer Institute Cooperative Early Lung Cancer Detection Program. Summary and conclusions. *Am Rev Respir Dis* 130:565, 1984.

144. Nohl HC. An investigation into the lymphatic and vascular spread of carcinoma of the bronchus. *Thorax* 11:172, 1956.

145. O'Bryan RM, et al. Dose-response evaluation of adriamycin in human neoplasia. *Cancer* 39:1940, 1977.

146. Oswald NC, et al. The diagnosis of primary lung cancer with special reference to sputum cytology. *Thorax* 26:623, 1971.

147. Otto TL, Zaslonka J, Lukianski M. Experience with mediastinoscopy. *Thorax* 27:463, 1972.

148. Pancoast HK. Superior pulmonary sulcus tumor: Tumor characterized by pain, Horner's syndrome, destruction of bone and atrophy of hand muscles. *JAMA* 99:1391, 1932.

149. Paris F, et al. Mediastinoscopy in the surgical management of lung carcinoma. *Thorax* 30:146, 1975.

150. Pastorino U, et al. Effect of chronic cardiopulmonary disease on survival after resection of stage I lung cancer. *Thorax* 37:680, 1982.

151. Paulson DL. Selection of patients for surgery for bronchogenic carcinoma. *Am Surg* 39:1, 1973.

152. Paulson DL. The survival rate in superior sulcus tumors treated by presurgical irradiation. *JAMA* 196:23, 1966.

153. Paulson DL, et al. Bronchoplastic procedures for bronchogenic carcinoma. *J Thorac Cardiovasc Surg* 59:38, 1970.

154. Payne CR, et al. Diagnostic accuracy of cytology and biopsy in primary bronchial carcinoma. *Thorax* 34:294, 1979.

155. Pearson FG. Discussion minisymposium on surgery for N2 disease. World Conference on Lung Cancer. *Chest* 89:339S, 1986.

156. Pearson FG, et al. Significance of positive superior mediastinal nodes identified at mediastinoscopy in patients with resectable cancer of the lung. *J Thorac Cardiovasc Surg* 83:1, 1982.

157. Pearson FG, et al. The role of mediastinoscopy in the selection of treatment of superior mediastinal lymph nodes. *J Thorac Cardiovasc Surg* 64:382, 1972.

158. Pilotti S, et al. Fine needle aspiration biopsy cytology of primary and metastatic pulmonary tumors. *Acta Cytol* 26:661, 1982.

159. Rainio P, Sutinen S, Sutinen SH. Ultrastructural Typing of Adenocarcinoma of the Lung: Correlation with Histology and Biologic Behavior (Abstract). In *Proceedings of the 2nd World Conference on Lung Cancer.* Copenhagen: International Association for the Study of Lung Cancer, 1980.

160. Rainio P, Sutinen S, Vaananen R. A scanning and transmission electron microscopic study of pulmonary adenocarcinoma with histological correlation. *Acta Pathol Microbiol Scand [A]* 90:463, 1982.

161. Ries LG, Pollack ES, Young JL. Cancer patient survival: Surveillance, epidemiology, and end results program, 1973–79. *J Natl Cancer Inst* 70:693, 1983.

162. Robert F, Omura G, Bartolucci AA. Combination chemotherapy with cyclophosphamide, adriamycin, intermediate-dose methotrexate and folinic acid rescue (CAMF) in advanced lung cancer. *Cancer* 45(1):1, 1980.

163. Royal College of Physicians. *Smoking and Health.* London: Pitman, 1962.

164. Rubin P. (Ed). *Radiation Biology and Radiation Pathology Syllabus.* Chicago: American College of Radiology, 1975. Pp 132–141, 158–187.

165. Ruckdeschel JC, et al. Chemotherapy for inoperable, non-small-cell bronchogenic carcinoma: EST 2575, generation II. *Cancer Treat Rep* 65(11):965, 1981.

166. Saba SR, et al. Dual differentiation in small-cell carcinoma (oat-cell carcinoma) of the lung. *Ultrastruct Pathol* 2:131, 1981.

167. Saba SR, et al. Carcinomas of the lung: An ultrastructural and immunocytochemical study. *Am J Clin Pathol* 80:6, 1983.

168. Sackner MA. Bronchofiberoscopy. *Am Rev Respir Dis* 111:62, 1975.
169. Saijo N, et al. Effect of ACNU on primary lung cancer, mesothelioma, and metastatic pulmonary tumors. *Cancer Treat Rep* 62(1):139, 1978.
170. Samson MK, et al. Mitomycin C in advanced adenocarcinoma and large-cell carcinoma of the lung. *Cancer Treat Rep* 62(1):163, 1978.
171. Sandler MA, et al. Computed tomographic evaluation of the adrenal gland in the preoperative assessment of bronchogenic carcinoma. *Radiology* 145:733, 1982.
172. Selawry O. The role of chemotherapy in the treatment of lung cancer. *Semin Oncol* 1(3):259, 1974.
173. Selawry O, et al. Methotrexate compared with placebo in lung cancer. *Cancer* 40:4, 1977.
174. Shields TW. Natural history of patients after resection of a bronchial carcinoma. *Surg Clin North Am* 61:1279, 1981.
175. Shields TW, et al. Relationship of cell type and lymph node metastasis to survival after resection of bronchial carcinoma. *Ann Thorac Surg* 20:501, 1975.
176. Sidhu GS. The ultrastructure of malignant epithelial neoplasms of the lung. *Pathol Annu* 17:235, 1982.
177. Siegelman SS, et al. CT of the solitary pulmonary nodule. *AJR* 135:1, 1980.
178. Silverberg E, Lubera J. Cancer statistics, 1987. *CA* 37:2, 1987.
179. Smyth JF, Ford HT. Methotrexate in the chemotherapy of lung cancer. *Cancer Treat Rep* 65:161, 1981.
180. Sorenson S. Treatment of small-cell carcinoma of the lung. *Eur J Respir Dis* 62:315, 1981.
181. Spencer H. *Pathology of the Lung.* Oxford: Pergamon, 1977.
182. Spiro SG. The Diagnosis and Staging of Lung Cancer. In JF Smith (Ed), *The Management of Lung Cancer.* London: Edward Arnold, 1984.
183. Stemmer EA, et al. Parasternal mediastinal exploration to evaluate resectability of thoracic neoplasms. *Ann Thorac Surg* 12:375, 1971.
184. Sunderman FW Jr. Recent advances in metal carcinogenesis. *Ann Clin Lab Sci* 14:93, 1984.
185. Tager IB, et al. Longitudinal study of the effects of maternal smoking on pulmonary function in children. *N Engl J Med* 309:699, 1983.
186. The Lugwig Lung Cancer Study Group: Patterns of failure in patients with resected stage I and II non-small cell carcinoma of the lung. *Ann Surg* 205:67, 1987.
187. The Lung Cancer Study Group: Effects of postoperative mediastinal radiation on completely resected stage II and III epidermoid cancer of the lung. *N Engl J Med* 315:1377, 1986.
188. Thomlinson RH, Gray LH. The histological structure of some human lung cancers and the possible implications for radiotherapy. *Br J Cancer* 9:539, 1955.
189. Tornyos K, Faust H. Oral high-dose methotrexate with citrovorum factor rescue in metastatic squamous cell carcinoma of the lung. *Cancer* 41:400, 1978.
190. Trell E, et al. Arylhydrocarbon hydroxylase inducibility and laryngeal carcinomas. *Lancet* 2:140, 1976.
191. Trell E, et al. Aryl hydrocarbon hydroxylase inducibility and carcinoma of oral cavity. *Lancet* 1:109, 1976.
192. Trichopoulos D, et al. Lung cancer and passive smoking. *Int J Cancer* 27:1, 1981.
193. Trovo MG, et al. Combined radiotherapy and chemotherapy with cyclophosphamide, Adriamycin, methotrexate, procarbazine (CAMP) in 64 consecutive patients with epidermoid carcinoma, limited disease: A prospective study. *Int J Radiat Oncol Biol Phys* 8:1051, 1982.
194. United States Public Health Service. *The Health Consequences of Smoking: A Report of the Surgeon General.* Rockville, Md: United States Department of Health, Education and Welfare, Health Services and Mental Health Administration, 1971.
195. United States Public Health Service. *The Health Consequences of Smoking—Cancer: A Report of the Surgeon General.* Rockville, Md: United States Department of Health and Human Services, Office on Smoking and Health, 1982.
196. United States Public Health Service. *The Health Consequences of Smoking for Women: A Report of the Surgeon General.* Rockville, Md: United States Department of Health and Human Services, Office on Smoking and Health, 1980.
197. United States Public Health Service. *Smoking and Health: Report of the Advisory Committee to the Surgeon General of the Public Health Service.* Rockville, Md: United States Department of Health, Education and Welfare, Centers for Disease Control, 1964.
198. United States Public Health Service. *Smoking and Health: A Report of the Surgeon General.* Rockville, Md: United States Department of Health, Education and Welfare, Public Health Service, Office on Smoking and Health, 1979.
199. van Houtte P, et al. Postoperative radiation therapy in lung cancer: A controlled trial after resection of curative design. *Int J Radiat Oncol Biol Phys* 6:983, 1980.
200. Vijayalaxmi Evans HJ. In vivo and in vitro effects of cigarette smoke on chromosomal damage and sister-chromatid exchange in human peripheral blood lymphocytes. *Mutat Res* 92:321, 1982.
201. Vincent RG, et al. The changing histopathology of lung cancer: A review of 1682 cases. *Cancer* 39:1647, 1977.
202. Warram J. Preoperative irradiation of cancer of the lung: Final report of a therapeutic trial—A collaborative study. *Cancer* 36(3):914, 1975.

203. Warren S. Effects of radiation on normal tissues. *Arch Pathol* 34:917, 1924.

204. Warren WH, Memoli VA, Gould VE. Immunohistochemical and ultrastructural analysis of bronchopulmonary neuroendocrine neoplasms: carcinoids. *Ultrastruct Pathol* 6:15, 1984.

205. Weiss RB. Small-cell undifferentiated lung carcinoma: Therapeutic management. *Ann Intern Med* 88:522, 1978.

206. Weiss W, Boucot K, Seidman H. The Philadelphia pulmonary neoplasm research project. *Clin Chest Med* 3:243, 1982.

207. White JR, Froeb HF. Small-airways dysfunction in nonsmokers chronically exposed to tobacco smoke. *N Engl J Med* 302:720, 1980.

208. Whitfield AGW, Bond WH, Arnott WM. Radiation reactions in the lung. *Q J Med* 25:67, 1956.

209. Wilkins EW, Scannell JG, Craver JG. Four decades of experience with resections for bronchogenic carcinoma at the Massachusetts General Hospital. *J Thorac Cardiovasc Surg* 76:364, 1978.

210. Williams DE, et al. Survival of patients with surgically treated for stage I lung cancer. *J Thorac Cardiovasc Surg* 82:70, 1981.

211. Willis RA, (Ed). Epithelial Tumours of the Trachea, Bronchi and Lung. In *Pathology of Tumours*. London: Butterworth, 1948.

212. Wolf J. Nitrosoureas as single agents in the treatment of pulmonary cancer. *Cancer Treat Rep* 60:753, 1976.

213. Yesner R. Small-cell tumors of the lung. *Am J Surg Pathol* 7:775, 1983.

214. Yoneda S, et al. Synergic effect of cis-platin, Adriamycin and cyclophosphamide combination chemotherapy and radiotherapy in nonsmall cell lung cancer. *Oncology* 42:1, 1985.

215. Yoshimura K. A clinical statistical study of lung cancer patients in Japan with special reference to the staging system of TNM classification: A report from the Japan Joint Committee of Lung Cancer associated with the TNM system of clinical classification (UICC). *Radiat Med* 1:186, 1983.

216. Young JL, Percy CL, Asire AJ. (Eds). *Surveillance, Epidemiology, End Results: Incidence and Mortality Data 1973–1977* (National Cancer Institute Monograph 57). Bethesda, Md: United States Department of Health and Human Services, Public Health Service, 1981.

217. Zavala DC. Diagnostic fiberoptic bronchoscopy: Techniques and results of biopsy in 600 patients. *Chest* 68:12, 1975.

218. Zerhouni EA. CT of the pulmonary nodule: Initial results of a cooperative study. Presented at the annual assembly of the Radiological Society of North America, Washington, DC, November 1984.

219. Zerhouni EA, et al. A standard phantom for quantitative analysis of pulmonary nodules by CT. *Radiology* 149:767, 1983.

54

Tumors of the Lung Other Than Bronchogenic Carcinoma

Scot H. Merrick   Noel H. Fishman

Excluding bronchial carcinoid and bronchoalveolar carcinoma, the pulmonary tumors to be discussed in this chapter are exceedingly rare, and collectively comprise approximately 2 percent of all lung tumors. Many of these tumors are benign, some are malignant, and others exhibit locally aggressive behavior.

With the introduction of electron microscopy, immunohistology, and cell culture techniques (and with some ongoing controversy), the commonly accepted World Health Organization classification of these tumors [2] has undergone major changes. One of the more useful classification schemes, devised by Spencer [115], segregates these tumors according to the cell of origin, as far as possible, as follows:

1. Tumors of amine precursor uptake and decarboxylation (APUD) cells, neural cells, or of unknown origin
   a. Bronchial carcinoid tumor
   b. Neurofibroma and neurofibrosarcoma of the lung
   c. Myoblastoma of the bronchus
   d. Malignant melanoma of the bronchus
   e. Pulmonary "chemodectoma"
   f. Benign clear-cell tumor of the lung
2. Tumors derived from bronchial epithelium or bronchial mucous glands
   a. Bronchial papillomatous tumors
   b. Bronchial cystadenoma, monomorphic and pleomorphic
   c. Pleomorphic bronchial gland adenomas
   d. Oncocytic bronchial gland adenoma
   e. Bronchial mucoepidermoid adenoma
   f. Adenoid cystic carcinoma of the bronchus
   g. Mucinous, multilocular cyst carcinoma of the bronchus
3. Tumors of pulmonary connective-tissue origin
   a. Chondroma of the bronchus
   b. Bronchial and subpleural lipomatous tumors
   c. Fibroma and myxoma of the lung
   d. Pulmonary fibroleiomyoma
   e. Pulmonary sarcoma
   f. Pulmonary rhabdomyosarcoma
   g. Embryonal pulmonary sarcoma
   h. Intravascular and sclerosing bronchoalveolar tumor
   i. Tumors of vascular origin
      (1) Angioma
      (2) Lymphangioma
4. Lung tumors of chronic granulomatous or uncertain origin
   a. Plasma cell granuloma, benign and malignant
   b. Sclerosing angioma
5. Hamartomas of the lung
   a. Chondromatous
   b. Fibroleiomyomatous
6. Blastoma and teratoma of the lung
7. Pulmonary reticuloses
   a. Lymphoid hyperplasia
   b. Hodgkin's disease
   c. Lymphosarcoma and histiocytic sarcoma
   d. Plasmacytoma of the lung
   e. Leukemia
   f. Giant intrathoracic lymph nodes
   g. Histiocytosis X disease

The term *bronchial adenoma* has been used for some time to describe fleshy, polypoid tumors of the tracheobronchial tree. Recently, however, in recognition of their malignant potential, the most common types of adenomas have undergone name changes. Cylindromas are now called *ade-*

noid cystic carcinoma, mucoepidermoid tumors are now called *mucoepidermoid carcinoma*, and a suggestion has been made to change the name of bronchial carcinoid tumors to *low-grade APUD carcinoma* or *Kulchitzky-cell carcinoma*. Bronchoalveolar cell carcinoma is also discussed in this chapter. The illustrative reviews of Dail and Hammar [22] and Mackay and colleagues [77] are recommended for further reading.

In general, tumors that originate within a bronchus tend to be discovered earlier because of signs and symptoms of bronchial stenosis and obstruction: wheezing, cough, atelectasis, obstructive pneumonitis, and distal bronchiectasis. Tumors originating in the periphery of the lung, on the other hand, may attain a large size before they produce symptoms. They are discovered either incidentally on routine chest x-ray films or when they have involved adjacent structures within the chest, at which point they may be inoperable.

Careful bronchoscopy, fine-needle biopsy, computed tomography (CT), and magnetic resonance imaging (MRI) may provide useful information in the evaluation of these tumors. However, in some cases the diagnosis will only be made postoperatively by the pathologist, since (lipomas and chondromatous hamartomas excepted) there are no diagnostic roentgenologic signs and even bronchoscopic biopsy can be misleading. With few exceptions, surgery is the treatment of choice to remove potentially lethal lesions and to relieve symptoms. In general, conservative resection is the rule, employing modern bronchoplastic techniques. Many lesions can now be resected thoracoscopically, without formal thoracotomy [70].

Bronchoalveolar Cell Carcinoma of the Lung

Bronchoalveolar cell carcinoma is a primary tumor of the lung, arising within alveoli and terminal bronchioles and spreading along the surface of the airways to involve other parts of the lung. It is also called *alveolar cell carcinoma, bronchiolar cell carcinoma, bronchioloalveolar cell carcinoma,* and *pulmonary adenomatosis* because of a controversy concerning the cell of origin. Previously this tumor comprised approximately 5 percent of all lung tumors [119], although recent evidence suggests that the incidence may be much higher [2]. Formerly, the production of mucus by these tumors suggested bronchiolar cell origin, but it has been subse-

quently shown that alveolar cells also can differentiate into cells capable of mucus secretion. It is now agreed that the tumor arises from type II alveolar pneumocytes and Clara cells. Clinically, two separate entities have been described [33]. *Focal* bronchoalveolar carcinoma usually presents as a solitary peripheral nodule, characterized by slow growth (tumor doubling time approximately 300 days) and infrequent regional lymph node metastases (Fig. 54-1). A *diffuse* form of the disease is less common but more aggressive and is characterized by multiple nodules or consolidation (Fig. 54-2). Prognosis for focal disease treated by complete resection is excellent [48]; however, if left untreated, some of these cases may progress to the diffuse form, presumably by aerogenous dissemination.

The etiology is unknown, but bronchoalveolar cell carcinoma bears a striking resemblance histologically and in mode of spread to an infectious (presumably viral) disease of animals (primarily sheep) in South Africa, called *jaagsiekte*.

Fig. 54-1. Asymptomatic, focal bronchoalveolar carcinoma of the left lower lobe (*arrow*). (Courtesy of Dr. Gordon Honda, Department of Pathology, University of California, San Francisco)

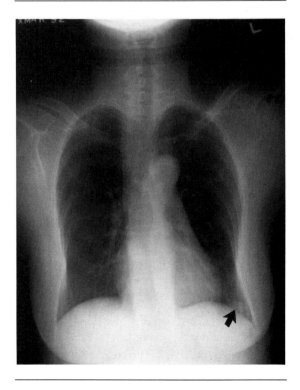

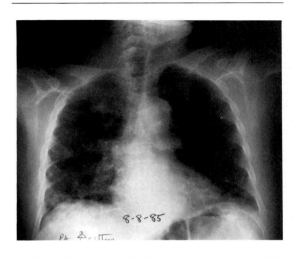

Fig. 54-2. Diffuse or pneumonic form of bronchoalveolar carcinoma, with bilateral, patchy tumor infiltrates. (Courtesy of Dr. Gordon Honda, Department of Pathology, University of California, San Francisco)

Fig. 54-3. Bronchoalveolar carcinoma showing tall, columnar cells and small nests of tumor floating within mucin (*arrow*) (H&E, × 50). (Courtesy of Dr. Gordon Honda, Department of Pathology, University of California, San Francisco)

The hallmark of the histologic diagnosis is the pattern of the growth of flat or columnar malignant cells along alveolar and bronchiolar walls, with frequent intraalveolar projections, but with preservation of the general interstitial framework of the lung [47,107] (Fig. 54-3). Electron microscopy commonly shows dense cytoplasmic granules and nuclear inclusions [77] (Fig. 54-4). By immunohistochemical techniques, these inclusions have been shown to represent a portion of the surfactant molecule [114].

Compared to bronchogenic carcinoma, bronchoalveolar tumors are less likely to be associated with smoking or chronic lung disease. Approximately 40 percent of patients present with advanced disease (TMN stages III and IV) and are usually symptomatic [51]. Cough, copious watery sputum, dyspnea, and constitutional symptoms and signs such as malaise, fatigue, and clubbing are characteristic of this disease. The diagnosis can occasionally be made by sputum cytology and more often bronchoscopic brushing and biopsy. The results of fine-needle biopsy are positive in 75 to 80 percent of patients [32,51].

The treatment of bronchoalveolar cell carcinoma is surgical, and lobectomy is the procedure of choice. Data from the Lung Cancer Study

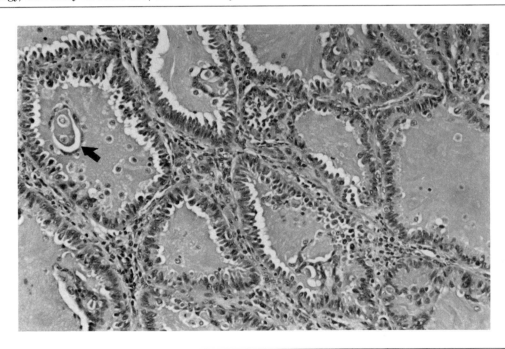

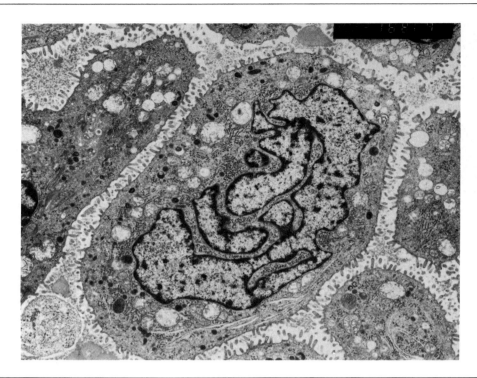

Fig. 54-4. Electron micrograph of bronchoalveolar cell carcinoma of the Clara-cell type. Note the prominent electron-dense granules, which are characteristic. (Courtesy of Dr. Gordon Honda, Department of Pathology, University of California, San Francisco)

Group has shown a 5-year survival rate of approximately 60 percent following surgical resection [48]. For tumors more advanced than T1N0, the yearly recurrence rate may exceed 20 percent. Since the disease spreads by local extension, the plane of a segmentectomy or wedge resection is likely to cut across invisible extensions of tumor, making conservative surgery inappropriate. Even for more-advanced disease, lobectomy or pneumonectomy should be considered (provided that there is no evidence of spread to the opposite lung), because there is no other suitable treatment. The tumor is not particularly responsive to chemotherapy or radiation therapy. Although the disease tends to spread slowly, untreated bronchoalveolar carcinoma proceeds inexorably to pulmonary insufficiency and death by inanition.

Bronchial Carcinoid

Although originally classified as bronchial adenomas, bronchial carcinoids should now be categorized as neuroendocrine neoplasms of the lung, which include tumorlets and small-cell carcinoma. Carcinoids comprise approximately 2 percent of primary lung tumors and usually present in the fifth decade of life as a reddish polypoid mass within view of a bronchoscope, occurring in a main, lobar, segmental, or subsegmental bronchus. Peripheral tumors may occur in 20 percent of cases [17,117] and rare tracheal occurrences have been reported [35]. Because of their location and tendency to expand into the bronchial lumen, carcinoids frequently produce partial or complete bronchial obstruction (Fig. 54-5). Wheezing and hemoptysis are common signs and intermittent lobar or segmental atelectasis is a hallmark of the tumor. Mucopurulent sputum and distal bronchiectasis occur in cases of long-standing obstruction. The majority of patients are symptomatic, but as many as 20 percent may present with an asymptomatic pulmonary nodule [17,117]. Smoking, occupation, and environmental factors do not appear to play a role in the genesis of this tumor.

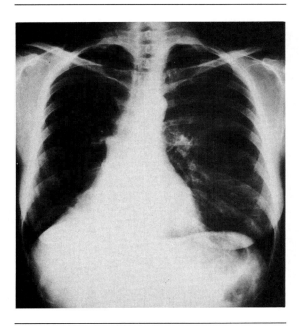

Fig. 54-5. Bronchial carcinoid tumor causing complete atelectasis of the lower lobe of the right lung. (Courtesy of Dr. Gordon Gamsu, Department of Radiology, University of California, San Francisco.)

Cytologic examination of the sputum, bronchial washings, and brushings is not productive, as the tumor is enveloped by normal mucosa [17]. However, fine-needle biopsy may be useful in a small number of cases [77]. Because the tumor is highly vascular, direct biopsy has been avoided in the past for fear of major bleeding (even fatal hemorrhage [5]). Today, with use of a "microbiopsy" forceps through a fiberoptic bronchoscope, direct biopsy can be performed safely with a diagnostic sensitivity of 60 to 80 percent [17,109].

Many hormones have been reported to be secreted by bronchial carcinoids, including corticotropin (ACTH), antidiuretic hormone (ADH), gastrin, somatostatin, calcitonin, and growth hormone. The most common is 5-hydroxytryptamine, or serotonin, but only a very small fraction of patients with bronchial carcinoids exhibit the carcinoid syndrome, and only when hepatic metastases have occurred for practical purposes [101].

The tumor usually presents as a polypoid mass, but the base of the polypoid lesion varies from a pedicle to a broad attachment. In fact, the stalk invariably penetrates through the bronchial wall to the extent that the bulk of the tumor is extrabronchial. Endobronchial resection is therefore not a definitive treatment, although in extremely poor-risk patients it may be reasonable to restore airway patency by laser resection [109].

Microscopically, the typical carcinoid tumor is made up of small, uniform argyrophilic cells with central nuclei and eosinophilic cytoplasm within a vascular stroma (Fig. 54-6). The cells may form clusters, cords, or tubules or grow in solid sheets [26]. They arise from Kulchitsky cells which belong to the APUD system [97]. These cells, which contain neurosecretory granules as seen under the electron microscope, also give rise to small-cell carcinoma of the lung. Previously thought to originate from neural crest cells [6], Kulchitsky cells are now believed to originate from bronchial germinal epithelium [115]. Immunohistochemical studies may be very useful, as bronchial carcinoids have been shown to express a number of epithelial and endocrine markers such as cytokeratin, neurofilament proteins, neuron-specific enolase, and chromogranins. Of these, chromogranin is the most useful marker, being demonstrated in 86 percent of specimens [77].

The *typical* carcinoid tumor is relatively benign. Mitoses are rare in the tissue, regional lymph node metastases are almost never present at the time of thoracotomy, and the 5-year survival rate approaches 95 percent [17,37,94,109, 117].

The *atypical* carcinoid tumor, on the other hand, is characterized histologically by mitoses, cell necrosis, and pleomorphism [22]. An aneuploid DNA content is more common [31] and a high percentage are in stage II or III at the time of surgery. Paladugu and colleagues [95] suggested a new designation for these tumors based on the cell of origin, the *Kulchitsky-cell carcinoma* (KCC). They would call typical carcinoids KCC-I, atypical carcinoids KCC-II, and small-cell carcinoma KCC-III.

The treatment of *typical* carcinoids is conservative resection, sparing pulmonary parenchyma where feasible unless the lung has been destroyed by bronchiectasis beyond the point of bronchial obstruction. Bronchoplastic procedures and sleeve resections can be performed even with surgical margins close to the tumor. *Atypical* carcinoids, on the other hand, should be treated in the same way as one would treat a bronchogenic carcinoma, by lobectomy or pneumonectomy with more adequate margins and lymph node excision. For these tumors and for

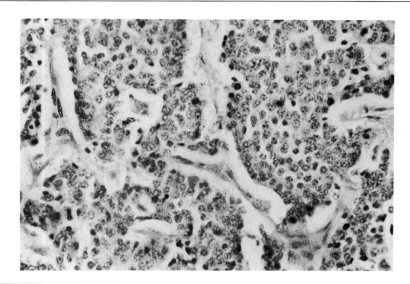

Fig. 54-6. Bronchial carcinoid tumor. Nests of uniform cells are separated by a delicate connective-tissue stroma. There are round nuclei with evenly dispersed, coarse chromatin and pale cytoplasm (H&E, × 400). (Courtesy of Dr. Miriam Lurie, Department of Pathology, Carmel Hospital, Haifa, Israel.)

any carcinoid with mediastinal lymph node involvement, the 5-year survival rate falls to 40 percent [117].

Neurogenic Tumors

Primary neurogenic tumors of the lung, which include benign neurofibromas, neurilemmomas, and neurofibrosarcomas, are quite rare, with fewer than 100 cases reported. Intrapulmonary neurofibromas are the most common, and are more likely to occur in association with von Recklinghausen's disease [77]. In this situation, the lung tumors may be multiple, causing significant arteriovenous shunting and hypoxemia [90]. Benign neurilemmomas (schwannomas) are more likely to arise sporadically.

These tumors are consistently related to a bronchus, either within the lumen (more commonly) or outside the bronchial wall [3]. Both neurofibroma and neurilemmomas originate from nerve sheath cells; however, their histology may be confused with that of neuroblastomas, leiomyomas, fibromas, and mesotheliomas. Immunostaining for neuron-specific enolase and protein S-100 will help establish nerve sheath origin [10,61]. Most primary neurogenic tumors of the lung are asymptomatic and therefore may attain a large size over a long period of time. Cough and hemoptysis are caused when a bronchus becomes obstructed within or compressed by the mass of a large tumor. Endobronchial lesions

may appear as polypoid lesions projecting into the lumen of a bronchus and can be resected successfully with yttrium-argon-garnet (YAG) laser [34]. Parenchymal lesions can be cured by conservative resections and recurrences are rare [61].

Malignant schwannomas (neurosarcomas, neurofibrosarcomas) are often accompanied by the finding of benign neurofibromas in other parts of the tumor. Invasiveness, hemorrhage, and necrosis of the tumor are characteristic. These tumors may grow very large and metastasize late in their natural history. Many patients have been cured by surgical resection, and adjuvant chemotherapy, particularly with doxorubicin (Adriamycin), may be useful for extensive tumors [34].

Granular Cell Tumor of the Bronchus

Although granular cell tumors occur in nearly all anatomic sites, they are found predominantly in the tongue and skin and are extremely rare in the lungs [24]. Previously termed *myoblastoma*, this tumor is now believed to originate from

Schwann's cells [22]. The tumor is found in the lung as a benign sessile or polypoid growth within the trachea or a central bronchus and is usually associated with obstructive pneumonitis. Ulceration of pedunculated lesions may produce hemoptysis. The tumor may be multicentric; coexisting lesions outside of the respiratory tract may be frankly malignant. Histologically, the tumor is composed of clusters of polygonal cells with small hyperchromatic nuclei and abundant cytoplasm containing numerous fine, acidophilic granules. These granules appear similar to lysosomes under electron microscopy.

Although benign, it is locally invasive and is associated with squamous metaplasia, simulating a malignant tumor of the bronchus [24]. Larger lesions may have extensive submucosal infiltration, making bronchoscopic or laser removal useful only for palliation. Definitive treatment is by surgical resection, with sleeve resection or a bronchoplastic procedure where feasible.

Oncocytomas and oncocytic carcinoids can be confused with granular cell tumors. Immunohistochemical stains for protein S-100 may be useful in differentiating ambiguous cases [50].

Malignant Melanoma of the Bronchus

Cutaneous and ocular malignant melanomas frequently spread to the lungs, presenting as multiple, bilateral parenchymal nodules. Approximately 2 percent of malignant melanomas will metastasize to the bronchus [22]. The diagnosis of *primary* malignant melanoma of the bronchus is one of exclusion, since a complete examination to exclude all other possible primary sites can only be done postmortem (Figs. 54-7 and 54-8) [104]. Nevertheless, several authors have suggested the following diagnostic criteria [22,64]: (1) absence of past or present atypical or malignant pigmented skin lesions from any site, (2) a solitary lung lesion centered on a bronchus with no evidence of other organ involvement, and (3) in situ melanocytic change of bronchial mucosa adjacent to or overlying the major tumor mass (the so-called junctional or lentiginous change). Using these criteria, a small number of reported cases may benefit from surgical resection [64].

Pulmonary Chemodectoma

Minute, multiple tumors are occasionally found at autopsy in patients who have died from cardio-

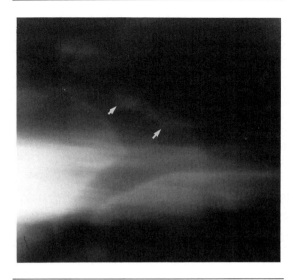

Fig. 54-7. Lung tomogram showing adenoid cystic carcinoma of the right mainstem bronchus (*arrows*). (Courtesy of Dr. Gordon Honda, Department of Pathology, University of California, San Francisco)

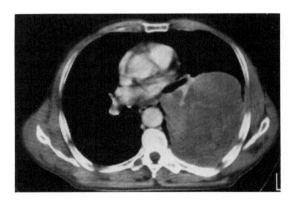

Fig. 54-8. Primary fibrosarcoma arising from the left mainstem bronchus. (Courtesy of Dr. Gordon Honda, Department of Pathology, University of California, San Francisco)

vascular disease, especially pulmonary thromboembolism. Over 80 percent of cases occur in women [22]. Grossly, these tumors appear as 1- to 3-mm nodules on the pleura or within the pulmonary parenchyma [39]. Microscopically, the tumors consist of nests of large cells in the interstitial tissues near or surrounding small veins

[18]. The tumor cells are large, spindled, or elongated with regular nuclei, eosinophilic cytoplasm, and indistinct cell borders. Immunohistochemical stains for epithelial membrane antigen and vimentin are usually positive [39,123]. Chemodectomas were formerly thought to have developed from chemoreceptor cells in the lung, but Churg and Warnock [18] failed to find neurosecretory granules ultrastructurally, as would have been expected in paraganglion cells. They suggested that these tumors have characteristics related to meningiomas.

Benign Clear-Cell Tumors of the Lung

Also known as sugar tumors, because of their high glycogen content, these tumors present as isolated, asymptomatic, solitary pulmonary nodules on chest x-ray films. They are exceedingly rare, occurring mainly in middle-aged adults [40]. Successful diagnosis by fine-needle aspiration has been reported [89]. Grossly, the tumors are not encapsulated. Nevertheless, they remain distinct from surrounding tissue. They are not associated with bronchi. Histologically, these tumors resemble clear-cell carcinoma of the kidney and so are confused with metastatic lesions [74]. However, frequent mitoses should be observed in the latter. In general, immunohistochemical stains may be helpful [42]. Conservative resection should be considered curative.

Bronchial Papillomatous Tumors

These are benign lesions of the larynx, trachea, and bronchi, usually multiple and only rarely solitary. The tumors are multicentric, and are usually caused by human papilloma virus [22]. In children and infants, the disease is self-limiting, and extends beyond the larynx in only 2 percent of cases. During the course of cellular proliferation, however, airway obstruction may occur from the florid overgrowth. Disease extending into the bronchopulmonary tree is more virulent, often presenting with symptoms and signs of obstruction and requiring multiple resections for recurrent disease. Endobronchial resection, conventional or laser, is life-saving.

In adults, the prognosis is poorer, especially in the form that spreads to the parenchyma [35]. According to Felson [35], laryngotracheal papillomas always appear first, followed by progressively lower airway involvement. In cases of bronchoalveolar spread, nodules form in the lung and then cavitate to form cysts. Distal bronchiectasis is common and frank lymphangitic invasion has been described [22]. The lesions tend to increase in number and size with time, and these patients usually die of progressive pulmonary insufficiency. Bronchoscopic and laser resections are the mainstays of therapy; good results have also been reported with photodynamic therapy [65] and interferon alfa [73].

Microscopically, a connective-tissue stroma is covered by a cuboidal or squamous epithelium in varying degrees of differentiation and keratinization. Because of cytologic atypia, papillomas may be difficult to distinguish from squamous cell carcinoma.

Bronchial Mucoepidermoid Adenoma

Mucoepidermoid tumors of the bronchus are the third most common type of bronchial adenoma, but comprise only 0.1 percent of all lung tumors as a whole [22]. This is a pedunculated polypoid tumor arising from excretory duct reserve cells of mucous glands [77]. It is usually located in the lobar or mainstem bronchi, and rarely in the trachea. The tumor is coated with mucus and is capable of producing a large mucocele beyond the point where it causes bronchial obstruction. Histologically, the tumor consists of large cells growing in sheets (epidermoid, without keratinization), scattered among which are numerous mucus-containing glands [15]. Tonofibrils and mucin granules are common ultrastructural findings [77]. These tumors have been found in virtually all age groups, characteristically producing symptoms of cough, wheezing, hemoptysis, and recurrent pneumonias [55].

There appears to be a spectrum of mucoepidermoid tumors ranging from benign and completely curable to a malignant and highly lethal variety. The latter are characterized by cytologic atypia, pleomorphic cells, greater mitotic activity, and infiltration into adjacent lung parenchyma. Although exceptions have been reported [110], in general the disease is nearly always benign in children. Therefore, an operation such as a sleeve resection should always be considered [87]. A sleeve resection allows a lobectomy, for example, to be substituted for a pneumonectomy. In adults, on the other hand, Turnbull and colleagues [125] found many of these tumors to be highly malignant histologically and very aggressive clinically, with a tendency to local invasiveness and early metastases. Conservative lung resection for *low-grade* tumors has been suggested [12,54], with no evidence of recurrent disease at a mean follow-up of 4.7 years. *High-grade* lesions, which may be difficult to distinguish from poorly differentiated squamous cell carcinomas, are typically unresectable and survival is less than 2 years [54].

Bronchial Oncocytomatous Adenoma

This is a rare benign polypoid tumor that arises from bronchial mucous glands and ducts. Oncocytes are epithelial cells with abundant eosinophilic cytoplasm and small nuclei. Ultrastructurally, they contain abundant mitochondria but no neurosecretory granules, which distinguishes them from the carcinoid tumor cells they may resemble histologically [21]. Demonstration of chromogranin by immunostaining may be useful in the distinction [77]. These tumors rarely exceed 4 cm in size [25].

Mucous Gland Adenoma

These rare benign tumors of the bronchial glands can produce obstructive symptoms or asthma. This tumor, which has also been found in the trachea [36], has also been termed *bronchial cystadenoma* and *adenomatous polyp* [22,77]. The basic histology is that of mucus-filled spaces lined by well-differentiated bronchial gland epithelium [22]. Several subtypes have been proposed (tubular, papillary, mucoepidermoid-type; monomorphic, pleomorphic) based on the predominant cell type [77,116]. Conservative resection is the treatment of choice.

Adenoid Cystic Carcinoma of the Bronchus

These tumors originate from mucous glands throughout the body. In the tracheobronchial tree, adenoid cystic carcinoma occurs primarily in the trachea or mainstem bronchus, more central than carcinoid tumors in general (see Fig. 54-7). Whereas adenoid cystic carcinomas constitute a small proportion of all primary bronchial neoplasms, they account for approximately 40 percent of primary tumors of the trachea [35]. Most patients are in their fourth decade.

These are sessile growths, and like other bronchial tumors, they may present as obstructing lesions often causing atelectasis of an entire lung.

Histologically, the tumor is composed of duct-lining cells of mucous glands which form into ductlike tubules (hence the older name *cylindroma*) and glands and cysts that contain mucin [76]. The stroma is also myxomatous. This tumor typically immunostains for keratin and vimentin [77].

These tumors are low-grade adenocarcinomas that spread by local extension through the tracheal wall and metastasize to lymph nodes. Perineural invasion is characteristic [76].

Treatment is by local wide excision, dictated by anatomic constraints. In some circumstances, sleeve resection of the trachea or of the main bronchus or a bronchoplastic procedure may be feasible. In other instances, tracheal-carinal resection or standard lobectomy or pneumonectomy may be required. Even though adenoid cystic carcinoma is relatively radioresistant, postoperative radiation should be administered when lymph node metastases have occurred or invasion of perineural lymphatics has been demonstrated in the surgical specimen.

Chondroma of the Bronchus

A chondroma grows directly from bronchial or tracheal cartilage into the lumen of the airway as a purely cartilaginous mass [133], unlike hamartomas which, in addition, contain other elements from the tissues of the bronchial wall. A chondroma has a very smooth, lobulated surface and may grow to be very large. It may be removed by local excision (through a bronchotomy incision) or preferably, by sleeve resection.

Sarcomas of the Lung

The most common sarcoma of the lung is metastatic. In general, these tumors are small, multiple lesions that may arise after a long interval from primary-site diagnosis and treatment. Removal of metastatic lung sarcomas may carry a favorable prognosis, which is discussed in a later section.

In contrast, primary sarcomas of the lung are rare as a group, and some of the varieties are exceedingly rare. These tumors may account for 0.2 to 0.4 percent of all lung cancer cases [22], and are usually large, solitary, and asymptomatic. The most common types are malignant fibrous histiocytoma (MFH), fibrosarcoma, and leiomyosarcoma [49,77]. Kaposi's sarcoma of the lung, associated with acquired immunodeficiency syndrome (AIDS), is being encountered with increasing frequency [44]. Chondrosarcomas, liposarcomas, myxosarcomas, and rhabdomyosarcomas also occur in the lung. Often the tumor is undifferentiated and referred to simply as a sarcoma or spindle-cell sarcoma of the lung. Differentiation of these tumors from carcinosarcomas may be difficult; immunohistochemistry (particularly CEA and cytokeratin) may be a useful diagnostic tool [20,63].

Pulmonary sarcomas may originate within a bronchus (usually in the mainstem or lobar bronchus [49]) (see Fig. 54-8), peripherally within the pulmonary parenchyma, or may arise from major vessels. Fine-needle biopsy and fiberoptic bronchoscopy may be diagnostic for some lesions (e.g., MFH and Kaposi's sarcoma, respectively) and CT or MRI scans may be useful for others. In general, a generous biopsy specimen is needed to secure the diagnosis.

MFH of the lung is usually found in middle-aged men and may occur more frequently in patients who have undergone radiation therapy. The tumor is characterized by a mixture of fibroblasts and histiocytes, with giant cells and inflammatory cells interspersed. Approximately 50 percent of patients have local or distant metastases and the recurrence rate may approach 40 percent. Not surprisingly, the prognosis is poor; a combination of surgery, radiotherapy, and chemotherapy may improve survival [81,130].

Endobronchial fibrosarcomas and leiomyosarcomas have a much better prognosis than their intrapulmonary counterparts, probably because they produce symptomatic bronchial obstruction relatively early in their course and are therefore smaller when resected. Intrapulmonary sarcomas tend to have a highly malignant histologic appearance and metastasize early to hilar and mediastinal lymph nodes [49,98]. Paradoxically, some fibrosarcomas attain a very large size without metastases, but the great majority of these are inoperable because of involvement of adjacent intrathoracic structures [49].

Chondrosarcomas are rarer. Despite the presence of radiographic calcification, these lesions are not benign. An intrabronchial chondrosarcoma may appear benign on bronchoscopic biopsy, only to be found to be invasive at surgery [136]. Intrabronchial chondrosarcomas also have a better prognosis than intraparenchymal tumors. However, the overall prognosis is poor, with most patients surviving only 6 to 12 months from the time of diagnosis [22].

Pulmonary rhabdomyosarcomas may become extremely large and invasive. They compress the surrounding parenchyma into a fibrous pseudo-capsule. Histologically, rhabdomyosarcomas consist of straplike cells with cross-striations. There are also undifferentiated round and spindle-shaped cells with cross-striations and nonstriated giant cells [28]. The presence of desmin by immunohistochemical staining is diagnostic. The origin of striated muscle cells in the lung is a source of speculation [126].

Kaposi's sarcoma can be a particularly virulent tumor. Spontaneous occurrence in the lung is rare; however, it has been estimated that 35 percent of patients with AIDS will develop pulmonary involvement [91]. Many patients present with hemoptysis and may have a bloody pleural effusion. Approximately 50 percent of patients will have a coexisting opportunistic infection. Rapid progression is not uncommon, although chemotherapy may reverse fulminant respiratory failure [44].

Lipomas of the Bronchus and Lung

These are among the least common of benign tumors, consisting of lobules of mature fat cells supported by a delicate fibrous stroma arising from the submucosal [134] or interstitial adipose tissue. They can occur anywhere along the entire tracheobronchial tree [30,108]. For unknown reasons, these tumors typically occur in middle-aged men.

Many patients present with obstructive symptoms. The diagnosis is difficult to establish by bronchoscopy because the pliable capsule resists the biopsy forceps. A CT scan, however, can make the diagnosis accurately based on the density coefficient of fat [83]; distal bronchiectasis may be seen in long-standing bronchial obstruction [60].

Removal of the tumor through the bronchoscope may be hazardous because the bronchial wall may be perforated in the process. Bronchotomy or sleeve resection is preferable.

Even more rare is the subpleural lipoma, a tumor that may attain a large size [115].

Pulmonary Fibroma and Myxoma

Fibromas of the lung are rare and may occur endobronchially, extrabronchially, or within the lung itself [67]. They are composed of fibrous connective tissue and may become large enough to cause bronchial obstruction, either intraluminally or by extrinsic compression. In children, fibromas may be found in the cervical trachea [35].

Recurrences may occur after endoscopic removal [22].

Pulmonary myxomas are extraordinarily rare. They look like fibromas grossly but have a gelatinous and glistening appearance on cut section. Microscopically, there is abundant extracellular mucin between stellate cells [75].

Pulmonary Leiomyoma

These tumors are some of the most common soft-tissue tumors found in the lungs. In order of frequency, the tumors are found in the peripheral lung, small bronchi, central bronchi, and trachea [135]. Parenchymal tumors are usually asymptomatic and may attain a large size before discovery. Lesions of the airway tend to produce obstructive symptoms and bronchiectasis. The consistency of the peripheral tumor is similar to that of a hamartoma; it is tough and fibrous and is readily "shelled out" of the parenchyma. Histologically, spindle-shaped cells containing smooth muscle are seen, but immunohistochemical studies and electron microscopy may be necessary to distinguish these tumors from fibromas, neurofibromas, and neurilemmomas [41]. In general, conservative resection using bronchoscopic, laser, or sleeve resection is curative.

There have been many reports of pulmonary leiomyomas occurring in women with similar tumors of the uterus [14,22,128]. Whether or not the pulmonary lesions represent so-called benign metastases is subject to controversy, as low-grade smooth-muscle metastases and primary leiomyomas are difficult to distinguish. Nevertheless, in women with pulmonary leiomyomas, a careful pelvic examination is recommended.

Epithelioid Hemangioendothelioma

Previously known as *intravascular bronchioloalveolar tumor*, this rare malignant tumor usually presents as small, asymptomatic, bilateral pulmonary nodules. Over 80 percent of patients are female, and most are less than 40 years old [22,77]. Most patients are asymptomatic, although alveolar and intrapleural hemorrhage may occur [16,118] (Fig. 54-9). The results of sputum cytology are usually negative although findings by fine-needle biopsy may be suggestive of the diagnosis. Tumor cells typically demonstrate reactivity for factor VIII–related antigen by immunohistochemistry, and pinocytotic vesicles are seen by electron microscopy. Hence, most believe this

tumor to be derived from the endothelial cell (Fig. 54-10).

These tumors tend to have an indolent but progressive course. Intrapulmonary spread is not uncommon and extension of tumor to the pleura and pericardium may occur. No effective therapy

Fig. 54-9. Epithelioid hemangioendothelioma in a 39-year-old woman presenting with hemoptysis and intrapleural hemorrhage. (Courtesy of Dr. Gordon Honda, Department of Pathology, University of California, San Francisco)

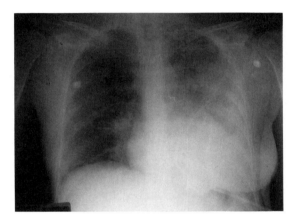

Fig. 54-10. Epithelioid hemangioendothelioma exhibiting irregular nests of large cells showing hyperchromatic nuclei and frequent mitotic activity. Hemorrhagic, cystic cavities are present (*arrows*); immunostaining for factor VIII was positive (H&E × 1000). (Courtesy of Dr. Gordon Honda, Department of Pathology, University of California, San Francisco)

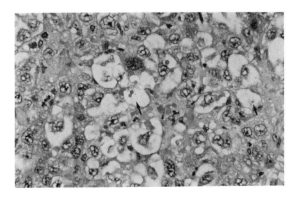

is available, although radiotherapy may provide some palliation. Hormonal therapy has been suggested, but efforts to substantiate expression of estrogen and progesterone receptors in this tumor have not been successful [92].

Pulmonary Angioma (Arteriovenous Fistula)

These are congenital lesions of mesodermal origin. Developmentally, this tumor may be a vascular type of pulmonary hamartoma [72]. In 30 to 40 percent of cases, hereditary telangiectasia (Rendu-Osler-Weber syndrome) is present. In a number of cases, the pulmonary lesions are multiple and bilateral [68]. These tumors have a predilection for the lower lobes and are highly variable in size, ranging from minute telangiectasis to cavernous aneurysms with a large right-to-left intrapulmonary shunt (with dyspnea, cyanosis, clubbing, and polycythemia). Diagnostic evaluation should include CT and angiography [27].

As a result of intrapulmonary shunting, systemic thromboembolism and cerebral abscesses may occur [115]. Furthermore, the lesions tend to increase in size with time [121]; subpleural aneurysm formation may result in free intrapleural rupture [71]. Surgical resection should be conservative (wedge resection or segmentectomy) because other lesions may manifest later [72]. Multiple lesions have been successfully treated by angiographic embolization [27,68].

There is an acquired form of pulmonary arteriovenous fistula owing to the development of abnormal vessels in chronic liver disease and in AIDS in the form of Kaposi's tumors around the walls of intrapulmonary blood vessels [115].

Pulmonary Hemangiopericytoma

Less than 100 cases of this tumor have been reported in the literature. They tend to occur in older patients and affect both sexes with equal frequency [137]. Approximately one-third of patients are asymptomatic; radiographic manifestations are nonspecific, although these tumors tend to be found in the left lower lobe and have sharp contours (probably owing to the presence of a fibrous capsule in many patients) (Fig. 54-11).

This tumor arises from pericytes within the basement membranes of capillaries. Microscopically, "antler-like" vascular spaces are characteristic (Fig. 54-12). The usual size is less than 5 cm;

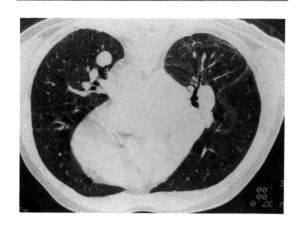

Fig. 54-11. Asymptomatic hemangiopericytoma of the left lower lobe in a 70-year-old man. (Courtesy of Dr. Gordon Honda, Department of Pathology, University of California, San Francisco)

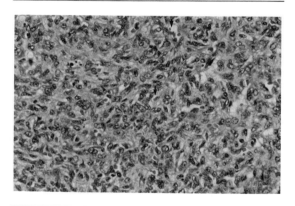

Fig. 54-12. Hemangiopericytoma exhibiting a fairly uniform population of spindle cells, arranged in small whorls and fascicles. Intricate vascular channels that stain positive for factor VIII are present (*arrows*). (Courtesy of Dr. Gordon Honda, Department of Pathology, University of California, San Francisco)

larger tumors tend to have extensive central necrosis [129]. Necrotic tumors over 5 cm in size, with a mitotic rate over 3 per 10 high-power fields and the presence of pleural, bronchial, or vascular invasion, are predictive of a poor prognosis [113]. Surgical resection is the treatment of choice, as radiation and chemotherapy are ineffective. The differential diagnosis should include pulmonary fibromas, metastatic sarcomas, and bronchial carcinoids.

Glomus Tumor

This interesting tumor is usually seen in the extremities (particularly, the nail beds) and is thought to be derived from cells of a special arteriovenous shunt [22]. Several cases have been documented in the lung and trachea [77]. Microscopically, the tumor appears similar to carcinoids and hemangiopericytomas. Electron microscopy is helpful, as neurosecretory granules are absent [53].

Pulmonary Plasma Cell Granulomas (Histiocytomas)

Most authorities agree that this entity, also known as inflammatory pseudotumor, xanthoma, fibroxanthoma, and mast cell granuloma, is not a neoplastic growth, but rather a reactive lesion [22]. Nearly half of the patients with this disease have a history of lung infections [22,127]. Men and women of all ages tend to be afflicted with equal frequency. The lesions are usually solitary and asymptomatic and commonly appear either as a circumscribed nodule or as an ill-defined mass on chest x-ray films. Bronchoscopy and fine-needle biopsy are not useful [122,127]. Rarely, these lesions may become very large and invade the pleura, mediastinum, diaphragm, chest wall, or vertebral bodies [127]. Metastases do not occur.

Microscopically, plasma cell granulomas contain mature plasma cells and lymphocytes within a framework of granulation tissue. Mast cells may also be present but true giant cells are rare. Although plasma cell granuloma has been associated with multiple myeloma, immunohistochemical studies show a polyclonal infiltrate [22,58].

Treatment is primarily surgical, although some lesions have been known to regress spontaneously [127]. Conservative resection is curative and recurrences are rare [23,62].

Sclerosing Hemangioma of the Lung

This rare but fascinating tumor has been reviewed extensively by Dail and Hammar [22]. It is a benign lesion that usually presents as a solitary, nodular density, less than 5 cm in diameter in 90 percent of cases, with some predilection for the lower lobes. Over 80 percent of the patients are female and the majority are asymptomatic [77]. Hemoptysis is the most common presenting sign. There are no specific radiographic features.

Grossly, these tumors are well circumscribed and can be "shelled out" from adjacent lung parenchyma. Microscopically, the pattern may be variable, but most commonly consists of tumor surrounded by extensive fibrosis and dilated vascular spaces that are filled with blood. Cholesterol clefts and hemosiderin-laden macrophages may also be seen. Originally, this histology led to a theory of endothelial cell origin. However, many immunohistochemical and electron microscopic studies do not support endothelial differentiation [22]. Instead, many of these studies demonstrated the presence of surfactant apoprotein in the tumor cells, and most now believe this tumor to be epithelial in nature, originating from type II pneumocytes [88,106,138]. In the past, sclerosing angioma has been confused with plasma cell granulomas (histiocytoma), which are also called *fibroxanthomas* because of fibrosclerotic tissue, cholesterol spaces, and fat-filled macrophages. These degenerative changes occur in both tumors. The difference is the absence of plasma cells in sclerosing angiomas [8].

Sclerosing hemangiomas may involve adjacent lymph nodes but they do not metastasize. As a rule, conservative resection is curative and recurrences are unusual.

Pulmonary Reticuloses

Lymphoproliferative disorders usually involve the lung secondarily. Primary lesions do occur [115] (Fig. 54-13), as the lung contains an extensive system of lymphoid tissue. Although generalization is difficult, one concept proposes that the lung is a part of a specific, mucosal associated lymphoid tissue (MALT), which has the capacity to form low-grade, indolent lymphomas [1,22,56]. Primary lymphomas of the lung may be more common in patients with AIDS [43]. Symptoms, signs, and radiographic features are nonspecific. Examination of sputum cytology or fine-needle aspirates for various immunologic markers may be diagnostic. Grossly, primary lung lymphomas usually do not involve the hilar lymph nodes and tend to be surrounded by cytologically benign infiltrates. Large lesions usually exhibit extensive necrosis. Solitary, circumscribed lung lesions may respond to resection with excellent long-term survival [66].

Some reported cases of successfully resected so-called lymphosarcomas followed by long-term disease-free survival were later reclassified as pseudolymphomas [59]. Pseudolymphomas have true lymphoid germinal centers within a massive

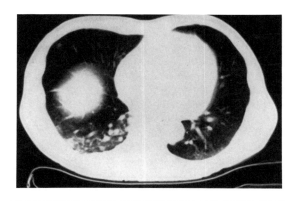

Fig. 54-13. Primary pulmonary lymphoma presenting as a bilateral, nodular infiltrate in the lower lobes. (Courtesy of Dr. Gordon Honda, Department of Pathology, University of California, San Francisco)

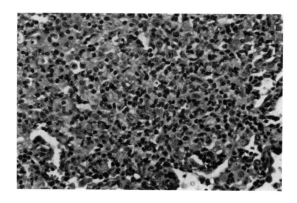

Fig. 54-14. Open lung biopsy specimen showing pulmonary lymphoma of a mixed small cleaved and large cell type (material from patient in Fig. 54-13). (Courtesy of Dr. Gordon Honda, Department of Pathology, University of California, San Francisco)

infiltrate of well-differentiated lymphocytes and other inflammatory cells. The bronchus is spared, leading to characteristic air bronchograms on chest x-ray films. Lymphomas, on the other hand, show a uniform cellular infiltrate of poorly differentiated lymphocytes without true germinal centers (Fig. 54-14).

Subpleural lymph nodes may become enlarged (lymphoid hyperplasia) occasionally enough to be seen on chest x-ray films. The presence of dust-laden histiocytes suggests an environmental etiology. A rare form of diffuse benign intrapulmonary lymphoid hyperplasia also has been described [11].

Giant intrathoracic lymph nodes occasionally arise at the pulmonary hilum without coexisting pulmonary or mediastinal disease [115]. They may be associated with fever or anemia. In the past, they have been mistaken for thymomas on chest x-ray films and histologically.

The lung is also frequently involved with other generalized diseases of the reticuloendothelial system, such as leukemia and histiocytosis X. The latter has a characteristic ring-appearance on high-resolution chest CT [120]. Lung biopsy may be required to establish the diagnosis in these conditions.

Hamartomas of the Lung

A pulmonary hamartoma is a noninvasive malformation originating from elements normally found in lung tissue [111]. Although the histogenesis is unclear, most investigators believe that hamartomas are not congenital and are true neoplasms [22]. As a group, these tumors are perhaps the most common benign tumors of the lung, accounting for over 60 percent of benign lesions in one series [84], and estimated to be present in 0.25 percent of the general population [22]. Males are afflicted more commonly than females and over 80 percent are asymptomatic [105]. These tumors are usually found in the periphery of the lung; radiographically, their borders are lobulated and sharp and speckled calcifications may be seen, giving the appearance of popcorn. Some 20 percent may be endobronchial, resulting in obstructive symptoms [9] (Figs. 54-15 and 54-16). Chest CT scans may be useful by demonstrating fat within the tumor and fine-needle aspiration is diagnostic in a high percentage of cases [29].

The typical hamartoma contains a mixture of cartilage, fat, smooth-muscle, epithelial, and mesenchymal cells (Fig. 54-17). Growth is slow, with an estimated doubling time of 14 years [77]. While malignant transformation has been reported, it is exceptional [4]. Excision is recommended if carcinoma cannot be excluded. Most tumors tend to "shell out" spontaneously when the overlying lung tissue is incised.

There is a special instance of a very aggressive tumor, *adenomatous hamartoma of infancy,* also known as *cystic adenomatoid malformation,* in which an entire lobe or lung is filled with

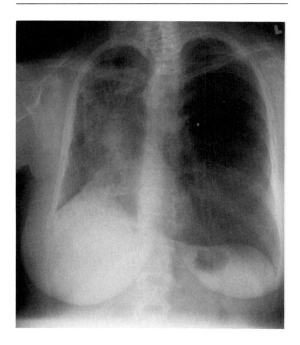

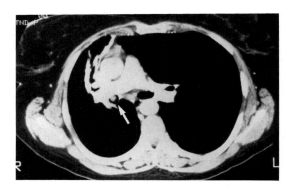

Fig. 54-16. Endobronchial hamartoma occupying the right mainstem bronchus (*arrow*). (Courtesy of Dr. Gordon Honda, Department of Pathology, University of California, San Francisco)

Fig. 54-15. Endobronchial hamartoma originating in the right middle lobe, resulting in near-complete obstruction of the right mainstem bronchus. (Courtesy of Dr. Gordon Honda, Department of Pathology, University of California, San Francisco)

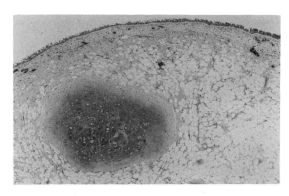

cystic spaces lined with bronchiolar epithelium, with a disorganized arrangement of dilated bronchioles and alveolar spaces [57]. Air trapping within cysts may produce dramatic distension of the involved lung. Pulmonary resection is urgently indicated in these infants.

Pulmonary Blastoma (Embryoma)

Pulmonary blastomas are rare malignant tumors of mixed epithelial and mesenchymal composition that are believed to recapitulate the fetal lung at 10 to 16 weeks of gestation. A bimodal age distribution is apparent, with an initial peak occurring during the first decade and a later peak in the seventh decade [38]. The tumor may be found in a peripheral or central location, with occasional endobronchial extension. Over 40 percent of patients are asymptomatic [69], and radiographic findings are not specific. Diagnosis by fine-needle aspiration has been described [19].

Grossly, these tumors are usually sharply circumscribed, but may contain areas of extensive

Fig. 54-17. Section of an endobronchial hamartoma showing typical features of epithelial border, and smooth-muscle and fat cells. A focus of cartilage is seen centrally (H&E, × 100). (Courtesy of Dr. Gordon Honda, Department of Pathology, University of California, San Francisco)

necrosis. Histologically, the tumor consists of undifferentiated embryonic connective tissue lined by vacuolated columnar epithelium, simulating fetal bronchioles. The epithelial component may form cell balls or morulae, and appears similar to squamous metaplasia. Theories of histogenesis must explain how these tumors involve two germ cell lines. Most pathologists believe that the tumor arises from a single cell type, which then differentiates in several directions [22].

The overall prognosis is poor, with only 16 percent of patients surviving 5 years [38,82]. Most patients die of extrathoracic metastases. Combination chemotherapy may be useful in pediatric patients [93].

Intrapulmonary Teratomas (Dermoid Cysts of the Lung)

True, primary intrapulmonary teratomas are exceedingly rare; one must first exclude direct extension from the mediastinum or metastasis from germ cell tumors in other locations (particularly, the testes). Most lesions are found in the left upper lobe and growth is very slow. They may be solid or cystic and contain tissue derived from all germ layers. They contain hair, sebum, pancreatic, and other tissue [22]. One-third to one-half of these tumors have been classified as malignant on the basis of histologically immature cells [45]. However, pulmonary teratomas rarely behave aggressively.

Carcinosarcoma

Carcinosarcoma is a rare tumor composed of both carcinomatous and sarcomatous elements. The tumor is usually found in older men, commonly in the upper lobes [13]. Many patients present with evidence of metastatic disease in patterns similar to traditional lung carcinoma. Endobronchial spread is very common [22].

Histologically, the epithelial component is usually squamous cell carcinoma under which there is a cellular, spindle-celled stroma with bone or cartilage [115]. The prognosis is poor, with death occurring within a year of initial diagnosis in the majority of patients.

Tumors Metastatic to the Lungs

The lungs are the most frequent site of metastases from nearly all organs [85], and up to 20 percent of patients dying of pulmonary metastases have no tumor noted elsewhere [103]. Carcinoma of the colon, kidney, breast, testis, uterus, head and neck, and ovary, as well as sarcomas and melanomas, are especially prone to metastasize to the lungs [79]. Except for abdominal visceral organs whose venous drainage is directly through the portal system, the lungs are the first organ to filter venous metastases. Blood-borne metastases account for the majority of secondary pulmonary malignancies. Tumor also may reach the lungs through lymphatic spread or by direct extension.

Over 80 percent of patients are asymptomatic; typically, peripheral lung nodules are found on screening chest films obtained during follow-up of the original tumor [86]. The tumors are commonly multiple and bilateral. However, isolated lesions may occur and it is important to distinguish these from benign lesions and/or primary bronchogenic carcinoma. Fine-needle biopsy can be helpful in these situations, but sputum cytology, bronchoscopy, and mediastinoscopy are usually of low yield. In general, new solitary lesions found in patients with a history of breast or head and neck cancers are most likely primary lung carcinomas. New lung lesions in patients with previous colon cancer are equally likely to represent primary lung carcinoma or metastatic disease [79], whereas new lung nodules in patients with prior sarcomas or melanomas are almost always metastatic [103]. Rarely, tumors of the breast, colon, or kidney may present as endobronchial metastases, producing obstructive symptoms.

In order to consider resection of metastatic pulmonary nodules, one must first establish that the primary tumor is under control. Second, there must be no evidence of extrapulmonary metastases and third, resection must not severely compromise lung function. Once these criteria have been satisfied, a chest CT scan should be obtained to investigate the number and laterality of the lesions (see Figs. 54-16 and 54-17). Although the number of metastatic lesions, the disease-free interval, tumor histology, and tumor doubling time have been positively correlated with overall survival [100,102,132], patient selection should not be absolutely dependent on these factors. The overall 5-year survival rate following resection of pulmonary metastases is approximately 35 percent [86].

Because one-third of patients with unilateral disease on chest CT scan are found to have bilateral nodules during surgery, many investigators recommend a median sternotomy approach so that both lungs can be evaluated [96,112]. Functional disability may be less with this incision and it may facilitate resection of future recurrences. However, overall survival is not affected by the type of incision [103]. Wedge resection of the metastatic deposits is satisfactory in the majority of patients. Should recurrent disease develop, some patients, particularly those with metastatic soft-tissue sarcomas, may benefit from repeat resection [99].

Approximate 5-year survival rates according to tumor histology are presented in Table 54-1 [52,80,86,102,131]. One particularly interesting metastatic tumor is the so-called benign metastasizing giant-cell tumor. This lesion usually contains a mixture of mononucleated and multinucleated giant cells and is characteristically found in the distal part of the radius [124]. Although histologically benign, the tumor may spread to the lungs, particularly after a local recurrence of the primary lesion [78] (Figs. 54-18 and 54-19). Spontaneous regression of the pulmonary lesions has been reported [7]; however, surgical resection is indicated for definitive diagnosis and to prevent complications of local growth [78].

Table 54-1. Actuarial survival rates according to tumor histology

Histology	5-year survival rate (%)
Teratoma	84
Uterus	54
Kidney	54
Head and neck cancer	47
Osteosarcoma	46
Soft-tissue sarcoma	33
Breast	27
Carcinoma	24
Colon	23
Melanoma	4

Fig. 54-18. Well-circumscribed focus of metastatic giant-cell tumor originating from the olecranon process. (Courtesy of Dr. Gordon Honda, Department of Pathology, University of California, San Francisco)

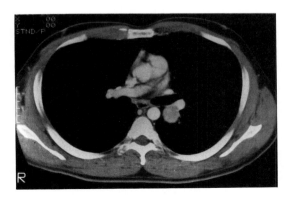

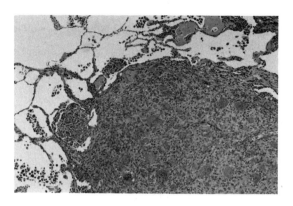

Fig. 54-19. Metastatic pulmonary giant-cell tumor showing prominent multinucleated cells within a benign architecture. (Courtesy of Dr. Gordon Honda, Department of Pathology, University of California, San Francisco)

Despite optimistic results for several tumors, surgical resection should still be considered palliative. Most patients will die of local recurrence or systemic spread of the primary lesion [102]. The role of adjuvant chemotherapy is not yet clearly defined, but patients with metastatic osteosarcoma may benefit [46].

References

1. Addis BJ, Hyjek E, Isaacson PG. Primary pulmonary lymphoma: A re-appraisal of its histogenesis and its relationship to pseudolymphoma and lymphoid interstitial pneumonia. *Histopathology* 13:1, 1988.
2. Auerbach O, Garfinkel L. The changing pattern of lung carcinoma. *Cancer* 68:1973, 1991.
3. Bartley TD, Arean VM. Intrapulmonary neurogenic tumors. *J Thorac Cardiovasc Surg* 50:114, 1965.
4. Basile A, et al. Malignant change in a benign pulmonary hamartoma. *Thorax* 44:232, 1989.
5. Batson JF, Gale JW, Hickey RC. Bronchial adenoma. *Arch Surg* 92:623, 1966.
6. Bensch KG, et al. Oat-cell carcinoma of the lung: Its origin and relationship to bronchial carcinoid. *Cancer* 22:1163, 1968.
7. Bertoni F, et al. Giant-cell tumor of bone with pulmonary metastases. Six case reports and a review of the literature. *Clin Orthop* 237:275, 1988.
8. Bhandori M, Liebow AA. Plasma cell granulomas of the lung. *Cancer* 31:191, 1973.
9. Borro JM, et al. Endobronchial hamartoma. Report of 7 cases. *Scand J Thorac Cardiovasc Surg* 23:285, 1989.

10. Bosch X, et al. Primary intrapulmonary benign schwannoma. A case with ultrastructural and immunohistochemical confirmation. *Eur Respir J* 3:234, 1990.

11. Brandes WW, Cook RA, Osborne MP. Bronchiolar lymphoid hyperplasia as a cause of emphysema: Report of a case. *Arch Pathol* 36:465, 1943.

12. Breyer RH, et al. Mucoepidermoid carcinoma of the trachea and bronchus: The case for conservative resection. *Ann Thorac Surg* 29:197, 1980.

13. Cabarcos A, Gomez DM, Lobo BJ. Pulmonary carcinosarcoma: A case study and review of the literature. *Br J Dis Chest* 79:83, 1985.

14. Canzonieri V, et al. Uterine benign-appearing smooth muscle tumor "metastatic" to the lungs: A case report. *Tumori* 76:513, 1990.

15. Carter D, Eggleston JC. *Tumors of the Lower Respiratory Tract.* Washington, DC: Armed Forces Institute of Pathology, 1980.

16. Carter EJ, et al. Alveolar hemorrhage with epithelioid hemangioendothelioma. A previously unreported manifestation of a rare tumor. *Am Rev Respir Dis* 142:700, 1990.

17. Chapleau D, et al. Bronchial carcinoids: Long-term prognostic factors. *Can J Surg* 34:111, 1991.

18. Churg AM, Warnock M. So-called "minute pulmonary chemodectoma": A tumor not related to paragangliomas. *Cancer* 37:1759, 1976.

19. Cosgrove MM, Chandrasoma PT, Martin SE. Diagnosis of pulmonary blastoma by fine-needle aspiration biopsy: Cytologic and immunocytochemical findings. *Diagn Cytopathol* 7:83, 1991.

20. Cupples J, Wright J. An immunohistological comparison of primary lung carcinosarcoma and sarcoma. *Pathol Res Pract* 186:326, 1990.

21. Cwierzyk TA, et al. Pulmonary oncocytoma: Report of a case with cytologic, histologic and electron microscopic study. *Acta Cytol* 29:620, 1985.

22. Dail DH, Hammar SP. *Pulmonary Pathology.* New York: Springer-Verlag, 1988.

23. Daudi FA, Lees GM, Higa TE. Inflammatory pseudotumours of the lung: Two cases and a review. *Can J Surg* 34:461, 1991.

24. De Clercq D, van der Straeten M, Roels H. Granular cell myoblastoma of the bronchus. *Eur J Respir Dis* 64:72, 1983.

25. De Jesus MG, Poon TP, Chung KY. Pulmonary oncocytoma. *NY State J Med* 89:477, 1989.

26. de Lima R. Bronchial adenoma: Clinicopathologic study and results of treatment. *Chest* 77:81, 1980.

27. Dines DE, Seward JB, Bernatz PE. Pulmonary arteriovenous fistulas. *Mayo Clin Proc* 58:176, 1983.

28. Drennan JM, McCormack RJM. Primary rhabdomyosarcoma of the lung. *J Pathol Bacteriol* 79:147, 1960.

29. Dunbar F, Leiman G. The aspiration cytology of pulmonary hamartomas. *Diagn Cytopathol* 5:174, 1989.

30. Eastridge CE, Young JM, Steplock AL. Endobronchial lipoma. *South Med J* 77:759, 1984.

31. El NA, et al. Typical and atypical bronchopulmonary carcinoids. A clinicopathologic and flow cytometric study. *Am J Clin Pathol* 95:828, 1991.

32. Elson CE, Moore SP, Johnston WW. Morphologic and immunocytochemical studies of bronchioloalveolar carcinoma at Duke University Medical Center, 1968–1986. *Anal Quant Cytol Histol* 11:261, 1989.

33. Epstein DM. Bronchioloalveolar carcinoma. *Semin Roentgenol* 25:105, 1990.

34. Feldhaus RJ, Anene C, Bogard P. A rare endobronchial neurilemmoma (schwannoma). *Chest* 95:461, 1989.

35. Felson B. Neoplasms of the trachea and main stem bronchi. *Semin Roentgenol* 18:23, 1983.

36. Ferguson CJ, Cleeland JA. Mucous gland adenoma of the trachea: Case report and literature review. *J Thorac Cardiovasc Surg* 95:347, 1988.

37. Francioni F, et al. Low grade neuroendocrine tumors of the lung (bronchial carcinoids)—25 years experience. *Eur J Cardiothorac Surg* 4:472, 1990.

38. Francis D, Jacobsen M. Pulmonary blastoma. *Curr Top Pathol* 73:265, 1983.

39. Gaffey MJ, Mills SE, Askin FB. Minute pulmonary meningothelial-like nodules. A clinicopathologic study of so-called minute pulmonary chemodectoma. *Am J Surg Pathol* 12:167, 1988.

40. Gaffey MJ, et al. Clear cell tumor of the lung. A clinicopathologic, immunohistochemical, and ultrastructural study of eight cases. *Am J Surg Pathol* 14:248, 1990.

41. Gal AA, Brooks JS, Pietra GG. Leiomyomatous neoplasms of the lung: A clinical, histologic, and immunohistochemical study. *Mod Pathol* 2:209, 1989.

42. Gal AA, et al. An immunohistochemical study of benign clear cell ('sugar') tumor of the lung. *Arch Pathol Lab Med* 115:1034, 1991.

43. Gibson PG, et al. Pulmonary manifestations of the acquired immunodeficiency syndrome. *Aust NZ J Med* 17:551, 1987.

44. Gill PS, et al. Pulmonary Kaposi's sarcoma: Clinical findings and results of therapy. *Am J Med* 87:57, 1989.

45. Gonzalez-Cruzzi F. *Extragonadal Teratomas.* Washington, DC: Armed Forces Institute of Pathology, 1982. P 184.

46. Goorin AM, et al. Changing pattern of pulmonary metastases with adjuvant chemotherapy in patients with osteosarcoma: Results from the multiinstitutional osteosarcoma study. *J Clin Oncol* 9:600, 1991.

47. Greco RJ, et al. Bronchoalveolar cell carcinoma of the lung. *Ann Thorac Surg* 41:652, 1986.
48. Grover FL, Piantadosi S. Recurrence and survival following resection of bronchioloalveolar carcinoma of the lung—The Lung Cancer Study Group experience. *Ann Surg* 209:779, 1989.
49. Guccion JG, Rosen SH. Bronchopulmonary leiomyosarcoma and fibrosarcoma. *Cancer* 30:836, 1972.
50. Guillou L, et al. Bronchial granular-cell tumor. Report of a case with preoperative cytologic diagnosis on bronchial brushings and immunohistochemical studies. *Acta Cytol* 35:375, 1991.
51. Harpole DH, et al. Alveolar cell carcinoma of the lung: A retrospective analysis of 205 patients. *Ann Thorac Surg* 46:502, 1988.
52. Harpole DJ, et al. Analysis of 945 cases of pulmonary metastatic melanoma. *J Thorac Cardiovasc Surg* 103:743, 1992.
53. Heard BE, et al. One very rare and one new tracheal tumor and acinic cell tumor resembling carcinoid tumors by light microscopy. *Thorax* 37:97, 1982.
54. Heitmiller RF, et al. Mucoepidermoid lung tumors. *Ann Thorac Surg* 47:394, 1989.
55. Helin I, et al. Mucoepidermoid tumor of the bronchus. *Int J Pediatr Otorhinolaryngol* 7:289, 1984.
56. Hernandez JA, Sheehan WW. Lymphomas of the mucosa-associated lymphoid tissue. Signet ring cell lymphomas presenting in mucosal lymphoid organs. *Cancer* 55:592, 1985.
57. Holder TM, Christy MG. Cystic adenomatoid malformation of the lung. *J Thorac Cardiovasc Surg* 47:590, 1964.
58. Hong HY, Castelli MJ, Walloch JL. Pulmonary plasma cell granuloma (inflammatory pseudotumor) with invasion of thoracic vertebra. *Mt Sinai J Med* 57:117, 1990.
59. Hutchinson WB, Friedenberg MJ, Saltzstein S. Primary pulmonary pseudolymphoma. *Radiology* 82:48, 1964.
60. Iannicello CM, et al. Endobronchial lipoma: Report of three cases. *Can J Surg* 30:430, 1987.
61. Imaizumi M, et al. A case of primary intrapulmonary neurilemoma and review of the literature. *Jpn J Surg* 19:740, 1989.
62. Ishida T, et al. Inflammatory pseudotumor of the lung in adults: Radiographic and clinicopathological analysis. *Ann Thorac Surg* 48:90, 1989.
63. Ishida T, et al. Carcinosarcoma and spindle cell carcinoma of the lung: Clinicopathologic and immunohistochemical studies. *J Thorac Cardiovasc Surg* 100:844, 1990.
64. Jennings TA, et al. Primary malignant melanoma of the lower respiratory tract. Report of a case and literature review. *Am J Clin Pathol* 94:649, 1990.
65. Kavuru MS, Mehta AC, Eliachar I. Effect of pho-
66. Kennedy JL, et al. Pulmonary lymphomas and other pulmonary lymphoid lesions. A clinicopathologic and immunologic study of 64 patients. *Cancer* 56:539, 1985.
67. Kinas HY, Garcia RL, Lugo E. Fibroma of the lung. *NY State J Med* 85:37, 1985.
68. Knight WB, et al. Multiple pulmonary arteriovenous fistulas in childhood. *Int J Cardiol* 23:105, 1989.
69. Koss MN, Hochholzer L, O'Leary T. Pulmonary blastomas. *Cancer* 67:2368, 1991.
70. Landreneau RJ, et al. Video-assisted thoracic surgery: Basic technical concepts and intercostal approach strategies. *Ann Thorac Surg* 54:800, 1992.
71. Laroche CM, Wells F, Shneerson J. Massive hemothorax due to enlarging arteriovenous fistula in pregnancy. *Chest* 101:1452, 1992.
72. Le Roux BT. Pulmonary hamartoma. *Thorax* 19:236, 1964.
73. Leventhal BG, et al. Long-term response of recurrent respiratory papillomatosis to treatment with lymphoblastoid interferon alfa-N1. Papilloma Study Group. *N Engl J Med* 325:613, 1991.
74. Liebow AA, Castleman B. Benign clear cell tumors of the lung. *Am J Pathol* 43:13, 1963.
75. Littlefield JB, Drash EC. Myxoma of the lung. *J Thorac Cardiovasc Surg* 37:745, 1959.
76. Lozowski MS, Mishriki Y, Solitare GB. Cytopathologic features of adenoid cystic carcinoma: Case report and literature review. *Acta Cytol* 27:317, 1983.
77. Mackay B, Lukeman JM, Ordonez NG. *Tumors of the Lung.* Philadelphia: Saunders, 1991.
78. Maloney WJ, et al. Benign metastasizing giant-cell tumor of bone. Report of three cases and review of the literature. *Clin Orthop* 243:208, 1989.
79. Mark JBD. Surgical Management of Metastatic Neoplasms to the Lungs. In DC Sabiston, FC Spencer (Eds), *Gibbon's Surgery of the Chest.* Philadelphia: Saunders, 1990. P 604.
80. McCormack P. Surgical resection of pulmonary metastases. *Semin Surg Oncol* 6:297, 1990.
81. McDonnell T, et al. Malignant fibrous histiocytoma of the lung. *Cancer* 61:137, 1988.
82. McKay MJ, Yung T, Langlands AO. Pulmonary blastoma. *Clin Oncol (R Coll Radiol)* 2:173, 1990.
83. Mendelsohn SL, Fagelman D, Zwanger-Mendelsohn S. Endobronchial lipoma demonstrated by CT. *Radiology* 148:790, 1983.
84. Mitsudomi T, et al. Benign tumors and tumor-like lesions of the lung. *Int Surg* 75:155, 1990.
85. Morgan WKC. Tumors of the Lung Other Than Bronchogenic Carcinoma. In GL Baum, E Wol-

insky (Eds), *Textbook of Pulmonary Disease.* Boston: Little, Brown, 1983.

86. Mountain CF, McMurtrey MJ, Hermes KE. Surgery for pulmonary metastasis: A 20-year experience. *Ann Thorac Surg* 38:323, 1984.

87. Mullins JD, Barnes RP. Childhood bronchial mucoepidermoid tumors. *Cancer* 44:315, 1979.

88. Nagata N, et al. Sclerosing hemangioma of the lung: Immunohistochemical characterization of its origin as related to surfactant apoprotein. *Cancer* 55:116, 1985.

89. Nguyen GK. Aspiration biopsy cytology of benign clear cell ("sugar") tumor of the lung. *Acta Cytol* 33:511, 1989.

90. ODonohue WJJ, et al. Multiple pulmonary neurofibromas with hypoxemia. Occurrence due to pulmonary arteriovenous shunts within the tumors. *Arch Intern Med* 146:1618, 1986.

91. Ognibene FP, et al. Kaposi's sarcoma causing pulmonary infiltrates and respiratory failure in the acquired immunodeficiency syndrome. *Ann Intern Med* 102:471, 1985.

92. Ohori NP, et al. Estrogen and progesterone receptors in lymphangioleiomyomatosis, epithelioid hemangioendothelioma, and sclerosing hemangioma of the lung. *Am J Clin Pathol* 96:529, 1991.

93. Ozkaynak MF, et al. Role of chemotherapy in pediatric pulmonary blastoma. *Med Pediatr Oncol* 18:53, 1990.

94. Pal V, Frigyes K, Attila C. Surgical treatment of bronchial carcinoid tumours. Radical surgery-prognosis. *Int Surg* 76:98, 1991.

95. Paladugu RR, et al. Bronchopulmonary Kulchitzky cell carcinomas: A new classification scheme for typical and atypical carcinoids. *Cancer* 55:1303, 1985.

96. Pastorino U, et al. Median sternotomy and multiple lung resections for metastatic sarcomas. *Eur J Cardiothorac Surg* 4:477, 1990.

97. Pearse AGE. The cytochemistry and ultrastructure of polypeptide hormone producing cells of the APUD series and the embryologic, physiologic and pathologic implications of the concept. *J Histochem Cytochem* 17:303, 1969.

98. Pedersen VM, et al. Primary pulmonary leiomyosarcoma: Review of the literature and report of a case. *Scand J Thorac Cardiovasc Surg* 18:251, 1984.

99. Pogrebniak HW, et al. Reoperative pulmonary resection in patients with metastatic soft tissue sarcoma. *Ann Thorac Surg* 52:197, 1991.

100. Putnam JBJ, et al. Analysis of prognostic factors in patients undergoing resection of pulmonary metastases from soft tissue sarcomas. *J Thorac Cardiovasc Surg* 87:260, 1984.

101. Ricci C, Patrassi N, Massa R. Carcinoid syndrome in bronchial adenoma. *Am J Surg* 126:671, 1973.

102. Roberts DG, et al. Long-term follow-up of op-erative treatment for pulmonary metastases. *Eur J Cardiothorac Surg* 3:292, 1989.

103. Roth JA. Resection of Pulmonary Metastases. In JA Roth, JC Ruckdeschel, TH Weisenburger (Eds), *Thoracic Oncology.* Philadelphia: Saunders, 1989. P 619.

104. Salm RA. Primary malignant melanoma of the bronchus. *J Pathol Bacteriol* 85:121, 1963.

105. Salminen US. Pulmonary hamartoma. A clinical study of 77 cases in a 21-year period and review of literature. *Eur J Cardiothorac Surg* 4:15, 1990.

106. Satoh Y, et al. Pulmonary sclerosing hemangioma of the lung. A type II pneumocytoma by immunohistochemical and immunoelectron microscopic studies. *Cancer* 64:1310, 1989.

107. Schraufnagel D, et al. Differentiating bronchioloalveolar carcinoma from adenocarcinoma. *Am Rev Respir Dis* 125:74, 1982.

108. Schraufnagel DE, Morin JE, Wang NS. Endobronchial lipoma. *Chest* 75:97, 1979.

109. Schreurs AJM, et al. A twenty-five-year follow-up of ninety-three resected typical carcinoid tumors of the lung. *J Thorac Cardiovasc Surg* 104:1470, 1992.

110. Seo IS, et al. Mucoepidermoid carcinoma of the bronchus in a 4-year-old child: A high-grade variant with lymph node metastases. *Cancer* 53:1600, 1984.

111. Shah JP, et al. Hamartomas of the lung. *Surg Gynecol Obstet* 136:406, 1973.

112. Shimizu N, et al. Transsternal thoracotomy for bilateral pulmonary metastasis. *J Surg Oncol* 50:105, 1992.

113. Shin MS, Ho KJ. Primary hemangiopericytoma of the lung: Radiology and pathology. *Am J Radiol* 133:1077, 1979.

114. Singh G, Katyal SL, Torikata C. Carcinoma of type II pneumocytes: PAS staining as a screening test for nuclear inclusions of surfactant-specific apoprotein. *Cancer* 50:946, 1982.

115. Spencer H. *Pathology of the Lung* (4th ed). Oxford: Pergamon, 1985.

116. Spencer H, Dail DH, Arneaud J. Noninvasive bronchial epithelial tumors. *Cancer* 45:1486, 1980.

117. Stamatis G, Freitag L, Greschuchna D. Limited and radical resection for tracheal and bronchopulmonary carcinoid tumour. Report on 227 cases. *Eur J Cardiothorac Surg* 4:527, 1990.

118. Struhar D, et al. Alveolar haemorrhage with pleural effusion as a manifestation of epithelioid haemangioendothelioma. *Eur Respir J* 5:592, 1992.

119. Swan LL. Pulmonary adenomatosis in man. *Pathology* 47:517, 1949.

120. Taylor DB, et al. Cavitating pulmonary nodules in histiocytosis-X high resolution CT demonstration. *Australas Radiol* 34:253, 1990.

121. Teragaki M, et al. Hereditary hemorrhagic telan-

giectasia with growing pulmonary arteriovenous fistulas followed for 24 years. *Am J Med Sci* 295:545, 1988.

122. Thunnissen FB, et al. Fine needle aspiration cytology of inflammatory pseudotumor of the lung (plasma cell granuloma). Report of four cases. *Acta Cytol* 33:917, 1989.

123. Torikata C, Mukai M. So-called minute chemodectoma of the lung. An electron microscopic and immunohistochemical study. *Virchows Arch A Pathol Anat Histopathol* 417:113, 1990.

124. Tubbs WS, et al. Benign giant-cell tumor of bone with pulmonary metastases: Clinical findings and radiologic appearance of metastases in 13 cases. *AJR* 158:331, 1992.

125. Turnbull AD, et al. Mucoepidermoid tumor of bronchial glands. *Cancer* 28:539, 1971.

126. Ueda K, et al. Rhabdomyosarcoma of lung arising in congenital cystic malformation. *Cancer* 40:383, 1977.

127. Urschel JD, Horan TA, Unruh HW. Plasma cell granuloma of the lung. *J Thorac Cardiovasc Surg* 104:870, 1992.

128. Uyama T, et al. Pulmonary leiomyomatosis showing endobronchial extension and giant cyst formation. *Chest* 94:644, 1988.

129. Van Damme H, et al. Primary pulmonary hemangiopericytoma: Early local recurrence after perioperative rupture of the giant tumor mass (two cases). *Surgery* 108:105, 1990.

130. Venn GE, et al. Malignant fibrous histiocytoma in thoracic surgical practice. *J Thorac Cardiovasc Surg* 91:234, 1986.

131. Venn GE, Sarin S, Goldstraw P. Survival following pulmonary metastasectomy. *Eur J Cardiothorac Surg* 3:105, 1989.

132. Vogt MI, et al. Results of surgical treatment of pulmonary metastases. *Eur J Cardiothorac Surg* 2:224, 1988.

133. Walsh TJ, Healey TM. Chondroma of the bronchus. *Thorax* 24:327, 1969.

134. Watts CF, Clagett OT, MacDonald JR. Lipoma of the bronchus: Discussion of benign neoplasms and report of a case of endobronchial lipoma. *J Thorac Cardiovasc Surg* 15:132, 1946.

135. Yellin A, Rosenman Y, Lieberman Y. Review of smooth muscle tumours of the lower respiratory tract. *Br J Dis Chest* 78:337, 1984.

136. Yellin A, et al. Chondrosarcoma of the bronchus: Report of a case and review of the literature. *Chest* 84:224, 1983.

137. Yousem SA, Hochholzer L. Primary pulmonary hemangiopericytoma. *Cancer* 59:549, 1987.

138. Yousem SA, et al. So-called sclerosing hemangiomas of lung. An immunohistochemical study supporting a respiratory epithelial origin. *Am J Surg Pathol* 12:582, 1988.

55

Tumors of the Mediastinum, Pleura, Chest Wall, and Diaphragm

Scot H. Merrick   *Noel H. Fishman*

Tumors and Cysts of the Mediastinum

The embryologic development of the mediastinum produces a number of closely opposed structures of different germ layer origins. Mediastinal masses may therefore have distinctly different histologies and a predilection to specific locations. There are also major differences in the patterns of occurrence between adults and children. Advances in radiographic imaging techniques, isotope scanning, and tumor markers have made important contributions to the management of mediastinal masses over the past decade.

The mediastinum consists of all structures between the two pleural cavities and is bounded superiorly by the thoracic inlet and inferiorly by the diaphragm. For purposes of discussion, it is customary, by drawing lines on a lateral chest x-ray film, to divide the mediastinum into three compartments (Fig. 55-1). This compartmentalization is clinically useful because of the predilection of certain tumors to arise within circumscribed areas. The posterior compartment is delineated by a line drawn along the posterior pericardial border and continued upward along the anterior borders of the thoracic vertebral bodies. A second line can be drawn along the anterior pericardial border and continued upward along the anterior surface of the tracheal air shadow in order to create two additional compartments, the anterior mediastinum and the middle mediastinum. In some texts, the anterior mediastinum is further subdivided into superior and inferior subcompartments, but the overlap of tumors such as thymomas between these subdivisions is so great as to limit the usefulness of this refinement.

The anterior compartment contains the thymus, ascending aorta, innominate artery and vein, superior vena cava, fat, and lymph nodes. Over 50 percent of mediastinal masses occur in this compartment [24]. The middle mediastinum contains the heart, pericardium, aortic arch and branches, bronchi, upper esophagus, trachea, and mediastinal lymph nodes. The posterior mediastinum contains the lower esophagus, descending aorta, sympathetic chain, and intercostal nerves and accounts for 25 percent of all mediastinal masses.

The most common lesions of the anterior mediastinum are thymic neoplasms, lymphomas, and germ cell tumors. They account for nearly 60 percent of tumors in this compartment. It is not uncommon for these tumors to enlarge and occupy the middle compartment as well. Masses in the middle mediastinum are primarily cystic; 25 percent of lesions are metastatic malignancies to lymph nodes (lymphoma, carcinoma). In most reports, 70 percent of lesions within the posterior compartment are either neurogenic in origin or cystic [25,88]. In children, neurogenic tumors and lymphomas are more common and thymomas are rare.

Approximately 30 percent of mediastinal masses are malignant [99], with lymphomas, primary carcinomas, malignant thymomas, and malignant germ cell tumors representing the majority. Malignant lesions are more common in children and between the ages of 20 to 40; several authors have reported increasing numbers of malignant mediastinal lesions coinciding with the increased incidence of lymphomas [18,25]. The presence of symptoms is also predictive of malignancy.

Approximately 60 percent of patients with

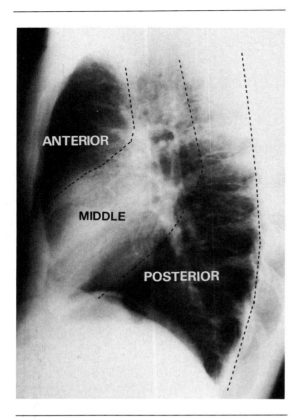

Fig. 55-1. Lateral chest x-ray film demonstrating the three compartments of the mediastinum. (Reproduced from DC Sabiston Jr, HN Oldham Jr. *The Mediastinum.* In DC Sabiston Jr, FC Spencer (Eds), *Gibbon's Surgery of the Chest* (4th ed.). Philadelphia: Saunders, 1983.

a mediastinal mass will have symptoms [25]. Nevertheless, in a large proportion of patients, benign lesions will be discovered on routine x-ray studies [11]. Chest pain, dyspnea, cough, and fever are the most common presenting symptoms. Many tumors will produce systemic syndromes as the result of hormone secretion. For example, excessive corticotropin (ACTH) production by mediastinal carcinoids can produce Cushing's disease, and mediastinal pheochromocytoma can produce hypertension. In addition, thymomas have a poorly understood association with myasthenia gravis, red cell aplasia, and collagen vascular disorders.

In addition to a careful history and physical examination, patients with a suspected mediastinal mass should undergo routine chest radiography and contrast-enhanced computed tomography (CT). These two studies will identify the size, location, and composition of the lesion in the majority of patients [13,76,130]. Magnetic resonance imaging (MRI) may help distinguish vascular from soft-tissue masses in some cases. Several radioisotope scans may accurately localize occult, functional mediastinal tumors. Examples include the use of ^{131}I-metaiodobenzylguanidine (MIBG) to detect pheochromocytomas and technetium-thallium studies for the localization of ectopic parathyroid adenomas. Numerous mediastinal tumor markers have been reported, but only alpha-fetoprotein (nonseminomatous germ cell tumors) and human chorionic gonadotropin (teratomas) are clinically useful [8].

Although fine-needle biopsy has been used with accuracy to diagnose mediastinal masses [111,137], it is not likely to alter therapy. Occasionally, mediastinoscopy is required to provide sufficient tissue for definitive diagnosis (e.g., lymphoma) [10]. In selected patients, video-assisted thoracoscopy may be diagnostic and therapeutic [59,62].

Although they also occur within the boundaries of the mediastinum, tumors and aneurysms of the thoracic aorta, trachea, esophagus, and heart are traditionally discussed as separate topics.

Classification of Mediastinal Tumors

Davis, Oldham, and Sabiston [24] classify mediastinal tumors according to tissues of origin as follows:

1. Neurogenic tumors
   a. Neurofibroma
   b. Neurilemmoma
   c. Neurosarcoma
   d. Ganglioneuroma
   e. Ganglioneuroblastoma
   f. Neuroblastoma
   g. Chemodectoma
   h. Pheochromocytoma
2. Thymomas
   a. Benign
   b. Malignant
3. Lymphomas
   a. Hodgkin's disease
   b. Lymphocytic lymphoma
   c. Lymphocytic/histiocytic lymphoma
   d. Histiocytic lymphoma
   e. Undifferentiated lymphoma

4. Teratodermoid tumors
   a. Benign
   b. Malignant
5. Germ cell tumors
   a. Seminoma
   b. Embryonal carcinoma
   c. Choriocarcinoma
6. Primary carcinomas
7. Mesenchymal tumors
   a. Fibroma/fibrosarcoma
   b. Lipoma/liposarcoma
   c. Myxoma
   d. Mesothelioma
   e. Leiomyoma/leiomyosarcoma
   f. Rhabdomyosarcoma
   g. Xanthogranuloma
   h. Mesenchymoma
   i. Hemangioma
   j. Hemangioendothelioma
   k. Hemangiopericytoma
   l. Lymphangioma
   m. Lymphangiomyoma
   n. Lymphangiopericytoma
8. Endocrine tumors
   a. Intrathoracic thyroid
   b. Parathyroid adenoma
   c. Carcinoid
9. Cysts
   a. Pericardial
   b. Bronchogenic
   c. Enteric
   d. Thymic
   e. Thoracic duct
   f. Nonspecific

A number on nonneoplastic lesions, particularly of the middle and posterior compartments, must be considered in the differential diagnosis of mediastinal masses. These include hiatal hernias, esophageal diverticula, meningoceles, and infections (mediastinitis, paravertebral abscess). An accurate differentiation should be possible in the majority of cases.

Neurogenic Tumors

Tumors that arise from intercostal nerve sheaths (neurilemmoma, neurofibroma), autonomic ganglia (ganglioneuroma, ganglioneuroblastoma), and the paraganglionic nervous system (chemodectoma, pheochromocytoma) account for 20 to 25 percent of all mediastinal tumors in adults [2,25,92,93] and 50 percent of mediastinal tumors in children [123]. The etiology of these tumors is unknown, and most are thought to occur spontaneously. However, approximately 25 to 40 percent of patients with neurofibromas will have von Recklinghausen's disease. Ninety percent of neurogenic tumors arise in the posterior mediastinum, typically along the paravertebral gutter where the sympathetic chains and the origin of intercostal nerves are located. Seventy-five percent of all posterior mediastinal tumors are neurogenic.

Although the great majority of neurogenic tumors in adults are benign, approximately 1 to 4 percent are malignant [41,92]. In contrast, most neurogenic tumors in children are malignant [24].

Approximately half of all benign and malignant neurogenic tumors are asymptomatic, being discovered incidentally on chest x-ray films. The classic appearance is that of a round, smooth, homogeneous mass with sharp margins lying in the posterior mediastinum abutting the vertebral bodies [76,130] (Fig. 55-2). The part that reaches the chest wall is flattened, lending a D shape to the tumor, a feature that is best appreciated on the lateral or appropriate oblique projection. The benign forms of these tumors usually increase in size slowly over a long period, whereas the malignant tumors tend to enlarge rapidly. Pain and cough are symptoms of local extension and compression. Some tumors enlarge sufficiently to cause dyspnea (Fig. 55-3). Catecholamine secretion from paraganglionic tumors may produce hypertension, headaches, sweating, and palpitations. Secretion of vasoactive intestinal polypeptide by ganglioneuromas and neuroblastomas may produce profuse, watery diarrhea.

Approximately 10 percent of neurogenic tumors will extend medially through the intervertebral foramen to form "dumbbell" tumors (Fig. 55-4). These are almost always symptomatic [46,96], with back pain, intercostal radicular pain, or signs of spinal compression. Typically, a CT scan will demonstrate erosion of the intervertebral neuroforamen, pedicles, and facets. In this situation, MRI is indicated as it will more effectively demonstrate intraspinal extension of tumor and spinal cord involvement [96]. If MRI is not available, then myelography should be performed. Current treatment of dumbbell tumors consists of a single-stage combined laminectomy and thoracotomy for complete removal of the tumor [3,46].

Neurofibromas and *neurilemmomas* account for the great majority of all neurogenic tumors. The former is thought to represent a metaplastic derivative of Schwann cells; it occurs sporadi-

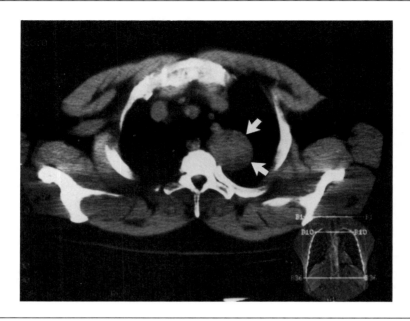

Fig. 55-2. Chest computed tomography scan showing a neurilemmoma of the posterior mediastinum (*arrows*) in a 44-year-old man with back pain.

cally and in association with phakomatoses (von Recklinghausen's disease, tuberous sclerosis, von Hippel-Lindau disease, etc.) [19] and may arise from any nerve in the thorax [23]. Neurofibromas contain all of the elements of the nerve trunk, including axons and connective tissue. Grossly, a true capsule is usually absent and on histologic examination, cellular palisading is absent.

Fig. 55-3. Operative photograph of a large ganglioneuroma, occupying most of the pleural space and producing dyspnea.

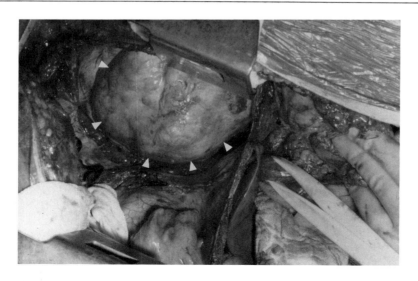

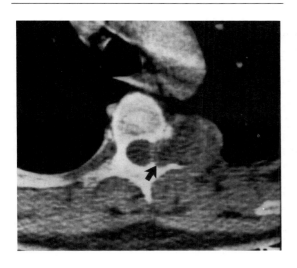

Fig. 55-4. Chest computed tomography scan showing a neurogenic tumor extending into the intervertebral foramen, forming a "dumbbell" (*arrow*).

Fig. 55-5. Neurilemmoma showing Antonio type A (*large arrow*) and type B (*small arrow*) features. Palisading nuclei are prominent (*open arrow*) (H&E stain, × 660). (Courtesy of Dr. Gordon Honda, Department of Pathology, University of California, San Francisco.)

Immunohistochemical stains will demonstrate S-100 protein, indicating a nerve sheath origin. Because of the propensity for continued, slow growth and malignant potential, surgical resection is recommended for all neurofibromas. Complete removal should be considered curative; a plexiform variant may be locally aggressive and difficult to control.

Neurilemmomas are derived from Schwann cells that encase each axon cylinder of peripheral nerves. In addition to von Recklinghausen's disease, this lesion is also associated with Noonan's syndrome. Histologically, two separate morphologies have been described. Antonio type A is characterized by palisading nuclei within a dense cytoplasmic stroma. Antonio type B typically reveals a loose, myxomatous stroma with areas of hemorrhage [123] (Fig. 55-5). As with neurofibromas, surgical resection is recommended and the prognosis is excellent.

Rarely, malignant degeneration of either neurofibromas or neurilemmomas occurs, giving rise to a neurosarcoma (malignant schwannoma). This lesion may synthesize an insulin analogue capable of producing hypoglycemia. Even with complete resection, only 30 to 60 percent of patients will be cured [19]; adjuvant radiotherapy may improve survival [3,11].

Ganglioneuromas are common benign tumors that arise from peripheral nerve cells of the sympathetic chain (Fig. 55-6). They occur more frequently in children. Microscopically, they consist of ganglion cells with three or four nuclei within

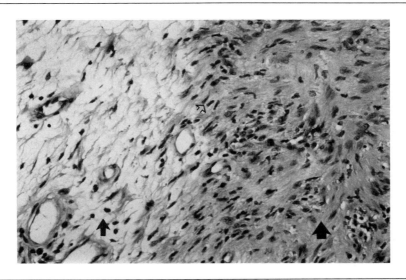

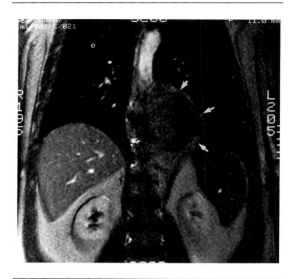

Fig. 55-6. Magnetic resonance image of a large, symptomatic ganglioneuroma (*arrows*) in a 47-year-old man. Figure 55-3 shows the operative picture.

a stroma of medullated and nonmedullated nerve fibers, connective tissue, and Schwann cells [77] (Fig. 55-7). Ganglioneuromas may undergo malignant degeneration either into a partially differentiated *ganglioneuroblastoma*, which contains immature sympathetic nerve cells and mature ganglion cells, or into a completely undifferen-

tiated *neuroblastoma*, which is composed of small lymphocyte-like cells frequently arranged into rosettes [24]. Neurosecretory granules are present on electron microscopy. While both lesions are seen most often in children, neuroblastomas are much more common, accounting for 15 percent of annual pediatric cancer deaths. However, only a minority of patients have disease confined to the chest at the time of presentation. In addition to cough, pain, and dyspnea, neuroblastomas can produce catecholamines (which cause hypertension and sweating) and vasoactive intestinal polypeptide (resulting in watery diarrhea), and have been associated with an autoimmune condition known as *opsoclonus-polymyoclonus syndrome*. Serum ferritin levels correlate with the presence of active tumor [19].

The treatment of minimally invasive ganglioneuroblastomas is primarily surgical, with an expected 5-year survival rate of nearly 90 percent. For neuroblastomas, prognosis is dependent on the age of the patient, histologic grade of the tumor, tumor location (better prognosis for disease limited to the chest), and tumor DNA content. For early-stage lesions, resection can effect a cure; only 10 percent of patients with dissemi-

Fig. 55-7. Ganglioneuroma showing prominent ganglion cells (*arrows*) within a background of loose connective tissue stroma (H&E stain, × 500). (Courtesy of Dr. Gordon Honda, Department of Pathology, University of California, San Francisco.)

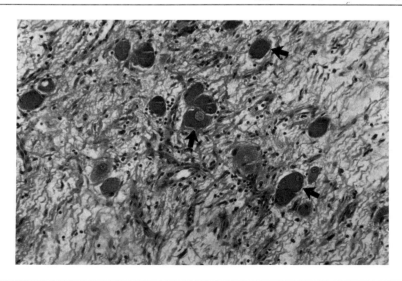

nated neuroblastoma will be disease-free at 2 years [47]. Combination chemotherapy and radiotherapy can achieve good response rates for advanced disease [72]. On rare occasions, neuroblastomas regress spontaneously [109].

Mediastinal *paragangliomas* are rare lesions, accounting for approximately 1 percent of all mediastinal tumors. Included in this group are carotid body tumors, chemodectomas, glomus tumors, and pheochromocytomas. All are capable of storing catecholamines intracellularly; pheochromocytomas are best known for secretory function as well. Multiple lesions may be present in 10 percent of patients, associated with the multiple endocrine neoplasia syndrome (MEN types II and III). Pathologically, these tumors are quite vascular and immunohistochemical staining will distinguish them from neurogenic tumors. For secretory lesions, symptoms of catecholamine excess are characteristic. Measurement of urinary catecholamines will establish the diagnosis. Chest CT scans and ^{131}I-MIBG scans will localize the majority of pheochromocytomas. Surgical resection is curative for benign paragangliomas; even with benign histology, some lesions will behave aggressively and the 5-year survival rate approaches 50 percent [108].

Thymoma

Several neoplastic conditions including thymoma, thymic carcinoma, and carcinoid may involve the thymus gland. Of these, thymoma is by far the most common. The normal thymus gland is composed of a mixture of epithelial cells and lymphocytes. Although the great majority of thymomas contain a mixture of these cell types, and even though at times the lymphocytes are predominant, only the epithelial cells are neoplastic [51]. It is true that a lymphoma also may occur in the thymus gland as a primary tumor or as a part of systemic disease, but in those cases the lymphocytes and not the epithelial elements are neoplastic. Several schemes have been proposed for the classification of thymomas, based on the degree of invasion (stages I to IV) (Table 55-1) and histology (cortical, medullary, mixed) (Table 55-2). The former is most widely accepted, but both have prognostic utility.

Thymomas comprise 10 to 20 percent of all mediastinal tumors [129]. Rare in childhood, the incidence of thymomas in adults increases with age. There is an equal sex distribution. Most of these tumors are located centrally in the anterior mediastinum (Fig. 55-8), but they also may occur laterally in the middle mediastinum when a tu-

Table 55-2. **Staging of thymoma based on tumor histopathology**

Histopathology	Proportion of patients (%)	5-year survival rate (%)
Cortical	41	52
Medullary	12	100
Mixed	46	85

Source: From references 56 and 93.

Table 55-1. **Staging system for thymoma based on tumor spread**

Stage	Description	Proportion of cases*	5-year survival rate (%)†
I	Completely encapsulated tumor without evidence of capsular invasion	40	90–93
II	Gross, or microscopic extracapsular extension of tumor into adjacent fat or pleura	14	70–95
III	Gross invasion of adjacent organs (pericardium, great vessels, etc.)	34	58–72
IVa	Diffuse, metastatic disease involving the pleura or pericardium	9	50–60
IVb	Distant metastases	3	24

*From reference 68.
†From references 64, 89, 128, 134.

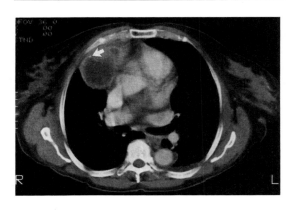

Fig. 55-8. Invasive thymoma in a patient with chest pain and arthralgias. Calcium is present within the mass (*arrow*).

mor in the inferior pole of the gland enlarges and descends along the border of the pericardium.

Fifty percent of patients are asymptomatic. Approximately 25 percent have cough, dyspnea, or chest pain. Obstruction of the superior vena cava is usually a sign of malignancy. Approximately 25 to 35 percent have an associated systemic syndrome and myasthenia gravis is the most frequent [86].

Ten to 50 percent of thymomas are associated with myasthenia gravis, whereas approximately 10 to 15 percent of patients with myasthenia will be found to have a thymoma at surgery [24, 129,134]. In the past, the occurrence of myasthenia in patients with a thymoma was thought to have a negative impact on survival. With improvement in drug therapy and plasmapheresis, this is no longer true [64]. Myasthenia has been observed more frequently with certain histologic types of thymoma [94]. A number of other autoimmune or immune phenomena have been associated with thymomas. Among the more common are red cell hypoplasia (virtual absence of erythroblasts and reticulocytes in the bone marrow), hypogammaglobulinemia, systemic lupus erythematosus, and Cushing's syndrome [99]. Red cell hypoplasia occurs in 5 percent of patients with a thymoma. However, 50 percent of all cases of red cell hypoplasia are associated with thymoma. Hypogammaglobulinemia occurs in a smaller percentage of patients with a thymoma, but approximately 10 percent of patients with this condition also have a thymoma. Cushing's syndrome is associated with carcinoid tumors of the thymus [133].

Standard chest radiographs in patients with thymomas typically show a smooth, lobulated mass located in the anterior mediastinum. Calcification within the mass may be present. Retrospective examination of serial roentgenograms suggests that thymomas usually enlarge slowly over a long period. Thymomas associated with myasthenia gravis are usually smaller than average. In fact, many are discovered incidentally during thymectomy intended for the relief of myasthenic symptoms. MRI is useful in determining the relationship of large tumor to the great vessels; a lobulated internal architecture may be associated with malignancy [106].

Grossly, thymomas are encapsulated, lobulated tumors. Degenerative changes including focal hemorrhage, calcification, and cyst formation are often found [129]. On cut section, the grayish-tan tumor is frequently compartmentalized by fibrous septa. Although commonly adherent to adjacent structures, frank invasion occurs in only 20 to 40 percent of patients.

Microscopically, a mixture of epithelial cells and lymphocytes may be found. The epithelial cells are either round, oval, or elongated, with vesicular nuclei and indistinct cell margins (Fig. 55-9), whereas the lymphocytes are normal in appearance. Rosettes are formed in 20 percent of cases, and Hassall's corpuscles (keratinized epithelial cells) are frequently present. With a predominance of epithelial cells, the lesion is called an *epithelial thymoma;* when the epithelial cells assume a fusiform shape, the lesion is termed a *spindle cell thymoma;* a predominance of lymphocytes is termed a *lymphocytic thymoma.* These groups occur with equal frequency; however, myasthenia is more commonly seen in patients with lymphocytic thymomas and red cell hypoplasia is more common in those with spindle lesions [73].

Surgical resection is recommended for most thymomas. En bloc removal of the tumor and surrounding tissue through a sternotomy incision is the most common practice. Often, the distinction between a benign and malignant lesion is made at operation, with the finding of tumor invasion. Even without gross evidence, microscopic invasion is seen in 20 percent of tumors [129]. The 5-year survival rate for stage I disease is approximately 90 percent (see Table 55-1). Several studies have shown that certain oncogene protein expression [78], or tumor DNA content [91] may predict outcome. However, the most accurate indicator of long-term prognosis is the degree of tumor invasion [68,89,134]. For advanced lesions

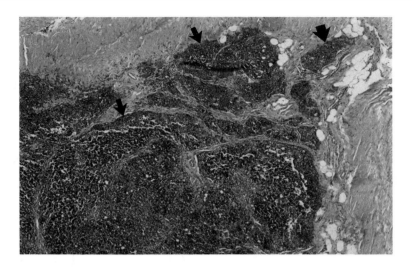

Fig. 55-9. Invasive, lymphocytic thymoma showing characteristic tumor lobules (*small arrows*). A focus of invasive tumor is seen (*large arrow*) (H&E stain, × 132). (Courtesy of Dr. Gordon Honda, Department of Pathology, University of California, San Francisco.)

or recurrences, radiotherapy, chemotherapy, or both can extend survival [39,40,121,122,128]. Thymectomy improves the symptoms of myasthenia in approximately 25 percent of patients with thymomas; nearly twice as many myasthenic patients without thymomas will improve with thymectomy [99]. Red cell hypoplasia is rarely helped by thymectomy, and hypogammaglobulinemia never is.

Lymphomas

As a group, the lymphomas represent approximately 20 percent of all adult mediastinal malignancies; this number doubles in children [117]. The incidence of malignant mediastinal lesions has increased, primarily due to an increase in the number of lymphomas [18,25]. The majority of mediastinal lymphomas are found in the anterior and middle compartments, arising from nodal tissue [31] as a part of systemic disease. Occasionally, the primary tissue of origin may be the thymus, thyroid, or heart. The classification of lymphomas is based on the cell of origin (B cell, T cell), cellular histology, degree of maturation, and cell-surface antigen markers [31]. Hodgkin's

lymphoma, lymphoblastic lymphoma, and diffuse large-cell non-Hodgkin's lymphoma account for 90 percent of primary mediastinal lymphomas [114]. The tumor biology, clinical presentation, and response to therapy vary according to the type of lymphoma [87].

The mediastinum is usually involved as part of a generalized systemic lymphoma. These patients suffer from fever, fatigue, weight loss, lymphadenopathy, hepatosplenomegaly, and so on. The diagnosis can be made by biopsy of lymph nodes or bone marrow and by study of the peripheral blood.

However, approximately 10 percent of patients with lymphomas present with disease apparently confined to the mediastinum (Figs. 55-10 and 55-11). In addition to systemic symptoms, mediastinal lymphomas can cause pain, cough, and dyspnea. In advanced stages, involvement of adjacent structures may result in pleural and pericardial effusions, tracheal obstruction, and obstruction of the superior vena cava [24].

There are no specific radiographic features that define mediastinal lymphomas. However, CT and MRI scans are essential to determine the extent of disease and invasion into contiguous structures and to establish a baseline for therapeutic response. Thymomas, germ cell tumors, and Castleman's disease (a benign lymph node hyperplasia seen in the mediastinum) should be considered in the differential diagnosis.

Because many lymphomas require electron microscopy and immunohistochemical stains for differentiation, open biopsy techniques are frequently required to provide sufficient tissue for examination. Anterior mediastinal masses can be accessed by mediastinoscopy [37,67]. Middle and posterior lesions can be biopsied using thoracoscopy. There are no serum markers specific for lymphomas, although serum lactate dehydrogenase levels may be elevated in many patients.

The treatment of patients with mediastinal lymphomas is based on primary radiotherapy (stage I and II Hodgkin's disease) or radiation with combination chemotherapy (non-Hodgkin's lymphomas). Patients with early-stage Hodgkin's disease have a 10-year survival rate of over 90 percent. Modern cure rates for non-Hodgkin's

lymphomas are approximately 50 percent [24, 117,135]. Recurrences are more frequent with "bulky" mediastinal disease. Although surgical resection of isolated lesions and tumor "debulking" have been reported with good results [95], this approach has limited application.

Germ Cell Tumors

These tumors can be divided into benign *teratodermoid tumors* and malignant tumors, which include seminomas, embryonal carcinomas, choriocarcinomas, and endodermal sinus (yolk sac) tumors. Germ cell tumors are thought to originate during an abnormal migration of germ cells during embryogenesis. Less than 1 percent represent metastases from a gonadal primary tumor [80]. Approximately 50 to 70 percent of all extragonadal germ cell tumors occur in the anterior mediastinum; other locations include the pineal gland, retroperitoneum, and sacrococcygeal areas. Germ cell tumors are more common in males with Klinefelter's syndrome [22,79].

TERATODERMOID TUMORS
The term *teratoma* indicates that a tumor is composed of tissues derived from all three germ lay-

Fig. 55-10. Anterior mediastinal Hodgkin's lymphoma in a 24-year-old woman.

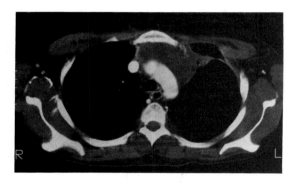

Fig. 55-11. Typical Hodgkin's lymphoma showing a background of benign lymphocytes and prominent Reed-Sternberg cells (*arrows*) (H&E stain, × 600). (Courtesy of Dr. Gordon Honda, Department of Pathology, University of California, San Francisco.)

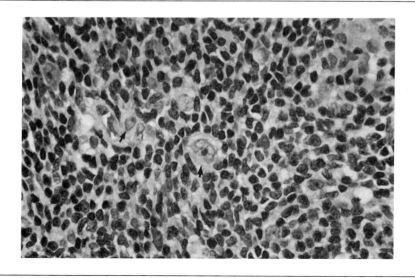

ers and that all those tissues are foreign to the organ in which they are found. *Dermoid cysts*, the name applied to the simplest form of teratoma, is a misnomer because tissue elements other than skin are also present in the cyst lining.

Approximately 10 percent of mediastinal tumors are teratomas [26,104]; this lesion also represents the most common germ cell neoplasm of the mediastinum. Essentially all mediastinal teratomas develop within the anterior compartment in connection with the thymus gland and sometimes within it.

Mostly asymptomatic, they are usually discovered on routine chest x-ray films as a mass in the anterior mediastinum projecting into one hemithorax or the other. Symptoms of pain and dyspnea are related to the compressive effects of a large tumor. In infants and children, compressive symptoms occur earlier because there is less space for tumor enlargement. Occasionally, these tumors erode, by pressure necrosis or infection, into adjacent organs such as the lung, pericardium, pleura, and superior vena cava, into which the cyst's contents may be discharged. A patient may, for example, cough up hair from a cyst that has eroded into the lung [66]. Typically, chest CT scans show a cystic structure that may contain calcium, bone, and fat [14,80] (Fig. 55-12).

Benign teratomas tend to be smooth and rounded, whereas their counterparts are usually lobulated. Grossly, most benign mediastinal teratomas are multicystic, whereas the malignant forms tend to be solid [98]. Microscopically, benign teratomas contain many cystic structures lined by tall mucus-secreting cells and a large

number of different types of tissue attempting to form organs. Teratomas may be extremely complex and contain a great variety of tissue, including skin, hair, teeth, sebum, muscle, bone, cartilage, fat, respiratory epithelium, pancreas, nerve tissue, and others in various stages of embryologic development [26,49,80].

Eighty percent of teratomas are composed of mature tissue elements and are therefore considered benign. Immature tissue elements in a teratoma constitute a sign of malignancy, especially in an adult.

Except for areas of inflammatory reaction or malignant invasion, teratomas have no real tissue attachment and can practically be shelled out of the mediastinum once the overlying pleura has been incised. Since the diagnosis is usually not known beforehand, it is probably good practice to approach the tumor through a median sternotomy, regardless of whether it projects more to one side than the other, and to remove the contiguous thymus en bloc with the tumor. All fistulous connections to other organs (e.g., bronchocystic fistulas) must be interrupted and properly sealed. Care must be exercised to avoid damaging the phrenic nerve, which is frequently stretched over the tumor. Resection of benign teratomas should be considered curative. For malignant lesions, chemotherapy may prolong survival [63].

SEMINOMA

Seminoma, also known as *dysgerminoma*, is a rare primary malignant tumor that almost invariably arises in the anterior mediastinum. It occurs almost exclusively in men between the ages of 20 to 40 years, and accounts for half of all mediastinal germ cell tumors. Chest pain, cough, dyspnea, and hoarseness are the most common symptoms. The superior vena cava syndrome may be present in 10 to 20 percent of patients [24,49]. Typically, a large, homogeneous anterior mediastinal mass is seen on chest CT, but there are no specific radiographic signs; metastatic spread tends to be local into the adjacent lung, great vessels, or both. A small number of patients will have elevations of beta-human chorionic gonadotropin (β-HCG) [53]. This tumor is histologically identical to seminoma of the testis, but the testicular tumor rarely metastasizes to the anterior mediastinum. In the absence of testicular enlargement and retroperitoneal adenopathy on CT scan, a seminoma in the mediastinum may be considered to be a primary extragonadal germ cell tumor.

Fig. 55-12. Teratoma of the anterior mediastinum with central calcium deposits.

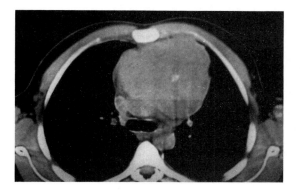

Seminomas are solid, nonencapsulated tumors adjacent to the thymus and sometimes enclosed within the gland. On cut section, they are homogeneous, pale tan to yellow, and firm in consistency. On microscopic examination, the tumor is typically divided into numerous islands by fine reticulum fibers [61]. The cells have large, dense nuclei, and the abundant cytoplasm contains glycogen (in contrast to thymomas, which they may resemble) [24]. Noncaseating granulomas are also frequently found in the tumor.

The primary treatment for seminomas is megavoltage radiotherapy, since the tumor is usually very sensitive [55,66,80]. Approximately 60 percent of patients will be cured with this approach [49]. For large, bulky lesions and in patients with extrathoracic spread or recurrence, the addition of cisplatin-based combination chemotherapy can produce complete remission rates of 80 to 90 percent [80].

NONSEMINOMATOUS GERM CELL TUMORS

Embryonal carcinoma, choriocarcinoma, and teratocarcinoma of the mediastinum are quite rare, and endodermal sinus (yolk sac) tumor of the mediastinum is extremely rare. As a group, they comprise approximately 3 to 10 percent of all mediastinal tumors [49]. Nonseminomatous germ cell tumors of the mediastinum almost always occur in men between the ages of 20 and 50. Rapid growth and invasive behavior are the rule. Symptoms include pain, cough, hemoptysis, dyspnea, fever, and weight loss. Approximately 20 percent of patients develop signs of superior vena cava obstruction. Gynecomastia develops in a significant percentage of patients with nonseminomatous germ cell tumors and is associated with high levels of β-HCG. β-HCG and alpha-fetoprotein are produced by the majority of these tumors [32,80]. Assays of these biomarkers are an extremely useful way to assess the efficacy of chemotherapy.

Almost all patients with nonseminomatous germ cell tumors have one or more foci of metastatic disease at the time of diagnosis [49]. Tumors tend to be large, with invasion into local structures, and the response to radiotherapy is poor. Multiagent cisplatin-based chemotherapy is the treatment of choice. With this approach, approximately 50 to 70 percent of patients will achieve complete remission and half may be long-term survivors [54,80]. A significant number of patients will have normalization of tumor markers, but residual disease is visible on x-ray studies. In this situation, surgical resection of the remaining tumor may be of benefit [43,54,80,120].

Mesenchymal Tumors

Mesenchymal tumors may arise from connective tissue, muscle, blood vessels, fat, and lymphatic tissue. As a group, they account for approximately 6 percent of all mediastinal tumors, and about half are benign [25,93]. These tumors include fibroma (benign mesothelioma), lipoma, and liposarcoma. Myxoma, leiomyoma, leiomyosarcoma, rhabdomyosarcoma, xanthogranuloma, and mesenchymoma are also listed in texts but occur so rarely that there are few recent reports. In addition, there are tumors of vascular and lymphatic origin; these include hemangiopericytoma, lymphangioma, cystic hygroma, and lymphangiomyoma (lymphangiopericytoma). All these are relatively more common in other parts of the body than in the mediastinum. Some of these tumors are of a mixed type. Swanson [118] provided a comprehensive review of these tumors.

Treatment of mesenchymal tumors is by surgical resection. The malignant forms are virtually all resistant to radiation and chemotherapy [24].

Fibromas occur more frequently in the pleura (benign pleural mesothelioma) than in the mediastinum. Some mediastinal fibromas have been associated with hypoglycemia and may degenerate into fibrosarcomas. Lipomas account for 2 percent of all primary mediastinal tumors and are found predominantly in the anterior mediastinum [93]. They must be differentiated from mediastinal lipomatosis, the excessive fat accumulation caused by excessive corticosteroid stimulation, herniated omentum, and thymolipoma. The diagnosis of a lipoma can be made on CT scan by the low specific coefficient of attenuation (-30 to -100 Hounsfield units) of fat. Lipomas in the lower mediastinum are usually asymptomatic, but large cervicomediastinal lipomas can produce tracheal obstruction. Approximately 50 cases of liposarcoma of the mediastinum have been reported [29]. Typically, this lobulated tumor may become quite large and infiltrate soft tissues and organs, producing symptoms of airway compression and chest pain.

Lesions of vascular origin, hemangiomas, hemangioendotheliomas, and angiosarcomas are extremely rare in the mediastinum [61]. They may arise anywhere in the mediastinum. Thirty percent are malignant and may erode into bone. Hemangiomas may be extremely vascular and may rupture freely into a pleural space. Complete resection may be difficult, but is usually curative [118].

Mediastinal lymphangiomyoma (lymphangiopericytoma) is a noninvasive benign tumor closely associated with the thoracic duct, derived from perilymphatic smooth muscle of the lung. The tumor oozes chyle and produces chylothorax. Discovery is usually made at surgery intended to ligate the thoracic duct [61].

The majority of mediastinal lymphangiomas begin in the neck ("cystic hygroma") and descend into the mediastinum. They are composed of multilocular, thin-walled cysts lined by endothelium and filled with clear fluid [118]. These tumors are surrounded by a vascular and fibrous reaction and grow in a budding fashion, making surgical resection difficult. Nevertheless, recurrence is rare following nearly complete removal.

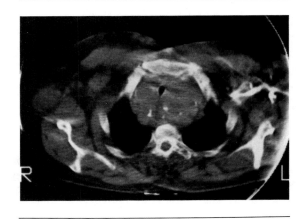

Fig. 55-13. Computed tomography scan of a large, intrathoracic thyroid causing severe airway compression and stridor.

Intrathoracic Thyroid

Intrathoracic thyroid is a common lesion, estimated to occur in 0.02 percent of the general population. More frequent in women, the intrathoracic goiter frequently arises as an extension from the isthmus or inferior pole of the cervical thyroid gland and descends into the mediastinum between the trachea and prevertebral fascia [75]. The mass may present either anterior to the trachea or in the posterior mediastinum partially overlying the trachea [21]. Approximately half of patients complain of respiratory distress. Typically, inspiratory stridor or a choking sensation is aggravated by leaning forward. Venous engorgement of the neck and arm may result from compression of the innominate vein. Hyperthyroidism may be present in 13 percent of patients [75]. On the chest x-ray films, the trachea is usually displaced laterally and the lumen is reduced. Esophageal compression can be appreciated on barium swallow studies. Findings of chest CT scan are characteristic, and consist of a nonhomogeneous mass with distinct borders, containing course calcifications (Fig. 55-13). Prolonged enhancement of the mass after injection of an iodinated contrast agent is typical [21,75,76]. Findings on radioactive iodine scans (^{131}I) are invariably positive.

Histologically, intrathoracic thyroid tumors are usually multinodular goiters. Follicular adenoma may be present on occasion and approximately 3 to 5 percent will contain occult carcinoma [21,75,132].

True ectopic thyroid tissue is a very uncommon condition. The tissue is usually found in the anterior mediastinum adjacent to the thymus. The blood supply is from the mediastinum rather than from the neck. Symptoms are infrequent. Rarely does this tissue represent the only functioning thyroid tissue in the body.

The use of L-thyroxine to suppress an intrathoracic goiter will do little to change the size of the mass. Because of the propensity for airway compromise and the possibility of occult carcinoma, most clinicians recommend surgical resection [75,107]. This can be accomplished through a cervical incision in most cases.

Intrathoracic Parathyroid Adenoma

Approximately 10 percent of parathyroid adenomas are found in the anterior mediastinum [20, 24], where they produce symptoms only by parathormone secretion. These adenomas are often embedded within the thymic tissue because each share a common embryologic origin (third branchial cleft). They are rarely visible on chest x-ray films and are usually the subject of an intensive search in a patient with persistent or recurrent hyperparathyroidism. High-resolution CT scanning, MRI, ultrasonography, thallium-technetium scintigraphy, and selective venous sampling in combination will localize the lesion in 80 to 90 percent of patients [21,93]. Angiographic ablation may provide long-term control in 60 percent of patients [30]; however, surgical removal is curative.

Thymic Cysts

These cysts develop as a result of a persistent thymopharyngeal duct and therefore may be found anywhere from the mandible to the lower anterior mediastinum, often in the lateral region of the neck [93]. An acquired inflammatory process may be required to produce cyst formation in ductal epithelium [116]. They are usually discovered incidentally, although they occasionally produce tracheal compression.

These cysts are round in the mediastinum and tubular in the neck. They have a thin fibrous wall and a smooth inner lining, and are filled with straw-colored fluid. They are prone to hemorrhage and hence may contain old blood and cholesterol crystals.

Microscopically, they are lined by columnar, cuboidal, or stratified squamous epithelium. In order to make the diagnosis of thymic cysts, it is necessary to identify thymic tissue in the wall of the cyst, which may be difficult in an atretic thymus gland. The differential diagnosis should include a cystic thymoma or lymphoma, making resection of all thymic cysts advisable.

Thoracic Duct Cysts

Thoracic duct cysts are very uncommon. Although usually asymptomatic, the larger cysts may compress the esophagus or adjacent structures. A fatty meal may exacerbate symptoms [93]. The principal diagnostic feature is the observation that the thoracic duct enters and leaves the cystic mass. Symptomatic lesions are usually excised, but chylothorax may result [97].

Enteric Cysts

Also known as *enterogenous cysts, reduplication cysts, inclusion cysts,* and *gastric cysts,* these cysts originate from the *dorsal* foregut that develops into the gastrointestinal tract. Approximately 25 percent of all mediastinal cysts are enteric in origin [18], and are more frequent in children. They may be found at any level in the posterior mediastinum [93] (Fig. 55-14).

Although most patients are asymptomatic, children frequently present with cough, dyspnea, and recurrent pulmonary infections [5,24]. In adults, dysphagia from esophageal compression is the most common symptom.

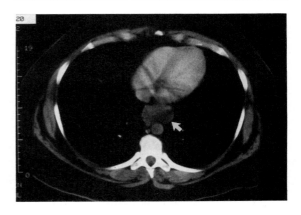

Fig. 55-14. Enteric cyst of the posterior mediastinum (*arrow*) causing dyspnea and chronic cough in a 32-year-old woman.

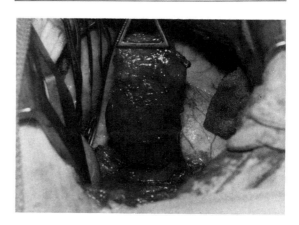

Fig. 55-15. Operative photograph of the woman shown in Figure 55-14, showing the cyst originating from the esophageal wall.

Grossly, enteric cysts are smooth-walled structures attached to the wall of the esophagus or completely embedded within the muscle (Fig. 55-15). Characteristically, a two-layer muscularis is present (Fig. 55-16). The mucosa may resemble that of the esophagus, stomach, or small intestine. Gastric mucosa is capable of acid secretion and may result in peptic ulceration with perforation into adjacent esophagus or bronchus. Rarely, adenocarcinoma may arise from chronic cysts [81].

There are no specific radiographic findings, although technetium-pertechnetate scans may lo-

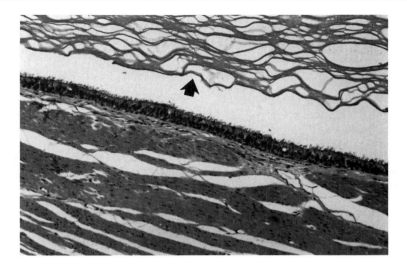

Fig. 55-16. Enteric cyst with ciliated columnar epithelium, bands of smooth muscle, and mucous debris (*arrow*) (H&E stain, × 500). (Courtesy of Dr. Gordon Honda, Department of Pathology, University of California, San Francisco.)

calize gastric mucosa [5]. Endoscopic and thoracoscopic decompression of these cysts has been described [5,62], but recurrence is likely if the cyst wall remains intact. Complete excision is the treatment of choice in symptomatic patients and to prevent the complications of infection and hemorrhage.

Bronchogenic Cysts

Originating as duplication cysts of the ventral foregut that forms the respiratory system, bronchogenic cysts are usually located in the lung parenchyma (most common) or in the mediastinum (immediately posterior to the carina) [5] (Fig. 55-17). They account for approximately 10 percent of mediastinal tumors and represent the most frequent mediastinal cyst [18,93]. They are round, frequently multilocular, and lined by pseudostratified ciliated columnar epithelium. The cyst wall may contain cartilage, smooth muscle, fibrous tissue, and mucous glands. Communication with the tracheobronchial tree is uncommon, but they are nearly always attached either intimately or by a cartilaginous band to the trachea.

In the most recent series [5,28,113], the majority of patients were symptomatic from bronchial

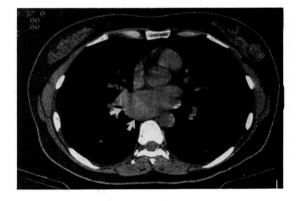

Fig. 55-17. Chest computed tomography scan showing a mediastinal bronchogenic cyst (*arrows*), posterior and inferior to the carina.

or tracheal compression or cyst infection. In infants and children, these symptoms may be life-threatening. Hemorrhage, rupture, and malignant degeneration of bronchogenic cysts have been reported. Therefore, excision of these lesions is recommended.

Pericardial Cysts

Pericardial cysts are round, usually unilocular, fluid-filled cysts that sit on the diaphragm in con-

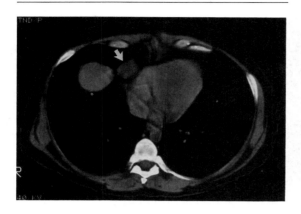

Fig. 55-18. Pericardial cyst located in the right cardiophrenic angle (*arrow*).

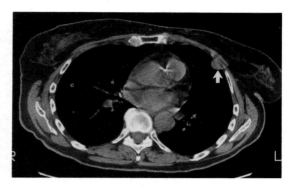

Fig. 55-19. Chest computed tomography scan of an asymptomatic fibrous mesothelioma (*arrow*) arising from the visceral pleura.

tact with the pericardium and anterior chest wall [24]. Embryologically, they represent a failure of fusion of the mesodermal elements that form the pericardium. The majority of pericardial cysts are located in the right cardiophrenic angle and are asymptomatic [93]. Occasionally, such a cyst has been observed to change in size under fluoroscopy during respiration. This correlates with the finding at surgery in approximately 5 percent of patients of a communicating tunnel between the cyst and the pericardium through which the cyst contents are reducible [61]. On CT scans, pericardial cysts classically have smooth borders and a water density [76] (Fig. 55-18). The differential diagnosis includes hydatid cyst, localized anterior exenteration of the diaphragm, pleural tumors, peripheral right-middle-lobe or lingular tumors, foramen of Morgagni hernias, and extraperitoneal fat hernias [61]. Large cysts have been managed successfully with needle aspiration.

Tumors of the Pleura

The majority of pleural tumors are metastatic, with carcinoma of the lung, breast, and lymphoma accounting for 75 percent of cases. Benign primary tumors such as lipomas, endotheliomas, and cysts do occur, but are very rare. The most common and clinically important primary pleural neoplasms are mesotheliomas. Chest films, chest CT scans, cytologic analysis of pleural fluid, and pleural biopsy should lead to a diagnosis in most patients with pleural tumors [27].

Mesothelioma

Pleural mesotheliomas are tumors derived from the serosal surface of the lung. They may be classified as benign or malignant; malignant forms can be further classified as localized or diffuse [50]. Benign lesions, also known as *pleural fibromas*, tend to be pedunculated tumors attached by a narrow stalk to the visceral or parietal pleural surface of the lung (Figs. 55-19 and 55-20). They represent approximately 10 percent of all mesotheliomas and may become very large before producing symptoms [27]. Grossly, these tumors consist of fibrous tissue and are well encapsulated [34]. Patients may present with pulmonary osteoarthropathy or hypoglycemia. These symptoms resolve after resection of the tumor.

Malignant mesothelioma is a rare tumor, accounting for 1 percent of cancer deaths [50]. The majority are of the diffuse form and are unilateral [101]. This disease usually presents between the ages of 50 to 70 years and is seen more frequently in men [127]. Shortness of breath and nonpleuritic chest pain are the most common complaints, and a pleural effusion is often present and may cause significant compression of the lung.

Malignant mesothelioma may develop at the site of pleural injury from a number of causes. The inhalation of asbestos fibers, especially crocidolite, is carcinogenic and is associated with the development of mesothelioma in 5 to 7 percent of exposed workers [131]. A latent period of 20 to 40 years between the time of exposure and

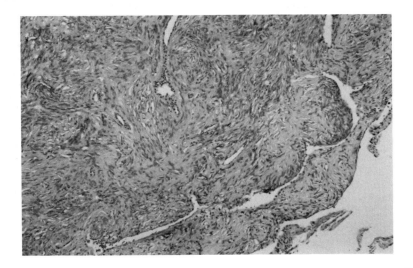

Fig. 55-20. Fibrous mesothelioma, characterized by bland spindle cells without mitoses (H&E stain, × 250). (Courtesy of Dr. Gordon Honda, Department of Pathology, University of California, San Francisco.)

the development of disease is not uncommon. Inhalation of other mineral fibers, such as zeolites, had been associated with mesothelioma.

Grossly, the entire lung often becomes encased within a mass of fibrous tissue, which also invades the chest wall, diaphragm, and mediastinum (Fig. 55-21). Some areas of the tumor are hard, like scar tissue, and other areas may be soft and gelatinous or necrotic. Histologically, mesotheliomas are classified with soft-tissue sarcomas, although a number of types (epithelial, sarcomatoid, transitional) are described. Distinguishing between the epithelial type (most common) and metastatic adenocarcinoma is often difficult, and requires electron microscopy and immunohistochemical stains (particularly cytokeratin and carcinoembryonic antigen) [100,127].

Cytologic diagnosis from pleural fluid is frequently inadequate; usually only hyperplastic mesothelial cells are retrieved. Needle biopsy of the pleura is equally unrewarding for lack of sufficiently cellular material; seeding of the biopsy tract with tumor is a recognized problem [60]. Thoracoscopy or thoracotomy is often required to obtain sufficient material for analysis [124] (Fig. 55-22).

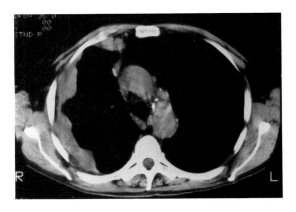

Fig. 55-21. Diffuse, malignant mesothelioma showing the characteristic lobulated pleural mass.

At the present time, the treatment of malignant pleural mesothelioma is only palliative. Conservative strategies include chemical pleurodesis for control of pleural effusions. Aggressive radiation, chemotherapy, or both have some success in controlling symptoms, but no survival benefit has been documented [6,69,101]. Similarly, radical pleurectomy and extrapleural pneumonectomy have not been shown to significantly alter the survival time, which averages 8 to 12 months [1,102,115].

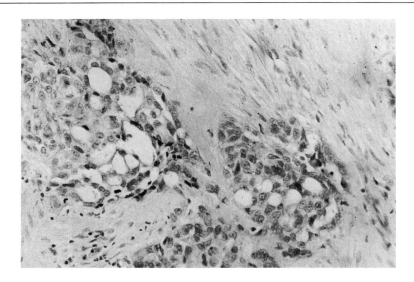

Fig. 55-22. Malignant pleural mesothelioma, mixed type, showing mesothelial and spindle cells (H&E stain, × 400). (Photomicrograph courtesy of Dr. Miriam Lurie, Department of Pathology, Carmel Hospital, Haifa, Israel.)

Endometriosis of the Lung and Pleura

Endometriosis is a very rare condition characterized by extragenital deposits of endometrial tissue on the visceral or parietal pleural surfaces. Symptoms of hemoptysis and pleuritic chest pain tend to be cyclical and more pronounced during menses [9,48,52]. Some cases have been associated with recurrent pneumothorax and hemorrhagic pleural effusions, with endometrial cells in the pleural fluid samples [35]. Treatment with synthetic androgens or gonadotropin-releasing hormone agonists may be useful [35].

Tumors of the Chest Wall

Tumors may originate in the soft tissue (skin, subcutaneous tissue, muscles, nerves, and blood vessels) or in the bony skeleton of the thoracic cage. Signs and symptoms depend on the location, size, and degree of malignancy of the neoplasm. In general, chest-wall tumors usually present as a slowly enlarging mass causing localized, dull pain [4,83,105]. Radicular pain indicates intercostal nerve involvement. Occasionally, an asymptomatic mass is palpated by the patient or seen incidentally on a routine chest x-ray film. A chest-wall tumor also may project inward and involve the lung as it expands. Approximately 60 percent of chest-wall tumors are malignant [33,83,85,105].

Benign tumors include chondroma, fibrous dysplasia, osteoblastoma, eosinophilic granuloma, lipoma, giant-cell tumor, fibroma, neurofibroma, osteochondroma, desmoid tumor, hemangioma, cystic hygroma, lymphangioma, and pigmented nevus. Aneurysmal bone cysts are benign lesions found in the ribs, but are generally thought to represent a nonneoplastic response to injury. Malignant tumors include fibrosarcoma, chondrosarcoma, solitary plasmacytoma, Ewing's sarcoma, liposarcoma, osteogenic sarcoma, reticulum cell sarcoma, rhabdomyosarcoma, hemangiopericytoma, and melanoma.

It should be noted that 40 to 50 percent of chest-wall tumors are metastatic in origin [36, 83,103]. Tumors of the genitourinary tract, thyroid, and colon and soft-tissue sarcomas are particularly likely to spread to the chest wall. Also, the chest wall may be invaded by direct extension from intrathoracic and extrathoracic tumors such as a superior sulcus tumor, bronchogenic carcinoma, breast carcinomas, and pleural mesotheliomas.

The evaluation of patients with a chest-wall tumor should include conventional chest radiographs as well as CT. The latter is particularly important in delineating the pleural, mediastinal, and pulmonary involvement of the lesion. Bone scans should be performed if metastatic disease is suspected. There is little utility in fine-needle or incisional biopsy for *primary* chest-wall lesions, as the tissue is usually insufficient for diagnosis [83].

Benign Tumors

Chondromas, also known as *enchondromas*, are the most common benign lesion of the chest wall, occurring at the costochondral or sternochondral junctions [4,33,105]. They usually present between the ages of 35 and 55. These tumors are rubbery and multicystic, with a gelatinous center [38]. On x-ray film, the medullary mass thins but does not penetrate the cortex [112]. These tumors may undergo malignant degeneration into chondrosarcomas. Hence, radical excision is warranted [4].

Fibrous dysplasia (osteitis fibrosa) accounts for approximately 15 percent of benign chest-wall tumors. They are usually situated in the posterior or lateral part of the rib. The rib appears locally expanded and filled with small cysts (Fig. 55-23). This tumor can become very large and may be locally aggressive. Histologically, the lesion consists of fibrous tissue and incompletely mineralized bone lacking a rim of osteoblasts [105] (Fig. 55-24). Osteochondroma is a small, hard, painless tumor. In the rib it appears as an excrescence of cartilage with a calcified cap projecting out of the rib [105,112]. Lipomas are usually found superficially in the chest wall. Neurofibromas occur as isolated sessile or pedunculated skin tumors or as part of generalized neurofibromatosis (von Recklinghausen's disease).

Osteoblastoma is a benign lytic lesion originating in the medulla of bones, affecting the ribs in 4 percent of patients. The great majority occur in patients less than 30 years old. Characteristically, CT scans show a lytic lesion with a thin bony shell, which concentrates technetium on bone scans [7,42,57] (Fig. 55-25). Abundant osteoblasts and giant cells may be present on light microscopy (Fig. 55-26). Resection is curative [7,105].

Eosinophilic granulomas are well-defined, lytic lesions that can occur in the ribs. They represent 10 percent of benign chest-wall lesions [105,125]. These tumors are composed of histiocytes and eosinophils with occasional giant cells, fibroblasts, and plasma cells [105]. Surgical resection is curative.

Desmoid tumors are slow-growing, hard masses occurring most often in the soft tissues of the abdomen and extremities; approximately 20 to 50 percent have occurred on the chest wall [12]. Females are affected more frequently [58]. These tu-

Fig. 55-23. Standard x-ray film of the rib showing fibrous dysplasia (*arrows*). The cortex is expanded and a lytic core is prominent.

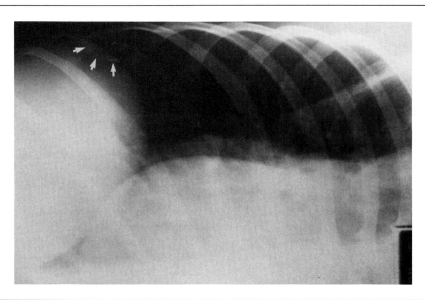

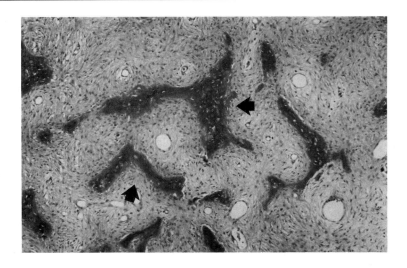

Fig. 55-24. Fibrous dysplasia showing the characteristic "Chinese characters" pattern (*arrows*) of bone formation. A background of bland fibrous reaction has replaced the marrow tissue (H&E stain, × 250). (Courtesy of Dr. Gordon Honda, Department of Pathology, University of California, San Francisco.)

mors are low-grade fibrosarcomas, but lack cellular pleomorphism and mitotic activity. Because tumor cells tend to infiltrate along muscle bundles, recurrence after surgical resection is a significant problem, averaging 30 percent [12, 45,74].

Cystic hygromas originate in the neck but may extend into the axilla. Lymphangiomas are more extensive, growing through the muscles of the chest wall into the mediastinum and lung [38]. They cause pleural effusions and occasionally, chylothorax (for which thoracic duct ligation may be required). Hemangiomas are seen in infancy and early childhood and spontaneously regress after the first 2 years of life [38].

Malignant Tumors

Fibrosarcomas usually occur in young adults and frequently near the scapula. It is the most common soft-tissue sarcoma of the chest wall and may account for 20 to 50 percent of all malignant chest-wall neoplasms [83,85,103,125]. These tumors are slow-growing and metastasize to regional lymph nodes and to the lungs. Wide local resection is the treatment of choice, although local recurrence may develop in a significant number of patients. Prognosis depends on the grade of the tumor; in general, a 5-year survival rate of 50 to 60 percent can be expected [45,90]. For high-grade lesions, large tumors, and incomplete resection, the addition of adjuvant chemotherapy, radiotherapy, or both may be beneficial [126,136].

In most reports, chondrosarcoma is the most common chest-wall neoplasm [4,36,103,105,125]. In order of frequency, these tumors are found in the ribs, scapula, and sternum. Most patients are over 40 years old. A presumptive diagnosis can often be made radiographically, with the finding of a large, lobulated mass with poorly defined margins and cortical bone destruction. Mottled calcification of the mass is commonly seen [85,112]. These are indolent lesions characterized by slow growth and local recurrence (Fig. 55-27). Patients with recurrent tumors often have metastatic disease involving local lymph nodes and the lung. Prognosis depends on tumor size, location, and grade as well as the extent of primary resection [70]. Complete resection should achieve a 60 to 70 percent 5-year survival rate [15,70]. Incomplete resection, recurrence, or both are ominous, as there is no effective role for chemotherapy or radiation.

Solitary plasmacytomas are uncommon in general, but account for approximately 30 percent of malignant chest-wall neoplasms [16,105,125]. Most patients complain of a mass or pain in the ribs and the characteristic radiographic finding is that of a punched-out, lytic lesion. Grossly and

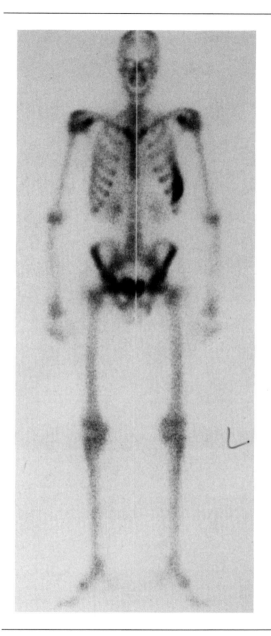

Fig. 55-25. Technetium bone scan of osteoblastoma involving the right ninth rib.

microscopically, this disease is indistinguishable from multiple myeloma. Local control of solitary plasmacytoma can be achieved with radiotherapy or chemotherapy in the majority of patients, with an expected 5-year survival rate of 40 percent [16]. However, most patients eventually develop multiple myeloma, which is usually fatal despite effective chemotherapy.

Ewing's sarcoma occurs during the first three decades of life [16,103] and involves the ribs, scapula, clavicle, or vertebrae. Approximately 7 percent will involve the ribs primarily. The disease usually presents as a painful mass and is associated with fever and leukocytosis. X-ray films typically show evidence of rib destruction or bone lysis. Occasionally, there is widening and sclerosis of the bony cortex with multiple layers of new bone formation, producing an "onion peel" appearance [103,105]. Histologically, Ewing's sarcoma requires electron microscopy to distinguish it from other round-cell tumors such as neuroblastoma and lymphoma. Disease located primarily in the chest wall is more aggressive than primary tumors of the extremities, probably because of a higher incidence of metastatic disease at presentation [16,85]. Treatment for isolated rib lesions is surgical resection; the combination of chemotherapy and radiation has been used successfully for more advanced lesions [16,136]. Five-year survival rates of 50 percent have been recently reported [16].

Osteogenic sarcoma is one of the rarest tumors of the ribs and sternum [103]. Patients usually complain of a painful mass and a significant number have received previous radiation for treatment of other diseases [15]. The x-ray film typically shows dense cortical sclerosis with radiating calcified subperiosteal spicules, producing a "sunburst" effect (Fig. 55-28). Thirty percent of patients will have synchronous metastases, usually to the lung. The overall 5-year survival rate following surgical resection for primary chest-wall lesions is 15 percent. Unlike primary lesions of the extremities, adjuvant or neoadjuvant chemotherapy does not appear to alter survival [15].

Rhabdomyosarcomas are rare and highly malignant [103]. The tumor spreads along fascial planes and metastasizes early by hematogenous spread. It is resistant to irradiation; surgical resection should be combined with adjuvant chemotherapy to achieve the best survival [45]. Liposarcomas, in contrast to benign lipomas which are superficial, tend to develop in deep fascial planes [58]. Resection of low-grade lesions is followed by excellent survival [45]. Reticulum cell sarcoma and hemangiopericytoma occur extremely rarely in the chest wall [45,110].

The mainstay of treatment of malignant tumors of the chest wall, especially fibrosarcomas and chondrosarcomas, is wide local excision. Maintaining 4-cm margins around the tumor will provide the lowest recurrence rates and best survival [82,105,125]. Tumors of the sternum should be re-

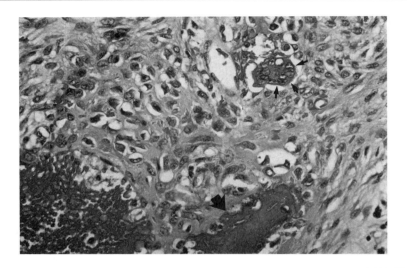

Fig. 55-26. Osteoblastoma, characterized by osteoblasts, prominent giant cells (*small arrows*), and osteoid formation (*large arrow*). (H&E stain, × 500). (Courtesy of Dr. Gordon Honda, Department of Pathology, University of California, San Francisco.)

garded as malignant. In lesions involving the manubrium, the head of the clavicle and costal cartilages also should be removed. Reconstruction of a large chest wall may be accomplished by the use of muscle flaps, myocutaneous flaps, rib grafts, Marlex mesh, and molded acrylic plates [82,85]. Operative mortality is less than 5 percent in most series and there is little effect on pulmonary function.

Fig. 55-27. Chondrosarcoma, showing a lobular tumor with a hypercellular matrix (H&E stain, × 250). (Courtesy of Dr. Gordon Honda, Department of Pathology, University of California, San Francisco.)

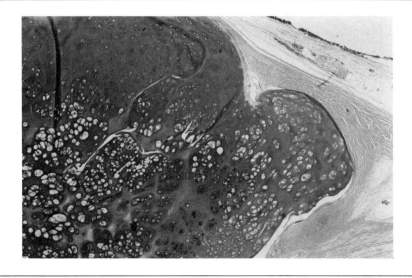

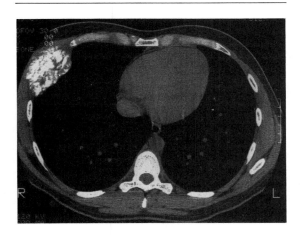

Fig. 55-28. Osteosarcoma of the rib showing the classic "sunburst" pattern.

Tumors of the Diaphragm

Although the diaphragm is frequently invaded by tumors arising from adjacent stomach, esophagus, liver, colon, ribs, and vertebrae, primary tumors of the diaphragm are extremely rare. Less than 100 cases have been reported; of those, approximately 60 percent are malignant [65].

The benign tumors include lipoma, fibroma, mesothelioma, angiofibroma, neurofibroma, and neurilemmoma [71]. Congenital and acquired cysts also have been found in the diaphragm [119].

The malignant tumors are primarily of mesenchymal origin: fibrosarcoma (most common), liposarcoma, rhabdomyosarcoma, and neurogenic sarcomas. A few leiomyosarcomas have also been reported [65,84].

Benign lesions are usually asymptomatic [65]. Malignant lesions give rise to pain in the lower chest and flank. Phrenic nerve involvement causes cough, hiccups, and shoulder pain [44]. Large tumors may produce dyspnea. Clubbing has occasionally been noted.

The differential diagnosis includes peripheral pulmonary parenchymal tumors, an elevated portion of hemidiaphragm, loculated subpulmonic pleural effusions, and hiatal hernia. A subdiaphragmatic mass may indent a portion of the diaphragm, which consequently protrudes above the remainder, simulating a tumor of the diaphragm itself.

Diagnostic tests to differentiate between these entities include CT scan and artificially induced pneumothorax and pneumoperitoneum. CT scanning is particularly useful in diagnosing lipomas, which have a very low specific coefficient of attenuation [17].

Diaphragmatic tumors should be excised. The resulting diaphragmatic defect can be repaired either directly with sutures or with a prosthetic patch, if necessary.

References

1. Achatzy R, et al. The diagnosis, therapy and prognosis of diffuse malignant mesothelioma. *Eur J Cardiothorac Surg* 3:445, 1989.
2. Adkins RB, Maples MD, Hainsworth JD. Primary malignant mediastinal tumors (current review). *Ann Thorac Surg* 38:648, 1984.
3. Akwari OE, et al. Dumbbell neurogenic tumors of the mediastinum. *Mayo Clin Proc* 53:353, 1978.
4. Ala-Kulju K, et al. Primary tumors of the ribs. *Scand J Thorac Cardiovasc Surg* 22:97, 1988.
5. Allen MS, Payne WS. Cystic foregut malformations in the mediastinum. *Chest Surg Clin North Am* 2:89, 1992.
6. Ball DL, Cruickshank DG. The treatment of malignant mesothelioma of the pleura: Review of a 5-year experience, with special reference to radiotherapy. *Am J Clin Oncol* 13:4, 1990.
7. Beauchamp CP, et al. Osteoblastoma: Experience with 23 patients. *Can J Surg* 35:199, 1992.
8. Benfield JR, Sawyer RW. Tumor markers. *Chest Surg Clin North Am* 2:213, 1992.
9. Bergqvist A. Extragenital endometriosis. A review. *Eur J Surg* 158:7, 1992.
10. Best LA, et al. The contribution of anterior mediastinotomy in the diagnosis and management of diseases of the mediastinum and lung. *Ann Thorac Surg* 43:78, 1987.
11. Blegvad S, et al. Mediastinal tumours. A report of 129 cases. *Scand J Thorac Cardiovasc Surg* 24:39, 1990.
12. Brodsky JT, et al. Desmoid tumors of the chest wall. A locally recurrent problem. *J Thorac Cardiovasc Surg* 104:900, 1992.
13. Brown K, et al. Current use of imaging in the evaluation of primary mediastinal masses. *Chest* 98:466, 1990.
14. Brown LR, et al. Computed tomography of benign mature teratomas of the mediastinum. *J Thorac Imaging* 2:66, 1987.
15. Burt M, et al. Primary bony and cartilaginous sarcomas of chest wall: Results of therapy. *Ann Thorac Surg* 54:226, 1992.
16. Burt M, et al. Medical tumors of the chest wall: Solitary plasmacytoma and Ewing's sarcoma. *J Thorac Cardiovasc Surg* 105:89, 1993.
17. Castillo M, Shirkhoda A. Computed tomography

of diaphragmatic lipoma. *J Comput Assist Tomogr* 9:167, 1985.

18. Cohen AJ, et al. Primary cysts and tumors of the mediastinum. *Ann Thorac Surg* 51:378, 1991.

19. Cohen PS, Israel MA. Biology and Treatment of Thoracic Tumors of Neural Crest Origin. In JA Roth, JC Ruckdeschel, TH Weisenburger (Eds), *Thoracic Oncology.* Philadelphia: Saunders, 1989. P 520.

20. Conn JM, et al. The mediastinal parathyroid. *Am Surg* 57:62, 1991.

21. Creswell LL, Wells SA. Mediastinal masses originating in the neck. *Chest Surg Clin North Am* 2:23, 1992.

22. Curry W, et al. Klinefelter's syndrome and mediastinal germ cell tumors. *J Urol* 125:127, 1981.

23. Davis CJ, Butchart EG, Gibbs AR. Neurilemmoma of the intrathoracic vagus nerve. *Eur Respir J* 4:508, 1991.

24. Davis RD, Oldham HN, Sabiston DC. The Mediastinum. In DC Sabiston Jr, FC Spencer (Eds), *Gibbon's Surgery of the Chest* (5th ed.). Philadelphia: Saunders, 1990. P 498.

25. Davis RJ, Oldham HJ, Sabiston DJ. Primary cysts and neoplasms of the mediastinum: Recent changes in clinical presentation, methods of diagnosis, management, and results. *Ann Thorac Surg* 44:229, 1987.

26. Dehner LP. Germ cell tumors of the mediastinum. *Semin Diagn Pathol* 7:266, 1990.

27. DeMeester TR, LaFontaine E. The Pleura. In DC Sabiston Jr, FC Spencer (Eds), *Gibbon's Surgery of the Chest* (5th ed.). Philadelphia: Saunders, 1990. P 444.

28. Di LM, et al. Bronchogenic cysts. *J Pediatr Surg* 24:988, 1989.

29. Dogan R, Ayrancioglu K, Aksu O. Primary mediastinal liposarcoma: A report of a case and review of the literature. *Eur J Cardiothorac Surg* 3:367, 1989.

30. Doherty GM, et al. Results of a multidisciplinary strategy for management of mediastinal parathyroid adenoma as a cause of persistent primary hyperparathyroidism. *Ann Surg* 215:101, 1992.

31. Dutcher JP, Wiernik PH. Lymphomas Involving the Mediastinum and Lungs. In JA Roth, JC Ruckdeschel, TH Weisenburger (Eds), *Thoracic Oncology.* Philadelphia: Saunders, 1989. P 448.

32. Economou JS, et al. Management of primary germ cell tumors of the mediastinum. *J Thorac Cardiovasc Surg* 83:643, 1982.

33. Eng J, et al. Primary bony chest wall tumours. *J R Coll Surg Edinb* 35:44, 1990.

34. England DM, Hochholzer L, McCarthy MJ. Localized benign and malignant fibrous tumors of the pleura. A clinicopathologic review of 223 cases. *Am J Surg Pathol* 13:640, 1989.

35. Espaulella J, et al. Pulmonary endometriosis: Conservative treatment with GnRH agonists. *Obstet Gynecol* 78:535, 1991.

36. Farley JH, Seyfer AE. Chest wall tumors: Experience with 58 patients. *Mil Med* 156:413, 1991.

37. Ferguson MK, et al. Selective operative approach for diagnosis and treatment of anterior mediastinal masses. *Ann Thorac Surg* 44:583, 1987.

38. Fonkalsrud EW. Abnormalities of the Chest Wall. In WWL Glenn et al (Eds), *Thoracic and Cardiovascular Surgery* (4th ed.). New York: Appleton-Century-Crofts, 1983.

39. Fornasiero A, et al. Chemotherapy of invasive thymoma. *J Clin Oncol* 8:1419, 1990.

40. Fornasiero A, et al. Chemotherapy for invasive thymoma. A 13-year experience. *Cancer* 68:30, 1991.

41. Gale AW, et al. Neurogenic tumors of the mediastinum. *Ann Thorac Surg* 17:434, 1974.

42. Gentry JF, Schechter JJ, Mirra JM. Case report 574. Periosteal osteoblastoma of rib. *Skel Radiol* 18:551, 1989.

43. Ginsberg RJ. Mediastinal germ cell tumors: The role of surgery. *Semin Thorac Cardiovasc Surg* 4:51, 1992.

44. Glenn WWL. The Diaphragm. In WWL Glenn et al (Eds), *Thoracic and Cardiovascular Surgery* (4th ed.). New York: Appleton-Century-Crofts, 1983.

45. Gordon MS, et al. Soft tissue sarcomas of the chest wall. Results of surgical resection. *J Thorac Cardiovasc Surg* 101:843, 1991.

46. Grillo HC, et al. Combined approach to "dumbbell" intrathoracic and intraspinal neurogenic tumors. *Ann Thorac Surg* 36:402, 1983.

47. Grosfeld JL, Baehner RL. Neuroblastoma: An analysis of 160 cases. *World J Surg* 4:29, 1980.

48. Guidry GG, George RB, Payne DK. Catamenial hemoptysis: A case report and review of the literature. *J La State Med Soc* 142:27, 1990.

49. Hainsworth JD, Greco FA. Mediastinal Germ Cell Neoplasms. In JA Roth, JC Ruckdeschel, TH Weisenburger (Eds), *Thoracic Oncology.* Philadelphia: Saunders, 1989. P 478.

50. Hammar SP, Bolen JW. Pleural Neoplasms. In DH Dail, SP Hammar (Eds), *Pulmonary Pathology.* New York: Springer, 1988. P 973.

51. Hammond EH, Flinner RL. The diagnosis of thymoma: A review. *Ultrastruct Pathol* 15:419, 1991.

52. Horsfield K. Catamenial pleural pain. *Eur Respir J* 2:1013, 1989.

53. Jain KK, et al. The treatment of extragonadal seminoma. *J Clin Oncol* 2:820, 1984.

54. Kay PH, Wells FC, Goldstraw P. A multidisciplinary approach to primary nonseminomatous germ cell tumors of the mediastinum. *Ann Thorac Surg* 44:578, 1987.

55. Kersh CR, et al. Primary malignant extragonadal germ cell tumors. An analysis of the effect of radiotherapy. *Cancer* 65: 2681, 1990.

56. Kirchner T, et al. Evaluation of prognostic features in thymic epithelial tumors. *Thymus* 14: 195, 1989.

57. Kroon HM, Schurmans J. Osteoblastoma: Clinical and radiologic findings in 98 new cases. *Radiology* 175:783, 1990.

58. Kyriakos M. Tumors and Tumorlike Conditions of the Soft Tissue. In JM Kissane (Eds), *Anderson's Pathology* (9th ed.). St. Louis: Mosby, 1990. P 1838.

59. Landreneau RJ, et al. Thoracoscopic resection of an anterior mediastinal tumor. *Ann Thorac Surg* 54:142, 1992.

60. Law MR, Hodson ME, Turner-Warwick M. Malignant mesothelioma of the pleura: Clinical aspects and symptomatic treatment. *Eur J Respir Dis* 65:162, 1984.

61. Le Roux BT, Kalichurum S, Shama DM. Mediastinal cysts and tumors. *Curr Probl Surg* 21:1, 1984.

62. Lewis RJ, Caccavale RJ, Sisler GE. Imaged thoracoscopic surgery: A new thoracic technique for resection of mediastinal cysts. *Ann Thorac Surg* 53:318, 1992.

63. Mackintosh JF, et al. Cisplatinum-based chemotherapy in malignant mediastinal teratoma. *Aust NZ J Surg* 59:399, 1989.

64. Maggi G, et al. Thymoma: Results of 241 operated cases. *Ann Thorac Surg* 51:152, 1991.

65. Mandal AK, Lee H, Salem F. Review of primary tumors of the diaphragm. *J Natl Med Assoc* 80:214, 1988.

66. Mandelbaum I. Germ cell tumors of the mediastinum. *Chest Surg Clin North Am* 2:203, 1992.

67. Mark JB. Management of anterior mediastinal tumors. *Semin Surg Oncol* 6:286, 1990.

68. Masaoka A, et al. Follow-up study of thymomas with special reference to their clinical stages. *Cancer* 48:2485, 1981.

69. Mattson K, et al. Multimodality treatment programs for malignant pleural mesothelioma using high-dose hemithorax irradiation. *Int J Radiat Oncol Biol Phys* 24:643, 1992.

70. McAfee MK, et al. Chondrosarcoma of the chest wall: Factors affecting survival. *Ann Thorac Surg* 40:535, 1985.

71. McClenathan JH, Okada F. Primary neurilemoma of the diaphragm. *Ann Thorac Surg* 48: 126, 1989.

72. McGuire WA, et al. Stage II neuroblastoma: Does adjuvant irradiation contribute to cure? *Med Pediatr Oncol* 13:117, 1985.

73. McKenna WG, et al. Malignancies of the Thymus. In JA Roth, JC Ruckdeschel, TH Weisenburger (Eds), *Thoracic Oncology*. Philadelphia: Saunders, 1989. P 466.

74. McKinnon JG, et al. Management of desmoid tumors. *Surg Gynecol Obstet* 169:104, 1989.

75. Mitchell JD, Donnelly RJ. Retrosternal thyroid. *Semin Thorac Cardiovasc Surg* 4:34, 1992.

76. Moore EH. Radiologic evaluation of mediastinal masses. *Chest Surg Clin North Am* 2:1, 1992.

77. Morgan WKC, Andrews CE. Tumors of the Mediastinum, Pleura, Chest Wall and Diaphragm. In GL Baum, E Wolinsky (Eds), *Textbook of Pulmonary Diseases*. Boston: Little, Brown, 1983.

78. Mukai K, et al. Expression of ras p21 protein by thymoma. *Virchows Arch B Cell Pathol* 59:11, 1990.

79. Nichols C, et al. Klinefelter's syndrome associated with mediastinal germ cell neoplasms. *J Clin Oncol* 5:1290, 1987.

80. Nichols CR. Mediastinal germ cell tumors. *Semin Thorac Cardiovasc Surg* 4:45, 1992.

81. Olsen JB, Clemmensen O, Andersen K. Adenocarcinoma arising in a foregut cyst of the mediastinum. *Ann Thorac Surg* 51:497, 1991.

82. Pairolero PC. Surgical Management of Neoplasms of the Chest Wall. In DC Sabiston Jr, FC Spencer (Eds), *Gibbon's Surgery of the Chest* (5th ed.). Philadelphia: Saunders, 1990. P 437.

83. Pairolero PC, Arnold PG. Chest wall tumors: Experience with 100 consecutive patients. *J Thorac Cardiovasc Surg* 90:367, 1985.

84. Parker MC. Leiomyosarcoma of the diaphragm: A case report. *Eur J Surg Oncol* 11:171, 1985.

85. Pass HI. Primary and Metastatic Chest Wall Tumors. In JA Roth, JC Ruckdeschel, TH Weisenburger (Eds), *Thoracic Oncology*. Philadelphia: Saunders, 1989. P 546.

86. Patterson GA. Thymomas. *Semin Thorac Cardiovasc Surg* 4:39, 1992.

87. Payne CM, Grogan TM, Spier CM. Lymphomas of the mediastinum. *Ultrastruct Pathol* 15:439, 1991.

88. Pearson FG. Mediastinal tumors. *Semin Thorac Cardiovasc Surg* 4:1, 1992.

89. Percarmona E, et al. Analysis of prognostic factors and clinicopathological staging of thymoma. *Ann Thorac Surg* 50:534, 1990.

90. Perry RR, et al. Survival after surgical resection for high-grade chest wall sarcomas. *Ann Thorac Surg* 49:363, 1990.

91. Pollack A, et al. Thymoma. The prognostic significance of flow cytometric DNA analysis. *Cancer* 69:1702, 1992.

92. Reed JC, Hallett KK, Feigen DS. Neural tumors of the thorax: Subject review from the AFIP. *Radiology* 126:9, 1978.

93. Rice TW. Benign neoplasms and cysts of the mediastinum. *Semin Thorac Cardiovasc Surg* 4:25, 1992.

94. Ricci C, et al. Correlations between histological

type, clinical behaviour, and prognosis in thymoma. *Thorax* 44:455, 1989.

95. Ricci C, et al. Surgical approach to isolated mediastinal lymphoma. *J Thorac Cardiovasc Surg* 99:691, 1990.

96. Ricci C, et al. Diagnostic imaging and surgical treatment of dumbbell tumors of the mediastinum. *Ann Thorac Surg* 50:586, 1990.

97. Rodriguez-Perez D, Ramirez de Arellano G. Chylous cysts of the mediastinum: Report of a case and review of the literature. *Bol Assoc Med P R* 83:333, 1991.

98. Rosado DE, et al. From the archives of the AFIP. Mediastinal germ cell tumors: Radiologic and pathologic correlation. *Radiographics* 12: 1013, 1992.

99. Rosenberg JC. Neoplasms of the Mediastinum. In JA Roth, JC Ruckdeschel, TH Weisenburger (Eds), *Thoracic Oncology*. Philadelphia: Saunders, 1989. P 599.

100. Ruffie P. Pleural mesothelioma. *Curr Opin Oncol* 4:334, 1992.

101. Ruffie PA. Pleural mesothelioma. *Curr Opin Oncol* 3:328, 1991.

102. Rusch VW, Piantadosi S, Holmes EC. The role of extrapleural pneumonectomy in malignant pleural mesothelioma. A Lung Cancer Study Group trial. *J Thorac Cardiovasc Surg* 102:1, 1991.

103. Ryan MB, McMurtrey MJ, Roth JA. Current management of chest-wall tumors. *Surg Clin North Am* 69:1061, 1989.

104. Saabye J, Elbirk A, Andersen K. Teratomas of the mediastinum. *Scand J Thorac Cardiovasc Surg* 21:271, 1987.

105. Sabanathan S, et al. Primary chest wall tumors. *Ann Thorac Surg* 39:4, 1985.

106. Sakai F, et al. MR imaging of thymoma: Radiologic-pathologic correlation. *AJR* 158:751, 1992.

107. Sanders LE, et al. Mediastinal goiters. The need for an aggressive approach. *Arch Surg* 127:609, 1992.

108. Scott HW, et al. Clinical experience with malignant pheochromocytoma. *Surg Gynecol Obstet* 154:801, 1982.

109. Seeger RC, Siegel SE, Sidell N. Neuroblastoma: Clinical perspectives, monoclonal antibodies and retinoic acid. *Ann Intern Med* 97:873, 1982.

110. Sellke FW, et al. Hemangiopericytoma of the sternum. *Arch Pathol Lab Med* 115:242, 1991.

111. Sherman ME, Black SS. Diagnosis of thymoma by needle biopsy. *Acta Cytol* 34:63, 1990.

112. Stelzer P, Gay WA Jr. Tumors of the chest wall. *Surg Clin North Am* 60:779, 1980.

113. St-Georges R, et al. Clinical spectrum of bronchogenic cysts of the mediastinum and lung in the adult. *Ann Thorac Surg* 52:6, 1991.

114. Strickler JG, Kurtin PJ. Mediastinal lymphoma. *Semin Diagn Pathol* 8:2, 1991.

115. Sugarbaker DJ, et al. Extrapleural pneumonectomy, chemotherapy, and radiotherapy in the treatment of diffuse malignant pleural mesothelioma. *J Thorac Cardiovasc Surg* 102:10, 1991.

116. Suster S, et al. Multilocular thymic cysts with pseudoepitheliomatous hyperplasia. *Hum Pathol* 22:455, 1991.

117. Sutcliff SB. Primary mediastinal malignant lymphoma. *Semin Thorac Cardiovasc Surg* 4:55, 1992.

118. Swanson PE. Soft tissue neoplasms of the mediastinum. *Semin Diagn Pathol* 8:14, 1991.

119. Tarver RD, Godwin JD, Putnam CE. The diaphragm. *Radiol Clin North Am* 22:615, 1984.

120. Toner GC, et al. Extragonadal and poor risk nonseminomatous germ cell tumors. Survival and prognostic features. *Cancer* 67:2049, 1991.

121. Urgesi A, et al. Role of radiation therapy in locally advanced thymoma. *Radiother Oncol* 19: 273, 1990.

122. Urgesi A, et al. Aggressive treatment of intrathoracic recurrences of thymoma. *Radiother Oncol* 24:221, 1992.

123. Wain JC. Neurogenic tumors of the mediastinum. *Chest Surg Clin North Am* 2:121, 1992.

124. Wakabayashi A. Expanded applications of diagnostic and therapeutic thoracoscopy. *J Thorac Cardiovasc Surg* 102:721, 1991.

125. Waller DA, Newman RJ. Primary bone tumours of the thoracic skeleton: An audit of the Leeds regional bone tumour registry. *Thorax* 45:850, 1990.

126. Wallner KE, et al. Adjuvant brachytherapy for treatment of chest wall sarcomas. *J Thorac Cardiovasc Surg* 101:888, 1991.

127. Walz R, Koch HK. Malignant pleural mesothelioma: Some aspects of epidemiology, differential diagnosis and prognosis. Histological and immunohistochemical evaluation and follow-up of mesotheliomas diagnosed from 1964 to January 1985. *Pathol Res Pract* 186:124, 1990.

128. Wang LS, et al. Malignant thymoma. *Cancer* 70:443, 1992.

129. Warren WH, Gould VE. Epithelial neoplasms of the thymus. *Chest Surg Clin North Am* 2:137, 1992.

130. Weisbrod GL, Herman SJ. Mediastinal masses: Diagnosis with non-invasive techniques. *Scand J Thorac Cardiovasc Surg* 4:3, 1992.

131. Whitwell F, Scott J, Grimshaw M. Relationship between occupation and asbestos fiber content of the lungs in patients with pleural mesothelioma, lung cancer and other diseases. *Thorax* 32:377, 1977.

132. Wick MR. Mediastinal cysts and intrathoracic thyroid tumors. *Semin Diagn Pathol* 7:285, 1990.

133. Wick MR, Rosai J. Neuroendocrine neoplasms

of the mediastinum. *Semin Diagn Pathol* 8:35, 1991.

134. Wilkins EJ, et al. Maxwell Chamberlain Memorial Paper. Role of staging in prognosis and management of thymoma. *Ann Thorac Surg* 51:888, 1991.

135. Yellin A. Lymphoproliferative diseases. *Chest Surg Clin North Am* 2:107, 1992.

136. Young MM, et al. Treatment of sarcomas of the chest wall using intensive combined modality therapy. *Int J Radiat Oncol Biol Phys* 16:49, 1989.

137. Yu CJ, et al. Evaluation of ultrasonically guided biopsies of mediastinal masses. *Chest* 100:399, 1991.

56

Extrapulmonary Syndromes Associated with Tumors of the Lung

Catherine B. Niewoehner

Unexpected adrenal hyperactivity in a patient with lung carcinoma was reported by Brown in 1928 [28]. Additional case reports of hormone activity associated with lung cancer followed, but it was not until 1941 that a possible mechanism for the association was suggested. Albright and Reifenstein discussed a patient with hypercalcemia resulting from a renal cell carcinoma, and proposed that tumors might secrete hormone-like substances producing clinical syndromes usually associated with endocrine tissues [1]. This was confirmed when high adrenocorticotropin (ACTH) concentrations were discovered in the plasma of patients with adrenal hyperactivity and bronchogenic carcinoma [23,36]. Syndromes resulting from the production of unexpected or "inappropriate" substances by tissues not normally associated with hormone production were termed *ectopic hormonal syndromes* [123].

Initially, ectopic hormone secretion was thought to be a rare event. However, careful application of new cell culture methods, more sensitive bioassays and immunoassays, new tissue immunostaining techniques, sensitive methods of extraction of hormones from tissues, and advances in molecular genetics revealed that ectopic peptide production is characteristic of all cancers [147]. Recent studies have shown that these peptides also are produced by the normal tissues from which the tumors are derived. Thus, increased peptide hormone production by lung neoplasms is quantitatively abnormal, but not truly ectopic [11,12]. Many of the hormones are secreted as inactive large-molecular-weight polypeptide precursors, due to either abnormal post-translational modification or an alternate process of secretion. Recognizable clinical syndromes result only if neoplastic tissue is able to metabolize the precursor to a bioactive hormone [145].

The highest reported incidence of tumor expression of neuroendocrine peptides occurs in lung cancers, particularly in small-cell carcinomas and bronchial carcinoid tumors [11]. However, increases in ectopic hormone concentrations are associated with diseases other than neoplasia, and evidence that the circulating hormone actually is produced by the tumor has not always been obtained. Criteria for establishing tumor hormone production are the following: (1) the presence of both the tumor and a hormonal syndrome or elevated blood or urine concentrations of the hormone, (2) failure of normal feedback mechanisms to suppress hormone levels in plasma or urine, (3) demonstration of the polypeptide in tumor tissue or tissue extracts, (4) increasing hormone concentrations across the tumor capillary bed, (5) decreased hormone concentrations if therapy directed toward the tumor is successful, (6) demonstration of hormone synthesis and release by the tumor in vitro, (7) cell-free translation of tumor peptide messenger RNA (mRNA), and (8) exclusion of other sites of significant hormone production [152]. Obviously, it is not always possible to satisfy these criteria, since several require an invasive procedure and a research laboratory.

Recognition that a wide array of peptide hormones is produced by normal and neoplastic tissues has provided new insight into the pathogenesis of neoplasia in general. Neuroendocrine properties of small-cell carcinomas of the lung have been known for some time. These neoplasms originally were thought to arise from cells derived from the neural crest in common with other normal and neoplastic cells demonstrating amine precursor uptake and decarboxylation (APUD cells) [154]. However, when hormone production was demonstrated to be a common property of all lung neoplasms, new hypotheses concerning tumor pathogenesis were required. It is unlikely that hormone production by tumors occurs as a result of random activation of areas of the genome that normally are repressed. This concept does not account for the strong association of some hormonal syndromes with specific lung and other carcinomas. Baylin and coworkers [11,12,72] developed an elegant model suggesting that the different types of bronchogenic carcinoma arise through a continuum of differentiation events occurring in cells of common cellular origin.

The true incidence of hormone production associated with lung carcinomas is difficult to determine. Surveys probably reflect the minimum incidence of abnormal hormone production. Tumors secrete peptides sporadically, and changes in tumor metabolism and peptide production occur with time [11,12], but tumor markers frequently are measured only once. Metastases may produce peptides that are different from those in the primary neoplasm. Excess hormone secretion frequently occurs only in response to a stimulus, and provocative tests for hormone responsiveness usually are not done. Finally, the presence of a hormone usually is assessed by radioimmunoassay, and the antibodies used vary from laboratory to laboratory.

Many tumors produce an array of peptide hormones, and no peptide is specific for a given bronchogenic carcinoma. This is as expected if different neoplasms arise from common precursors. However, peptide monitoring has been reported to help make the diagnosis of mesothelioma versus bronchial adenocarcinoma [68]. Some investigators reported that fluctuations in the concentration of peptides elaborated by bronchogenic carcinomas reflect the clinical course of these tumors [80,109,233], but this often has not been the case [19,81,89–91,113,138]. Although a decrease in peptide concentration frequently is observed following tumor resection or chemotherapy, peptide concentrations do not consistently reflect tumor progression or recurrence. Peptide production may be better correlated with the state of tumor differentiation than with tumor mass [11,12]. Nevertheless, monitoring tumor peptide concentrations may provide information about changes in tumor metabolism or malignant potential. It also is important to recognize peptide-induced extrapulmonary syndromes in order to avoid unnecessary evaluation or procedures and to provide appropriate treatment if possible.

In the discussion that follows, the extrapulmonary syndromes associated with lung tumors have been divided into categories as follows: (1) hormonal and metabolic, (2) neuromyopathic, (3) connective tissue and osseous, (4) vascular, (5) hematologic, (6) cutaneous, and (7) gastrointestinal.

Hormonal and Metabolic Syndromes

Adrenocorticotropin and Corticotropin-Releasing Hormone

ACTH production by neoplasms in lung and other tissues has been studied extensively. In 1974 Gewirtz and Yalow [67] reported that tissue extracts from lung carcinomas of all types contain an ACTH-like material recognizable by immunoassay. They also demonstrated that this material was a large-molecular-weight, biologically inactive form of ACTH (pro-ACTH) which could be converted to bioactive ACTH by trypsin [66].

Subsequently, others have shown that normal lung and all lung carcinomas contain the precursor peptide pro-opiomelanocortin (POMC) and its component peptides—pro-ACTH and beta lipotropin, a hormone with weak lipotrophic and melanocyte-stimulating activity [46,146,177,228]. In normal lung, the concentration of POMC mRNA is only 0.008 to 0.080 percent of that in the pituitary gland and smaller forms of POMC mRNA predominate. These do not code for a signal sequence, so the POMC peptides cannot be secreted. The ACTH concentration in normal lung is only 0.000003 to 0.000050 percent of that in the pituitary gland [46]. However, lung carcinomas contain larger amounts of full-length POMC mRNA, and POMC-derived peptides can be secreted in sufficient quantities to produce clinical syndromes. In nonpituitary tumors, more POMC is cleaved to smaller peptides including melanocyte-stimulating peptide fragments, beta endorphin, and corticotropin-like intermediate lobe peptide (CLIP), which has no known function [46,221,228].

Elevated plasma levels of pro-ACTH were found in 72 percent of patients hospitalized with an abnormal-appearing chest roentgenogram who were shown subsequently to have lung cancer [235]. Plasma ACTH was reported to be elevated in 27 to 60 percent of patients with lung cancers of all histologic types [144]. The predominance of pro-ACTH indicates either that tumors are unable to process pro-ACTH effectively or that the normal regulation of pro-ACTH secretion fails. Immunoradiometric assays using monoclonal antibodies now make it possible to measure plasma levels of other POMC-related peptides, especially CLIP, but this has not been done in a large group of patients with bronchogenic carcinoma.

In some patients with high plasma ACTH concentrations there are no clinical manifestations, even though morning cortisol concentrations are high and the normal diurnal variation of cortisol is absent. Plasma 11-deoxycorticosterone and dehydroepiandrostanedione sulfate concentrations and urinary free cortisol, 17-hydroxycorticosteroid, and 17-ketosteroid concentrations also are increased [144]. In these patients, either the circulating cortisol concentrations are not high enough to produce symptoms or death ensues before there is sufficient time for symptoms and signs of hypercortisolism to develop.

Although only 5 to 10 percent of cases of Cushing's syndrome are produced by nonadrenal, nonpituitary tumors [142], 50 percent are due to lung carcinoma. Clinically evident ACTH excess occurs most often in patients with bronchial carcinoid tumors, but is found in 2.5 to 7.0 percent of patients with small-cell carcinoma [90,112], and occasionally in patients with undifferentiated large-cell carcinoma or adenocarcinoma. It virtually never is seen in patients with squamous cell carcinoma [144]. Plasma ACTH and cortisol concentrations are not suppressed normally by dexamethasone administration [113,151]. However, partial suppression has been observed [139,206], and differentiating pulmonary tumor ACTH production from pituitary tumor ACTH production (Cushing's disease) can be difficult. Results of metyrapone and corticotropin-releasing hormone (CRH) stimulation tests also may be compatible with Cushing's disease [131,206,207]. Since excess CLIP is produced by lung carcinomas but not by pituitary tumors, the CLIP/CLIP + ACTH ratio has been used to confirm ectopic origin of the ACTH [117].

The effects of ectopic ACTH on electrolyte flux develop more rapidly than the effects on lipid and carbohydrate metabolism. Thus, the most common clinical manifestations are muscle weakness and polyuria due to hypokalemic alkalosis (serum bicarbonate usually $\geq$ 30 mmol/liter and pH $\geq$ 7.45), which may be very resistant to treatment. Hyperpigmentation (Fig. 56-1) results from the excess lipotropin or the melanocyte-stimulating fragments of POMC [144]. Patients with more slowly progressive tumors develop classic features of Cushing's syndrome including moon facies, truncal obesity, purple abdominal striae, hirsutism, psychosis, hypertension, edema, os-

teoporosis, and glucose intolerance (Fig. 56-2). These seldom are seen in patients with small-cell carcinoma, since progression of this disease is so rapid. Opportunistic infections are a well-known complication of cortisol excess, and three simultaneous infections have occurred in a patient with an oat cell carcinoma and ectopic ACTH production [192].

Occasionally, adrenocortical hyperactivity becomes clinically evident before the tumor is recognized. The appearance of Cushing's syndrome after the primary tumor has been successfully removed indicates development of ACTH-secreting metastases. Monitoring central nervous system metastases by measuring ACTH concentrations in cerebrospinal fluid has been attempted, but the results have been disappointing [156].

By the time excess ACTH production becomes clinically apparent in patients with small-cell carcinoma, the prognosis is poor. Potassium and spironolactone can be given to control hypokalemia. In more indolent tumors, inhibitors of steroid biosynthesis such as metyrapone and aminoglutethimide can be used. Both have severe side effects that may be diminished by using combination therapy with lower doses of each. Ketoconazole, another inhibitor of steroid biosynthesis, also has been used for the treatment of ectopic Cushing's syndrome [187]. The adrenocorticolytic drug o,p'-DDD is less useful owing to the slow onset of action; several weeks usually are required to control cortisol secretion. Severe gastrointestinal and central nervous system side effects also accompany its use. Bromocryptine has been reported to suppress ACTH production in a bronchial carcinoid tumor [168]. Bilateral adrenalectomy is effective if medical therapy fails.

Why so many tumors, especially lung carcinomas, produce excess pro-ACTH, ACTH, and other POMC-derived peptides remains an enigma. Luster and coworkers [127] found that the ACTH produced by a small-cell carcinoma induced an increased rate of growth of the tumor in vitro and suggested that ACTH might play an autocrine role. If so, early suppression of tumor ACTH might be important [175,228]. The role of other POMC-derived peptides secreted by lung tumors is unknown.

CRH has been found in bronchial carcinoid tumors and in small-cell carcinomas of the lung. Rare cases of Cushing's syndrome due to bronchial carcinoid corticotropin-releasing factor (CRF)–induced pituitary hyperstimulation and bilateral adrenal hyperplasia have been reported [219,239].

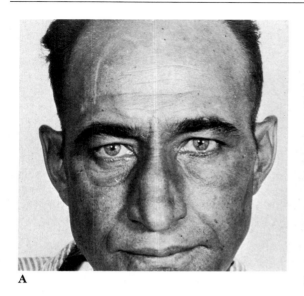

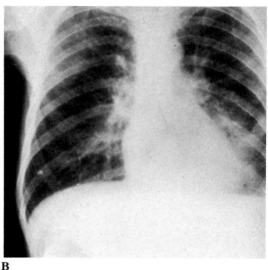

A   **B**

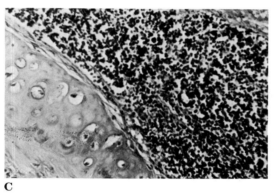

C

Antidiuretic Hormone (Arginine Vasopressin) and Atrial Natriuretic Factor

In 1938 Winkler and Crankshaw [234] described a patient with lung cancer, hyponatremia, and excessive urinary sodium loss. Schwartz and colleagues [185] later described two similar patients and observed that despite an increased extracellular fluid volume and hypotonic plasma, the urine of these patients was hypertonic. They postulated that the fluid and electrolyte imbalance seen in these patients was a consequence of inappropriate secretion of antidiuretic hormone (ADH, arginine vasopressin [AVP]). Further evidence to support this hypothesis came from the demonstration of significant amounts of this hormone, or a closely related substance, in extracts

Fig. 56-1. A. This patient with carcinoma of the lung complained of darkening of the skin. Note the hyperpigmentation under his eyes and around his mouth. B. The chest film revealed an area of infiltration along the left cardiac border. Examination of a scalene node biopsy specimen demonstrated anaplastic carcinoma. The patient had increased levels of 17-ketosteroids, total 17-ketogenic steroids, and 17-hydroxycorticosteroids, but no clinical Cushing's syndrome. C. Small-cell anaplastic carcinoma arising in the left-lower-lobe bronchus was found at postmortem examination. Note the marked variation in the size and shape of the deeply staining nuclei ($\times$ 450).

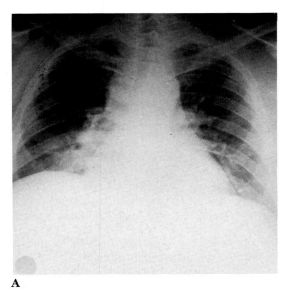

A

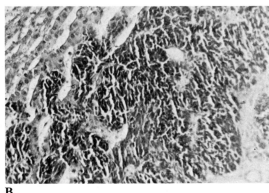

B

Fig. 56-2. A. Chest roentgenogram showing an area of increased density along the right cardiac border. The patient was a 34-year-old man with truncal obesity, edema, hypertension, hypokalemic alkalosis, polycythemia, and the typical urinary steroid values of Cushing's syndrome. B. A liver biopsy specimen was obtained at abdominal exploration. A large nest of anaplastic carcinoma cells metastatic from the lung is seen adjacent to cords of liver cells ($\times$ 450).

of lung tumors and plasma [2,10,24,65,87,119]. Tumor-associated ADH is indistinguishable chemically and immunologically from ADH released from the posterior pituitary gland. Pituitary ADH is stored attached to a neurophysin (a single-chain, 10,000-molecular-weight polypeptide), and ADH and its neurophysin are secreted concomitantly. Pulmonary neoplasms also synthesize ADH and neurophysin but neurophysin has not been detected in all tumor extracts [135].

Elevated or inappropriate ADH concentrations have been reported in 50 to 68 percent of patients with small-cell carcinoma [40,135]. Winkelmann [223] found inappropriately high plasma ADH concentrations in 27 of 58 patients with small-cell carcinoma, 4 of 10 patients with large-cell carcinoma, 5 of 11 patients with adenocarcinoma, and 12 of 41 patients with squamous cell carcinoma. Inappropriate ADH secretion may precede evidence of the tumor mass by several months. The highest and most persistent ADH concentrations have occurred in patients with extensive or rapidly progressing tumors, but neither plasma nor cerebrospinal ADH concentrations can be used to assess progression of disease or response to therapy [125,155].

The clinical response to tumor ADH depends on the degree of water loading. Hyponatremia also may be exacerbated by chemotherapy or radiation therapy [125]. Most patients are asymptomatic, particularly if the serum sodium concentration is 120 mmol/liter or higher. If the serum sodium falls further, patients may develop headache, lethargy, generalized weakness, confusion, and somnolence. When severe hyponatremia develops rapidly, the initial symptoms may be nausea and vomiting. If the serum sodium falls below 110 mmol/liter, the risk of seizures, hypothermia, coma, and death is markedly increased.

No treatment usually is needed if the serum sodium remains above 120 mmol/liter. If the patient becomes symptomatic or hyponatremia worsens, fluid restriction to an intake less than insensible water loss will restore the sodium concentration. Pharmacologic doses of fludrocortisone may be used in conjunction with fluid restriction if more rapid correction is necessary. If the hyponatremia is severe, hypertonic saline infusion can be coupled with furosemide administration and replacement of urinary electrolyte losses. Once the serum sodium concentration has increased, maintenance can be achieved with fluid restriction. Demeclocycline can be added if fluid restriction alone is not sufficient or tolerated.

In some lung cancer patients with hyponatremia, neither increased plasma nor tumor ADH can be found. However, some tumors and tumor cell lines from these patients express abundant atrial natriuretic factor (ANF) mRNA [15]. Peptide analysis has confirmed mRNA expression. The effects of sustained supraphysiologic tumor ANF concentrations on serum sodium are unknown, and it is impossible to determine from these studies whether tumor production of ANF was the primary cause of the hyponatremia.

Gonadotropins

Human chorionic gonadotropin (HCG), follicle-stimulating hormone (FSH), and luteinizing hormone (LH) are glycoproteins composed of a common alpha subunit and a unique beta subunit. Both subunits are required for biologic activity. The added carbohydrate is not, but without the carbohydrate the protein is degraded so rapidly that activity essentially is lost. HCG was once thought to be a specific marker for tumors derived from trophoblast tissue. However, an HCG-like substance has been found in extracts from a wide range of normal tissues, including the lung [25,236]. Extracts of all types of carcinomas contain a material indistinguishable from HCG [232]. Tumors may contain primarily alpha or beta subunits or both. Fukiyama and coworkers [61] suggested on the basis of immunohistochemical studies that alpha subunits are present primarily in small-cell carcinomas and carcinoids and that beta subunits are present primarily in non–small-cell carcinomas of the lung. They also suggest that the subunits are regulated by independent mechanisms and that further study of this regulation may provide insight into the mechanisms of differentiation and carcinogenesis.

Serum HCG concentrations are elevated in only one-third of patients with lung cancer [147]. Since tumor-associated HCG is poorly glycosylated, secreted HCG may be degraded too rapidly to be measured in most patients [80,235,237]. Gropp and coworkers [80] found elevated HCG levels in 17 of 51 patients with oat cell carcinoma, in 7 of 37 patients with squamous cell carcinoma, and in 5 of 19 with large-cell carcinoma at the time the lung cancer was diagnosed. Measurable HCG was not found in the 6 patients with adenocarcinoma. The HCG concentration did not reflect the extent of disease. Testosterone levels were lower in the cancer patients than in the control group; estrogen concentrations were not measured in this study. None of the patients with elevated HCG had gynecomastia [80], the only clinical sign associated with an elevated HCG concentration in adults. Increased estradiol concentrations, which were correlated with tumor mass and HCG concentration, were reported by Kirschner and coworkers [110]. Tumor HCG is not suppressed by the administration of androgens, estrogens, or progestins [152].

Faiman and coworkers [54] reported a step-up in the arteriovenous gradient of FSH but not LH across a bronchogenic carcinoma capillary bed. Serum concentrations of both FSH and LH were elevated prior to tumor resection and decreased postoperatively. In all other cases in which lung tumors have been associated with gonadotropin production, either the gonadotropin proved to be HCG or the immunoassay was not sufficiently specific that cross-reactivity with HCG could be excluded. No increase in circulating inhibin, a polypeptide hormone that suppresses FSH secretion by the pituitary gland, was found in a survey of cancer patients [189].

Human Placental Lactogen and Prolactin

Human placental lactogen (HPL) production also has been reported in 2 to 5 percent of patients with bronchogenic carcinoma [80]. In an immunohistochemical study of tumor antigens, Harach and coworkers [92] found HPL in 20 percent of primary lung tumors. Prolactin production by lung cancers also has been described [218]. No clinical consequences of either HPL or prolactin have been observed.

Hormones Regulating Growth

Small amounts of human growth hormone (HGH) have been found in extracts of all normal human tissues [116] and in extracts of lung carcinomas of all histologic types [199,201]. Classic acromegaly due to bronchial carcinoid tumors produced by growth hormone–releasing hormone (GHRH) has been well described [60,137]. The clinical features and the pattern of growth hormone secretion do not differentiate between hypothalamic and tumor secretion of GHRH, and many of the patients with tumor secretion of GHRH also have an intrasellar mass. When pituitary histology has been examined in these cases, the results have been consistent with either somatotroph hyperplasia or an adenoma as a consequence of hyperstimulation by carcinoid GHRH. Clinical improvement has been reported after carcinoid tumor resection [18]. Treatment of disseminated GHRH-producing bronchial carcinoid with chemotherapy (CCNU and 5-fluorouracil) [94], bromocryptine, or the somatostatin analogue octreotide [115,118,137] has been reported to decrease circulating HGH, somatomedin C, and GHRH concentrations and to reduce symptoms and signs of acromegaly. Such treatment may not affect the size of the tumor mass.

Somatostatin, a tetradecapeptide secreted by pancreatic islet D cells and widely distributed throughout the nervous system, inhibits release of many hormones, including growth hormone, insulin, glucagon, and bombesin. Somatostatin has been found in all bronchial carcinoid tumors and 25 to 40 percent of small-cell carcinomas [118,157,167,208]. Paracrine and autocrine effects of somatostatin production have been proposed, that is, inhibition of bombesin which is thought to be a local growth factor for tumor cells. No clinical sequelae resulting from tumor somatostatin production have been described. Initially somatostatin receptors were thought to be expressed only in bronchial carcinoid tumors and small-cell carcinomas, but non–small-cell carcinomas and their metastases also express somatostatin receptors, albeit fewer of them. Thus, scintographic labeling of the somatostatin receptor cannot be used clinically for identification of tumor type. Efforts are being made to develop this technique for identification of occult tumor metastases [118].

Gastrointestinal Hormones

Several gastrointestinal hormones have been found in bronchogenic carcinomas by immunohistochemical staining. The watery diarrhea-hypokalemia-achlorhydria syndrome caused by vasoactive intestinal peptide has occurred in patients with small-cell carcinomas [96,176]. Gastrin also has been identified in small-cell carcinomas and in bronchial carcinoid tumors [76,96].

Bombesin, a tetradecapeptide first found in amphibians, is the mammalian equivalent of the 27–amino acid gastrin-releasing peptide (GRP). Both peptides have a wide range of bioactivity resulting in hypothermia, hyperglycemia, and release of gastrointestinal peptides including gastrin and glucagon [27,29]. Peak levels in pulmonary neuroendocrine cells occur shortly after birth, indicating a role for bombesin in fetal lung development [164,215]. A role for bombesin/GRP as an autocrine stimulator of small-cell carcinoma of the lung also has been proposed. Bom-

besin/GRP stimulates clonal growth and DNA synthesis in small-cell carcinoma cell lines in vitro, and an antibody directed against the bombesin/GRP-binding site prevented growth of tumor cells. Antagonists to bombesin/GRP have been developed and their effects on tumor growth are being tested [175]. Most small-cell carcinomas produce bombesin/GRP, although only 5 percent of patients with small-cell carcinoma have elevated serum levels [175]. Bombesin/GRP also is found in carcinoid tumors and adenocarcinomas [174]. No clinical manifestations of bombesin/GRP produced by a bronchogenic carcinoma have been reported.

Calcium Metabolism and Bronchogenic Carcinoma: Humoral Hypercalcemia of Malignancy

The association of hypercalcemia with malignancy was first described in 1924 [240]. Hypercalcemia and hypophosphatemia in the absence of bony metastases were reported in a patient with bronchogenic carcinoma in 1936 [85]. Subsequently, hypercalcemia without evidence of bony metastases has been found in association with tumors of many kinds, and the syndrome is known as *humoral hypercalcemia of malignancy* (HHM). In the lung, HHM is associated primarily with squamous cell tumors and less often with adenocarcinomas and bronchial carcinoid tumors [197]. HHM has been confirmed in the presence of small-cell tumors [98,180,238], but most earlier reports of hypercalcemia associated with small-cell carcinoma probably reflected unidentified bone marrow metastases or concomitant parathyroid hyperplasia or adenoma [195,197, 238]. A prospective Swedish study of 245 patients with bronchogenic carcinoma found that 25 percent had at least mild hypercalcemia at the time of presentation, and 38 percent were given this diagnosis at some time during the course of the disease [195].

Humoral hypercalcemia of malignancy results primarily from increased bone resorption, which is uncoupled from bone formation, but also from increased tubular resorption of calcium. Both of these are mediated by parathyroid hormone (PTH)–related protein (PTHrP). The N-terminal region that binds to the receptor is shared by both PTHrP and PTH, but the remaining structure of each is unique. PTHrP is produced by normal tissues and benign tumors in which its role is uncertain; concentrations are especially high in epidermis and breast milk. PTHrP also may be an important regulator of fetal calcium homeostasis. Both PTHrP and PTH secretion results in osteoclastic activity and similar histologic changes in bone, increased nephrogenous cyclic adenosine monophosphate (AMP), renal phosphate wasting, and calcium resorption. In most cases of HHM, the levels of immunoreactive PTH are low. Circulating levels of 1,25-dihydroxyvitamin D also are low, intestinal calcium absorption is decreased, and a hypokalemic alkalosis may be present [26,30,31,108,114,133,141,163,179,195,204].

Tumor-derived growth factors such as transforming growth factor alpha and beta and interleukin-1 (osteoclast-activating factors), platelet-derived growth factor, prostaglandins, and vitamin D analogues have been implicated as mediators of bone resorption, but it is clear that these are not responsible for most of the hypercalcemia accompanying bronchogenic carcinomas [141]. Decreased mobility and chemotherapeutic drugs toxic to bone cells also contribute to increased bone resorption in patients with bronchogenic cancer.

A serum calcium concentration of 10.5 mg/dl or higher in patients with bronchogenic carcinoma has been associated with large tumor masses and a poor outcome [34,38,71,197]. Surgical cure was not obtained in these patients, although temporary normocalcemia was achieved in some following tumor resection. Most patients with mild hypercalcemia are asymptomatic. Even serum calcium concentrations of 12 to 13 mg/dl or more often are associated with only mild anorexia, constipation, myalgias, or lethargy. However, when hypercalcemia is severe, patients may experience nausea and vomiting, abdominal pain, and polyuria, and develop dehydration, weakness, confusion, or obtundation. Band keratitis, uremia, and renal calculi are uncommon because of the short duration of the hypercalcemia. The encephalogram and electromyogram often show nonspecific abnormalities [203].

If treatment is required, intravenous saline and furosemide can be used to lower serum calcium acutely. Dietary calcium restriction, oral phosphate, glucocorticoids, indomethacin, and calcitonin are effective only transiently, if at all. Mithramycin (plicamycin) is cytotoxic for bone cells and inhibits osteoclastic bone resorption within 24–48 hours. Repeated doses may be required every few days, and use is limited by renal and hepatic toxicity and bone marrow suppression. Bisphosphonates impair osteoclast activity by mechanisms which are still uncertain and, in conjunction with hydration and diuresis, have been safe and effective in lowering the serum calcium concentration for 5–14 days [17,20,84,93,95,105, 153,190,196,211]. The two bisphosphonates which are available at the present time are etidronate disodium, given intravenously for 3–7 days, and pamidronate, given intravenously over 24 hours. Fever, asymptomatic hypocalcemia, hypophosphatemia, hypomagnesemia and small increases in creatinine occur in some patients. Effectiveness of repeated doses for recurrent hypercalcemia is uncertain [211].

Gallium nitrate also inhibits bone resorption and has been shown safely to lower serum calcium when administered as a continuous infusion for five days with concomitant hydration and diuresis [22,63,225,226]. The effect of retreatment with gallium nitrate has not been examined in controlled studies.

In clinical trials pamidronate was more effective in lowering serum calcium than etidronate disodium [84] and plicamycin [213]. Gallium nitrate also was more effective than etidronate disodium [225]. Small studies have shown more rapid reduction of hypercalcemia with combined calcitonin and bisphosphonate therapy [55,210].

Calcitonin and Calcitonin Gene–Related Peptide

Calcitonin inhibits bone resorption and decreases renal tubular resorption of calcium and phosphorus, resulting in calciuria and phosphaturia in animal studies and in vitro. Pharmacologic doses of calcitonin inhibit secretion of pancreatic enzymes and induce central nervous system effects including analgesia. The precise role of calcitonin in normal human physiology is unknown. Although the highest concentration of calcitonin is found in the parafollicular cells of the thyroid gland, calcitonin is produced by neuroendocrine cells in many tissues. Indeed, the lungs contain more calcitonin than the thyroid gland. Calcitonin is synthesized as a high-molecular-weight precursor, which then undergoes further processing that depends on its tissue of origin [35,52,173]. Serum calcitonin is increased in smokers and in patients with chronic obstructive pulmonary disease (COPD) as well as in those with other lung diseases [13,209]. Calcitonin has been found in extracts of neoplasms of all types, particularly lung carcinoma. In vivo catheterization studies in patients with bronchogenic carcinoma have shown that the calcitonin may originate either in the tumor or in the thyroid gland [41,82,194].

In a prospective study, increased serum calcitonin was found in 19 of 49 patients with bronchogenic carcinoma of all types [184] but has been reported most frequently in patients with small-cell carcinoma. Luster and coworkers [128] found increased calcitonin concentrations in 57 percent of patients with small-cell carcinoma, but in only 10 percent of patients with squamous cell carcinoma. An increased calcitonin response to pentagastrin has been observed in lung cancer patients whose basal calcitonin concentrations were normal [178]. Both increased serum [128] and urine [14] calcitonin concentrations have been reported to be correlated positively with lack of tumor differentiation and increased disease activity. Calcitonin concentrations decreased in patients who responded to therapy and increased in association with relapse or tumor progression.

Alternative intranuclear splicing of mRNA yields the mRNA either for calcitonin or for calcitonin gene–related peptide (CGRP). CGRP is a potent vasodilator and is found in pulmonary neuroendocrine cells. CGRP mRNA has been detected in lung tumor cell lines by several groups [52,103,142,172], but Hoppener and coworkers [103] could not detect CGRP mRNA in any bronchogenic carcinoma tissue or lung tumor metastasis. They suggested that CGRP production is a function of lung tumor cell lines but not of lung tumor cells in vivo.

No adverse consequences of bronchogenic carcinoma CGRP or calcitonin production are known. Serum calcium, inorganic phosphate, and vitamin D concentrations remain normal.

Renin

Most tumors secreting renin are of renal origin. The renin usually is secreted in the form of a large, inactive precursor, suggesting that the tumor is unable to carry out normal posttranslational processing. However, rare bronchial carcinoid and small-cell carcinomas of the lung have been reported to secrete enough active renin to produce hypertension and hyperkalemia. Hypertension may be severe and poorly responsive to treatment, including treatment with beta blockers and angiotensin-converting enzyme inhibitors [175].

Hypoglycemic Factors

Most cases of tumor-associated hypoglycemia have occurred in patients with large retroperitoneal tumors, but hypoglycemia has been reported with intrathoracic tumors, including rhabdomyosarcomas, fibrosarcomas, neurofibromas, and bronchogenic carcinoma [130,214]. Although these tumors are large, increased glucose utilization by the tumor mass cannot account for the hypoglycemia. Non–beta cell tumors producing immunoreactive and bioactive insulin have been described [166], but in most cases of tumor-associated hypoglycemia, circulating insulin concentrations are low. Insulin-like growth factors (IGF-I and IGF-II) that have weak insulin-like activity and other peptides with insulin-like bioactivity that is not suppressible by antibodies directed against insulin may be responsible for the hypoglycemia of malignancy in some patients. These seldom have been associated with bronchogenic carcinoma [152], and the mechanism responsible for most hypoglycemia associated with bronchogenic carcinoma is unknown. Hypoglycemia usually develops when patients are fasting. Food ingestion may not be sufficient to relieve symptoms in patients with very severe disease.

Hormonal Syndromes Associated with Bronchial Carcinoid Tumors

Carcinoid tumors are neuroendocrine tumors that arise from a heterogeneous population of enterochromaffin cells. They were first documented in the small intestine and were shown to originate from the Kulchitsky cells in the crypts of Lieberkühn. They can be found scattered throughout the body but occur principally in the submucosa of the intestine and the bronchi. Carcinoids have been classified according to the part of the primitive gut from which they are derived and by whether or not they reduce silver salts and produce 5-hydroxytryptamine (5-HPT). Carcinoid tumors arising in tissues derived from the primitive foregut usually produce 5-HPT. They may produce a wide array of peptides and amines and have receptors for numerous peptide hormones and neurotransmitters. Both bronchial carcinoids and small-cell carcinomas contain secretory granules that are typical of polypeptide-secreting endocrine tissues. Carcinoid tumors arising from primitive midgut usually produce 5-hydroxytryptophan (5-HT) which is converted to 5-HPT in other tissues. Tumors arising from the hindgut secrete neither 5-HPT nor 5-HT.

The carcinoid syndrome, which was first described by Scholte [181] and later by Thorson and coworkers [212], refers to the clinical manifestations that may occur if sufficient quantities of vasoactive substances from the carcinoid tumor reach the systemic circulation. The syndrome is characterized by episodic flushing, diarrhea, paroxysmal bronchospasm, and valvular disease of the right side of the heart. These are attributed to overproduction of serotonin and its metabolites, and possibly to prostaglandins and substance P, a decapeptide distributed in gut and brain. Severe tryptophan depletion may occur due to excessive diversion of tryptophan into 5-HPT synthesis. Although most bronchial carcinoid tumors contain 5-HPT, the carcinoid syndrome occurs in association with 10 percent or less of these.

Other hormonally mediated clinical syndromes also have been associated with bronchial carcinoid tumors. Production of ACTH [122,123] or CRH [49] or both [182] has resulted in Cushing's syndrome. ACTH and melanocyte-stimulating hormone have produced hyperpigmentation (Nelson's syndrome). Acromegaly has been reported to be due to secretion of growth hormone or GHRH [18,45,199]. Hypercalcemia also has been attributed to a bronchial carcinoid tumor [220]. Immunoperoxidase staining has revealed production of additional peptide hormones which were not accompanied by clinical syndromes: calcitonin, HCG, somatostatin [217], gastrin [76], vasoactive intestinal peptide [76], and bombesin [174]. Immunologic evidence for GHRH and the alpha subunit in bronchial carcinoids also has been reported [224]. Although as many as 8 to 10 hormones may be found in a single bronchial carcinoid tumor, most or all of these may not be secreted [76].

Bronchial carcinoid tumors have been classified either as typical carcinoids, which are centrally located, have classic morphologic features, numerous secretory granules, and little pleomorphism, and have a benign course, or as atypical carcinoids, which may be peripherally located, are more pleomorphic, are more likely to metastasize, and have fewer, smaller secretory granules. Although both types of bronchocarcinoid tumors show positive immunochemical staining for multiple hormones, clinical syndromes resulting from ectopic hormone secretion are reported to occur almost exclusively with the atypical tumors [76].

If the carcinoid tumor cannot be removed, treatment is directed toward the systemic manifestations. Nicotinamide supplementation may be necessary to counteract tryptophan depletion. The somatostatin analogue octreotide does not reduce tumor size but inhibits flushing, diarrhea, and bronchoconstriction [73], and is the treatment of choice. Flushing occasionally responds temporarily to phenoxybenzamine, and diarrhea may be ameliorated by serotonin antagonists such as cyproheptadine. Chemotherapy results in response rates of less than 25 percent for single agents or combinations, and even then remissions usually last only a few months. Anesthetics, surgery, and chemotherapy can precipitate a carcinoid crisis—severe flushing with hypotension. This can be treated with octreotide or methoxamine or angiotensin. Other pressors should be avoided [134].

Additional Peptide/Protein Products of Bronchogenic Carcinomas

ONCOFETAL ANTIGENS

Several glycoproteins normally are found in high concentrations in the developing fetus but in low concentrations in tissues in adults. Increased carcinoembryonic antigen (CEA) has been found in patients with all types of lung tumors as well as in smokers and in patients with nonneoplastic pulmonary disease [68,92,138,217]. Attempts have been made to use scintographic localization of CEA to examine tumor location [47], to use CEA concentrations to follow tumor progression [81,113,138], to differentiate benign from malignant pleural effusions [217,223], and to differentiate adenocarcinomas from mesotheliomas [43,101]. However, in most cases measurement of CEA is not helpful in following an individual patient.

Alpha fetoprotein is seldom produced by lung tumors. Immunoreactivity for this antigen has been found in only 0 to 2.7 percent of patients with bronchogenic cancer [217].

NEURON-SPECIFIC ENOLASE

Neuron-specific enolase (NSE) is found in normal neurons and in neuroendocrine cells, all of which contain secretory granules and store and secrete peptides and biogenic amines. Carcinoid tumors and small-cell carcinomas, which are derived from these cells, contain secretory granules and express NSE [33,217]. NSE levels also have been reported to be correlated with the tumor burden in patients with small-cell carcinoma [107,188]. The transient rise in serum NSE following initial chemotherapy is thought to reflect tumor cell destruction [22,56]. Trump and coworkers [217] proposed that NSE may be a useful marker both for detecting and monitoring small-cell carcinoma and for separating atypical carcinoid tumors from epidermoid tumors, large-cell tumors, and adenocarcinomas. NSE has been reported to be elevated in less than 15 percent of patients with non–small-cell lung carcinomas [106,107].

ADDITIONAL PROTEINS
High levels of creatine kinase BB have been reported in 25 to 62 percent of patients with small-cell cancer and have been reported to provide prognostic information about patient survival [22,88,106]. Alkaline phosphatase, amylase, thymidine kinase, ferritin, pancreatic oncofetal antigen, calmodulin, beta microglobulin, keratin and other cytoskeletal markers, and calmodulin all have been reported to be elevated in association with bronchogenic carcinoma. However, their concentrations are too erratic and too nonspecific to be used as tumor markers [3,138,217].

Neuromyopathic Syndromes

In 1948 Denny-Brown [48] first described a sensory neuromyopathy associated with bronchogenic carcinoma. Since then nonmetastatic neurologic syndromes that may accompany lung cancer have been shown to be singularly varied and not as rare as was originally believed [99]. Most of the neuromyopathic syndromes have been described in conjunction with small-cell lung carcinoma. Croft and Wilkinson [44] observed that 16 percent of 250 consecutive male patients with bronchogenic carcinoma had some evidence of neuromyopathy; well-developed signs were present in 40 percent of these. More than one syndrome may coexist in the same patient. Since the same syndromes develop in patients with and those without cancer, the relationship of the neurologic syndrome to the malignancy usually is based on the increased frequency of the association. The neurologic disorders often are discovered before the tumor becomes evident and, in contrast to the hormonal syndromes, most neurologic syndromes do not remit if the malignancy is removed. Furthermore, there is little correlation between the size of the tumor burden or the rate of progression of the tumor and the severity of the neurologic disease [98].

Three different mechanisms for the development of these syndromes have been proposed: (1) viral infection, (2) circulating neurotoxins secreted by the carcinoma, and (3) immunity directed against nervous system antigens due to either a viral agent or cross-reactivity between the tumor and elements of the nervous system

[51,162]. As yet, no specific viral agent or neurotoxin has been identified in association with lung carcinomas. However, some role for the immune system for a few syndromes seems well established, based on a strong association between the syndrome and the tumor, and identification of a specific immune mechanism in cancer patients but not the controls [7]. Paraneoplastic syndromes can involve any part of the central or peripheral nervous system. Those most frequently associated with bronchogenic carcinoma are described below.

Central Nervous System

ENCEPHALOMYELITIS
A group of paraneoplastic syndromes that may occur in isolation or combined under the umbrella term *encephalomyelitis* include limbic encephalitis, brainstem encephalitis, myoclonus-opsoclonus, and cerebellar degeneration. These disorders are characterized by target tissue inflammation in addition to neuronal degeneration and are associated mainly with small-cell carcinoma. The clinical presentation may include a variety of psychiatric disorders, dementia, loss of memory, and seizures. Brainstem encephalitis may result in ophthalmoplegia, bulbar palsy, involuntary movements, evidence of bilateral pyramidal tract lesions, and so on, depending on the location involved [51]. Opsoclonus is characterized by involuntary, chaotic eye movements. Cerebellar disease presents first with ataxia and may be mild or severe, localized or diffuse. "Anti-Hu" antibodies to a 35,000- to 40,000-kd neuronal nucleoprotein that also cross-react with small-cell carcinoma tumor cell homogenates have been detected in the serum of patients with paraneoplastic encephalitis [7,51,162], but whether these are responsible for the development of the encephalitis or are an epiphenomenon is not certain.

CEREBELLAR DEGENERATION
Paraneoplastic cerebellar degeneration (PCD) has been reported in association with small-cell carcinoma, although it is seen much more frequently in association with breast carcinoma. There is diffuse degeneration of Purkinje cells coupled with thinning of other molecular layers, but few inflammatory lesions are found. The clinical presentation usually begins with ataxia, but nystagmus, dysmetria, tremor, and dysarthria may develop. PCD is associated with specific serum and cerebrospinal fluid immunoglobulins

that bind to Purkinje cell cytoplasm and proximal dendrites in a characteristic pattern. A group of cerebellar proteins that react with the anticerebellar antibodies have been identified. Neither the proteins nor the antibody recognition have been found in patients with cerebellar degeneration who do not have a malignancy. The gene coding for one of the PCD target antigens has been cloned and its mRNA identified in cerebellar tissue and in the RNA isolated from tumor tissue. These experiments support the concept that paraneoplastic neurologic syndromes are the end result of shared brain-tumor antigens [51].

CANCER-ASSOCIATED RETINOPATHY

A syndrome characterized by rapid loss of binocular vision has been described in association with small-cell carcinoma. Circulating antibodies to retinal cells, optic nerve, and the cancer tissue have been found in these patients [170]. However, these antibodies also have been found in normal controls, indicating that antibodies to neurofilaments may not be the cause of this syndrome [6].

NECROTIZING MYELOPATHY

Necrotizing myelopathy is a rare paraneoplastic syndrome found in patients with small-cell carcinoma. The syndrome presents with subacute bilateral loss of motor, sensory, and sphincter function but little pain. Most patients deteriorate rapidly, developing an ascending level of flaccid paralysis and numbness. Necrotizing myelopathy has been associated with antibodies that react with the spinal cord and the tumor, but the etiologic significance of these is uncertain [51].

Peripheral Nervous System

SUBACUTE SENSORY NEUROPATHY

The paraneoplastic syndrome of subacute sensory neuropathy (SSN) also is associated with small-cell carcinoma and is found more frequently in women. SSN may occur alone or in combination with encephalomyelitis. The most common initial complaints are symmetric numbness and paresthesias, especially in the lower limbs, but painful dysesthesias develop later. All sensory modalities are involved, although vibration and position senses are often the most impaired. Later in the course, patients frequently are unable to walk due to pain and loss of proprioception. Pathologic findings include loss of sensory neurons of the dorsal root ganglia and degenerative changes in the remaining cells. The

anti-Hu neuronal antinuclear antibodies are associated with this syndrome and have been found in tumor extracts and cultured cell lines from patients with small-cell carcinoma. However, there is as yet no direct evidence that SSN results when these antibodies are directed against common tumor and neuron antigens. There has been no clinical improvement following immunosuppressive therapy [7,51,170].

PERIPHERAL SENSORIMOTOR NEUROPATHY

A heterogeneous group of sensorimotor peripheral neuropathies are found in association with a wide variety of malignancies. These paraneoplastic syndromes, like all of the others, may occur alone or in combination with other types and may antedate the diagnosis of malignancy. An axonal form is seen most often in patients with small-cell carcinoma. Lower neuron symptoms and signs predominate and are symmetric; symptoms progress at a variable rate. The etiology is unknown.

NEUROMUSCULAR JUNCTION SYNDROMES

Lambert-Eaton Syndrome. The Lambert-Eaton syndrome (LES) is the best understood of all of the paraneoplastic neurologic syndromes. Most of the well-documented cases have occurred in association with lung cancer, especially with small-cell carcinoma [150]. The incidence of LES in patients with this tumor is estimated to be 3 to 5 percent [97]. A presynaptic defect in the calcium-dependent release of acetylcholine from nerve terminals is thought to be the primary defect in LES. Patients complain of easy fatigability and weakness that affects the pelvic girdle and shoulder girdle muscles more than distal strength and bulbar function. Fifty to 75 percent of patients are reported to have clinical evidence of autonomic cholinergic dysfunction [51]. In contrast to the findings in myasthenia gravis, muscle strength improves with exercise and the response to edrophonium chloride is poor [100].

Autoimmunity is thought to underlie LES on the basis of the association with other autoimmune disorders; association with the histocompatibility antigens HLA-B8 and -DR3; the presence of antinuclear antibodies, antiparietal cell and antithyroid antibodies, or rheumatoid factors in 15 to 40 percent of patients with LES; and improvement with treatment with corticosteroids or other immunosuppressive drugs or plasmapheresis. Antibodies to the voltage-gated calcium channel complex of small-cell lung cancer cell lines have been found twice as often in patients with LES who had lung cancer than those who did not [121]. The best evidence for the role of the immune system comes from passive transfer experiments in which the syndrome was transferred to mice by administration of purified IgG from the sera of LES patients with and those without a malignancy [62,122].

AUTONOMIC DYSFUNCTION

Intestinal pseudoobstruction with evidence of sympathetic and parasympathetic postganglionic dysfunction has been attributed to a neoplastic syndrome associated with small-cell carcinoma (see Gastrointestinal Syndromes).

PARANEOPLASTIC VASCULITIC NEUROPATHY

Paraneoplastic vasculitic neuropathy (PVN) has been described as a distinct paraneoplastic syndrome relatively recently [79,149]. The syndrome is characterized by an asymmetric sensorimotor peripheral neuropathy. Nerve conduction studies reveal either no response or slowed conduction, indicating axonal disease. In most cases the sedimentation rate is high. In contrast to the other paraneoplastic neurologic syndromes with which it often occurs, spinal fluid protein is high. The diagnosis is confirmed by nerve biopsy, which reveals microvasculitis and axonal degeneration. In only one case has improvement been reported following therapy (cyclophosphamide) directed against the vasculitis [149]. PVN has been described in association with both small-cell carcinoma and adenocarcinoma of the lung.

Connective-Tissue and Osseous Syndromes

Hypertrophic Osteoarthropathy and Clubbing

Hypertrophic osteoarthropathy (HOA, Bamberg-Marie syndrome [9,132]) occurs primarily in association with thoracic malignancies, especially squamous cell carcinoma. Adenocarcinoma, large-cell carcinoma, and other thoracic malignancies also are associated with HOA, but small-cell carcinoma very rarely causes this syndrome [229]. The syndrome consists of a bilateral, symmetric periosteal reaction producing subperiosteal new bone formation along the bone shaft and tenderness and swelling over the joints and the ends of the long bones. Joints develop chronic synovitis with plasma and round-cell infiltrations, osteoporosis, and periarticular

thickening. Moderate-size, noninflammatory joint effusions are common. The knees, ankles, wrists, and metacarpophalangeal joints are most commonly affected (Fig. 56-3). The syndrome frequently presents with a constant dull ache in the ends of the long bones or with arthralgia. Later, overt signs of arthritis may be florid enough to suggest acute rheumatoid arthritis.

Clubbing of the fingers and toes is a painless, symmetric uniform swelling of the soft tissues at the ends of the digits which usually accompanies HOA. The earliest changes occur at the base of the nail, where the skin becomes shiny and tense, and the nail rocks more easily on its bed. Later the nail becomes curved, and the angle between the nail and the soft tissues at the base increases to over 180 degrees. At a more advanced stage, soft-tissue hypertrophy develops. The transverse diameter of the distal phalanx is increased (referred to as *acropachy*) and the digit resembles a drumstick. Histologic examination of the clubbed digits reveals dilated, engorged vessels in the nail bed, edema, and deposition of new collagen [231]. Both HOA and clubbing may develop before the underlying tumor manifests. Although clubbing almost always accompanies HOA, the reverse is not true. Digital clubbing is associated

Fig. 56-3. Roentgenogram of knees shows pulmonary hypertrophic osteoarthropathy. Note the periosteal thickening along the distal portion of the femoral shaft and proximal parts of the tibial and fibular shafts.

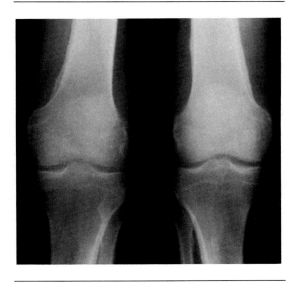

with a number of nonmalignant diseases. When clubbing does occur with HOA, the time of onset may be quite different and the severity may not be proportional to the bone and joint changes. It is likely that clubbing is due to a different process but one that usually occurs when HOA develops [191]. When HOA and clubbing are associated with long-standing disease, the alterations in bone are more extensive than those seen in patients with bronchogenic carcinoma whose long-term survival rate is lower [159,160].

In a few patients, HOA is accompanied by thickened, deeply furrowed, oily facial skin, broadening of the nose, and prominent nasolabial folds. When this occurs in the setting of malignancy, the condition is termed *pachydermoperiostitis*. A similar condition also can be inherited as a dominant trait; in these cases there is no association with malignancy and the correct term is *pachydermoperiostosis*.

Although the structural and functional changes in clubbing and pulmonary osteoarthropathy have been well described, the underlying mechanism is uncertain. Digital clubbing and HOA are characterized by increased blood flow through the long bones, digits, the nose, and rarely, periauricular tissues [69,126]. The increased flow is believed to pass mainly through dilated arteriovenous anastomoses. Vascularity can be reduced by combined alpha- and beta-adrenergic blockade [191]. Tumor production of a vasodilator is considered unlikely, because studies in dogs and humans have shown that either vagotomy alone or removal of the lung tumor decreases peripheral blood flow and abolishes HOA [102]. Blood flow was not altered by paralyzing the motor fibers of the vagus nerve with atropine. The increased blood flow is thought to be mediated through a reflex arc, the afferent fibers of which travel via the vagus nerve. Since the bronchogenic carcinomas, fibromas, or pulmonary metastases causing HOA usually are large and necrotic and/or impinge on the pleura, a pleural or subpleural origin for the afferent reflex arc has been suggested [191]. The site and type of receptors mediating such an afferent pathway do not appear to involve any of the known chemoreceptor reflexes in the lung [39]. The efferent pathway mediating the development of HOA is unknown. Vasoactive substances produced by the central nervous system or by the pituitary have been suggested [16,161]. In recent years it has become clear that vasodilators (i.e., nitric oxide, which acts via generation of cyclic guanosine monophosphate) are produced by vascular endothelium in response to nonadrenergic, noncholinergic neurotransmitters. One or more of these may be involved in the efferent pathway [83,165].

Increased estrogen excretion and gynecomastia have been documented in patients with osteoarthropathy and bronchogenic carcinoma (Fig. 56-4) [9,69,70,83,161]. However, increased estrogen secretion has not been found when HOA is associated with nonpulmonary diseases [191]. Increased growth hormone and gonadotropin secretion also have been documented in some, but not all patients with HOA [78,203]. In a recent study, plasma growth hormone concentrations were higher in patients with bronchogenic carcinoma and clubbing than in patients with carcinoma but no clubbing, but there was marked overlap between the values for the two groups [75]. Furthermore, the digital changes of acromegaly are different from those associated with clubbing and HOA.

HOA is seen (rarely) in association with cyanotic congenital heart disease [50,86,159]. This may be due to the presence of a circulating vasodilator. However, it is possible that the lungs remove some substance from mixed venous blood that is capable of dilating arteriovenous anastomoses. The inflammatory changes resulting in damage to the microvasculature that have been seen with electron microscopy may be important and may explain the response of HOA symptoms to prostaglandin synthetase inhibitors such as indomethacin and aspirin [120,186] and to glucocorticoid therapy [202]. Pineda and coworkers [159] pointed out that 25 centuries after Hippocrates described clubbing, there is still debate over its morphologic characteristics. Thesame can be said about the underlying mechanism(s).

Vascular Syndromes

Venous Thrombosis

The association of venous thrombosis and malignancy has been reported repeatedly [57,74,124,200] since it was first described in 1868 [216]. Thrombosis is associated particularly with mucin-producing adenocarcinomas of the gastrointestinal tract, pancreas, and ovaries but also with bronchogenic carcinoma [58]. Pulmonary embolism is a frequent complication of venous thrombosis; large thrombi also may cause gangrene or priapism (Fig. 56-5). Thrombophlebitis migrans [124,143] and pulmonary embolism with or without overt deep vein thrombosis [74] may precede

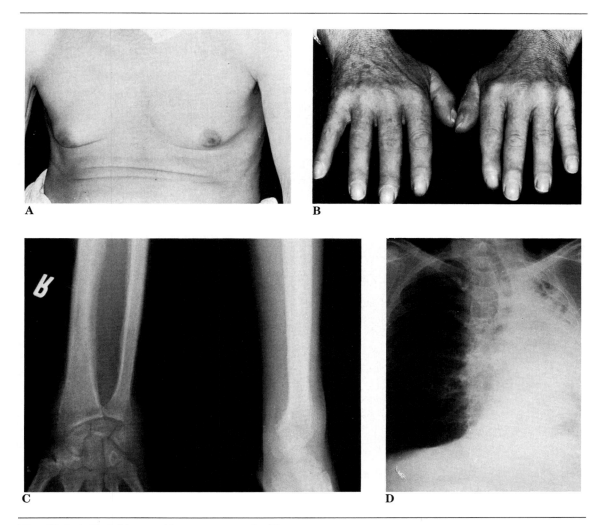

Fig. 56-4. A, B. A 64-year-old man presented with dyspnea, gynecomastia (A), clubbing of the fingers (B), and tender wrists. C. Roentgenogram of the forearm and wrist shows hypertrophic osteoarthropathy. Note the periosteal thickening of the long bones. D. Chest roentgenogram shows complete atelectasis of the left lung. A scalene node biopsy was positive for anaplastic carcinoma.

appearance of the neoplasm by as much as 18 months. In addition to mechanical obstruction by the tumor, thrombocytosis, and increased platelet adhesiveness, possible mechanisms include accelerated thromboplastin regeneration due to an antihemophilic globulin-like factor [5], activation of coagulation factor X by a serine protease from tumor cells [158,227], hypercalcemia, and decreased antithrombin III [200]. Treatment is dif-

ficult if the tumor cannot be removed. Anticoagulants may be effective in acute situations and can be used to prevent pulmonary emboli [42].

Nonbacterial Endocarditis

Nonbacterial endocarditis is characterized by the formation of sterile vegetations due to accumulation of fibrin on the mitral and aortic valves in patients with a variety of wasting illnesses, including bronchogenic carcinoma [4,129]. MacDonald and Robbins [129] found evidence of nonbacterial thrombotic endocarditis in 78 of 18,486 consecutive postmortem examinations. This was associated with carcinoma in 24 patients, 4 of whom had bronchogenic carcinoma [129].

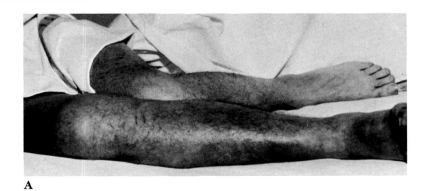

A

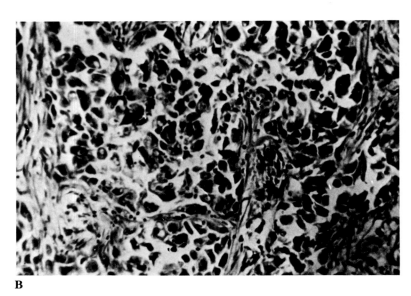

B

Fig. 56-5. A 60-year-old man was admitted with thrombophlebitis of the right leg. A. Gangrene of the entire leg developed rapidly. Within 3 months the same brawny induration had developed in the other three extremities. Chest roentgenograms appeared normal. At postmortem examination after his sudden death, a small tumor was found in the right mainstem bronchus. The cause of death was acute myocardial infarction. B. Histologic section of the tumor showed anaplastic carcinoma (× 900).

Fibrinogen Deficiency

Fibrinogen deficiency has been reported in patients with bronchogenic carcinoma, although this is seen more commonly with prostatic carcinoma [59]. Fibrinogen deficiency may be due to widespread intravascular clotting, but elaboration of a circulating fibrinolysin by the tumor also has been proposed.

Hematologic Syndromes

Anemia

Anemia in the absence of blood loss is common in malignancy. The anemia usually is normo-chromic and normocytic. Low serum iron without chronic blood loss, and high serum iron with decreased utilization and impaired erythrocyte formation are found most frequently [140]. Hemolytic anemia occurs in response to tumor production of hemolysins.

Leukemoid and Leukoerythroblastic Reactions

Leukemoid and leukoerythroblastic reactions also are associated with bronchogenic carcinoma [37]. Profound eosinophilia may occur [77], especially with tumor necrosis [8,111].

Cutaneous Syndromes

Acanthosis Nigricans

Adult acanthosis is characterized by bilateral, soft, symmetric, darkly pigmented, verrucous lesions situated in the axillae, in flexural areas, in body folds, around the neck, around the umbilicus, and in the perianal region. The mucous membranes also may be involved. Histologic examination reveals thickened layers of the epidermis with an increase in the pigmented basal layers. The more common forms not associated with an underlying malignancy may be associated with insulin resistance and other endocrine disorders. In the so-called malignant forms, the associated tumor is usually intraabdominal, but about 5 percent of patients have an adenocarcinoma of the lung. Although detection of acanthosis nigricans may precede detection of the underlying tumor, both the tumor and the skin disorder tend to progress concomitantly. Removal of the tumor may lead to regression of the cutaneous changes [53,171].

Dermatomyositis

The association of dermatomyositis and cancer has been recognized for many years [21,170,230]. Approximately 15 percent of persons with dermatomyositis have an underlying malignancy [193]. The percentage is higher in persons over 50 years old, especially in males. Cutaneous manifestations usually precede the overt appearance of the tumor. Classic findings include a violaceous rash on the face, heliotrope eyelids, and proximal muscle weakness and atrophy. The mechanism underlying the development of this disorder is unknown.

Erythema Gyratum Repens

This is a rare condition usually found in association with breast cancer or an oat cell tumor of the bronchus [64]. Erythema gyratum repens is an erythematous gyrate macular eruption that gives the skin a knotty-pine appearance. The tumor is present when the skin changes appear, and resection of the tumor results in disappearance of the cutaneous stigmata. This condition is thought to develop in response to altered organ proteins produced by tumor necrosis.

Additional Cutaneous Conditions Associated with Malignancy

A number of nonspecific dermatitides may occur, ranging from hyperpigmentation to bullous and eczematous rashes [32,136]. Intense nocturnal pruritus, usually of the lower limbs, may be the first symptom of thoracic lymphoma or bronchogenic carcinoma [233]. Ichthyosis and hypertrichosis also may be presenting signs of bronchogenic cancer [104].

Gastrointestinal Syndromes

Intestinal Pseudoobstruction

Chronic intestinal pseudoobstruction is characterized by early satiety, nausea and vomiting, constipation, abdominal pain, and delayed gastric emptying. Pseudoobstruction can be produced by degeneration of neurons in the myenteric plexus within the gut or by disruption anywhere within the brain-neural axis extrinsic to the gut. The association of chronic intestinal pseudoobstruction and malignancy was first described in 1948 [148]. Since then, several cases have been documented in patients who had small-cell carcinoma or developed small-cell carcinoma weeks to months later [183,198]. Some, but not all, had other signs of abnormal autonomic nervous system function. In only one patient was there evidence of brain metastases and preganglionic as well as postganglionic sympathetic dysfunction. In some cases, treatment of the tumor with chemotherapy or radiation therapy resulted in resolution of the motility disorder, but shrinkage of the tumor burden did not always ameliorate the symptoms. In the few cases for which data are available, autopsy studies of the gut reveal axonal degeneration, infiltration of plasma cells and lymphocytes, and proliferation of Schwann cells of the myenteric plexus. These findings are similar to those in other paraneoplastic neurologic syndromes. Although it is not possible to rule out a parallel disorder of the gastrointestinal tract occurring in conjunction with small-cell carcinoma, current data are consistent with the occurrence of chronic intestinal pseudoobstruction as a paraneoplastic syndrome.

References

1. Albright F, Reifenstein EC (Eds), *The Parathyroid Glands and Metabolic Bone Disease—Selected Studies*. Baltimore: Williams & Wilkins, 1948.
2. Amatruda TT Jr, et al. Carcinoma of the lung with inappropriate antidiuresis: Demonstration of antidiuretic-hormone-like activity in the tumor extract. *N Engl J Med* 269:544, 1963.
3. Ammann RW, et al. Hyperamylasemia with carcinoma of the lung. *Ann Intern Med* 78:521, 1973.
4. Amromin GD, Wang SK. Degenerative verrucal endocardiosis and myocardial infarction: Report of two cases associated with mucus-producing bronchogenic carcinoma. *Ann Intern Med* 50:1519, 1959.
5. Amundsen MA, et al. Hypercoagulability associated with malignancy and post-operative state (abstract). *Ann Intern Med* 56:683, 1962.
6. Anderson NE. Anti-neuronal autoantibodies and neurological paraneoplastic syndromes. *Aust NZ J Med* 19:379, 1989.
7. Antel JP, Moumdjian R. Paraneoplastic syndromes: A role for the immune system. *J Neurol* 236:1, 1989.
8. Ascensao JL, et al. Leukocytosis and large cell lung cancer. *Cancer* 60:903, 1987.
9. Bamberger E. Ueber Knochenveranderungen bei chronischem Lungen und Herzkrankheiten. *A Klin Med* 18:193, 1891.
10. Barraclough MA, Jones JJ, Lee J. Production of vasopressin by anaplastic oat-cell carcinoma of the bronchus. *Clin Sci* 31:135, 1966.
11. Baylin SB, et al. Neuroendocrine-related biochemistry in the spectrum of human lung cancers. *Exp Lung Res* 3:209, 1982.
12. Baylin SB, Mendelsohn G. Ectopic (inappropriate) hormone production by tumors: Mechanisms involved and the biological and clinical implications. *Endocr Rev* 1:45, 1980.
13. Becker KL. The Endocrine Lung. In KL Becker (Ed), *Principles and Practice of Endocrinology and Metabolism*. Philadelphia: Lippincott, 1990. Pp 1343–1347.
14. Becker KL, et al. Urine calcitonin levels in patients with bronchogenic carcinoma. *JAMA* 243:670, 1980.
15. Bliss DP, et al. Expression of the atrial natriuretic factor gene in small cell lung cancer tumors and tumor cell lines. *J Am Cancer Inst* 82:305, 1990.
16. Bloom W. Pituitary implications in hypertrophic pulmonary osteoarthropathy. *Ann Intern Med* 29:361, 1948.
17. Body J-J, et al. Dose/response study of aminohydroxypropylidene bisphosphonate in tumor associated hypercalcemia. *Am J Med* 82:957, 1987.
18. Boizel R, et al. Acromegaly due to a growth hormone-releasing hormone-secreting bronchogenic carcinoid tumor: Further information on the abnormal responsiveness of the somatotroph cells and their recovery after successful treatment. *J Clin Endocrinol Metab* 64:304, 1987.
19. Bondy PK, Gilby ED. Endocrine function in small cell undifferentiated carcinoma of the lung. *Cancer* 50:2147, 1982.
20. Bonjour J, Rizzoli R. Clodronate in hypercalcemia of malignancy. *Calcif Tissue Int* 46 (Suppl):S20, 1990.
21. Bonnetblanc JM, Bernard P, Fayol J. Dermatomyositis and malignancy: A multicenter cooperative study. *Dermatologica* 180:212, 1990.
22. Bork E, et al. Early detection of response in small cell bronchogenic carcinoma by changes in serum concentrations of creatine kinase, neuron-specific enolase, calcitonin, ACTH, seratonin and gastrin releasing peptide. *Eur J Cancer Clin Oncol* 24:1033, 1988.
23. Bornstein P, Nolan JP, Bernanke D. Adrenocortical hyperfunction in association with anaplastic carcinoma of the respiratory tract. *N Engl J Med* 264:363, 1961.
24. Bower BF, Mason DM, Forsham PH. Bronchogenic carcinoma with inappropriate antidiuretic activity in plasma and tumor. *N Engl J Med* 271:934, 1964.
25. Braunstein GD, et al. Varying bioactive to immunoreactive ratios of the human chorionic gonadotropin-like substance in normal human tissues. *J Clin Endocrinol Metab* 58:170, 1984.
26. Broadus AE, et al. Humoral hypercalcemia of cancer. *N Engl J Med* 319:556, 1988.
27. Brown MR. Bombesin, somatostatin, and related peptides: Actions on thermoregulation. *Fed Proc* 40:2765, 1981.
28. Brown WH. A case of pluriglandular syndrome: "Diabetes of bearded women." *Lancet* 2:1022, 1928.
29. Bruzzone R, et al. Effects of bombesin on plasma insulin, pancreatic glucagon, and gut glucagon in man. *J Clin Endocrinol Metab* 56:643, 1983.
30. Budayr AA, et al. Increased serum levels of a parathyroid hormone-like protein in malignancy-associated hypercalcemia. *Ann Intern Med* 111:807, 1989.
31. Burstis WJ, et al. Immunochemical characterization of circulating parathyroid hormone-related peptide in patients with humoral hypercalcemia of malignancy. *N Engl J Med* 322:1106, 1990.
32. Callen JP. Skin Signs of Internal Malignancy. In JP Callen (Ed), *Cutaneous Aspects of Internal Disease*. Chicago: Year Book, 1981. P 207.
33. Carney DN, et al. Serum neuron-specific enolase: A marker for disease extent and response to therapy of small-cell lung cancer. *Lancet* 1:583, 1982.

34. Case records of the Massachusetts General Hospital. *N Engl J Med* 270:898, 1964.

35. Cate CC, Pettengill OS, Sorenson GD. Biosynthesis of procalcitonin in small cell carcinoma of the lung. *Cancer Res* 46:812, 1986.

36. Christy NP. Adrenocorticotrophic activity in the plasma of patient with Cushing's syndrome associated with pulmonary neoplasms. *Lancet* 1:85, 1961.

37. Clarke B, Carr AC, Hasleton PS. Malignant hypercalcemia and leukocytosis associated with carcinoma of the bronchus. *Thorax* 38:474, 1983.

38. Coggeshall J, et al. Implications of hypercalcemia with respect to diagnosis and treatment of lung cancer. *Am J Med* 80:325, 1986.

39. Coleridge JCG, Coleridge HM. Cardiovascular afferents involved in regulation of peripheral vessels. *Annu Rev Physiol* 42:413, 1980.

40. Comis RL, Miller M, Ginsberg SJ. Abnormalities in water homeostasis in small cell anaplastic lung cancer. *Cancer* 45:2414, 1980.

41. Coombes RC, et al. Plasma-immunoreactive-calcitonin in patients with nonthyroid tumors. *Lancet* 1:1080, 1974.

42. Cooper T, Barker NW. Recurrent venous thrombosis: Early complications of the obscure visceral carcinoma. *Minn Med* 27:31, 1944.

43. Corson JM, Pinkus GS. Mesothelioma, profile of keratin proteins, and carcioembryonic antigen. An immunoperoxidase study of 20 cases and comparison with pulmonary adenocarcinomas. *Am J Pathol* 108:80, 1982.

44. Croft PB, Wilkinson M. Carcinomatous neuromyopathy: Its incidence in patients with carcinoma of the lung and carcinoma of the breast. *Lancet* 1:184, 1963.

45. Dabek JT. Bronchial tumor with acromegaly in two patients. *J Clin Endocrinol Metab* 38:329, 1974.

46. DeBold CR, et al. Proopiomelanocortin gene is expressed in many normal human tissues and in tumors not associated with ectopic adrenocorticotropin syndrome. *Mol Endocrinol* 2:862, 1988.

47. Deland FH, Kim EE, Goldenberg DM. Lymphoscintography with radionuclide-labelled antigens to carcinoembryonic antigen. *Cancer Res* 40:2984, 1980.

48. Denny-Brown D. Primary sensory neuropathy with muscular changes associated with carcinoma. *J Neurol Neurosurg Psychiatry* II:73, 1948.

49. DeStephano DB, Lloyd RV, Schteingart DE. Cushing's syndrome produced by a bronchial carcinoid tumor. *Hum Pathol* 15:890, 1984.

50. Dorney ER, Fowler NO, Mannix EP. Unilateral clubbing of the fingers due to absence of the aortic arch. *Am J Med* 18:150, 1955.

51. Dropcho EJ. The remote effects of cancer on the nervous system. *Neurol Clin* 7:579, 1989.

52. Edbrooke MR, et al. Expression of the human calcitonin/CGRP gene in lung and thyroid carcinoma. *EMBO J* 4:715, 1985.

53. Ellenbogen BK. Acanthosis nigricans associated with bronchial carcinoma: Report of 2 cases. *Br J Dermatol* 61:251, 1949.

54. Faiman C, et al. Gonadotropin secretion from a bronchogenic carcinoma: Demonstration by radioimmunoassay. *N Engl J Med* 277:1395, 1967.

55. Fatemi S, Singer FR, Rude RK. Effect of salmon calcitonin and etidronate on hypercalcemia of malignancy. *Calif Tissue Int* 50:107, 1992.

56. Fischbach W, Schwarz-Wallrauch C, Jany B. Neuron-specific enolase and thymidine kinase as an aid to diagnosis and treatment monitoring of small-cell lung cancer. *Cancer* 63:1143, 1989.

57. Fisher ER, Baird WF. The nature of arteriolar and capillary occlusion in patients with carcinoma. *Am J Pathol* 32:1185, 1956.

58. Fisher MM, Hochberg LA, Wilensky ND. Recurrent thrombophlebitis in obscure malignant tumor of the lung: Report of 4 cases. *JAMA* 147:1213, 1951.

59. Fountain JR, Holman RL. Acquired fibrinogen deficiency associated with carcinoma of the bronchus. *Ann Intern Med* 52:459, 1960.

60. Frohman LA, et al. Partial purification and characterization of a peptide with growth hormone releasing activity from extrapituitary tumors in patients with acromegaly. *J Clin Invest* 65:43, 1980.

61. Fukiyama M, et al. Human chorionic gonadotropin in lung tumors. Immunochemical study on unbalanced distribution of subunits. *Lab Invest* 55:433, 1986.

62. Fukunaga H, et al. Lambert-Eaton myasthenic syndrome with IgG from man to mouse depletes the presynaptic membrane active zones. *Proc Natl Acad Sci USA* 80:7636, 1983.

63. Gallium nitrate. *Med Lett* 33:41, 1991.

64. Gammel JA. Erythema gyratum repens: Skin manifestations in patients with carcinoma of breast. *Arch Dermatol Syph* 66:494, 1952.

65. George JM, Capen CC, Phillips AS. Bio-synthesis of vasopressin *in vitro* and ultrastructure of bronchogenic carcinoma. Patient with the syndrome of inappropriate secretion of antidiuretic hormone. *J Clin Invest* 51:141, 1972.

66. Gewirtz G, et al. Big-ACTH conversion to biologically active ACTH by trypsin. *J Clin Endocrinol Metab* 38:227, 1974.

67. Gewirtz G, Yalow RS. Ectopic ACTH production in carcinomas of the lung. *J Clin Invest* 53:1022, 1974.

68. Gibbs AR, et al. Comparison of tumor markers in malignant mesothelioma and pulmonary adenocarcinoma. *Thorax* 40:91, 1985.

69. Ginsburg J. Observations on the peripheral circulation in hypertrophic pulmonary osteoarthropathy. *Q J Med* 27:335, 1958.

70. Ginsburg J, Brown JB. Increased oestrogen ex-

ertion in hypertrophic pulmonary osteoarthropathy. *Lancet* 2:1274, 1961.

71. Gislason T, Palmer M, Nou E. Serum calcium in bronchial carcinoma: A population-based study. *Eur J Respir Dis* 70:8, 1987.

72. Goodwin G, et al. Analysis of cell surface proteins delineates a differentiation pathway linking endocrine and nonendocrine human lung cancers. *Proc Natl Acad Sci USA* 80:3807, 1983.

73. Gorden P, et al. Somatostatin and somatostatin analogue (SMNS 201-995) in treatment of hormone-secreting tumors of the pituitary and gastrointestinal tract and non-neoplastic diseases of the gut. *Ann Intern Med* 110:35, 1989.

74. Gore JM, et al. Occult cancer in patients with acute pulmonary embolism. *Ann Intern Med* 96:556, 1982.

75. Gosney MA, Gosney JR, Lye M. Plasma growth hormone and digital clubbing in carcinoma of the bronchus. *Thorax* 45:545, 1990.

76. Gould VE, et al. Neuroendocrine components of the bronchopulmonary tract: Hyperplasias, dysplasias, and neoplasms. *Lab Invest* 49:519, 1983.

77. Greenberg E, Divertie MB, Woolner LB. A review of unusual systemic manifestations associated with carcinoma. *Am J Med* 36:106, 1964.

78. Greenberg PB, et al. Synthesis and release of human growth hormone from lung carcinoma in cell culture. *Lancet* 1:350, 1972.

79. Greer JM, et al. Vasculitis associated with malignancy. Experience with 13 patients and literature review. *Medicine* 67:220, 1988.

80. Gropp C, Havemann K, Scheuer A. Ectopic hormones in lung cancer patients at diagnosis and during therapy. *Cancer* 46:347, 1980.

81. Gropp C, Havemann K, Scheuer A. The use of carcinogenic antigen and peptide hormones to stage and monitor patients with lung cancer. *Int J Radiat Oncol Biol Phys* 6:1047, 1980.

82. Gropp C, Luster W, Havemann K. Salmon and human calcitonin-like material in lung cancer. *Br J Cancer* 51:897, 1985.

83. Gruetter CA, et al. Relaxation of bovine coronary artery and activation of coronary arterial guanine cyclase by nitric oxide, nitroprusside, and a carcinogenic nitrosoamine. *J Cyclic Nucleotide Res* 5:211, 1979.

84. Gucalp R, et al. Comparative study of pamidronate disodium and etidronate disodium in the treatment of cancer-related hypercalcemia. *Clin Oncol* 10:134, 1992.

85. Gutman AB, Tyson TL, Gutman EB. Serum calcium inorganic phosphorus and phosphatase activity in hyperparathyroidism, Paget's disease, multiple myeloma and neoplastic disease of the bones. *Arch Intern Med* 57:379, 1936.

86. Hall GH. The cause of digital clubbing: Testing a new hypothesis. *Lancet* 1:750, 1959.

87. Hamilton BPM, Upton GV, Amatruda TT Jr. Evidence for the presence of neurophysin in tumors producing the syndrome of inappropriate antidiuresis. *J Clin Endocrinol Metab* 35:764, 1972.

88. Hansen M. Paraneoplastic syndromes and tumor markers for small cell and non-small cell lung cancer. *Curr Opin Oncol* 2:345, 1990.

89. Hansen M, Bork E. Peptide hormones in patients with lung cancer. *Recent Results Cancer Res* 99:180, 1985.

90. Hansen M, Hammer M, Hummer L. ACTH, ADH, and calcitonin concentrations as markers of response and relapse in small-cell carcinoma of the lung. *Cancer* 46:2062, 1980.

91. Hansen M, Pedersen AG. Tumor markers in patients with lung cancer. *Chest* 89(Suppl):219S, 1986.

92. Harach HR, Skinner M, Gibbs AR. Biological markers in human lung carcinomas. An immunopathological study of six antigens. *Thorax* 35:937, 1983.

93. Harinck HIJ, et al. Role of bone and kidney in tumor-induced hypercalcemia and its treatment with bisphosphonate and sodium chloride. *Am J Med* 82:1133, 1987.

94. Harris PE, et al. Successful treatment by chemotherapy for acromegaly associated with ectopic growth hormone releasing hormone secretion from a carcinoid tumor. *Clin Endocrinol (Oxf)* 32:315, 321, 1990.

95. Hasling C, Charles P, Moskilde L. Etidronate disodium in the management of malignancy-related hypercalcemia. *Am J Med* 82(Suppl 2A): 51, 1987.

96. Havemann K, et al. Peptide production associated with small cell lung cancer. *Recent Results Cancer Res* 97:65, 1985.

97. Hawley RJ, et al. The carcinomatous neuromyopathy of oat cell lung cancer. *Ann Neurol* 7:65, 1980.

98. Hayward ML, et al. Hypercalcemia complicating small cell carcinoma. *Cancer* 48:1643, 1981.

99. Henson RA, Russell DS, Wilkinson M. Carcinomatous neuropathy and myopathy: A clinical and pathologic study. *Brain* 77:82, 1954.

100. Hildebrand J. Signs, symptoms, and significance of paraneoplastic neurological syndromes. *Oncology* 3:57, 1989.

101. Holden J, Churg A. Immunohistochemical staining for keratin and carcinoembryonic antigen in the diagnosis of malignant mesothelioma. *Lab Invest* 50:26A, 1984.

102. Holling HE, Brodey RS, Boland HC. Pulmonary hypertrophic osteoarthropathy. *Lancet* 2:1269, 1961.

103. Hoppener JWM, et al. Detection of mRNA encoding calcitonin, calcitonin gene related peptide and proopiomelanocortin in human tumors. *Mol Cell Endocrinol* 47:125, 1986.

104. Hovenden AL. Acquired hypertrichosis lanuginosa associated with malignancy. *Arch Intern Med* 147:2013, 1987.

105. Jacobs T, et al. Neoplastic hypercalcemia: Phys-

iologic response to intravenous etidronate disodium. *Am J Med* 82(Suppl 2A):42, 1987.

106. Jaques G, et al. Prognostic value of pretreatment carcinoembryonic antigen, neuron-specific enolase, and creatine kinase-BB levels in sera of patients with small-cell lung cancer. *Cancer* 62:125, 1988.

107. Jorgensen LGM, et al. The prognostic influence of serum neuron-specific enolase in small cell lung cancer. *Br J Cancer* 58:805, 1988.

108. Kao PC, et al. Parathyroid hormone-related peptide in plasma of patients with hypercalcemia and malignant lesions. *Mayo Clin Proc* 65:1399, 1990.

109. Kasurinen J, Syrjanen KJ. Peptide hormone reactivity and prognosis in small-cell carcinoma of the lung. *Respiration* 49:61, 1986.

110. Kirschner MA, Cohen FB, Jesperson D. Estrogen production and its origin in men with gonadotropin-producing neoplasms. *J Clin Endocrinol Metab* 39:112, 1974.

111. Kodama T, et al. Large cell carcinoma of the lung associated with marked eosinophilia. *Cancer* 54:2313, 1984.

112. Kohler PC, Trump DL. Ectopic hormone syndromes. *Cancer Invest* 4:543, 1986.

113. Krauss S, Macy S, Ichiki AT. A study of immunoreactive calcitonin (CT), adrenocorticotropic hormone (ACTH) and carcinoembryonic antigen (CEA) in lung cancer and other malignancies. *Cancer* 47:2485, 1981.

114. Kukreja SC, et al. Elevated nephrogenous cyclic AMP with normal serum parathyroid hormone levels in patients with lung cancer. *J Clin Endocrinol Metab* 51:167, 1980.

115. Kvols LK, et al. Treatment of the malignant carcinoid syndrome. Evaluation of a long-acting somatostatin analogue. *N Engl J Med* 315:663, 1986.

116. Kyle CV, Evans MC, Odell WD. Growth hormone-like material in normal human tissues. *J Clin Endocrinol Metab* 53:1138, 1981.

117. Lalau JD, et al. A case of pseudo-Nelson's syndrome: Cure of ACTH hypersecretion by removal of a bronchial carcinoid tumor responsible for Cushing's syndrome. *J Endocrinol Invest* 13:531, 1990.

118. Lamberts WJ, Kreunning EP, Reubi J-C. The role of somatostatin and its analogs in the diagnosis and treatment of tumors. *Endocr Rev* 12:450, 1991.

119. Lee J, Jones JJ, Barraclough MA. Inappropriate secretion of vasopressin. *Lancet*. 2:792, 1964.

120. Leung FW, Williams AJ, Fan P. Indomethacin therapy for hypertrophic pulmonary osteoarthropathy in patients with bronchogenic carcinoma. *West J Med* 142:345, 1985.

121. Leys K, et al. Calcium channel antibodies in Lambert-Eaton myasthenic syndrome. *Lancet* 2:1107, 1989.

122. Liddle GW, et al. Cushing's syndrome caused by recurrent malignant bronchial carcinoid. *Arch Intern Med* 111:471, 1963.

123. Liddle GW, et al. Clinical and laboratory studies of ectopic hormones. *Rec Prog Horm Res* 25:283, 1969.

124. Lieberman JS, et al. Thrombophlebitis and cancer. *JAMA* 177:542, 1961.

125. List AF, et al. The syndrome of inappropriate secretion of antidiuretic hormone (SIADH) in small-cell cancer. *J Clin Oncol* 4:1191, 1986.

126. Logan JS, et al. Changes in hand circulation in a case of pulmonary osteoarthropathy. *Ir J Med Sci* 6:127, 1954.

127. Luster W, et al. *Recent Results Cancer Res* 99:117, 1985.

128. Luster W, et al. Demonstration of immunoreactive calcitonin in sera and tissues of lung cancer patients. *Eur J Cancer Clin Oncol* 18:1275, 1982.

129. MacDonald RA, Robbins SL. The significance of nonbacterial thrombotic endocarditis: An autopsy and clinical study of 78 cases. *Ann Intern Med* 117:57, 1966.

130. Maier HC, Barr D. Intrathoracic tumors associated with hypoglycemia. *J Thorac Cardiovasc Surg* 44:321, 1962.

131. Malchoff CD, et al. Ectopic ACTH syndrome caused by a bronchial carcinoid tumor responsive to dexamethasone, metyrapone and corticotropin-releasing factor. *Am J Med* 84:760, 1988.

132. Marie P. De l'osteo-arthropathie hypertrophilante pneumique. *Rev Med (Paris)* 10:1, 1890.

133. Martin TJ, Suva LJ. Parathyroid hormone-related protein in hypercalcemia of malignancy. *Clin Endocrinol (Oxf)* 31:631, 1989.

134. Maton PN. The Carcinoid Tumor and the Carcinoid Syndrome. In KL Becker (Ed), *Principles and Practice of Endocrinology and Metabolism*. Philadelphia: Lippincott, 1990. Pp 1640–1643.

135. Mauer LH, et al. Human neurophysins in carcinoma of the lung: Relation to histology, disease stage, response rate, survival, and syndrome of inappropriate antidiuretic hormone secretion. *Cancer Treat Rep* 76:971, 1983.

136. McLean DJ, Haynes HA. Cutaneous Manifestations Associated with Malignant Internal Disease. In TB Fitzpatrick, et al (Eds), *Dermatology in General Medicine* (3rd ed). New York: McGraw-Hill, 1987.

137. Melmed S, et al. Medical management of acromegaly due to ectopic production of growth hormone-releasing hormone by a carcinoid tumor. *J Clin Endocrinol Metab* 67:395, 1988.

138. Merrill WW, Bondy PK. Production of biochemical marker substances by bronchogenic carcinomas. *Clin Chest Med* 3:307, 1982.

139. Metzler C, Flink EB. Adrenal cortical hyperfunction associated with metastatic carcinoma. *Lancet (Minn)* 76:242, 1956.

140. Miller A, et al. Studies of the anemia and iron metabolism in cancer. *J Clin Invest* 35:1248, 1956.

141. Mundy GR. Incidence and pathophysiology of hypercalcemia. *Calcif Tissue Int* 46(Suppl):G3, 1990.

142. Nelkin BD, et al. Structure and expression of a gene encoding human calcitonin and calcitonin gene related peptide. *Biochem Biophys Res Commun* 123:648, 1984.

143. Nusbacher J. Migratory venous thrombosis and cancer: Mechanisms and clinical manifestations. *Prog Clin Cancer* 3:151, 1967.

144. Odell WD. Humoral Manifestations of Cancer. In JD Wilson, DW Foster (Eds), *Williams Textbook of Endocrinology.* Philadelphia: Saunders, 1981. Chap. 36.

145. Odell WD, Wolfsen AR. Ectopic Hormone Secretion by Tumors. In F Becker (Ed), *Cancer. A Comprehensive Treatise.* New York: Plenum, 1975. P 81.

146. Odell WD, et al. Ectopic production of lipotropin by cancer. *Am J Med* 66:631, 1979.

147. Odell WD, Wolfsen AR, Yoshimoto Y. Ectopic peptide synthesis: A universal concomitant of neoplasia. *Trans Assoc Am Physicians* 40:204, 1977.

148. Ogilvie H. Large intestine colic due to sympathetic deprivation, a new clinical syndrome. *Br Med J* 2:671, 1948.

149. Oh SJ, Slaughter R, Harrell L. Paraneoplastic vasculitic neuropathy: A treatable neuropathy. *Muscle Nerve* 14:152, 1991.

150. O'Neill JH, Murray NMF, Newson-Davis J. The Lambert-Eaton myasthenic syndrome. *Brain* 111:577, 1988.

151. O'Riordan JLH, et al. Corticotrophin-secreting carcinomas. *Q J Med* 35:137, 1966.

152. Orth DN. Ectopic Hormone Production. In P Felig, JD Baxter, AE Broadus, LA Frohman (Eds). *Endocrinology and Metabolism.* New York: McGraw-Hill, 1981. Chap. 27.

153. Pamidronate. *Med Lett* 34:1, 1992.

154. Pearse AGE. The cytochemistry and ultrastructure of polypeptide hormone producing cells of the APUD series and the embryologic, physiologic, and pathologic implications of the concept. *J Histochem Cytochem* 17:303, 1969.

155. Pederson AG, et al. Cerebrospinal fluid vasopressin as a marker of central nervous system metastases from small-cell bronchogenic carcinoma. *J Clin Oncol* 3:48, 1985.

156. Pedersen AG, et al. Cerebrospinal fluid ACTH as a marker of central nervous system metastases from small cell carcinoma of the lung. *Cancer* 56:2476, 1985.

157. Penman E, et al. Somatostatin secretion by lung and thymic tumors. *Clin Endocrinol (Oxf)* 13:613, 1980.

158. Pinea GF, et al. Tumors, mucus production, and hypercoagulability. *Ann NY Acad Sci* 230:262, 1974.

159. Pineda CJ, et al. The skeletal manifestations of clubbing: A study in patients with cyanotic congenital heart disease and hypertrophic osteoarthropathy. *Semin Arthritis Rheum* 14:263, 1985.

160. Pineda CJ, et al. Periostitis in hypertrophic osteoarthropathy. *AJR* 148:773, 1987.

161. Polak JM, Bloom SR. Neuropeptides of the gut; a newly discovered major control system. *World J Surg* 3:393, 1979.

162. Posner JB, Furneaux HM. Paraneoplastic Syndromes. In BH Waksman (Ed), *Immunologic Mechanisms in Neurologic and Psychiatric Disease.* New York: Raven, 1990. Pp 187–215.

163. Powell D, et al. Nonparathyroid hypercalcemia in patients with neoplastic diseases. *N Engl J Med* 289:176, 1974.

164. Price J, et al. Characterization of bombesin-like immunoreactivity in human fetal lung. *Regul Pept* 7:315, 1983.

165. Rajfer J, et al. Nitric oxide as a mediator of relaxation of the corpus cavernosum in response to nonadrenergic, noncholinergic neurotransmission. *N Engl J Med* 326:90, 1992.

166. Rees LH, Ratcliffe JG. Ectopic hormone production by non-endocrine tumors. *Clin Endocrinol (Oxf)* 3:263, 1974.

167. Reichlin S. Somatostatin. *N Engl J Med* 309: 1495, 1556, 1983.

168. Reith P, Monnot EA, Bathija PJ. Prolonged suppression of a corticotropin-producing bronchial carcinoid by oral bromocriptine. *Arch Intern Med* 147:989, 1987.

169. Richardson GE, Johnson BE. Paraneoplastic syndromes in thoracic malignancies. *Curr Opin Oncol* 3:320, 1991.

170. Richardson JB, Callen JP. Dermatomyositis and malignancy. *Med Clin North Am* 73:1211, 1989.

171. Rigel DS, Jacobs MI. Malignant acanthosis nigricans: A review. *J Dermatol Surg Oncol* 6:923, 1980.

172. Riley JH, Edbrooke MR, Craig RK. Ectopic synthesis of high-Mr calcitonin by the BEN lung carcinoma cell line reflects aberrant proteolytic processing. *FEBS Lett* 198:71, 1986.

173. Roos BA, et al. Plasma immunoreactive calcitonin in lung cancer. *J Clin Endocrinol Metab* 50:659, 1980.

174. Roth KA, et al. Gastrin-releasing peptide-related peptides in a human malignant lung carcinoid tumor. *Cancer Res* 43:5411, 1983.

175. Russell PJ, O'Mara SM, Raghavan D. Ectopic hormone production by small cell undifferentiated carcinomas. *Mol Cell Endocrinol* 71:1, 1990.

176. Said SE. Evidence for secretion of vasoactive intestinal peptide by tumors of the pancreas,

adrenal medulla, thyroid and lung: Support for the unifying APUD concept. *Clin Endocrinol (Oxf)* 5(Suppl):201, 1983.

177. Saito ER, Odell WD. Corticotropin/lipotropin common precursor-like material in normal rat extrapituitary tissues. *Proc Natl Acad Sci USA* 80:3792, 1983.

178. Samaan NA, et al. Serum calcitonin after pentagastrin stimulation in patients with bronchogenic in breast cancer compared to that in patients with medullary thyroid carcinoma. *J Clin Endocrinol Metab* 51:237, 1980.

179. Scheinman SJ, Mitnick ME, Steewart AF. Quantitative evaluation of anticalciuretic effects of synthetic parathyroid hormonelike peptides. *J Bone Miner Res* 5:653, 1990.

180. Schmelzer HJ, Hesch RD, Mayer H. Parathyroid hormone and PTH mRNA in a small cell lung cancer. In K Havemann, G Sorenson, C Gropp (Eds), *Peptide Hormones in Lung Cancer.* Berlin: Springer-Verlag, 1985. P 83.

181. Scholte AJ. Ein Fall von Angioma Telangectaticum Cutis mit chronischer Endocarditis und malignum Dunndarmcarcinoid. *Beitr Pathol Anat* 86:440, 1931.

182. Schteingart DE, et al. Cushing's syndrome secondary to ectopic corticotropin-releasing hormone-adrenocorticotropin secretion. *J Clin Endocrinol Metab* 63:770, 1986.

183. Schuffler MD, et al. Intestinal pseudoobstruction as the presenting manifestation of small cell carcinoma of the lung: A paraneoplastic neuropathy of the gastrointestinal tract. *Ann Intern Med* 98:129, 1983.

184. Schwartz KE, Wolfsen A, Forster B. Calcitonin in nonthyroidal cancer. *J Clin Endocrinol Metab* 49:438, 1979.

185. Schwartz WB, Tassel D, Bartter FC. Further observations of hyponatremia and renal sodium loss probably resulting from inappropriate secretion of antidiuretic hormone. *N Engl J Med* 262:743, 1960.

186. Segal AM, Mackenzie AH. Hypertrophic osteoarthropathy: A 10 year retrospective analysis. *Semin Arthritis Rheum* 12:220, 1982.

187. Shepherd FA, et al. Ketoconazole: Use in the treatment of ectopic adrenocorticotropic hormone production and Cushing's syndrome in small-cell lung cancer. *Arch Intern Med* 145:863, 1985.

188. Sheppard MN, et al. Immunocytochemical localization of neuron specific enolase in small cell carcinomas and carcinoid tumors of the lung. *Histopathology* 8:171, 1984.

189. Sheth NA, et al. Circulating levels of inhibin in cancer. *Neoplasma* 31:3, 1984.

190. Shevrin DH, et al. Treatment of cancer-associated hypercalcemia with mithramycin and oral etidronate disodium. *Clin Pharm* 4:204, 1985.

191. Shineerson JM. Digital clubbing and hypertrophic osteoarthropathy: The underlying mechanisms. *Br J Dis Chest* 75:113, 1981.

192. Sieber SC, et al. Three opportunistic infections associated with ectopic corticotropin syndrome. *Arch Intern Med* 149:2589, 1989.

193. Sigurgeirsson B, et al. Risk of cancer in patients with dermatomyositis or polymyositis. *N Engl J Med* 326:363, 1992.

194. Silva OL, et al. Hypercalcitonemia in bronchogenic cancer: Evidence for thyroid origin of the hormone. *JAMA* 234:183, 1975.

195. Simpson EL, et al. Absence of parathyroid hormone messenger RNA in nonparathyroid tumors associated with hypercalcemia. *N Engl J Med* 309:325, 1983.

196. Singer FR, et al. Treatment of hypercalcemia of malignancy with intravenous etidronate. *Arch Intern Med* 151:471, 1991.

197. Skrabanek P, McPartlin J, Powell D. Tumor hypercalcemia and "ectopic parathyroidism." *Medicine* 59:262, 1980.

198. Sodhi N, et al. Autonomic function and motility in intestinal pseudoobstruction caused by paraneoplastic syndrome. *Dig Dis Sci* 34:1937, 1989.

199. Soenkson PH, et al. Acromegaly caused by bronchial carcinoid tumors. *Clin Endocrinol (Oxf)* 5:503, 1976.

200. Sons HU. Pulmonary embolism and cancer; predisposition to venous thrombosis and embolism as a paraneoplastic syndrome. *J Surg Oncol* 40:100, 1989.

201. Sparagana M, et al. Ectopic growth hormone syndrome associated with lung cancer. *Metabolism* 20:730, 1971.

202. Stein HB, Little HA. Localized hypertrophic osteoarthropathy in the presence of an abdominal aortic prosthesis. *Can Med J Assoc* 118:947, 1978.

203. Steiner H, Dahlback O, Waldenstrom J. Ectopic growth hormone production and osteoarthropathy in carcinoma of the bronchus. *Lancet* 1:783, 1968.

204. Stewart AF, et al. Identification of adenylate cyclase-stimulating activity and cytochemical glucose-6-phosphate dehydrogenase-stimulating activity in extracts of tumors from patients with humoral hypercalcemia of malignancy. *Proc Natl Acad Sci USA* 80:1454, 1983.

205. Strickland NJ, Bold AM, Medd WE. Bronchial carcinoma with hypercalcaemia simulating cerebral metastases. *Br Med J* 3:590, 1967.

206. Strott CA, Nugent CA, Tyler FH. Cushing's syndrome caused by bronchial adenomas. *Am J Med* 44:97, 1968.

207. Suda T, et al. Ectopic adrenocorticotropin syndrome caused by lung cancer that responded to corticotropin-releasing hormone. *J Clin Endocrinol Metab* 63:1047, 1986.

208. Szabo M, et al. Ectopic production of somatostatin-like immuno- and bioactivity by cultured

human pulmonary small cell carcinoma. *J Clin Endocrinol Metab* 51:978, 1980.

209. Tabassian AR, et al. Evidence for cigarette smoke-induced calcitonin secretion from lungs of man and hamster. *Life Sci* 42:2323, 1988.

210. Thiebaud D, Jacqunet AF, Burckhardt P. Fast and effective treatment of malignant hypercalcemia. *Arch Int Med* 150:2125, 1990.

211. Thiebaud D, Jaeger P, Burckhardt P. Response to treatment of malignant hypercalcemia with the bisphosphonate AHPrBP (APD): Respective role of kidney and bone. *J Bone Miner Res* 5:221, 1990.

212. Thorson A, et al. Malignant carcinoid of the small intestine with metastases to the liver, valvular disease of the right side of the heart (pulmonary stenosis and tricuspid regurgitation without septal defects), peripheral vasomotor symptoms, bronchoconstriction, and an unusual type of cyanosis: A clinical and pathologic syndrome. *Am Heart J* 47:795, 1954.

213. Thurlimann B, et al. Plicamycin and pamidronate in symptomatic tumor-related hypercalcemia: a prospective randomized crossover trial. *Ann Oncol* 3:619, 1992.

214. Touyz R, Plitt M, Rumbak M. Hypoglycemia associated with a lung mass. *Chest* 89:289, 1986.

215. Track N, Cutz E. Bombesin-like immunoreactivity in developing human lung. *Life Sci* 30:1553, 1982.

216. Trousseau A. Phlegmasia alba dolens. In *Clinique Medicale de l'Hotel Dieu de Paris* vol 3. Paris: JB Balliese, 1868. P 95.

217. Trump BF, et al. Preneoplasia and neoplasia of the bronchus, esophagus, and colon: The use of markers in determining phenotypes and classification. *Monogr Pathol* 26:101, 1985.

218. Turkington RW. Ectopic production of prolactin. *N Engl J Med* 285:1455, 1971.

219. Upton GV, Amatruda TT Jr. Evidence for the presence of tumor peptides with corticotropin-releasing factor-like activity in the ectopic ACTH syndrome. *N Engl J Med* 285:419, 1971.

220. uz Zafar MS, et al. Acromegaly associated with a bronchial carcinoid tumor: Evidence for ectopic production of growth hormone-releasing activity. *J Clin Endocrinol Metab* 48:66, 1979.

221. Vieau D, et al. Corticotropin-like intermediary lobe peptide as a marker of alternate pro-opiomelanocortin processing in ACTH-producing non-pituitary tumors. *Clin Endocrinol (Oxf)* 31:691, 1989.

222. Vincent A, Lang B, Newsom-Davis J. Autoimmunity to the voltage-gated calcium channel underlies the Lambert-Eaton myasthenic syndrome, a paraneoplastic disorder. *Trends Neurosci* 12:496, 1989.

223. Vladutiu AO, Brason FW, Adler RH. Differential diagnosis of pleural effusions: Clinical usefulness of cell marker quantitation. *Chest* 79:297, 1981.

224. Wahlstrom T, Seppala M. Immunological evidence for the occurrence of luteinizing hormone-releasing factor and the alpha subunit of glycoprotein hormones in carcinoid tumors. *J Clin Endocrinol Metab* 53:209, 1981.

225. Warrell RP. Clinical trials of gallium nitrate in patients with cancer-related hypercalcemia. *Sem Oncol* 18:26, 1991.

226. Warrell RP, et al. Gallium nitrate for acute treatment of cancer-related hypercalcemia. *Ann Intern Med* 108:669, 1988.

227. Wessler S, Yin ET. Experimental hypercoagulable state induced by factor X: Comparison of the activated and nonactivated forms. *J Lab Clin Med* 72:256, 1968.

228. White A, Clarj AJL, Stewart MF. The synthesis of ACTH and related peptides by tumours. *Ballieres Clin Endocrinol Metab* 4:1, 1990.

229. Wierman WH, Clagett OT, McDonald JR. Articular manifestations in pulmonary diseases: An analysis of their occurrence in 1,024 cases in which pulmonary resection was performed. *JAMA* 155:1459, 1954.

230. Williams RC Jr. Dermatomyositis and malignancy: A review of the literature. *Ann Intern Med* 50:1174, 1959.

231. Wilson GM. Local circulatory changes associated with clubbing of fingers and toes. *Q J Med* 21:201, 1952.

232. Wilson TS, et al. Elaboration of human chorionic gonadotropin by lung tumors. *Arch Pathol Lab Med* 105:169, 1981.

233. Winkelmann RK. Dermatologic clinics: I. Comments on pruritus related to systemic disease. *Mayo Clin Proc* 36:187, 1961.

234. Winkler AW, Crankshaw OF. Chloride depletion in conditions other than Addison's disease. *J Clin Invest* 17:1, 1938.

235. Wolfsen AR, Odell WD. Pro-ACTH: Use for early detection of lung cancer. *Am J Med* 66:765, 1979.

236. Yoshimoto Y, Wolfsen AR, Odell WD. Human chorionic gonadotropin-like substance in non-endocrine tissues of normal subjects. *Science* 197:575, 1977.

237. Yoshimoto Y, Wolfsen AR, Odell WD. Glycosylation: A variable in hCG production by cancers. *Am J Med* 76:414, 1979.

238. Yoshimoto K, et al. Ectopic production of parathyroid hormone by small cell lung cancer in a patient with hypercalcemia. *J Clin Endocrinol Metab* 68:976, 1989.

239. Zarate A, et al. ACTH and CRF-producing bronchial carcinoid associated with Cushing's syndrome. *Clin Endocrinol (Oxf)* 24:699, 1986.

240. Zondek H, Petow H, Siebert W. Die Bedeutung der Kalzium Bestimmung im Blut fur Diagnose der Niereninsuffizienz. *Z Klin Med* 99:129, 1924.

IX

Pulmonary Manifestations in Systemic Diseases

As well as being subject to assault and damage from inhaled substances and organisms in the atmosphere, the respiratory system, perhaps more often than any other organ system, frequently bears the brunt of injury initiated by diseases that are primarily nonpulmonary in origin. In many of these diseases, pulmonary manifestations are the first indication of multisystem disease. The mechanisms by which such involvement occurs are almost as diverse as the diseases themselves.

The most common and best-documented mechanism of lung injury is the inhalation of pathogenetic substances including dusts, gases, smoke, microorganisms, and various types of antigens and chemicals. Injuries arising from these usually appear in the conducting airways or pulmonary parenchyma as infections, bronchitis, emphysema, asthma, bronchogenic carcinoma, malignant mesothelioma, or pneumoconioses.

Changes in the lung vasculature may accompany widespread disease of the systemic blood vessels or be caused by various pulmonary or extrapulmonary conditions. Leakage of protein molecules or red blood cells from capillaries into the extravascular and alveolar spaces can occur by mechanisms that are not well understood. This is exemplified by the intraalveolar hemorrhage of Goodpasture's syndrome, in which circulating anti–basement membrane antibody is present, and the alveolar bleeding is a dramatic indication of underlying glomerulonephritis. A second example is the nonhydrostatic pulmonary edema of the respiratory distress syndrome, which may be due to a wide variety of insults ranging from the hypoperfusion of the shock state to amniotic fluid embolism and pancreatitis. In contrast, the intraalveolar hemorrhage of Wegener's granulomatosis, systemic lupus erythematosus, and hypersensitivity angiitis results from the necrotizing vasculitis of small vessels, which occurs in these diseases as part of the damage caused by deposition of circulating immune complexes. Auscultatory and roentgenographic changes due to pulmonary arteriovenous fistulas may be early indications of hereditary hemorrhagic telangiectasia, and bleeding from the lesions can be severe enough to threaten life. Chemical mediators produced at a nonpulmonary site may enter pulmonary circulation and cause respiratory problems, as exemplified by the bronchospasm noted in patients with extrapulmonary carcinoid that produces serotonin.

The lung interstitium is involved in a number of heritable diseases. Defective collagen synthesis is believed to be a significant factor in the abnormalities of the Marfan and Ehlers-Danlos syndromes, and in both disorders tissue fragility may predispose to spontaneous pneumothorax. In some cases of tuberous sclerosis, smooth muscle replaces normal alveolar interstitial tissue to such an extent that gas exchange is rendered ineffective and irreversible respiratory failure is produced. Interstitial fibrosis observed in collagen disorders such as rheumatoid arthritis, scleroderma, and polymyositis may have underlying autoimmune mechanisms.

More commonly, the lung parenchyma is a site of pathologic changes that represent infiltration by acquired disease processes. Prominent among these are the lymphoproliferative disorders, characterized by multiplication and aberration of lymphocytes and histiocytes, and their precursors and derivatives. Similar mechanisms are responsible for lung involvement in uncommon diseases such as eosinophilic granuloma, Gaucher's disease, and plasma cell dyscrasia. Diffuse infiltrative changes, both microscopic and roentgenographic, occur in acute and chronic leukemias, whether lymphocytic or nonlymphocytic. More nodular changes are seen in the tumor masses of Hodgkin's and non-Hodgkin's lymphomas, but pulmonary involvement by myeloma or Waldenström's macroglobulinemia is distinctly rare. These conditions and histiocytosis X, whose generic designation covers several patterns of histiocytosis, lack specific radiographic features that would permit ready diagnosis in the absence of microscopic proof. In all of them, pulmonary involvement may be an early or late feature. These statements are also true of the noncaseous granulomas of sarcoidosis, which may be recognized first in lung parenchyma without the presence of the characteristic hilar and paratracheal adenopathy. In both these diseases, deposition of collagen often follows the inflammatory changes in the lungs, which are themselves only one part of a more generalized process. A similar progression can occur from a hypersensitivity or dose-related lung reaction to certain drugs.

The pulmonary system is the most common site of infection in immunosuppressed patients. Not infrequently, respiratory infection may alert the clinician to the possibility of immunosuppression. Pneumocystic pneumonia, for instance, in patients with undiagnosed acquired immunodeficiency syndrome (AIDS), may alert the clinician to the possibility of underlying disease. In patients with sickle cell anemia, there is a high incidence of pulmonary infection by streptococci. The pathogenesis has been attributed to impaired splenic function and concomitant pulmonary damage due to vaso-occlusion by abnormal erythrocytes.

The lungs may be affected in an unusual manner, as exemplified by the neurogenic pulmonary edema following damage to the brain, aspiration penumonia as a result of incompetent lower esophageal sphincter, respiratory distress syndrome following acute pancreatitis, or pulmonary calcification noted in patients on long-term hemodialysis.

Even in a single disease entity, there can be a multitude of intrathoracic manifestations. In rheumatoid arthritis, for example, the pulmonary system may demonstrate any or many of the following: pleural effusion, pulmonary nodules, interstitial pneumonitis and fibrosis, laryngeal nodules, bronchiolitis obliterans, or pulmonary vasculitis. The examples provided in the following chapters are not exhaustive but are sufficient to illustrate that the respiratory system provides a valuable indication of the presence and progress of many important systemic diseases. The diseases and chapters are arranged on the basis of subspecialty orientation in the practice of internal medicine. Many diseases overlap subspecialty or organ-system boundaries. These are included under the subspecialty area where they are commonly handled in clinical practice. The chapters on rheumatologic diseases and vasculitides are new additions to this section. I gratefully acknowledge my colleague and friend Thomas V. Colby, MD, for providing many of the photomicrographs.

Udaya B. S. Prakash

57

Rheumatologic Diseases

Udaya B. S. Prakash

The terms *rheumatologic diseases, connective tissue diseases, collagenoses,* and *autoimmune diseases* are employed synonymously in clinical medicine. As a group, the rheumatologic diseases have no known etiologic factors, even though the inflammatory process in most of these diseases is immunologically mediated, as displayed by the presence of autoantibodies, rheumatoid factor, immune complexes, elevated erythrocyte sedimentation rate, and certain clinical characteristics. For the most part, the histologic changes are nonspecific in all the rheumatologic diseases. These diseases are a diverse group of disorders generally involving multiple organs by various degrees of inflammation. In disorders such as systemic lupus erythematosus, multiple criteria are used to make the diagnosis [44,226,229]. Although secondary vasculitis is present in the pathologic specimens obtained from patients with these disorders, they are not usually considered primary vasculitides. At times, however, it becomes difficult to separate the vasculitides from rheumatologic diseases.

In each rheumatologic disorder, it is common to see one major organ system affected to a greater extent than others. It is not uncommon to see pulmonary manifestation as the presenting symptom or sign in many of these disorders; pulmonary aspects often assume a major role [112,242]. This chapter will describe the pulmonary manifestations observed in rheumatoid arthritis (RA), systemic lupus erythematosus (SLE), scleroderma or progressive systemic sclerosis (PSS), polymyositis-dermatomyositis (PM-DM), mixed connective tissue disease (MCTD), Sjögren's syndrome, and relapsing polychondritis (RPC). For detailed definitions, criteria for classification, and nonpulmonary manifestations of various rheumatologic diseases, the reader is referred to a standard textbook of rheumatology or

the *Primer on Rheumatic Diseases* published by the Arthritis Foundation [198].

Systemic Lupus Erythematosus

SLE is a disease of unknown etiology characterized by immunologically mediated inflammation that affects multiple organs, including the skin, musculoskeletal, renal, and central nervous systems, and by the presence of multiple autoantibodies in the serum. Clinical criteria necessary to establish the diagnosis of SLE have been published by the American Rheumatologic Association [121]. Pleuropulmonary complications occur in 50 to 60 percent of patients with SLE, a higher percentage than in any other rheumatologic disease [112,230]. Intrathoracic manifestations of SLE include pleurisy with or without pleural effusion, lupus pneumonitis, atelectatic pneumonitis, interstitial pneumonitis and fibrosis, pulmonary hemorrhage, diaphragmatic dysfunction, infections, pulmonary edema, obstructive lung disease, and pulmonary vasculitis. Histopathologic abnormalities in pleuropulmonary tissues are nonspecific [96]. Many of the pathologic lesions are not caused by SLE itself but by secondary factors, such as congestive cardiac failure, infection, aspiration, and drug-induced pulmonary complications [96].

Pleural Involvement

Pleurisy is the most common and often the presenting manifestation of SLE and has been found in 50 to 83 percent of patients at necropsy [56,84]. Nonspecific pathologic changes in the pleura include infiltration by lymphocytes, mononuclear cells, and plasma cells, along with various degrees of fibrosis [14,186,230,231]. Painful pleurisy occurs in 41 to 51 percent of patients, and pleuritic pain may be the first symptom in many [187,246]. All young women who present with the new onset of pleurisy or pleural effusion should be evaluated for SLE. Another important differential diagnosis in such patients is the possibility of pulmonary embolism, because patients with SLE are at higher risk of thromboembolic phenomena. Pleuritic pain may be unilateral or bilateral and is usually located at the costophrenic margins. Pleural effusions usually are small to moderate, bilateral in nearly 50 percent of patients, occasionally associated with small pericardial effusion, and frequently accompanied by dyspnea, cough, and fever (Fig. 57-1) [76]. Massive effusions are rare in SLE [76,94,246]. The pleural effusions may occur as a complication of lupus-induced nephrotic syndrome or an infectious process.

Thoracentesis often is not necessary unless the cause of pleural effusion is uncertain. The pleural fluid is clear or serosanguineous [76,246]; grossly bloody effusions are uncommon [163,177]. The fluid is almost always an exudate with varying numbers of leukocytes. The differential leukocyte count in SLE-associated pleural effusion is nonspecific [32,76]. The glucose level in patients with SLE is usually normal (greater than 60 mg/dl) or high [32,76,111]. Decreased levels of total hemolytic complement as well as of C3 and C4 components, and increased immune complexes in the pleural fluid have been used as diagnostic

Fig. 57-1. Chest roentgenogram demonstrates a large pericardial effusion, blunting of left costophrenic angle, and patchy pulmonary infiltrates in a patient with systemic lupus erythematosus.

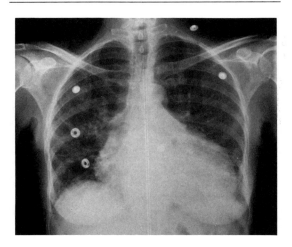

tests of SLE-related pleurisy. Decreased levels and, occasionally, undetectable levels of complement components, observed in nearly 80 percent of lupus effusions, have been used to corroborate the diagnosis of lupus pleuritis, but they are not diagnostic because similar findings have been described in rheumatoid pleural effusion and other disorders [17,76,88,110,111]. The presence of antinuclear antibody in the pleural fluid is nondiagnostic [187]. Likewise, the nature of immune complexes in SLE-induced pleural effusion is unclear. Lupus erythematosus cells have been found in zero to more than 85 percent of lupus effusions [17,32,76,175]. The presence of in vivo lupus cells in pleural effusion (but not in blood) is characteristic of SLE and has not been described in other conditions except in drug-induced SLE [32,64,76,175], in which pleural effusions are also common [111].

Acute Lupus Pneumonitis

Although the clinical syndrome of acute lupus pneumonitis has been described in several publications [29,147,178,179,199], it is distinctly uncommon. In two large series of 150 and 207 patients, the incidence of acute lupus pneumonia was 9.3 and 1.4 percent, respectively [51,137]. The immediate postpartum period is considered to be a time of increased risk for acute lupus pneumonitis [133,165,242]. This disorder is characterized by acute onset of dyspnea, high fever, and cough with occasional hemoptysis. Physical findings are minimal unless hypoxia is severe enough to cause cyanosis. Leukocytosis, an elevated erythrocyte sedimentation rate, and significant hypoxemia may be apparent. Chest roentgenograms may reveal unilateral or bilateral localized, diffuse, or patchy lung infiltrates, predominantly in the lower-lung zones with small pleural effusions (Fig. 57-2). Histologically, lupus pneumonitis reveals nonspecific changes that may include interstitial pneumonia, edema, and arteriolar thrombi. Vasculitis of major vessels is uncommon [96, 112,147,197,230]. Culture of lung tissue for pathogenic organisms is negative; however, because infections and other nonspecific pulmonary parenchymal abnormalities are more common in these patients, the diagnosis of lupus pneumonitis is one of exclusion [113,147,179,186].

Pulmonary Hemorrhage

Pulmonary hemorrhage is a rare but often fatal manifestation of SLE. A Mayo Clinic study in

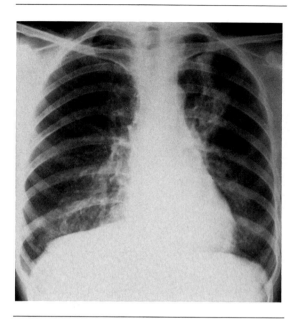

Fig. 57-2. Lupus pneumonitis involving left upper-lobe segment. This entity is very rare.

1955 reported a high incidence of pulmonary hemorrhage discovered during autopsy examinations of patients with SLE [186]. However, the clinical significance of this has been recognized only during the past decade [35,48,77,144,158, 159]. Even though pulmonary hemorrhage was observed in 1.6 percent of 750 patients with SLE, it was the primary cause of death in 14.4 percent of 76 autopsy cases of SLE collected over a period of 20 years [1]. In another series of 57 patients with SLE, pulmonary hemorrhage was the cause of death in 10.5 percent [159]. It is now clear that acute pulmonary alveolar hemorrhage is a common cause of mortality in these patients [48,147]. Pulmonary hemorrhage may be mediated by activation of the complement system and leukocytes, which are attracted by immune complex deposits in the lungs that cause disruption of alveolar and capillary basement membrane integrity [24]. Uremia, bleeding diathesis, oxygen toxicity, and infection may increase the risk of pulmonary hemorrhage [48]. Pathologic analysis of the lungs in cases of hemorrhage has shown abnormalities similar to those in lupus pneumonitis [48] as well as distinctive vasculitis of small vessels [164].

Pulmonary hemorrhage may vary from subclinical to massive. Chronic subclinical pulmonary alveolar hemorrhage may lead to a clinical and pathologic picture of pulmonary hemosiderosis [1,27,129]. Significant hemoptysis is noted in 8 to 15 percent of patients [48,159,186]. The prognosis of massive pulmonary hemorrhage in SLE patients is grave. The mortality of pediatric patients with pulmonary hemorrhage has been reported to be 50 percent [157]. The onset of hemoptysis and progressive respiratory distress can be abrupt, and the clinical presentation frequently resembles that of acute lupus pneumonitis [35,48, 77,144,147,157–159,210]. Chest roentgenograms usually reveal bibasal, patchy, alveolar infiltrates (Fig. 57-3). The mortality from lupus-induced pulmonary alveolar hemorrhage is in excess of 50 percent, with many patients dying within several days of the onset of hemoptysis [144,159].

Interstitial Pneumonitis

Extensive interstitial fibrosis, as observed in patients with RA and PSS, is seldom seen in SLE. The prevalence of a diffuse interstitial process in SLE has been calculated to be approximately 3 percent [49]. Patchy and irregular areas of nonspecific interstitial pneumonitis and fibrosis develop in 15 to 45 percent of patients with SLE (Fig. 57-4) [25,49,84,96,104,108]. Immunofluorescent staining for IgG may show patchy and lumpy staining of the alveolar wall (Fig. 57-5). The most common presentation is an insidious onset of chronic, nonproductive cough, dyspnea on exertion, and a history of recurrent pleuritic pain. Less commonly, the diffuse process may develop

Fig. 57-3. Pulmonary alveolar hemorrhage in a patient with systemic lupus erythematosus and severe renal involvement. Alveolar infiltrates are basal and patchy in distribution.

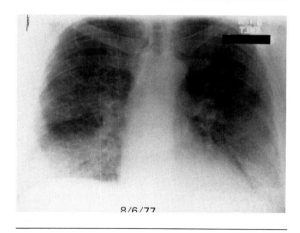

8/6/77

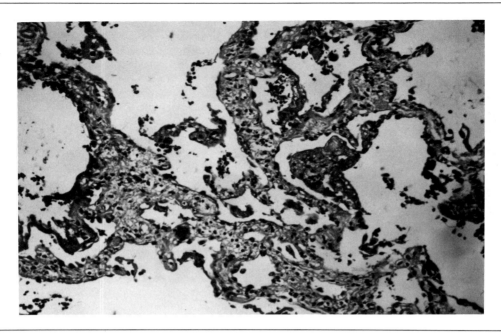

Fig. 57-4. Lung changes in systemic lupus erythematosus showing edema and thickening of alveolar septa, fibrinous exudate, and hyaline membrane formation in the alveoli.

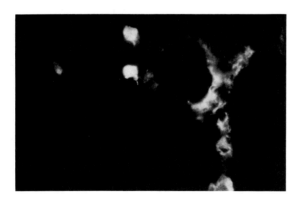

Fig. 57-5. Immunofluorescence of lung specimen for IgG in systemic lupus erythematosus shows patchy staining of alveolar wall as well as a few intraalveolar cells.

after a bout of acute lupus pneumonitis. Clinical manifestations of diffuse interstitial process are similar to those of RA and PSS. In a study of 18 patients with SLE-induced diffuse lung disease, the mean age was 45.7 years and the mean duration of the disease was 10.3 years; pulmonary symptoms were present for a mean of 6 years [49]. Pulmonary function tests in patients with diffuse lung disease demonstrate a restrictive pattern and diminished diffusing capacity for carbon monoxide. The clinical course is similar to that of diffuse lung disease associated with RA or PSS [241].

Platelike or discoid atelectatic areas are more common and usually occur in the lower two-thirds of lung fields (Fig. 57-6) [49]. Infectious processes, particularly in patients who are on immunosuppressive therapy for SLE, are the most common cause of pulmonary parenchymal infiltrates [96]. Sepsis and renal disease are more frequent causes of mortality in these patients than are pulmonary complications.

Pulmonary Thromboembolism

Thrombophlebitis has been described in 5 to 12 percent of patients with SLE [187]. The factors that predispose patients with SLE to thrombophlebitis and pulmonary embolism include chronic low-grade disseminated intravascular coagulation, small-vessel angiitis, prolonged bed rest, and increased thromboplastin generation [187]. More recently, it has been recognized that venous and arterial thromboses are associated paradoxically with circulating lupus anticoagu-

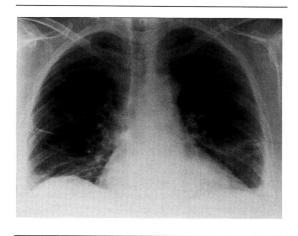

Fig. 57-6. Discoid or platelike atelectasis, also called *atelectatic pneumonitis*, is perhaps the most common chest roentgenologic finding in patients with chronic systemic lupus erythematosus. Diffuse interstitial process is distinctly uncommon.

lants and antiphospholipid antibodies. The lupus anticoagulant syndrome is characterized by a prolonged activated partial thromboplastin time, in association with otherwise normal clotting and platelet counts, anticardiolipin antibody, and a false-positive VDRL test [50]. Recurrent thromboembolism and pulmonary emboli complicated by pulmonary hypertension have been described in patients with lupus anticoagulant syndrome [11,22]. Long-term anticoagulant therapy is required in these patients [10]. Symptomatic pulmonary hypertension is relatively rare in SLE, although mild subclinical cases are not uncommon [141,143,178,199]. The pathology of pulmonary hypertension in SLE is not well understood. Vasculitis of pulmonary vasculature rarely is seen. Potential mechanisms underlying it include progressive hypoxemia from interstitial fibrosis, chronic alveolar hemorrhage syndrome, vasculitis of small vessels, and recurrent pulmonary embolism.

Diaphragmatic Dysfunction

Elevated diaphragms with diminished diaphragmatic function have been described in some patients with SLE [71,103,146,247]. The clinical significance of this finding is unclear, although this phenomenon may be responsible for the unexplained dyspnea in the absence of pulmonary parenchymal abnormalities in some patients with

SLE [55]. The term *shrinking lung syndrome* has been used to describe this complex [103]. The mechanisms responsible for the diaphragmatic weakness are unknown but may include recurrent episodes of diaphragmatic pleurisy, basal atelectasis, and steroid myopathy. Most patients with lung involvement from SLE will demonstrate restriction on pulmonary function tests. Diaphragm dysfunction does not appear to respond to corticosteroid therapy [242].

Other Complications

Obstruction to airflow is rare in SLE, although severe airway obstruction has been reported in a small number of patients [75,108,120]. The airflow obstruction may be attributable to bronchiolitis, which is noted in some patients, [148,179]. Several cases of upper airway involvement from laryngeal inflammation have been described [242].

Lung biopsies from patients with SLE may demonstrate areas of vasculitis. However, vasculitis is not characteristic of all lupus-induced pleuropulmonary processes. Nevertheless, vasculitic lesions of large vessels and capillaries of the lung have been observed in nearly 50 percent of patients [55,84,96,186]. Still, not all pleuropulmonary lesions in SLE are caused by vasculitis [242].

Pulmonary function testing in patients with SLE usually reveals a restrictive type of dysfunction with diminished lung volumes [107]. The diffusing capacity of carbon monoxide in the lung (D_LCO) is characteristically reduced, and the test is a reliable method to monitor patients with pulmonary parenchymal disease. Unless the diaphragmatic weakness is significant, maximal inspiratory and expiratory pressures may not exhibit severe abnormalities.

Drug-Induced SLE and the Lung

Drug-induced SLE is a clinically important syndrome, and the number of drugs known to cause SLE continues to increase [42,91]. Pleural and pulmonary involvement are common in drug-induced lupus. Pleural disease is more common with certain drugs such as procainamide and hydralazine. The pleural fluid in this group of patients shows biochemical characteristics similar to the classic form of lupus. Withdrawal of the offending chemical usually results in resolution of symptoms and signs within days or weeks [242].

Treatment and Prognosis

Pleural effusion responds favorably to systemic corticosteroid therapy, with an occasional large effusion being refractory [14,118]. Lupus pneumonitis and alveolar hemorrhage syndrome may respond to high-dose corticosteroid therapy. *Cytotoxic agents* have been used in patients refractory to corticosteroid therapy, but there is little evidence to suggest improved efficacy of the former [48,147,148]. Sepsis and progressive renal dysfunction are the most frequent causes of mortality in patients with SLE, but acute pulmonary alveolar hemorrhage is also important. In patients with lupus pneumonitis, dramatic response can be expected following systemic corticosteroid therapy, although a review of 12 cases of lupus pneumonitis noted a mortality of approximately 50 percent [242].

Rheumatoid Arthritis

RA is a chronic systemic inflammatory process characterized by nonsuppurative arthritis involving the diarthrodial joints, with frequent involvement of tendons, ligaments, fascia, muscle, and bone. The American Rheumatism Association has described the criteria that establish the diagnosis of RA [198]. The pleuropulmonary complications of this disease are somewhat peculiar:

Although the pleuropulmonary involvement is more common in those with active RA, the respiratory findings may precede the onset of skeletal symptoms. Middle-aged men are more likely than women to be affected by pulmonary complications, even though RA is much more common in women. The prevalence of pleuropulmonary involvement in RA varies from 1.6 percent using chest roentgenography alone to 47 percent utilizing DlCO [112].

Pleural Involvement

Pleural involvement is the most common intrathoracic manifestation of RA (Fig. 57-7). In a study of 309 patients with RA, chest roentgenographic evidence of pleural involvement was observed in 24 percent of men and 16 percent of women [117]. Autopsy studies have demonstrated pleural involvement in nearly 50 percent [112,207]. In contrast to the common occurrence of painful pleurisy encountered in patients with SLE, one-third of patients with rheumatoid pleurisy are asymptomatic [246]. Patients with active RA are more likely to develop pleurisy with effusion than those with inactive disease. Pleural

Fig. 57-7. Pleuropulmonary interphase (upper right) in rheumatoid arthritis. Virtually all patients with rheumatoid arthritis show evidence of pleural thickening at autopsy.

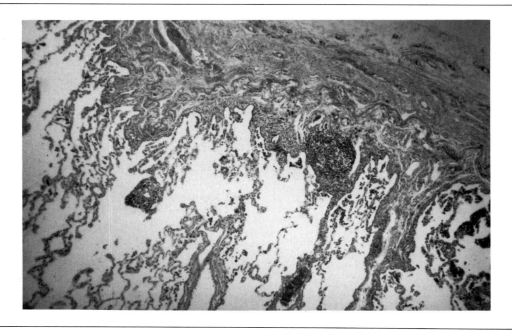

effusion may precede the onset of arthritic symptoms by months [207]. The effusions are usually unilateral, small, persistent, or recurrent, and chronic effusions that persist for months to years are not uncommon. One-third of rheumatoid pleural effusions are associated with other lung processes [112].

Pleural fluid in RA is typically an exudate, usually yellow, and occasionally bloody [33,54,112]. Chronic effusions may appear opalescent green due to high cholesterol content (pseudochylothorax). The glucose content is very low (<30 mg/dl) in more than 80 percent of patients [33,112,207]. An extremely low level of glucose in rheumatoid pleural fluid results both from selective blockage of glucose transport into the pleural space and from increased glucose use by the inflamed and metabolically active pleural mesothelial cells. Pleural fluid hypoglycemia is nonspecific, occurring in pleural effusions secondary to empyema, malignant mesothelioma, and tuberculosis. In some patients, the low pH of some rheumatoid pleural effusions results from localized acidosis caused by blockage to the efflux of the end products (lactate and CO_2) of glucose metabolism within the pleural space. Total complement levels in pleural fluid are low in 40 percent of patients [111]. The presence of rheumatoid factor and the so-called RA cell (monocytes containing cytoplasmic inclusions representing phagocytized IgM in immune complex form) are not specific in the diagnosis of rheumatoid pleural effusion [54,112,207]. High cholesterol levels, including some of the highest ever recorded, are common in chronic pleural effusions associated with RA [212].

Rheumatoid Lung

Rheumatoid lung is defined as diffuse interstitial pneumonitis or fibrosis associated with RA (Figs. 57-8, 57-9), and it is perhaps the most serious pulmonary complication of RA [112]. A diffuse pulmonary process is observed in 1.6 to 4.5 percent of chest roentgenograms in patients with RA [112,117,190]. Restrictive pulmonary dysfunction can be demonstrated in more than one-third of patients with rheumatoid lung disease [112,190]. Clinically, physiologically, and morphologically, the respiratory involvement in RA is identical to that in idiopathic pulmonary fibrosis [125]. Cough and dyspnea are common symptoms, and clubbing has been observed in up to 70 percent [190]. Chest roentgenograms generally demonstrate a bibasilar interstitial process or micro-

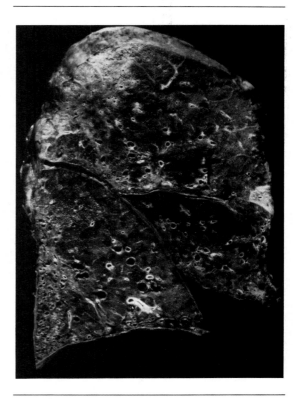

Fig. 57-8. Gross photograph of chronic interstitial pneumonia in rheumatoid arthritis. Zones of honeycombing can be seen in the posterior subpleural regions. Some contraction and thickening of the lung also is noted along with pleural thickening.

nodules. Honeycombing occurs in late stages of the disease. Fewer than 6 percent of patients with RA have been shown to develop a bilateral upper-lobe process, similar to the pulmonary abnormalities in ankylosing spondylitis [140,150,190]. The diffuse interstitial disease caused by RA typically results in restrictive lung dysfunction. The earliest physiologic abnormality is diminished DLCO.

Histologic findings in diffuse rheumatoid lung disease may consist of several abnormalities, depending on the stage of the disease [249,250]. However, the pathologic changes by themselves are nonspecific without clinical correlates. One study of 40 patients with RA and active pulmonary process described five histologic patterns of pulmonary disease: rheumatoid nodules, nonspecific interstitial pneumonitis, bronchiolitis obliterans with patchy organizing pneumonia, lymphoid hyperplasia, and cellular interstitial infiltrates (Figs. 57-9, 57-10, 57-11) [249]. Bron-

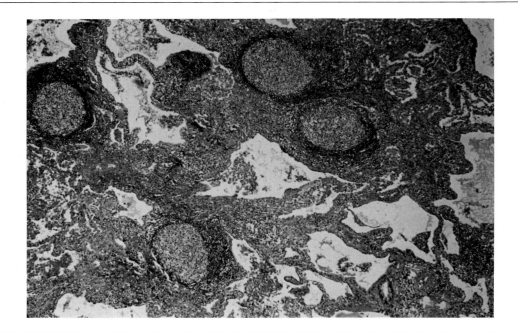

Fig. 57-9. Chronic fibrosing interstitial pneumonia with associated lymphoid hyperplasia and germinal centers in rheumatoid arthritis. Alveolar architecture is somewhat preserved.

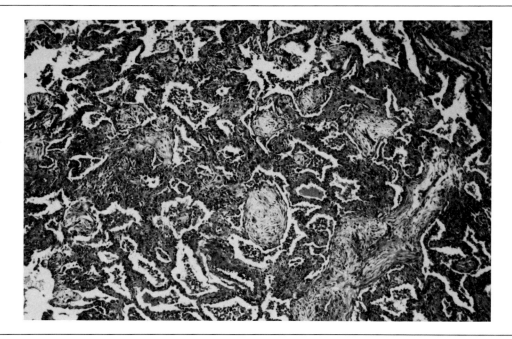

Fig. 57-10. Bronchiolitis obliterans with patchy organizing pneumonia in rheumatoid arthritis. Several pale rounded polyps of edematous granulation tissue are seen within the airspace, between which mildly thickened alveolar septa with a mild chronic inflammatory infiltrate can be seen.

choalveolar lavage in patients with rheumatoid lung disease has revealed abnormalities identical to those in idiopathic pulmonary fibrosis [62, 63,72,240]. Even though it has been suggested that increased lymphocytosis of bronchoalveolar lavage fluid is associated with a good pulmonary prognosis [235], this has yet to be confirmed by further studies. Systemic corticosteroid therapy in its early stages may reverse the lung process.

Necrobiotic Rheumatoid Nodules

Necrobiotic rheumatoid pulmonary nodules are different from the nodules observed in Caplan's syndrome. Necrobiotic nodules occur within the lung parenchyma and are histologically similar to subcutaneous rheumatoid nodules [207]. They are more common in men than in women and in those with seropositive RA. Necrobiotic nodules are known to precede the arthritic symptoms [26,109,112,170,236]. The pulmonary nodules produce minimal symptoms and often are discovered incidentally. They measure from a few millimeters to several centimeters in diameter and are usually bilateral (Fig. 57-11), occur near pleural surfaces, cavitate in two-thirds, and may rupture into pleural space to produce pneumothorax or empyema [47,140,155,183]. Aspergilloma is a complication of rheumatoid nodules [151]. The necrobiotic nodules usually wax and wane with activity of the RA [112], although they

Fig. 57-11. Multiple bilateral rheumatoid nodules in the lower lung zones. Cavitation is not seen clearly in this computed tomographic image, even though one-third of the nodules cavitate.

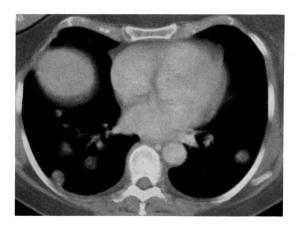

may resolve spontaneously despite continuously active RA.

Rheumatoid Pneumoconiosis (Caplan's Syndrome)

Caplan's syndrome denotes the presence of rheumatoid nodules in association with pneumoconiosis. Originally described in coal workers with rheumatoid arthritis, Caplan's syndrome now encompasses persons with silicosis, asbestosis, aluminosis, and the like [8,30,80]. The syndrome is uncommon in North America, so most reports have been from Europe [242]. It is characterized by pulmonary parenchymal nodules that measure 1 to 5 cm in diameter, evolve rapidly, may undergo cavitation, appear in crops, and frequently are associated with other lung lesions. Histologic analysis will demonstrate features identical to those of rheumatoid nodules as well as the presence of pneumoconiotic material in the center [207]. Occasionally, the nodules remain quiescent and heal by fibrosis.

Obstructive Airways Disease

Obstructive airways disease is now a well-recognized complication of RA, having been documented in several prospective studies. Nearly one-third of patients (nonsmokers) with RA exhibit obstructive lung dysfunction [41,65–67,100, 101,162,177,196]. In one study of patients with active rheumatoid lung disease, 23 percent were found to have obstructive dysfunction secondary to rheumatoid bronchiolitis; others had follicular bronchiolitis and bronchitis in RA [249]. Mucociliary clearance may be diminished in some patients with RA [218]. The combination of RA and smoking is associated with a much higher prevalence of obstructive lung disease than is either of these factors alone. Genetic predisposition to obstructive lung disease has been proposed as a contributing factor. Several studies have shown that patients with RA and pulmonary involvement have a 50 percent incidence of non-MM (that is, MZ and MS) phenotypes of alpha$_1$-antitrypsin [67,155,190]. Penicillamine and gold salts are used to treat RA, and since these drugs are known to cause bronchiolitis obliterans, this potentiality should be considered in patients with RA who present with symptoms of airways obstruction. High-resolution computed chest tomography may show pulmonary parenchymal "ground-glass" type alveolar infiltrates (Fig. 57-12).

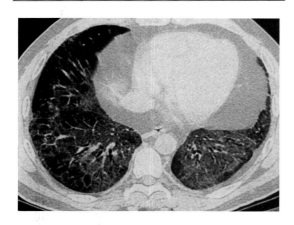

Fig. 57-12. High-resolution computed tomographic image of basal regions of lungs in bronchiolitis obliterans associated with rheumatoid arthritis. Diffuse but patchy "ground-glass" type of infiltrates are well seen.

Other Complications

Rheumatoid nodules may occur occasionally in the laryngeal region. Although cricoarytenoid arthritis is acknowledged clinically in 25 to 35 percent of cases [131], it is present in the majority of autopsies performed on patients with RA [19,139]. This feature is clinically manifested by chronic persistent sore throat and hoarseness. Both inspiratory and expiratory difficulty may result from fixed obstruction at the laryngeal level. Laryngoscopy may demonstrate edema and erythema of the vocal apparatus, abnormal motion of vocal cords, and dysfunction of the arytenoids.

Pulmonary hypertension is rare, although several case reports have been published [124,202]. Alveolar hemorrhage is uncommon in RA, but the association has been described in six patients [132,166,172,200,209]. Pulmonary vasculitis also is uncommon, although several cases have been reported and the presence of vasculitic lesions within the pulmonary capillaries may explain the alveolar hemorrhage [132,200]. Goodpasture's syndrome has also been reported in association with RA [166].

Treatment and Prognosis

Corticosteroid therapy in the early phases of rheumatoid lung disease may reverse the acute inflammatory process and thwart progression to the irreversible fibrotic stage. The prognosis is poor when the interstitial process is advanced. In one large series, such patients had a median survival of 3.5 years and a 5-year survival rate of 39 percent [87]. Rheumatoid bronchiolitis carries a poor prognosis. Corticosteroid and cytotoxic agents have been tried, but the response in chronic cases is unsatisfactory. Certain cytotoxic agents, such as gold, methotrexate, and cyclophosphamide, used to treat RA can produce pulmonary toxicity.

Progressive Systemic Sclerosis or Scleroderma

PSS is a systemic connective tissue disease characterized by a vascular disorder and excessive deposition of collagen and other matrix proteins in the skin and internal organs [135]. The major pathologic attributes of PSS include vascular changes, immune dysfunction, and increased collagen synthesis [36]. Pulmonary involvement is common in patients with PSS [174,213,214]. Up to 80 percent have abnormal pulmonary histology at necropsy, even though the patients remain minimally symptomatic during life [43,238]. Intrathoracic involvement may include pulmonary fibrosis, pulmonary hypertension with or without cor pulmonale, diffuse pulmonary calcification, aspiration pneumonia as a result of esophageal involvement, chest wall restriction from skin involvement, and scar cancer related to long-term fibrosis.

Pulmonary Fibrosis

Chronic progressive interstitial pulmonary fibrosis is the most common pulmonary complication of PSS and develops in up to two-thirds of patients. The frequency of roentgenographic interstitial fibrosis is increased in patients with serum anti-Scl-70 antibody and decreased in those with anticentromere antibody [198]. The histologic appearances are analogous to those of idiopathic pulmonary fibrosis [92]. In the beginning stages, alveolar edema with lymphocytic and monocytic infiltrates are noted. Later, severe fibrosis with honeycombing, cyst formation, and increased incidence of pneumothorax occurs (Fig. 57-13). Although only one-third of patients with PSS have abnormal chest roentgenographic findings, more than 50 percent complain of dyspnea on exertion and exhibit diminished DLCO. Evidence of subclinical alveolitis as judged by bronchoalveolar lavage findings has been noted in asymptomatic patients with PSS [93,235]. Further studies have shown that increased pulmonary vascular leak-

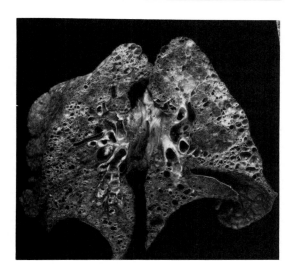

Fig. 57-13. Gross appearance of lungs in a patient with severe scleroderma. Lungs show extensive honeycombing.

Fig. 57-14. Pulmonary hypertension in scleroderma, with marked thickening of the muscular wall of small pulmonary arteries.

age and neutrophilic alveolitis may be the beginning features of interstitial lung disease in PSS and that these abnormalities often are associated with indicating enhanced lung type II collagen synthesis [92]. Pulmonary involvement is more severe in patients with the CREST (*c*alcinosis, *R*aynaud's phenomenon, *e*sophageal involvement, *s*clerodactyly, and *t*elangiectasia) variant of PSS.

PSS patients as a group have undergone extensive pulmonary function testing. The most common abnormality is the slow but relentlessly progressive restrictive dysfunction with diminished DLCO, which is the earliest aberration. The DLCO is also an important predictor of mortality [12,173]. Studies have shown that the presence of Raynaud's phenomenon is associated with a lower DLCO [182,233].

Pulmonary Hypertension

Pulmonary hypertension is common in patients with PSS and is a major cause of morbidity and mortality [135]. It usually develops as a result of medial hypertrophy of the pulmonary arteries (35 to 60 percent of patients with PSS) (Fig. 57-14) [192,216,248]. Patients with the CREST syndrome are at higher risk of developing pulmonary hypertension [216,233,238,248]. Another cause of pulmonary hypertension is chronic hypoxemia

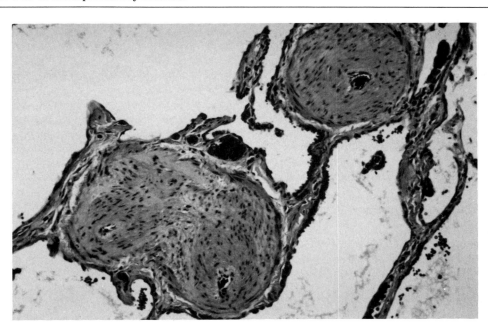

incited by pulmonary fibrosis. A progressive decrease in the diffusing capacity of carbon monoxide is the earliest indicator of pulmonary hypertension in PSS. The overall results of treatment, using vasodilators, have been discouraging [61,74,168,171]. The incidence of renovascular pathology is high among patients with pulmonary vascular involvement.

Aspiration Pneumonia

There is esophageal involvement in more than 90 percent of patients with PSS. Distal esophageal motor dysfunction is the most common manifestation of internal involvement, and it leads to esophageal dysfunction and acid reflux. Aspiration of gastric contents secondary to esophageal reflux is hypothesized to be one of the etiologic factors causing pulmonary fibrosis [115].

Other Complications

Miscellaneous pulmonary complications of PSS include diffuse pulmonary calcification in some patients with the CREST syndrome, resorption of ribs in chronic cases, and rare instances of pleural thickening. Even though diffuse alveolar hemorrhage is encountered in patients with SLE and several vasculitides, it has been described in only 2 cases of PSS [83,119].

Chronic PSS is associated with an increased risk of lung cancer [180,191,224,225]. Some have reported that the risk for developing bronchoalveolar carcinoma is increased [228], but other histologic types including small-cell carcinoma have also been described in patients with chronic PSS [195,213,214,245]. It is not clear whether these cancers represent the so-called scar cancers or just incidental findings [153].

Other uncommon thoracic manifestations of PSS reported in the literature include diaphragmatic dysfunction [34,45], hemoptysis due to telangiectasia of the airways [126], and a syndrome resembling pulmonary hemosiderosis [155].

Treatment and Prognosis

Systemic corticosteroid therapy has had no effect on the prognosis in patients with PSS. D-Penicillamine has been used to prevent progression of the pulmonary complications [45,152,214]. When patients with PSS develop hypoxemia, supplemental oxygen therapy is the only treatment that relieves the dyspnea.

Polymyositis-Dermatomyositis

Polymyositis and dermatomyositis are idiopathic myopathies characterized by inflammation of skeletal muscles with resultant weakness of proximal muscles and a characteristic skin rash (heliotrope hue). The autoimmune type of PM-DM, discussed here, is different from the idiopathic or paraneoplastic type, the latter being associated, in 5 to 10 percent of cases, with bronchogenic carcinoma and other malignancies [28, 130,142]. When elderly patients present with PM-DM, an underlying malignancy must be excluded before the diagnosis of autoimmune PM-DM is considered [181]. The autoimmune inflammatory myopathies are very uncommon, with no more than 5 to 10 cases per million persons per year in the USA [181]. The disease is more common in women. The diagnosis is by clinical features, elevation of creatine phosphokinase and aldolase, electromyographic studies, and muscle biopsy. Pulmonary involvement has been described in up to 5 percent of patients with PM-DM [23,60,112]. In approximately one-third of patients, the respiratory manifestations may precede the musculocutaneous signs and symptoms [23]. A relationship between the severity and progression of the myositis and the severity of respiratory disease is lacking [242].

Interstitial Pneumonitis and Fibrosis

The most common pulmonary complication is interstitial pneumonitis and fibrosis, which occurs in 5 to 10 percent of patients [181,193]. The process is basal in distribution and may present as acute pneumonitis with alveolar or mixed alveolar-interstitial infiltrates. The pathogenesis of the interstitial pneumonitis and fibrosis in PM-DM is unknown, but hypersensitivity may play a role. Morphologic examination may show nonspecific fibrosis and bronchiolitis and desquamation of alveolar lining cells (Fig. 57-15). Pulmonary dysfunction is present in more than half the patients and consists of decreased volumes, D_LCO, and arterial oxygenation. Not all patients with PM-DM will demonstrate the anti-Jo-1 antibody in their serum. However, more than 50 percent of patients with this antibody exhibit interstitial pulmonary disease [9,18,102,181,237]. Bronchoalveolar lavage studies have not identified any diagnostic characteristics [82,181]. Pulmonary disease precedes the dermatologic or myopathic manifestations by 1 to 24 months in nearly one-

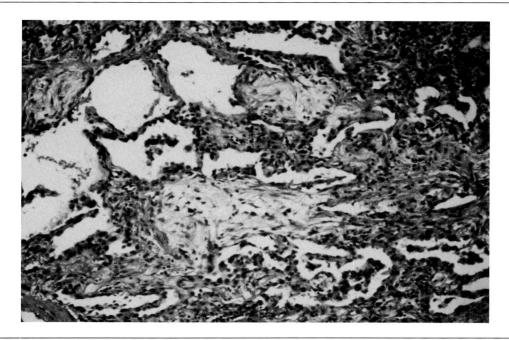

Fig. 57-15. Bronchiolitis obliterans with patchy organizing pneumonia in polymyositis-dermatomyositis. Two rounded edematous masses of intraalveolar fibrous connective tissue can be seen in the center of the figure.

third of patients. Pulmonary disease may present with dyspnea, cough, and hypoxemia; symptoms related to gastroesophageal reflux may be the initial manifestation in some. Chest roentgenography may reveal an alveolar process in the basal lung segments.

Hypoventilation

Weakness of the respiratory muscles due to the myopathic process results in progressive hypoventilation and respiratory failure. Increasing hypercapnia is a poor prognostic sign in these patients. Muscle weakness may severely compromise the respiratory bellows mechanism, thereby worsening the basal atelectasis. An ineffective cough increases the risk of bacterial pneumonia.

Aspiration Pneumonitis

Patients with PM-DM commonly exhibit esophageal involvement in the form of uncoordinated peristalsis, esophageal reflux, odynophagia, and delayed gastric emptying [106]. Bulbar involve-

ment and dysfunction of the muscles of deglutition often lead to recurrent aspiration problems. Poor cough strength as a result of respiratory muscle weakness contributes to the development and progression of aspiration pneumonia. Aspiration pneumonia is often the cause of death in these patients [21,154,193].

Treatment and Prognosis

Many treatment programs consisting of corticosteroids, azathioprine, methotrexate, total body irradiation, and thymectomy have been tried, with varying rates of success [181]. The pulmonary involvement in PM-DM is usually progressive, and long-term response to corticosteroid therapy is poor even though the initial response may be good [97]. Patients receiving high-dose therapy (prednisolone, 1 to 2 mg/kg/day) have shown less morbidity [23,31,60,244].

Mixed Connective Tissue Disease

Physicians use the terms, *overlap syndrome, undifferentiated connective tissue disease, sclerodermatomyositis, RUPUS* (RA and SLE), or *lupoderma* (SLE and PSS) when confronted with a patient who demonstrates clinical features of more than one of the rheumatologic diseases [15,73]. The term *mixed connective tissue disease* was introduced in 1972 based on the recognition that many patients with clinical features of SLE, PSS, and PM-DM had unusually high titers of a specific circulating antibody to an extractable nuclear ribonucleoprotein antigen (ENA) [205]. The presence of high titers of antibody to ENA and the absence of antibodies to Sm antigen are believed to be specific for MCTD, although this has been questioned [4]. A review of the literature reveals that clinicians are accepting MCTD as a distinct entity [3,134,136,189,203,204]. The etiology and prevalence of MCTD is unknown, but it is more common than PM-DM and less common than SLE. The majority of patients are women, and the average age at time of diagnosis is 37 years. Renal disease occurs in 10 to 20 percent, and some patients may require aggressive or prolonged pharmacologic therapy [78,169, 185,217,243]. Pleuropulmonary involvement has been described in 20 to 80 percent of patients with MCTD [90,234]. Many of these manifestations, both clinical and pathophysiologic, are similar to those observed in SLE, PSS, and PM-DM [185,234].

Interstitial Fibrosis

Morphologic features analogous to idiopathic pulmonary fibrosis and characterized by alveolar septal infiltration by lymphocytes, plasma cells, and type III collagen have been demonstrated in patients with MCTD [114,206,243]. Generally, the degree of fibrosis tends to be severe if the predominant clinical feature is that of PSS [184]. Abnormal pulmonary function tests and chest roentgenograms have been noted in 69 percent of patients without respiratory symptoms [90]. In a multicenter study of 100 patients with MCTD, impaired DLCO was noted in 67 percent, and restrictive lung volumes were observed in 50 percent [206].

Chest roentgenographic changes are similar to those in idiopathic pulmonary fibrosis if the clinical profile is predominantly scleroderma-like [90,208]. Mixed infiltrates can be seen in those with primarily PM-DM-like features. In a retrospective study of 81 patients, respiratory symptoms included dyspnea (16 percent), chest pain and tightness (7 percent), and cough (5 percent). Chest roentgenograms revealed abnormalities in 21 percent, the most common being an interstitial process in both lower lung fields. Pulmonary function testing demonstrated a restrictive type

of defect in 69 percent [185]. DLCO is the most sensitive single parameter in evaluating pulmonary dysfunction in MCTD [46].

Pleural Effusion

Pleurisy is one of the common manifestations of MCTD. Nearly 40 percent of patients in a prospective study were noted to have pleuritic pain [217]. Pleural fluid shows the same characteristics as that in SLE. The effusions are usually small and resolve spontaneously [105].

Pulmonary Hypertension

Progressive pulmonary hypertension is the most severe pulmonary complication of MCTD. This phenomenon may be accompanied by severe vasculitic lesions [6,90,116,243]. In a prospective evaluation of 34 patients, significant pulmonary hypertension was noted in 67 percent of the 15 patients studied [217]. Examination of lung biopsy tissue has revealed muscular hypertrophy of small pulmonary arteries. Plexogenic angiopathy and chronic intimal thickening of medium-size pulmonary arteries have been observed in patients with MCTD [127,243], and fatal pulmonary hypertension has been reported in a number of patients [79,232].

Aspiration Pneumonitis

Patients with MCTD have been found to exhibit abnormal esophagograms and esophageal manometric readings [185]. Hypotonicity and dilatation of the esophagus, similar to that in PSS, are responsible for the reflux and aspiration pneumonia. This aspect of MCTD has received little attention.

Other Complications

Several cases of MCTD with circulating lupus anticoagulant, recurrent thromboemboli complicated by pulmonary embolism, and pulmonary hypertension have been described [6,86,116]. The clinical features of these patients are similar to those with SLE.

Pulmonary hemorrhage, a recognized complication of SLE, has been reported in MCTD [68]. Localized pulmonary lesions are uncommon, but cavitated pulmonary nodules have been noted in five patients [239]. Even though generalized lymphadenopathy has been observed in 50 percent of patients with MCTD [217], mediastinal lymphadenopathy has been described in only two [85,239]. Systemic corticosteroid and immuno-suppressive therapy for MCTD increases the risk of opportunistic infections [16].

If the characteristics of PM-DM are prominent in a patient with MCTD, significant proximal muscle weakness may cause hypoventilatory respiratory failure. Diaphragmatic weakness has been described in a patient with MCTD [145].

Treatment and Prognosis

Although early reports on MCTD implied that corticosteroids were effective [15,205], accumulated experience has shown that most patients do not respond to corticosteroid or immunosuppressive agents. Pleurisy generally responds well to corticosteroid therapy, whereas pulmonary hypertension does not. In a prospective study of 34 patients with MCTD, a favorable response to corticosteroids was noted in two-thirds of the patients [217], though patients with predominantly PSS-like disease respond poorly [185]. In a retrospective study of 81 patients, a 5-year follow-up observed six deaths due to carcinoma of the esophagus, aspiration pneumonia, pulmonary hypertension, cardiorespiratory arrest, and myocardial infarction [185].

Sjögren's Syndrome

Sjögren's syndrome, a chronic inflammatory and autoimmune disorder, is characterized by diminished lacrimal and salivary gland secretion (sicca complex) resulting in keratoconjunctivitis sicca and xerostomia [219,222]. Original description of the syndrome consisted of a triad of dry eyes, dry mouth, and rheumatoid arthritis. It is now known that other connective tissue diseases—for example, SLE, PSS, and polymyositis—may be present in place of rheumatoid arthritis and that the sicca complex can exist as a primary pathologic entity with no associated disorder. Only 50 percent of patients referred for suspected Sjögren's syndrome have an autoimmune disease. Approximately half the patients with secondary Sjögren's syndrome have rheumatoid arthritis, whereas smaller percentages have other connective tissue disorders accompanying the sicca complex. Sjögren's syndrome should be considered a lymphoproliferative disorder because the incidence of lymphoma is increased 44-fold [220]. Additionally, patients with Sjögren's syndrome are at high risk for developing non-Hodgkin's lymphoma, which may affect the lungs. However, a wide spectrum of lymphoproliferation can be seen. Lymphocytic infiltration of the exocrine glands, reticuloendothelial system, kidneys, muscles, and other organs is present in approximately one-fourth of the patients. When lymphoid tumors occur that have not met the histologic criteria for malignancy, the term *pseudolymphoma* has been used [5], although many pseudolymphomas have recently been reclassified as low-grade lymphomas on the basis of immunologic proof of clonality.

Pulmonary complications are seen in both primary and secondary forms of Sjögren's syndrome and are reported to occur in 1.5 to 75 percent of patients [20,39,40,59,112,122,176,215]. In a Mayo Clinic study of 343 patients with the syndrome, 9 percent were found to have respiratory involvement [215]. The pulmonary manifestations described in the literature include diffuse interstitial pneumonitis, desiccation of the upper respiratory tract (xerotrachea), an obstructive process involving both large and small airways, localized infiltrates, diffuse pulmonary fibrosis, pneumonic patches, discoid atelectasis, localized pulmonary nodules, bronchitis, asthma, recurrent tracheobronchitis, bronchiectasis, pleurisy, pleural effusion, pulmonary hypertension, amyloidosis, vasculitis, and diaphragmatic myopathy.

Airway Disease

The term *xerotrachea* has been used to describe the dryness of airways encountered in patients with Sjögren's syndrome [39]. This phenomenon is more common in those with the primary extraglandular form [176]. However, there is no convincing evidence of diminished mucosal secretions or ciliary dysfunction. Nonproductive cough despite normal chest roentgenogram and pulmonary function tests is noted in 17 percent of patients [39,176].

Pulmonary function tests have demonstrated obstructive lung disease in 2.5 to 35 percent of patients with both primary and secondary forms of Sjögren's syndrome [39,53,57,167,176,201,215]. Up to 40 percent of patients with both RA and Sjögren's syndrome are more likely to demonstrate obstructive lung disease [13,188]. Lymphocytic bronchitis is partly responsible for the obstructive lung disease observed in these patients, even though studies have reported mononuclear cell infiltrates around small airways [167]. Invasion of bronchial mucosa by lymphocytes has been considered a benign process but, without special immunohistologic studies, it is difficult to differentiate low-grade lymphomatous involvement of the bronchial mucosa [89].

Diffuse Interstitial Process

Nearly 15 percent of patients with Sjögren's syndrome develop a diffuse interstitial pulmonary process [201]. However, one group investigated the prevalence of interstitial lung disease in this syndrome using chest roentgenography and pulmonary function tests and reported diffuse interstitial disease in 37.5 percent [176]. The lung process may represent nonspecific interstitial pneumonia and fibrosis or lymphocytic interstitial pneumonitis. Bronchoalveolar lavage has revealed increased percentages of lymphocytes and neutrophils [95], which suggests a high frequency of subclinical alveolitis in Sjögren's syndrome. The physiologic dysfunction is usually mild. The clinical problem is one of differentiating lymphocytic interstitial pneumonitis from nonlymphocytic interstitial pneumonitis without lung biopsy because of the clinical implications (see the next sections).

Lymphocytic Interstitial Pneumonitis

Lymphocytic interstitial pneumonitis is characterized by parenchymal infiltrates consisting predominantly of small lymphocytes, with variable numbers of plasma cells and transformed lymphocytes (Fig. 57-16) [81,138,221,223]. Chest roentgenograms in lymphocytic interstitial pneumonitis usually show a diffuse interstitial process, which is predominantly basal in distribution [2]. Among the 343 patients with Sjögren's syndrome reported from the Mayo Clinic, there were 8 (2.3 percent) patients who developed lymphoproliferative pathology in the lungs; 3 had lymphocytic interstitial pneumonitis, 2 had pseudolymphoma, and 3 were found to have lymphoma [215]. Although this earlier study from the Mayo Clinic suggested that this entity generally represents a benign process, many of these are actually low-grade lymphomas [89]. Some patients with lymphocytic interstitial pneumonitis eventually develop disseminated lymphoma, which has led to the theory that lymphocytic interstitial pneumonitis is prelymphomatous [69,211].

Pseudolymphoma

Localized lymphoid infiltrates may expand to form pseudolymphomas, which may be clinically

Fig. 57-16. Chronic bronchiolitis in Sjögren's syndrome with marked chronic inflammation in the wall of the bronchiole associated with lymphoid hyperplasia with germinal centers (right).

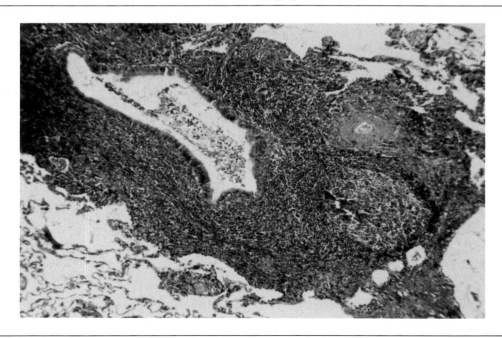

and histologically difficult to distinguish from lymphoma [7]. These peculiar lesions probably represent the middle portion of the spectrum from a benign lymphocytic process to malignant lymphoma, and pseudolymphomas are believed to develop in patients with secondary Sjögren's syndrome alone. Histologically, pseudolymphomas exhibit highly heterogeneous infiltrates consisting of large and small lymphocytes, plasma cells, or reticulum cells. Chest roentgenograms may demonstrate rounded mass lesions or nodular lesions. Recent studies have used immunohistochemical techniques to show that most pseudolymphomas of lung are lymphomas, and so prior reports of pseudolymphoma and lymphocytic interstitial pneumonitis in this syndrome must be viewed in this light; probably many would have proved to be monoclonal had they been studied [20,53]. These lesions are generally detected on chest roentgenograms of patients with chronic Sjögren's syndrome who are usually without symptoms. The lesions may be well defined, rounded, and usually solitary, and measure from 1.5 to 6 cm. Current concepts indicate that most pseudolymphomas are probably indolent, well-differentiated lymphocytic and lymphoplasmacytic lymphomas, and the majority demonstrate a benign clinical course, whereas only a few are aggressive [52,58,89,194]. Studies using polyclonalities suggest that pseudolymphoma in Sjögren's syndrome results from the infiltration of salivary glands and extraglandular tissues by nonneoplastic helper T cells, and the chronic stimulation of B cells by the T cells leads to eventual escape of a malignant B-cell clone and development of frank malignant lymphoma [2,58]. Whereas some pseudolymphomas and even low-grade lymphomas regress spontaneously or with systemic corticosteroids, others may develop into malignant lymphomas.

Pulmonary Lymphoma

A study from the National Institutes of Health ascertained the risk of malignancy in 136 women with Sjögren's syndrome who were followed for an average period of 8 years [123]. Non-Hodgkin's lymphoma occurred in seven and Waldenström's macroglobulinemia in three patients. This was 43.8 times the incidence expected from the rates of malignancy prevailing among the women of the same age range in the general population during this time. Patients with a history of parotid enlargement, splenomegaly, and lymphadenopathy were particularly at risk. Others have ob-

served clinical evidence of lymphoproliferation in 17 percent of 36 men with Sjögren's syndrome and concluded that men are at the same risk as women for the development of lymphoma [161]. The overwhelming majority of malignant lymphomas reported in patients with this syndrome have been monoclonal B-cell neoplasms.

Pulmonary involvement by lymphoma is more likely to occur in those with systemic lymphoma. A Mayo Clinic study of 50 patients with Sjögren's syndrome and associated lymphoma revealed pulmonary involvement in 10 patients [89]. The mean age of the 10 patients was 59.7 years, and 8 were women; the mean duration of the syndrome was 7.2 years, and the mean interval between the onset of the syndrome and lymphoma was 5.4 years. Of the 10 patients, 4 died from 8 to 48 months after lymphoma was diagnosed. Lung biopsies revealed a spectrum of low-grade to high-grade lymphomas.

Some patients may receive an initial diagnosis of benign lymphocytic interstitial pneumonitis, but further pathologic examination may reveal low-grade lymphomas [89,98]. In an extensive review of the topic, it was concluded that some published cases of lymphocytic interstitial pneumonitis may represent malignant lymphoma [37,38]. Some investigators have concluded that *all* cases of lymphocytic interstitial pneumonitis are actually low-grade lymphomas [98]. Although it is difficult to differentiate lymphocytic interstitial pneumonitis from malignant lymphoma when the chest roentgenogram reveals an interstitial process, the presence of multiple nodular lesions suggests lymphoma [81,89]. Hilar lymphadenopathy or masses should also suggest a high likelihood of lymphoma. Patients with low-grade lymphomas fare significantly better than those with high-grade lymphomas. Patients with pulmonary lymphomas are believed to have a better prognosis [194].

Treatment and Prognosis

The treatment of the lymphomas in Sjögren's syndrome depends on the grade of the tumor; low-grade lymphoma may not require chemotherapy. Because of the potential of these tumors to assume the status of high-grade malignancy, close surveillance is indicated. Because most patients with Sjögren's syndrome do not have disabling pulmonary symptoms, only symptomatic therapy is indicated. The treatment of lymphoma should be designed according to the cell type and aggressiveness of the tumor.

Relapsing Polychondritis

RPC is a relatively rare, often episodic form of inflammatory disease of unknown etiology characterized by potentially destructive lesions commonly involving organs of special sense, laryngotracheal structures, the cardiovascular system, and joints. Clinical manifestations include iritis, episcleritis, hearing deficit, cataract, aortic valvular insufficiency, anemia, elevated erythrocyte sedimentation rate, and liver function abnormalities. The majority of cases present in patients between the ages of 40 and 60 years, with equal distribution between the sexes. The disease primarily affects Caucasians.

One of the difficulties in establishing whether the disease is idiopathic is related to the fact that in approximately one-third of reported cases, RPC coexists with other diseases including Wegener's granulomatosis, RA, SLE, Sjögren's syndrome, ankylosing spondylitis, Reiter's syndrome, Behçet's disease, hypothyroidism, Graves' disease, chronic ulcerative colitis, cryptogenic cirrhosis, cryoglobulinemia, and hydralazine therapy [99]. Malignancies occur on occasion, particularly in older patients. In many patients, these diseases precede the onset of polychondritis by months to years. Another problem is that even the biopsy of affected cartilage may show only nonspecific findings. There are no specific serologic or other tests to aid in the diagnosis. Nonetheless, if three of the following six metabolic diseases are diagnosed in the proper clinical setting, the diagnosis of RPC is considered to be established: auricular chondritis; nonerosive inflammatory polyarthritis; nasal chondritis; ocular inflammation (conjunctivitis, keratitis, scleritis, episcleritis, uveitis); laryngeal, tracheal, or bronchial chondritis; and cochlear or vestibular damage [149].

Fig. 57-17. Tomogram showing severely narrowed trachea as determined by the size of the air tracheogram in relapsing polychondritis. Anteroposterior view (A) and lateral view (B) delineate the normal dimensions of the trachea.

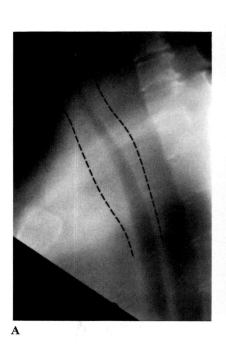

A

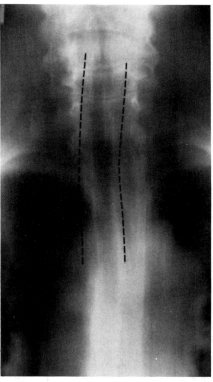

B

Pulmonary Disease

Recurrent inflammation of the nasal cartilage causes structural damage and results in the typical "saddle-nose" deformity. More than 50 percent of patients with RPC develop respiratory tract abnormalities [70,99,156]. Involvement of the laryngotracheal region is considered a poor prognostic sign [156]. The major abnormalities in the airways include thickening of the mucosa, loss of elasticity, and development of stenotic segments. When multiple cartilaginous segments become affected, the structural integrity of the tracheobronchial tree may be lost and result in severe expiratory collapse of the airway (Fig. 57-17). As a result, coughing becomes ineffective and this, combined with recurrent infections due to inability to clear mucus, may cause bronchiectasis. Pulmonary function testing with flow-volume curves in patients with significant respiratory symptoms will demonstrate the plateau patterns of maximal inspiratory or expiratory flows [69,128,160].

Tracheal tomography and cine-computed tomography may provide further insight into the abnormal anatomy of the major airways [227]. Bronchoscopy is also helpful in assessing the dynamic aspects of major airways.

Treatment and Prognosis

Treatment is mainly symptomatic, with nonsteroidal antiinflammatory drugs. Systemic corticosteroids (prednisolone, 30 to 60 mg/dl) often effectively suppress acute manifestations. In refractory cases, cytotoxic agents (cyclophosphamide, 6-mercaptopurine, and azathioprine), cyclosporin A, and dapsone have been tried [99].

Involvement of major airways may require tracheobronchial stent therapy or resection if the strictures are localized and amenable to surgery. Tracheostomy may actually aggravate the expiratory collapse. Nasal continuous positive airway pressure or similar physiologic "stenting" may help some patients.

Earlier series of patients with RPC reported respiratory tract disease to be the cause of death in more than 50 percent [149]. In a comprehensive review of 112 patients from the Mayo Clinic, death was noted in 37 percent; the median survival period was 11 years from the time of diagnosis. Seven of 41 deaths were attributed primarily to pneumonia or laryngotracheal chondritis. The 5- and 10-year probabilities of survival were 74 and 55 percent, respectively [156].

References

1. Abud-Mendoza C, Diaz-Jouanen E, Alarcón-Segovia D. Fatal pulmonary hemorrhage in systemic lupus erythematosus. Occurrence without hemoptysis. *J Rheumatol* 12:558, 1985.
2. Adamson T, et al. Immunohistologic analysis of lymphoid infiltrates in primary Sjögren's syndrome monoclonal antibodies. *J Immunol* 130:203–208, 1983.
3. Alarcón-Segovia D. Mixed connective tissue disease—a decade of growing pains. *J Rheumatol* 8:535, 1981.
4. Alarcón-Segovia D, Palacios R. Human post-thymic precursor cells in health and disease: IV. Abnormalities in immunoregulatory T cell circuits in mixed connective tissue disease. *Arthritis Rheum* 24:1486, 1981.
5. Alexander M. Clinical aspects of Sjögren's syndrome. *South Med J* 79:857–862, 1986.
6. Alpert MA, et al. Cardiovascular manifestations of mixed connective tissue disease in adults. *Circulation* 68:1182, 1983.
7. Anderson LG, Talal N. The spectrum of benign to malignant lymphoproliferation in Sjögren's syndrome. *Clin Exp Immunol* 10:199–221, 1972.
8. Anttila S, et al. Rheumatoid pneumoconiosis in a dolomite worker: A light and electron microscopic and x-ray microanalytical study. *Br J Dis Chest* 78:195, 1984.
9. Arnett FC, et al. The Jo-1 antibody system in myositis: Relationships to clinical features and HLA. *J Rheumatol* 8:925, 1981.
10. Asherson RA, et al. Anticardiolipin antibody, recurrent thrombosis, and warfarin withdrawal. *Ann Rheum Dis* 44:823, 1985.
11. Asherson RA, et al. Pulmonary hypertension in systemic lupus erythematosus. *Br Med J* 287:1024, 1983.
12. Bagg LR, Hughes TD. Serial pulmonary function tests in progressive systemic sclerosis. *Thorax* 34:224, 1979.
13. Begin R, et al. Airway disease in a subset of nonsmoking rheumatoid arthritis patients. *Am J Med* 72:743, 1982.
14. Bell R, Lawrence DS. Chronic pleurisy in systemic lupus erythematosus treated with pleurectomy. *Br J Dis Chest* 73:314, 1979.
15. Bennett RM. Mixed Connective Tissue Disease and Other Overlap Syndromes. In WN Kelley et al (Eds), *Textbook of Rheumatology* (2nd ed, vol 1). Philadelphia: Saunders, 1985. P 1115.
16. Bennett RM, O'Connell DJ. Mixed connective tissue disease: A clinicopathologic study of 20 cases. *Semin Arthritis Rheum* 10:25, 1980.
17. Berendes J, Miehlke A. A rare ankylosis of the cricoarytenoid joints. *Arch Otolaryngol* 98:63, 1973.
18. Bernstein RM, et al. Anti-Jo-1 antibody: A

marker for myositis with interstitial lung disease. *Br Med J* 289:151, 1984.

19. Bienenstock H, Ehrich GE, Freyberg RH. Rheumatoid arthritis of the cricoarytenoid joint: A clinicopathologic study. *Arthritis Rheum* 6:48, 1963.

20. Boch KJ, Buchanan WW, Wohl MG. Sjögren's syndrome: A clinical, pathological, and serological study of 63 cases. *Medicine* 44:187, 1965.

21. Blumbergs PC, Byrne E, Kakulas BA. Polymyositis presenting with respiratory failure. *J Neurol Sci* 65:221, 1984.

22. Boey ML, et al. Thrombosis in systemic lupus erythematosus: Striking association with the presence of circulating lupus anticoagulant. *Br Med J* 287:1021, 1983.

23. Bohan A, Peter JB. Polymyositis and dermatomyositis. *N Engl J Med* 292:344, 1975.

24. Brentjens J, et al. Disseminated immune deposits in lupus erythematosus. *Arthritis Rheum* 20:962, 1977.

25. Bulgrin JG, Dubois EL, Jacobson G. Chest roentgenographic changes in systemic lupus erythematosus. *Radiology* 74:42, 1960.

26. Burke GW, Carrington CB, Grinnan R. Pulmonary nodules and rheumatoid factor in the absence of arthritis. *Chest* 72:538, 1977.

27. Byrd RB, Trunk G. Systemic lupus erythematosus presenting as pulmonary hemosiderosis. *Chest* 64:128, 1973.

28. Callen JP. Dermatomyositis and malignancy. *Clin Rheum Dis* 8:369, 1982.

29. Cannon G, Zimmerman G, (Eds). Rheumatologic diseases. The lung in rheumatic diseases. *Lung Biol Health Dis* 45:545, 1990.

30. Caplan A. Certain unusual radiological appearances in the chest of coal-miners suffering from rheumatoid arthritis. *Thorax* 8:29, 1953.

31. Carpenter JR, et al. Survival in polymyositis: Corticosteroids and risk factors. *J Rheumatol* 4:207, 1977.

32. Carr DT, Lillington GA, Mayne JG. Pleural-fluid glucose in systemic lupus erythematosus. *Mayo Clin Proc* 45:409, 1970.

33. Cervantes-Perez P, Toro-Perez AH, Rodriguez-Jurado P. Pulmonary involvement in rheumatoid arthritis. *JAMA* 243:1715, 1980.

34. Chausow AM, et al. Reversible hypercapnic respiratory insufficiency in scleroderma caused by respiratory muscle weakness. *Am Rev Respir Dis* 130:142, 1984.

35. Churg A, et al. Pulmonary hemorrhage and immune-complex deposition in the lung: Complications in a patient with systemic lupus erythematosus. *Arch Pathol Lab Med* 104:388, 1980.

36. Claman HN. On scleroderma: Mast cells, endothelial cells, and fibroblasts. *JAMA* 262:1206, 1989.

37. Colby TV, Carrington CB. Pulmonary lymphomas: Current concepts. *Hum Pathol* 14:884, 1983.

38. Colby TV, Carrington CB. Lymphoreticular tumors and infiltrates of the lung. *Pathol Annu* 18:27, 1983.

39. Constantopoulos SH, et al. Xerotrachea and interstitial lung disease in primary Sjögren's disease. *Respiration* 46:310, 1984.

40. Constantopoulos SH, Papadimitriou CS, Moutsopoulos HM. Respiratory manifestations in primary Sjögren's syndrome. A clinical, functional, and histologic study. *Chest* 88:226, 1985.

41. Corrin B. Bronchiolitis obliterans: A new form of rheumatoid lung (letter)? *Chest* 73:244, 1978.

42. Cush JJ, Goldings EA. Southwestern Internal Medicine Conference. Drug-induced lupus: Clinical spectrum and pathogenesis. *Am J Med Sci* 290:36, 1985.

43. D'Angelo WA, et al. Pathologic observations in systemic sclerosis (scleroderma): A study of fifty-eight autopsy cases and fifty-eight matched controls. *Am J Med* 46:428, 1969.

44. Davis P, et al. Criteria for classification of SLE. *Br Med J* 3:88, 1973.

45. de Clerck LS, et al. D-Penicillamine therapy and interstitial lung disease in scleroderma: A long-term follow up study. *Arthritis Rheum* 30:643, 1987.

46. Derderian SS, et al. Pulmonary involvement in mixed connective tissue disease. *Chest* 88:45, 1985.

47. Dumas LW, Gregory RL, Ozer FL. Case of rheumatoid lung with cavity formation. *Br Med J* 1:383, 1963.

48. Eagen JW, et al. Pulmonary hemorrhage in systemic lupus erythematosus. *Medicine* 57:545, 1978.

49. Eisenberg H, et al. Diffuse interstitial lung disease in systemic lupus erythematosus. *Ann Intern Med* 79:37, 1973.

50. Espinoza LR, Hartmann RC. Significance of the lupus anticoagulant. *Am J Hematol* 22:331, 1986.

51. Estes D, Christian CL. The natural history of systemic lupus erythematosus by prospective analysis. *Medicine* 50:85, 1971.

52. Faguet GB, et al. Immunologically diagnosed malignancy in Sjögren's pseudolymphoma. *Am J Med* 5:424, 1978.

53. Fairfax AJ, et al. Pulmonary disorders associated with Sjögren's syndrome. *Q J Med* 50:279, 1981.

54. Faurschou P. Decreased glucose in RA-cell-positive pleural effusion: Correlation of pleural glucose, lactic dehydrogenase and protein concentration to the presence of RA-cells. *Eur J Respir Dis* 65:272, 1984.

55. Fayemi AO. Pulmonary vascular disease in systemic lupus erythematosus. *Am J Clin Pathol* 65:284, 1976.

56. Fayemi AO. The lung in systemic lupus erythematosus: A clinico-pathologic study of 20 cases. *Mt Sinai J Med* 42:110, 1975.

57. Forman MB, et al. Severe airway obstruction associated with rheumatoid arthritis and Sjögren's syndrome. A case report. *S Afr Med J* 61:674, 1982.

58. Fox RI, et al. Lymphocyte phenotype and function in pseudolymphoma associated with Sjögren's syndrome. *J Clin Invest* 72:52, 1983.

59. Fox RI, et al. Primary Sjögren's syndrome: Clinical and immunopathologic features. *Semin Arthritis Rheum* 14:77, 1984.

60. Frazier AR, Miller RD. Interstitial pneumonitis in association with polymyositis and dermatomyositis. *Chest* 65:403, 1974.

61. Fudman EJ, Kelling DG Jr. Transient effect of nifedipine on pulmonary hypertension of systemic sclerosis. *J Rheumatol* 12:1191, 1985.

62. Garcia JGN, et al. Bronchoalveolar lavage fluid evaluation in rheumatoid arthritis. *Am Rev Respir Dis* 133:450, 1986.

63. Garcia JGN, et al. Lower respiratory tract abnormalities in rheumatoid interstitial lung disease: Potential role of neutrophils in lung injury. *Am Rev Respir Dis* 136:811, 1987.

64. Garnet RF Jr, et al. Rapid screening for lupus erythematosus cells using cytocentrifuge-prepared buffy coat monolayers. *Am J Clin Pathol* 67:537, 1977.

65. Geddes DM, et al. Progressive airway obliteration in adults and its association with rheumatoid disease. *Q J Med* 46:427, 1977.

66. Geddes DM, et al. α1-Antitrypsin phenotypes in fibrosing alveolitis and rheumatoid arthritis. *Lancet* 2:1049, 1977.

67. Geddes DM, Webley M, Emerson PA. Airways obstruction in rheumatoid arthritis. *Ann Rheum Dis* 38:222, 1979.

68. Germain MJ, Davidman M. Pulmonary hemorrhage and acute renal failure in a patient with mixed connective tissue disease. *Am J Kidney Dis* 3:420, 1984.

69. Gibbs AR, Seal RME. Primary lymphoproliferative conditions of the lung. *Thorax* 33:140, 1978.

70. Gibson GJ, Davis P. Respiratory complications of relapsing polychondritis. *Thorax* 29:726, 1974.

71. Gibson GJ, Edmonds JP, Hughes GRV. Diaphragm function and lung involvement in systemic lupus erythematosus. *Am J Med* 63:926, 1977.

72. Gilligan DM, et al. Bronchoalveolar lavage in patients with mild and severe rheumatoid lung disease. *Thorax* 45:591, 1990.

73. Ginsburg WW, et al. Comparison of clinical and serologic markers in systemic lupus erythematosus and overlap syndrome: A review of 247 patients. *J Rheumatol* 10:235, 1983.

74. Glikson M, et al. Nifedipine and prazosin in the management of pulmonary hypertension in CREST syndrome. *Chest* 98:759, 1990.

75. Gold WM, Jennings DB. Pulmonary function in

76. Good JT Jr, et al. Lupus pleuritis: Clinical factors and pleural fluid characteristics with special reference to pleural fluid antinuclear antibodies. *Chest* 84:714, 1983.

77. Gould DB, Soriano RZ. Acute alveolar hemorrhage in lupus erythematosus. *Ann Intern Med* 83:836, 1975.

78. Grant KD, Adams LE, Hess EV. Mixed connective tissue disease—a subset with sequential clinical and laboratory features. *J Rheumatol* 8:587, 1981.

79. Graziano FM, Friedman LC, Grossman J. Pulmonary hypertension in a patient with mixed connective tissue disease: Clinical and pathologic findings, and review of literature. *Clin Exp Rheumatol* 1:251, 1983.

80. Greaves IA. Rheumatoid "pneumoconiosis" (Caplan's syndrome) in an asbestos worker: A 17 years' follow-up. *Thorax* 34:404, 1979.

81. Greenberg SD, Heisler JG, Gyorkey F. Pulmonary lymphoma versus pseudolymphoma: A perplexing problem. *South Med J* 65:775, 1972.

82. Greene NB, Solinger AM, Baughman RP. Patients with collagen vascular disease and dyspnea: The value of gallium scanning and bronchoalveolar lavage in predicting response to steroid therapy and clinical outcome. *Chest* 91:698, 1987.

83. Griffin MT, Robb JD, Martin JR. Diffuse alveolar haemorrhage associated with progressive systemic sclerosis. *Thorax* 45:903, 1990.

84. Gross M, Esterly JR, Earle RH. Pulmonary alterations in systemic lupus erythematosus. *Am Rev Respir Dis* 105:572, 1972.

85. Guit GL, et al. Mediastinal lymphadenopathy and pulmonary arterial hypertension in mixed connective tissue disease. *Radiology* 154:305, 1985.

86. Hainaut P, et al. Circulating lupus type anticoagulant and pulmonary hypertension associated with mixed connective tissue disease. *Clin Rheumatol* 5:96, 1986.

87. Hakala M. Poor prognosis in patients with rheumatoid arthritis hospitalized for interstitial lung fibrosis. *Chest* 93:114, 1988.

88. Halla JT, Schrohenloher RE, Volanakis JE. Immune complexes and other laboratory features of pleural effusions: A comparison of rheumatoid arthritis, systemic lupus erythematosus, and other diseases. *Ann Intern Med* 92:748, 1980.

89. Hansen LA, Prakash UBS, Colby TV. Pulmonary lymphoma in Sjögren's syndrome. *Mayo Clin Proc* 64:920, 1989.

90. Harmon C, et al. Pulmonary involvement in mixed connective tissue disease (MCTD) (abstract). *Arthritis Rheum* 19:801, 1976.

91. Harmon CE, Portanova JP. Drug-induced lupus:

patients with systemic lupus erythematosus. *Am Rev Respir Dis* 93:556, 1966.

Clinical and serological studies. *Clin Rheum Dis* 8:121, 1982.

92. Harrison NK, et al. Evidence for protein oedema, neutrophil influx, and enhanced collagen production in lungs of patients with systemic sclerosis. *Thorax* 45:606, 1990.

93. Harrison NK, et al. Pulmonary involvement in systemic sclerosis: The detection of early changes by thin section CT scan, bronchoalveolar lavage and 99mTc-DTPA clearance. *Respir Med* 83:403, 1989.

94. Harvey AM, et al. Systemic lupus erythematosus: Review of the literature and clinical analysis of 138 cases. *Medicine* 33:291, 1954.

95. Hatron P, et al. Subclinical lung inflammation in primary Sjögren's syndrome. *Arthritis Rheum* 30:1226, 1987.

96. Haupt HM, Moore GW, Hutchins GM. The lung in systemic lupus erythematosus: Analysis of the pathologic changes in 120 patients. *Am J Med* 71:791, 1981.

97. Henriksson KG, Sandstedt P. Polymyositis—treatment and prognosis: A study of 107 patients. *Acta Neurol Scand* 65:280, 1982.

98. Herbert A, et al. Lymphocytic interstitial pneumonia identified as lymphoma of mucosa associated lymphoid tissue. *J Pathol* 146:129, 1985.

99. Herman JH. Polychondritis. In HR Schumacher Jr (Ed), *Primer on Rheumatic Diseases* (9th ed). Atlanta: Arthritis Foundation, 1988.

100. Herzog CA, Miller RR, Hoidal JR. Bronchiolitis and rheumatoid arthritis. *Am Rev Respir Dis* 124:636, 1981.

101. Hills EA, Davies S, Geary M. Frequency dependence of dynamic compliance in patients with rheumatoid arthritis. *Thorax* 34:755, 1979.

102. Hochberg MC, et al. Antibody to Jo-1 in polymyositis/dermatomyositis: Association with interstitial pulmonary disease. *J Rheumatol* 11:663, 1984.

103. Hoffbrand BI, Beck ER. "Unexplained" dyspnoea and shrinking lungs in systemic lupus erythematosus. *Br Med J* 1:1273, 1965.

104. Holgate ST, et al. Respiratory involvement in systemic lupus erythematosus: A clinical and immunological study. *Clin Exp Immunol* 24:385, 1976.

105. Hoogsteden HC, et al. Bilateral exudative pleuritis, an unusual pulmonary onset of mixed connective tissue disease. *Respiration* 48:164, 1985.

106. Horowitz M, et al. Abnormalities of gastric and esophageal emptying in polymyositis and dermatomyositis. *Gastroenterology* 90:434, 1986.

107. Huang C-T, Hennigar GR, Lyons HA. Pulmonary dysfunction in systemic lupus erythematosus. *N Engl J Med* 272:288, 1965.

108. Huang C-T, Lyons HA. Comparison of pulmonary function in patients with systemic lupus

erythematosus, scleroderma, and rheumatoid arthritis. *Am Rev Respir Dis* 93:865, 1966.

109. Hull S, Mathews JA. Pulmonary necrobiotic nodules as a presenting feature of rheumatoid arthritis. *Ann Rheum Dis* 41:21, 1982.

110. Hunder GG, et al. Pleural fluid complement, complement conversion, and immune complexes in immunologic and nonimmunologic diseases. *J Lab Clin Med* 90:971, 1977.

111. Hunder GG, McDuffie FC, Hepper NGG. Pleural fluid complement in systemic lupus erythematosus and rheumatoid arthritis. *Ann Intern Med* 76:357, 1972.

112. Hunninghake GW, Fauci AS. Pulmonary involvement in the collagen vascular diseases. *Am Rev Respir Dis* 119:471, 1979.

113. Hunter T, Arnott JE, McCarthy DS. Features of systemic lupus erythematosus and sarcoidosis occurring together. *Arthritis Rheum* 23:364, 1980.

114. Hurst DJ, Baker WM, Gilbert G. Lung collagen synthesis and type analysis in patients with mixed connective tissue disease (abstract). *Clin Res* 28:744A, 1980.

115. Johnson DA, et al. Pulmonary disease in progressive systemic sclerosis: A complication of gastroesophageal reflux and occult aspiration? *Arch Intern Med* 149:589, 1989.

116. Jones MB, et al. Fatal pulmonary hypertension and resolving immune-complex glomerulonephritis in mixed connective tissue disease: A case report and review of the literature. *Am J Med* 65:855, 1978.

117. Jurik AG, Davidsen D, Graudal H. Prevalence of cardiac and aortic enlargement in rheumatoid arthritis and its relationship to some characteristics of the patients: A radiological and clinical study. *Rheumatol Int* 5:15, 1984.

118. Kaine JL. Refractory massive pleural effusion in systemic lupus erythematosus treated with talc poudrage. *Ann Rheum Dis* 44:61, 1985.

119. Kallenbach J, Prinsloo I, Zwi S. Progressive systemic sclerosis complicated by diffuse pulmonary haemorrhage. *Thorax* 32:767, 1977.

120. Kallenbach J, Zwi S, Goldman HI. Airways obstruction in a case of disseminated lupus erythematosus. *Thorax* 33:84, 1978.

121. Kalunian KC. Definition, Classification, and Activity Indices. In DJ Wallace, BH Hahn (Eds), *Dubois' Lupus Erythematosus* (4th ed). Philadelphia: Lea & Febiger, 1993. Pp 57–63.

122. Karlish AJ. Lung changes in Sjögren's syndrome. *Proc R Soc Med* 62:1042, 1969.

123. Kassan SS, Thomas TL, Moutsopoulos HM. Increased risk of lymphoma in sicca syndrome. *Ann Intern Med* 89:888, 1978.

124. Kay JM, Banik S. Unexplained pulmonary hypertension with pulmonary arteritis in rheumatoid disease. *Br J Dis Chest* 71:53, 1977.

125. Keogh BA, Crystal RG. Chronic Interstitial Lung

Disease. In DH Simmons (Ed), *Current Pulmonology.* Chichester, NY: Wiley, 1981. Pp 237–240.

126. Kim JH, et al. Endobronchial telangiectasias and hemoptysis in scleroderma. *Am J Med* 84:173, 1988.

127. Kobayashi H, et al. Mixed connective tissue disease with fatal pulmonary hypertension. *Acta Pathol Jpn* 32:1121, 1982.

128. Krell WS, Staata BA, Hyatt RE. Pulmonary function in relapsing polychondritis. *Am Rev Respir Dis* 133:1120, 1986.

129. Kuhn C. Systemic lupus erythematosus in a patient with ultrastructural lesions of the pulmonary capillaries previously reported in the review as due to idiopathic pulmonary hemosiderosis. *Am Rev Respir Dis* 106:931, 1972.

130. Lakhanpal S, et al. Polymyositis-dermatomyositis and malignant lesions: Does an association exist? *Mayo Clin Proc* 61:645, 1986.

131. Lawry GV, et al. Laryngeal involvement in rheumatoid arthritis: A clinical, laryngoscopic, and computerized tomographic study. *Arthritis Rheum* 27:873, 1984.

132. Leatherman JW, Sibley RK, Davies SF. Diffuse intrapulmonary hemorrhage and glomerulonephritis unrelated to anti-glomerular basement membrane antibody. *Am J Med* 72:401, 1982.

133. Leikin JB, Arof HM, Pearlman LM. Acute lupus pneumonitis in the postpartum period: A case history and review of the literature. *Obstet Gynecol* 68:29S, 1986.

134. Lemmer JP, et al. Clinical characteristics and course in patients with high titer anti-RNP antibodies. *J Rheumatol* 9:536, 1982.

135. LeRoy EC. Scleroderma (Systemic Sclerosis). In WN Kelley (Ed), *Textbook of Rheumatology* (Vol 2). Philadelphia: Saunders, 1981. P 1211.

136. LeRoy EC, Maricq HR, Kahaleh MB. Undifferentiated connective tissue syndromes. *Arthritis Rheum* 23:341, 1980.

137. Levin AS. Proper interpretation of pulmonary roentgen changes in systemic lupus erythematosus. *Am J Roentgenol* 11:511, 1971.

138. Liebow AA, Carrington CB. Diffuse pulmonary lymphoreticular infiltrations associated with dysproteinemia. *Med Clin North Am* 57:809, 1973.

139. Lofgren RH, Montgomery WW. Incidence of laryngeal involvement in rheumatoid arthritis. *N Engl J Med* 267:193, 1962.

140. Macfarlane JD, Franken CK, van-Leeuwen AWFM. Progressive cavitating pulmonary changes in rheumatoid arthritis: A case report. *Ann Rheum Dis* 43:98, 1984.

141. Mahowald ML, et al. Pulmonary hypertension in systemic lupus erythematosus: Effect of vasodilators on pulmonary hemodynamics. *J Rheumatol* 12:773, 1985.

142. Manchul LA, et al. The frequency of malignant neoplasms in patients with polymyositis-dermatomyositis: A controlled study. *Arch Intern Med* 145:1835, 1985.

143. Marchesoni A, et al. Pulmonary hypertension and systemic lupus erythematosus. *Clin Exp Rheumatol* 1:247, 1983.

144. Marino CT, Pertschuk LP. Pulmonary hemorrhage in systemic lupus erythematosus. *Arch Intern Med* 141:201, 1981.

145. Martens J, Demedts M. Diaphragm dysfunction in mixed connective tissue disease: A case report. *Scand J Rheumatol* 11:165, 1982.

146. Martens J, et al. Respiratory muscle dysfunction in systemic lupus erythematosus. *Chest* 84:170, 1983.

147. Matthay RA, et al. Pulmonary manifestations of systemic lupus erythematosus: Review of twelve cases of acute lupus pneumonitis. *Medicine* 54:397, 1975.

148. Matthay RA, Hudson LD, Petty TL. Acute lupus pneumonitis: Response to azathioprine therapy. *Chest* 63:117, 1973.

149. McAdam LP, et al. Relapsing polychondritis: Prospective study of 23 patients and a review of the literature. *Medicine* 55:193, 1976.

150. McCann BG, et al. Obliterative bronchiolitis and upper-zone pulmonary consolidation in rheumatoid arthritis. *Thorax* 38:73, 1983.

151. McConnochie K, et al. *Aspergillus* colonization of pulmonary rheumatoid nodule. *Respir Med* 83:157, 1989.

152. Medsger TA, Jr. D-Penicillamine treatment of lung involvement in patients with systemic sclerosis (scleroderma). *Arthritis Rheum* 30:832, 1987.

153. Medsger TA Jr. Systemic sclerosis and malignancy—are they related? *J Rheumatol* 12:1041, 1985.

154. Medsger TA Jr, Robinson H, Masi AT. Factors affecting survivorship in polymyositis: A life-table study of 124 patients. *Arthritis Rheum* 14:249, 1971.

155. Michalski JP, et al. Alpha$_1$-antitrypsin phenotypes, including M subtypes, in pulmonary disease associated with rheumatoid arthritis and systemic sclerosis. *Arthritis Rheum* 29:586, 1986.

156. Michet CJ, et al. Relapsing polychondritis: Survival and predictive role of early disease manifestation. *Ann Intern Med* 104:74, 1986.

157. Miller RW, et al. Pulmonary hemorrhage in pediatric patients with systemic lupus erythematosus. *J Pediatr* 108:576, 1986.

158. Millman RP, et al. Systemic lupus erythematosus complicated by acute pulmonary hemorrhage: Recovery following plasmapheresis and cytotoxic therapy (letter). *J Rheumatol* 8:1021, 1981.

159. Mintz G, et al. Acute massive pulmonary hem-

orrhage in systemic lupus erythematosus. *J Rheumatol* 5:39, 1978.

160. Mohsenifar Z, et al. Pulmonary function in patients with relapsing polychondritis. *Chest* 81: 711, 1982.

161. Molina R, et al. Primary Sjögren's syndrome in men: Clinical, serologic, and immunologic features. *Am J Med* 80:23, 1986.

162. Mountz JD, et al. Rheumatoid arthritis and small airways function: Effects of disease activity, smoking, and α1-antitrypsin deficiency. *Arthritis Rheum* 27:728, 1984.

163. Mulkey D, Hudson L. Massive spontaneous unilateral hemothorax in systemic lupus erythematosus. *Am J Med* 56:570, 1974.

164. Myers JL, Katzenstein A-LA. Microangiitis in lupus-induced pulmonary hemorrhage. *Am J Clin Pathol* 85:552, 1986.

165. Myers SA, Podczaski E, Freese U. Acute lupus pneumonitis in the puerperium: A case report and literature review. *J Reprod Med* 25:285, 1980.

166. Naschitz JE, et al. Recurrent massive alveolar hemorrhage, crescentic glomerulonephritis, and necrotizing vasculitis in a patient with rheumatoid arthritis. *Arch Intern Med* 149:406, 1989.

167. Newball HH, Brahim SA. Chronic obstructive airway disease in patients with Sjögren's syndrome. *Am Rev Respir Dis* 115:295, 1977.

168. Niarchos AP, et al. Hemodynamic effects of captopril in pulmonary hypertension of collagen vascular disease. *Am Heart J* 104:834, 1982.

169. Nimelstein SH, et al. Mixed connective tissue disease: A subsequent evaluation of the original 25 patients. *Medicine* 59:239, 1980.

170. Nüsslein HG, et al. Multiple peripheral pulmonary nodules preceding rheumatoid arthritis. *Rheumatol Int* 7:89, 1987.

171. O'Brien JT, Hill JA, Pepine CJ. Sustained benefit of verapamil in pulmonary hypertension with progressive systemic sclerosis. *Am Heart J* 109:380, 1985.

172. Ognibene AJ, Dito WR. Rheumatoid disease with unusual pulmonary manifestations: Pulmonary hemosiderosis, fibrosis, and concretions. *Arch Intern Med* 116:567, 1965.

173. Owens GR, et al. Pulmonary function in progressive systemic sclerosis: Comparison of CREST syndrome variant with diffuse scleroderma. *Chest* 84:546, 1983.

174. Owens GR, Follansbee WP. Cardiopulmonary manifestations of systemic sclerosis. *Chest* 91:118, 1987.

175. Pandya MR, Agus B, Grady RF. In vivo LE phenomenon in pleural fluid (letter). *Arthritis Rheum* 19:962, 1976.

176. Papathanasiou M, et al. Reappraisal of respiratory abnormalities in primary and secondary Sjögren's syndrome. A controlled study. *Chest* 90:370, 1986.

177. Passero FC, Myers AR. Hemopneumothorax in systemic lupus erythematosus. *J Rheumatol* 7:183, 1980.

178. Perez HD, Kramer N. Pulmonary hypertension in systemic lupus erythematosus: Report of four cases and review of the literature. *Semin Arthritis Rheum* 11:177, 1981.

179. Pertschuk LP, et al. Acute pulmonary complications in systemic lupus erythematosus: Immunofluorescence and light microscopic study. *Am J Clin Pathol* 68:553, 1977.

180. Peters-Golden M, et al. Incidence of lung cancer in systemic sclerosis. *J Rheumatol* 12:1136, 1985.

181. Plotz PH, et al. Current concepts in the idiopathic inflammatory myopathies: Polymyositis, dermatomyositis, and related disorders. *Ann Intern Med* 111:143, 1989.

182. Ploysongsang Y, Foad BSI. Lung function tests in connective tissue diseases associated with Raynaud's phenomenon. *Respiration* 46:222, 1984.

183. Portner MM, Gracie WA Jr. Rheumatoid lung disease with cavitary nodules, pneumothorax and eosinophilia. *N Engl J Med* 275:697, 1966.

184. Prakash UBS. Pulmonary manifestations in mixed connective tissue disease. *Semin Respir Med* 9:318, 1988.

185. Prakash UBS, Luthra HS, Divertie MB. Intrathoracic manifestations in mixed connective tissue disease. *Mayo Clin Proc* 60:813, 1985.

186. Purnell DC, Baggenstoss AH, Olsen AM. Pulmonary lesions in disseminated lupus erythematosus. *Ann Intern Med* 42:619, 1955.

187. Quisimorio FP. Pulmonary manifestations (in systemic lupus erythematosus). In DJ Wallace, BH Hahn (Eds), *Dubois' Lupus Erythematosus* (4th ed). Philadelphia: Lea & Febiger, 1993. Pp. 343–355.

188. Radoux V, et al. Airways disease in rheumatoid arthritis patients. One element of a general exocrine dysfunction. *Arthritis Rheum* 30:249, 1987.

189. Reichlin M. Problems in differentiating SLE and mixed connective-tissue disease (editorial). *N Engl J Med* 295:1194, 1976.

190. Roschmann RA, Rothenberg RJ. Pulmonary fibrosis in rheumatoid arthritis: A review of clinical features and therapy. *Semin Arthritis Rheum* 16:174, 1987.

191. Rossi GA, et al. Evidence for chronic inflammation as a component of the interstitial lung disease associated with progressive systemic sclerosis. *Am Rev Respir Dis* 131:612, 1985.

192. Salerni R, et al. Pulmonary hypertension in the CREST syndrome variant of progressive systemic sclerosis (scleroderma). *Ann Intern Med* 86:394, 1977.

193. Salmeron G, Greenberg SD, Lidsky MD. Polymyositis and diffuse interstitial lung disease: A

review of the pulmonary histopathologic findings. *Arch Intern Med* 141:1005, 1981.

194. Saltzstein SL. Pulmonary malignant lymphomas and pseudolymphomas: classification, therapy, and prognosis. *Cancer* 16:928, 1963.

195. Sarma DP, Weilbaecher TG. Systemic scleroderma and small cell carcinoma of the lung. *J Surg Oncol* 29:28, 1985.

196. Sassoon CS, et al. Small airways function in nonsmokers with rheumatoid arthritis. *Arthritis Rheum* 27:1218, 1984.

197. Schleissner LA, Sheehan WW, Orselli RC. Lupus erythematosus in a patient with amyloidosis, adrenal insufficiency, and subsequent immunoblastic sarcoma: Demonstration of the LE phenomenon in the lung. *Arthritis Rheum* 19: 249, 1976.

198. Schumacher HR (Ed). *Primer on Rheumatic Diseases* (9th ed). Atlanta: Arthritis Foundation, 1988.

199. Schwartzberg M, et al. Systemic lupus erythematosus and pulmonary vascular hypertension. *Arch Intern Med* 144:605, 1984.

200. Scott DGI, Bacon PA, Tribe CR. Systemic rheumatoid vasculitis: A clinical and laboratory study of 50 cases. *Medicine* 60:288, 1981.

201. Segal IE, et al. Pulmonary function abnormalities in Sjögren's syndrome and the sicca complex. *Thorax* 36:286, 1981.

202. Sharma S, Vaccharajani A, Mandke J. Severe pulmonary hypertension in rheumatoid arthritis. *Int J Cardiol* 26:220, 1990.

203. Sharp GC. Anti-nRNP and anti-Sm antibodies. *Arthritis Rheum* 25:757, 1982.

204. Sharp GC, Anderson PC. Current concepts in the classification of connective tissue diseases: Overlap syndromes and mixed connective tissue disease (MCTD). *J Am Acad Dermatol* 2: 269, 1980.

205. Sharp GC, et al. Mixed connective tissue disease—an apparently distinct rheumatic disease syndrome associated with a specific antibody to an extractable nuclear antigen (ENA). *Am J Med* 52:148, 1972.

206. Sharp GC, Singsen BH. Mixed Connective Tissue Disease. In DJ McCarty (Ed), *Arthritis and Allied Conditions: A Textbook of Rheumatology* (10th ed). Philadelphia: Lea & Febiger, 1985. P 962.

207. Shiel WC Jr, Prete PE. Pleuropulmonary manifestations of rheumatoid arthritis. *Semin Arthritis Rheum* 13:235, 1984.

208. Silver TM, et al. Radiological features of mixed connective tissue disease and scleroderma–systemic lupus erythematosus overlap. *Radiology* 120:269, 1976.

209. Smith BS. Idiopathic pulmonary haemosiderosis and rheumatoid arthritis. *Br Med J* 1:1403, 1966.

210. Someren AO, et al. Massive asphyxiating pulmonary hemorrhage and glomerulonephritis in a 41-year-old woman. *South Med J* 76:775, 1983.

211. Spencer H. *Pathology of the Lung* (3rd ed). Oxford: Pergamon Press, 1977. Pp. 937–938.

212. Staats BA, et al. The lipoprotein profile of chylous and nonchylous pleural effusions. *Mayo Clin Proc* 55:700, 1980.

213. Steen VD, et al. The effect of D-penicillamine on pulmonary findings in systemic sclerosis. *Arthritis Rheum* 28:882, 1985.

214. Steen VD, et al. Pulmonary involvement in systemic sclerosis (scleroderma). *Arthritis Rheum* 28:759, 1985.

215. Strimaln CV, et al. Pulmonary manifestations of Sjögren's syndrome. *Chest* 70:354, 1976.

216. Stupi AM, et al. Pulmonary hypertension in the CREST syndrome variant of systemic sclerosis. *Arthritis Rheum* 29:515, 1986.

217. Sullivan WD, et al. A prospective evaluation emphasizing pulmonary involvement in patients with mixed connective tissue disease. *Medicine* 63:92, 1984.

218. Sutton PP, et al. Lung mucociliary clearance in rheumatoid disease. *Ann Rheum Dis* 41:47, 1982.

219. Talal N. Sjögren's Syndrome. In N Rose, I Mackay (Eds), *The Autoimmune Diseases.* New York: Academic, 1985. Pp 145–159.

220. Talal N. Sjögren's Syndrome. In HR Schumacher (Ed), *Primer on the Rheumatic Diseases.* Atlanta: Arthritis Foundation, 1988. P 136.

221. Talal N, Bunim JJ. The development of malignant lymphoma in the course of Sjögren's syndrome. *Am J Med* 36:529, 1964.

222. Talal N, Moustopoulos H, Kassan S (Eds). *Sjögren's Syndrome: Clinical and Immunologic Aspects.* Berlin: Springer-Verlag, 1987.

223. Talal N, Sokoloff L, Barth WF. Extrasalivary lymphoid abnormalities in Sjögren's syndrome (reticulum cell sarcoma, "pseudolymphoma," macroglobulinemia). *Am J Med* 43:50, 1967.

224. Talbott JH, Barrocas M. Carcinoma of the lung in progressive systemic sclerosis: A tabular review of the literature and a detailed report of the roentgenographic changes in two cases. *Semin Arthritis Rheum* 9:191, 1980.

225. Talbott JH, Barrocas M. Progressive systemic sclerosis (PSS) and malignancy, pulmonary and non-pulmonary. *Medicine* 58:182, 1979.

226. Tan EM, et al. The 1982 revised criteria for the classification of systemic lupus erythematosus. *Arthritis Rheum* 25:1271, 1982.

227. Tanoue LT. Pulmonary involvement in collagen vascular disease: A review of the pulmonary manifestations of the Marfan syndrome, ankylosing spondylitis, Sjögren's syndrome, and relapsing polychondritis. *J Thorac Imaging* 7:62, 1992.

228. Tesluk H. Progressive systemic sclerosis and

pulmonary cancer [letter]. *Arch Pathol Lab Med* 108:7, 1984.

229. Trimble RB, et al. Preliminary criteria for the classification of systemic lupus erythematosus (SLE): Evaluation in early diagnosed SLE and rheumatoid arthritis. *Arthritis Rheum* 17:184, 1974.

230. Turner-Stokes L, Turner-Warwick M. Intrathoracic manifestations of SLE. *Clin Rheum Dis* 8:229, 1982.

231. Turner-Warwick M. Immunological aspects of systemic diseases of the lungs. *Proc R Soc Med* 67:541, 1974.

232. Ueda N, et al. Mixed connective tissue disease with fatal pulmonary hypertension and a review of literature. *Virchows Arch* [A] 404:335, 1984.

233. Ungerer RG, et al. Prevalence and clinical correlates of pulmonary arterial hypertension in progressive systemic sclerosis. *Am J Med* 75:65, 1983.

234. Vitali C, et al. Lung involvement in Sjögren's syndrome: A comparison between patients with primary and with secondary syndrome. *Ann Rheum Dis* 44:455, 1985.

235. Wallaert B, et al. Subclinical alveolitis in immunological systemic disorders. Transition between health and disease? *Eur Respir J* 3:1206, 1990.

236. Walters MN-I, Ojeda VJ. Pleuropulmonary necrobiotic rheumatoid nodules: A review and clinicopathological study of six patients. *Med J Aust* 144:648, 1986.

237. Wasicek CA, Reichlin M, Montes M, Raghu G. Polymyositis and interstitial lung disease in a patient with anti-Jo-1 prototype. *Am J Med* 76:538, 1984.

238. Weaver AL, Diverite MB, Titus JL. Pulmonary scleroderma. *Dis Chest* 54:490, 1968.

239. Webb WR, Gamsu G. Cavitary pulmonary nodules with systemic lupus erythematosus: Differential diagnosis. *AJR* 136:27, 1981.

240. Weiland JE, et al. Neutrophil collagenase in rheumatoid interstitial lung disease. *J Appl Physiol* 62:628, 1987.

241. Weinrib L, Sharma OP, Quismorio FP Jr. A long term study of interstitial lung disease in systemic lupus erythematosus. *Semin Arthritis Rheum* 16:479, 1990.

242. Wiedemann HP, Matthay RA. Pulmonary manifestations of the collagen vascular diseases. *Clin Chest Med* 10:677, 1989.

243. Wiener-Kronish JP, et al. Severe pulmonary involvement in mixed connective tissue disease. *Am Rev Respir Dis* 124:499, 1981.

244. Winkelmann RK, et al. Course of dermatomyositis polymyositis: Comparison of untreated and cortisone-treated patients. *Mayo Clin Proc* 43:545, 1968.

245. Winkelmann RK, Flach DB, Unni KK. Lung cancer and scleroderma. *Arch Dermatol Res* 280 (Suppl):S15, 1988.

246. Winslow WA, Ploss LN, Loitman B. Pleuritis in systemic lupus erythematosus: Its importance as an early manifestation in diagnosis. *Ann Intern Med* 49:70, 1958.

247. Worth H, et al. Lung function disturbances versus respiratory muscle fatigue in patients with systemic lupus erythematosus. *Respiration* 53:81, 1988.

248. Young RH, Mark GJ. Pulmonary vascular changes in scleroderma. *Am J Med* 64:998, 1978.

249. Yousem SA, Colby TV, Carrington CB. Follicular bronchitis/bronchiolitis. *Hum Pathol* 16:700, 1985.

250. Yousem SA, Colby TV, Carrington CB. Lung biopsy in rheumatoid arthritis. *Am Rev Respir Dis* 131:770, 1985.

58

Pulmonary Vasculitides

Udaya B. S. Prakash

The primary vasculitides are a heterogeneous group of disorders characterized by degrees of inflammation and necrosis of the arteries. Similar processes may affect the veins and capillaries in some of the vasculitides. Depending on the type of vasculitis, arteries and veins of all sizes and capillaries in different locations throughout the body may become involved. Etiologic factors for most of the primary vasculitides are not known. Secondary vasculitides are caused by collagenoses, immunologic aberrations, absence or deficiency of certain chemical mediators in the body, and mycoses, especially from *Aspergillus* and *Mucor* species.

There is no satisfactory clinical classification of vasculitides. However, the diagnostic criteria for various vasculitides by the American College of Rheumatology (ACR), published in 1990, provides a proper perspective regarding the incidence of different vasculitides in the 1980s [4, 9,16,65,88,89,110,119,123,127,132,133]. This study gathered data on 1020 patients with various types of vasculitides from 48 centers in the United States and Canada over a 5-year period. Only 807 patients met the criteria established for the diagnosis of several types of primary vasculitides. Interestingly, the majority of the remainder had vasculitis secondary to rheumatologic diseases. This chapter will discuss the respiratory manifestations in primary vasculitides. In addition, certain disorders such as lymphomatoid granulomatosis and eosinophilia-myalgia syndrome are included in the discussion because the vasculitic processes and clinical features often resemble those of other primary vasculitic syndromes.

Wegener's Granulomatosis

Wegener's granulomatosis is a systemic vasculitis characterized by necrotizing granulomatous vasculitis of the upper and lower respiratory tract, glomerulonephritis, and variable degrees of small-vessel vasculitis involving arteries and veins [29,58,60,110,120,184]. Some consider Wegener's granulomatosis to be a necrotizing granulomatous disorder rather than a true vasculitis [119]. The Wegener's triad to establish the diagnosis consists of necrotizing granulomas of the upper or lower respiratory tract or both, generalized focal necrotizing vasculitis of arteries and veins in lungs (Fig. 58-1) and other organs, and focal necrotizing glomerulitis [71]. The term *limited Wegener's granulomatosis* has been used to describe Wegener's granulomatosis involving the respiratory system without glomerulonephritis [19], but the nomenclature is misguided because many patients with limited Wegener's granulomatosis develop renal involvement in the course of their disease, and kidney biopsy obtained in these patients will show typical morphology. Renal involvement with focal segmental glomerulonephritis remains a hallmark of Wegener's granulomatosis. Histologic features include discrete or confluent granulomatosis and necrotizing granuloma with vasculitis (Fig. 58-2). Fibrinoid necrosis, microabscesses, focal vasculitis, thrombosis, and fibrous obliteration of vascular lumen may be seen (Figs. 58-3, 58-4).

Only 10.5 percent of 807 patients with various vasculitides studied by the ARC had Wegener's granulomatosis. The mean age at onset of symptoms of the disease was 45.2 years. Men outnumbered women by a ratio of 2 : 1, and 91 percent were Caucasians [110]. Initially, patients present with nonspecific symptoms, including fever, malaise, weight loss, arthralgias, and myalgias [58]. Focal segmental glomerulonephritis is a hallmark of Wegener's granulomatosis. The incidence of the involvement of other organs is as follows: skin, 40 to 50 percent; eyes, 43 percent; arthralgias, 58 percent; arthritis, 28 percent; and neurologic involvement, 25 percent [58,60,82,137,146,

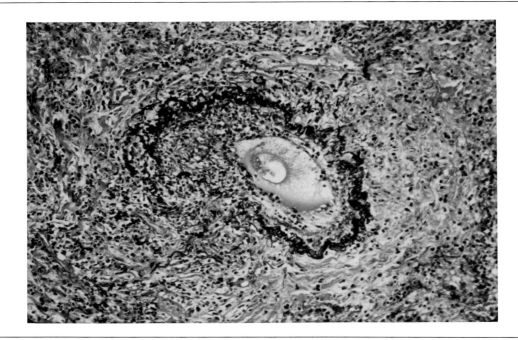

Fig. 58-1. Wegener's granulomatosis with vasculitis involving a medium-size vein. Inflammatory infiltrate is eccentric and segmental and is associated with destruction of the vascular elastica.

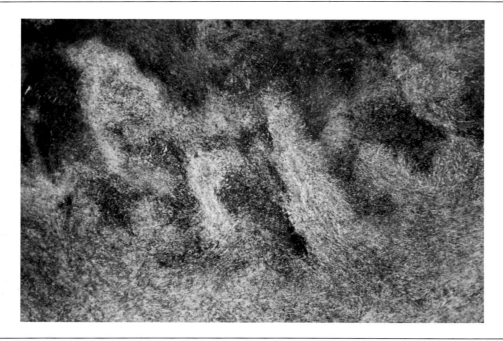

Fig. 58-2. Geographically dark irregular zones of necrosis in Wegener's granulomatosis are seen that involve the upper portion of the lung.

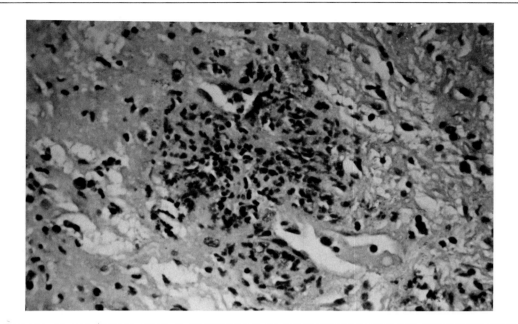

Fig. 58-3. An early microscopic granuloma in Wegener's granulomatosis manifests as a cluster of cells, often centered on a capillary, with central neutrophilia and surrounding histiocytes. Such a lesion ultimately would enlarge to form the characteristic geographic necrotic granulomas of Wegener.

190]. The cardiovascular system may also be involved.

The presence of antineutrophil cytoplasmic antibodies (ANCAs) in the blood has been used to confirm the diagnosis [39,97,153,163,164,179], but the ACR studies did not include these tests in the diagnostic classification of Wegener's granulomatosis [56,94]. Of the two main patterns of cytoplasmic fluorescence recognized—namely, cytoplasmic ANCA (c-ANCA) or, more specifically, Pr3 antibodies, and perinuclear ANCA (p-ANCA)—c-ANCA seems specific for Wegener's granulomatosis, whereas p-ANCA is associated with other vasculitides, rheumatoid arthritis, ulcerative colitis, Crohn's disease, autoimmune chronic active hepatitis, primary biliary cirrhosis, and sclerosing cholangitis [97]. c-ANCA is present in more than 90 percent of patients with Wegener's granulomatosis associated with respiratory, renal, and systemic vasculitis, whereas in those with so-called limited Wegener's granulomatosis the positive rate is in the range of 67 to 86 percent [97]. The overall sensitivity is approx-

imately 81 percent, and the specificity of c-ANCA for Wegener's granulomatosis is reported to be 98 percent [97]. The titers and sensitivity of the test for c-ANCA correlate with activity of the disease, whereas the specificity of the test depends on the nature of the controls chosen for analysis [110, 153]. There is in vitro evidence that ANCAs are directly involved in the pathogenesis of ANCA-associated diseases [95]. Titers of c-ANCA can be used to follow disease activity in patients with Wegener's granulomatosis and related disorders.

The presence of c-ANCA is not limited to patients with only classic Wegener's granulomatosis. It has been noted also in approximately 50 percent of patients with necrotizing (pauciimmune) glomerulonephritis in combination with systemic small-vessel vasculitis but without granulomatous inflammation. This entity has been named *microscopic polyarteritis* [153,154]. In fact, some patients who initially manifest microscopic polyarteritis develop features of Wegener's granulomatosis during a relapse of their disease [97]. Some patients with systemic necrotizing vasculitis involving medium-size arteries but without pathologic proof of Wegener's granulomatosis are positive for c-ANCA and frequently have signs of upper airway disease and thus fulfill the ACR criteria for the diagnosis of Wegener's granulomatosis [35,97,110]. The term *polyangiitis* has been used to describe syn-

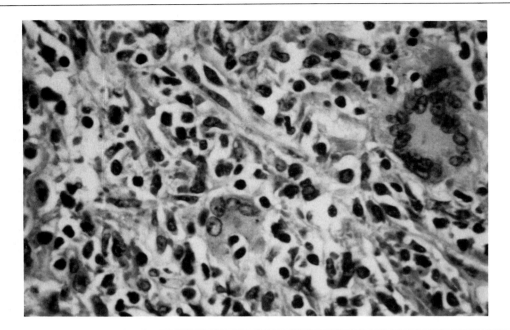

Fig. 58-4. Background inflammatory infiltrate in Wegener's granulomatosis includes mixed chronic inflammatory cells, usually with numerous plasma cells and occasional eosinophils, as well as scattered giant cells. Sarcoid-like granulomas and nonnecrotizing granulomas are lacking.

dromes in which patients demonstrate overlapping clinical features of polyarteritis nodosa, Wegener's granulomatosis, Churg-Strauss syndrome, and vasculitides [111]. A majority of the patients with polyangiitis appear to be positive for c-ANCA [97].

More recently, ANCAs with myeloperoxidase specificity (MPO-ANCAs) have been used in the diagnosis of vasculitic syndromes. The MPO-ANCAs have been identified in up to 87 percent of patients with p-ANCA but not in those with c-ANCA [13]. The presence of MPO-ANCA is reported to recognize patients with idiopathic and polyarteritis nodosa–associated necrotizing and crescentic glomerulonephritis, and these antibodies have also been detected in 30 percent of patients with a proved diagnosis of antiglomerular basement membrane disease [13].

Laboratory tests in patients with Wegener's granulomatosis may reveal mild to moderate normochromic normocytic anemia, mild leukocytosis, mild thrombocytosis, elevated erythrocyte sedimentation rate (often exceeding 100 mm/hr), positive rheumatoid factor, and elevations of immunoglobulins IgG and IgA and circulating immune complexes [60]. Peripheral blood eosinophilia is not a feature of Wegener's granulomatosis even though eosinophilic infiltrates are seen in tissue samples. All of these abnormalities are nonspecific and indicate a systemic inflamma-

tory disease [58]. Urinalysis is an important test, as abnormalities such as hematuria, proteinuria, and red cell casts are observed in 80 percent of patients [60]. Pulmonary function tests, particularly flow-volume curves, are helpful in assessing major airway involvement in Wegener's granulomatosis.

Acute Airways Disease

Symptoms referable to the head and neck are noted initially by more than 85 percent of patients. Rhinorrhea, purulent or bloody nasal discharge, nasal mucosal drying and crust formation, epistaxis, and otitis media are common. Deep facial pain from paranasal sinus involvement, nasal septal perforation, and ulceration of the vomer are important signs of Wegener's granulomatosis [130]. The incidence of bacterial infection is increased in Wegener's granulomatosis due to a disruption in the mucosal barrier and the failure to clear secretions. Superinfection particularly from *Staphylococcus aureus* is common. Other clinical signs include aphthous lesions of the nasal and oral mucosa and inflammation and destruction of the nasal cartilages leading to a so-called saddle-nose deformity, which is usually a subacute or, more often, a chronic complication. Ulcerated lesions of the larynx and trachea are present in 30 percent of untreated cases. Hemoptysis in such cases may arise from mucosal ulcerations in the tracheobronchial tree, and bronchoscopic examination usually reveals extremely friable mucosa that bleeds profusely on instrumentation.

Pulmonary Parenchymal Disease

Although only one-third of patients with Wegener's granulomatosis manifest symptoms of lower respiratory tract involvement, the lower respiratory tract is involved in nearly all patients [59]. The term *limited Wegener's granulomatosis* has been applied to isolated involvement of the lower respiratory tract [19]. When lungs are affected, symptoms include hemoptysis, dyspnea, cough, and chest pain. Hemoptysis, the most common symptom, was noted in 98 percent of patients studied by the ARC [110]. Overall, pulmonary involvement was seen in 94 percent, paranasal disease in 91 percent, and nasal and pharyngeal involvement in 64 percent of patients.

Chest pain, which also is common, may be caused by pleural effusion, which is described in 5 to 55 percent of cases of Wegener's granulomatosis [150]. The clinical presentation can vary from subacute nonspecific respiratory illness to rapidly progressive respiratory failure. Pulmonary symptoms are almost always associated with chest roentgenographic abnormalities [58, 112]. The ACR study noted abnormal chest roentgenograms in 65 percent of patients [110]. An analysis of 80 patients reported from three separate studies observed the following chest roentgenographic abnormalities: unilateral, 55 percent; bilateral, 45 percent; infiltrates, 63 percent; nodules, 31 percent; infiltrates with cavitation, 8 percent; and nodules with cavitation, 10 percent [128]. The nodules usually are rounded, range from a few millimeters to several centimeters in diameter, and commonly are bilateral (Fig. 58-5). One-third contain cavities, which are irregular in outline, thick-walled, and possess a shaggy inner lining (Fig. 58-6). Solitary nodules occur in 30 to 40 percent of patients with Wegener's granulomatosis [192]. Unusual manifestations of the disease include diffuse pulmonary infiltrates (Fig. 58-7), lymphadenopathy, pneumonic infiltrates, lobar consolidation, and

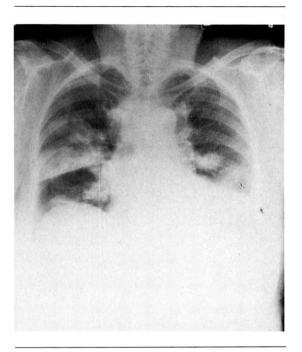

Fig. 58-5. Bilateral multiple nodular as well as masslike lesions in Wegener's granulomatosis.

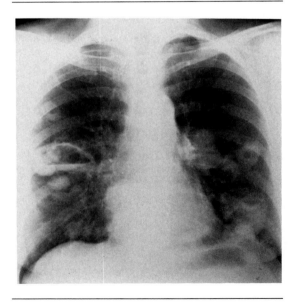

Fig. 58-6. Bilateral multiple cavitated nodules of varying sizes in Wegener's granulomatosis.

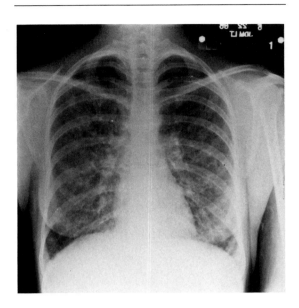

Fig. 58-7. Diffuse micronodular infiltrates in Wegener's granulomatosis.

pleural effusions [113,150]. Pure interstitial infiltrates are uncommon. Diffuse alveolar infiltrates may indicate alveolar hemorrhage.

Before the diagnosis of Wegener's granulomatosis can be firmly established, vasculitis secondary to infectious processes and collagenoses must be excluded. Mycobacteria, fungi, and helminths can cause systemic illness, pulmonary infiltrates, and histologic evidence of granulomatous vasculitis [58,112]. The ACR classification criteria for Wegener's granulomatosis included four features: nasal inflammation, abnormal chest roentgenogram, abnormal urinary sediment, and granulomatous inflammation on biopsy. However, in the absence of biopsy, hemoptysis was used as a "surrogate criterion" based on the high incidence (in 98 percent) of hemoptysis [110]. Currently, the diagnosis should be based on clinical features, the presence of c-ANCA, exclusion of other causes of vasculitis, and biopsy if the diagnosis remains doubtful [144].

A study of the histologic features in 87 open-lung biopsies from 67 patients (72 percent of whom had classic Wegener's granulomatosis with renal involvement and 28 percent of whom had so-called limited disease) reported the following findings: Interstitial fibrosis appeared in 26 percent; alveolar hemorrhage in 49 percent; tissue eosinophilia in 100 percent; organizing intralu-

minal fibrosis in 70 percent; endogenous lipoid pneumonia in 59 percent; lymphoid aggregates in 37 percent; and a variety of bronchial or bronchiolar lesions including acute and chronic bronchiolitis in 51 and 64 percent, respectively, follicular bronchiolitis in 28 percent, and bronchiolitis obliterans in 31 percent [175].

Alveolar Hemorrhage

Wegener's granulomatosis is among the causes of alveolar hemorrhage syndromes (see Chapter 61) and so should be considered in the differential diagnosis [109]. Massive pulmonary alveolar hemorrhage is occasionally seen in Wegener's granulomatosis and often presents as a life-threatening problem [135,173,174]. Diffuse pulmonary hemorrhage from necrotizing capillaritis occurs in 5 to 45 percent of biopsy or necropsy cases [36,110,173]. As cited previously, alveolar hemorrhage was noted in 49 percent of 87 open-lung biopsies from 67 patients [175]. In the presence of renal dysfunction and urinary sediment abnormalities, differentiating Wegener's granulomatosis from antiglomerular antibody disease becomes difficult. Biopsy and special immunofluorescent studies may be necessary to establish the diagnosis.

Tracheobronchial Stenosis

Endotracheal or endobronchial involvement with Wegener's granulomatosis occurs in a significant number of patients [10]. Subglottic stenosis is seen in 5 to 8 percent of treated patients, whereas benign-appearing stenoses of the tracheobronchial tree are more likely in chronic cases and in patients whose disease is stable. The National Institutes of Health study reported that 14 percent of 85 patients had endobronchial disease at some point during their illness, and subglottic stenosis was present in 7 percent [58]. The symptoms tend to be insidious in onset. Inspiratory and expiratory flow-volume loops may aid in assessing the impairment of the upper airway as well as in the follow-up of these patients [149].

Treatment and Prognosis

Corticosteroids administered in combination with cyclophosphamide result in complete remission in more than 90 percent of patients [58]. The usual dosage of these is up to 2 mg/kg/day of each orally. In milder cases, corticosteroids alone may be sufficient, although some believe this is inadequate [186]. Some patients require prolonged treatment with smaller doses of corticosteroids or cyclophosphamide or both. The antimicrobial agent trimethoprim-sulfamethoxazole has been reported to be effective in maintaining remission [45]. As observed earlier, "limited" Wegener's granulomatosis may not be a distinct entity because most patients with obvious respiratory involvement also have clinically undetectable renal lesions. Although the original description of the limited disease reported that these patients have an excellent prognosis [19], it is important to treat them aggressively.

Nd : YAG laser therapy followed by stent dilatation or bronchoscopic balloon dilatation has been used to treat large tracheal granuloma caused by Wegener's granulomatosis [144]. Others have used CO_2 laser to treat subglottic stenosis [166]. Symptomatic subglottic stenosis may require surgical therapy [44]. Relapse of pulmonary Wegener's granulomatosis usually is associated with viral or bacterial infections. If such infections go untreated, Wegener's granulomatosis may ensue within 1 year [186].

Fig. 58-8. Lymphomatoid granulomatosis showing angiocentric infiltration by dense lymphoid infiltrates. Cytologically, this case had features of a diffuse large-cell lymphoma.

Lymphomatoid Granulomatosis

Lymphomatoid granulomatosis is a lymphoproliferative disorder and not a primary vasculitis. Clinically and roentgenologically, lymphomatoid granulomatosis mimics Wegener's granulomatosis [91,120]. Earlier terms for lymphomatoid granulomatosis include *polymorphic reticulosis, midline malignant reticulosis, midline granuloma,* and *Stewart's granuloma* [46,51,90,165, 185]. Some have suggested a newer name, *angiocentric malignant lymphoma* [185].

Lymphomatoid granulomatosis is a destructive angiocentric process of unknown etiology characterized by prominent vascular infiltrates and necrosis of medium and small blood vessels with formation of granulomas (Fig. 58-8) [57,99]. Histologic analysis of tissues may show a spectrum of benign-appearing lymphocytic interstitial pneumonitis to overtly malignant lymphoma in the same patient. Although a retrospective study documented progression to non-Hodgkin's lymphoma in only 12 percent of patients [99], a prospective study reported the occurrence of lymphoma in 50 percent [40]. Impairment of the immune system due to unknown causes may predispose patients with lymphomatoid granulomatosis to develop anergy and, eventually, lymphoma [78]. Lymphomas occurring in patients

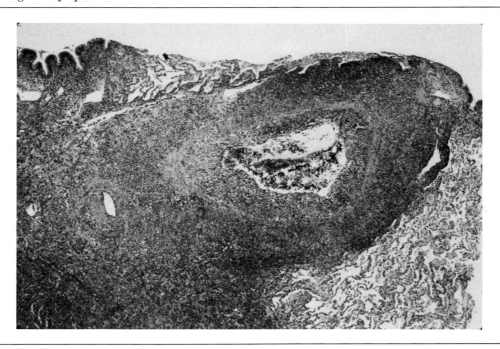

with lymphomatoid granulomatosis are malignant lymphomas of T-lymphocytic identity [185].

Lymphomatoid granulomatosis is an uncommon disease, with approximately 200 cases reported in the literature [128]. The disease usually presents during middle age, and there is a slightly higher prevalence in men. The presenting symptoms of lymphomatoid granulomatosis are nonspecific. Systemic symptoms of fewer, malaise, and weight loss are common. Lymphomatoid granulomatosis can affect any organ system, but the disease is found with particular frequency in the central nervous system, skin, kidney, and lymphatic system [99,121]. Nearly one-fourth of patients demonstrate involvement of the central nervous system [121]. Ataxia, hemiparesis, blindness, and dizziness may be the presenting symptoms. Almost half of patients with lymphomatoid granulomatosis develop skin lesions in the form of erythematous, macular, or plaquelike lesions over the extremities [121].

Laboratory tests are not helpful in the diagnosis. Leukocytosis (in 30 percent of patients), leukopenia (in 20 percent of patients), mild to moderate elevation of the erythrocyte sedimentation rate, and mild elevations of IgG or IgM may be present [99]. Urinalysis usually is normal in patients with lymphomatoid granulomatosis because the glomerulus is characteristically spared.

The diagnosis of this disease requires biopsy examination of the affected tissue, usually lung, skin, kidney, or head and neck lesions. Affected lung tissue in lymphomatoid granulomatosis is characterized by an angiocentric angiodestructive infiltration of atypical lymphocytoid and plasmacytoid cells (see Fig. 58-8).

Pulmonary Disease

As in Wegener's granulomatosis, pulmonary involvement is present in virtually all patients. Along with the systemic symptoms, cough and dyspnea are prominent respiratory symptoms [57,91,99,121]. If head and neck areas are involved, patients may present with symptoms similar to those of Wegener's granulomatosis. Hemoptysis is more likely in those with cavitated lung lesions. Chest roentgenograms most frequently disclose nodular infiltrates. Nodular densities may cavitate and are more common in the lower lung zones. Multiple nodules with poorly defined borders were observed in 88 percent of patients, with cavitation in 25 percent in one series [183]. Occasionally, alveolar infiltrates are noted. Pleural effusions may be seen in approximately one-third of cases [192]. Pleural effusion has been noted in 25 percent of patients [183]. One review of 173 patients collected from two separate series noted the following chest roentgenologic abnormalities: multiple bilateral nodules in 80 percent of patients; cavitation of nodules in 30 percent; air bronchograms in 35 percent; pleural effusion in 33 percent; atelectasis in 30 percent; pneumonitis or masslike lesions in 30 percent; and pneumothorax in 5 percent (Figs. 58-9, 58-10) [128].

Presence of hilar or mediastinal lymphadenopathy usually signifies lymphomatous transformation. Unilateral or bilateral large pulmonary masses measuring more than 10 cm in diameter often signal the presence of lymphoma [57].

Airway involvement is unusual but can be extensive. Pathologic findings described include bronchiolitis obliterans, bronchial ulceration, and destruction and occlusion of bronchioles by masses of inflammatory cells and fibrous tissue [99,121].

Treatment and Prognosis

A definitive therapy for lymphomatoid granulomatosis is not available. In most patients, a therapeutic approach similar to that for highly malignant lymphoma must be considered [57,112,114]. Adequate clinical staging and multiple biopsies to assess properly the degree of malignancy is necessary before commencing multiple-drug therapy [114]. Multiple chemotherapeutic agents with a

Fig. 58-9. Bilateral multiple nodular lesions in lymphomatoid granulomatosis.

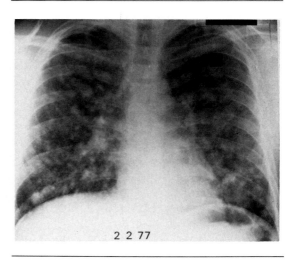

2 2 77

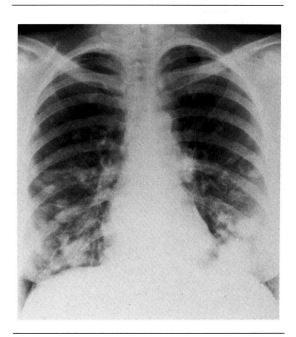

Fig. 58-10. Bilateral multiple nodules of varying sizes in lymphomatoid granulomatosis. Several nodules are cavitated.

corticosteroid may be needed in patients who demonstrate highly malignant features. Localized lesions in the head and neck area may respond to irradiation. Progressive respiratory involvement, usually due to lymphoma and related complications, is the most frequent cause of death [99, 121]. Fever, leukopenia, cutaneous anergy, and hepatomegaly have been reported to portend poor prognosis [27,57].

Churg-Strauss Syndrome

Churg-Strauss syndrome, also known as *allergic granulomatosis and angiitis*, is separate from hypersensitivity vasculitis and polyarteritis nodosa. A significant amount of confusion exists in the definition of this syndrome. The original report described 13 cases of severe asthma with a "strikingly uniform clinical picture including fever, hypereosinophilia, and vascular abnormality in various organ systems." The records of 11 patients who died were located through autopsy files, and in all 11 the original diagnosis was polyarteritis nodosa [30]. In 1981, the syndrome was redefined to include eosinophilic pneumonitis, eosinophilic nonnecrotizing angiitis, bronchocentric granulomatosis, allergic granuloma, and nec-

rotizing angiitis [31]. Further, some characterize Churg-Strauss syndrome as an overlap syndrome that includes hypereosinophilic disease (Löffler's syndrome), systemic vasculitides (polyarteritis nodosa and hypersensitivity vasculitis), and Wegener's granulomatosis [107]. In many patients, the clinical and pathologic features overlap those of Wegener's granulomatosis and polyarteritis nodosa [119]. The confusion is exacerbated by the associations made among Churg-Strauss syndrome and bacterial endocarditis, chronic active hepatitis, leukemia, lymphoma, myeloma, rheumatoid arthritis, systemic lupus erythematosus, and ulcerative colitis [62].

Despite multiple reports on the topic, Churg-Strauss syndrome is an uncommon disease. In the ACR study of 807 patients with various vasculitides, Churg-Strauss syndrome constituted only 2.5 percent of cases [9]. At the Mayo Clinic, only 30 cases were identified between 1950 and 1974 [28].

The two diagnostically essential lesions of Churg-Strauss syndrome are granulomatous or nongranulomatous angiitis and extravascular necrotizing granulomas, usually with eosinophilic infiltrates [119]. The angiitis is disseminated and involves pulmonary and systemic arteries and veins (Fig. 58-11). Unlike Wegener's granulomatosis, extrapulmonary lesions are found more commonly in the gastrointestinal tract, spleen, and heart than in the kidney [119]. Thus, renal failure seldom is seen in Churg-Strauss syndrome [28]. Other characteristic features include pulmonary and systemic vasculitis, extravascular granulomas, and eosinophilia occurring almost exclusively in patients with asthma or a history of allergy. The so-called limited Churg-Strauss syndrome occurs in isolated organs or tissues and in some patients with collagenoses or autoimmune disorders [119]. The Churg-Strauss granulomas of cutaneous and subcutaneous tissues lack diagnostic specificity because approximately 50 percent of these lesions occur in systemic diseases other than Churg-Strauss syndrome [118]. Hypereosinophilia in peripheral blood and elevation of serum IgE are common [29,30,180].

Upper Airways Disease

The 20 patients studied by the ACR had a mean age of 50 years at the onset of Churg-Strauss syndrome [127]. Nasal symptoms such as allergic rhinitis, nasal polyps, nasal mucosal crusting, and septal perforation are seen in more than 70 per-

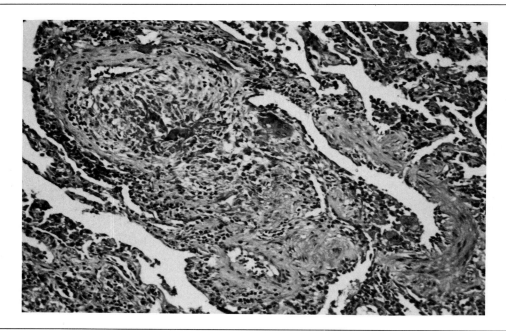

cent of patients [29,30,180]. Nasal polyps are the major clinical finding. All 20 patients in the ACR study had chronic paranasal sinus pain or tenderness, 18 had seasonal allergy, and 14 had opacification of paranasal sinuses [127]. In contrast to Wegener's granulomatosis, major airway involvement seldom is seen in Churg-Strauss syndrome.

Pulmonary Disease

The major pulmonary symptom in Churg-Strauss syndrome is related to underlying asthma, which is believed to be present in all patients [30, 44,107], although the syndrome has been described in the absence of asthma in a 38-year-old man [26]. In the ACR report on 20 patients, 19 had asthma, and all had transitory pulmonary infiltrates on the chest roentgenogram, peripheral blood eosinophilia, and mononeuritis or polyneuritis multiplex [127]. The 15 patients in the Mayo Clinic series who died from Churg-Strauss syndrome had asthma for a mean interval of only 3 years prior to the onset of vasculitis; the mean duration of asthma among the remaining 15 survivors was 13 years [28]. A phasic pattern of Churg-Strauss syndrome has been described, beginning with allergic rhinitis, evolving into asthma, followed by peripheral blood eosinophilia and eosinophilic tissue infiltrates, and ultimately developing to vasculitis [107].

Fig. 58-11. Churg-Strauss syndrome involving the lung shows mixed inflammatory infiltrates including occasional giant cells (upper center) as well as a necrotic granuloma with central eosinophilic debris involving a vessel wall (upper left).

In one study of 154 patients, 84 of whom were male, the mean ages were 28 years at the onset of allergic rhinitis, 35 years at the onset of asthma, and 38 years when vasculitis was diagnosed [107]. The mean peak eosinophil count was 12.9×10^9/liter. Anemia was present in 83 percent, granulomas in 40 percent, tissue eosinophilia in approximately 50 percent, and vasculitis in more than 70 percent. The patients surviving longer than 1 year had a mean interval of 6.6 years, whereas those who died within 1 year of onset of vasculitis had a mean interval of 4.2 years between the onset of asthma and vasculitis. Lung failure was the cause of death in only 2 percent, although 8 percent died from status asthmaticus. The main causes of mortality were heart failure (48 percent), renal failure (18 percent), cerebral hemorrhage (16 percent), and gastrointestinal hemorrhage (8 percent) [107]. Massive pulmonary alveolar hemorrhage is described in Churg-Strauss syndrome but is rare [33].

Chest roentgenographic abnormalities are present in more than 60 percent of patients. The findings may include patchy and occasionally diffuse

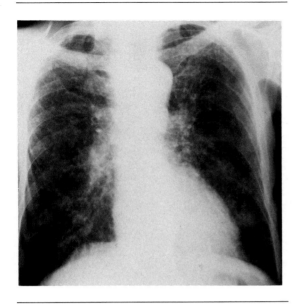

Fig. 58-12. Diffuse fine nodular infiltrates in Churg-Strauss syndrome. Note the relative sparing of lower lung zones and the hyperinflation from asthma.

alveolar-interstitial infiltrates in the perihilar area with a propensity for the upper two-thirds of the lung fields (Fig. 58-12) [28]. Areas of cavitation occur rarely. Nodular changes seen in Wegener's granulomatosis are uncommon in Churg-Strauss syndrome, though pleural effusion can occur [54].

Treatment and Prognosis

None of the 20 patients described in the ACR report died from Churg-Strauss syndrome [127]. Dramatic response can be expected from high-dose systemic corticosteroid therapy, which should be instituted as soon as the diagnosis is made.

Giant-Cell Arteritis

Giant-cell arteritis, also known as *temporal arteritis, cranial arteritis*, and *granulomatous arteritis*, was the most common form of vasculitis, observed in 26.5 percent of 807 patients with various types of vasculitides studied by the ACR [9]. Giant-cell arteritis is a vasculitis of unknown etiology and, although morphologic findings are variable, the characteristic findings consist of lymphocytic infiltration with fragmentation of the internal elastic lamina, granulomatous in-

flammation, histiocytes, and multinucleate giant cells. The classic pathologic features of giant-cell arteritis are seen in approximately 60 percent of temporal artery biopsies [119]. Although giant-cell arteritis has been described in association with polymyalgia rheumatica, the relationship between these two entities remains uncertain [34]. Giant-cell arteritis usually affects middle-aged or older persons. There has been an increase in the annual incidence of giant-cell arteritis, with rates of 24.1 cases per 100,000 persons per year reported in the mid-1980s [87,88].

The onset of arteritis and blindness may be sudden, but usually the clinical illness has a gradual onset, with the development of nonspecific systemic symptoms such as low-grade fever, malaise, and weight loss. Headache, variable but often severe, is the most common symptom in giant-cell arteritis. The generalized symptoms may be followed by more specific symptoms such as jaw claudication and sudden loss of vision. Amaurosis fugax is observed in 20 percent and visual loss in 10 percent of cases [20]. There are no specific laboratory tests available to diagnose giant-cell arteritis, though a moderate elevation of erythrocyte sedimentation rate is common.

Pulmonary Involvement

Pulmonary complications of giant-cell arteritis were first recognized in 1984 when a report from the Mayo Clinic described 16 patients with giant-cell arteritis and observed that 9 percent of patients had prominent respiratory tract symptoms and that the presenting symptoms originated from the respiratory tract in 4 percent [108]. The respiratory symptoms, which included cough, sore throat, and hoarseness, were the initial findings in 10 patients and resolved quickly when corticosteroids were given. A population-based study of patients with giant-cell arteritis noted respiratory symptoms in up to 30 percent of 94 patients [126]. Therefore, giant-cell arteritis should be considered in any older patient with a new cough or throat pain without obvious cause.

Isolated small airways disease has been detected in 46.2 percent of patients with giant-cell arteritis, but the abnormalities have not been significantly different from those of the controls; chest roentgenograms in those with abnormal pulmonary function tests have been normal [2]. However, pulmonary nodules, interstitial infiltrates, and occlusion and aneurysms of the pulmonary artery have been described [14,43,70, 104]. Multinodular pulmonary lesions in one patient and a diffuse interstitial pattern in another have both resolved following corticosteroid therapy [104]. Individual case reports of giant-cell arteritis in association with asthma, eosinophilic interstitial infiltrates, and small nodules [3], pulmonary vascular disease [47], and focal necrosis as well as granulomatous inflammation of large and medium pulmonary arteries [105], and giant-cell arteritis limited to large pulmonary arteries [104] have been published.

Treatment and Prognosis

Virtually all patients respond favorably to systemic corticosteroids. Uniform resolution of pulmonary complications were reported following corticosteroid therapy among the patients in the literature just cited.

Behçet's Disease

Behçet's disease is a chronic, relapsing multisystemic inflammatory disorder characterized by aphthous stomatitis along with two or more of the following: aphthous genital ulcerations, uveitis, cutaneous nodules or pustules, synovitis, or meningoencephalitis [8,106,138]. Major and minor diagnostic criteria have been established [134]. The prevalence rates in Japan (1 : 16,000) are approximately equivalent to those in the United States (1 : 20,000). However, the disease runs a more severe course in the Japanese and in patients from the eastern Mediterranean [138]. HLA-B5 and its subtype B51 are three to six times more common, and the presence of B51 antigen indicates a severe course [138]. Histologic examination of mucocutaneous lesions is nonspecific. When present, the vasculitic lesions may exhibit varying severity with lymphocytic and plasma cell infiltration and deposition of IgM and C3 in the dermal vessels [138]. Both arteries and veins are involved by the vasculitis.

Occlusion of major vessels and aneurysms occurs in 10 to 37 percent of patients [42,106,138]. Thrombosis of superficial and deep veins of both upper and lower extremities and superior and inferior vena cavae develops in 7 to 37 percent of patients [23,98,138]. Renal involvement is uncommon.

Pulmonary Involvement

The most serious respiratory complication is the occurrence of significant to massive hemoptysis. An earlier review of the literature noted pulmo-

nary involvement in only 13 patients, 4 of whom developed massive hemoptysis [141]. A more recent review of Behçet's disease with pulmonary complications observed a definite clinical pattern of hemoptysis, fever, chest pain, and dyspnea in all 28 patients [50]. Lung involvement was characteristically associated with active disease at other sites, and patients often complained of hemoptysis. Thrombophlebitis and hemoptysis seemed to be more common in men. Serious hemoptysis, initially responsive to corticosteroid therapy, showed a propensity to recur. Significant hemoptysis was common and was the cause of death in 39 percent, and all deaths from hemoptysis occurred within 6 years of the onset of disease.

Another report on 49 patients with respiratory involvement noted that recurrent dyspnea, cough, chest pain, and hemoptysis were the primary clinical signs, particularly in young men, and appeared 3.6 years after the initial presentation of Behçet's disease [145]. Fever, elevated erythrocyte sedimentation rate, and anemia were common, and chest roentgenograms demonstrated pulmonary infiltrates, pleural effusions, and prominent pulmonary arteries (Fig. 58-13). Aneurysms of the pulmonary artery were detected in 7 of 13 patients who underwent angiography [145].

A recent publication described the clinical findings in 12 patients with Behçet's disease and lung involvement [53]: The male-to-female ratio was 11 : 1, and mean age was 35.3 ± 8.8 years. Vasculitic involvement of at least four other organs was recorded either in the patients' history or during the period of respiratory involvement. The chief complaint was hemoptysis of varying degree in 11 of the 12 patients. Chest roentgenographic abnormalities included unilateral hilar enlargements, elevated diaphragm, horizontally or obliquely oriented linear opacities, diffuse ill-defined infiltrates in the upper and lower zones, wedge-shaped peripheral opacities, and bilateral pleural effusion. Computed tomography of the thorax in 9 patients with Behçet's disease and pulmonary involvement showed aneurysms, narrowing, and cutoffs of the main, lobar, segmental, or peripheral branches of the pulmonary artery and irregular configuration of other pulmonary vessels. Pulmonary angiography revealed amputation of branches of the pulmonary artery and aneurysmal dilatations [54].

Pathologic analysis of lung tissue has shown vasculitis of pulmonary vessels of various sizes, thrombosis, pulmonary embolism, destruction

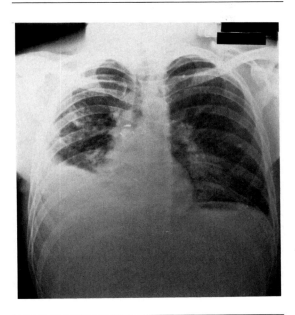

Fig. 58-13. Behçet's disease showing loss of lung volume on the right due to right lower lobectomy to treat a bronchoarterial fistula that caused massive hemoptysis. Small infiltrates seen in both lungs were caused by minor intraalveolar bleeding.

of the elastic laminae, aneurysms, aphthous lesions of the tracheobronchial tree, and arterialbronchial fistulae [145]. Other abnormalities described include mucoid degeneration and intimal thickening of larger elastic pulmonary arteries, with medial hyperplasia, intimal fibroplasia, and angiomatoid lesions in muscular pulmonary arteries [41]. Recurrent pneumonia [141] and bronchial obstruction from mucosal involvement have also been reported [68]. Immunopathologic studies indicate that pulmonary vasculitis is a result of circulating immune complexes [67].

Aneurysms of the pulmonary artery communicating with the bronchial tree (bronchovascular anastomosis) should be considered in patients with Behçet's disease and hemoptysis [7,79,117, 145,161]. Because of the high incidence of deep vein thrombosis of the extremities and the vena cavae, pulmonary embolism may occur in these patients [23,98,106,138]. Ventilation-perfusion scans are misleading, and anticoagulant therapy for presumed pulmonary embolism can be catastrophic [68,138]. Pulmonary angiography is diagnostic [145]. Computed tomography has been suggested as a less invasive test to detect pulmonary artery aneurysms [188].

Chest roentgenograms may show patchy interstitial infiltrates, rounded opacities, and lobar consolidations. Cavitation and pleural involvement are uncommon. Proximal perihilar densities or opacities are usually due to the lobular or segmental pulmonary artery aneurysms [74,141]. Tuberculosis has been reported in patients with Behçet's disease [49].

Treatment and Prognosis

Corticosteroids are palliative. However, sudden deaths in corticosteroid-treated patients have indicated that corticosteroid alone may be inadequate [138]. Drugs such as colchicine, chlorambucil, methotrexate, and azathioprine may be needed for chronic therapy. Anticoagulant therapy should be avoided in the presence of pulmonary arteritis [138]. The prognosis is poor in those who develop significant hemoptysis or diffuse pulmonary infiltrates [15]. A review of 49 patients with respiratory involvement from Behçet's disease recorded 16 deaths, 15 from fatal pulmonary hemorrhage; 80 percent died within 2 years after the onset of lung disease [145].

Takayasu's Arteritis

Takayasu's arteritis, also described as *pulseless disease, aortic arch syndrome,* or *reversed coarctation,* is a chronic inflammatory disease of unknown etiology that primarily affects the aorta and its major branches (including the proximal coronary arteries and renal arteries) and the elastic pulmonary arteries [65,76,119,170]. Among the 807 patients with various vasculitides studied by the ACR, 7.8 percent met the criteria for Takayasu's arteritis [9].

The disease primarily occurs in young adults of Asian descent, although it has been described in the population in the West. The female-to-male ratio is 8.5 : 1, and 80 percent of patients are between 11 and 30 years of age [125]. Pulseless disease and aortic arch syndrome are classic manifestations, but claudication and renovascular hypertension may be the more disabling complications of the disease. Initial or acute clinical features of Takayasu's arteritis include fever, malaise, weight loss, arthralgias, and night sweats lasting for 4 to 6 weeks [160]. Chronic disease is the result of ischemia of affected organs.

Pulmonary Involvement

Although clinically not apparent, involvement of the pulmonary artery is common. Up to 50 percent of all patients with Takayasu's arteritis develop lesions generally localized to medium and large pulmonary arteries [81,119,124]. One report described three patients with disease involving the aorta and its major branches, and all exhibited a unique small pulmonary arteriopathy characterized by the deficiency of the outer media, with capillary ingrowth and thickened, fibrosed intima; other histologic features included granulomatous arteritis, transmural inflammation, patchy destruction of the medial musculoelastic lamellae, and lymphoplasmacytic infiltrates confined to the media with a variable number of giant cells [119]. These abnormalities lead to pulmonary arterial occlusion and stenoses, which are found in the majority of cases.

A retrospective study of 180 perfusion lung scans of 120 patients with Takayasu's arteritis showed abnormalities in 76 percent of the patients. Initial anomalies developed in the upper lobes, whereas the middle and lower lobes were affected at later stages of the disease. There was a poor correlation between these abnormalities and results of spirometric and arterial blood gas analysis [177]. In another study, intravenous digital subtraction angiography in 42 patients with Takayasu's arteritis showed involvement of the pulmonary artery in 14.3 percent of patients, even though the respiratory problem was not suspected clinically in any patient and the chest roentgenograms were abnormal in only two [159]. A comparison study of 59 patients with temporal arteritis showed that although chest roentgenograms were abnormal in 68 percent, pulmonary angiography revealed arterial occlusions in 86 percent [191].

There are in the literature case reports of diffuse unilateral involvement of the right pulmonary artery associated with fistulas between the right coronary artery and the right pulmonary artery and between the right bronchial artery and the right pulmonary artery, pulmonary artery–bronchial artery fistula, pulmonary hypertension as the presenting manifestation, and interstitial pulmonary fibrosis [73,75,77,86,87,147].

Treatment and Prognosis

Corticosteroid therapy has resulted in symptomatic remission within days to weeks [76]. Patients with significant vascular disease may require sur-

gical treatment [24,93]. Death is usually the result of vascular complications such as rupture of an aneurysm, myocardial infarction, congestive cardiac failure, or cerebrovascular accident [76]. Pulmonary involvement signifies a poor prognosis [12].

Henoch-Schönlein Purpura

Henoch-Schönlein purpura, also known as *anaphylactoid purpura* or *allergic purpura*, is a syndrome characterized by acute purpura, arthritis, colicky abdominal pain, and nephritis [83,155]. Although Henoch-Schönlein purpura is more common in children younger than age 10, an adult form of the disease exists [38,156]. Among the 807 cases of various vasculitides studied by the ARC, Henoch-Schönlein purpura constituted 10.5 percent of cases [9]. The mean age of the patients was 17.4 years, and nearly two-thirds were younger than 16 [132]. The male-to-female ratio was approximately equal [132].

Pathologic features include acute arteriolitis and venulitis in the superficial dermis and the bowel. Proliferative and necrotizing glomerulonephritis usually is mild [119]. A similar type of renal lesion is seen in patients with infective endocarditis, Wegener's granulomatosis, systemic lupus erythematosus, Goodpasture's syndrome, and polyarteritis nodosa [66,72,139]. Immunofluorescence microscopy exhibits large deposits of IgA in the skin and kidney, but the presence of this immunoglobulin as a diagnostic indicator is questionable [115,116]. Adults with Henoch-Schönlein purpura exhibit elevations in serum IgA and IgG-containing complexes.

Palpable purpura, usually distributed over the buttocks and lower extremities, and fever are generally the first signs of Henoch-Schönlein purpura. The purpura may precede, accompany, or follow arthralgias and abdominal colic. The triad of purpura, arthritis, and abdominal pain is present in approximately 80 percent of patients. Joint involvement is typically monoarticular and transient, involves large joints, and causes pain out of proportion to objective evidence of synovitis [132]. Peritonitis and melena are common.

Pulmonary Involvement

A personal review of the English literature revealed that lung involvement is rare in Henoch-Schönlein purpura. However, several pulmonary complications have been described. Perihilar patchy opacities, reticulonodular changes, and pulmonary alveolar hemorrhage have been recorded [48,61,92,139,140]. Among the 85 cases of Henoch-Schönlein purpura studied by the ARC, not a single respiratory complication was described [132].

Treatment and Prognosis

High-dose corticosteroid therapy (0.5 to 1.0 mg/kg/day) results in full recovery. However, relapse of purpura, abdominal pain, and arthritis may occur for 3 to 6 weeks before the disease resolves completely [132].

Urticarial Vasculitis

Urticarial vasculitis is a systemic disorder characterized by urticarial wheals or papules similar to those in the usual urticaria, itching and arthralgias in 60 percent of cases, arthritis in 28 percent, abdominal pain in 25 percent, and glomerulonephritis in 5 percent. Angioedema, fever, uveitis, episcleritis, and seizures may also occur [69]. Urticarial vasculitis with or without hypocomplementemia can also occur in systemic lupus erythematosus [182]. The erythrocyte sedimentation rate is elevated in 66 percent of patients, and hypocomplementemia is seen in 38 percent [1,69,96]. The hypocomplementemic form of urticarial vasculitis has been associated with pulmonary complications.

Vasculitis of the pulmonary vasculature is not characteristic of this disease. However, obstructive pulmonary disease occurs in many of these patients. Airways disease is believed to result from a combination of smoking and an immunological process that has yet not been identified [5,157]. Up to 62 percent of patients with hypocomplementemic urticarial vasculitis develop chronic obstructive pulmonary disease [152,157]. Tobacco smoking may have contributed to this high incidence in some series. Nevertheless, one report on 16 patients with hypocomplementemic urticarial vasculitis reported severe obstructive airways disease in 8 of 10 smokers studied, 1 of whom died of lung disease. Severe obstructive pulmonary disease developed in three patients at a young age after smoking cigarettes for a relatively low number of pack-years. A recent review of 72 cases of biopsy-proved urticarial vasculitis revealed that 32 percent had hypocomplementemia and 21 percent had obstructive lung disease [131].

Leukocytoclastic Vasculitis

Leukocytoclastic vasculitis is characterized by necrotizing vasculitis and fibrinoid necrosis of the vessel walls, with leukocytoclasis of the inflammatory cells in the wall of the vessel [69]. Leukocytoclastic vasculitis may occur in association with inflammatory, autoimmune, and malignant disease. It commonly presents as palpable purpura.

Several respiratory complications have been described. Patchy pneumonitis secondary to biopsy-proved leukocytoclastic vasculitis of the pulmonary venous system, manifested by hemoptysis and pleuritic chest pains, has been described in a patient who also exhibited obstructive airways disease [55]. Metformin-induced leukocytoclastic vasculitis has been reported in one patient [102].

Mixed Cryoglobulinemia

Mixed cryoglobulinemia is manifested by recurrent purpura, arthralgias, and systemic involvement and, frequently, elevated cryoglobulin and rheumatoid factor. Biopsy of vascular structures reveals findings similar to those in leukocytoclastic vasculitis. The most serious complication is glomerulonephritis from deposition of immune complexes. Lung function tests in 19 patients (17 of whom were female, with a mean age of 49.6 years) showed diminished diffusing capacity of carbon monoxide in the lung and maximal expiratory flow at 50 percent of forced vital capacity, total lung capacity, and functional residual capacity [11,181]. Respiratory complications described include bronchiectasis, pulmonary fibrosis, pulmonary insufficiency, and Sjögren's syndrome–like illness with lung involvement [25,52,162]. Severe pulmonary hemorrhage has also been described in cryoglobulinemia [64].

Polyarteritis Nodosa

Polyarteritis nodosa is characterized by a necrotizing arteritis of small and medium muscular arteries, affecting multiple organ systems [123]. The ACR study of 807 patients with various vasculitic syndromes recorded polyarteritis in 14.6 percent [9,123]. Differentiating polyarteritis from Churg-Strauss syndrome can be difficult [122]. This confusion is exacerbated by the fact that many include Churg-Strauss syndrome, classic polyarteritis, and other vasculitic syndromes under the umbrella *polyarteritis nodosa group* of systemic vasculitides [189].

It is important to recognize that polyarteritis seldom involves the lungs. In the ACR study of 118 patients with polyarteritis, pulmonary complications were not observed in a single patient [9,123]. The earlier literature cited vasculitis in the bronchial and pulmonary vessels, but many of the patients exhibited granulomatous lesions with eosinophilic infiltrates [148,168,187]. In retrospect, it appears that the majority of the patients in whom pulmonary polyarteritis was diagnosed indeed had Churg-Strauss syndrome [144]. Nevertheless, recent reports have continued to describe patients with respiratory involvement in polyarteritis [18,80,103,136]. When polyarteritis is widespread, pulmonary pathologic changes may include fibrinoid necrosis of the pulmonary artery with an infiltrate rich in neutrophils [37].

Eosinophilia-Myalgia Syndrome

The eosinophilia-myalgia syndrome is a multisystem inflammatory disease with characteristic features of myalgia and eosinophilia [22,63,84,176]. This syndrome occurred in epidemic proportions in the United States during 1989, affecting more than 1500 persons and causing approximately 30 deaths [21,22,142,169]. Cases of the eosinophilia-

myalgia syndrome have been reported from Canada, Europe, and other countries [85].

Epidemiologic studies have demonstrated that the eosinophilia-myalgia syndrome is the result of ingestion of L-tryptophan, used by lay people as a remedy for insomnia, depression, premenstrual syndrome, and other health disorders. Several contaminants—3-(phenylamino)alanine, 1,1′-ethylidenebis(tryptophan), and 3-anilino-L-alanine—involved in the manufacturing of L-tryptophan have been implicated as the causative agents of both the eosinophilia-myalgia syndrome and the Spanish toxic oil syndrome [129].

The clinical manifestations resemble those of the Spanish toxic oil syndrome, caused by ingestion of adulterated rapeseed oil [100,101,172]. Among these are myalgias, fatigue, muscle weakness, arthralgias, edema of the extremities, skin rash, oral and vaginal ulcers, scleroderma-like changes, fasciitis, ascending neuropathy, and profound eosinophilia [6,21,22,32,167,171,174].

Respiratory complications were observed in approximately 60 percent of patients with the eosinophilia-myalgia syndrome [21]. Pulmonary manifestations have included pulmonary infil-

Fig. 58-14. Pulmonary involvement in L-tryptophan-induced eosinophilia-myalgia syndrome. A mixed inflammatory infiltrate involving a septal vein. There is marked intimal proliferation and infiltration by cells that include relatively numerous eosinophils.

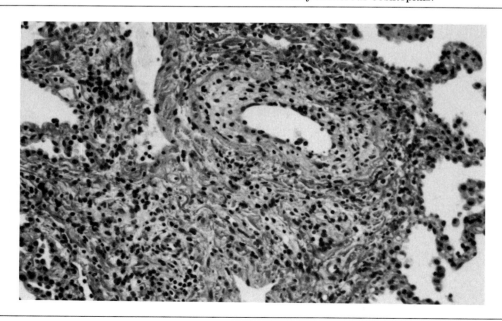

trates associated with severe respiratory distress and progressive hypoxemia, pleural effusion, diffuse bilateral reticulonodular infiltrates, and pulmonary hypertension [6,21,176]. In a study of five cases of pathologically proved eosinophilia-myalgia syndrome, all patients were women ranging in age from 34 to 65 years, and all presented with pulmonary symptoms that began after 1 to 9 months of L-tryptophan therapy. Four patients exhibited peripheral eosinophilia and bilateral interstitial infiltrates (one had a normal chest roentgenogram). Lung specimens revealed vasculitis and perivasculitis associated with eosinophilia and mild interstitial pneumonitis. Clinical or morphologic evidence of pulmonary hypertension was noted in three, and one patient had a follicular bronchiolitis. Whereas four patients responded promptly to discontinuation of L-tryptophan ingestion and systemic corticosteroids, one patient showed only minimal symptomatic improvement [171].

Other histologic changes described in the lungs of patients with the eosinophilia-myalgia syndrome have included alveolar exudate made up of eosinophils and histiocytes, changes characteristic of hypersensitivity pneumonitis, interstitial and perivascular infiltrates, and fibrointimal hyperplasia of small pulmonary vessels (Fig. 58-14) [6,21,167,176].

Secondary Vasculitis

Many of the rheumatologic diseases, discussed in Chapter 57, may exhibit secondary vasculitic processes in the organs involved [17,143]. Infectious processes, particularly secondary to *Aspergillus* and *Mucor* species, invade vascular structures and produce secondary vasculitis. Certain drugs and chemicals also can induce vasculitis [158, 178]. Other uncommon secondary vasculitic entities include benign lymphocytic angiitis and granulomatosis, bronchocentric granulomatosis, and necrotizing sarcoid angiitis. Whether these are distinct entities or represent uncommon phases of the vasculitides discussed in this chapter is unclear [151].

References

1. Aboobaker J, Greaves MW. Urticarial vasculitis. *Clin Exp Dermatol* 11:436, 1986.
2. Acritidis NC, et al. Pulmonary function of non-smoking patients with giant cell arteritis and/or polymyalgia rheumatica; a controlled study. *Clin Rheumatol* 7:231, 1988.
3. Amato MB, et al. Concurrent Churg-Strauss syndrome and temporal arteritis in a young patient with pulmonary nodules. *Am Rev Respir Dis* 139:1539, 1989.
4. Arend, WP, et al. The American College of Rheumatology 1990 criteria for the classification of Takayasu arteritis. *Arthritis Rheum* 33:1129, 1990.
5. Baer AN, et al. Evidence for immunologically mediated pulmonary injury in the hypocomplementemic urticarial vasculitis syndrome (letter). *J Am Acad Dermatol* 13:509, 1985.
6. Banner AS, Borochovitz D. Acute respiratory failure caused by pulmonary vasculitis after L-tryptophan ingestion. *Am Rev Respir Dis* 143:661, 1991.
7. Barberis M, Casadio C, Borghini U. Massive haemoptysis in Behçet syndrome: Case report. *Respiration* 52:303, 1987.
8. Behçet H. Über rezidivierende, aphthöse, durch ein Virus vesursachte Geschwüre am Mund, am Auge und an den Genitalien. *Dermatol Wochenschr* 105:1152, 1937.
9. Bloch DA, et al. The American College of Rheumatology 1990 criteria for the classification of vasculitis: Patients and methods. *Arthritis Rheum* 33:1068, 1990.
10. Bohlman ME, Ensor RE, Goldman SM. Pulmonary Wegener's granulomatosis of the trachea: Radiologic manifestations. *South Med J* 77:1318, 1984.
11. Bombardieri S, et al. Lung involvement in essential mixed cryoglobulinemia. *Am J Med* 66:748, 1979.
12. Bonventure MV. Takayasu's disease revisited. *NY State J Med* 74:1960, 1970.
13. Bosch X, et al. Anti-myeloperoxidase autoantibodies in patients with necrotizing glomerular and alveolar capillaritis. *Am J Kidney Dis* 20:231, 1992.
14. Bradley JD, et al. Giant cell arteritis with pulmonary nodules. *Am J Med* 77:135, 1984.
15. Cadman EC, Lundberg WB, Mitchell MS. Pulmonary manifestations in Behçet syndrome: Case report and review of the literature. *Arch Intern Med* 136:944, 1976.
16. Calabrese LH, et al. The American College of Rheumatology 1990 criteria for the classification of hypersensitivity vasculitis. *Arthritis Rheum* 33:1108, 1990.
17. Cannon G, Zimmerman G (Eds). The lung in rheumatic diseases. *Lung Biol Health Dis* 45: 545 1990.
18. Carratalá J, et al. Polyarteritis nodosa associated with idiopathic pulmonary fibrosis: Report of two cases (letter). *Ann Rheum Dis* 48:876, 1989.
19. Carrington CB, Liebow AA. Limited forms of angiitis and granulomatosis of Wegener's type. *Am J Med* 41:497, 1966.
20. Caselli RJ, Hunder GG, Whisnant JP. Neurologic

disease in biopsy-proven giant cell (temporal) arteritis. *Neurology* 38:352, 1988.

21. Catton CK, et al. Pulmonary involvement in the eosinophilia-myalgia syndrome. *Chest* 99:327, 1991.

22. Centers for Disease Control. Eosinophilia-myalgia syndrome—New Mexico. *MMWR* 38(45): 765, 1989.

23. Chajek T, Fainaru M. Behçet's disease. Report of 41 cases and review of the literature. *Medicine* 54:179, 1975.

24. Chauvaud S, et al. Takayasu's arteritis with bilateral pulmonary artery stenosis: Successful surgical correction. *J Thorac Cardiovasc Surg* 94:246, 1987.

25. Chejfec G, et al. Respiratory insufficiency in a patient with mixed cryoglobulinemia. *Ultrastruct Pathol* 2:295, 1981.

26. Chen KR, et al. Churg-Strauss syndrome: Report of a case without preexisting asthma. *J Dermatol* 19:40, 1992.

27. Chen KT. Abdominal forms of lymphomatoid granulomatosis. *Hum Pathol* 8:99, 1977.

28. Chumbley LC, Harrison EG Jr, DeRemee RA. Allergic granulomatosis and angiitis (Churg-Strauss syndrome): Report and analysis of 30 cases. *Mayo Clin Proc* 52:477, 1977.

29. Churg A. Pulmonary angiitis and granulomatosis revisited. *Hum Pathol* 14:868, 1983.

30. Churg J, Strauss L. Allergic granulomatosis, allergic angiitis, and periarteritis nodosa. *Am J Pathol* 27:277, 1951.

31. Churg J, Strauss L. Case 46-1980: Interstitial eosinophilic pneumonitis, pleuritis, and angiitis (letter). *N Engl J Med* 304:611, 1981.

32. Clauw DJ, et al. Tryptophan-associated eosinophilic connective-tissue disease: A new clinical entity? *JAMA* 263:1502, 1990.

33. Clutterbuck EJ, Pusey CD. Severe alveolar haemorrhage in Churg-Strauss syndrome. *Eur J Respir Dis* 71:158, 1987.

34. Cohen MD, Ginsburg WW. Polymyalgia rheumatica. *Rheum Dis Clin North Am* 16:325, 1990.

35. Cohen-Tervaert JW, et al. Detection of autoantibodies against myeloid lysosomal enzymes: A useful adjunct to classification of patients with biopsy proven necrotizing arteritis. *Am J Med* 91:59, 1991.

36. Colby TV. Diffuse pulmonary hemorrhage in Wegener's granulomatosis. *Semin Respir Med* 10:136, 1989.

37. Colby TV, et al. *Atlas of Pulmonary Surgical Pathology.* Philadelphia: Saunders, 1991. P 323.

38. Cream JJ, Gumpel JM, Peachy RDG. Schönlein-Henoch purpura in the adult: A study of anaphylactoid or Schönlein-Henoch purpura. *Q J Med* 39:461, 1970.

39. Cross CE, Lillington GA. Serodiagnosis of Wegener's granulomatosis: Pathobiologic and clinical implications. *Mayo Clin Proc* 64:119, 1989.

40. Cupps TR, Fauci AS. *The Vasculitides.* Philadelphia: Saunders, 1981. Pp 1–211.

41. Davies JD. Behçet's syndrome with haemoptysis and pulmonary lesions. *J Pathol* 109:351, 1973.

42. Decroix AG. Thoracic manifestations of Behçet's syndrome (abstract). *Thorax* 24:380, 1969.

43. Dennison AR, Watkins RM, Gunning AJ. Simultaneous aortic and pulmonary artery aneurysms due to giant cell arteritis. *Thorax* 40:156, 1985.

44. DeRemee RA. Wegener's Granulomatosis. In JP Lynch III, RA DeRemee (Eds), *Immunologically Mediated Pulmonary Diseases.* Philadelphia: Lippincott, 1991. P 250.

45. DeRemee RA, McDonald TJ, Weiland LH. Wegener's granulomatosis: Observations on treatment with antimicrobial agents. *Mayo Clin Proc* 60:27, 1985.

46. DeRemee RA, Weiland LH, McDonald TJ. Polymorphic reticulosis, lymphomatoid granulomatosis (two diseases or one?). *Mayo Clin Proc* 53:634, 1978.

47. Doyle L, McWilliam L, Hasleton PS. Giant cell arteritis with pulmonary involvement. *Br J Dis Chest* 82:88, 1988.

48. Drogendijk AC. Schlesinger FG. Anatomical findings in a case of Schöenlein-Henoch syndrome. *Acta Med Scand* 169:525, 1961.

49. Efthimiou J, et al. Pulmonary tuberculosis in Behçet's syndrome. *Br J Dis Chest* 82:300, 1988.

50. Efthimiou J, et al. Pulmonary disease in Behçet's syndrome. *Q J Med* 58:259, 1986.

51. Eichel BS, et al. Primary lymphoma of the nose including a relationship to lethal midline granuloma. *Am J Surg* 112:597, 1966.

52. Erhardt CC, Mumford P, Maini RN. The association of cryoglobulinaemia with nodules, vasculitis and fibrosing alveolitis in rheumatoid arthritis and their relationship to serum C1q binding activity and rheumatoid factor. *Clin Exp Immunol* 38:405, 1979.

53. Erkan F, Cavdar T. Pulmonary vasculitis in Behçet's disease. *Am Rev Respir Dis* 146:232, 1992.

54. Erzurum SC, et al. Pleural effusion in Churg-Strauss syndrome. *Chest* 95:1357, 1989.

55. Falk DK. Pulmonary disease in idiopathic urticarial vasculitis. *J Am Acad Dermatol* 11:346, 1984.

56. Falk RJ, et al. Clinical course of anti-neutrophil cytoplasmic autoantibody-associated glomerulonephritis and systemic vasculitis. *Ann Intern Med* 113:656, 1990.

57. Fauci AS, et al. Lymphomatoid granulomatosis. Prospective clinical and therapeutic experience for 10 years. *N Engl J Med* 306:68, 1982.

58. Fauci AS, et al. Wegener's granulomatosis: Prospective clinical and therapeutic experience with 85 patients for 21 years. *Ann Intern Med* 98:76, 1983.

59. Fauci AS, Haynes BF, Katz P. The spectrum of vasculitis. Clinical, pathologic, immunologic, and therapeutic considerations. *Ann Intern Med* 89:660, 1978.

60. Fauci AS, Wolff SM. Wegener's granulomatosis: Studies in eighteen patients and a review of the literature. *Medicine* 52:535, 1973.

61. Fiegler VW, Siemoneit KD. Schöenlein-Henoch syndrome. *Fortschr Geb Rontgenstr Nuklearmed* 134:269, 1981.

62. Finan MC, Winkelmann RK. The cutaneous extravascular necrotizing granuloma (Churg-Strauss granuloma) and systemic disease: A review of 27 cases. *Medicine* 62:142, 1983.

63. Flannery MT, et al. A case of the eosinophilia-myalgia syndrome associated with use of L-tryptophan product. *Ann Intern Med* 112:300, 1990.

64. Frankel AH, et al. Type II essential mixed cryoglobulinaemia: Presentation, treatment and outcome in 13 patients. *Q J Med* 82:101, 1992.

65. Fries JF, et al. The American College of Rheumatology 1990 criteria for the classification of vasculitis: Summary. *Arthritis Rheum* 33:1135, 1990.

66. Furlong TJ, Ibels LS, Eckstein RP. The clinical spectrum of necrotizing glomerulonephritis. *Medicine* 66:192, 1987.

67. Gamble CN, et al. The immune complex pathogenesis of glomerulonephritis and pulmonary vasculitis in Behçet's disease. *Am J Med* 66:1031, 1979.

68. Gibson JM, et al. Bronchial obstruction in a patient with Behçet's disease. *Eur J Respir Dis* 63:356, 1982.

69. Gibson LE, Su WPD. Cutaneous vasculitis. *Rheum Dis Clin North Am* 16:309, 1990.

70. Glover MU, et al. Pulmonary artery obstruction due to giant cell arteritis. *Chest* 91:924, 1987.

71. Godman GC, Churg J. Wegener's granulomatosis: Pathology and review of the literature. *Arch Pathol* 58:533, 1954.

72. Goldstein J, Weil J, Liel Y. Intrapulmonary hemorrhages and immune complex glomerulonephritis masquerading as Goodpasture's syndrome. *Hum Pathol* 17:754, 1986.

73. Greene NB, Baughman RP, Kim CK. Takayasu's arteritis associated with interstitial lung disease and glomerulonephritis. *Chest* 89:605, 1986.

74. Grenier P, et al. Pulmonary involvement in Behçet disease. *AJR* 137:565, 1981.

75. Haas A, Stiehm ER. Takayasu's arteritis presenting as pulmonary hypertension. *Am J Dis Child* 140:372, 1986.

76. Hall S, Buchbinder R. Takayasu's arteritis. *Rheum Dis Clin North Am* 16:411, 1990.

77. Halon DA, et al. Coronary artery to bronchial artery anastomosis in Takayasu's arteritis. *Cardiology* 74:387, 1987.

78. Hammar SP, et al. Lymphomatoid granulomatosis: Association with retroperitoneal fibrosis and evidence of impaired cell-mediated immunity. *Am Rev Respir Dis* 115:1045, 1977.

79. Hamza M. Large artery involvement in Behçet's disease. *J Rheumatol* 14:554, 1987.

80. Haworth SJ, et al. Pulmonary haemorrhage complicating Wegener's granulomatosis and microscopic polyarteritis. *Br Med J [Clin Res]*, 290: 1775, 1985.

81. Hayashi K, et al. Initial pulmonary artery involvement in Takayasu arteritis. *Radiology* 159: 401, 1986.

82. Haynes BF, et al. The ocular manifestations of Wegener's granulomatosis: Fifteen years experience and review of the literature. *Am J Med* 63:131, 1977.

83. Henoch EH. Uber ein eigenthumliche form von purpura. *Berl Klin Wochenschr* 11:641, 1874.

84. Hertzman PA, et al. Association of the eosinophilia-myalgia syndrome with the ingestion of tryptophan. *N Engl J Med* 322:869, 1990.

85. Hertzman PA, et al. The eosinophilia-myalgia syndrome: The Los Alamos Conference. *J Rheumatol* 18:867, 1991.

86. Horimoto M, et al. Unilateral diffuse pulmonary artery involvement in Takayasu's arteritis associated with coronary-pulmonary artery fistula and bronchial-pulmonary artery fistula: A case report. *Angiology* 42:73, 1991.

87. Hunder GG. Giant cell (temporal) arteritis. *Rheum Dis Clin North Am* 16:399, 1990.

88. Hunder GG, et al. The American College of Rheumatology 1990 criteria for the classification of vasculitis: Introduction. *Arthritis Rheum* 33:1065, 1990.

89. Hunder GG, et al. The American College of Rheumatology 1990 criteria for the classification of giant cell arteritis. *Arthritis Rheum* 33:1122, 1990.

90. Ishi F, et al. Nasal T-cell lymphoma as a type of so-called "lethal midline granuloma." *Cancer* 50:2336, 1982.

91. Israel HL, Patchefsky AS, Saldana MJ. Wegener's granulomatosis, lymphomatoid granulomatosis, and benign lymphocytic angiitis and granulomatosis of lung, recognition and treatment. *Ann Intern Med* 87:691, 1977.

92. Jacome AF. Pulmonary hemorrhage and death complicating anaphylactoid purpura. *South Med J* 60:1003, 1967.

93. Jakob H. Surgical correction of a severely obstructed pulmonary artery bifurcation in Takayasu's arteritis. *Eur J Cardiothorac Surg* 4: 456, 1990.

94. Jennette JC, Falk RJ. Antineutrophil cytoplasmic autoantibodies and associated diseases: A review. *Am J Kidney Dis* 15:517, 1990.

95. Jennette JC, Falk RJ. Disease associations and pathogenic role of antineutrophil cytoplasmic

autoantibodies in vasculitis. *Curr Opin Rheumatol* 4:9, 1992.

96. Jones RR, et al. Urticaria and vasculitis: A continuum of histological and immunopathological changes. *Br J Dermatol* 108:695, 1983.

97. Kallenberg CGM, Mulder AHL, Tervaert JWC. Antineutrophil cytoplasmic antibodies: A still-growing class of autoantibodies in inflammatory disorders. *Am J Med* 93:675, 1992.

98. Kansu E, et al. Behçet's syndrome with obstruction of the venae cavae. *Q J Med* 41:151, 1972.

99. Katzenstein ALA, Carrington DB, Liebow AS. Lymphomatoid granulomatosis: A clinicopathologic study of 152 cases. *Cancer* 43:360, 1979.

100. Kilbourne EM, et al. Toxic oil syndrome: A current clinical and epidemiologic summary, including comparisons with the eosinophilia-myalgia syndrome. *J Am Coll Cardiol* 18:711, 1991.

101. Kilbourne EM, et al. Clinical epidemiology of toxic oil syndrome: Manifestations of a new illness. *N Engl J Med* 309:1408, 1983.

102. Klapholz L, Leitersdorf E, Weinrauch L. Leucocytoclastic vasculitis and pneumonitis induced by metformin. *Br Med J [Clin Res]* 293:483, 1986.

103. Komadina KH, Houk RW. Polyarteritis nodosa presenting as recurrent pneumonia following splenectomy for hairy-cell leukemia. *Semin Arthritis Rheum* 18:252, 1989.

104. Kramer MR, et al. Pulmonary manifestations of temporal arteritis. *Eur J Respir Dis* 71:430, 1987.

105. Ladanyi M, Fraser RS. Pulmonary involvement in giant cell arteritis. *Arch Pathol Lab Med* 111:1178, 1987.

106. Lakhanpal S, et al. Pathologic features of Behçet's syndrome: A review of Japanese autopsy registry data. *Hum Pathol* 16:790, 1985.

107. Lanham JG, et al. Systemic vasculitis with asthma and eosinophilia: A clinical approach to the Churg-Strauss syndrome. *Medicine* 63:65, 1984.

108. Larson TS, et al. Respiratory tract symptoms as a clue to giant cell arteritis. *Ann Intern Med* 101:594, 1984.

109. Leatherman JW, Davies SF, Hoidal JR. Alveolar hemorrhage syndromes: Diffuse microvascular lung hemorrhage in immune and idiopathic disorders. *Medicine* 63:343, 1984.

110. Leavitt RY, et al. The American College of Rheumatology 1990 criteria for the classification of Wegener's granulomatosis. *Arthritis Rheum* 33:1101, 1990.

111. Leavitt RY, Fauci AS. Polyangiitis overlap syndrome. Classification and prospective clinical experience. *Am J Med* 81:79, 1986.

112. Leavitt RY, Fauci AS. Pulmonary vasculitis. *Am Rev Respir Dis* 134:149, 1986.

113. Leavitt RY, Fauci AS. Less common manifestations and presentations of Wegener's granulomatosis. *Curr Opin Rheumatol* 4:16, 1992.

114. Letendre L. Treatment of lymphomatoid granulomatosis: Old and new perspectives. *Semin Respir Med* 10:178, 1989.

115. Levinsky RJ, Barratt TM. IgA immune complexes in Henoch-Schönlein purpura. *Lancet* 2:1100, 1979.

116. Lie JT. Systemic and isolated vasculitis: A rational approach to classification and pathologic diagnosis. *Pathol Annu* 24:25, 1988.

117. Lie JT. Cardiac and pulmonary manifestations of Behçet syndrome. *Pathol Res Pract* 183:347, 1988.

118. Lie JT. The classification of vasculitis and a reappraisal of allergic granulomatosis and angiitis (Churg-Strauss syndrome). *Mt Sinai J Med* 53:429, 1986.

119. Lie JT, Members and Consultants of the American College of Rheumatology Subcommittee on Classification of Vasculitis. Illustrated histopathologic classification criteria for selected vasculitis syndromes. *Arthritis Rheum* 33:1074, 1990.

120. Liebow AA. Pulmonary angiitis and granulomatosis. *Am Rev Respir Dis* 108:1, 1973.

121. Liebow AA, Carrington CB, Friedman PJ. Lymphomatoid granulomatosis. *Hum Pathol* 3:457, 1972.

122. Lightfoot RW Jr. Churg-Strauss syndrome and polyarteritis nodosa. *Curr Opin Rheumatol* 3:3, 1991.

123. Lightfoot, RW Jr, et al. The American College of Rheumatology 1990 criteria for the classification of polyarteritis nodosa. *Arthritis Rheum* 33:1088, 1990.

124. Lupi E, et al. Pulmonary artery involvement in Takayasu's arteritis. *Chest* 67:69, 1975.

125. Lupi-Herrera E, et al. Takayasu's arteritis: Clinical study of 107 cases. *Am Heart J* 93:94, 1977.

126. Machado EBV, et al. Trends in incidence and clinical presentation of temporal arteritis in Olmsted County, Minnesota, 1950–1985. *Arthritis Rheum* 31:745, 1988.

127. Masi AT, et al. The American College of Rheumatology 1990 criteria for the classification of Churg-Strauss syndrome (allergic granulomatosis and angiitis). *Arthritis Rheum* 33:1094, 1990.

128. Matthews S, Cupps TR. Systemic vasculitis. *Lung Biol Health Dis* 45:329, 1990.

129. Mayeno AN, et al. (Phenylamino)alanine, a novel aniline-derived amino acid associated with the eosinophilia-myalgia syndrome: A link to toxic oil syndrome? *Mayo Clin Proc* 67:1134, 1992.

130. McDonald TJ, et al. Nasal manifestations of Wegener's granulomatosis. *Laryngoscope* 84:2101, 1974.

131. Mehregan DR, Hall MJ, Gibson LE. Urticarial

vasculitis: A histopathologic and clinical review of 72 cases. *J Am Acad Dermatol* 26:441, 1992.

132. Mills JA, et al. The American College of Rheumatology 1990 criteria for the classification of Henoch-Schonlein purpura. *Arthritis Rheum* 33:1114, 1990.

133. Mills JA, et al. The American College of Rheumatology 1990 criteria for the classification of vasculitis: Summary. *Arthritis Rheum* 33:1135, 1990.

134. Momoi H, Inaba G, Mimura Y. Guidance for Diagnosis of Behçet's Disease. In G Inaba (Ed), *Guidance as to Diagnosis and Treatment for Behçet's Disease.* Tokyo: Behçet's Disease Research Committee of Japan, Ministry of Welfare, 1982. Pp 1–10.

135. Myers JL, Katzenstein ALA. Wegener's granulomatosis presenting with massive pulmonary hemorrhage and capillaritis. *Am J Surg Pathol* 11:895, 1987.

136. Nguyen VD. A rare cause of splenic infarct and fleeting pulmonary infiltrates: Polyarteritis nodosa. *Comput Med Imaging Graph* 15:61, 1991.

137. Noritake DT, et al. Rheumatic manifestations of Wegener's granulomatosis. *J Rheumatol* 14:949, 1987.

138. O'Duffy JD. Vasculitis in Behçet's disease. *Rheum Dis Clin North Am* 16:423, 1990.

139. Parfrey PS, et al. The spectrum of diseases associated with necrotizing glomerulonephritis and its prognosis. *Am J Kidney Dis* 6:387, 1985.

140. Payton CD, Allison MEM, Boulton-Jones JM. Henoch-Schonlein purpura presenting with pulmonary haemorrhage. *Scott Med J* 32:26, 1987.

141. Petty TL, Scoggin CH, Good JT. Recurrent pneumonia in Behçet's syndrome: Roentgenographic documentation during 13 years. *JAMA* 238:2529, 1977.

142. Philen RM, et al. Eosinophilia-myalgia syndrome: A clinical case series of 21 patients. *Arch Intern Med* 151:533, 1991.

143. Prakash UBS. Rheumatological diseases. *Lung Biol Health Dis* 59:385, 1992.

144. Prakash UBS. Vasculitides. *Lung Biol Health Dis* 59:431, 1992.

145. Raz I, Okon E, Chajek-Shaul T. Pulmonary manifestations in Behçet's syndrome. *Chest* 95:585, 1989.

146. Reed WB, et al. The cutaneous manifestations in Wegener's granulomatosis. *Acta Derm Venereol* (Stockh) 43:250, 1963.

147. Rose AG, Halper J, Factor SM. Primary arteriopathy in Takayasu's disease. *Arch Pathol Lab Med* 108:644, 1984.

148. Rose GA, Spencer H. Polyarteritis nodosa. *Q J Med* 26:43, 1957.

149. Rosenberg DM, et al. Functional correlates of lung involvement in Wegener's granulomatosis: Use of pulmonary function tests in staging and follow-up. *Am J Med* 69:387, 1980.

150. Sahn SA. Pathogenesis of pleural effusions and pleural lesions. *Lung Biol Health Dis* 45:27, 1990.

151. Saldana MJ, Israel HL. Necrotizing granulomatosis, benign lymphocytic angiitis, and granulomatosis: Do they exist? *Semin Respir Med* 10:182, 1989.

152. Sanchez NP, et al. The clinical and histopathologic spectrums of urticarial vasculitis: Study of forty cases. *J Am Acad Dermatol* 7:599, 1982.

153. Savage COS, et al. Prospective study of radioimmunoassay for antibodies against neutrophil cytoplasm in diagnosis of systemic vasculitis. *Lancet* 1:1389, 1987.

154. Savage COS, et al. Microscopic polyarteritis: Presentation, pathology, and prognosis. *Q J Med* 56:467, 1985.

155. Schönlein H. *Allgemeine und Specielle Pathologie und Therapie*(3rd ed. vol. 2). Wurzburg: Herisau, 1837.

156. Schönlein-Henoch purpura in adults (editorial). *Br Med J* I:436, 1971.

157. Schwartz HR, et al. Hypocomplementemic urticarial vasculitis: Association with chronic obstructive pulmonary disease. *Mayo Clin Proc* 57:231, 1982.

158. Seiden MV, et al. Vasculitis with recurrent pulmonary hemorrhage in a long-term survivor after autologous bone marrow transplantation. *Bone Marrow Transplant* 6:345, 1990.

159. Sharma S, et al. The incidence and patterns of pulmonary artery involvement in Takayasu's arteritis. *Clin Radiol* 42:177, 1990.

160. Shelhamer JH, et al. Takayasu's arteritis and its therapy. *Arch Intern Med* 103:121, 1985.

161. Shimizu T, et al. Behçet disease (Behçet syndrome). *Semin Arthritis Rheum* 8:223, 1979.

162. Singer DRJ, et al. Cryoglobulinaemia: Clinical features and response to treatment. *Ann Med Interne* (Paris) 137:251, 1986.

163. Specks U, DeRemee RA. Granulomatous vasculitis: Wegener's granulomatosis and Churg-Strauss syndrome. *Rheum Dis Clin North Am* 16:377, 1990.

164. Specks U, et al. Anticytoplasmic autoantibodies in the diagnosis and follow-up of Wegener's granulomatosis. *Mayo Clin Proc* 64:28, 1989.

165. Stewart JP. Progressive lethal granulomatous ulceration of the nose. *J Laryngol* 48:657, 1933.

166. Strange C, et al. Subglottic stenosis in Wegener's granulomatosis: Development during cyclophosphamide treatment with response to carbon dioxide laser therapy. *Thorax* 45:300, 1990.

167. Strumpf IJ, et al. Acute eosinophilic pulmonary disease associated with the ingestion of L-tryptophan-containing products. *Chest* 99:8, 1991.

168. Sweeney AR, Baggenstoss AH. Pulmonary le-

sions in periarteritis nodosa. *Proc Staff Meet Mayo Clin* 24:35, 1949.

169. Swygert LA, et al. Eosinophilia-myalgia syndrome: Results of national surveillance. *JAMA* 264:1698, 1990.

170. Takayasu M. Case with unusual changes of the central vessels in the retina. *Acta Soc Ophthalmol.* 12:554, 1908.

171. Tazelaar HD, et al. Pulmonary disease associated with L-tryptophan-induced eosinophilic myalgia syndrome: Clinical and pathologic features. *Chest* 97:1032, 1990.

172. Toxic Epidemic Syndrome Study Group. Toxic epidemic syndrome, Spain, 1981. *Lancet* 2:697, 1982.

173. Travis WD, Carpenter HA, Lie JT. Capillaritis and pulmonary hemorrhage in Wegener's granulomatosis (letter). *Am J Surg Pathol* 13:78, 1989.

174. Travis WD, et al. A clinicopathologic study of 34 cases of diffuse pulmonary hemorrhage with lung biopsy confirmation. *Am J Surg Pathol* 14:1112, 1990.

175. Travis WD, et al. Surgical pathology of the lung in Wegener's granulomatosis: Review of 87 open lung biopsies from 67 patients. *Am J Surg Pathol* 15:315, 1991.

176. Travis WD, et al. Hypersensitivity pneumonitis and pulmonary vasculitis with eosinophilia in a patient taking an L-tryptophan preparation. *Ann Intern Med* 112:301, 1990.

177. Umehara I, et al. Comprehensive analysis of perfusion scintigraphy in Takayasu's arteritis. *Clin Nucl Med* 16:352, 1991.

178. Vaillant L, et al. Iododerma and acute respiratory distress with leucocytoclastic vasculitis following the intravenous injection of contrast medium. *Clin Exp Dermatol* 15:232, 1990.

179. Van der Woude FJ, et al. Autoantibodies to neutrophils and monocytes: A new tool for diagnosis and a marker of disease activity in Wegener's granulomatosis. *Lancet* 2:425, 1985.

180. Varriale P, Minogue WF, Alfenito JC. Allergic granulomatosis: Case report and review of literature. *Arch Intern Med* 113:235, 1964.

181. Viegi G, et al. Lung function in essential mixed cryoglobulinemia: A short-term follow-up. *Clin Rheumatol* 8:331, 1989.

182. Wallace DJ. Cutaneous Manifestations of SLE. In DJ Wallace, BH Hahn (Eds), *Dubois' Lupus Erythematosus.* Philadelphia: Lea & Febiger, 1993. Pp 356–369.

183. Wechsler RJ, et al. Chest radiograph in lymphomatoid granulomatosis: Comparison with Wegener's granulomatosis. *AJR* 142;79, 1984.

184. Wegener F. Über generalisierte, septische Gefäßerkrankungen. *Verh Dtsch Ges Pathol* 29:202, 1936.

185. Weiland LH, McDonald TJ, DeRemee RA. Relationship of polymorphic reticulosis to lymphomatoid granulomatosis. *Semin Respir Med* 10: 173, 1989.

186. Weiner SR, Paulus HE. Treatment of Wegener's granulomatosis. *Semin Respir Med* 10:156, 1989.

187. Wilson KS, Alexander HL. The relationship of periarteritis nodosa to bronchial asthma and other forms of human hypersensitiveness. *J Lab Clin Med* 30:195, 1945.

188. Winer-Muram HT, Gavant ML. Pulmonary CT findings in Behcet disease. *J Comput Assist Tomogr* 13:346, 1989.

189. Wolfe CA, Hunninghake GW. Vasculitides of the Polyarteritis Nodosa Group. In Immunologically Mediated Pulmonary Diseases. Philadelphia: Lippincott, 1991. Pp 234–249.

190. Wolff SM, et al. Wegener's granulomatosis. *Ann Intern Med* 81:513, 1974.

191. Yamato M, et al. Takayasu arteritis: Radiographic and angiographic findings in 59 patients. *Radiology* 161:329, 1986.

192. Young KR Jr. Pulmonary-renal syndromes. *Clin Chest Med* 10:655, 1989.

59

Immunodeficiency Diseases

Udaya B. S. Prakash

Immunodeficiency diseases are encountered in different forms, often in association with other diseases. Disorders of immunodeficiency, whether total or partial, can be congenital or acquired. These disease states are the consequences of impaired function in one or more components of the immune system, including both B and T lymphocytes, phagocytes, and the complement system. Regardless of the nature of the immunodeficiency syndrome, the immunocompromised host or patient is immunologically compromised as a result of an acquired state. The patient develops immunodeficiency as a sequel of malignancy, long-term corticosteroid therapy, cytotoxic chemotherapy, malnutrition, or alteration of the helper-suppressor T-lymphocyte ratio, as seen in the acquired immunodeficiency syndrome (AIDS). Because the clinical features of immunodeficiency states are not highly specific and vary from one entity to another, definitive diagnosis often is delayed. Normally, these immunodeficiency syndromes are recognized when a subject develops a predisposition to unusual or recurrent infections. The majority of these infections occur in the respiratory system and are the most common cause of morbidity and mortality.

In this chapter, immunodeficiency syndromes, noninfectious pulmonary complications in AIDS and etiologic and diagnostic evaluation of the immunocompromised patient are discussed. Certain immunodeficiency diseases (the Chediak-Higashi syndrome, chronic granulomatous disease of childhood, and severe combined immunodeficiency syndrome) are discussed in Part X.

Immunodeficiency Syndromes

Congenital Agammaglobulinemia

Bruton's infantile X-linked agammaglobulinemia is an inherited disease characterized by the ab-

sence, in the blood and blood-forming tissues, of fully developed B lymphocytes and plasma cells [22]. Synthesis and secretion of immunoglobulins and antibodies are deficient or absent. Allergic rhinitis and asthma occur at a higher rate than in the normal population. Undue susceptibility to bacterial infections is seen usually after the first year of life. An important clue to the diagnosis is a unique susceptibility to infection with encapsulated pyogenic organisms, including *Streptococcus pneumoniae, Streptococcus pyogenes, Hemophilus influenzae, Pseudomonas aeruginosa*, and staphylococci. This phenomenon probably reflects a requirement for specific opsonization of these bacteria before efficient phagocytic cell ingestion is possible. Recurrent purulent sinusitis, bronchitis, and pneumonia, if untreated, may develop into progressive bronchiectasis and secondary respiratory failure. *Pneumocystis carinii* pneumonia, although rare in agammaglobulinemia, has been described in congenital agammaglobulinemia. There is no evidence of increased susceptibility to viral infections of the respiratory system, but these patients are prone to viral central nervous system infections. Restrictive lung disease and lymphocytic interstitial pneumonitis are the other long-term complications.

In a multicenter study involving 96 patients (53 familial and 43 nonfamilial) with X-linked agammaglobulinemia, pulmonary infections were observed in 65 percent, pneumonitis in 56 percent, bronchitis in 9 percent, and bronchiolitis in 5 percent [97]. Bacterial cultures of sputum were available for 33 patients with chronic or recurrent pneumonia. Multiple bacterial species isolated included *H. influenzae* in 82 percent, *S. aureus* in 27 percent, and *S. pneumoniae* in 21 percent. Chronic pulmonary disease was the most frequent long-term complication, occurring in 46 percent of all patients. The prevalence of lung disease was age-related, present in 13 percent of those younger than 10 years and 76 percent of those older than 20.

High-dose intravenous immunoglobulin therapy has been shown to prevent severe complications in patients with X-linked agammaglobulinemia [102].

Acquired Agammaglobulinemia

Acquired agammaglobulinemia, also known as common-variable immunodeficiency, is one of the most frequently seen primary immunodeficiency disorders. It occurs in both sexes, may have its onset at any age, and manifests as loss of all immunoglobulin subclasses and diminished antibody production. Most patients with this disorder have immunoglobulin-bearing B cells in their blood and lymphoid tissue but lack mature plasma cells. A primary defect in B-cell maturation has been demonstrated. The role of immunologic defense mechanisms in the development of acute or recurrent or chronic sinusitis is obviously important, but the incidence of such immune problems is unknown [106].

Pulmonary disease seems to be more common and more severe in patients with common-variable immunodeficiency than in those with X-linked agammaglobulinemia [206]. Sinopulmonary infections begin in the second or third decade. Chronic complications include bronchitis, cystic bronchiectasis, patchy pulmonary fibrosis, and interstitial pneumonitis. Chest roentgenographic features may include atelectasis, bronchiectasis (Fig. 59-1), and homogeneous and heterogeneous segmental opacities. Patients with late-onset agammaglobulinemia and recurrent pulmonary infections have occasionally presented with pulmonary hypertrophic osteoarthropathy. In a brief review of patients who developed pneumonia or empyema due to infection from *Moraxella catarrhalis*, nearly one-third were found to have immunoglobulin abnormalities [37]. Bronchiolitis obliterans–organizing pneumonitis is another complication described in common-variable immunodeficiency [87].

Prophylactic treatment using immunoglobulin replacement is indicated for patients with primary agammaglobulinemia, common-variable hypogammaglobulinemia, and the antibody deficiencies that accompany chronic lymphocytic leukemia, multiple myeloma, and the hypogammaglobulinemia found in very low-birth-weight newborns who have not received adequate transplacental IgG from their mothers [15].

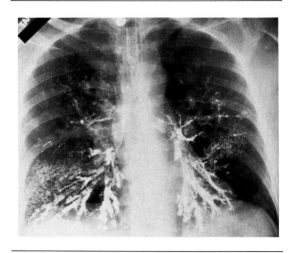

Fig. 59-1. Bronchography demonstrating bronchiectasis of both lower lobes in a patient with acquired agammaglobulinemia.

Selective Immunoglobulin Deficiencies

Selective deficiencies of one or more, but not all, immunoglobulin subclasses are characterized as *dysgammaglobulinemias*. The most common is that due to the absence of IgA. The estimated incidence of selective IgA deficiency ranges from 1 in 700 to 1 in 1000, with most occurring sporadically, although some persons inherit it as an autosomal dominant or a recessive trait. Many patients are asymptomatic, whereas others develop atopic asthma, repeated respiratory infections, bronchiectasis, sinusitis, and otitis media. Pulmonary hemosiderosis has been described in some patients [4]. A study that evaluated 29 patients with IgA deficiency and recurrent upper and lower respiratory infections showed decreased levels of IgG2 and IgG3 in 21 percent. Low levels of IgG2 and IgG3 were significantly related to abnormal lung functions. These studies suggest that there may be a causal relationship between low levels of IgG subclasses and deterioration in lung function, implying that patients with combined IgA and IgG subclass deficiencies may benefit from immunoglobulin prophylaxis [17].

A prospective study of 43 children reported that the probability of developing asthma was much higher in those without any measurable IgA and elevated IgE [24]. Variable deficiencies of IgG and IgA in children have been associated with lymphoid interstitial pneumonitis. The factors responsible for the B-lymphocyte dysfunction and lymphoid infiltrations in the pulmonary parenchyma are unknown.

Selective deficiencies of IgM and IgG are less common. Deficiencies of minor IgG subclasses may be obscured by measuring only the major IgG class and should be specifically sought in clinically suspicious cases [106]. Recurrent bacterial infections of the lungs and upper respiratory tract are common in these patients. Selective IgG subclass (IgG1, IgG2, IgG3, and IgG4) deficiencies predispose patients to recurrent infections of the ears, upper respiratory tract, and lungs. Encapsulated bacteria such as *S. pneumoniae* and *H. influenzae* are responsible for these infections. Deficiencies of IgG, especially those of subclasses IgG2 and IgG4 (often in combination with IgA) or IgG4 alone, correlate well with upper respiratory tract infections and chronic bronchial inflammation contributing to bronchiectasis [139,146,215]. Asthma has been noted in some patients with this disorder [43]. Deficiency of IgG3 and poor response to pneumococcal antigen 7 was demonstrated in more than 50 percent of 61 pediatric patients with refractory sinusitis [190]. Isolated IgG4 deficiency appears to be associated with impaired respiratory tract defenses and may occur in the absence of an easily definable antibody deficiency state [130]. Acquired hypogammaglobulinemia rarely is associated with obstructive lung disease, and the pathogenesis of lung disease may be related to an associated increase in elastase load and a reduction in protease inhibitor function [48].

Functional deficiency of IgG may come to light in patients who present with recurrent pulmonary infections, but such patients may have normal serum levels of IgG. For instance, IgG2 contains an important group of antibodies against common bacteria such as *S. pneumoniae* and *H. influenzae*, and patients with this isolated deficiency may develop recurrent sinopulmonary infections despite normal serum levels of total IgG. Patients with community-acquired pneumonia of bacterial or unknown cause generally demonstrate decreased concentrations of serum IgG2 subclass at the time of admission, after recovery, and 9 months later [75]. After immunization with pneumococcal vaccine, the increases in serum concentrations of IgG subclass and antipneumococcal antibodies in patients do not differ from those in control subjects. Combined deficiencies of IgG2 subclass and IgG- and IgM-specific antibodies may be associated with normal serum immunoglobulin concentrations. In patients with recurrent lung infections and bronchiectasis who show normal serum concentrations of immunoglobulins, it is important to determine both IgG subclasses and antibody production because immunoglobulin replacement has been shown to be beneficial in these patients [157]. Other functional deficiencies of IgG are due to an absence of IgG antibody response to polysaccharide antigens [3] and antibody deficiency because of IgG degradation, such as that found in cystic fibrosis [49]. IgG subclass deficiencies, particularly IgG1, appear to be related to long-term, low-dose corticosteroid therapy in patients with obstructive lung disease [88].

Familial deficiency of serum IgE, presumably an autosomal dominant trait with variable penetrance, associated with sinopulmonary infections has been described. Examination of sera from 23 family members, of whom 14 were symptomatic, revealed very low levels (less than 5 IU/ml) of serum IgE in 12 of the symptomatic group [184].

Hyperimmunoglobulinemia E

Hyperimmunoglobulinemia E, or Job's syndrome, is a rare disorder of phagocyte function characterized by poor antibody and cell-mediated responses to new antigens, high serum IgE (often more than 4000 IU/ml) and IgD levels, blood and sputum eosinophilia, and normal concentrations of IgG, IgA, and IgM. Occasionally also called *Buckley's syndrome*, more than 100 cases of this disorder have been described, mostly in young children [35,100].

Clinically, the syndrome may include eczematoid dermatitis, dysmorphic syndrome with retarded growth, coarse facies, prognathism, osteogenesis imperfecta, and axial osteoporosis. Respiratory complications include sinusitis, pneumonia, and bronchiectasis caused by *S. aureus*, *S. pneumoniae*, gram-negative bacilli, *Candida albicans*, and *Aspergillus* species, pneumatoceles, and chronic dermatitis. Asthma has been reported in approximately 10 percent of patients [100]. The frequency of pneumatoceles is remarkably high, and surgical therapy often is necessary (Fig. 59-2). The primary chest roentgenologic abnormalities are recurrent alveolar lung disease and pneumatoceles. Pneumothorax may occur occasionally [52].

Hypogammaglobulinemia with Hyperimmunoglobulinemia M

Hypogammaglobulinemia with hyperimmunoglobulinemia M is an uncommon syndrome that

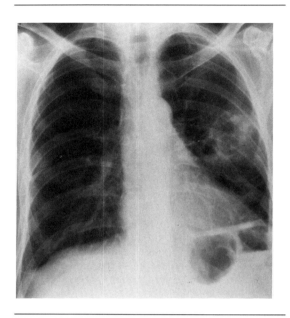

Fig. 59-2. Hyperimmunoglobulinemia E syndrome (Job's syndrome) with left lung abscess caused by *Staphylococcus aureus.* Beginning stages of pneumatoceles, a common complication in this syndrome, can be seen.

has been described as both an X-linked and an autosomal recessive disease. Occasional sporadic cases occur in later life. The cellular immunity tests are normal, but abnormalities in immunoglobulin production are believed to be the result of dysfunctional B-cell regulation by defective T cells [50]. Patients with this syndrome usually exhibit elevated levels of IgM and IgD but an inability to make IgG and IgA antibodies. Patients with hypogammaglobulinemia with hyperimmunoglobulinemia M demonstrate a propensity to pyogenic infections of the respiratory and gastrointestinal tracts as well as a predisposition to develop lymphoproliferative diseases, severe neutropenia, and autoimmune thrombocytopenia.

Congenital Thymic Aplasia (DiGeorge's Syndrome)

Congenital thymic aplasia, also called *DiGeorge's syndrome,* is manifested by the absence of a thymic shadow on the chest roentgenogram, failure of the development of parathyroid glands, T lymphopenia, neonatal hypocalcemia and tetany, and cardiac defects, including tetralogy of Fallot,

right-sided aortic arch, and truncus arteriosus [92]. Serum immunoglobulin concentrations usually are normal, but IgG and IgA antibody responses frequently are impaired. Lymphocyte counts are normal, but all lymphocytes are B cells. Oral and cutaneous candidiasis, viral and bacterial infections, and interstitial pneumonitis can be overwhelming in infants with this disorder. Other pulmonary abnormalities reported include hypoplastic lungs with abnormal lobation and hypoplastic pulmonary artery [44].

Wiskott-Aldrich Syndrome

The Wiskott-Aldrich syndrome is a rare X-linked immunologic disorder characterized by eczema, profound thrombocytopenia, progressive immunodeficiency, and recurrent infections. Deficiency of IgM, elevated levels of IgA and IgG, and very high levels of IgE are seen frequently. Otitis media followed by pneumonia is a common complication. These patients are also susceptible to herpes simplex, cytomegalovirus, *P. carinii,* and varicella infections. Gram-positive and gram-negative bacterial infections are common [33]. Pulmonary vasculitis with features typical of lymphomatoid granulomatosis has been described [78]. Nearly 10 percent of these patients develop malignant neoplasms, and more than 80 percent of these lesions are leukemias and lymphoreticular tumors [11].

Ataxia-Telangiectasia

Transmitted as an autosomal recessive disease, hereditary ataxia-telangiectasia is characterized by progressive cerebellar ataxia followed by choreoathetoid movements and, several years later, development of ocular and cutaneous telangiectasia. Dysfunctional helper T cells may account for the underlying B-cell activity. Lack of both serum and secretory fractions of IgA is noted in more than 80 percent of patients, and serum IgA is absent in approximately 50 percent. Deficiency of IgG2 is a common occurrence in this group of patients [145]. Isolated deficiency of IgG4, with normal levels of total IgG and other subclasses, may lead to severe recurrent sinopulmonary infections and bronchiectasis. This has been observed in children as well as in adults [12]. Repeated infections of the sinuses and lungs from viral agents and bacteria are common (Fig. 59-3). Chest roentgenograms have demonstrated a prominent, symmetric thicket-like pattern in the

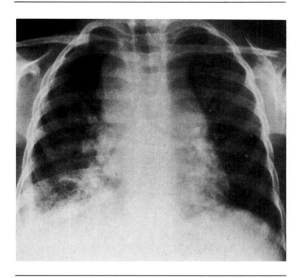

Fig. 59-3. Bilateral lower-lobe infiltrates in a child with ataxia-telangiectasia. This patient has recurrent pulmonary infections caused by *Hemophilus influenzae*.

lungs. One study of 160 patients with ataxia-telangiectasia reported recurrent sinopulmonary infections in 66 percent of patients and low or absent serum IgA in 51 percent [45].

Patients with ataxia-telangiectasia have a marked propensity to develop lymphoma and acute lymphocytic leukemia, and more than 10 percent succumb to malignancy [18,73].

Nezelof's Syndrome

Nezelof's syndrome denotes thymic dysplasia with normal immunoglobulins. It is an inherited disorder characterized by lymphopenia, diminished lymphoid tissue, abnormal architecture of thymus, and normal or elevated immunoglobulin levels. Flawed function of interleukin-2 has been observed in several patients. Deficiency of T-cell function is the main abnormality in these patients, although Nezelof's syndrome sometimes is discussed in conjunction with the severe combined immunodeficiency syndrome [68]. Although a disease of children, several adult cases have been described [137,207]. Recurrent respiratory infections secondary to bronchiectasis and sinusitis are common. Fatal bronchiolitis caused by cytomegalovirus has been described in a child [208].

Hyposplenism

Decreased or absent splenic function occurs in congenital aplasia, splenectomy, hyposplenism due to hemolytic states, malignancy involving the spleen, and chronic sickle cell disease. Phagocytosis of encapsulated bacteria is dependent on normal splenic function. Hyposplenism results in loss of protection against encapsulated organisms such as *S. pneumoniae* and *H. influenzae*. Pneumococcal vaccine and prompt treatment of infections are important.

Acquired Immunodeficiency Syndrome

Since it was first described in 1981, AIDS has become *the* disease of major concern worldwide. The loss of human life from AIDS is staggering because of the near-total mortality in those with advanced disease with its many attendant complications. AIDS is caused by the human immunodeficiency virus (HIV), previously known as the human T-lymphotropic virus III/lymphadenopathy-associated virus (HTLV-III/LAV).

The severe immunodeficiency in AIDS is caused by HIV infecting the CD4(T4) T lymphocyte. Cellular susceptibility to HIV is controlled primarily in the cell membrane. The hallmark of the immunodeficiency in AIDS is the qualitative and quantitative defect of CD4 T lymphocytes (helper T lymphocytes). The loss of function of these cells adversely affects the function of all immune-effector cells [188]. HIV is transmitted through sexual contact, both homosexual and heterosexual, through blood, and maternofetally. The four major groups who have a particularly high risk of developing AIDS include homosexual men, intravenous drug abusers, Haitians, and hemophiliacs.

Decreases in T helper-inducer T lymphocytes to below-normal levels (normal values for helper T lymphocytes are 493 to 1191 cells/liter, or 34 to 67 percent; values for suppressor T lymphocytes are 182 to 785 cells/liter, or 10 to 41.9 percent) and of helper-inducer (OKT4+) to suppressor-cytotoxic (OKT8+) T lymphocyte levels to 0.8 (normal exceeds 1.0) are noted in almost all patients. Laboratory evidence of HIV infection, such as serologic activity, is required by the Centers for Disease Control (CDC) for AIDS case definition in any patient with opportunistic infections with coexistent immunodeficiency from other causes, disseminated histoplasmosis or coccidioidomycosis, chronic symptomatic isosporiasis, Kaposi's sarcoma, primary brain lymphoma in individuals younger than 60 years, high-grade non-T-cell lymphoma, extrapulmonary tuberculosis, and recurrent *Salmonella* septicemia [28]. Pulmonary tuberculosis is now included in the case definition of AIDS [151].

Detection of antibodies to HIV by enzyme-linked immunoassay (ELISA) and the Western blot technique have become nearly universal for screening blood and organ donors. HIV-positive individuals are assumed to be viremic for an indefinite period [112,182]. False-positive ELISA reactivity can be seen in patients with other immunodeficiency diseases, including chronic hepatitis B, hematologic malignancy, acute viral infections, multiple myeloma, primary biliary cirrhosis, alcoholic hepatitis, and primary sclerosing cholangitis; in multiparous women; in those who received multiple transfusions; and in patients with sera positive for rheumatoid factor, antinuclear antibody, and other autoantibodies.

Transmission of HIV may or may not result in infection. Among those who are infected, as determined by serologic tests, many remain asymptomatic for several years. The risk for AIDS is closely associated with the duration of HIV infection [65,85]. Approximately 10 to 20 percent become symptomatic, with fever, rash, lymphadenopathy, aseptic meningitis, and hematologic changes that resemble infectious mononucleosis. Some of these (6 to 10 percent) revert to an asymptomatic state. The AIDS-related complex (ARC) may follow, in both symptomatic and asymptomatic subjects. Although ARC lacks a standard definition, it is clinically characterized by lengthy febrile illness, weight loss, persistent diarrhea, multidermatomal herpes zoster, oral candidiasis, and leukoplakia. Most patients with ARC and persistent lymphadenopathy and an increasing number of asymptomatic carriers develop AIDS. Generally, patients with AIDS are men in their midthirties, and they may present with profound weight loss, nonproductive cough, and significant dyspnea.

Noninfectious Pulmonary Complications in AIDS

Pulmonary involvement is the major cause of morbidity and mortality in patients with AIDS [115,131,223]. The noninfectious pulmonary complications of AIDS are listed in Table 59-1. The infectious pulmonary complications of AIDS are discussed in Chapter 19.

Table 59-1. Noninfectious pulmonary complications of the acquired immunodeficiency syndrome (AIDS)

Diffuse interstitial pulmonary disease
  Idiopathic interstitial pneumonitis
  Lymphocytic interstitial pneumonitis
Alveolar disease
  Pulmonary cystic lesions
  Emphysema
  Lymphocytic alveolitis
  Pulmonary alveolar (phospholipo)proteinosis
Pleural disease
  Pneumothorax
  Pleural effusion
Pulmonary vascular disease
  Pulmonary hypertension
AIDS-related malignancies
  Kaposi's sarcoma
  Non-Hodgkin's lymphoma
  Hodgkin's lymphoma (see text)
  Other neoplasia (see text)
Miscellaneous complications
  Pulmonary dysfunction
  Lactic acidosis
  Pulmonary thromboembolism
  Pulmonary malakoplakia

INTERSTITIAL PNEUMONITIS

Nonspecific interstitial pneumonitis is being recognized more commonly in patients with AIDS [200,205]. During a 4.4-year period, workers at the National Institutes of Health (NIH) observed this entity among 38 percent of 110 patients with AIDS. Interstitial pneumonitis accounted for 32 percent of all episodes of clinical pneumonitis in these patients. Although diffuse alveolar damage was the typical feature of the nonspecific interstitial pneumonitis, neither lung biopsy nor diagnostic bronchoalveolar lavage detected a pathogen. More than 25 percent of these patients had concurrent Kaposi's sarcoma, previous experimental therapies, or a history of *P. carinii* pneumonia or drug abuse. The clinical features were similar to those of patients with *P. carinii* pneumonia. Histopathologic features of the lung in interstitial pneumonitis associated with AIDS may include varying degrees of edema, fibrin deposition, and interstitial inflammation with lymphocytes and plasma cells (Fig. 59-4). Extensive upper-lobe pulmonary calcification has been described in a patient receiving aerosolized pentamidine [199].

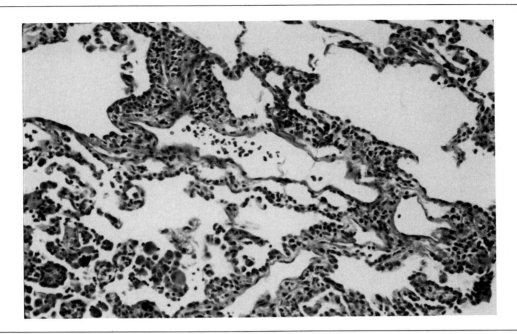

Fig. 59-4. Nonspecific interstitial pneumonia in AIDS. Mild diffuse alveolar infiltrate of chronic inflammatory cells seen. No infections were identified, and the lesion responded to corticosteroid therapy.

LYMPHOCYTIC INTERSTITIAL PNEUMONITIS

Lymphocytic interstitial pneumonitis, a disorder characterized by pulmonary infiltration with mature polyclonal B lymphocytes and plasma cells, is seen in lymphoproliferative disorders and autoimmune diseases [129,210]. It is a well-recognized complication of AIDS, having occurred in the children of mothers in groups at high risk for AIDS [144], in Haitians [183], and in patients with AIDS [129]. Whereas lymphocytic interstitial pneumonitis is nonspecific in adults, its presence is diagnostic of AIDS when it occurs in a child younger than 13 years with a positive HIV antibody test [131].

Pulmonary lymphoid hyperplasia has been reported in 40 percent of children with AIDS [180]. These children were older and had digital clubbing, parotid gland enlargement, and elevated serum IgG levels. Results of serologic assays and lung tissue analysis were suggestive of persistent Epstein-Barr virus (EBV) infection exclusively in patients with pulmonary lymphoid hyperplasia. Although rare in patients with AIDS, EBV and HIV are potential etiologic agents in the causation of lymphocytic interstitial pneumonitis

[70,223]. High titers of EBV antibodies have been demonstrated in adult patients with lymphocytic interstitial pneumonitis associated with AIDS [91,214]. Recognition of the clinical and laboratory findings characteristic of *P. carinii* pneumonia and lymphocytic interstitial pneumonitis in children may assist in the differential diagnosis without the need for surgical biopsy [180].

The chest roentgenogram in lymphocytic interstitial pneumonitis may show fine or coarse reticular or reticulonodular infiltrates and patchy alveolar infiltrates (Fig. 59-5). Histologic examination reveals lymphocytes, plasma cells, and reticulum cells aggregated about the small arteries and compressing the distal airways (Fig. 59-6). Diffuse lymphoid hyperplasia in the lung is the pulmonary analogue of diffuse lymphoid hyperplasia of lymph nodes in ARC (Fig. 59-7). One study of 16 patients with AIDS and biopsy-proved lymphocytic interstitial pneumonitis reported that the chest roentgenologic findings remained stable for several months [27].

LYMPHOCYTIC ALVEOLITIS

Lymphocytic alveolitis is the term used to distinguish a subset of HIV-positive patients with high levels of viremia [34,105]. Most patients with lymphocytic alveolitis have had minimal respiratory symptoms, physiologic abnormalities, or roentgenologic changes. Bronchoalveolar lavage has

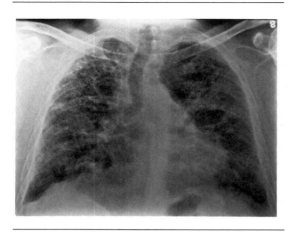

Fig. 59-5. Diffuse interstitial infiltrates in AIDS. Even though lung biopsy showed lymphocytic interstitial pneumonitis, *Pneumocystis carinii* and cytomegalovirus were also present in the bronchoalveolar lavage.

shown a marked increase in both the absolute number and percentage (up to 70 percent) of T lymphocytes in the absence of detectable infections or malignancies; T lymphocytosis appears early and then gradually disappears as the HIV-related disease evolves [71]. The relationship between lymphocytic alveolitis and lymphocytic interstitial pneumonitis, a nonspecific interstitial process, and non-Hodgkin's lymphoma is unclear at this time.

PULMONARY HYPERTENSION

The occurrence of pulmonary hypertension in AIDS has provided some insight into the pathogenesis of primary pulmonary hypertension. Pulmonary hypertension with typical features of the primary disorder has been described in approximately 30 cases of AIDS [120,159,198]. A prospective evaluation of 74 HIV-infected individuals with cardiopulmonary complaints revealed pulmonary hypertension in 8 percent and, when analyzed with a cohort of 1200 HIV-infected subjects, an incidence of 0.5 percent was recorded [198]. This is strikingly high, considering that primary pulmonary hypertension is rare. Although the patients with AIDS have many pulmonary anomalies (chronic hypoxemia, interstitial process, pulmonary embolism, etc.) that may contribute to the development of secondary pulmonary hypertension, there have been no predisposing factors in most reported cases.

In contrast to the female preponderance in primary pulmonary hypertension, almost all pa-

tients who developed pulmonary hypertension in association with AIDS have been male. The mean age of these patients was 37.5 years, and pulmonary artery systolic pressures ranged from 50 to 106 mmHg [159].

Chronic hypoxemia has not been a feature, thereby excluding this as a cause of pulmonary hypertension. Plexogenic pulmonary arteriopathy, regarded as a feature of primary pulmonary hypertension, has been the most common pathologic finding. The mechanism of pulmonary hypertension in patients with AIDS remains unknown. It has been speculated that HIV or another virus may produce the primary damage to pulmonary endothelium or secondary injury through the release of a mediator [120,159,198]. Testing for HIV infection should be considered in patients who present with pulmonary hypertension or who demonstrate a diminished diffusing capacity for carbon monoxide in the lung (DLCO) in the absence of roentgenologic or computed tomographic abnormalities.

PULMONARY EMPHYSEMA AND CYSTIC LESIONS

Pulmonary parenchymal cystic as well as emphysematous lesions have been described in patients with AIDS [38,214]. The mechanism by which these lesions are produced is unknown, although most of the patients described had received therapy for *P. carinii* pneumonia. The HIV itself may have a direct cytotoxic effect on the alveolar walls and pulmonary capillaries [38]. A computed tomographic study of 55 patients with AIDS revealed bullous lung disease in 42 percent [95]. Pulmonary function tests in such patients have shown signs of air trapping, hyperinflation, and a markedly decreased DLCO, but only mild signs of airway disease [38]. Pneumatoceles complicating *P. carinii* pneumonia have been described [80]. Pulmonary emphysema should be considered in the differential diagnosis of HIV-infected patients presenting with dyspnea and normal chest roentgenograms.

PNEUMOTHORAX

The occurrence of pneumothorax in patients with AIDS is a well-recognized pulmonary complication, with more than 100 cases reported. In a prospective cohort study of 1030 patients, 2 percent developed this complication [189]. Although the mechanism is unclear in most cases, an overwhelming majority of patients with AIDS who develop pneumothorax have an underlying *P. carinii* infection [14,172]. Other associations de-

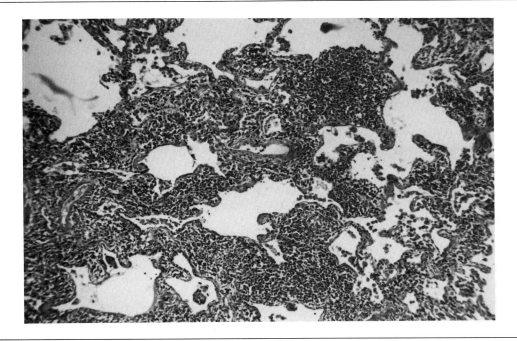

Fig. 59-6. Lymphocytic interstitial pneumonitis in AIDS with diffuse dense interstitial infiltrate of mononuclear cells. No infection was identified.

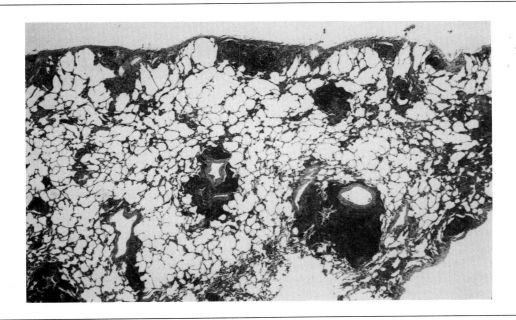

Fig. 59-7. Diffuse lymphoid hyperplasia in AIDS, with germinal centers found in the pleura and along bronchovascular bundles. This lesion is the pulmonary analogue of diffuse lymphoid hyperplasia of lymph nodes in AIDS-related complex (ARC).

scribed include pulmonary Kaposi's sarcoma [55] and toxoplasmosis [101] and *P. carinii* pneumonia [172]. Pulmonary emphysema and cystic lesions may also contribute to the occurrence of pneumothorax. Because transbronchoscopic lung biopsy is frequently performed in patients with AIDS and a pulmonary process, the possibility of iatrogenic pneumothorax should be included in the etiologic possibilities.

One study of 48 patients who were administered aerosolized pentamidine for treatment of *P. carinii* pneumonia found bilateral pneumothoraces in 10 percent [172]. Patients with AIDS who are at the highest risk for developing pneumothorax are those with a history of *P. carinii* pneumonia who are receiving aerosolized pentamidine prophylaxis but who nevertheless develop pneumonia [189]. This may occur because of synergistic relation between aerosolized pentamidine and a history of *P. carinii* pneumonia. Mortality is higher in those who develop pneumothoraces. Interestingly, a low DLCO before aerosolized pentamidine therapy is associated with an increased risk of bilateral pneumothoraces [172].

PLEURAL EFFUSION

Pleural effusion has been observed in more than 62 to 89 percent of patients with pulmonary Kaposi's sarcoma [36,138]. Pleural effusions tend to occur as a late manifestation of extensive pulmonary parenchymal involvement by this condition. Analysis of pleural fluid from patients with pulmonary Kaposi's sarcoma has revealed the fluid to be a serosanguineous, mononuclear cell–predominant exudate, blood-tinged and occasionally chylous [138]. Hypoalbuminemic patients may develop transudates. Closed needle biopsy of the pleura seldom is diagnostic as parietal pleural involvement by Kaposi's sarcoma is very uncommon. Pleural effusion can also result from pulmonary infections, non-Hodgkin's lymphoma, and pneumothorax [86,110,203].

Progressive pleural effusions lead to significant morbidity and mortality. Large pericardial effusions occur in patients with AIDS. In a study of 50 consecutive patients undergoing pericardiocentesis, the most common underlying cause (28 percent) was AIDS, and tuberculosis was the etiology in 57 percent of this group [173].

ALVEOLAR (PHOSPHOLIPO)PROTEINOSIS

Primary pulmonary alveolar (phospholipo)proteinosis is an uncommon disease of unknown etiology characterized by the deposition of lipo-

proteinaceous material in the alveoli [166]. Secondary alveolar proteinosis occurs in many pulmonary disorders, including infectious processes such as *P. carinii*. The finding of pulmonary alveolar (phospholipo)proteinosis in the lung specimens of patients with AIDS is most likely related to an underlying infection rather than a primary process [79].

PULMONARY DYSFUNCTION

Because of the various pulmonary complications related to AIDS, pulmonary function tests in AIDS patients may demonstrate abnormalities. A study evaluated the factors responsible for the reduction in DLCO in 474 HIV-positive patients over an 18-month period and noted that the DLCO was reduced in patients with persistent generalized lymphadenopathy, ARC, nonpulmonary Kaposi's sarcoma, and pulmonary infections [125]. Serial measurements over 18 months showed no change in the DLCO, nor did zidovudine therapy affect this measure. The reasons for diminished DLCO in these patients may be related to emphysematous and cystic lesions and pulmonary hypertension. Low DLCO has been recorded in HIV-positive subjects with normal roentgenograms and high-resolution computed tomograms of the chest [59]. Other studies have shown that low DLCO before aerosolized pentamidine therapy is associated with an increased risk of bilateral pneumothoraces [172]. Studies of the long-term effects of aerosolized pentamidine therapy have failed to show clinically significant changes in pulmonary function [213].

Abnormal airway function, responsive to bronchodilator therapy, has been reported in nearly one-third of patients with AIDS [140]. Some patients who are HIV-positive but who do not have AIDS develop an inability to perform physical activities even when there is no apparent indication of pulmonary disease. Cardiopulmonary exercise testing in 32 such patients has shown that HIV-seropositive subjects have impaired maximum exercise capacity without evidence of ventilatory limitation and, therefore, the authors speculate that the limitation may be secondary to occult cardiac disease [81]. The presence of occult pulmonary hypertension in these patients may also contribute to the decreased exercise capacity.

LACTIC ACIDOSIS

Lactic acidosis, either aerobic or anaerobic, is characterized by metabolic acidosis and a blood lactate level higher than 5 mmol/liter. The aerobic type of lactic acidosis, in which tissue hypoxia is not a feature, may be associated with malignancy, myopathies, and glycogen storage diseases. Aerobic lactic acidosis has been described in seven HIV-infected patients seen during a 2-year period [31]. These patients presented with nausea, emesis, anorexia, weight loss, fever, malaise, and dyspnea. Detailed studies showed no evidence of hypoxia, metabolic acidosis, or mixed acid-base disorder. The onset of lactic acidosis was sudden and without obvious cause. Increased production of lactate may also have been associated with zidovudine myopathy.

KAPOSI'S SARCOMA

Kaposi's sarcoma is the most common malignancy in patients with AIDS. The mechanisms responsible for the development of Kaposi's sarcoma in AIDS patients are unclear. This neoplasm occurs with much greater frequency in homosexuals with AIDS than in AIDS patients in the other risk groups. Garay and associates [60] studied 318 patients with AIDS and Kaposi's sarcoma over a 4-year period and detected Kaposi's sarcoma in approximately 20 percent of patients, all of whom were homosexual men, and all but one of whom presented with cutaneous or visceral Kaposi's sarcoma. Previous or concurrent pulmonary opportunistic infections were noted in 79 percent.

Pulmonary involvement is encountered in 20 to 40 percent of patients with Kaposi's sarcoma (Fig. 59-8) [141,155,230]. The diagnostic yields from fiberoptic bronchoscopy and open-lung biopsy were 24 and 56 percent, respectively, in the series by Garay and associates [60]. At autopsy, pulmonary involvement has been reported in as many as 47 percent of patients with Kaposi's sarcoma [117,223], which is frequently preceded by cutaneous lesions. Although the lungs often are involved when the neoplasm becomes disseminated, rarely is the initial diagnosis made by lung biopsy. However, there have been patients in whom Kaposi's sarcoma was present in lung biopsy specimens and in whom there was no other systemic evidence of the neoplasm [135]. Zibrak and associates [230] noted that in a group of 61 patients with AIDS, 25 (41 percent) had Kaposi's sarcoma of the skin and mucosa, and the respiratory system was involved in 8 of these.

Pulmonary Kaposi's sarcoma is less cellular than the cutaneous lesion, and the tumor consists of loosely aggregated spindle cells often containing atypical nuclei with occasional mitotic figures surrounding small bronchi and vessels and extending into the interstitium (Fig. 59-9). Endo-

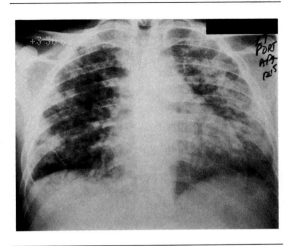

Fig. 59-8. Pulmonary Kaposi's sarcoma in AIDS, showing extensive nodular infiltrates.

bronchial tumors reveal tumor cells in tight bundles beneath the respiratory epithelium [60]. Occult alveolar hemorrhage has been noted in pulmonary Kaposi's sarcoma [77].

Clinically, pulmonary Kaposi's sarcoma is indistinguishable from opportunistic pneumonia. In the series of 318 patients with Kaposi's sarcoma described earlier [60], nonpulmonary Kaposi's sarcoma was diagnosed 8 months before the pulmonary involvement. Cough is a common symptom, but hemoptysis is an uncommon complication of pulmonary or tracheobronchial Kaposi's sarcoma [123,135]. This is most likely due to parenchymal involvement by the neoplasm, as endobronchial Kaposi's sarcoma usually does not produce hemoptysis, although there have been cases with hemoptysis due to nodular Kaposi's sarcoma of the tracheobronchial tree [155]. Tracheobronchial involvement by the sarcomatous process has been described in 8 to 79 percent of patients with Kaposi's sarcoma associated with AIDS [60,123,126,161]. Endobronchial involvement is particularly common in patients with cutaneous Kaposi's sarcoma.

Histologic diagnosis from bronchial biopsy often is difficult because of the submucous involvement of endobronchial tumor. Tracheobronchial Kaposi's sarcoma has a typical appearance—red or violaceous, multiple flat or raised discrete plaques similar in appearance to dermal Kaposi's sarcoma [57,60,155]. Impending airways obstruction due to bulky laryngeal and subglottic nodules and wheezing and shortness of breath

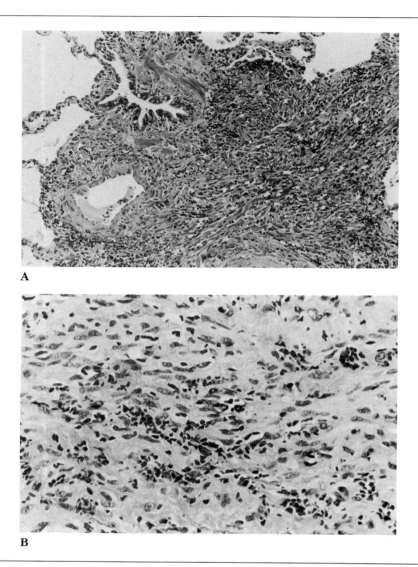

Fig. 59-9. Lung biopsy exhibiting pulmonary Kaposi's sarcoma in AIDS. (A) There is a spindle-cell infiltrate of Kaposi's sarcoma adjacent to and partially surrounding a bronchiole and its accompanying pulmonary artery. (B) The infiltrate is pulmonary Kaposi's sarcoma, composed of spindle cells with cleftlike spaces containing extravasated erythrocytes.

from lobar and segmental bronchial lesions have been reported [230].

Chest roentgenograms may exhibit the typical nodular infiltrates in a very small number of patients (fewer than 10 percent) [60]. However, the slightly more nodular (as opposed to interstitial) pattern and the rather slow evolution of lung infiltrates in Kaposi's sarcoma are different from the relatively rapid involvement in *P. carinii* pneumonia [230]. A review of chest roentgenograms and postmortem pathologic findings in 24 patients with AIDS and autopsy-proved intrathoracic Kaposi's sarcoma revealed that premortem radiographic visualization of pulmonary lesions

of Kaposi's sarcoma depended on the extent of involvement and the presence of concomitant disease. In 3 patients (13 percent), the chest roentgenograms showed nodular opacities that corresponded in size and configuration to nodules seen at autopsy. In 21 patients (87 percent), the lesions were not radiographically identifiable, in some cases because they were obscured by infection. Findings with a high positive predictive value for the diagnosis of pulmonary Kaposi's sarcoma included parenchymal nodular and reticular opacities (100 percent), pleural effusions (89 percent), and hilar or mediastinal lymphadenopathy (92 percent). None of these findings was specific, but the presence of any one in a patient with AIDS should increase the possibility of intrathoracic involvement by Kaposi's sarcoma.

Hilar and mediastinal lymphadenopathy has been observed in more than 26 percent of patients with pulmonary Kaposi's sarcoma, and this may be associated with perihilar parenchymal infiltrates that progress to diffuse bilateral infiltrates over a period of months. Computed tomography is reported to show abnormal hilar densities characteristically extending into the adjacent pulmonary parenchyma along distinctly perivascular and peribronchial pathways [133]. Other pulmonary manifestations of Kaposi's sarcoma include chylothorax [19,167], upper airway obstruction [179], and fulminant respiratory failure [181].

Pulmonary irradiation may result in both subjective and objective responsiveness of Kaposi's sarcoma in AIDS patients and may be utilized for palliative treatment in some patients with AIDS and Kaposi's sarcoma [136]. Therapy for Kaposi's sarcoma is not curative [84,127]. Chemotherapy has been tried, but the median duration of survival once the pulmonary involvement occurs in 6 months [60].

NON-HODGKIN'S LYMPHOMA
As with the incidence of Kaposi's sarcoma, the incidence of non-Hodgkin's lymphoma seems to be increasing. Non-Hodgkin's lymphomas occur with increasing frequency in chronically immunosuppressed patients, in patients who are on chemotherapy to prevent rejection of transplanted organs [149,222], and in those with AIDS [98,99,211,231,232]. Non-Hodgkin's lymphomas seen in AIDS are Burkitt-like lymphomas, B-cell lymphomas, or B-cell immunoblastic sarcomas, with or without plasmacytoid features [98,99, 231,232]. They also tend frequently to be extranodal. Lymphomas in organ transplant recipients may be oligoclonal or polyclonal in origin [32] and may be related to the use of cyclosporin A [132].

Non-Hodgkin's lymphoma limited to the lung is uncommon in AIDS and has rarely been reported [99,231]. In the report by Ziegler and associates [231] on 90 homosexual men (median age, 37 years) with non-Hodgkin's lymphoma secondary to AIDS, 62 percent of the lymphomas were high-grade, 29 percent intermediate-grade, and 7 percent low-grade. All were B-cell lymphomas, and all but two were of extranodal origin. Central nervous system, bone marrow, bowel, and the mucocutaneous area were most commonly involved. Lungs were affected in 8 percent, but no further details were published regarding the type of pulmonary involvement. Kaposi's sarcoma was present in 20 patients before the diagnosis of non-Hodgkin's lymphoma was made and developed in another 3 patients after the diagnosis of non-Hodgkin's lymphoma was made.

Di Carlo and associates [39] reported on 29 homosexual men and 1 thalassemic woman with AIDS and non-Hodgkin's lymphoma. The median age of the patients was 42 years; 90 percent of the lymphomas were extranodal, 67 percent exclusively so. Nearly 50 percent constituted diffuse, large follicular center-cell types. Lung involvement was observed in only two patients. Another publication observed a 10 percent incidence of pulmonary involvement among 40 patients with non-Hodgkin's lymphoma related to AIDS [158].

Chest roentgenographic findings have included patchy nodular infiltrates, multiple nodules, and interstitial infiltrates. A high incidence of opportunistic infections and Kaposi's sarcoma prior to the diagnosis of non-Hodgkin's lymphoma has been observed [98].

Approximately half the patients with non-Hodgkin's lymphoma occurring in AIDS have responded to chemotherapy, radiation, or both, with relapse in 50 percent. The median survival, even with therapy, is approximately 8 months.

HODGKIN'S LYMPHOMA
Kaposi's sarcoma, non-Hodgkin's lymphoma, and primary lymphoma of the brain are currently included in the case definition of AIDS. More recently, a higher incidence of Hodgkin's lymphoma has been reported among intravenous drug users infected with HIV. In a study of 6704 homosexual men in the San Francisco Clinic cohort study, 8 cases of Hodgkin's lymphoma and 90 cases of non-Hodgkin's lymphoma were identified [76]. The incidence of Hodgkin's lymphoma in men with HIV infection was estimated to be 19.3 cases per 100,000 person-years, and the incidence of non-Hodgkin's lymphoma was 240 cases per 100,000 person-years. The excess Hodgkin's lymphoma cases attributable to HIV infection were 19.3 cases per 100,000 person-years [76]. Further

studies are necessary to determine whether Hodgkin's lymphoma should be considered an HIV-related malignancy.

OTHER PULMONARY NEOPLASIAS

Multiple leiomyomas and leiomyosarcomas mainly involving the lungs and gastrointestinal tract have been described in children with AIDS [29]. A case of lymphomatoid granulomatosis (polymorphic reticulosis or lethal midline granuloma) has been reported in a patient with AIDS [66]. Six patients with AIDS and primary lung cancer have also been described [20].

OTHER NONINFECTIOUS PULMONARY COMPLICATIONS

Aerosolized pentamidine has been associated with respiratory disturbances. Bronchospasm has been reported to occur in as many as 34 percent of patients on aerosolized pentamidine therapy [168,212]. Direct effect of nebulized particles as well as histamine-mediated bronchial reaction may be involved in this side effect. Bronchospasm following intravenous pentamidine therapy has also been reported in a patient; the mechanism of this adverse reaction is unclear [62]. The use of trimethoprim-sulfamethoxazole for treatment of P. carinii has been associated with the onset of new pulmonary infiltrates and hypoxia that recurred when the drug was reintroduced [193].

There is some indication that thromboembolism and pulmonary embolism may be more common in patients with AIDS [26,153]. Bronchiolitis obliterans–organizing pneumonitis has been described in a patient with AIDS [2]. In contrast to neutrophilic predominance in bronchiolitis obliterans–organizing pneumonitis in non-AIDS patients, bronchoalveolar lavage in this patient demonstrated 48 percent lymphocytes; clinical and chest roentgenographic abnormalities resolved with corticosteroid therapy [2].

Pulmonary malakoplakia is an unusual inflammatory condition characterized pathologically by accumulations of benign macrophages that are associated with deposition of typical intracellular and extracellular calcispherites. Pulmonary malakoplakia has been described in 7 patients with AIDS [187].

There have been several case reports of sarcoidosis occurring in patients with AIDS. As both diseases are more common in the age group of 25 to 40 years, the association may represent chance occurrence. However, further experience may shed new light on this association.

Pulmonary Diagnostic Procedures in AIDS

A chest roentgenogram is the initial diagnostic procedure for known HIV-positive patients. A normal chest roentgenogram does not exclude pulmonary disease because up to 14 percent of patients subsequently found to have respiratory disease will not exhibit chest roentgenographic abnormalities [121]. The various roentgenologic abnormalities observed in pulmonary complications of AIDS were described in the preceding sections.

Induced sputum analysis is an excellent technique to identify P. carinii. In a patient with AIDS who is suspected of having P. carinii pneumonia, examination of induced sputum should be considered before bronchoscopy. The diagnostic sensitivity of induced sputum examination in detecting P. carinii is approximately 55 percent [16,122,156], and the diagnostic yield is dependent on the technique of sputum induction. Indirect immunofluorescent staining using monoclonal antibodies to P. carinii is reported to have a diagnostic yield of 92 percent [90]. The development of DNA probes specific for P. carinii is likely to further increase the sensitivity.

Fiberoptic bronchoscopy with diagnostic bronchoalveolar lavage is a safe procedure with a high diagnostic yield in patients with AIDS and lung disease. Stover and associates [200] evaluated the effectiveness of fiberoptic bronchoscopy with the addition of diagnostic bronchoalveolar lavage in 72 patients with AIDS and parenchymal pulmonary disease and reported a diagnostic yield of 94 percent for P. carinii, 67 percent for cytomegalovirus, and 62 percent for M. avium-intracellulare. Both transbronchial biopsy and diagnostic bronchoalveolar lavage provided high independent yields (88 and 85 percent, respectively) for P. carinii pneumonia, but combining the procedures gave the best yield. Overall, the yield of bronchoscopy for all pathogens was 65 percent [200].

Marchevsky and associates [109] reviewed pulmonary complications in 70 patients with AIDS and reported that P. carinii pneumonia, present in 67 percent of the patients, was diagnosed by fiberoptic bronchoscopy with transbronchial biopsies in all the patients except two adults, who required open-lung biopsy, and two children, in whom the infection was detected only at autopsy. Other opportunistic infections, such as cytomegalovirus pneumonitis, mycobacterial infections, invasive candidiasis, toxoplasmosis, cryptococcosis, and histoplasmosis, were more difficult to diagnose by fiberoptic bronchoscopy.

Bronchoalveolar lavage in 63 patients with AIDS, reported by Venet and coworkers [217], revealed *P. carinii* in 63 percent, cytomegalovirus in 62 percent, and mycobacteria in 22 percent. Overall, bronchoalveolar lavage yielded at least one opportunistic agent in 94 percent of patients who presented with clinical or roentgenographic pulmonary disease and in 80 percent of patients who presented with fever only. In a report on 32 patients suspected of having AIDS, 25 were found to have *P. carinii* pneumonia. A double-lumen lavage catheter used through an endotracheal tube, without a bronchoscope, has detected opportunistic infection in 43 percent of patients with AIDS [108]. Bronchoalveolar lavage can also be used to recover HIV but not to detect the HIV p24-antigen [103]. Transbronchoscopic lung biopsy and multiple bronchial brushings are reported to be noncontributory to the diagnosis of pulmonary complications in AIDS [119,124].

Barrio and colleagues [9] reported on 286 patients with AIDS who had repeat fiberoptic bronchoscopies performed for the diagnosis of persistent pulmonary infiltrates. The repeat bronchoscopy was performed within 30 days in one group and after 60 days in a second group. Repeat bronchoscopy yielded a new treatable diagnosis (*P. carinii*, *M. tuberculosis*, *M. avium-intracellulare*) in 5 percent of the former group and 59 percent of the latter. *P. carinii* pneumonia was the most common diagnosis in both groups on initial evaluation, being found in 55 percent of all patients. In both groups, nondiagnostic bronchoscopies were common (29 percent overall). The most commonly missed bronchoscopic diagnoses (proved by open-lung biopsy) were cytomegalovirus pneumonia and Kaposi's sarcoma, and neither had much therapeutic implication. In patients with AIDS who have persistent or worsening pulmonary infiltrates despite therapy, repeat bronchoscopy after a short interval (i.e., less than 30 days) is unlikely to have therapeutic implications. In contrast, those patients whose pulmonary involvement resolves initially may benefit from an aggressive diagnostic approach if new pulmonary infiltrates appear.

Open-lung biopsy in patients with AIDS is likely to be useful diagnostically when bronchoscopy could not be safely performed or when a preceding bronchoscopic procedure was nondiagnostic. However, open-lung biopsies in patients whose conditions continue to deteriorate despite treatment for disorders established bronchoscopically are not likely to yield therapeutically useful information [53].

In patients with pulmonary Kaposi's sarcoma, the diagnostic yields from fiberoptic bronchoscopy and open-lung biopsy were 24 and 56 percent, respectively, in the series by Garay and associates [60]. Of the 11 cases of documented Kaposi's sarcoma in the lung parenchyma reported by Stover and colleagues [200], none was diagnosed bronchoscopically, although characteristic endobronchial lesions were seen in 6 patients. However, others have reported diagnostic yields of 34 to 56 percent with bronchoscopy, biopsy of bronchial lesions, and transbronchial lung biopsy [57,72].

Finally, the exploration of AIDS risk factors and a few easily detectable physical signs are the most important clues to the correct clinical diagnosis. Once AIDS is suspected, an aggressive and rapid approach for diagnosis is justified. Selected individually for each patient, the most commonly successful tests include bronchoscopy with bronchoalveolar lavage or transbronchial lung biopsy (or both); bone marrow, lymph node, or liver biopsy with both microbiologic and pathologic processing of the material; blood (and, often, spinal fluid) cultures for fungal organisms; cranial computed tomographic scan; and *Toxoplasma* serology.

There is no curative treatment for HIV infection or AIDS [224]. However, zidovudine (azidothymidine [AZT]) was the first drug therapy approved for AIDS. A thymidine analogue, zidovudine is an inhibitor of the in vitro replication of some viruses, including HIV [128]. The data in 281 patients treated for an average duration of 4.5 months in the United States have shown that opportunistic infections and deaths continued to occur; however, the efficacy of zidovudine in prolonging survival for most patients was evident for an additional 5 months of treatment [51,56,174]. Further, zidovudine also significantly reduced the risk of acquiring an AIDS-defining infection, such as *P. carinii* pneumonia, after the first 4 to 6 months of treatment. Bone marrow suppression with pancytopenia is the major toxicity of this drug [63].

In a 4-year study of 130 patients with AIDS, the overall mortality from respiratory causes identified during the study was 41 percent, but this statistic varied markedly with the etiologic agent. Respiratory failure, however, carried a 100 percent mortality despite the underlying cause [201]. Mortality is nearly 100 percent in patients who have AIDS for more than 1 year and 70 percent in those diseased for less than 1 year. Despite some symptomatic responses to therapy for pulmonary infections, the mortality in AIDS seems to be unaffected by appropriate therapy for the pulmonary manifestations of this disease.

Organ Transplantation and the Lung

After organ transplantation, pulmonary complications can be related to infection, transfusion of blood products, and immunosuppressive drugs. Pulmonary infections are the most common cause of death in patients with organ transplants [41,185,186]. Some complications are more commonly encountered with certain types of organ transplants, whereas others are nonspecific and occur in most organ recipients, irrespective of the organ transplanted.

The following is a brief discussion of the common pulmonary complications among recipients of solid-organ transplants. The pulmonary complications of bone marrow transplantation and the graft-versus-host disease are discussed in Chapter 60.

Infectious Pulmonary Complications

VIRAL INFECTIONS
Cytomegalovirus, EBV, herpes simplex virus, and varicella-zoster virus have been implicated in pulmonary infections and may be related to immunosuppression or corticosteroid therapy after transplantation [7]. Respiratory syncytial virus, adenovirus, and other viruses also cause pneumonitis in the transplant recipient.

BACTERIAL INFECTIONS
Approximately 4 percent of recipients of solid-organ transplants in the United States develop bacterial pneumonia, often in the first 3 months following transplantation. The incidence of bacterial pneumonia is highest in recipients of heart-lung (22 percent) and liver transplants (17 percent), intermediate in recipients of heart transplants (5%), and lowest in renal transplants (1 to 2 percent) [118]. Particular risk factors for developing bacterial infections include pulmonary cytomegalovirus infection, graft rejection, antirejection therapy, the use of corticosteroids, azathioprine, or antilymphocyte globulin, the presence of OKT3, and splenectomy. In addition to the usual gram-positive and gram-negative bacteria, uncommon bacteria such as *Legionella pneumophila* should be considered in recipients

of solid-organ transplants, particularly kidney. *Legionella* pneumonia tends to occur within several weeks after transplantation and frequently coincides with episodes of rejection [5,82]. Pulmonary infection by *P. aeruginosa* should be considered in all patients hospitalized for more than 48 hours. The crude mortality secondary to bacterial pneumonia in solid-organ transplantation exceeds 40 percent [118]. Gram-negative bacilli, *S. aureus*, and *Legionella* predominate in the first 3 months after transplantation and are associated with mortality rates in excess of 60 percent. Bacterial pneumonias after 3 months are caused by *S. pneumoniae* and *H. influenzae* and are associated with considerably lower mortality.

FUNGAL INFECTIONS
Fungal pneumonia is an infrequent but devastating complication of solid-organ transplantation [229]. A patient's present or immediate past areas of residence and underlying or concomitant diseases influence the type of fungal organism involved in the infection. A high incidence of pulmonary fungal infections from *Candida*, *Cryptococcus neoformans*, and zygomycetes is associated with diabetes mellitus. *Nocardia asteroides* is an important pathogen in solid-organ transplant recipients, and the infection presents as lung disease in 80 to 90 percent of infected transplant patients [30].

PROTOZOAL INFECTIONS
P. carinii pneumonia is an uncommon problem, occurring in fewer than 5 percent of patients. The infection most commonly presents from 2 to 56 months after transplantation with symptoms of dyspnea, fever, and dry cough lasting from a few days to a few weeks [42].

Noninfectious Pulmonary Complications

BRONCHIOLITIS OBLITERANS
Bronchiolitis obliterans has emerged as the most important and problematic long-term complication of heart-lung transplantation, occurring in 10 to 50 percent of patients who left the hospital with normal cardiopulmonary function [23,47,113]. The obliterative bronchiolitis after heart-lung transplantation may be related to airway-directed chronic rejection modulated by upregulation of class II major histocompatibility complex antigens on bronchial epithelium. Although bronchiolitis obliterans may appear as early as 2 months and as late as 4 years posttransplantation, the mean time has been 8 to 12

months [113]. Treatment with immunosuppressive agents in the initial stages may retard the rate of progression [64].

Even though the ventilatory response to exercise is significantly improved after heart transplantation [111], the gradual deterioration in pulmonary function tests indicates the possibility of bronchiolitis obliterans. The earliest physiologic abnormality is the reduction in forced expiratory flow during the middle half of exhalation (FEF_{25-75}. When bronchiolitis obliterans is suspected, the diagnosis should be confirmed by lung biopsy if possible. Bronchoalveolar lavage can diagnose opportunistic infections in these patients, but it is not diagnostic for bronchiolitis obliterans. Azathioprine and cyclosporine are currently the main drugs used to treat acute rejection and thus prevent bronchiolitis obliterans.

RESPIRATORY FAILURE, PULMONARY EDEMA, AND ATELECTASIS

The major noninfectious pulmonary complications after kidney transplantation are pulmonary edema and pulmonary embolism, seen in approximately 15 percent of patients and accounting for nearly one-third of all pulmonary complications [170,194,221]. Pulmonary edema is the result of the rejection process, fluid retention, and hypervolemia. Pulmonary edema after renal transplantation usually develops within the first postoperative month, and the clinical presentation often mimics infectious pulmonary disease. Nearly one-fourth of readmissions to the intensive care unit after liver transplantations are due to respiratory failure [46]. Adult respiratory distress syndrome, occurring within the first postoperative week, is noted in 4.5 to 17.5 percent of liver transplant recipients and is associated with a mortality of 80 percent [46]. Sepsis is most often the cause of adult respiratory distress syndrome in these patients. Pulmonary edema is common in the immediate postoperative period after heart transplantation.

Patchy atelectasis in the immediate postoperative period is common after liver and renal transplantations, being encountered in 25 percent of renal transplant recipients. Extensive manipulation of diaphragms and subdiaphragmatic spaces intraoperatively contributes to this problem. Atelectasis can be expected in 65 to 90 percent of patients undergoing heart transplantation and, although nearly 50 percent of patients develop bilateral atelectasis, the vast majority exhibit atelectasis of the left lower lobe [47]. Left hemidiaphragmatic dysfunction due to paresis or paralysis is the result of hypothermic cardioplegia and can last from weeks to months. Chest physiotherapy and therapeutic bronchoscopy may be required to treat atelectasis and improve ventilation and oxygenation.

DRUG-INDUCED PULMONARY INJURY

Cytotoxic drugs that are used as immunosuppressive agents to minimize graft rejection are capable of causing pulmonary damage. Interstitial pneumonitis [13,25,93] and noncardiogenic edema [8,197] have been observed in patients treated with azathioprine and orally administered cyclosporine, respectively. Administration of cyclosporine through the central veins 5 days after liver transplantation has resulted in fatal acute respiratory distress syndrome in 2 of 12 patients [160], whereas cyclosporine administration through peripheral veins has not been reported to cause pulmonary abnormalities [8,160]. Blood loss during liver transplantation may necessitate substantial transfusions, which can lead to noncardiogenic and cardiogenic pulmonary edema [216].

PLEURAL EFFUSION

Pleural effusion is nearly universal in recipients of liver transplantation. These effusions are almost exclusively right-sided, occur within the first week of transplantation, are often large, and usually are transudative [46]. The presence of ascites before transplantation may contribute to the accumulation of pleural fluid. Most effusions resolve spontaneously within a few weeks. Pleural effusion, atelectasis, and diaphragmatic dysfunction contribute to prolonged mechanical ventilation.

Pleural effusions also occur in up to 78 percent of patients who undergo heart transplantation. The etiologies are multifactorial. Most effusions are small, bilateral, and often associated with atelectasis. Collection of fluid or blood in the mediastinum may be seen in heart transplant recipients [47].

PULMONARY MALIGNANCY

Posttransplantation pulmonary malignancy is the result of chronic immunosuppressive therapy employed in most recipients of organ transplants. Such pulmonary malignancies have been described more commonly in renal transplant recipients, and the types of neoplasms have included B-cell non-Hodgkin's lymphoma, Kaposi's sarcoma, and metastatic renal cell cancer in which the primary originated in the donor kidney. The introduction of cyclosporine as an antirejection drug has greatly increased the risk of developing these malignancies [148]. As discussed earlier, the role of EBV has been considered in the etiology of the neoplasms. The incidence of Kaposi's sarcoma in the renal transplant population is estimated to be increased 400- to 500-fold over that in the general population, but pulmonary involvement is rare [46]. The incidence of developing malignancy after heart transplantation is approximately 7 percent, the majority being lymphoproliferative disorders [47].

OTHER NONINFECTIOUS PULMONARY COMPLICATIONS

Pulmonary thromboembolism is one of the most common complications following renal transplantation. In a review of 227 renal transplant patients, pulmonary embolism is the most common pulmonary complication, occurring in 60 percent of patients [170]. Intraoperative manipulation of pelvic veins, immunosuppressive agents, and prolonged preoperative immobility contribute to a high incidence of deep vein thrombosis in these patients [21,170].

After liver transplantation, right hemidiaphragmatic dysfunction is common but reversible [46,94]. The resulting atelectasis of the right lower lobe may persist as long as 3 months after transplantation.

Pulmonary calcification can occur after renal or liver transplantation. It is a dystrophic calcification similar to that seen in patients on chronic hemodialysis and, although often asymptomatic, respiratory failure has been reported [46].

Mediastinitis, usually caused by bacteria, is a serious complication of cardiac surgery and should be considered in any patient who presents with fever, leukocytosis, inflammation, or instability of the sternal wound after cardiac transplantation.

Pulmonary Disease in the Immunocompromised Patient

Although the term *immunocompromised patient* or *compromised host* generally describes a patient whose defense mechanisms are impaired, thereby rendering him or her more susceptible to infections, the pulmonary abnormalities noted in these patients do not always represent an infectious process. The etiologic possibilities for the abnormal chest roentgenogram in the immunocompromised patient are varied because the lungs are involved in most of the complications

in such a patient [176,177,225,226]. If the pulmonary involvement is diffuse, the mortality approaches 50 percent [134,195].

Most immunocompromised patients with diffuse pulmonary infiltrates exhibit typical clinical features: fever, nonproductive cough, dyspnea, abnormal chest roentgenograms, anemia, normal or low leukocyte count, decreased platelet count, and hypoxemia of varying degree. The chest roentgenogram rarely is helpful in making a definitive diagnosis [226]. Faced with a rapidly deteriorating immunocompromised patient with progressive chest roentgenographic abnormalities, the clinician is forced to consider quickly a myriad of diagnoses. Simplifying the possibilities by grouping the differential diagnoses in such a patient is extremely helpful in planning the appropriate diagnostic procedures and treatment (Table 59-2). The abnormal chest roentgenogram in the immunocompromised patient may indicate one or more of the following diagnoses: (1) extension of the basic disease process, (2) opportunistic infection, (3) drug-induced lung disease, (4) nonspecific interstitial pneumonitis, (5) lymphocytic interstitial pneumonitis, (6) B-cell neoplasia associated with chronic immunosuppression, (7) a new pulmonary problem unrelated to the preceding diagnoses, or (8) a combination of two or more of the preceding diagnoses.

Up to one-third of immunocompromised patients have two or more complications. The most common types of impairment of defense mechanisms are reductions in the number of granulocytes, B lymphocytes, and T lymphocytes. Nearly one-fourth of the pulmonary complications in these patients are noninfectious. The increasing use of chemotherapeutic agents, with consequently more frequent remissions and relapses of the basic disease process and more frequent cy-

Table 59-2. **Differential diagnosis of pulmonary disease in the immunocompromised patient**

Extension of basic disease process into the lungs

Opportunistic infection

Drug-induced lung disease

Nonspecific interstitial pneumonitis

Lymphocytic interstitial pneumonitis

Pulmonary malignancy associated with chronic immunosuppression

New pulmonary problem unrelated to immunodeficiency

Combination of two or more of the preceding

totoxic pulmonary reactions to the chemotherapy, has made it increasingly difficult to pinpoint the cause of a pulmonary abnormality in a compromised host. Because some of the respiratory problems are associated with a rapid downhill clinical course, it is imperative that diagnostic consideration of an abnormal pulmonary process include the following steps: (1) recognition of the patient as an immunocompromised host, (2) definition of the derangement of the host defense mechanism, (3) categorization of chest roentgenographic abnormalities, (4) assessment of the degree of urgency with regard to various diagnostic procedures, and (5) determination and performance of the most productive diagnostic procedure.

Recognition that the patient is at added risk of infection is the first important step toward diagnosis of the pulmonary process. The various immunodeficiency syndromes that may be seen in immunocompromised patients were discussed earlier. Additionally, local mechanical factors predispose these patients to special problems. In this group of underlying problems are included diseases of the airways, mucociliary clearance defects, deficiency of secretory IgA, absence of surfactant from acute lung injury, and preexisting pulmonary structural damage such as bullous lesion, bronchiectasis, ancient cavities, and a fibrotic process. The etiologic factors of pulmonary abnormalities seen in compromised hosts are outlined in Tables 59-3 and 59-4. Each of the

---

Table 59-3. **Etiologic classification of pulmonary complications in the immunocompromised patient**

Extension of basic disease process into lungs
  Lymphomas, Hodgkin's and non-Hodgkin's
  Leukemias
  Plasma cell neoplasms
  Carcinomatosis, primary and metastatic
  Collagenoses
  Vasculitides
Opportunistic infections
  Viruses
    Herpes simplex
    Varicella zoster
    Cytomegalovirus
  Bacteria*
    Gram-positive bacteria
    Gram-negative bacteria
    Anaerobes
  Mycobacteria
    M. tuberculosis
    M. avium-intracellulare
    M. kansasii
  Fungi
    Aspergillus species
    Candida species
    Zygomycetes (Mucorales) species
    Cryptococcus neoformans
    Histoplasma capsulatum
    Blastomyces dermatitidis
    Coccidioides immitis
    Trichosporon species
    Nocardia asteroides
  Protozoa
    Pneumocystis carinii
    Toxoplasma gondii
    Cryptosporidium species
  Parasites
    Strongyloides stercoralis

Drug-induced pulmonary disease
  Pulmonary cytotoxic drugs
  Oxygen toxicity
  Radiation pneumonitis and fibrosis
  Transfusion-related acute lung injury
Nonspecific interstitial pneumonitis
  Viral infections
  Graft-versus-host disease
  Acquired immunodeficiency syndrome (AIDS)
  Organ transplant recipients
  Bronchiolitis obliterans
  Pulmonary alveolar hemorrhage
  Pulmonary edema
Lymphocytic interstitial pneumonitis
  Viral infections
  AIDS
  Graft-versus-host disease
  Agammaglobulinemia
Pulmonary malignancy associated with
    immunosuppression
  Non-Hodgkin's lymphoma
  Kaposi's sarcoma
  Carcinoma of lung
New pulmonary process unrelated to
    immunodeficiency
  Pulmonary embolism
  Aspiration pneumonia
  Community-acquired pneumonia
  Nosocomial pneumonia
  Congestive cardiac failure
  Renal failure
  Malignant disease
Combination of two or more of the preceding: More
    than two-thirds of the immunocompromised
    patients belong to this group.

*Unusual organisms include *Branhamella, Legionella, Cunninghamella, Listeria, Salmonella,* and *Serratia* species.

Table 59-4. Factors predisposing the host to opportunistic pulmonary infection

Basic disease process (see Table 59-3)

Congenital and acquired immunodeficiency states

Altered physical barriers
    Indwelling catheters
    Nebulizers and ventilators
    Local mechanical disruption by tumor and the like
    Ciliary dysfunction
    Bronchospastic disease
    Intubation or tracheostomy

Altered indigenous microbial flora
    Systemic illnesses (diabetes mellitus, alcoholism, etc.)
    Surgery
    Malnutrition
    Aspiration
    Hospitalization
    Broad-spectrum antibiotic therapy
    Change in virulence of microbial flora
    Intubation or tracheostomy

Leukopenia
    Basic disease process
    Decreased migration
    Defective phagocytosis
    Decreased bactericidal activity
    Cytotoxic drug therapy
    Protein-calorie malnutrition

Impaired lymphocyte-mediated immunity
    Corticosteroid therapy
    Cytotoxic drug therapy
    Radiation
    Transplantation
    Acquired immunodeficiency syndrome
    Protein-calorie malnutrition

Underlying pulmonary pathology
    Obstructive pulmonary disease
    Bronchiectasis
    Ancient cavitary disease
    Secretory IgA deficiency
    Surfactant deficiency

broad categories of diagnostic possibilities will be briefly described here.

Differential Diagnosis

PULMONARY EXTENSION OF BASIC DISEASE PROCESS

The basic disease processes listed in Table 59-3 often are associated with various degrees of suppression of immune defense mechanisms. In the present context, patients with such disorders may be considered as compromised hosts. When presented with pulmonary problems in such a patient, the clinician must ascertain whether the pulmonary manifestations represent extension of the basic disease into the lungs or opportunistic infection. Intrathoracic spread of primary pulmonary and extrapulmonary malignancies together constitute the most common cause of pulmonary extension of the basic disease process. Hematologic malignancies (especially leukemias) and lymphomas are more likely to produce chest roentgenographic abnormalities than are other systemic neoplastic processes (Fig. 59-10). Leukemias as a group produce mediastinal and hilar lymphadenopathy in 50 percent of cases at autopsy and pulmonary involvement in 25 percent. Occasionally, patients may present with acute respiratory distress from extensive leukemic infiltrates in the lungs [165]. Roentgenographically, mediastinal lymphadenopathy is found in 50 percent of patients with Hodgkin's lymphoma, whereas pulmonary parenchymal involvement occurs in approximately 30 percent. Non-Hodgkin's lymphoma exhibits mediastinal lymphadenopathy in 35 percent of cases. Primary pulmonary lymphoma may present as an alveolar infiltrate or as a homogeneous mass. In such cases, elaborate diagnostic investigations may be necessary to rule out an extrapulmonary focus of the lymphoma. (A detailed discussion of the pulmonary manifestations in hematologic malignancies is provided in Chapter 60.) Lung involvement is more common in untreated lymphoproliferative diseases than in myeloproliferative diseases.

Fig. 59-10. Pulmonary extension of non-Hodgkin's lymphoma refractory to chemotherapy. Diffuse alveolar infiltrates are seen in both lungs.

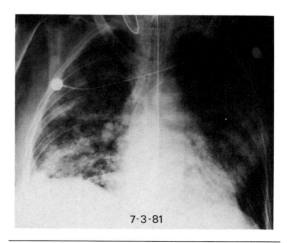

Opportunistic infections are the most common cause of morbidity and mortality in these patients. A clinically important point is that opportunistic infections of lungs are very uncommon in patients with hematologic malignancies who have no history of chemotherapy, radiation therapy, or malnutrition. Lymphangitic metastases from nonhematologic malignancies should be included in the differential diagnosis of lung infiltrates in this group.

Collagenoses and vasculitides are often associated with pulmonary manifestations [162,163]. Untreated rheumatologic entities such as rheumatoid arthritis, systemic lupus erythematosus, progressive systemic sclerosis or scleroderma, polymyositis-dermatomyositis, Sjögren's syndrome, mixed connective tissue disease, Wegener's granulomatosis, temporal arteritis, and Churg-Strauss vasculitis are well-known to produce pulmonary complications. Pulmonary manifestations of these disorders are discussed at length in Chapters 57 and 58. As in the case of malignancies, pulmonary opportunistic infections are uncommon in these patients unless they have received prolonged immunosuppressive therapy for their disease.

OPPORTUNISTIC PULMONARY INFECTIONS

Overwhelming pneumonias remain an important cause of morbidity and mortality. Many of these infections progress rapidly and are fatal. An immunocompromised patient is prone to develop pulmonary infections caused by viruses, bacteria, mycobacteria, fungi, protozoa, and parasites. In the setting of immunocompromise, the clinical manifestations of viral pneumonitis are variable. Fever may be impressive or absent. Cough and dyspnea are present in most patients, as are varying degrees of hypoxia and chest roentgenographic abnormalities. Cytomegalovirus and herpes zoster virus infections are seen in patients with a wide variety of underlying problems. Hematologic malignancies, corticosteroid therapy, and broad-spectrum antibiotics may predispose patients to primary varicella pneumonia. A study of 20 patients with herpes simplex pneumonia disclosed that 18 of the patients had hematologic malignancy [169].

Because most immunocompromised patients are hospitalized, hospital-acquired pneumonitis is a major threat to their lives. Infections caused by gram-positive, gram-negative, and anaerobic bacteria are common causes of infection in immunocompromised patients. The pathophysiology of respiratory tract colonization by bacteria in ill patients is unknown. Oropharyngeal colonization by gram-negative organisms is increased in patients with chronic alcoholism, chronic obstructive pulmonary disease, diabetes mellitus, congestive cardiac failure, immunologic diseases, bronchiectasis, azotemia, intubation, tracheostomy, and malnutrition, and in those on chronic antimicrobial therapy and corticosteroid therapy [147]. Carrier rates for aerobic gram-negative rods in pharyngeal secretions have been found to be higher for alcoholics and diabetics [107]. Patients with malignant disease are frequently at risk of developing a wide variety of infections as a result of their immunosuppressed state. *Moraxella catarrhalis*, a gram-negative bacterium, has emerged as an opportunistic organism. Nearly one-third of the cases of pneumonia and empyema caused by *M. catarrhalis* have occurred in patients with various immunologic abnormalities.

Fungal infections, particularly aspergillosis and candidiasis, are common in leukemic patients, in debilitated individuals, and in those receiving long-term antimicrobial therapy. Immunocompromised patients, especially those with severe and sustained granulocytopenia, have a high propensity to develop potentially fatal *Aspergillus* and *Candida* infections. *Candida* epiglottitis has been described in these patients either as a localized lesion or as a source of *Candida* bronchopneumonia [220]. Infection with *C. neoformans* may be seen in patients with Hodgkin's disease, those receiving corticosteroid therapy for sarcoidosis, and in patients with chronic pulmonary disease. *Aspergillus* exists commonly as a saprophyte. Invasive and disseminated aspergillosis, however, is almost always seen in patients with malignancy or severe immunosuppression [228]. Granulocytopenic and leukemic patients in relapse are also more susceptible. *N. asteroides* becomes an opportunistic invader in patients with chronic diseases, especially those receiving corticosteroid therapy [58].

P. carinii is a relatively common and well-recognized pulmonary pathogen in immunocompromised patients, especially those receiving immunosuppressive therapy, and in those with underlying diseases, including hematologic malignancies, solid tumors, organ transplants, and collagen-vascular diseases. The most common disease associated with *P. carinii* infection is AIDS. Coexisting pulmonary infection is a major negative prognostic factor in patients with *P. carinii* pneumonia [152]. *P. carinii* is the most common cause of interstitial pneumonia in immuno-suppressed patients [67].

PULMONARY CYTOTOXIC REACTIONS TO DRUGS

The lungs exhibit various reactions to a wide range of drugs, among which the chemotherapeutic agents employed in the treatment of neoplastic diseases are notable (see Chapter 30). Diagnosis of a pulmonary process becomes a formidable challenge when the patient is receiving such treatment. In addition to excluding the possibilities of extension into the lungs of the basic disease and the presence of an opportunistic infection, one has to rule out a drug-induced pulmonary response (Fig. 59-11).

Busulfan (Myleran), a chemotherapeutic agent used in the treatment of chronic granulocytic leukemia, is known to cause diffuse interstitial pulmonary fibrosis. Bleomycin, cyclophosphamide, methotrexate, and melphalan are some of the

Fig. 59-11. Cytotoxic pulmonary damage secondary to busulfan in the immunocompromised patient. (A) Chest roentgenogram shows diffuse alveolar-interstitial infiltrates. (B) Lung biopsy demonstrates inflammatory changes, fibrosis, and hypertrophy of alveolar lining cells following busulfan therapy.

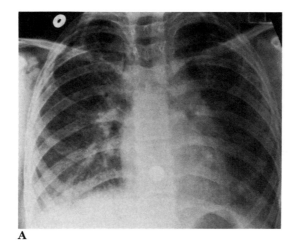

A

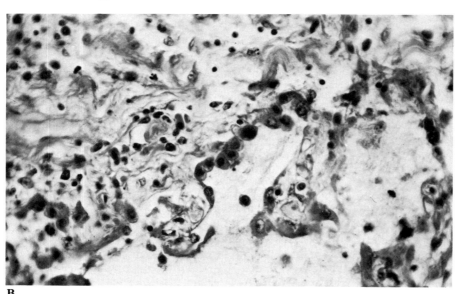

B

other drugs used to treat neoplastic diseases and implicated in the genesis of pulmonary fibrosis. Radiation-induced pneumonitis can confuse the issue, particularly in a patient with an intrathoracic neoplasm.

Systemic corticosteroid therapy is a well-known risk factor for the development of opportunistic infections. The predisposition to opportunistic infections is the result of panlymphopenia. As little as 2.5 mg prednisone given every 6 hours has the ability to depress the helper–suppressor T-cell ratio [74]. Corticosteroid-induced lymphopenia is maximal 4 to 6 hours after a single administration of the drug but disappears within 24 hours [23,96,218]. The decrease in the helper–suppressor T-cell ratio is due to a disproportionate decrease in the number of helper-inducer T cells [196]. B lymphocytes are less affected than the T cells [192]. Long-term administration of corticosteroids is likely to produce prolonged lymphopenia and thus to expose the patient to the risk of opportunistic infections.

Protein-calorie malnutrition adversely affects more or less all immunocompetent cells. It results in the impaired function of phagocytes and decreases both the quantity and quality of lymphocytes. Protein-calorie malnutrition is generally considered the most frequent cause of immunodepression [61].

NONSPECIFIC INTERSTITIAL PNEUMONITIS

Nonspecific pathologic changes are common in the lung tissue of immunocompromised patients with a diffuse pulmonary process (Fig. 59-12). In a study of 70 immunosuppressed patients with diffuse lung disease who underwent open-lung biopsy, the procedure provided diagnostic accuracy in 97 percent [178]. However, 45 percent of the diagnoses were nonspecific (fibrosis), and there was no significant difference in mortality between those with a specific diagnosis and those without, nor between those whose biopsy diagnosis caused an alteration of their therapy and those for whom it did not. In contrast, a study from Stanford noted a recovery rate of only 25 percent in those without a specific diagnosis following lung biopsy [69]. In patients in whom a treatable problem had been diagnosed, the overall recovery rate was 70 percent.

High-dose whole-body irradiation is commonly included in conditioning regimens for bone marrow transplantation for treatment of patients with hematologic malignancies. Interstitial pneumonitis is a major complication after bone marrow transplantation, and nearly one-fourth of all bone marrow transplant patients die from this

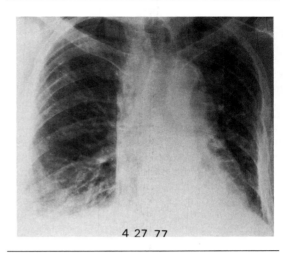

Fig. 59-12. Nonspecific interstitial pneumonitis in an immunocompromised patient who developed dyspnea and cough after thoracic radiation and multiple courses of chemotherapy for Hodgkin's lymphoma. Open-lung biopsy revealed nonspecific inflammation and fibrosis.

complication. In approximately half these patients, an infectious agent, particularly cytomegalovirus, is involved. Additional factors such as remission-induction chemotherapy, cyclophosphamide, methotrexate, cyclosporin A, and graft-versus-host disease combine to cause interstitial lung disease in these patients. Lymphocytic interstitial pneumonitis associated with bone marrow transplantation is considered in Chapter 61. Idiopathic interstitial pneumonitis in patients with AIDS was discussed earlier.

Occult pulmonary hemorrhage can occur in immunocompromised patients [40,83,202]. However, the clinical significance of this phenomenon is unclear as a small number (fewer than 5 percent) will have pulmonary hemorrhage as the sole pulmonary manifestation. An overall incidence of 27 percent has been reported in a series of 52 immunocompromised patients with pulmonary infiltrates [83]. A significant association exists between thrombocytopenia and *Aspergillus* infection and pulmonary hemorrhage. Close to 50 percent of patients with severe pulmonary hemorrhage may have documented aspergillosis.

LYMPHOCYTIC INTERSTITIAL PNEUMONITIS

The differential diagnosis of lymphocytic interstitial pneumonitis is discussed in Chapter 61. In the immunocompromised patient, the etiology for lymphocytic interstitial pneumonitis includes viral infections, AIDS (discussed earlier), graft-versus-host disease, and agammaglobulinemia. Because many of the diseases associated with lymphocytic interstitial pneumonitis involve lymphoma, immunocompromised patients with lymphocytic interstitial pneumonitis should be closely observed for the possibility of lymphoproliferative disease.

MALIGNANT PULMONARY NEOPLASIA ASSOCIATED WITH IMMUNODEFICIENCY

Non-Hodgkin's lymphomas occur with increasing frequency in immunocompromised patients as a result of iatrogenic immunosuppressive therapy in cardiac and renal transplantation [149,222]. Lymphomas in organ transplant recipients may be oligoclonal or polyclonal in origin [32] (Fig. 59-13) and may be related to the use of cyclosporin A [132]. In contrast, non-Hodgkin's lymphomas seen in AIDS are Burkitt-like lymphomas, B-cell lymphomas, or B-cell immunoblastic sarcoma, with or without plasmacytoid features [98,99, 231,232]. They tend frequently to be extranodal.

As a result of successful treatment with radiation, chemotherapy, or both, patients with lymphoma are living longer. Long-term follow-up of these patients has shown an increased incidence

Fig. 59-13. B-cell lymphoma developing in right upper lobe in a patient on chronic immunosuppressive therapy following renal transplantation.

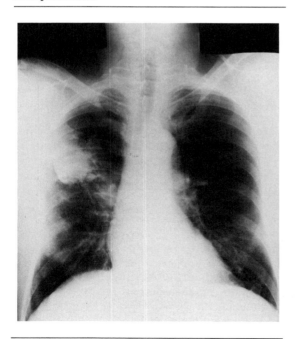

of lung carcinoma [89]. Patients treated for Hodgkin's and non-Hodgkin's lymphoma accrue a relative risk two to three times that of the normal population for developing newer malignancies [1]. Previous radiation therapy also may increase the risk of developing pulmonary nonlymphomatous malignancies.

Small-cell carcinoma is the predominant histologic type of lung cancer in both smoking and nonsmoking irradiated patients [104]. However, patients with Hodgkin's lymphoma who receive supradiaphragmatic irradiation or combined-modality therapy may be at higher risk for developing non-small-cell carcinoma of the lung. In a study of such patients, the risk ratio for the development of lung cancer among Hodgkin's lymphoma patients was 5.6 times that expected in the general population [104]. The median age at diagnosis of Hodgkin's lymphoma and lung carcinoma was 39 and 45 years, respectively. The interval between the diagnosis of Hodgkin's lymphoma and metachronous lung cancer averaged 7 years but appeared to vary inversely with age, thus emphasizing the need for close long-term observation [104].

NEW PULMONARY PROBLEM UNRELATED TO IMMUNODEFICIENCY

The immunocompromised patient is more susceptible to the medical processes that affect nonimmunocompromised subjects. An abnormal chest roentgenogram in an immunocompromised patient may represent cardiac or noncardiac pulmonary edema, pulmonary embolism, community-acquired pulmonary infections, aspiration pneumonitis, or the delayed effects of thoracic irradiation. More than one-third of immunocompromised patients will demonstrate a combination of two or more of these complications.

Diagnostic Approach to Pulmonary Problems in the Compromised Host

As outlined earlier, when one is confronted with a compromised host with an abnormal chest roentgenogram, various etiologic factors must be considered (see Tables 59-3 and 59-4). A detailed history and complete physical examination will provide important clues toward the diagnosis. Routine laboratory procedures—blood counts, cultures of blood and urine, and other analyses—when used appropriately, will provide additional help. The choice of diagnostic approach depends on the expertise available in one's own institution, the sensitivity of the procedure for the diagnosis of likely processes in the differential diagnoses, the severity of the patient's illness, and the rapidity with which the illness is progressing [191].

Chest roentgenograms are essential for characterizing the abnormalities present and for narrowing the spectrum of possible diagnoses. However, it should be stressed that the typical roentgenographic features produced by isolated disease entities may not manifest their classic form in the case of a compromised host because of the effect of various factors on the lung, including opportunistic infections, cytotoxic changes, and radiation pneumonitis. Additional roentgenographic procedures such as lateral decubitus films and computed tomography may aid in making the diagnosis.

Assessing the degree of clinical urgency is of great importance in these patients, for in the absence of a specific diagnosis and proper therapy, many follow a rapid downhill course. The selection and prompt application of an appropriate investigative procedure will aid in reaching the proper decisions and instituting the correct therapeutic regimen. When routine blood tests, cultures from extrapulmonary sources, and biopsies fail to yield a specific answer, the course of diagnostic procedures is shown in Fig. 59-14.

Fig. 59-14. Diagnostic approach to the immunocompromised patient with an abnormal chest roentgenogram. *Empiric therapy should be individualized and may include antiviral, antibacterial, and antifungal drugs and trimethoprim-sulfamethoxazole against *Pneumocystis carinii.* It may also include systemic corticosteroids, discontinuation of cytotoxic drugs, and therapy for pulmonary edema. †Cultures should be individualized depending on the clinical situation and chest roentgenographic abnormalities, but may include blood and other easily obtainable body fluids and secretions and bone marrow, as well as bronchoalveolar lavage and transbronchial lung biopsy.

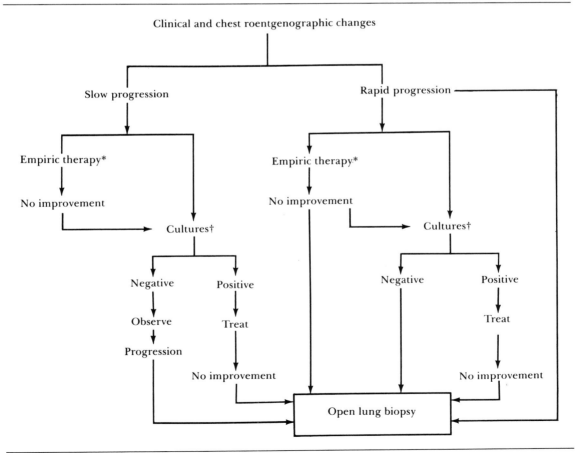

When the battery of routine tests is exhausted without providing a clue to the etiology of the pulmonary process, consideration should be given to direct examination of material from the lungs. Possibilities include (1) study of easily obtainable secretions and fluid (sputum, gastric washings, and pleural fluid), (2) transtracheal aspiration, (3) percutaneous (transthoracic) needle aspiration and needle biopsy of pleura and lung, (4) bronchoscopic brushing and aspirations or transbronchoscopic lung biopsy, (5) diagnostic bronchoalveolar lavage, (6) thoracoscopic biopsy of pleura and lung, and (7) thoracotomy and open biopsy of pleura and lung.

As emphasized earlier, the degree of diagnostic urgency and the appropriateness of a given procedure should be weighed against the potential effect of delay on the subsequent outcome. The procedures just listed have varying yields and complication rates. The following is a brief summary of these aspects.

STUDY OF EASILY OBTAINABLE SECRETIONS AND FLUIDS

Sputum cultures usually are of limited value in diagnosing bacterial infections in the immunosuppressed host. However, induced sputum is valuable in the detection of *P. carinii.* Overwhelming growth of saprophytic fungi in the oropharyngeal regions of these patients is a hindrance in isolating true pathogenic bacteria and fungi. Sputum examination is valuable in diagnosing mycobacterial infections and bronchogenic carcinoma. Gastric washings are helpful in the diagnosis of tuberculosis and certain fungal infections. Pleural fluid culture is very useful in diagnosing bacterial infections and malignancies. Minor pneumothoraces occur in fewer than 5 percent of thoracenteses and in fewer than 10 percent of pleural biopsies [164].

The role of transtracheal aspiration and transthoracic (percutaneous) needle aspiration and biopsy are discussed in Chapter 13.

BRONCHOSCOPY, BRONCHOALVEOLAR LAVAGE, AND TRANSBRONCHOSCOPIC LUNG BIOPSY

Fiberoptic bronchoscopy has become the procedure of choice for diagnosing opportunistic infections in patients with AIDS and in other immunocompromised patients. It is probably the safest of the invasive pulmonary diagnostic procedures. In several large series, the incidence of major complications has been reported to be less than 1 percent [6]. Both diagnostic bronchoalveolar lavage and transbronchial lung biopsy should be

considered, since the yield from these two procedures is complementary. Brush biopsy is least helpful. If the initial bronchoscopy is nondiagnostic and the patient's clinical condition is deteriorating, repeat bronchoscopy or open-lung biopsy should be considered [131]. Bronchoscopic brushings and biopsies (without bronchoalveolar lavage) have an accuracy rate of 60 to 75 percent in the diagnosis of *P. carinii*, bronchogenic carcinoma, and mycoses.

A higher diagnostic yield from bronchoscopy, particularly bronchoalveolar lavage, can be expected in immunocompromised patients [82,154]. Bilateral bronchoalveolar lavage has been shown to increase the diagnostic yield significantly in patients with opportunistic pulmonary infections [116]. An overall diagnostic yield from bronchoalveolar lavage and transbronchial lung biopsy in the diagnosis of *P. carinii* in immunocompromised hosts is 82 and 92 percent, respectively [142,200,202]. Cytomegalovirus can frequently be diagnosed from examination and culture of the diagnostic bronchoalveolar lavage fluid. Recovery of *M. avium-intracellulare* is highest with culture of both washings and lavage [200]. Bronchoalveolar lavage in patients with leukemia and pulmonary infiltrates is not helpful in diagnosing invasive aspergillosis, and it may not alter therapeutic options in a significant number of these patients.

Bronchoscopic examination is usually a nonsterile procedure, but use of a double-catheter brush system with telescoping cannulas and a distal occluding plug in the outer catheter can provide culture specimens uncontaminated by upper-airway organisms [10,209]. Relatively pure cultures of the lower respiratory tract can be obtained by this method [227]. Gram stain preparations from the bronchoscopic specimens correlate well with clinical assessment [54]. The indications for using this technique are similar to those for transtracheal aspiration. Bronchoscopy is a safe procedure in immunocompromised patients with respiratory distress and hypoxemia [143]. With supplemental oxygenation and appropriate preparation, the procedure can be performed even in patients with severe hypoxemia [219].

THORACOSCOPIC (PLEUROSCOPIC) BIOPSY

Thoracoscopy, which allows biopsy of pleura or lung under direct vision, is an excellent way to obtain material for culture as well as for histologic analysis, and it is gaining popularity. Rodgers and coworkers [175] have reported the results of thoracoscopic biopsy in 24 children, all of whom had underlying hematologic or neurologic malignancies and who had been receiving chemotherapy; one had Wilms' tumor, one had systemic lupus erythematosus, and one had received a renal transplant. *P. carinii* was identified in 18 patients, cytomegalovirus in 1, and fibrosis in 6. Complications included four pneumothoraces, two prolonged air leaks, and two instances of bleeding.

THORACOTOMY AND BIOPSY

Open-lung biopsy is the most effective, but also the most invasive, pulmonary diagnostic procedure available to detect the origin of the pulmonary process in a compromised host. This procedure yields the diagnosis in 90 to 95 percent of patients, and its mortality does not exceed that of needle biopsy *if* seriously ill patients are excluded [204]. It has demonstrated the presence of *P. carinii* in 97 percent of transplant recipients studied, whereas needle aspiration biopsy and transtracheal aspirates revealed *P. carinii* in 66 and 11 percent, respectively [171]. Open-lung biopsy provided a diagnostic accuracy of 100 percent in a study of 47 patients with lymphomas and leukemias who were receiving chemotherapy [150]. A retrospective study of 64 consecutive immunocompromised patients undergoing open-lung biopsy during a 5-year period noted that the procedure rarely missed a specific, treatable cause, if present [114]. However, the results from open-lung biopsy infrequently led to a change in the treatment that improved the patient's clinical course. With increasing use of bronchoalveolar lavage and thoracoscopy, the number of open-lung biopsies has been significantly reduced.

References

1. Abernathy D, Beltran G, Stuckey WJ. Lung cancer following treatment of lymphoma. *Am J Med* 81:215, 1986.
2. Allen JN, Wewers MD. HIV-associated bronchiolitis obliterans organizing pneumonitis. *Chest* 96:197, 1989.
3. Ambrosino DM, et al. An immunodeficiency characterized by impaired antibody responses to polysaccharides. *N Engl J Med* 316:790, 1987.
4. Ammann AJ, Hong R. Selective IgA deficiency: Presentation of 30 cases and a review of the literature. *Medicine* 50:223, 1971.
5. Ampel NM, Wing EJ. *Legionella* infection in transplant patients. *Semin Respir Infect* 5:30, 1990.
6. Andersen HA. Transbronchoscopic lung biopsy for diffuse pulmonary diseases: Result in 939 patients. *Chest* 73(Suppl):734, 1978.
7. Anderson DJ, Jordan MC. Viral pneumonia in recipients of solid organ transplants. *Semin Respir Infect* 5:38, 1990.
8. Barrett AJ, et al. Cyclosporin A as prophylaxis against graft-versus-host disease in 36 patients. *Br Med J* 285:162, 1982.
9. Barrio JL, et al. Value of repeat fiberoptic bronchoscopies and significance of nondiagnostic bronchoscopic results in patients with the acquired immunodeficiency syndrome. *Am Rev Respir Dis* 135:422, 1987.
10. Bartlett JG. Diagnosis of bacterial infections of the lung. *Clin Chest Med* 8:119, 1987.
11. Beard LJ, et al. Early bone marrow transplantation in an infant with Wiskott-Aldrich syndrome. *Am J Pediatr Hematol Oncol* 13:310, 1991.
12. Beck CS, Heiner DC. Selective immunoglobulin G4 deficiency and recurrent infections of the respiratory tract. *Am Rev Respir Dis* 124:94, 1981.
13. Bedrossian CWM, et al. Azathioprine-associated interstitial pneumonitis. *Am J Pathol* 82:148, 1984.
14. Beer MF, Sohn M, Swartz M. Recurrent pneumothorax in AIDS patients with *Pneumocystis carinii*. A clinicopathologic report of three cases and review of the literature. *Chest* 98:266, 1990.
15. Berger M, Gilbert I. Role of gamma globulin. *Semin Respir Infect* 4:272, 1989.
16. Bigby TD, et al. The usefulness of induced sputum in the diagnosis of *Pneumocystis carinii* pneumonia in patients with the acquired immunodeficiency syndrome. *Am Rev Respir Dis* 133:515, 1986.
17. Bjorkander JF, et al. Impaired lung function in patients with IgA deficiency and low levels of IgG2 or IgG3. *N Engl J Med* 313:720, 1985.
18. Boder E, Sedgwick RP. Ataxia-telangiectasia: A familial syndrome of progressive cerebellar ataxia, oculocutaneous telangiectasia, and frequent pulmonary infections. *Pediatrics* 21:526, 1958.
19. Bogner JR, et al. Chylothorax as fatal complication in fulminating Kaposi's sarcoma in a patient with AIDS. *Klin Wochenschr* 69:134, 1991.
20. Braun MA, et al. Lung cancer in patients seropositive for human immunodeficiency virus. *Radiology* 175:341, 1990.
21. Brunkwall J, et al. Postoperative deep venous thrombosis after renal transplantation. *Transplantation* 43:647, 1987.
22. Bruton OC. Agammaglobulinemia. *Pediatrics* 9:722, 1952.
23. Burke CM, et al. Lung immunogenicity, rejection, and obliterative bronchiolitis. *Chest* 92:547, 1987.

24. Calvo M, et al. Secretory IgA deficiency in pediatric patients: Clinical and laboratory follow-up. *Allergol Immunopathol (Madr)* 18:149, 1990.

25. Carmichael DJS, et al. Interstitial pneumonitis secondary to azathioprine in a renal transplant patient. *Thorax* 38:951, 1983.

26. Carson PJ, Goldsmith JC. Atypical pulmonary diseases associated with AIDS. *Chest* 100:675, 1991.

27. Castillo M, et al. HIV-associated lymphocytic interstitial pneumonia: Radiologic manifestations and pathologic correlation. *Radiology* 170:83, 1989.

28. Centers for Disease Control. Revision of the CDC surveillance case definition for acquired immunodeficiency syndrome. *MMWR* 36(Suppl.): 3S, 1987.

29. Chadwick EG, et al. Tumors of smooth-muscle origin in HIV-infected children. *JAMA* 263:3182, 1990.

30. Chapman SW, Wilson JP. Nocardiosis in transplant recipients. *Semin Respir Infect* 5:74, 1990.

31. Chattha G, et al. Lactic acidosis complicating the acquired immunodeficiency syndrome. *Ann Intern Med* 118:37, 1993.

32. Cleary ML, Sklar J. Lymphoproliferative disorders in cardiac transplant recipients are multifocal lymphomas. *Lancet* 2:489, 1984.

33. Cooper MD, et al. Wiskott-Aldrich syndrome: An immunologic deficiency disease involving the afferent limb of immunity. *Am J Med* 44:499, 1968.

34. Daar ES, et al. Transient high levels of viremia in patients with primary human immunodeficiency virus type 1 infection. *N Engl J Med* 324:961, 1991.

35. Daumling S, et al. The Buckley syndrome: Recurring, severe staphylococcal infections, eczema and hyperimmunoglobulinemia E. *Infection* 8:248, 1980.

36. Davis SD, et al. Intrathoracic Kaposi's sarcoma in AIDS patients: Radiographic-pathologic correlation. *Radiology* 163:495, 1987.

37. Diamond LA, Lorber B. *Branhamella catarrhalis* pneumonia and immunoglobulin abnormalities: A new association. *Am Rev Respir Dis* 129:876, 1984.

38. Diaz PT, Clanton TL, Pacht ER. Emphysema-like pulmonary disease associated with human immunodeficiency virus infection. *Ann Intern Med* 116:124, 1992.

39. Di Carlo EF, et al. Malignant lymphomas and the acquired immunodeficiency syndrome. *Arch Pathol Lab Med* 110:1012, 1986.

40. Drew WL, Finley TN, Golde DW. Diagnostic lavage and occult pulmonary hemorrhage in thrombocytopenic immune-compromised patients. *Am Rev Respir Dis* 116:215, 1977.

41. Drummer JS, et al. Early infections in kidney, heart, and liver transplant recipients on cyclosporine. *Transplantation* 36:259, 1983.

42. Dummer JS. *Pneumocystis carinii* infections in transplant recipients. *Semin Respir Infect* 5:50, 1990.

43. Ehtessabian R, et al. Common variable immunodeficiency with pernicious anemia, asthma, and reactions to gamma globulin: Treatment with plasma. *J Allergy Clin Immunol* 58:337, 1976.

44. el-Fouly MH, et al. DiGeorge anomaly in an infant with deletion of chromosome 22 and dup(9p) due to adjacent type II disjunction. *Am J Med Genet* 38:569, 1991.

45. Ersoy F, et al. Twenty-year follow-up of 160 patients with ataxia-telangiectasia. *Turk J Pediatr* 33:205, 1991.

46. Ettinger NA, Trulock EP. Pulmonary considerations of organ transplantation (part 1). *Am Rev Respir Dis* 143:1386, 1990.

47. Ettinger NA, Trulock EP. Pulmonary considerations of organ transplantation (part 3). *Am Rev Respir Dis* 144:433, 1991.

48. Fein AM, et al. COPD and endobronchial polyposis associated with hypogammaglobulinemia: Are proteolytic enzymes involved? *Chest* 82:127, 1982.

49. Fick RB, et al. Immunoglobulin-G subclasses in cystic fibrosis: IgG2 response to *Pseudomonas* polysaccharide. *Am Rev Respir Dis* 133:418, 1986.

50. Fiorilli M, et al. Hypogammaglobulinemia with hyper-IgM, severe T-cell defect, and abnormal recirculation of OKT4 lymphocytes in a girl with chronic lymphadenopathy. *Clin Immunol Immunopathol* 38:256, 1986.

51. Fischl MA, et al. The efficacy of azidothymidine (AZT) in the treatment of patients with AIDS and AIDS-related complex. *N Engl J Med* 317: 185, 1987.

52. Fitch SJ, et al. Hyperimmunoglobulinemia E syndrome: Pulmonary imaging considerations. *Pediatr Radiol* 16:285, 1986.

53. Fitzgerald W, et al. The role of open lung biopsy in patients with the acquired immunodeficiency syndrome. *Chest* 91:659, 1987.

54. Flatauer FE, Chabalko JJ, Wolinsky E. Fiberoptic bronchoscopy in bacteriologic assessment of lower respiratory tract secretions: Importance of microscopic examination. *JAMA* 244:2427, 1980.

55. Floris C, et al. Pneumothorax in pleuropulmonary Kaposi's sarcoma related to acquired immunodeficiency syndrome. *Am J Med* 87:123, 1989.

56. Food and Drug Administration. Special AIDS issue. *FDA Drug Bull* 17:14, 1987.

57. Fouret PJ, et al. Pulmonary Kaposi's sarcoma in

patients with acquired immunodeficiency syndrome: A clinicopathologic study. *Thorax* 42: 262, 1987.

58. Frazier AR, Rosenow EC III, Roberts GD. Norcardiosis: A review of 25 cases occurring during 24 months. *Mayo Clin Proc* 50:657, 1975.

59. French PD, et al. Low carbon monoxide transfer factor (T_LCO) in HIV-infected patients without lung disease. *Thorax* 86:253, 1992.

60. Garay SM, et al. Pulmonary manifestations of Kaposi's sarcoma. *Chest* 91:39, 1987.

61. Garre MA, Boles JM, Youinou PY. Current concepts in immune derangement due to undernutrition. *JPEN J Parenter Ent Nutr* 11:309, 1987.

62. Gearhart MO, Bhutani MS. Intravenous pentamidine-induced bronchospasm. *Chest* 102: 1891, 1992.

63. Gill PS, et al. Azidothymidine associated with bone marrow failure in the acquired immunodeficiency syndrome (AIDS). *Ann Intern Med* 107:502, 1987.

64. Glanville AR, et al. Obliterative bronchiolitis after heart-lung transplantation: Apparent arrest by augmented immunosuppression. *Ann Intern Med* 107:300, 1987.

65. Goedert JJ, et al. Three-year incidence of AIDS in five cohorts of HTLV-III-infected risk group members. *Science* 231:992, 1986.

66. Gold JE, et al. Angiocentric immunoproliferative lesion/T-cell non-Hodgkin's lymphoma and the acquired immune deficiency syndrome: A case report and review of the literature. *Cancer* 66:2407, 1990.

67. Goodell B, et al. *Pneumocystis carinii:* The spectrum of diffuse interstitial pneumonia in patients with neoplastic diseases. *Ann Intern Med* 72:337, 1970.

68. Gosseye S, Nezelof C. T system immunodeficiencies in infancy and childhood. *Pathol Res Pract* 171:142, 1981.

69. Greenman RL, Goodall PT, King D. Lung biopsy in immunocompromised hosts. *Am J Med* 59: 488, 1975.

70. Grieco MH, Chinoy-Acharya P. Lymphocytic interstitial pneumonia associated with the AIDS. *Am Rev Respir Dis* 131:952, 1985.

71. Guillon JM, et al. HIV-related lymphocytic alveolitis. *Chest* 94:1264, 1988.

72. Hanson PJV, et al. Fiberoptic bronchoscopy in diagnosis of bronchopulmonary Kaposi's sarcoma. *Thorax* 42:269, 1987.

73. Hecht F, Hecht BK. Cancer in ataxia-telangiectasia patients. *Cancer Genet Cytogenet* 46:9, 1990.

74. Hepburn B, Slade JD. Effect of divided daily dose prednisone therapy on circulating T-cell subsets. *J Rheumatol* 14:19, 1987.

75. Herer B, et al. Selective IgG subclass deficiencies and antibody responses to pneumococcal capsular polysaccharide antigen in adult community-acquired pneumonia. *Am Rev Respir Dis* 142:854, 1990.

76. Hessol NA, et al. Increased incidence of Hodgkin's disease in homosexual men with HIV infection. *Ann Intern Med* 117:309, 1992.

77. Hughes-Davies L, et al. Occult alveolar haemorrhage in bronchopulmonary Kaposi's sarcoma. *J Clin Pathol* 45:536, 1992.

78. Ilowite NT, et al. Pulmonary angiitis with atypical lymphoreticular infiltrates in Wiskott-Aldrich syndrome: Possible relationship of lymphomatoid granulomatosis and EBV infection. *Clin Immunol Immunopathol* 41:479, 1986.

79. Israel RH, Magnussen CR. Are AIDS patients at risk for pulmonary alveolar proteinosis? *Chest* 96:641, 1989.

80. Jacob CN, Henein S, Hill AR. AIDS-related *Pneumocystis* pneumonia complicated by diffuse pneumatocele formation. *NY State J Med* 92:20, 1992.

81. Johnson JE, et al. Exercise dysfunction in patients seropositive for the human immunodeficiency virus. *Am Rev Respir Dis* 141:618, 1990.

82. Johnson PC, Hogg KM, Sarosi GA. The rapid diagnosis of pulmonary infections in solid organ transplant recipients. *Semin Respir Infect* 5:2, 1990.

83. Kahn FW, Jones JM, England DW. Diagnosis of pulmonary hemorrhage in the immune-compromised host. *Am Rev Respir Dis* 136:155, 1987.

84. Kahn JO, Northfelt DW, Miles SA. AIDS-associated Kaposi's sarcoma. *AIDS Clin Rev* 2:261, 1992.

85. Kaslow RA, et al. Infection with the human immunodeficiency virus: Clinical manifestations and their relationship to immune deficiency. *Ann Intern Med* 107:474, 1987.

86. Katz AS, Niesenbaum L, Mass B. Pleural effusion as the initial manifestation of disseminated cryptococcosis in acquired immune deficiency syndrome. Diagnosis by pleural biopsy. *Chest* 96:440, 1989.

87. Kaufman J, Komorowski R. Bronchiolitis obliterans organizing pneumonia in common variable immunodeficiency syndrome. *Chest* 100: 552, 1991.

88. Klaustermeyer WB, et al. IgG subclass deficiency associated corticosteroids in obstructive lung disease. *Chest* 102:1137, 1992.

89. Konits PH, et al. Lung cancer as a complication of prolonged survival in patients with lymphoma. *Med Pediatr Oncol* 10:331, 1982.

90. Kovacs JA, et al. Diagnosis of *Pneumocystis carinii* pneumonia: improved detection in sputum with use of monoclonal antibodies. *N Engl J Med* 318:589, 1988.

91. Kramer MR, et al. High titers of Epstein-Barr virus antibodies in adult patients with lympho-

cytic interstitial pneumonitis associated with AIDS. *Respir Med* 86:49, 1992.

92. Kretschmer R, et al. Congenital aplasia of the thymus gland (DiGeorge's syndrome). *N Engl J Med* 279:1295, 1968.

93. Krowka MJ, Breuer RI, Kehoe TJ. Azathioprine-induced pulmonary dysfunction. *Chest* 83:696, 1983.

94. Krowka MJ, Cortese DA. Pulmonary aspects of chronic liver disease and liver transplantation. *Mayo Clin Proc* 60:407, 1985.

95. Kuhlman JE, et al. Premature bullous pulmonary damage in AIDS: CT diagnosis. *Radiology* 173:23, 1989.

96. Kuriyama K, et al. Reduced helper (OKT4+): suppressor (OKT8+) T-cell ratios in aplastic anaemia: Relation to immunosuppressive therapy. *Br J Haematol* 57:329, 1984.

97. Lederman HM, Winkelstein JA. X-linked agammaglobulinemia: An analysis of 96 patients. *Medicine* 64:145, 1985.

98. Levine AM, et al. Retrovirus and malignant lymphoma in homosexual men. *JAMA* 254:1921, 1985.

99. Levine AM, et al. Development of B-cell lymphoma in homosexual men: Clinical and immunological findings. *Ann Intern Med* 100:7, 1984.

100. L'Huillier JP, et al. The hyperimmunoglobulinaemia E and recurrent infections in an adult. *Thorax* 45:707, 1990.

101. Libanore M, et al. Pneumothorax during pulmonary toxoplasmosis in an AIDS patient (letter). *Chest* 100:1184, 1991.

102. Liese JG, et al. High- vs low-dose immunoglobulin therapy in the long-term treatment of X-linked agammaglobulinemia. *Am J Dis Child* 146:335, 1992.

103. Linnemann CC Jr, et al. Recovery of human immunodeficiency virus and detection of p24 antigen in bronchoalveolar lavage fluid from adult patients with AIDS. *Chest* 96:64, 1989.

104. List AF, Doll DC, Greco FA. Lung cancer in Hodgkin's disease: Association with previous radiotherapy. *J Clin Oncol* 3:215, 1985.

105. Longworth DL, et al. Lymphocytic alveolitis in primary HIV infection. *Cleve Clin J Med* 57:379, 1990.

106. Lund VJ, Scadding GK. Immunologic aspects of chronic sinusitis. *J Otolaryngol* 20:379, 1991.

107. Mackowiak PA, Martin RM, Smith JW. The role of bacterial interference in the increased prevalence of oropharyngeal gram-negative bacilli among alcoholics and diabetics. *Am Rev Respir Dis* 120:589, 1979.

108. Mann JM, et al. Nonbronchoscopic lung lavage for diagnosis of opportunistic infection in AIDS. *Chest* 91:319, 1987.

109. Marchevsky A, et al. Pulmonary complications of the acquired immunodeficiency syndrome: A clinicopathologic study of 70 cases. *Hum Pathol* 16:659, 1985.

110. Marshall BC, et al. Histoplasmosis as a cause of pleural effusion in the acquired immunodeficiency syndrome. *Am J Med Sci* 300:98, 1990.

111. Marzo KP, Wilson JR, Mancini DM. Effects of cardiac transplantation on ventilatory response to exercise. *Am J Cardiol* 69:547, 1992.

112. Mayer KH, et al. Human T-lymphotropic virus type III in high-risk, antibody-negative homosexual men. *Ann Intern Med* 104:194, 1986.

113. McCarthy PM, et al. Improved survival after heart-lung transplantation. *J Thorac Cardiovasc Surg* 99:54, 1990.

114. McKenna RJ Jr, Mountain CF, McMurtrey MJ. Open lung biopsy in immunocompromised patients. *Chest* 86:671, 1984.

115. McKenzie R, et al. The causes of death in patients with human immunodeficiency virus infection: A clinical and pathologic study with emphasis on the role of pulmonary diseases. *Medicine* 70:326, 1991.

116. Meduri GU, et al. Bilateral bronchoalveolar lavage in the diagnosis of opportunistic pulmonary infections. *Chest* 100:1272, 1991.

117. Mendini GV, et al. Pulmonary sarcoma in the acquired immunodeficiency syndrome: Pathological and clinical manifestations. *Am Rev Respir Dis* 131:A75, 1985.

118. Mermel LA, Maki DG. Bacterial pneumonia in solid organ transplantation. *Semin Respir Infect* 5:10, 1990.

119. Metersky ML, Harrell JH II, Moser KM. Lack of utility of bronchial brush biopsy in patients infected with the human immunodeficiency virus. *Chest* 101:680, 1992.

120. Mette SA, et al. Primary pulmonary hypertension in association with human immunodeficiency virus infection. A possible viral etiology for some forms of hypertensive pulmonary arteriopathy. *Am Rev Respir Dis* 145:1196, 1992.

121. Millar AB, Mitchell DM. Non-invasive investigation of pulmonary disease in patients positive for the human immunodeficiency virus. *Thorax* 45:57, 1990.

122. Miller RF, et al. Tests giving an aetiological diagnosis in pulmonary disease in patients infected with the human immunodeficiency virus. *Thorax* 45:62, 1990.

123. Miller RF, et al. Bronchopulmonary Kaposi's sarcoma in patients with AIDS. *Thorax* 47:721, 1992.

124. Miro AM, et al. The role of fiberoptic bronchoscopy for diagnosis of pulmonary tuberculosis in patients at risk for AIDS. *Chest* 101:1211, 1992.

125. Mitchell DM, et al. Pulmonary function in human immunodeficiency virus infection. A prospective 18-month study of serial lung function in 474 patients. *Am Rev Respir Dis* 146:745, 1992.

126. Mitchell DM, et al. Bronchopulmonary Kaposi's sarcoma in patients with AIDS. *Thorax* 47:726, 1992.
127. Mitchell DM, Miller RF. Recent developments in the management of the pulmonary complications of HIV disease. *Thorax* 47:381, 1992.
128. Mitsuya H, Broder S. Strategies for antiviral therapy in AIDS. *Nature* 325:773, 1987.
129. Morris JC, et al. Lymphocytic interstitial pneumonia in patients at risk for the acquired immunodeficiency syndrome. *Chest* 91:63, 1987.
130. Moss RB, Carmack MA, Esrig S. Deficiency of IgG4 in children: Association of isolated IgG4 deficiency with recurrent respiratory tract infection. *J Pediatr* 120:16, 1992.
131. Murray JF, et al. NHLBI workshop summary: Pulmonary complications of the acquired immunodeficiency syndrome. An update. Report of the second National Heart, Lung and Blood Institute workshop. *Am Rev Respir Dis* 135:504, 1987.
132. Nagington J, Gray J. Cyclosporin A immunosuppression, Epstein-Barr antibody and lymphoma. *Lancet* 1:536, 1980.
133. Naidich DP, et al. Kaposi's sarcoma. CT-radiographic correlation. *Chest* 96:723, 1989.
134. Nash G. Pathologic features of the lung in the immune-compromised host. *Hum Pathol* 13:841, 1977.
135. Nash G, Fligiel S. Kaposi's sarcoma presenting as pulmonary disease in the acquired immunodeficiency syndrome: Diagnosis by lung biopsy. *Hum Pathol* 15:999, 1984.
136. Nobler P. Pulmonary irradiation for Kaposi's sarcoma in AIDS. *Am J Clin Oncol* 8:441, 1985.
137. Novis BH, et al. Plasma cell infiltration of the small intestine, recurrent pulmonary infections, and cellular immunodeficiency (Nezelof's syndrome). *Am J Gastroenterol* 80:891, 1985.
138. O'Brien RF, Cohn DL. Serosanguineous pleural effusions in AIDS-associated Kaposi's sarcoma. *Chest* 96:460, 1989.
139. Ochs HD, Wedgwood RJ. IgG subclass deficiencies. *Annu Rev Med* 38:325, 1987.
140. O'Donnell CR, et al. Abnormal airway function in individuals with the acquired immunodeficiency syndrome. *Chest* 94:945, 1988.
141. Ognibene FP, Shelhamer JH. Kaposi's sarcoma. *Clin Chest Med* 9:459, 1988.
142. Ognibene FP, Shelhamer J, Gill V. The diagnosis of *Pneumocystis carinii* pneumonia in patients with the acquired immune deficiency syndrome using subsegmental bronchoalveolar lavage. *Am Rev Respir Dis* 129:929, 1984.
143. Olapade CS, Prakash UBS. Bronchoscopy in the Critical Care Unit. *Mayo Clin Proc* 64:1255, 1989.
144. Oleske J, et al. Immunodeficiency syndrome in children. *JAMA* 249:2345, 1983.
145. Oxelius VA, Berkel AI, Hanson LA. IgG2 deficiency in ataxia-telangiectasia. *N Engl J Med* 306:515, 1982.
146. Oxelius VA, et al. IgG subclasses in selective IgA deficiency: Importance of IgG2-IgA deficiency. *N Engl J Med* 304:1476, 1981.
147. Palmer LB. Bacterial colonization: Pathogenesis and clinical significance. *Clin Chest Med* 8:455, 1987.
148. Penn I. Lymphomas complicating organ transplantation. *Transplant Proc* 15:2790, 1983.
149. Penn I. Risk of lymphoma after cytotoxic therapy after transplantation. *Lancet* 2:1385, 1978.
150. Pennington JE, Feldman NT. Pulmonary infiltrates in patients with hematologic malignancy: Assessment of transbronchial biopsy. *Am J Med* 62:581, 1977.
151. Perronne C, et al. Should pulmonary tuberculosis be an AIDS-defining diagnosis in patients infected with HIV? *Tuberc Lung Dis* 73:39, 1992.
152. Peters SG, Prakash UBS. *Pneumocystis carinii* pneumonia: Review of 53 cases. *Am J Med* 82:73, 1987.
153. Pinilla J, Hill AR. Thromboembolism associated acquired immunodeficiency syndrome. *Chest* 102:1634, 1992.
154. Pisani RJ, Wright AJ. Clinical utility of bronchoalveolar lavage in immunocompromised hosts. *Mayo Clin Proc* 67:221, 1992.
155. Pitchenik AE, Fischl MA, Saldana MJ. Kaposi's sarcoma of the tracheobronchial tree. *Chest* 87:122, 1985.
156. Pitchenik AE, et al. Sputum examination for the diagnosis of *Pneumocystis carinii* pneumonia in the acquired immunodeficiency syndrome. *Am Rev Respir Dis* 133:226, 1986.
157. Plebani A, Duse M, Monafo V. Recurrent infections with IgG2 deficiency. *Arch Dis Child* 60:670, 1985.
158. Polish LB, et al. Pulmonary non-Hodgkin's lymphoma in AIDS. *Chest* 96:1321, 1989.
159. Polos PG, et al. Pulmonary hypertension and human immunodeficiency virus infection. Two reports and a review of the literature. *Chest* 101:474, 1992.
160. Powell-Jackson PR, et al. Acute respiratory distress syndrome and convulsions associated with administration of cyclosporine in liver transplant recipients. *Transplantation* 38:341, 1984.
161. Pozniak AL, et al. Pulmonary Kaposi's sarcoma in Africa. *Thorax* 47:730, 1992.
162. Prakash UBS. Rheumatological diseases. *Lung Biol Health Dis* 50:385, 1992.
163. Prakash UBS. Vasculitides. *Lung Biol Health Dis* 50:431, 1992.
164. Prakash UBS, Dines DE. Thoracentesis, pleural biopsy, and pleuroscopy. *Semin Respir Med* 3:42, 1981.
165. Prakash UBS, Divertie MB, Banks PM. Aggressive therapy in acute respiratory failure from

leukemic pulmonary infiltrates. *Chest* 75:345, 1979.

166. Prakash UBS, et al. Pulmonary alveolar phospholipoproteinosis: Experience with 34 cases and a review. *Mayo Clin Proc* 62:499, 1987.

167. Priest ER, Weiss R. Chylothorax with Kaposi's sarcoma (letter). *South Med J* 84:806, 1991.

168. Quieffin J, et al. Aerosol pentamidine-induced bronchoconstriction. *Chest* 100:624, 1991.

169. Ramsey PG, et al. Herpes simplex pneumonia: Clinical, viral, and pathologic features in 20 patients. *Ann Intern Med* 97:813, 1982.

170. Ramsey PG, et al. The renal transplant patient with fever and pulmonary infiltrates: Etiology, clinical manifestation, and management. *Medicine* 59:206, 1980.

171. Remington JS, Anderson SE Jr. Diagnosis and treatment of pneumocystosis and toxoplasmosis in the immunosuppressed host. *Transplant Proc* 5:1263, 1973.

172. Renzi PM, et al. Bilateral pneumothoraces hasten mortality in AIDS patients receiving secondary prophylaxis with aerosolized pentamidine. Association with a lower DcO prior to receiving aerosolized pentamidine. *Chest* 102:491, 1992.

173. Reynolds MM, et al. Large pericardial effusions in the acquired immunodeficiency syndrome. *Chest* 102:1746, 1992.

174. Richman DD, et al. The toxicity of azidothymidine (AZT) in the treatment of patients with AIDS and AIDS-related complex. *N Engl J Med* 317:192, 1987.

175. Rodgers BM, Moazam F, Talbert JL. Thoracoscopy: Early diagnosis of interstitial pneumonitis in the immunologically suppressed child. *Chest* 75:126, 1979.

176. Rosenow EC, III. The spectrum of drug-induced pulmonary disease. *Ann Intern Med* 77:977, 1972.

177. Rosenow EC III, Wilson WR, Cockerill FR III. Pulmonary disease in the immunocompromised host (part 1). *Mayo Clin Proc* 60:473, 1985.

178. Rossiter SJ, et al. Open lung biopsy in the immunosuppressed patient: Is it really beneficial? *J Thorac Cardiovasc Surg* 77:338, 1979.

179. Roy TM, Dow FT, Puthuff DL. Upper airway obstruction from AIDS-related Kaposi's sarcoma. *J Emerg Med* 9:23, 1991.

180. Rubinstein A, et al. Pulmonary disease in children with acquired immune deficiency syndrome and AIDS-related complex. *J Pediatr* 108:498, 1986.

181. Sadaghdar H, Eden E. Pulmonary Kaposi's sarcoma presenting as fulminant respiratory failure. *Chest* 100:858, 1991.

182. Salahuddin SZ, et al. HTLV-III in symptom-free seronegative persons. *Lancet* 2:1418, 1984.

183. Saldana MJ, Mones J, Buck BE. Lymphoid interstitial pneumonia in Haitian residents of Florida. *Chest* 84:347, 1983.

184. Schoettler JJ, Schleissner LA, Heiner DC. Familial IgE deficiency associated with sinopulmonary disease. *Chest* 96:516, 1989.

185. Schroter GPJ, et al. Fungus infections after liver transplantation. *Ann Surg* 186:115, 1977.

186. Schroter GPJ, et al. Infections complicating orthoptic liver transplantation: A study emphasizing graft-related septicemia. *Arch Surg* 111:1337, 1976.

187. Schwartz DA, et al. Pulmonary malakoplakia in a patient with the acquired immunodeficiency syndrome. Differential diagnostic considerations. *Arch Pathol Lab Med* 114:1267, 1990.

188. Seligmann M, et al. Immunology of human immunodeficiency virus infection and the acquired immunodeficiency syndrome: An update. *Ann Intern Med* 107:234, 1987.

189. Sepkowitz KA, et al. Pneumothorax in AIDS. *Ann Intern Med* 114:455, 1991.

190. Shapiro GG, et al. Immunologic defects in patients with refractory sinusitis. *Pediatrics* 87:311, 1991.

191. Shelhamer JH, et al. Respiratory disease in the immunocompromised patient. *Ann Intern Med* 117:415, 1992.

192. Silverman ED, Myones BL, Miller JJ III. Lymphocyte subpopulation alterations induced by intravenous megadose pulse methylprednisolone. *J Rheumatol* 11:287, 1984.

193. Silvestri RC, et al. Pulmonary infiltrates and hypoxemia in patients with the acquired immunodeficiency syndrome re-exposed to trimethoprim-sulfamethoxazole. *Am Rev Respir Dis* 136:1001, 1987.

194. Simmons RL, et al. Pulmonary complications in transplant recipients. *Arch Surg* 105:260, 1972.

195. Singer C, et al. Diffuse pulmonary infiltrates in immunosuppressed patients: Prospective study of 80 cases. *Am J Med* 66:110, 1979.

196. Slade JD, Hepburn B. Prednisone-induced alterations of circulating human lymphocyte subsets. *J Lab Clin Med* 101:479, 1983.

197. Sloane JP, et al. Histopathology of the lung after bone marrow transplantation. *J Clin Pathol* 36:546, 1983.

198. Speich R, et al. Primary pulmonary hypertension in HIV infection. *Chest* 100:1268, 1991.

199. Srivatsa SS, Burger CD, Douglas WW. Upper lobe pulmonary parenchymal calcification in a patient with AIDS and *Pneumocystis carinii* pneumonia receiving aerosolized pentamidine. *Chest* 101:266, 1992.

200. Stover DE, et al. Diagnosis of pulmonary disease in acquired immune deficiency syndrome (AIDS): Role of bronchoscopy and bronchoalveolar lavage. *Am Rev Respir Dis* 130:659, 1984.

201. Stover DE, et al. Spectrum of pulmonary diseases associated with the acquired immune deficiency syndrome. *Am J Med* 78:429, 1985.

202. Stover DE, et al. Bronchoalveolar lavage in the

diagnosis of diffuse pulmonary infiltrates in the immunocompromised host. *Ann Intern Med* 101:1, 1984.

203. Strazzella WD, Safirstein BH. Pleural effusions in AIDS. *N Engl J Med* 88:39, 1991.

204. Stulbarg MS, Golden JA. Open lung biopsy in the acquired immunodeficiency syndrome (AIDS) (editorial). *Chest* 91:639, 1987.

205. Suffredini AF, et al. Nonspecific interstitial pneumonitis: A common cause of pulmonary disease in the acquired immunodeficiency syndrome. *Ann Intern Med* 107:7, 1987.

206. Sweinberg SK, et al. Retrospective analysis of the incidence of pulmonary disease in hypogammaglobulinemia. *J Allergy Clin Immunol* 88:96, 1991.

207. Tan ST, Blake GB, Chambers S. Recurrent orf in an immunocompromised host. *Br J Plast Surg* 44:465, 1991.

208. Tanner DD, et al. Fatal cytomegalovirus bronchiolitis in a patient with Nezelof's syndrome. *Pediatrics* 65:98, 1980.

209. Teague RD, Wallace RJ Jr, Awe RJ. The use of quantitative sterile brush culture and gram stain analysis in the diagnosis of lower respiratory tract infection. *Chest* 79:157, 1981.

210. Teirstein AS, Rosen MJ. Lymphocytic interstitial pneumonia. *Clin Chest Med* 9:467, 1988.

211. Tirelli U, et al. Malignant lymphoma related to HIV infection in Italy: A report of 46 cases. *JAMA* 258:2064, 1987.

212. Toronto Aerosolized Pentamidine Study (TAPS) Group. Acute pulmonary effects of aerosolized pentamidine. *Chest* 98:907, 1990.

213. Tullis E, et al. The long-term effects of aerosol pentamidine on pulmonary function. The Toronto Aerosolized Pentamidine Study (TAPS) Group. *Clin Invest Med* 15:42, 1992.

214. Tung KT. Cystic pulmonary lesions in AIDS. *Clin Radiol* 45:149, 1992.

215. Umetsu DT, et al. Recurrent sinopulmonary infection and impaired antibody response to bacterial capsular polysaccharide antigen in children with selective IgG-subclass deficiency. *N Engl J Med* 313:1247, 1985.

216. Van Thiel DH, et al. Medical aspects of liver transplantation. *Hepatology* 4(Suppl):79, 1984.

217. Venet A, et al. Lung in acquired immune deficiency syndrome: Infectious and immunological status assessed by bronchoalveolar lavage. *Bull Eur Physiopathol Respir* 21:535, 1985.

218. Verbruggen G, et al. The effect of low doses of prednisolone on the traffic of T helper-inducer cells in rheumatoid arthritis. *Clin Rheumatol* 1:199, 1982.

219. Verra F, et al. Bronchoalveolar lavage in immunocompromised patients. Clinical and functional consequences. *Chest* 101:1215, 1992.

220. Walsh TJ, Gray WC. *Candida* epiglottitis in immune-compromised patients. *Chest* 91:482, 1987.

221. Webb WR, et al. Pulmonary complications of renal transplantation: A survey of patients treated by low-dose immunosuppression. *Radiology* 126:1, 1978.

222. Weintraub J, Warnke RA. Lymphoma in cardiac allotransplant recipients: Clinical and histological features and immunological phenotype. *Transplantation* 33:347, 1982.

223. White DA, Matthay RA. Noninfectious pulmonary complications of infection with the human immunodeficiency virus. *Am Rev Respir Dis* 140:1763, 1989.

224. White DA, Zaman MK. Medical management of AIDS patients. Pulmonary disease. *Med Clin North Am* 76:19, 1992.

225. Williams DM, Krick JA, Remington JS. Pulmonary infection in the compromised host (parts I and II). *Am Rev Respir Dis* 114:359, 593, 1976.

226. Wilson WR, Cockerill FR III, Rosenow EC III. Pulmonary disease in the immunocompromised host (part 2). *Mayo Clin Proc* 60:610, 1985.

227. Wimberly N, Faling LJ, Bartlett JG. Flexible fiberbronchoscopy technique to obtain uncontaminated lower airway secretion for bacterial culture. *Am Rev Respir Dis* 119:337, 1979.

228. Young RC, et al. Aspergillosis: The spectrum of the disease in 98 patients. *Medicine* 49:147, 1970.

229. Zeluff BJ. Fungal pneumonia in transplant recipients. *Semin Respir Infect* 5:80, 1990.

230. Zibrak JD, et al. Bronchoscopic and radiologic features of Kaposi's sarcoma involving the respiratory system. *Chest* 90:476, 1986.

231. Ziegler JL, et al. Non-Hodgkin's lymphoma in 90 homosexual men: Relation to generalized lymphadenopathy and the acquired immunodeficiency syndrome. *N Engl J Med* 311:565, 1984.

232. Ziegler JL, et al. Outbreak of Burkitt's-like lymphoma in homosexual men. *Lancet* 2:631, 1982.

60

Hematologic Diseases

Udaya B. S. Prakash

Tissue oxygenation depends as much on the erythropoietic system as on the respiratory system. Anemia, polycythemia, abnormal hemoglobins, and significant changes in blood volume frequently produce alterations in various respiratory functions. Additionally, myeloproliferative and lymphoproliferative disorders and other hematologic malignancies frequently affect the pulmonary system. Pulmonary complications are the most common cause of mortality in patients with hematologic malignancies. Respiratory manifestations in these disorders may be caused by pulmonary extension of the basic disease process, cytotoxic drug-induced pulmonary pathology, opportunistic infections, or a combination of these factors. This chapter will discuss the various intrathoracic manifestations described in hematologic diseases.

Hemoglobinopathies

A *hemoglobinopathy* is an abnormality of hemoglobin synthesis manifested by the production of globin with a structural abnormality [17,180]. More than 90 percent of these abnormalities are the result of single amino acid replacements. The clinically significant hemoglobinopathies, as far as the pulmonary system is concerned, include sickle syndromes, hemoglobinopathies with high oxygen affinity (familial erythrocytosis), hemoglobinopathies with low oxygen affinity (familial cyanosis), M hemoglobinopathies (familial cyanosis), and methemoglobinemia and sulfhemoglobinemia. Although cyanosis as a result of these disorders is rare in clinical practice, the possibility of abnormal hemoglobin should be considered in the differential diagnosis in a cyanotic patient (Table 60-1).

Hemoglobinopathies with High Oxygen Affinity

At least 116 human hemoglobin variants are known to exhibit increased oxygen affinity, and newer variants continue to be described [17,149]. By definition, these hemoglobins demonstrate a shift to the left of the whole-blood oxygen dissociation curve. The hemoglobinopathies with high oxygen affinity are due to amino acid substitution at sites crucial to hemoglobin function. These disorders are manifested in the heterozygous state and follow an autosomal codominant pattern of inheritance. A partial list of abnormal hemoglobins with increased affinity for oxygen include Chesapeake, J-Capetown, Malmo, Yakima, Kempsey, Ypsilanti, Hiroshe, Brigham, Rainier, Bethesda, Hiroshima, Little Rock, Olympia, Tarrant, Sureness, Helsinki, Creteil, Hotel Dieu, Radcliffe, Alberta, British Columbia, Heathrow, San Diego, Syracuse, York, and Cowtown.

Many of these hemoglobinopathies are manifested by secondary erythrocytosis. Most patients are asymptomatic, and the diagnosis is entertained when unexplained erythrocytosis is detected. Patients with hemoglobin variants with a marked increase in oxygen affinity may demonstrate cyanosis. Because of the defective hemoglobin function, the arterial blood is partially unsaturated despite normal oxygen tension, which results in elevated levels of deoxyhemoglobin in the blood—hence the cyanosis. However, the cyanosis is a cosmetic problem and warrants no specific therapy. Several individuals with high-affinity variants have had persistent leukocytosis, and an occasional subject has exhibited splenomegaly. Pulmonary fibrosis has been described in several members of a family with hemoglobin Malmo, but the occurrence seems coincidental [9].

Table 60-1. **Differential diagnosis of cyanosis**

Inadequate oxygenation of hemoglobin (common)
    Pulmonary diseases
    Cardiac and noncardiac right-to-left shunt
    Vascular collapse (shock)
    Low-oxygen-affinity hemoglobin variant
Methemoglobinemia (uncommon)
    Hereditary (congenital)
        Cytochrome b_5 reductase deficiency
        M hemoglobinopathies
    Acquired (toxic)
        Nitrites and nitrates: amyl nitrite, nitroglycer-
            ine, nitroprusside, silver nitrate, sodium
            nitrite
        Other drugs: acetanilid, benzocaine, lidocaine,
            phenazopyridine, phenacetin, procaine,
            sulfonamides
        Industrial and environmental toxins: aniline
            dyes, chlorate, etc.
Sulfhemoglobinemia (uncommon)
    Congenital (?)
    Acquired: acetaminophen, acetanilide, arylam-
        ines, phenacetin, sulfur, toxins, etc.
Pseudocyanosis
    Argyria
    Hemochromatosis
    Chloroma

Hemoglobinopathies with Low Oxygen Affinity

More than a dozen variants of hemoglobinopathies with low oxygen affinity have been described. A partial list includes Kansas, Beth Israel, St. Mande, Titusville, Connecticut, Bologna,
Rothschild, Mobile, Hope, J-Cairo, Raleigh, Van-
couver, Presbyterian, and Yoshizuka. Many affected family members exhibit slightly diminished hemoglobin levels. The shift to the right of
the oxyhemoglobin dissociation curve reduces
the erythropoietin-mediated stimulus to erythropoiesis. In hemoglobin Kansas, cyanosis in heterozygotes results from increased deoxyhemoglobin. The patients with hemoglobin Kansas
demonstrate a marked decrease in whole-blood
oxygen affinity. Despite the diminished oxygen
content of the arterial blood, the shift to the right
of the oxyhemoglobin dissociation curve allows
adequate oxygen release. The subjects with
hemoglobin Kansas may develop limited tolerance to strenuous muscular exercise, which depends on a greatly increased oxygen unloading.

In addition to hemoglobin Kansas, cyanosis
can be seen in hemoglobin variants Beth Israel

and St. Mande [133]. Both have amino acid substitutions at the same site as hemoglobin Kansas
(i.e., a substitution of threonine for asparagine at
102). Familial pulmonary hypertension has been
described in association with abnormal hemoglobin with low oxygen affinity [166].

M Hemoglobinopathies

The main group of hemoglobins that produce cyanosis are known as *M hemoglobinopathies.*
Hemoglobins M-Boston, M-Iwate, M-Saskatoon,
M-Hyde Park, and M-Milwaukee exhibit abnormal absorbance spectra owing to the oxidation of
the heme iron in the affected subunit. These hemoglobinopathies behave as autosomal codominant mutations. In the heterozygous state, they
produce methemoglobinemia, which results in
chronic cyanosis. The Bohr effect is markedly decreased to absent in the alpha-chain variants but
normal to only slightly decreased in variants of
the beta chain [73]. Thus hemoglobins Iwate and
Boston, both associated with alpha-chain alterations, show decreased oxygen affinity and decreased Bohr effect; hemoglobins Hyde Park and
Saskatoon, which exemplify beta-chain mutations, have essentially normal oxygen affinity and
Bohr effect [163].

The predominant characteristic of hemoglobin
M disorders is the presence of cyanosis from
early childhood. Subjects with alpha-chain variants (M-Boston and M-Iwate) are cyanotic at
birth, whereas those with beta-chain variants
(M-Saskatoon, M-Hyde Park, M-Milwaukee) do
not exhibit cyanosis until approximately 5 to 6
months of age, when fetal hemoglobin is replaced
by adult hemoglobin. Hemoglobin Freiburg resulting from a beta-chain mutation is associated
with mild cyanosis, whereas hemoglobin Seattle
is not associated with cyanosis but does show decreased oxygen affinity [181]. Despite the cyanosis in these hemoglobinopathies, there is no
evidence of cardiac disease or clubbing. Exertional dyspnea is not a feature of these hemoglobinopathies.

Methemoglobinemia and Sulfhemoglobinemia

Methemoglobinemia results when more than 1
percent of hemoglobin has been oxidized to fer-
ric form. When hemoglobin is oxidized to methemoglobin, the heme iron becomes Fe^{3+} and is
incapable of binding oxygen [17,86]. Methemoglobin content of normal red cells is less than 1

percent. When methemoglobin level exceeds 1.5 gm/dl (10 percent of total hemoglobin), clinically obvious cyanosis results. Both hereditary (congenital) and acquired forms of methemoglobinemia exist. Congenital methemoglobinemia results from either hereditary deficiency of the enzyme cytochrome b5 reductase (methemoglobin reductase) or the presence of one of the M hemoglobins. The major clinical feature is cyanosis without cardiopulmonary problems. In the methemoglobinemia due to methemoglobin reductase deficiency, oral administration of methylene blue (100 to 200 mg/day) or ascorbic acid (300 to 500 mg/day) will markedly reduce the level of methemoglobin. The benefit is purely cosmetic.

Acquired methemoglobinemia, also known as *toxic methemoglobinemia*, results when drugs or toxins oxidize hemoglobin directly in the circulation or facilitate its oxidation by molecular oxygen (see Table 60-1) [31,86]. Toxic methemoglobinemia may be acute or chronic. In the latter circumstance, chronic administration of the offending agent leads to an increased steady-state concentration of methemoglobin that results in asymptomatic cyanosis. Blood gas analysis usually reveals normal arterial oxygen tension with disproportionately low arterial oxygen saturation and increased levels of methemoglobin. Acute methemoglobinemia, especially when the level of methemoglobin exceeds half the total hemoglobin, may present a serious medical emergency. When the methemoglobin level exceeds 35 percent, the symptoms include headaches, weakness, and dyspnea. The severity of methemoglobinemia depends on the dose of the causative agent as well as on the susceptibility of the exposed individual. Levels in excess of 80 percent are incompatible with life. Severe toxic methemoglobinemia should be treated with intravenous methylene blue (2 mg/kg).

Sulfhemoglobinemia refers to the presence, in peripheral blood, of hemoglobin derivatives that poorly characterize chemically. Occasionally, subjects exposed to oxidant compounds will develop cyanosis that cannot be explained by simple hemoglobin oxidation. Because of its high absorbance in the red region of the visible spectrum, sulfhemoglobinemia causes more cyanosis than an equivalent percentage of methemoglobinemia. Congenital and acquired forms of sulfhemoglobinemia have been described [103,145]. A number of pharmacologic and other agents (see Table 60-1) are capable of producing sulfhemoglobinemia and cyanosis.

Sickle Cell Anemia

Sickle cell disease is caused primarily by hemoglobin SS, SC, or Sβ thalassemia. Sickle cell anemia is a chronic, hereditary hemolytic disease resulting from clinical expression of homozygosity for hemoglobin S. The affected persons are predominantly blacks who have inherited the mutant gene from both parents. Pulmonary complications are common in patients with sickle cell anemia (SS hemoglobin) but less so in patients with SC hemoglobin. Pulmonary complications are important causes of morbidity and mortality.

Pneumococcal pneumonia is a major cause of morbidity and mortality in children with sickle cell disease. Pneumonia, especially in children and probably in all age groups, is the most common lung disease encountered in sickle cell anemia, where its incidence is 20 times greater than in the normal population. The major factors that predispose these patients to infections include abnormal complement activity, poor splenic function, and a lack of type-specific pneumococcal antibody [104]. Local factors such as previous or concomitant pulmonary damage by vaso-occlusion probably play a role. In children with sickle cell disease, the incidence of pneumonia increases significantly after the age of 8 months [31]. In children, the pneumonia usually is due to *Streptococcus pneumoniae*, whereas in adults, *Staphylococcus aureus* or *Hemophilus* species predominate. The majority of suspected pneumonias in adults are due to pulmonary embolism, and the differentiation of infectious pneumonia from acute chest syndrome or pulmonary embolism is difficult [71,176]. Barrett-Connor [5] reported that 45 percent of 166 patients with sickle cell anemia were hospitalized because of acute bacterial pneumonia, and half of this group had positive bacterial cultures. However, in another study of 18 patients with acute chest syndrome, respiratory secretion was obtained via bronchoscopy, and the study concluded that bacterial pneumonia is uncommon in this group of patients [95]. Multilobar involvement is not uncommon, with the upper and middle lobes being involved more often than the others [5]. Administration of pneumococcal vaccine is mandatory in patients with sickle cell anemia.

Fungal infections are uncommon in patients with sickle cell anemia, although occasional cases of cryptococcal infection have been described [70]. A higher incidence of tuberculous infection in sickle cell anemia was reported by Weiss and Waife [202], but other studies have not substantiated this increased incidence of tuberculosis in sickle cell trait.

The acute chest syndrome (also called *sickle chest syndrome, chest crisis, pulmonary sickle crisis,* and *pulmonary infarction,* among other names) is seen in 15 to 35 percent of patients hospitalized with sickle cell disease. It is a common manifestation of sickling vaso-occlusive crises and accounts for a vast number of hospitalizations. The syndrome is characterized by fever, chest pain, and pulmonary infiltrates. Sudden onset of pleuritic chest pains, cough without hemoptysis, fever, and leukocytosis is common. Hypoxemia ($PaO_2 < 50$ mmHg) is present in up to 40 percent of patients. Dense bilateral lower-lung consolidations are common. A retrospective analysis of 100 hospitalized pediatric cases of sickle cell anemia revealed lower-lobe pulmonary infiltrates in 86 percent and upper- and middle-lobe infiltrates in 25 and 22 percent, respectively [178]. Pleural effusions were observed in 38 percent. Pulmonary hypertension and cor pulmonale are the expected late complications due to recurrent episodes of pulmonary vascular thromboembolism. Nevertheless, the incidence of these complications is low.

Pulmonary pathologic features include pulmonary vascular occlusion, capillary stasis, thrombus formation, infarction, alveolar wall necrosis, and emboli of necrotic bone marrow. These complications are more common in women, particularly during late pregnancy or shortly after delivery. Patients with hemoglobin SC disease may be at risk of in situ thrombosis of pulmonary vessels. The roentgenographic appearance of these lesions is no different from that produced by thromboemboli. Oppenheimer and Esterly [138], in a necropsy study of 36 older patients, identified thromboemboli in most, but pulmonary infarction is believed to be a much less frequent complication among younger patients. Although circulatory stasis may develop in situ, vascular occlusion by marrow embolus is probably a more common cause of pulmonary infarction and has been discovered at autopsy in 13 percent of patients with sickle cell disease [71]. In patients with sickle cell anemia, pulmonary hemosiderosis may result from repeated blood transfusions.

Pulmonary edema is another reported complication of sickle cell crisis. Vigorous hypotonic fluid replacement and parenteral analgesic therapy, commonly used in patients in sickle cell crisis, may contribute to the development of pulmonary edema [74]. Autopsy findings in patients who died from pulmonary edema are consistent with a diffuse pulmonary vaso-occlusive disease.

Sickle cell crisis may be precipitated by asthmatic attacks [147].

Decreased diffusing capacity has been demonstrated in sickle cell anemia and has been attributed to a loss of membrane area due to obstruction of pulmonary vessels [128]. Other physiologic studies [39,129] have shown a decreased vital capacity, normal maximal breathing capacity, arterial oxygen desaturation, and a widened alveolar-arterial oxygen tension difference in most patients with the disease. Both venoarterial shunting and abnormal ventilation-perfusion relationships play major roles in widening this tension difference. The arterial oxygen desaturation predisposes to in vivo sickling and its consequences. Earlier reports noted that the heterozygous state of sickle cell trait (hemoglobin AS) may lead to abnormal pulmonary function, as a result of sickling, at high altitudes. The sickling phenomenon can result in pulmonary thromboembolism and can further aggravate sickling, with resultant increasing hypoxemia. Short exposures to hypoxia at high altitudes do not acutely or cumulatively alter diffusing capacity or spirometric values in healthy persons with sickle cell trait [32,56].

Sickle cell disease and sarcoidosis are two disorders commonly affecting blacks [65]. Studies have shown the prevalence rates of hemoglobinopathies in sarcoid patients to be 18 to 20 percent, although sickle cell hemoglobinopathy was rare [61,83].

Beta-Thalassemia Major

Thalassemia major is characterized by an unbalanced synthesis of globin chain, resulting in ineffective hematopoiesis and severe anemia. Severe hemolytic anemia and ineffective erythropoiesis from infancy are the main characteristics of this disorder. The ability of these patients to increase their oxygen-carrying capacity during periods of physical exertion is limited. Patients succumb at a young age to congestive cardiac failure. Patients with thalassemia major who are chronically transfused exhibit a high cardiac output during exercise, regardless of hemoglobin concentration, and the mechanism for this phenomenon is unknown [60]. Cardiopulmonary evaluation of 35 patients with homozygous beta-thalassemia observed hypoxemia in 85 percent, reduced lung volumes and flow rates in 51 and 63 percent, respectively, and diminished diffusing capacity for carbon monoxide in 50 percent [63]. Pulmonary hypertension was present in 75 percent, and right ventricular dysfunction was more prevalent than left ventricular dysfunction. The possible causes for these complications may include left ventricular failure, iron deposits in the pulmonary vessels, and a hypercoagulable state with thrombotic obstruction of the pulmonary arteries. Transfusion-induced decreases in forced vital capacity and PaO_2 in the absence of pulmonary edema have been observed, but the mechanism is unclear [3].

Hemorrhagic Diseases

Pulmonary complications such as pulmonary embolism and alveolar hemorrhage can result from an underlying disorder of coagulation. Both hypercoagulable and hypocoagulable states may be associated with these complications. The presence of a hemorrhagic disorder predisposes to pulmonary bleeding, and the risk of bleeding is increased if the patient has a preexisting pulmonary lesion such as a tumor, bulla (Fig. 60-1), cyst, cavity, or bronchiectasis.

Hemophilia

Classic hemophilia is the result of functional deficiency of antihemophilic factor (factor VIII).

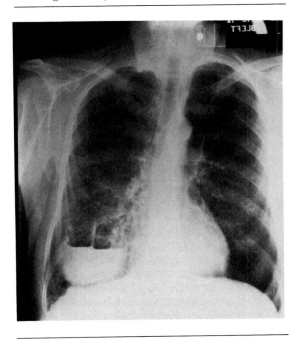

Fig. 60-1. Hemorrhage into a bullous lesion in the right lower lobe in a patient with excessive bleeding tendency secondary to coumarin therapy.

This abnormality is attributable to an X-linked recessive gene, for the disorder occurs almost exclusively in men. The most serious complication is the occurrence of the acquired immunodeficiency syndrome (AIDS) in those who were administered factor VIII contaminated by the human immunodeficiency virus. Pulmonary manifestations (unrelated to AIDS) are unusual but have included spontaneous pneumothorax, hemomediastinum, tracheal obstruction by a hematoma, and pleural hematomas [182,205]. By a review of chest roentgenograms, Putman and associates [159] discovered abnormalities in 26 of 33 adult hemophiliacs. Scarring, fibrosis, and pleural thickening were seen in 12 cases, and abnormalities of pulmonary vessels were seen in the remaining 14, of which 4 had evidence of hyperinflation. Several cases of primary pulmonary hypertension have been described in patients receiving factor VIII infusion [55]. Pulmonary hypertension is a well-recognized complication in patients with AIDS, and it is likely that the pathogenic mechanism of pulmonary hypertension in patients with hemophilia is similar to that in AIDS patients (see Chapter 59).

Disseminated Intravascular Coagulation

Pulmonary hemorrhage has been seen in patients with disseminated intravascular coagulation. Robbins and associates [168] estimated the incidence of pulmonary hemorrhage to be approximately 14 percent in this condition, and intrapulmonary hemorrhage was the immediate cause of 7 of the 10 deaths in their studies. The pulmonary hemorrhage syndrome has features in common with the adult respiratory distress syndrome, such as hyaline membrane formation and pulmonary hypoperfusion. Thrombocytopenia has been shown to lead to the development of pulmonary hematoma, hemothorax, and fatal pulmonary hemorrhage. Pulmonary infarction has been described in several patients with disseminated intravascular coagulation [194].

Myeloproliferative Disorders
Leukemia

Pulmonary involvement in leukemia occurs more often than is usually suspected. The reported mortality rate associated with pulmonary complications in leukemia is approximately 60 to 65 percent [177]. The respiratory complications depend on the type of leukemia, the nature and course of treatment, and the presence or absence of significant neutropenia [79]. Many of the complications are secondary to the immunocompromised status of leukemic patients, which is caused either by the leukemic state itself or by treatment.

Infectious pneumonia is a frequent and often fatal complication and is responsible for 60 to 75 percent of reported deaths in patients with acute leukemia [79]. In a series of 68 patients with pulmonary infiltrates, 82 percent of focal and 35 percent of diffuse infiltrates were the product of infectious causes [189]. Gram-negative organisms are the most common cause of pneumonia. The incidence of fungal pneumonia has been found to be as high as 25 percent, but a figure of approximately 12 percent is more representative [177,200]. *Pneumocystis carinii* pneumonia occurs less often in adults than in children with acute leukemia. In a review of 53 cases of *P. carinii* pneumonia, including 4 in children, leukemia was the underlying hematologic disorder in 28 percent [150]. Sickles and associates [177] observed 52 episodes of pneumonia among 68 leukemic patients. The agents were isolated in 37 cases (71 percent) but in only 27 antemortem (52 percent). Most were gram-negative bacilli, with a 25 percent incidence of fungal pneumonia. The overall mortality was a disturbing 65 percent. In childhood leukemia, viruses are more important as respiratory pathogens and are major causes of morbidity from pulmonary infections.

Granulocytopenia, hypogammaglobulinemia, and lymphocytic bronchitis in graft-versus-host disease may follow bone marrow transplantation and predispose to infectious complications in leukemic patients. Granulocytopenia in leukemic patients poses a significant risk of invasive aspergillosis and acute respiratory distress syndrome. Invasive pulmonary aspergillosis is a life-threatening complication in patients with prolonged granulocytopenia. The rapidity of bone marrow recovery markedly influences the clinical and roentgenographic course of the disease, and the risk for invasive aspergillosis is proportional to the duration of granulocytopenia. For patients with acute leukemia, granulocytopenia persisting longer than 3 weeks is the major risk factor for developing this life-threatening infection. In an observation of such patients, granulocyte recovery, with counts exceeding 500/mm^3, was followed by cavitary pulmonary aspergillosis in 73 percent [50]. Nearly one-third of the patients with malignancies who receive empiric antibiotic therapy during episodes of granulocytopenia develop pulmonary fungal infections. Massive hemoptysis may occur in some patients. Prognosis

has been uniformly poor, with mortality rates exceeding 65 to 70 percent in some series [78,124]. A study reported that early diagnosis of aspergillosis in leukemic patients on chemotherapy can be established by computed tomography, which will reveal a characteristic progression from multiple fluffy masses to cavitation or air crescent formation.

Hypogammaglobulinemia, related to inherent abnormalities of B-lymphocyte function and T-cell imbalances, is found in approximately 50 percent of patients with chronic lymphocytic leukemia. Infections, particularly with encapsulated microorganisms, are a frequent cause of morbidity and mortality.

Hairy-cell leukemia is an unusual hematologic malignancy involving splenomegaly, pancytopenia, and circulating mononuclear cells with prominent cytoplasmic projections. Infections are secondary to granulocytopenia and defects in cell-mediated immunity. Bacterial, fungal, and mycobacterial infections occur frequently. Disseminated infections caused by *Mycobacterium kansasii* and *Mycobacterium avium-intracellulare* may occur in patients with hairy-cell leukemia [79,111].

Autopsy studies reveal that noninfectious intrathoracic involvement by leukemia is a common late development. Mediastinal and hilar adenopathy is seen in 50 percent of cases, and pulmonary parenchyma is involved in approximately 25 percent. Acute myelogenous leukemias produce pulmonary parenchymal leukemic infiltrates more commonly than the chronic varieties, but among the chronic group, lymphocytic leukemia is more likely than the granulocytic type to invade pulmonary parenchyma (Figs. 60-2, 60-3). The usual roentgenographic abnormality within pulmonary parenchyma is a diffuse bilateral reticulonodular infiltration resembling that of lymphangitic metastasis (Fig. 60-4). This is not uncommon in the terminal stages of leukemia. However, several cases of acute leukemia presenting with diffuse pulmonary infiltrates and respiratory failure have been described [154]. In patients who are granulocytopenic, diffuse lung infiltrates should warn of the possibility of invasive aspergillosis (Fig. 60-5). Other presenting manifestations—namely, discrete nodules and infarcts—are very rare. Rapidly progressive pulmonary infiltrates have been noted as a major clinical problem in chronic myelogenous leukemia. The leukemic infiltrates may be parenchymal (focal or diffuse), pleural, peribronchial, or endobronchial. In the so-called Richter's trans-

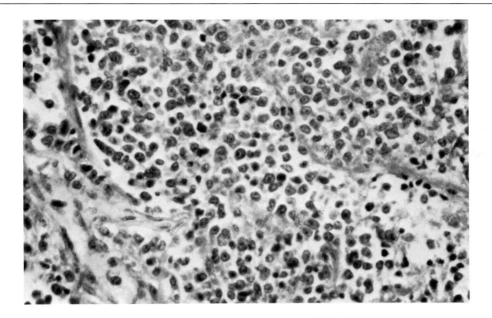

Fig. 60-2. Pulmonary infiltration by acute granulocytic leukemia.

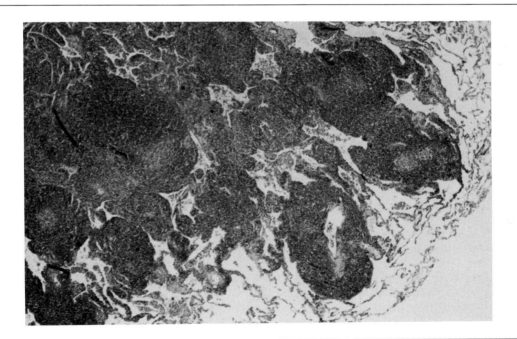

Fig. 60-3. Pulmonary involvement by chronic lymphocytic leukemia. A dense infiltrate of small lymphocytes can be seen around vessels and in alveolar septa.

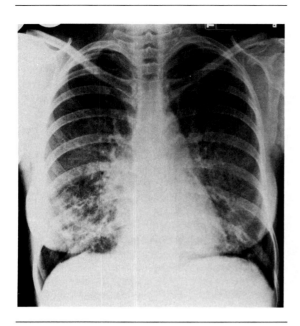

Fig. 60-4. Leukemic infiltrates in the lower lobes of both lungs in a patient with acute monomyelocytic leukemia.

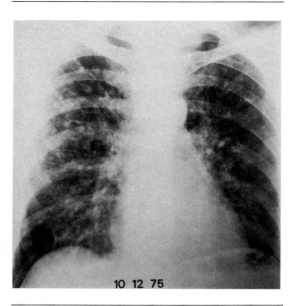

Fig. 60-5. Diffuse nodular-reticular infiltrates in a severely granulocytopenic patient on chemotherapy for acute monomyelocytic leukemia.

formation, chronic lymphocytic leukemia may convert from a low-grade histologic picture to high-grade non-Hodgkin's lymphoma and produce hilar or mediastinal lymphadenopathy [79]. Pleural effusion, usually unilateral, is second in frequency only to enlargement of mediastinal nodes and is seen in nearly 25 percent of cases.

Pulmonary alveolar hemorrhage often is found at autopsy in leukemic patients [189]. In a necropsy study of 50 patients with acute leukemia, pulmonary hemorrhage and leukemic pulmonary infiltrates were recorded in 54 and 64 percent, respectively [12]. Pulmonary hemorrhage usually is associated with thrombocytopenia and may be extensive. Another predisposing cause is invasive pulmonary aspergillosis. The majority of patients with pulmonary alveolar hemorrhage do not exhibit hemoptysis.

Respiratory failure may occur as a result of any of the complications just discussed. Additionally, *leukostasis* of the pulmonary vasculature, caused by severe leukocytosis (leukocyte count exceeding 200,000/μl), and *leukemic cell lysis pneumopathy* within 48 hours of chemotherapy initiation may cause respiratory failure [34,120,132]. Studies have shown that adult respiratory distress syndrome can also occur in the setting of severe

neutropenia [106,119,137]. The development of acute respiratory failure in patients with hematologic disorders is a life-threatening condition. Irrespective of the etiology of acute respiratory failure in this group of patients, the outcome is dismal, with a mortality rate of 80 percent [36].

In patients with leukemia, lung biopsy may suggest areas of pulmonary alveolar phospholipoproteinosis. The mechanism is secondary to the monocytopenia in leukemia. Alveolar macrophages are derived from monocytes, and the deficiency of monocytes in leukemia results in the inability of the limited number of alveolar macrophages to ingest intraalveolar phospholipids. In addition, opportunistic infections and cytotoxic drugs may affect the alveolar clearance of phospholipids and produce patchy areas of secondary pulmonary alveolar (phospholipo) proteinosis. However, this finding is clinically insignificant, and chest roentgenograms may or may not show patchy areas of alveolar infiltrates [8,155].

Pseudohypoxemia or spurious hypoxemia denotes low oxygen tension and normal oxygen saturation in arterial blood in the absence of clinical evidence of tissue hypoxemia [30]. This phenomenon occurs in patients with extreme degrees of leukocytosis. During the in vitro transportation of arterial blood sample from the patient to the laboratory, the leukocytes in the syringe consume significant amounts of oxygen and hence the measurement reveals a low PaO_2 (so-called leukocyte larceny) [46]. Pseudohypoxemia is seen also in patients with thrombocytosis.

Polycythemia

Defined as a sustained excess of red blood cell volume, *polycythemia* occurs in either a primary or a secondary form. Secondary polycythemia is a compensatory mechanism seen in various chronic hypoxemic states. The pulmonary manifestations in patients with such diseases are those of the underlying disease.

Primary polycythemia, or polycythemia rubra vera, is a chronic disease of unknown etiology characterized by hyperplasia of all the cellular elements of the bone marrow, nucleated red blood cells being more prominently involved. Chest roentgenographic abnormalities consist of accentuated vascular markings and minor infiltrates and, occasionally, nodular lesions in the midlung zones. Thrombosis, stasis, or infarction in pulmonary veins is believed to produce discrete lesions. Other abnormal roentgenographic findings include enlargement of hilar vessels and passive pulmonary congestion. Symptoms are those of pulmonary insufficiency from pulmonary edema. Acute airway obstruction caused by spontaneous retropharyngeal bleeding and hematoma formation has been described in a patient with polycythemia rubra vera [117].

Normal arterial oxygen saturation (equal to or greater than 92 percent) has been regarded as one of the findings that differentiates polycythemia vera from the secondary (hypoxemic) form, because almost all patients with primary polycythemia have normal arterial oxygen saturation. However, mild degrees of desaturation may occur with otherwise well-documented polycythemia vera in the absence of cardiopulmonary problems. The pathogenesis of this desaturation is not apparent.

Pulmonary function studies have shown that patients with polycythemia vera usually have normal vital capacity, airway resistance, and alveolar ventilation. Studies of pulmonary diffusing capacity have produced conflicting results. Pulmonary capillary blood volume and the size of the pulmonary vascular bed may be reduced in some patients, with resultant abnormalities in the ventilation-perfusion relationship.

Lymphoproliferative Disorders

Hodgkin's Disease

Intrathoracic involvement in Hodgkin's disease is common, occurring in 15 to 40 percent of patients, especially in those with advanced stage IIIB or IV disease, and every type of chest roentgenographic abnormality may be exhibited. Pleuropulmonary involvement is more common in Hodgkin's lymphoma than in other lymphomas. Pulmonary involvement may be seen in more than 50 percent of cases of Hodgkin's lymphoma in necropsy series [210]. A study of 300 consecutive patients with untreated Hodgkin's disease and non-Hodgkin's lymphoma indicated that intrathoracic involvement was twice as common with the Hodgkin's as with the non-Hodgkin's lymphoma [41]. The incidence of significant respiratory complications is directly related to the size of the mediastinal mass and the extent of the disease in Hodgkin's lymphoma [142].

Primary pulmonary Hodgkin's disease is a distinct entity and denotes involvement of the lung without hilar adenopathy or disseminated disease. As of 1990, 61 cases were reported [160]. This form of Hodgkin's lymphoma is more common in women, typically involves upper lung fields, and may appear as a solitary mass or a multinodular process with or without cavitation.

The abnormality seen most often on chest roentgenograms in Hodgkin's disease is enlargement of mediastinal lymph nodes, which is noted in 50 percent of cases. Bilateral lymph node enlargement is common, particularly if the paratracheal nodes are involved (Fig. 60-6). Enlargement also affects retrosternal nodes, posterior mediastinal nodes, and the diaphragmatic group of parietal lymph nodes. Intrapulmonary lymph node involvement may not be visible on the chest roentgenogram (Fig. 60-7).

Pulmonary parenchymal involvement is seen in up to 30 percent of patients (Figs. 60-8 through 60-10), especially those with the nodular sclerosing type of Hodgkin's disease, and is usually accompanied by mediastinal lymphadenopathy. However, in a study of 112 patients with advanced Hodgkin's disease, more than 25 percent were found to have parenchymal disease without adenopathy [203]. The parenchymal features include direct invasion of lung from regional lymph nodes (characterized by linear, feathery densities), massive homogeneous infiltrates with lymphadenopathy, nodular infiltrates, and generalized dissemination resembling miliary tuberculosis. Pulmonary parenchymal involvement ordi-

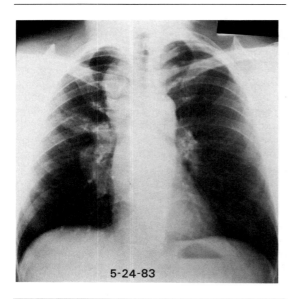

5-24-83

Fig. 60-6. Bilateral hilar and right paratracheal lymphadenopathy caused by Hodgkin's lymphoma.

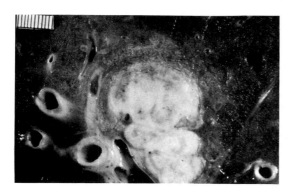

Fig. 60-7. Involvement of intrapulmonary peribronchial lymph node by Hodgkin's lymphoma, found at autopsy.

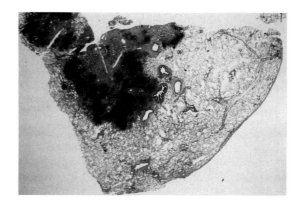

Fig. 60-8. Hodgkin's lymphoma presenting as a localized nodular lesion. The histologic pattern was nodular sclerosing Hodgkin's lymphoma. Some of the darker nodules of lymphoid tissue seem to be surrounded by a paler fibrous tissue indicative of a nodular sclerosing pattern.

narily is due to direct extension from mediastinal nodes along the lymphatics of bronchovascular sheaths. The parenchymal masses may develop cavities, and usually these are multiple and located in lower lobes. Cavitation of pulmonary nodules secondary to Hodgkin's disease is rare and has been noted in approximately 55 cases [174].

Endobronchial involvement occurs in nearly 5 percent of patients with Hodgkin's lymphoma. Lobar or segmental atelectasis, cough, and hemoptysis may result. Bronchial mucosal involvement from non-Hodgkin's lymphoma may become severe enough to cause airflow obstruction [142]. Extrinsic compression of the trachea and main stem bronchi by large mediastinal Hodgkin's lymphoma can lead to airway obstruction and respiratory failure. Patients may experience varying degrees of dyspnea in the supine posture [153].

Several cases of acute airway obstruction and respiratory failure during general anesthesia have been described [87,134]. During general anesthesia, the extrinsic airway compression is exacerbated due to diminished lung volumes secondary to reduced inspiratory muscle tone, relaxation of bronchial smooth-muscle tone and the resultant compressibility of airway, diminished expiratory flow rate, and severely diminished movement of the diaphragm [153]. Pulmonary function tests performed in 43 patients with Hodgkin's disease before mantle irradiation (total dose of 36 to 42 Gy) and at 3, 6, 9, 12, and 15 or more months thereafter have revealed only small variations in the functional indices [22].

Pleural effusion occurs in 30 percent of patients and usually is associated with other intrathoracic lesions. The main factor responsible for the collection of pleural fluid is the obstruction

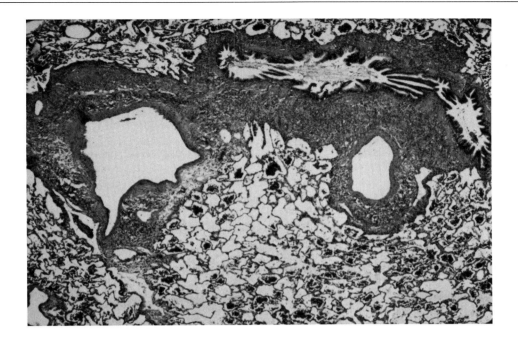

Fig. 60-9. Hodgkin's lymphoma in the lung as part of disseminated disease at presentation. The lung infiltrates were caused by a cellular proliferation around vessels and airway that have the cytologic features of Hodgkin's lymphoma.

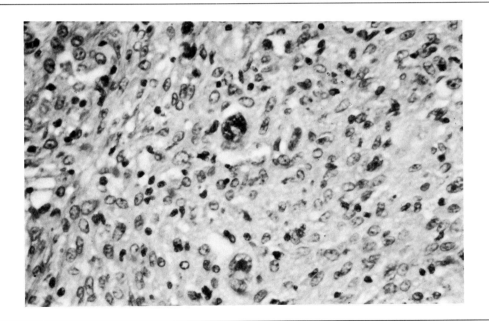

Fig. 60-10. Hodgkin's lymphoma replacing normal lung parenchyma. Reed-Sternberg cell is the center.

to lymphatics by the enlarged hilar lymph nodes. The pleural fluid is commonly an exudate, serous and chylous in one-third. *Chylothorax* is the accumulation of chyle in the pleural space due to disruption of the thoracic duct or a major lymphatic tributary. Intrathoracic malignancy is the most common cause of chylothorax, and lymphoproliferative disorders are responsible 75 percent of the time. In a study of 38 patients with chylous effusions, 20 effusions were due to lymphomas [179]. Diagnostic thoracentesis and needle biopsy of the pleura may aid in determining whether the pleural space or the pleura is involved with Hodgkin's or non-Hodgkin's lymphoma. However, the clinical correlation is extremely important in interpreting cytologic preparations. In one report, pleural biopsy was helpful in diagnosing non-Hodgkin's lymphoma in 9 of 10 patients [88]. In contrast, a large series from the Mayo Clinic demonstrated that the finding of lymphocytic pleuritis on biopsy or lymphocytosis of pleural fluid was nondiagnostic and that clinical correlation was essential to confirm the diagnosis [156]. Massive pleural effusions have occurred as a late complication of radiation therapy for Hodgkin's lymphoma, probably from impaired lymphatic drainage due to mediastinal fibrosis induced by radiation [169].

Spontaneous pneumothorax is an unusual complication in Hodgkin's disease. One study noted 17 episodes of pneumothorax in eight patients, seven with Hodgkin's lymphoma and one with non-Hodgkin's lymphoma [209]. The observed incidence of pneumothorax among 1977 patients with lymphoma was 10-fold higher than expected; this included a significantly higher incidence in patients younger than 30 years compared to those older than 30 years and a higher incidence in patients with Hodgkin's lymphoma than in those with non-Hodgkin's lymphoma. This study suggested a strong relation between radiation and pneumothorax. Other contributing factors included pulmonary involvement by lymphoma, radiation fibrosis, and infection. Pneumothorax associated with lymphoma is more complex and difficult to manage. Other unusual manifestations include thoracic cage involvement and diaphragmatic paralysis.

Non-Hodgkin's Lymphomas

The most common intrathoracic manifestation of non-Hodgkin's lymphoma is mediastinal lymph node enlargement, which is seen in nearly 35 percent of patients. Primary pulmonary lymphoma ordinarily presents as an alveolar infiltrate or a homogeneous mass. It is unusual to see bronchial obstruction or endobronchial involvement from this type of tumor.

When the lung is involved secondarily by non-Hodgkin's lymphoma, the typical roentgenographic pattern is that of solitary or multiple nodules 3 mm to several centimeters in diameter, more frequently in the lower lobes. Other manifestations are similar to those seen in Hodgkin's disease. Endobronchial recurrence of non-Hodgkin's lymphoma can be seen in patients who are unresponsive to therapy [84]. Diagnostic bronchoalveolar lavage in patients with pulmonary lymphoma may assist in diagnosis by subtyping lymphocytes with monoclonal antibodies.

Pleural effusions are also common in non-Hodgkin's lymphoma [88]. Indolent lymphomas may produce chylous pleural effusions [69]. Among 26 pleural effusions associated with non-Hodgkin's lymphomas, 20 were exudative and 5 were chylous. Cytologic examinations were positive in 86 percent of exudative effusions, whereas 61 percent of pleural biopsies were positive for the disease [208]. In a study of 19 patients with pleural effusion caused by non-Hodgkin's lymphoma, pleural tissue disclosed lymphoma in 17 patients, supporting the contention that pleural effusion in patients with non-Hodgkin's lymphoma is usually due to pleural lymphoma rather than to obstruction of mediastinal lymphatics [19]. Systemic chemotherapy results in resolution of pleural effusion in approximately half the patients; the prognosis tends to be poor in those with refractory effusions.

Patients treated for Hodgkin's and non-Hodgkin's lymphoma should be observed for the development of both hematologic and solid neoplasms. Studies have shown that these patients accrue a relative risk two to three times that of the normal population of developing newer malignancies [1]. Patients with Hodgkin's disease who receive supradiaphragmatic irradiation or combined-modality therapy may be at higher risk for developing non-small-cell lung cancer. In a study of such patients, the risk ratio for the development of lung cancer among Hodgkin's patients was 5.6 times that expected in the general population. The median ages at diagnosis of Hodgkin's disease and lung cancer were 39 and 45 years, respectively. The interval between the diagnoses of Hodgkin's disease and metachronous lung cancer averaged 7 years but appeared to vary inversely with age [115].

Primary Lymphoma of the Lung

Primary lymphomas of the lung are rare, representing fewer than 1 percent of all primary pulmonary malignancies. They are usually well-differentiated B-cell tumors of the IgM type, although a few cases of the IgG and IgA types have been described. Among 62 cases of primary lymphoma of lung, 58 were B-cell and 2 T-cell type, and 2 other cases could not be classified. The largest group (43 cases) consisted of low-grade B-cell lymphoma of the bronchus-associated lymphoid tissue (BALT) [110]. The histologic features were similar to low-grade B-cell lymphoma of the mucosa-associated lymphoid tissue (MALT) of the stomach. The definitive diagnosis of primary pulmonary lymphoma rests on the typical histopathologic and immunochemical staining pattern [109]. The low-grade lymphomas show a peak occurrence in the sixth decade of life, whereas the high-grade lymphomas occur most often in the seventh decade. There is a slight male predominance. Nearly 75 percent of the patients with low-grade B-cell lymphoma of BALT (*baltoma*) exhibit solitary or multiple sharply defined lung nodules. The prognosis is favorable in those without systemic symptoms [110].

The majority of primary extranodal lymphomas (not to be confused with primary lymphoma of lung) originate in MALT, and the term *maltoma* has been applied to them [121]. The maltomas seem to be associated with a good prognosis. In a study of 161 cases of non-Hodgkin's lymphomas and pseudolymphomas of lung, lymphomas were noted in 31.6 percent—plasmacytoid lymphocytic and small, cleaved, follicular center-cell lymphomas in 22.4 and 11.8 percent of cases, respectively. The remainder were follicular center-cell lymphomas and B-immunoblastic sarcomas [96]. Most patients were elderly and asymptomatic and, in most cases, a solitary nodule or infiltrate was seen on the chest roentgenogram. Hilar lymphadenopathy also was observed.

Mycosis Fungoides and Sézary Syndrome

Cutaneous T-cell lymphomas encompass a spectrum of diseases, including mycosis fungoides and Sézary syndrome, characterized by the malignant proliferation of phenotypically mature T lymphocytes with a propensity to infiltrate the skin. Microscopic infiltration of the lung parenchyma occurs in 43 to 56 percent of these patients [164,184]. Lung biopsy and sometimes the sputum cytology will show distinctive large and small mononuclear cells with an indented cerebri form and hyperchromatic nuclei. Lymphadenopathy precedes visceral involvement. Pulmonary manifestations may include diffuse basilar infiltrates, nodular densities, perihilar densities, pneumonic processes, consolidative lesions, and pleural effusion. Hemoptysis and hypoxemia are described. Rapid pulmonary dissemination can occur in Sézary syndrome.

Pseudolymphoma

Lymphoid tumors that do not fulfill the criteria for malignant lesions have been called *pseudolymphoma*, although many pseudolymphomas have been reclassified as indolent well-differentiated lymphocytic and lymphoplasmacytic lymphomas on the basis of immunologic proof of clonality [68]. Pseudolymphoma of the lung is characterized pathologically by the presence of a mixed cellular infiltrate (mature lymphocytes predominating), the presence of germinal centers, and regional lymph nodes free of lymphoma. Nonetheless, it often is difficult to distinguish pulmonary pseudolymphoma, lymphoma, and other lymphoid neoplasms and infiltrates by simple histologic examination [96,118]. In the study of 161 cases of primary non-Hodgkin's lymphomas of the lung, pseudolymphoma was observed in 14 percent [96]. Pulmonary manifestations consist of well-delineated nodules, segmental parenchymal consolidation, or diffuse interstitial infiltration. Pulmonary pseudolymphoma is distinguished microscopically from lymphoid interstitial pneumonia by the diffuse infiltrative nature of the latter [53]. Localized lesions are best treated by resection, whereas diffuse lesions may need immunosuppressive therapy.

Angioimmunoblastic Lymphadenopathy

Angioimmunoblastic lymphadenopathy mimics lymphomas. It is a disorder in which diffuse obliteration of the lymph node architecture occurs as a result of proliferation of small vessels and immunoblasts. Both an autoimmune mechanism and a T-cell defect leading to polyclonal B-cell activation have been suggested as possible mechanisms in angioimmunoblastic lymphadenopathy with dysproteinemia. The disease is systemic, and histopathologic features appear benign, although progression to lymphoma is not infrequent [49,116]. Angioimmunoblastic lymphadenopathy usually presents as generalized lymph-adenopathy with hepatosplenomegaly and constitutional symptoms and mimics Hodgkin's disease. Some differentiating features that are present are polyclonal gammopathy, autoimmune hemolytic anemia, and a predilection for men older than 50 years. The chest roentgenographic features are similar to those of Hodgkin's disease and include hilar lymphadenopathy, interstitial infiltrates, and pleural effusion [131,157]. Superior vena caval obstruction has been described [171].

Castleman's Disease

Originally reported as mediastinal lymph node hyperplasia resembling thymoma, Castleman's disease is also described by other terms, including *angiofollicular lymph node hyperplasia, giant lymph node hyperplasia, lymph node hamartoma, benign giant lymphoma, multifollicular lymph node hyperplasia* [173]. The two histologic types of Castleman's disease are the hyaline-vascular (proliferation of hyalinized blood vessels) and plasma-cell (abundance of plasma cells) types. The former accounts for 90 percent of cases and is usually asymptomatic, whereas the latter is associated with systemic manifestations. The disease has no predilection for age, sex, or race. It occurs in the thoracic cage in up to 70 percent of cases [122]. The most common clinical manifestation is the well-defined and lobulated enlargement of anterior mediastinal lymph nodes adjacent to thymus and tracheobronchial tree. Symptoms, when present, are caused by compression of the tracheobronchial tree by enlarged lymph nodes and may include cough, dyspnea, and hemoptysis. Intrapulmonary lesions, nodules, and pleural effusion are uncommon. Computed tomography has shown vascular lesions that are well rounded and lobulated. Surgical resection is curative if the disease is limited to resectable lymph nodes.

Confusion exists in the understanding of Castleman's disease and its relation to other syndromes. Crow-Fukase syndrome, also known as *POEMS syndrome* (*p*olyneuropathy, *o*rganomegaly, *e*ndocrinopathy, *m*onoclonal gammopathy, and *s*kin changes) has been described in association with Castleman's disease [52].

Lymphocytic Interstitial Pneumonitis

Lymphocytic interstitial pneumonitis is characterized by pulmonary parenchymal infiltrates that consist predominantly of small lymphocytes and variable numbers of plasma cells and transformed lymphocytes. Many patients with lymphocytic interstitial pneumonitis have eventually developed lymphomas. Some investigators now believe that all cases of lymphocytic interstitial pneumonitis represent low-grade lymphomas [77]. It is not clear whether the lymphocytic infiltrative lung diseases are premalignant, initially neoplastic, or due to a hypersensitivity reaction with neoplasia developing subsequently. They comprise a poorly defined group in which are included lymphocytic interstitial pneumonitis, immunoblastic lymphadenopathy, plasma cell interstitial pneumonitis, lymphomatoid granulomatosis, and benign lymphocytic angiitis and granulomatosis. The diseases associated with lymphocytic interstitial pneumonitis are listed in Table 60-2. Many of these demonstrate similar histologic features, but involvement of the central nervous system, skin, kidneys, and lymph nodes outside the thorax varies, with a course that may be slow or rapidly fatal.

The original description of lymphocytic interstitial pneumonitis included several cases of lym-

Table 60-2. Differential diagnosis of lymphocytic interstitial pneumonitis

Hodgkin's lymphoma
Non-Hodgkin's lymphoma
Lymphomatoid granulomatosis
Chronic lymphocytic leukemia
Waldenstrom's macroglobulinemia
Angioimmunoblastic lymphadenopathy
Sézary syndrome
Pseudolymphoma
Sjögren's syndrome
Acquired immunodeficiency syndrome (AIDS)
Children of mothers at high risk for AIDS
Graft-versus-host disease
Congenital agammaglobulinemia
Chronic active hepatitis
Primary biliary cirrhosis
Crohn's regional enteritis
Nontropical sprue
Myasthenia gravis
Autoimmune hemolytic anemia
Systemic lupus erythematosus
Chronic thyroiditis
Idiopathic

phoma. It is likely that many of the earlier cases diagnosed as lymphocytic interstitial pneumonitis are actually low-grade lymphomas [68]. Therefore, many disease entities that demonstrate lymphocytic interstitial pneumonitis (e.g., lymphomatoid granulomatosis, Sjögren's syndrome) should be considered lymphoproliferative disorders.

The occurrence of lymphocytic interstitial pneumonitis in patients with AIDS is well recognized. This pneumonitis occurs frequently in children of mothers who are at high risk for developing AIDS.

Plasma Cell Disorders

Many plasma cell disorders may present with monoclonal gammopathy and abnormal proliferation of plasma cells. Monoclonal gammopathies are found in patients with multiple myeloma, lymphoproliferative disorders, Waldenstrom's macroglobulinemia, and amyloidosis. Monoclonal gammopathy can be seen in other diseases, including infection and nonhematologic malignancies, and in healthy subjects older than 70 years. In a study of 52 patients (mean age, 64 years; range, 36 to 84 years) with monoclonal gammopathy, the presence of the monoclonal gammopathy led to the diagnosis of multiple myeloma or a lymphoproliferative disorder affecting the chest in 19 percent [26]. The plasma cell dyscrasias discussed here include amyloidosis, Waldenstrom's macroglobulinemia, multiple myeloma, and heavy-chain disease.

Amyloidosis

Amyloidosis is a plasma cell disease of unknown etiology, characterized pathologically by the extracellular deposition of acellular fibrils derived from the light chain of a monoclonal immunoglobulin. In primary amyloidosis, 35 to 70 percent of cases show roentgenographic evidence of amyloid deposition in the lung, whereas in secondary amyloidosis, pulmonary involvement is rare. A review, in 1983, of 126 reported cases of primary localized amyloidosis of the lower respiratory tract revealed the following pulmonary abnormalities: hilar or mediastinal lymphadenopathy in 5 percent, tracheobronchial multifocal submucosal plaques in 45 percent, tracheobronchial amyloid tumor-like masses in 8 percent, discrete nodules in the pulmonary parenchyma in 44 percent, and diffuse alveolar septal amyloidosis in 3 percent [192]. Hilar and mediastinal lymph-

adenopathy have been noted as well [193]. Pleural effusion is uncommon [91].

Pulmonary amyloidosis may be classified into several groups, as shown in Table 60-3. Macroglossia associated with amyloidosis has been reported to cause airway obstruction and sleep apnea [66]. Laryngeal and subglottic deposition of amyloid may contribute to the airway obstruction (Fig. 60-11). Diffuse tracheobronchial submucosal plaques result in generalized narrowing of the tracheobronchial tree with progressive stridor, dyspnea, cough, atelectasis, and hemoptysis

Table 60-3. Pulmonary amyloidosis

Type	Pulmonary symptoms
Macroglossia	Sleep apnea
Laryngeal and subglottic (localized, stenotic)	Stridor, dyspnea
Diffuse tracheobronchial (submucosal plaques)	Stridor, dyspnea, hemoptysis
Localized tracheobronchial (masslike lesions)	Stridor, dyspnea, hemoptysis
Diffuse nodular (parenchymal)	Mild symptoms, bronchiectasis, cavitation in 30 percent
Solitary nodular (parenchymal; amyloidoma)	Rare, minimal symptoms, incidental finding
Diffuse parenchymal (septal or interstitial)	Progressive dyspnea, hemoptysis
Mediastinal and hilar lymphadenopathy[a]	Seen in 5 percent of all amyloidoses
Tracheobronchopathia osteoplastica	Late sequelae of tracheobronchial submucosal amyloid, collapse of airways
Secondary[b]	Incidental (biopsy or autopsy finding, asymptomatic)
Senile	Incidental (autopsy or biopsy finding, asymptomatic)
Malignancy associated[c]	Incidental

[a]Sometimes associated with multiple myeloma.
[b]Associated with tuberculosis, syphilis, bronchiectasis, and hypergammaglobulinemia.
[c]Pulmonary malignancy, carcinoid, and amyloid associated with medullary thyroid carcinoma.

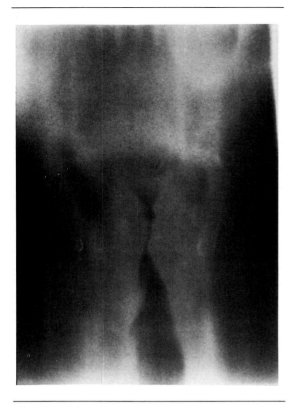

Fig. 60-11. Tracheal tomogram demonstrates amyloidosis involving subglottic and upper trachea.

[18,188]. Bronchoscopic examination will reveal submucosal elevation of the tracheobronchial mucosa, pale, shiny ridges, and areas of stenoses with various degrees of luminal narrowing. A deep submucosal bronchoscopic biopsy of the submucosal area will yield the diagnosis.

Tracheobronchial amyloidosis is an indolent form of disease. However, hemoptysis and stridor can pose life-threatening emergencies. In contrast to the submucosal variety, localized tracheobronchial amyloidosis will exhibit, on bronchoscopy, endobronchial tumor-like amyloid masses that are usually polypoid and solitary and occur only in major bronchi. Secondary changes may include atelectasis, obstructive emphysema, or obstructive pneumonitis or bronchiectasis [57,107]. Fatal bronchopulmonary hemorrhage has been described in a case of laryngotracheal amyloidosis [175].

The lower respiratory tract often is involved in systemic primary amyloidosis and, occasionally,

disease is restricted to that region. The lower respiratory involvement may manifest as nodular changes or diffuse infiltrations. Amyloid nodules in the pulmonary parenchyma tend to be peripheral and to grow slowly, may be solitary (amyloidoma) or multiple (Fig. 60-12), and cavitate in one-third of patients. In some cases, the nodules undergo cavitation or calcification [192].

The diffuse alveolar septal form of pulmonary parenchymal amyloidosis usually is associated with systemic amyloidosis and carries the worst prognosis of all types of pulmonary amyloidosis (Fig. 60-13) [81]. Impaired gas transfer and a progressively restrictive type of pulmonary function abnormality are common. Diffuse deposition of interstitial amyloid in autonomic nervous system alveolar walls can be demonstrated in lung biopsy (Fig. 60-14). Electron-microscopic studies show that the deposition of amyloid is confined to the interstitial space of alveolar septa and that capillaries are involved in the later stages [161]. Involvement of pulmonary vasculature in amyloidosis may cause hemoptysis as a result of medical dissection of pulmonary arteries [167].

Localized deposits of amyloid can occur in the lower respiratory tract. In the tumor-forming kind of amyloidosis, solitary or multiple nodules develop within pulmonary parenchyma [108]. A

Fig. 60-12. Localized amyloidosis (amyloidoma) of right lower lobe treated by surgical resection.

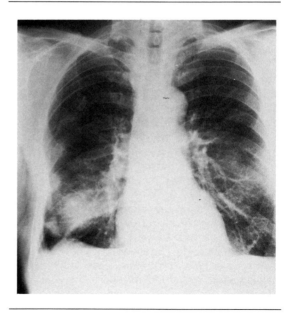

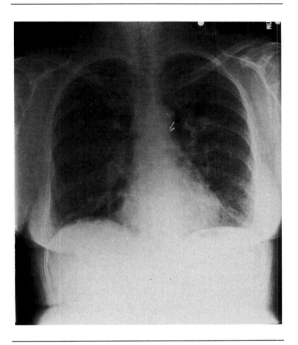

Fig. 60-13. Diffuse parenchymal amyloidosis showing basal interstitial infiltrates.

solitary amyloid nodule (amyloidoma) of the respiratory tract is very unusual, may grow very slowly, and may mimic lung cancer.

Systemic amyloidosis has an unfavorable prognosis, with median survivals of approximately 12 months. The degree of pulmonary embarrassment seems to be related to the amount of amyloid in the gas diffusion zones. Congestive cardiac failure with secondary pulmonary edema may contribute to the pulmonary infiltrations in these patients [27,51].

The prognosis is much better for the nodular pulmonary parenchymal type than for the tracheobronchial obstructive or diffuse interstitial forms of amyloidosis. The latter often leads to death from respiratory insufficiency. Localized tracheobronchial amyloidosis may respond to repeated bronchoscopic Nd : YAG or carbon dioxide laser photoresection [16,48]. However, diffuse involvement of the airway may pose a formidable problem.

Although it has been suggested that tracheobronchopathia osteoplastica is the end result of tracheal amyloidosis or other metabolic diseases, the literature fails to support this contention. Diaphragmatic myopathy from amyloidosis infiltration may result in respiratory failure [185].

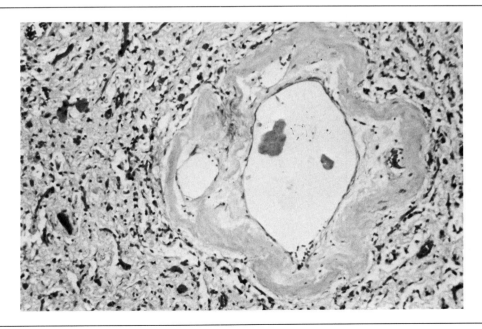

Fig. 60-14. Amyloid deposits surrounding pulmonary blood vessels in primary amyloidosis.

Secondary localized amyloidosis of the lower respiratory tract has been noted in tuberculosis, syphilis, hypogammaglobulinemia, malignancies (usually pulmonary), and carcinoid [192].

Waldenstrom's Macroglobulinemia

Waldenstrom's macroglobulinemia is an uncommon disorder characterized by monoclonal IgM gammopathy, anemia, and lymphocytic or plasmacytic infiltration of bone marrow. Pleuropulmonary involvement is relatively common in Waldenstrom's macroglobulinemia. Among a series of 20 cases, 5 exhibited abnormalities—pleural effusion in 1 and asymmetric nodular lesions in the other 4 [206]. Biopsies showed infiltration of lungs by lymphocytes and plasmacytes in four cases, and roentgenograms demonstrated significant radiographic clearing in three [206]. Characteristically, the chest roentgenogram shows a diffuse reticulonodular pattern and, occasionally, local homogeneous consolidation (Fig. 60-15). Other studies have shown that pleural effusion is present in nearly 50 percent of patients with Waldenstrom's macroglobulinemia. Whereas pleural effusion is common, chylothorax is a rare occurrence in this disease. Plasmapheresis can cause

Fig. 60-15. Bilateral lower-lung infiltrates associated with a large right pleural effusion in Waldenstrom's macroglobulinemia.

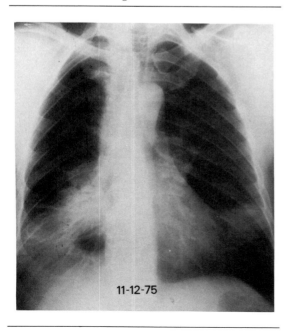

11-12-75

transudative pleural effusion in patients who were previously hemodynamically compensated at high levels of colloid oncotic pressure, as has been noted in a patient with Waldenstrom's macroglobulinemia.

In a literature review by Rausch and Herion [165], in 1980, of pulmonary complications of Waldenstrom's macroglobulinemia documented by biopsy of pleura or lung (or both) in 44 patients (26 men; ages 33 to 84 years; median age, 64 years), mass lesions were noted in 50 percent, infiltrates in 70 percent, and pleural effusions in 43 percent. Mediastinal lymphadenopathy was associated with pulmonary disease in 25 percent. Fifty-five percent of patients had two or more of these manifestations. Dyspnea (54 percent), nonproductive cough (33 percent), and chest pain (7 percent) were the main pulmonary symptoms, whereas 15 percent of patients were asymptomatic. Many had pulmonary manifestations at the time of initial disease. Respiratory involvement appeared 2 to 67 months after the diagnosis of Waldenstrom's macroglobulinemia in two-thirds [165].

Pulmonary manifestations respond to alkylating agents, corticosteroids, and radiation, and do not appear to affect prognosis adversely. Nineteen of the 31 patients responded to chlorambucil given alone or with corticosteroids. Bronchoalveolar lavage studies in a patient with diffuse pulmonary involvement from Waldenstrom's macroglobulinemia have shown abnormal plasma cells (10 to 47 percent), lymphocytes (60 percent), and myeloma protein in the lavage effluent [42,123].

Multiple Myeloma

Usually defined as a malignant neoplasm of plasma cells, multiple myeloma is manifested primarily by widespread skeletal destruction and frequently is associated with anemia, hypercalcemia, and impairment of renal function. Pulmonary manifestations are a rare initial feature of multiple myeloma. The chest roentgenographic finding of a plasmacytoma is typically that of a homogeneous mass associated with an osteolytic rib lesion, with the mass normally protruding into the thoracic cage (Fig. 60-16). Pulmonary parenchymal involvement by the abnormal plasma cells is a rare occurrence [94]. However, disseminated pulmonary infiltrates in a patient with lambda light-chain myeloma were shown, postmortem, to be the result of infiltration by neoplastic plasma cells with crystalline casts, similar to those found in myelomatous kidney [75].

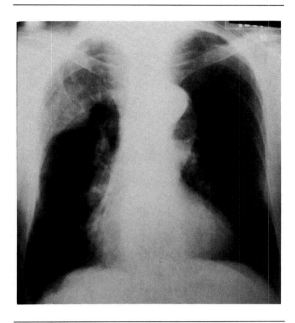

Fig. 60-16. Multiple myeloma involving right upper ribs with protrusion of the bony tumor into the chest cavity.

Solitary plasmacytoma of the upper respiratory tract or the pulmonary parenchyma may occur. Primary tracheal plasmacytoma, when present, appears as a solitary or multiple mass of homogeneous density. Unusual manifestations reported include nonosseous pleural lesions, pleural effusions, chylothorax, and pulmonary parenchymal calcification.

Pulmonary Complications in Bone Marrow Transplantation

Pulmonary complications occur in 40 to 60 percent of patients with bone marrow transplants and are serious and often life-threatening problems [20,37,190]. One of the contributing factors is that pulmonary functions usually are suboptimal even before bone marrow transplantation, owing to multiple episodes of infections, cytotoxic chemotherapy, and total-body irradiation. The pulmonary complications seen in bone marrow transplantation can be broadly classified as early and late (Table 60-4).

Infections

Pneumonia complicates approximately half of all bone marrow transplantations and, in approxi-

Table 60-4. Pulmonary complications following bone marrow transplantation

Clinical and roentgenographic features	Differential diagnosis
Early[a]	
Pulmonary edema	Fluid overload
	Myocardial injury
	Acute hemorrhagic edema (cyclosporine-toxicity)
	Transfusion reactions
Adult respiratory distress syndrome	Septicemia
	Pulmonary edema
	Idiopathic
Bronchopneumonia	Bacterial
	Fungal (aspergillosis, candidiasis)
	Viral (cytomegalovirus)
Interstitial pneumonitis	Idiopathic
	Infectious (*Pneumocystis carinii,* cytomegalovirus)
	Pulmonary embolism
	Veno-occlusive disease
Late[b]	
Bronchopneumonia	Bacterial
	Viral
	Fungal
	Protozoal (*Pneumocystis carinii*)
	Pulmonary embolism (fat embolism)
	Veno-occlusive disease
Interstitial pneumonitis	Nonspecific interstitial pneumonitis
	Bronchiolitis obliterans
	Lymphocytic interstitial pneumonitis

[a]Occurring within 100 days of transplantation.
[b]Occurring 100 days or more after transplantation.

mately one-third of the cases, no specific cause is identified [126]. The incidence of pneumonia is higher among older patients. Overall, 15 to 20 percent of all bone marrow transplant recipients develop cytomegalovirus pneumonia, generally between 50 to 60 days after transplantation. Pneumonia from cytomegalovirus carries a mortality rate of approximately 90 percent. Risk factors for developing cytomegalovirus pneumonia include advanced age of patients, seropositivity of patients, multiple blood transfusions, and presence of severe graft-versus-host disease. Cytomegalovirus pneumonia is uncommon in recipients of autologous or syngeneic bone marrow transplants. Early diagnosis and treatment using newer antiviral agents have shown some improvement in survival. Other viral infections, including herpes simplex, parainfluenza, and the respiratory syncytial viruses are uncommon in patients undergoing bone marrow transplantation. Bacterial pneumonias are common in these patients. Infection by *Chlamydia* species has been noted [127]. Unusual bacteria such as *Cunninghamella* and *Branhamella* species also are being recognized in these patients.

Bacterial pneumonia is uncommon during the early stages after bone marrow transplantation. However, the overall incidence of bacterial pneumonia in this group of patients is 20 to 50 percent [37]. During the early granulocytopenic period, gram-negative organisms predominate, although the possibility of gram-positive infections cannot be excluded. Most late cases of bacterial pneumonia (occurring more than 6 months after bone marrow transplantation) are encountered in patients with graft-versus-host disease. Routine prophylaxis with antibiotics is recommended to prevent these episodes.

The incidence of fungal infections after bone marrow transplantation has increased partly because of widespread use of antibiotics, high-dose corticosteroid therapy, and the prolonged duration of granulocytopenia induced by cytotoxic therapy. Fungal infections of the lung are more likely in neutropenic patients receiving broad-spectrum antibiotics. Infections caused by *Aspergillus* species are the most common and most lethal. Infections by *Candida albicans* and the zygomycetes as well as other fungi are also seen [11,37].

Among 271 consecutive patients treated with bone marrow transplantation during a 9-year interval, *Aspergillus* pneumonia was noted in 36 percent; the crude mortality for these patients was 95 percent [143]. Invasive aspergillosis may present with fever, dyspnea, cough, pleuritic chest pain, and hemoptysis. Chest roentgenologic abnormalities include diffuse or focal interstitial infiltrates, triangular peripheral infiltrates due to infarction, and cavitated lesions. Mortality in bone marrow transplant recipients approaches 80 to 90 percent. The diagnosis is established by documentation of fungal invasion of the pulmonary parenchyma, although the presence of

Aspergillus species in respiratory secretions in the appropriate clinical setting may be highly suggestive.

Tracheobronchial aspergillosis is another serious complication in neutropenic and other immunocompromised patients, including those with AIDS, and recipients of a lung or heart-lung transplant [24,35,82,97]. In the latter group, the tracheobronchial anastomotic sites seem particularly affected by the process. Clinically, cough, upper airway wheezes, and progressive dyspnea are present in most patients. Respiratory failure can result from tracheobronchial obstruction. Bronchoscopy is both diagnostic and initially therapeutic in the relief of dyspnea by removal of the obstructing pseudomembrane secondary to tracheobronchial aspergillosis.

Results of clinical trials in which aerosolized amphotericin B, in doses varying from 5 mg to 100 mg, or oral itraconazole has been used prophylactically suggest that in high-risk patients these treatments are well tolerated and efficacious in preventing disseminated tracheobronchial aspergillosis [35]. Various preparations of liposomal amphotericin B and newer agents such as fluconazole and itraconazole appear promising in improving the prognosis in patients predisposed to develop invasive and tracheobronchial aspergillosis.

Mycobacterial infections are uncommon after allogeneic bone marrow transplantation, although several cases of infections caused by *Mycobacterium avium-intracellulare* have been described [141]. The incidence of *P. carinii* pneumonia in bone marrow transplant recipients has significantly diminished, with only 4 percent of cases of interstitial pneumonitis in these patients being caused by *P. carinii*. Prophylactic administration of trimethoprim-sulfamethoxazole prior to bone marrow transplantation and after marrow engraftment has virtually eliminated *P. carinii* pneumonia in bone marrow recipients [125].

Pulmonary Edema

Pulmonary edema is perhaps the earliest and most common complication of bone marrow transplantation. This phenomenon is seen usually 2 to 3 weeks postoperatively. The etiology for the pulmonary edema includes fluid overload, cardiac dysfunction due to chemotherapy with doxorubicin hydrochloride (Adriamycin), transfusion-related acute lung injury, graft-versus-host disease, fat embolism syndrome, renal dysfunction and, occasionally, irradiation [72,93,98,151]. Congestive cardiomyopathy associated with the use of Adriamycin and daunorubicin is dose-dependent (550 mg/m²).

The pulmonary edema and cytomegalovirus pneumonia have similar chest roentgenographic appearances. Pulmonary edema, both cardiogenic and noncardiogenic, is rapid in onset and occurs between the second and third week posttransplantation, whereas cytomegalovirus infection is seen 4 to 6 weeks after transplantation. Hemorrhagic pulmonary edema is more likely in those receiving mismatched transplants and high doses of cyclosporine. It also may result from fluid retention, hypoalbuminemia, hypotension, and incipient renal failure. Pulmonary edema in bone marrow transplant patients is critically related to fluid balance and can be prevented by careful clinical examination, close monitoring of weight change, avoidance of fluid overload, and appropriate diuretic therapy.

Fig. 60-17. Idiopathic interstitial pneumonitis in a bone marrow transplant recipient has the pattern of diffuse alveolar damage. Mild thickening and inflammatory infiltrate of alveolar septa lined by type II pneumocytes as well as edema fluid, exudate, and macrophages are present in the alveoli.

Interstitial Pneumonitis

The most serious threat after bone marrow transplantation is nonspecific interstitial pneumonitis (Fig. 60-17), seen in 35 to 50 percent of recipients of allogeneic transplants and in approximately 20 percent of syngeneic or autologous bone marrow transplants, with an attendant mortality rate of nearly 75 percent [4,126,201]. In approximately 50 percent of these patients, an infectious agent, particularly cytomegalovirus, is involved. Progressive dyspnea, cough, end-inspiratory crackles, interstitial infiltrates on chest roentgenogram, and hypoxemia occurring 40 to 75 days after grafting should strongly suggest interstitial pneumonitis.

Computed tomography of the thorax is superior to regular chest roentgenography in evaluating pulmonary complications after bone marrow transplantation [59]. Active cytomegalovirus infection has been present in more than 50 percent of these patients and accounts for the majority of cases of interstitial pneumonitis after bone marrow transplantation.

Factors contributing to the development of this serious complication include the following: older patients for whom there is a long interval between primary diagnosis of leukemia and bone

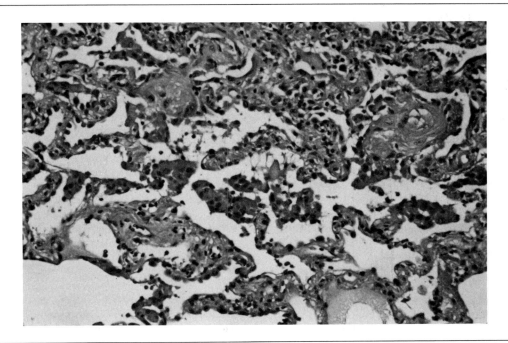

marrow transplantation and who are then treated with cyclosporine and develop graft-versus-host disease; HLA disparity; graft-versus-host disease; and combined chemotherapy and radiation therapy prior to transplantation [54,105]. The probability of developing interstitial pneumonitis from radiation during the first year is approximately 31 percent [100]. High-dose radiation therapy results in significantly reduced diffusing capacity for carbon monoxide for the first 3 months, followed by some improvement over a 2- to 3-year period [4].

Obstructive Lung Disease

Obstructive lung disease in bone marrow transplant patients is a well-recognized entity. Although airway problems usually are the result of the mucosal toxicity of the conditioning regimen, it is possible that different pathologic mechanisms contribute to the pathogenesis of obstructive lung disease in the setting of transplantation. Positive or borderline response to metacholine, seen in 20 percent of patients prior to bone marrow transplantation, is not associated with the development of either clinical or pathologically proved posttransplantation bronchiolitis obliterans [99].

Rapidly progressive obstructive pulmonary disease has developed 9 months to 2 years after bone marrow transplantation [23]. Sinusitis, bronchitis, and esophageal dysfunction are common in these patients, and lung biopsy has revealed obliterative bronchiolitis. Graft-versus-host disease is believed to be responsible for the airways pathology [89,162]. Lymphocytic bronchitis manifested by lymphocytic infiltration of the bronchial mucosa, loss of cilia and goblet cells, and occasional necrosis of mucosa and submucosa, and presenting with severe cough and dyspnea may be seen in more than 25 percent of posttransplantation patients. These features are the result of previous chemotherapy rather than graft-versus-host disease [135]. Obstructive lung disease seems to worsen with the passage of time, and a mortality rate of 65 percent at 3 years after transplantation has been noted [23].

Pretransplantation pulmonary dysfunction is a strong predictor and risk factor for the posttransplantation development of cytomegalovirus pneumonia and an interstitial process [85]. Pulmonary function tests performed before and after bone marrow transplantation in leukemic and aplastic anemic patients have shown that in leukemic patients, obstructive disorders of ventilation develop or, if already present, worsen. A case

series review of 1297 bone marrow transplant recipients observed that a decreased diffusing capacity for carbon monoxide in the lung and increased alveolar-arterial oxygen tension gradient before bone marrow transplantation carry a significantly increased risk of death after transplantation [28]. In addition, respiratory failure requiring assisted mechanical ventilation occurred in 23 percent [28].

Bronchiolitis Obliterans

Bronchiolitis obliterans, another form of obstructive lung disease, is now a recognized complication of bone marrow transplantation and occurs in up to 15 percent of all bone marrow transplant recipients (Fig. 60-18). Though it is believed to be more common after allogeneic bone marrow transplantation, bronchiolitis obliterans has occurred after autologous bone marrow transplantation [146]. Bronchiolitis obliterans was originally reported in the context of graft-versus-host disease, but the etiology may be multifactorial, including viral infection, other infections, irradiation, and recurrent gastroesophageal reflux. Bronchiolitis obliterans occurs within 5 months of bone marrow transplantation. Clinically, the patient develops dyspnea, cough, hyperinflation of the thoracic cage on chest roentgenogram, and reduced elastic recoil pressure. The clinical course is variable with a high mortality, although some patients may respond to corticosteroids and azathioprine [89,114,140,162].

Pulmonary Veno-Occlusive Disease

Although pulmonary vascular abnormalities are discovered histologically in as many as 50 percent of postmortem cases of bone marrow transplantation, the pathologic role such lesions play in causing pulmonary alveolar hemorrhage and other pulmonary processes is unclear. Pulmonary embolism is uncommon in bone marrow transplant recipients [37]. Pulmonary veno-occlusive disease has been observed in patients receiving chemotherapy and after bone marrow transplantation [144,196]. The other possible etiologic factors responsible for pulmonary veno-occlusive disease include irradiation, multiple high-dose chemotherapy, and acute graft-versus-host disease. Clinical features in these patients include progressive dyspnea along with signs of right-sided congestive cardiac failure. High-dose corticosteroids have been used with favorable results.

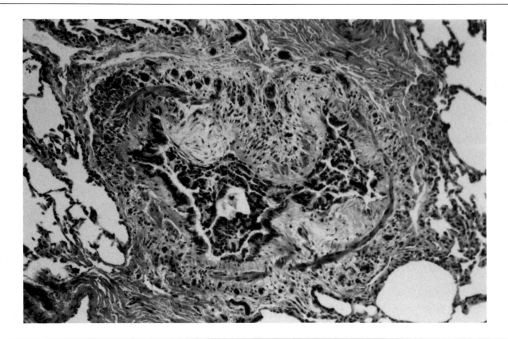

Fig. 60-18. Bronchiolitis obliterans–associated progressive airflow obstruction following bone marrow transplantation. Note fibrous thickening of the submucosa and distortion of the muscularis with resultant compromise in the bronchiolar lumen.

Graft-Versus-Host Disease

The graft-versus-host disease is peculiar to recipients of organ transplantation. Three requirements for the development of graft-versus-host disease are (1) histocompatibility of the host and the effector cells of this process (commonly introduced through transplantation of lymphohematologic tissues or transfusion of blood containing viable lymphocytes), (2) the immunocompetence of the host, and (3) the capability of effector cells to proliferate and attack host tissues protractedly in vivo [197,204]. Graft-versus-host disease is believed to result because donor T lymphocytes recognize the recipient's tissue as foreign and, therefore, mount an immune response and damage them. Both acute and chronic graft-versus-host disease can be seen. In recipients of bone marrow transplants, graft-versus-host disease is encountered in 35 to 75 percent of patients with leukemia [195,204], as compared to 50 percent of those with aplastic anemia [13,186]. In patients given bone marrow transplants from HLA-identical siblings and posttransplantation immunosuppression, approximately 50 percent develop moderate to severe graft-versus-host disease. Recipients of kidney, liver, heart, and other organs have a much lower risk of developing this problem.

Pulmonary involvement in graft-versus-host disease is less common than that of skin, gastrointestinal tract, and liver. Clinical features include dry nonproductive cough, symptoms of hyperreactive airways, obstructive or restrictive pulmonary dysfunction, and patchy interstitial infiltrates on chest roentgenograms. Lymphocytic bronchitis has been reported in 25 percent of allogeneic bone marrow transplant recipients at necropsy [10]. The lymphocytic bronchitis may be complicated by bronchopneumonia, frequently due to *Pseudomonas aeruginosa*. The latter is presumably a result of obstruction of bronchi from necrotic bronchial mucosa. Interstitial pneumonitis may include infiltrates made of lymphocytes, histiocytes, plasma cells, and immunoblasts. Lymphocytic interstitial pneumonitis is another late complication of bone marrow transplantation [148], but the relationship between lymphocytic interstitial pneumonitis and graft-versus-host disease is uncertain.

The time of onset of pulmonary symptoms and signs and chest roentgenographic abnormalities after bone marrow transplantation has diagnostic importance (see Table 60-4). During the first 2 postoperative weeks, pulmonary edema and some bacterial infections cause problems, whereas most cases of interstitial pneumonitis, including infections by cytomegalovirus and *P. carinii*, occur after 100 days. Pulmonary embolism from fat and bone fragments collected during bone marrow harvest cause embolic phenomena at the small pulmonary arterial level and produce transient hypoxemia. In addition, the endothelial damage from radiation therapy and cytotoxic chemotherapy also may predispose to thrombosis of pulmonary vasculature [196].

Alveolar Hemorrhage Syndrome

Diffuse pulmonary alveolar hemorrhage may occur in recipients of autologous bone marrow transplants. Among a group of 141 consecutive autologous bone marrow transplant recipients, pulmonary alveolar hemorrhage was detected in 21 percent [168]. Further details of this complication are discussed in Chapter 61.

Mediastinal Emphysema

Among 146 patients who underwent bone marrow transplantation over a 2-year period, six cases of mediastinal emphysema were reported; 5 of the latter group of patients had or eventually developed interstitial pneumonitis, and 5 died of respiratory failure [80]. None of the patients was mechanically ventilated prior to the development of mediastinal emphysema. However, they had received higher doses of radiation than the others during the conditioning procedure.

Transfusion and the Lung

The use of blood and blood products, even under the best circumstances, carries considerable risk for the recipient. Immediate pulmonary reactions include dyspnea, bronchospasm, and pulmonary edema. It should be emphasized that pulmonary edema following blood transfusion need not be the result of overloading the circulation. In addition to the blood and blood products, patients receive crystalloid solutions and other drugs via the intravenous route. Transfusion-related acute lung injury and the postperfusion syndrome are discussed here.

Transfusion-Related Acute Lung Injury

Transfusion-related acute lung injury (TRALI) is a form of noncardiogenic pulmonary edema. Earlier cases of transient pulmonary edema during blood transfusions were attributed to incompatibility of an undetermined nature, and further studies implicated increased capillary permeability due to leukoagglutinins in the pathogenesis of pulmonary edema [191,199]. Studies strongly support the concept that passive transfusion of granulocyte or lymphocyte antibodies, or both, in donor sera is the more common setting for this unusual reaction [151]. These antibodies in the donor serum may activate granulocytes and complements. The use of therapeutic or prophylactic granulocyte transfusion has been associated with the development of cytomegalovirus pneumonia. Granulocyte transfusion in association with amphotericin B or in the setting of endotoxemia has been associated with acute respiratory failure.

The incidence of TRALI may be underestimated. A review of 36 cases over a 2-year period at the Mayo Clinic indicated an incidence of 0.02 percent per unit and 0.16 percent per patient transfused. The clinical features are dramatic. Acute respiratory distress within 4 hours after transfusion (in most cases, after 2 hours) is the sine qua non of this syndrome. Other findings include acute onset of chills, fever, tachycardia, nonproductive cough, and blood eosinophilia [199]. Roentgenograms show patchy opacities in the perihilar and lower-lung regions (Fig. 60-19). Although recovery is rapid and complete in 81 percent, some form of respiratory support may be required in more than two-thirds of the patients. Pulmonary infiltrates and hypoxemia have persisted for 7 days in 17 percent of patients. Granulocyte antibodies in the serum of at least 1 unit of donor blood were demonstrated in 89 percent of cases, whereas lymphocytotoxic antibodies were present in 72 percent [199].

Postperfusion Syndrome

Pulmonary complications not uncommonly follow prolonged cardiopulmonary bypass. This postperfusion syndrome also is known as *pump lung, perfusion lung,* and *postperfusion atelectasis.* Although some investigations have suggested an immunologic mechanism, the exact etiology remains unknown. After prolonged maintenance on cardiopulmonary bypass, patients develop progressive pulmonary insufficiency that

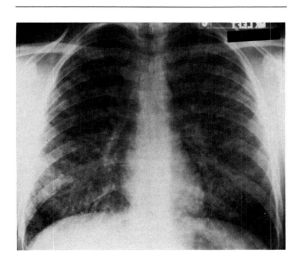

Fig. 60-19. Diffuse bilateral soft nodular infiltrates as a result of transfusion-related acute lung injury.

is manifested by cyanosis, hypoxemia, increased work of breathing due to severely diminished compliance, and widening of the alveolar-arterial oxygen tension gradient. Chest roentgenograms usually reveal patchy, diffuse alveolar infiltrates whose appearance resembles that of pulmonary edema. Pathologic changes are similar to those seen in the respiratory distress syndrome, which may complicate shock and hemorrhage.

Causes that contribute to the postperfusion lung syndrome include hypoxia, interruption of blood supply to pulmonary tissues (especially to alveolar cells), loss of surfactant, interaction of homologous blood with a pump gas exchanger, and an underlying pulmonary disease process.

Prevention of the postperfusion syndrome is very important, because treatment is not promising. Corticosteroids given early may help, but the results are similar to those seen in the respiratory distress syndrome from other causes.

Pulmonary Eosinophilic Granuloma (Histiocytosis X) and Other Histiocytic Reticulocytoses

Pulmonary eosinophilic granuloma, or primary pulmonary histiocytosis X, is a granulomatous disease of unknown etiology characterized by abnormal proliferation of histiocytes and an unpredictable natural history, although the disease usu-ally exhibits a slowly progressive course [152]. Pulmonary eosinophilic granuloma belongs to the group of diseases collectively known as *histiocytic reticulocytosis* or *histiocytic reticuloendotheliosis;* the latter category of disorders includes Letterer-Siwe disease (acute disseminated histiocytosis X), Hand-Schüller-Christian disease (chronic disseminated histiocytosis X), and localized histiocytosis X or eosinophilic granuloma [112]. Others have challenged this unitary concept and have recommended the term *multifocal eosinophilic granuloma* [113]. The Writing Group of the Histiocyte Society [207] has suggested that the syndromes belonging to the histiocytosis X family of diseases be called *Langerhans-cell histiocytosis.*

Pulmonary Eosinophilic Granuloma

HISTOPATHOLOGIC FEATURES
The origin of pulmonary eosinophilic granuloma is unknown. Presence of intramitochondrial crystalline inclusion bodies in the abnormal tissues has suggested a viral etiology, but there has been no documentation that the disease is caused by an infectious agent [158]. An immune mechanism has been suggested because of the presence of circulating immune complexes and granular IgG and complement components (C3) in alveolar walls and pulmonary capillaries. Some studies have reported immunodeficiency in the form of lack of histamine H2 surface receptors on T lymphocytes and deficiency of suppressor cell in some patients [139]. The most striking association, however, is between pulmonary eosinophilic granuloma and tobacco smoking: A history of tobacco smoking has been observed in more than 95 percent of patients with the disorder [25,47,67]. Observations using special staining techniques to diagnose this disorder strongly suggest an immune-mediated mechanism or mechanisms [38]. Macrophage colony-stimulating factor and platelet-derived factor may have a role in initiating and or maintaining pathologic lesions [6].

The effector cell responsible for the disease process originates in the mononuclear phagocyte system. These monocytes, generally referred to as *histiocytes,* are a combination of pigment-laden alveolar macrophages and histiocytosis X cells (H-X cells), which are closely related to Langerhans' cells in normal skin. A Langerhans' cell is seldom, if ever, seen in normal lungs. H-X cells are judged to be reactive or activated Langerhans' cells and, therefore, pulmonary eosinophilic granuloma is considered to represent a pathologic proliferation of Langerhans' cells [21, 92,102]. Electron microscopy shows a common marker organelle (X-body or Birbeck granule) in the H-X cell. These pentalaminar cytoplasmic inclusion bodies are not specific for pulmonary eosinophilic granuloma. They are present also in nearly one-fourth of patients with idiopathic pulmonary fibrosis and hypersensitivity pneumonitis but absent in inorganic pneumoconioses, pulmonary lymphangioleiomyomatosis, and sarcoidosis [152].

Bronchoalveolar lavage studies have observed that H-X cells are not normally present in the alveolar wall and rarely are seen in the bronchiolar wall but may constitute 2 to 20 percent of the effector cells in pulmonary eosinophilic granuloma [92]. Langerhans' cells express surface antigen identified by the monoclonal antibody OKT6 or positive immunoperoxidase staining for S-100 protein, but the latter is not specific for pulmonary eosinophilic granuloma [43,44]. A study utilized the monoclonal OKT6 antibody to label H-X cells obtained from bronchoalveolar lavage in patients with pulmonary eosinophilic granuloma, pulmonary sarcoidosis, and other pulmonary disorders, and noted that all patients with pul-

monary eosinophilic granuloma exhibited the presence of OKT6-reactive cells in their bronchoalveolar effluent.

Gross morphologic features in the early phase of the disease include widespread subpleural nodules that measure 2 to 10 mm or more and a varying number of small, irregular cystic lesions. The nodules contain a wide variety of cells, including cells with large vesicular nuclei, cells with vacuolated cytoplasm, giant cells, histiocytes, lymphocytes, eosinophils, and polymorphonuclear leukocytes, and the degree of lymphocytic and plasma cell infiltration, extent of eosinophilia, number of foam cells, and amount of necrosis or fibrosis vary considerably from lesion to lesion (Figs. 60-20, 60-21) [207]. The histiocytes fuse to form multinucleate giant cells, which results in the accumulation of so-called foam cells, vacuolated histiocytes with sudanophilic material in the cytoplasm. Langerhans' bodies and fibrils are apparent also in cytoplasm. The H-X cells are seen in large numbers in acute and active forms of the disease, decreasing in number as the disease becomes chronic. Fibrosis

Fig. 60-20. The earliest lesions of pulmonary eosinophilic granuloma are central lobular proliferations of cells along small bronchioles and alveolar ducts, seen here as a small parenchymal nodule.

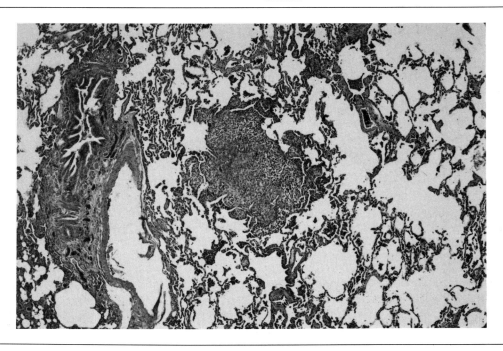

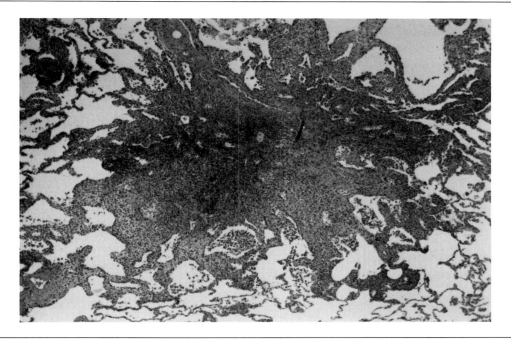

Fig. 60-21. In established cases of pulmonary eosinophilic granuloma, the classic lesion is a stellate nodule with central pigmentation and scarring and peripheral cellularity in which Langerhans' histiocytes can be found.

eventually replaces the granulomatous process, and formation of characteristic honeycomb cysts occurs. Nonspecific pulmonary fibrosis is the end result.

INCIDENCE AND CLINICAL AND LABORATORY FINDINGS

Pulmonary eosinophilic granuloma is usually a disease of adults and is more commonly limited to the lungs or the bones or both. More than 1000 cases have been reported, and more than 300 of these have displayed diffuse abnormalities on chest roentgenography and an interstitial pulmonary process on pathologic examination [152]. The incidence of the disease is unknown. Most patients are 20 to 40 years old, and the male-to-female ratio is approximately equal, although most series have shown a slight male predominance [25,47]. The disorder occurs most frequently in Caucasians, is rare in blacks, and is never reported in Asians. Familial incidence has been reported in one instance [25].

Nearly one-fourth of patients with pulmonary eosinophilic granuloma are asymptomatic, the disease being uncovered by a routine chest roentgenogram. One-third of patients have systemic symptoms such as fatigue, fever, and weight loss. A nonproductive cough is the commonest symptom, observed in nearly 65 percent. Dyspnea and chest pain are the complaints in 40 percent and 25 percent of patients, respectively. Chest pain may be secondary to a spontaneous pneumothorax or an osteolytic rib lesion.

Spontaneous pneumothorax caused by rupture of a subpleural cystic lesion occurs in approximately 10 to 20 percent of patients, and recurrent pneumothorax is observed in some [47]. Pleural effusion is rare and is caused by eosinophilic granuloma of the rib or chronic pneumothorax. Uncommon pulmonary symptoms include hemoptysis and wheezing. A case of endobronchial eosinophilic granuloma in the absence of pulmonary parenchymal disease or other manifestations of eosinophilic granuloma has been reported in a 12-year-old boy who presented with atelectasis of the left lung [136]. Isolated pulmonary eosinophilic granuloma is rare in children, although several cases have been described.

Nonpulmonary manifestations of eosinophilic granuloma described in the literature include diffuse maculopapular skin nodules, solitary or multiple bony lesions, diabetes insipidus (seen in 20 percent of patients), head and neck lesions, otologic involvement, periodontal disease, gynecologic disease, renal disease, hepatic nodules, and hepatic cirrhosis [152]. Two examples are reported of eosinophilic granuloma presenting as lymphadenopathy and apparently being confined to lymph nodes [45].

It is common to observe relatively good pulmonary function even when the chest roentgenogram reveals appreciable pulmonary abnormalities. Up to 15 percent of patients will demonstrate normal lung functions [7]. In contrast, 13 percent of children with pulmonary eosinophilic granuloma and normal chest roentgenograms have had abnormal pulmonary function tests [64]. When present, a restrictive type of pulmonary dysfunction with decreased lung volumes, normal flow rates, and diminished carbon monoxide diffusion capacity is the most common finding. Significant obstructive airways disease, however, is common in advanced cases and may be present in up to 20 percent of patients [47]. Tobacco smoking, peribronchial fibrosis and compression of airways by the cystic lesions, and obliterative bronchiolitis due to infiltration of bronchial walls by cells and granulomas may contribute to airways obstruction. Some patients may present with symptoms of severe airways disease.

Typically, chest roentgenologic abnormalities in pulmonary eosinophilic granuloma are diffuse, bilateral, and most pronounced in the upper two-thirds of the lung fields. Initial stages of the disease may produce a nodular pattern, with lesions ranging from 1 to 12 mm in diameter (Fig. 60-22) [101]. In the later stages of the disease, a reticulonodular pattern and honeycomb appearance, with cysts varying from 5 to 30 mm and averaging less than 1 cm, is typical. The honeycomb pattern, when located in upper lung zones, is highly suggestive of eosinophilic granuloma. Spontaneous pneumothorax may be the first indicator of this condition in 6 to 20 percent of patients (Fig. 60-23). The sparing of costophrenic angles is common, and this roentgenologic sign is considered to indicate good prognosis. Pleural reaction or thickening is uncommon, even in patients with recurrent pneumothoraces. Uncommon chest roentgenologic features reported in pulmonary eosinophilic granuloma include hilar prominence (in fewer than 25 percent), hilar vascular prominence, pulmonary arteries, alveolar consolidation, solitary nodules, cavitation of nodules, and solid mediastinal masses with development of cavitation within the mass, mass lesions

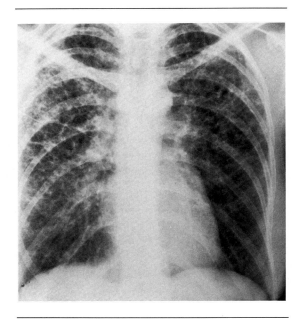

Fig. 60-22. Pulmonary eosinophilic granuloma with diffuse reticulonodular pattern and honeycombing. Upper-lung distribution of the infiltrates is noteworthy.

of the anterior chest wall, and a mass in the neck with tracheal involvement [14,40,152].

DIAGNOSIS

High-resolution computed tomography of the chest is very useful in diagnosing pulmonary eosinophilic granuloma (Fig. 60-24). A study of 18 patients by this technique revealed the following abnormalities: thin-walled cysts in 94 percent, nodules in 78 percent, cavitated nodules in 17 percent, thick-walled cysts in 39 percent, reticulation in 22 percent, ground-glass opacities in 22 percent, and irregular interfaces in 22 percent. The lesions were most often diffuse (89 percent), with a predominant distribution in the upper or middle lung zones in 9 patients (50 percent). Comparison of computed tomography and chest roentgenograms showed that small and large cysts and micronodules were better detected by computed tomography [15,130]. Longitudinal studies in some patients suggested that computed tomographic patterns progressed from nodules to cavitated nodules, thick-walled cysts to cysts, and distinct cysts to confluent cysts. Similar studies have shown that many small nodules are distributed in the centers of secondary

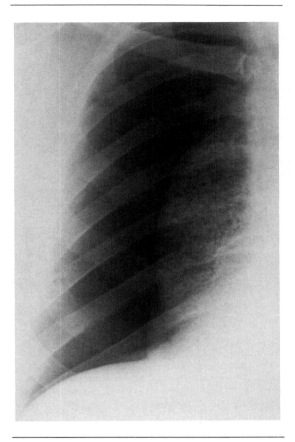

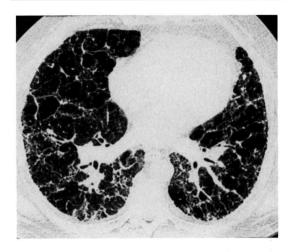

Fig. 60-24. High-resolution computed tomogram of lung in advanced stages of pulmonary eosinophilic granuloma shows extensive cystic changes.

Fig. 60-23. Spontaneous pneumothorax in pulmonary eosinophilic granuloma. Fine honeycombing can be seen in the partially collapsed lung.

lobules around small airways and that computed tomographic findings correlate better with the diffusing capacity than do the chest roentgenologic findings. Dynamic ultrafast high-resolution computed tomography has demonstrated air trapping [183].

The diagnosis of pulmonary eosinophilic granuloma is made on the basis of typical clinical features, chest roentgenologic findings, high-resolution computed tomography of the thorax, bronchoalveolar lavage, and transbronchoscopic lung biopsy. Not every patient requires each of the diagnostic procedures. In the proper clinical setting, many clinicians make the diagnosis on clinical grounds alone. For instance, a young adult man who presents with a spontaneous pneumothorax and in whom the chest roentgen-

ogram reveals diffuse honeycombing or a reticulonodular process is assumed to have pulmonary eosinophilic granuloma unless proved otherwise. The physical examination in patients with pulmonary eosinophilic granuloma may be normal, and therefore it is of little help. Clubbing may be observed in patients with advanced disease and chronic hypoxemia. Lymphadenopathy and hepatosplenomegaly are conspicuously absent in patients with isolated pulmonary eosinophilic granuloma. Routine hematologic and serologic data are generally normal, and sedimentation rate is either normal or only minimally elevated. Peripheral eosinophilia is not a feature of eosinophilic granuloma.

If clinical and roentgenologic features are atypical, bronchoscopy with bronchoalveolar lavage and transbronchoscopic lung biopsy may be necessary. The materials obtained can be subjected to a variety of special techniques to identify the Langerhans' cells (Fig. 60-25). The cells obtained from bronchoalveolar lavage can be studied for the presence of surface antigens using OKT6 monoclonal antibodies, antibodies to S-100 protein, or antibodies to the HLA-DR protein. Although none of these tests is specific for the diagnosis of pulmonary eosinophilic granuloma, the presence of OKT6 monoclonal antibody is most accurate. Presence of more than 5 percent

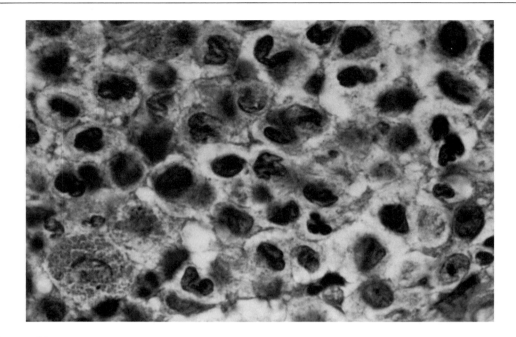

Fig. 60-25. Langerhans' cells of pulmonary eosinophilic granuloma have delicate folded and indented nuclei and are distinct from pulmonary alveolar macrophages. An eosinophil with cytoplasmic granules is seen at lower left.

CD1-positive cells in bronchoalveolar lavage is reported to indicate pulmonary eosinophilic granuloma [2]. As stated earlier, electron microscopy is useful to detect cytoplasmic Langerhans' cell inclusion bodies (Birbeck granules or X-bodies). Electron microscopy can be performed on biopsy material as well as lavage material. Lung biopsy, obtained by either the tracheobronchoscopic route or thoracoscopy or thoracotomy, is an excellent technique to establish the diagnosis.

Letterer-Siwe Disease

Letterer-Siwe disease is almost always encountered in infants and children. The disease becomes manifest before the age of 2 years and is characterized by extensive systemic dissemination and a fulminating, fatal course. However, Letterer-Siwe disease has been reported in 26 adult patients, with involvement of the lungs in half them [29]. If the symptoms appear after the age of 2 years, the 10-year survival rate is 85 percent, and in those who develop symptoms earlier, 10-year survival is 40 percent [62,198].

Hand-Schüller-Christian Disease

Patients with Hand-Schüller-Christian disease may manifest one or all of the classic three signs—exophthalmos, diabetes insipidus, and osteolytic lesions of the skull. The characteristic triad, however, is observed in only 10 percent of children with multifocal eosinophilic granuloma. Hand-Schüller-Christian disease usually becomes apparent during later childhood or adolescence and progresses slowly, so that most patients reach adulthood. Lieberman and associates [113], based on their experience with 113 cases, suggested that the Hand-Schüller-Christian triad is nonspecific and that the term *multifocal eosinophilic granuloma* should be used to describe the abnormalities observed in various organs.

Treatment and Prognosis

Pulmonary eosinophilic granuloma in adults demonstrates a fluctuating course and frequent tendency toward spontaneous resolution. Asymptomatic patients and those with stable chest roentgenologic abnormalities may be observed without specific therapy. Smoking cessation should be stressed [152]. Progressive disease may require prolonged high-dose corticosteroid therapy (prednisone, 0.75 to 1.0 mg/kg/day for 6 to 12 months). In refractory cases, a therapeutic trial of vinca alkaloids (vinblastine or vincristine) has been tried. In children, therapy using vinca alkaloids with or without corticosteroid has proved to be equally efficacious. Expanding or symptomatic bone lesions are treated with steroids, excision and curettage, or radiation. Radiation is not indicated in pulmonary eosinophilic granuloma.

The prognosis is poor in patients with large bullous type lesions, progressive obstructive airways disease, severe hypoxemia, secondary pulmonary hypertension, and involvement of the costophrenic angles on chest roentgenography. The overall prognosis, however, is good in adults with pulmonary eosinophilic granuloma, with mortality rates of less than 5 percent. Indicators of poor prognosis include extremes of age, multiple pneumothoraces, extensive multisystem disease, prolonged constitutional disturbance, extensive cysts or honeycombing on chest roentgenograms, and markedly decreased diffusing capacity for carbon monoxide. Radiation therapy and chemotherapy to treat histiocytosis X may be associated with nearly a 50 percent chance of inducing malignancy, particularly lung cancer and pulmonary lymphoma [62,170,195].

Miscellaneous Hematologic Disorders

Chronic anemia, in addition to its effects on cardiovascular hemodynamics, is known to produce a reduction in the pulmonary diffusing capacity for carbon monoxide. The diffusing capacity decreases approximately 7 percent for each gram per 100-ml decrease in hemoglobin [33]. Before using carbon monoxide diffusing capacity to evaluate lung function, a correction for significant anemia should be made. Studies in anemic patients have demonstrated higher extraction of oxygen from blood, presumably as a result of increased work by the heart.

Paroxysmal nocturnal hemoglobinuria is a hematopoietic stem cell disorder characterized by an increased sensitivity of blood cells to complement-mediated lysis. Vascular thrombosis of pulmonary vasculature and pulmonary hypertension have been described [76].

Autoimmune hemolytic anemia has been shown to be associated with fibrosing alveolitis in two patients, and a possible relationship between autoimmune hemolysis and fibrosing alveolitis has been suggested [172]. Four patients

with "primary" pulmonary hypertension in association with microangiopathic hemolytic anemia and thrombocytopenia have been described [90].

Bare lymphocyte syndrome is characterized by the absence of cell surface HLA-A, HLA-B, and sometimes HLA-C antigens, and is a form of immunodeficiency in infants. The adult form of this syndrome, complicated by chronic sinusitis and bronchiectasis, has been described [187].

Extramedullary hematopoiesis is rare. A case of hematopoiesis occurring in bronchus has been described [58].

References

1. Abernathy D, Beltran G, Stuckey WJ. Lung cancer following treatment of lymphoma. *Am J Med* 81:215, 1986.
2. Auerswald U, Barth J, Magnussen H. Value of CD-1-positive cells in bronchoalveolar lavage fluid for the diagnosis of pulmonary histiocytosis X. *Lung* 169:305, 1991.
3. Bacalo A, et al. Blood transfusion and lung function in children with thalassemia major. *Chest* 101:362, 1992.
4. Barrett A, Depledge MH, Powles RL. Interstitial pneumonitis following bone marrow transplantation after low dose rate total-body irradiation. *Int J Radiat Oncol Biol Phys* 9:1029, 1983.
5. Barrett-Connor E. Pneumonia and pulmonary infarction in sickle cell anemia. *JAMA* 224:997, 1973.
6. Barth J, et al. Increased expression of growth factor genes for macrophages and fibroblasts in bronchoalveolar lavage cells of a patient with pulmonary histiocytosis X. *Thorax* 46:835, 1991.
7. Basset F, et al. Pulmonary histiocytosis-X. *Am Rev Respir Dis* 118:811, 1978.
8. Bedrossian CWM, et al. Alveolar proteinosis as a consequence of immunosuppression: A hypothesis based on clinical and pathologic observations. *Hum Pathol* 11(Suppl):527, 1980.
9. Berglund S, Ohlsson NM. Radiologic pulmonary findings in haemoglobin Malmo and erythrocytosis. *Acta Radiol Diagn* (Stockh) 14:241, 1973.
10. Beschorner WE, et al. Lymphocytic bronchitis associated with graft-versus-host disease in recipients of bone marrow transplants. *N Engl J Med* 299,1030, 1978.
11. Bigby TD, et al. Clinical spectrum of pulmonary mucormycosis. *Chest* 89:435, 1986.
12. Bodey GP, et al. Pulmonary complications of acute leukemia. *Cancer* 19:781, 1966.
13. Bortin MM, Gale RP, Rimm AA. Allogeneic bone marrow transplantation for 144 patients with severe aplastic anemia. *JAMA* 245:1132, 1981.
14. Brambilla E, et al. Pulmonary histiocytosis X

with mediastinal lymph node involvement. *Am Rev Respir Dis* 142:1216, 1990.

15. Brauner MW, et al. Pulmonary histiocytosis X: Evaluation with high-resolution CT. *Radiology* 172:255, 1989.
16. Breuer R, et al. Tracheobronchial amyloidosis: Treatment by carbon dioxide laser photoresection. *Thorax* 40:870, 1985.
17. Bunn HF, Forget BG. *Hemoglobin: Molecular, Genetic, and Clinical Aspects.* Philadelphia: Saunders, 1986. Pp 595–622.
18. Carbone JE, Barker D, Stauffer JL. Sleep apnea in amyloidosis. *Chest* 87:401, 1985.
19. Celikoglu F, et al. Pleural effusion in non-Hodgkin's lymphoma. *Chest* 101:1357, 1992.
20. Chan CK, Hyland RH, Hutcheon MA. Pulmonary complications following bone marrow transplantation. *Clin Chest Med* 11:323, 1990.
21. Chollet S, et al. Diagnosis of pulmonary histiocytosis X by immunodetection of Langerhans cells in bronchoalveolar lavage fluid. *Am J Pathol* 115:225, 1984.
22. Cionini L, et al. Respiratory function tests after mantle radiation in patients with Hodgkin's disease. *Acta Radiol (Oncol)* 23:401, 1984.
23. Clark JG, et al. Obstructive lung disease after allogeneic marrow transplantation. Clinical presentation and course. *Ann Intern Med* 111:368, 1989.
24. Clarke A, Skelton J, Fraser RS. Fungal tracheobronchitis: Report of 9 cases and review of the literature. *Medicine* 70:1, 1991.
25. Colby TV, Lombard C. Histiocytosis X in the lung. *Hum Pathol* 14:847, 1983.
26. Cordier JF, et al. Monoclonal gammopathies in chest disease. *Thorax* 40:629, 1985.
27. Cordier JF, Loire R, Brune J. Amyloidosis of the lower respiratory tract: Clinical and pathological features in a series of 21 patients. *Chest* 90:827, 1986.
28. Crawford SW, Fisher L. Predictive value of pulmonary function tests before marrow transplantation. *Chest* 101:1257, 1992.
29. Crowe MJ, et al. Histiocytosis X with pulmonary and cutaneous manifestations (Letterer-Siwe disease) in an elderly woman. *Ir J Med Sci* 150:278, 1981.
30. Cuttner J, et al. Hyperleukocytosis in adult leukemia. *Cancer Treat Res* 26:263, 1985.
31. De Ceulaer K, et al. Pneumonia in young children with homozygous sickle cell disease: Risk and clinical features. *Eur J Pediatr* 144:255, 1985.
32. Dillard TA, et al. Pulmonary function in sickle cell trait. *Ann Intern Med* 106:191, 1987.
33. Dinakara P, et al. The effect of anemia on pulmonary diffusing capacity with deprivation of a correction equation. *Am Rev Respir Dis* 102:965, 1970.

34. Dombret H, et al. Acute lysis pneumopathy after chemotherapy for acute myelomonocytic leukemia with abnormal marrow eosinophils. *Cancer* 69:1356, 1992.
35. Edmonds LC, Prakash UBS. Lymphoma, neutropenia, and wheezing in a 70-year-old man. *Chest* 103:585,1993.
36. Estopa R, et al. Acute respiratory failure in severe hematologic disorders. *Crit Care Med* 12:26, 1984.
37. Ettinger NA, Trulock EP. Pulmonary considerations of organ transplantation (part 2). *Am Rev Respir Dis* 144:213, 1991.
38. Favara BE, McCarthy RC, Mierau GW. Histiocytosis-X. *Hum Pathol* 14:663, 1983.
39. Femi-Pearse D, Gazioglu KM, Yu PN. Pulmonary function studies in sickle cell disease. *J Appl Physiol* 28:574, 1970.
40. Fichtenbaum CJ, Kleinman GM, Haddad RG. Eosinophilic granuloma of the lung presenting as a solitary pulmonary nodule. *Thorax* 45:905, 1990.
41. Filly R, Blank N, Castellino RA. Radiographic distribution of intrathoracic disease in previously untreated patients with Hodgkin's disease and non-Hodgkin's lymphoma. *Radiology* 120:277, 1976.
42. Filuk RB, Warren PW. Bronchoalveolar lavage in Waldenstrom's macroglobulinemia with pulmonary infiltrates. *Thorax* 41:409, 1986.
43. Fithian E, et al. Reactivity of Langerhans cells with hybridoma antibody. *Proc Natl Acad Sci USA* 78:2541, 1981.
44. Flint A, et al. Pulmonary histiocytosis X. Immunoperoxidase staining for HLA-DR antigen and S100 protein. *Arch Pathol Lab Med* 110:930, 1986.
45. Fox F, et al. Eosinophilic granuloma of lymph nodes. *Histopathology* 1:31, 1977.
46. Fox MJ, et al. Leukocyte larceny: A cause of spurious hypoxemia. *Am J Med* 67:742, 1979.
47. Friedman PJ, Leibow AA, Sokoloff J. Eosinophilic granuloma of lung. Clinical aspects of primary pulmonary histiocytosis in the adult. *Medicine* 60:385, 1981.
48. Fukumura M, et al. Primary diffuse tracheobronchial amyloidosis treated by bronchoscopic Nd-YAG laser irradiation. *Jpn J Med* 29:620, 1990.
49. Ganesan TS, et al. Angioimmunoblastic lymphadenopathy: A clinical, immunological and molecular study. *Br J Cancer* 55:437, 1987.
50. Gerson SL, et al. Prolonged granulocytopenia: The major risk factor for invasive pulmonary aspergillosis in patients with acute leukemia. *Ann Intern Med* 100:345, 1984.
51. Gertz MA, Greipp PR. Clinical aspects of pulmonary amyloidosis. *Chest* 90:790, 1986.
52. Gherardi RK, Malapert D, Degos J-D. Castleman

disease–POEMS syndrome overlap. *Ann Intern Med* 114:520, 1991.

53. Gibbs AR, Seal RME. Primary lymphoproliferative conditions of lung. *Thorax* 33:140, 1978.
54. Ginsberg SJ, Comis RL. The pulmonary toxicity of antineoplastic agents. *Semin Oncol* 9:34, 1982.
55. Goldsmith GH, et al. Primary pulmonary hypertension in patients with classic hemophilia. *Ann Intern Med* 108:797, 1988.
56. Goodman RL, et al. Sickle cell trait and loss of pulmonary function of 5280 feet and sea level. *Thromb Diath Haemorrh* 53:91, 1974.
57. Gordon W. Amyloid deposits in the bronchi. *Br Med J* 1:825, 1955.
58. Gowitt GT, Zaatari GS. Bronchial extramedullary hematopoiesis preceding chronic myelogenous leukemia. *Hum Pathol* 16:1069, 1985.
59. Graham NJ, et al. Intrathoracic complications following allogeneic bone marrow transplantation: CT findings. *Radiology* 181:153, 1991.
60. Grant GP, et al. Cardiorespiratory response to exercise in patients with thalassemia major. *Am Rev Respir Dis* 136:92, 1987.
61. Greenberg S, Atwater J, Israel H. Frequency of hemoglobinopathies in sarcoidosis. *Ann Intern Med* 62:125, 1965.
62. Greenberger JS, Crocker AC, Vawter G. Results of treatment of 127 patients with systemic histiocytosis (Letterer-Siwe syndrome, Schuller-Christian syndrome and multifocal eosinophil granuloma). *Medicine* 60:311, 1981.
63. Grisaru D, et al. Cardiopulmonary assessment in thalassemia major. *Chest* 98:1138, 1990.
64. Ha SY, et al. Lung involvement in Langerhans' cell histiocytosis: Prevalence, clinical features, and outcome. *Pediatrics* 89:466, 1992.
65. Hall G, Carter J. Sarcoidosis and sickle cell disease. *Ann Intern Med* 118:157, 1993.
66. Hammerseley N, Moos KF. Primary amyloidosis causing macroglossia and respiratory symptoms. *Br J Oral Maxillofac Surg* 23:445, 1985.
67. Hance AJ, et al. Smoking and interstitial lung disease. The effect of cigarette smoking on the incidence of pulmonary histiocytosis X and sarcoidosis. *Ann NY Acad Sci* 465:643, 1986.
68. Hansen L, Prakash UBS, Colby TV. Pulmonary lymphoma in Sjogren's syndrome. *Mayo Clin Proc* 64:920, 1989.
69. Hansen RM, et al. Indolent diffuse histiocytic lymphoma with sclerosis and chylous effusions. *Cancer* 51:2144, 1983.
70. Hardy RE, et al. Cryptococcal pneumonia in a patient with sickle cell disease. *Chest* 89:892, 1986.
71. Haupt HM, et al. The lung in sickle cell disease. *Chest* 81:569, 1982.
72. Haupt HM, Hutchins GM, Moore GW. Ara-C

lung: Noncardiogenic pulmonary edema complicating cytosine therapy of leukemia. *Am J Med* 70:256, 1981.
73. Hayashi A, et al. Properties of hemoglobin M: Unequivalent nature of the alpha and beta subunits in the hemoglobin molecule. *Biochim Biophys Acta* 168:262, 1968.
74. Haynes J Jr, Allison RC. Pulmonary edema: Complication in the management of sickle cell pain crisis. *Am J Med* 80:833, 1986.
75. Hejfec G, Natarelli J, Gould VE. Myeloma lung: A previously unreported complication of multiple myeloma. *Hum Pathol* 14:558, 1983.
76. Heller PG, et al. Pulmonary hypertension in paroxysmal nocturnal hemoglobinuria. *Chest* 102:642, 1992.
77. Herbert A, et al. Lymphocytic interstitial pneumonia identified as lymphoma of mucosa associated lymphoid tissue. *J Pathol* 146:129, 1985.
78. Herbert PA, Bayer AS. Fungal pneumonia: IV. Invasive pulmonary aspergillosis. *Chest* 80:220, 1981.
79. Hildebrand FL Jr, et al. Pulmonary complications of leukemia. *Chest* 98:1233, 1990.
80. Hill G, et al. Mediastinal emphysema in marrow transplant recipients. *Bone Marrow Transplant* 2:315, 1987.
81. Himmelfarb E, Wells S, Rabinowitz JG. The radiologic spectrum of cardiopulmonary amyloidosis. *Chest* 72:327, 1977.
82. Hines DW, et al. Pseudomembranous tracheobronchitis caused by *Aspergillus*. *Am Rev Respir Dis* 143:1408, 1991.
83. Hirschman R, Johns C. Hemoglobin studies in sarcoidosis. *Ann Intern Med* 62:129, 1965.
84. Ho AD, et al. Respiratory distress as a primary symptom of relapse in a patient with non-Hodgkin's lymphoma. *Blut* 51:287, 1985.
85. Horak DA, et al. Pretreatment pulmonary function predicts cytomegalovirus-associated interstitial pneumonia following bone marrow transplantation. *Chest* 102:1484, 1992.
86. Jaffe EF. Methemoglobinemia. *Clin Hematol* 10:99, 1981.
87. Jeffery GM, Mead GM, Whitehouse JM. Life-threatening airway obstruction at the presentation of Hodgkin's disease. *Cancer* 67:506, 1991.
88. Jenkins PF, et al. Non-Hodgkin's lymphoma, chronic lymphocytic leukemia, and the lung. *Br J Dis Chest* 75:22, 1981.
89. Johnson FL, et al. Chronic obstructive airways disease after bone marrow transplantation. *J Pediatr* 105:370, 1984.
90. Jubelirer SJ. Pulmonary hypertension. Its association with microangiopathic hemolytic anemia and thrombocytopenia. *Arch Intern Med* 151:1221, 1991.

91. Kavuru MS, et al. Amyloidosis and pleural disease. *Chest* 98:20, 1990.
92. Kawanami O, et al. Pulmonary Langerhans' cells in patients with fibrotic lung disorders. *Lab Invest* 44:227, 1981.
93. Khouri NF, et al. Pulmonary interstitial changes following bone marrow transplantation. *Radiology* 133:587, 1979.
94. Kintzer JS, Rosenow EC III, Kyle RA. Thoracic and pulmonary abnormalities in multiple myeloma: A review of 958 cases. *Arch Intern Med* 138:727, 1978.
95. Kirkpatrick MB, Haynes J Jr, Bass JB Jr. Results of bronchoscopically obtained lower airway cultures from adult sickle cell disease patients with the acute chest syndrome. *Am J Med* 90:206, 1991.
96. Koss MN, et al. Primary non-Hodgkin's lymphoma and pseudolymphoma of the lung: A study of 161 patients. *Hum Pathol* 14:1024, 1983.
97. Kramer MR, et al. Ulcerative tracheobronchitis after lung transplantation: A new form of invasive aspergillosis. *Am Rev Respir Dis* 144:552, 1991.
98. Krowka MJ, Rosenow EC III, Hoagland HC. Pulmonary complications of bone marrow transplantation. *Chest* 87:237, 1985.
99. Krowka MJ, Staats BA, Hoagland HC. A prospective study of airway reactivity before bone marrow transplantation. *Mayo Clin Proc* 65:5, 1990.
100. Kurisu K, et al. Interstitial pneumonitis after allogeneic bone marrow transplantation following total body irradiation. *Radiat Med* 9:118, 1991.
101. Lacronique J, et al. Chest radiological features of pulmonary histiocytosis X: A report based on 50 adult cases. *Thorax* 37:104, 1982.
102. Lahey ME. Prognostic factors in histiocytosis-X. *Am J Pediatr Hematol Oncol* 3:57, 1981.
103. Lambert M, et al. Delayed sulfhemoglobinemia after acute dapsone intoxication. *Clin Toxicol* 19:45, 1982.
104. Landesman SH, Rao SP, Ahonkhai VI. Infections in children with sickle cell anemia: Special reference to pneumococcal and salmonella infections. *Am J Pediatr Hematol Oncol* 4:407, 1982.
105. Latini P, et al. Lung damage following bone marrow transplantation after hyperfractionated total body irradiation. *Radiother Oncol* 22:127, 1991.
106. Laufe MD, et al. Adult respiratory distress syndrome in neutropenic patients. *Am J Med* 80:1022, 1986.
107. Lee AB, Bogaars HA, Passero MA. Nodular pulmonary amyloidosis: A cause of bronchiectasis and fatal pulmonary hemorrhage. *Arch Intern Med* 143:603, 1983.
108. Lee SC, Johnson HA. Multiple nodular pulmonary amyloidosis: A case report and comparison with diffuse alveolar-septal pulmonary amyloidosis. *Thorax* 30:178, 1975.
109. Letourneau A, Andonin J, Garbe I. Primary pulmonary malignant lymphoma: Clinical and pathological findings, immunohistochemical and ultrastructural studies. *Hematol Oncol* 1:49, 1983.
110. Li G, et al. Primary lymphomas of the lung: Morphological, immunohistochemical and clinical features. *Histopathology* 16:519, 1990.
111. Libshitz HI, et al Pneumonias in hairy cell leukemia. *Radiology* 139:19, 1981.
112. Lichtenstein L. Histiocytosis X: Integration of eosinophilic granuloma of bone, "Letterer-Siwe disease," and "Schuller-Christian disease" as related manifestations of a single nosologic entity. *Arch Pathol* 56:84, 1953.
113. Lieberman PH, et al. A reappraisal of eosinophilic granuloma of bone, Hand-Schuller-Christian syndrome, and Letterer-Siwe syndrome. *Medicine* 48:375, 1969.
114. Link H, Reinhard D, Neithammer D. Obstructive ventilation disorder as a severe complication of chronic graft-versus-host disease after bone marrow transplantation. *Exp Hematol* 10:92, 1982.
115. List AF, Doll DC, Greco FA. Lung cancer in Hodgkin's disease: Association with previous radiotherapy. *J Clin Oncol* 3:215, 1985.
116. Lukes RJ, Tindle BH. Immunoblastic lymphadenopathy: A hyperimmune entity resembling Hodgkin's disease. *N Engl J Med* 292:1, 1975.
117. Mackenzie JW, Jellicoe JA. Acute airway obstruction: Spontaneous retropharyngeal haematoma in a patient with polycythemia rubra vera. *Anaesthesia* 41:57, 1986.
118. Marchevsky A, et al. Localized lymphoid nodules of lung: A reappraisal of the lymphoma vs. pseudolymphoma dilemma. *Cancer* 51:2070, 1983.
119. Maunder RJ, et al. Occurrence of the adult respiratory distress syndrome in neutropenic patients. *Am Rev Respir Dis* 133:313, 1986.
120. McKee LC Jr, Collins RD. Intravascular leukocyte thrombi and aggregates as a cause of morbidity and mortality in leukemia. *Medicine* 53:463, 1974.
121. Mead AM, Whitehouse JMA. Modern management of non-Hodgkin's lymphoma. *Br Med J* 293:577, 1986.
122. Meisel S, et al. Castleman's disease. An uncommon computed tomographic feature. *Chest* 93:1307, 1988.
123. Menashe P, et al. Bronchoalveolar lavage plasmacytosis in a patient with a plasma cell dyscrasia. *Chest* 95:226, 1989.
124. Meyer RD, et al. Aspergillosis complicating neoplastic disease. *Am J Med* 54:6, 1973.
125. Meyers JD. Infection in bone marrow transplant recipients. *Am J Med* 81(1A):27, 1986.

126. Meyers JD, Flournoy N, Thomas ED. Nonbacterial pneumonia after allogeneic marrow transplantation: A review of 10 years' experience. *Rev Infect Dis* 4:1119, 1982.

127. Meyers JD, Hackman RC, Stamm WE. *Chlamydia trachomatis* infection as a cause of pneumonia after human marrow transplantation. *Transplantation* 36:130, 1983.

128. Miller GJ, Serjeant GR. An assessment of lung volumes and gas transfer in sickle-cell anaemia. *Thorax* 26:309, 1971.

129. Milner PF. Oxygen transport in sickle cell anemia. *Arch Intern Med* 133:565, 1974.

130. Moore AD, et al. Pulmonary histiocytosis X: Comparison of radiographic and CT findings. *Radiology* 172:249, 1989.

131. Myers T, Cole S, Pastuszak W. Angioimmunoblastic lymphadenopathy: Pleural-pulmonary disease. *Cancer* 40:266, 1978.

132. Myers TJ Jr, et al. Respiratory failure due to pulmonary leukostasis following chemotherapy of acute nonlymphocytic leukemia. *Cancer* 51:1808, 1983.

133. Nagel RL, et al. Hemoglobin Beth Israel: A mutant causing clinically apparent cyanosis. *N Engl J Med* 295:125, 1976.

134. Neuman GG, et al. The anesthetic management of the patient with anterior mediastinal mass. *Anesthesiology* 60:144, 1984.

135. O'Brien KD, et al. Lymphocytic bronchitis unrelated to acute graft versus host disease in canine marrow graft recipients. *Transplantation* 37:233, 1984.

136. O'Donnell AE, et al. Endobronchial eosinophilic granuloma: A rare cause of total lung atelectasis. *Am Rev Respir Dis* 136:1478, 1987.

137. Ognibene FP, et al. Adult respiratory distress syndrome in patients with severe neutropenia. *N Engl J Med* 315:547, 1986.

138. Oppenheimer EH, Esterly JR. Pulmonary changes in sickle cell disease. *Am Rev Respir Dis* 103:858, 1971.

139. Osband ME, et al. Histiocytosis-X. Demonstration of abnormal immunity, T-cell histamine H2-receptor deficiency, and successful treatment with thymic extract. *N Engl J Med* 304:146, 1981.

140. Ostrow D, et al. Bronchiolitis obliterans complicating bone marrow transplantation. *Chest* 87:828, 1985.

141. Ozkaynak MF, et al. *Mycobacterium avium-intracellulare* infections after allogeneic bone marrow transplantation in children. *Am J Pediatr Hematol Oncol* 12:220, 1990.

142. Packe GE, Edwards CW, Cayton RM. Non-Hodgkin's lymphoma of the bronchial mucosa presenting with reversible airflow obstruction. *Thorax* 40:954, 1985.

143. Pannuti CS, et al. Nosocomial pneumonia in adult patients undergoing bone marrow transplantation: A 9-year study. *J Clin Oncol* 9:77, 1991.

144. Paradinas FJ, et al. Pulmonary fat embolisation after bone marrow transplantation. *Lancet* 1:715, 1983.

145. Park CM, Nagel RL. Sulfhemoglobinemia: Clincal and molecular aspects. *N Engl J Med* 310:1579, 1984.

146. Paz HL, et al. Bronchiolitis obliterans after autologous bone marrow transplantation. *Chest* 101:775, 1992.

147. Perin RJ, et al. Sickle cell disease and bronchial asthma. *Ann Allergy* 50:320, 1983.

148. Perreault C, et al. Lymphoid interstitial pneumonia after allogenic bone marrow transplantation. *Cancer* 55:1, 1985.

149. Perry MC, et al. Hemoglobin Columbia Missouri or α_2[88 (F9) Ala →Val]B$_2$: A new high-oxygen affinity hemoglobin that causes erythrocytosis. *Mayo Clin Proc* 66:5, 1991.

150. Peters SG, Prakash UBS. *Pneumocystis carinii* pneumonia: Review of 53 cases. *Am J Med* 82:73, 1987.

151. Popovsky MA, Moore SB. Diagnostic and pathogenetic considerations in transfusion-related lung injury. *Transfusion* 25:573, 1985.

152. Prakash UBS. Pulmonary Eosinophilic Granuloma. In: JP Lynch III, RA DeRemee (Eds), *Immunologic Pulmonary Diseases*. Philadelphia: Lippincott, 1991. Pp 432–448.

153. Prakash UBS, Abel MD, Hubmayr RD. Mediastinal mass and tracheal obstruction during general anesthesia. *Mayo Clin Proc* 63:1004, 1988.

154. Prakash UBS, Divertie MB, Banks PM. Aggressive therapy in acute respiratory failure from leukemic pulmonary infiltrates. *Chest* 75:345, 1979.

155. Prakash UBS, et al. Pulmonary alveolar phospholipoproteinosis: Experience with 34 cases and a review. *Mayo Clin Proc* 62:499, 1987.

156. Prakash UBS, Reiman HM. Comparison of needle biopsy with cytologic analysis for the evaluation of pleural effusion: Analysis of 414 cases. *Mayo Clin Proc* 60:158, 1985.

157. Price D, Dent RG. Pulmonary involvement in angio-immunoblastic lymphadenopathy. *Postgrad Med J* 59:728, 1983.

158. Prophet D. Primary pulmonary histiocytosis-X. *Clin Chest Med* 3:643, 1982.

159. Putman CE, et al. Radiographic chest abnormalities in adult hemophilia. *Radiology* 118:41, 1976.

160. Radin AI. Primary pulmonary Hodgkin's disease. *Cancer* 65:550, 1990.

161. Rajan VT, Kikkawa Y. Alveolar septal amyloidosis in primary amyloidosis: An electron microscopic study. *Arch Pathol* 89:521, 1970.

162. Ralph DD, et al. Rapidly progressive airflow obstruction in marrow transplant recipients: Possible association between bronchiolitis obliter-

ans and chronic graft-versus-host disease. *Am Rev Respir Dis* 129:641, 1984.

163. Ranney HM, et al. Oxygen equilibrium of hemoglobin M[cf16]Hyde Park. *Biochim Biophys Acta* 160:112, 1968.

164. Rappaport H, Thomas LB. Mycosis fungiodes: The pathology of extracutaneous involvement. *Cancer* 34:1198, 1974.

165. Rausch PG, Herion JC. Pulmonary manifestations of Waldenstrom's macroglobulinemia. *Am J Hematol* 9:201, 1980.

166. Rich S, Hart K. Familial pulmonary hypertension in association with an abnormal hemoglobin. Insights into the pathogenesis of primary pulmonary hypertension. *Chest* 99:1208, 1991.

167. Road JD, Jacques J, Sparling JR. Diffuse septal amyloidosis presenting with recurrent hemoptysis and medial dissection of pulmonary arteries. *Am Rev Respir Dis* 132:1368, 1985.

168. Robbins RA, et al. Diffuse alveolar hemorrhage in autologous bone marrow transplant recipients. *Am J Med* 87:511, 1989.

169. Rodriguez-Garcia JL, et al. Recurrent massive pleural effusion as a late complication of radiotherapy in Hodgkin's disease. *Chest* 100:1165, 1991.

170. Sadoun D, et al. Bronchogenic carcinoma in patients with pulmonary histiocytosis-X. *Chest* 101:1610, 1992.

171. Sanghvi S, et al. Angioimmunoblastic lymphadenopathy presenting as superior vena caval obstruction. *Chest* 100:1721, 1991.

172. Scadding JW. Fibrosing alveolitis with autoimmune haemolytic anaemia: Two case reports. *Thorax* 32:134, 1977.

173. Serour F, et al. Castleman's disease of the mediastinum: Misleading clinical and radiological characteristics. *Respir Med.* 83:509, 1989.

174. Shahar J, et al. Recurrent cavitary nodules secondary to Hodgkin's disease. *Chest* 91:273, 1987.

175. Shaheen NA, Salman SD, Nassar VH. Fatal bronchopulmonary hemorrhage due to unrecognized amyloidosis. *Arch Otolaryngol* 101:259, 1975.

176. Shapiro MP, Hayes JA. Fat embolism in sickle cell disease: Report of a case with a brief review of the literature. *Arch Intern Med* 144:181, 1984.

177. Sickles EA, et al. Pneumonia in acute leukemia. *Ann Intern Med* 79:528, 1973.

178. Sprinkle RH, et al. Acute chest syndrome in children with sickle cell disease: A retrospective analysis of 100 hospitalized cases. *Am J Pediatr Hematol Oncol* 8:105, 1986.

179. Staats BA, et al. The lipoprotein profile of chylous and nonchylous pleural effusions. *Mayo Clin Proc* 55:700, 1980.

180. Stamatoyannopoulos G, et al. Abnormal hemoglobins with high and low oxygen affinity. *Annu Rev Med* 22:221, 1971.

181. Stamatoyannopoulos G, Parer JT, Finch CA. Physiologic implications of a hemoglobin with decreased oxygen affinity (hemoglobin Seattle). *N Engl J Med* 281:915, 1969.

182. Stanievich JF, Marshak G, Stool SE. Airway obstruction in a haemophiliac child. *Ann Otol Rhinol Laryngol* 89:572, 1980.

183. Stern EJ, et al. Cystic lung disease associated with eosinophilic granuloma and tuberous sclerosis: Air trapping at dynamic ultrafast high-resolution CT. *Radiology* 182:325, 1992.

184. Stokar LM, et al. Clinical manifestations of intrathoracic cutaneous T-cell lymphoma. *Cancer* 56:2694, 1985.

185. Streeten EA, de la Monte SM, Kennedy TP. Amyloid infiltration of the diaphragm as a cause of respiratory failure. *Chest* 89:760, 1986.

186. Strob R, et al. Marrow transplantation in thirty "untransfused" patients with aplastic anemia. *Ann Intern Med* 92:30, 1980.

187. Sugiyama Y, et al. Progressive sinobronchiectasis associated with the "bare lymphocyte syndrome" in an adult. *Chest* 89:398, 1986.

188. Tariq SM, Morrison D, McConnochie K. Solitary bronchial amyloid presenting with haemoptysis. *Eur Respir J* 3:1230, 1990.

189. Tenholder MF, Hooper RG. Pulmonary infiltrates in leukemia. *Chest* 78:468, 1980.

190. Thomas ED, et al. Bone marrow transplantation. *N Engl J Med* 292:832, 1975.

191. Thompson JS, et al. Pulmonary "hypersensitivity" reactions induced by transfusion of non-HL-A leukoagglutinins. *N Engl J Med* 284:1120, 1971.

192. Thompson PJ, Citron KM. Amyloid and the lower respiratory tract. *Thorax* 38:84, 1983.

193. Thompson PJ, et al. Primary bronchopulmonary amyloid tumor with massive hilar lymphadenopathy. *Thorax* 38:153, 1983.

194. Thomson FJ, et al. Pulmonary infarction, myocardial infarction, and acute disseminated intravascular coagulation. *J Clin Pathol* 44:1034, 1991.

195. Tomashefski JF, Khiyami A, Kleinerman J. Neoplasms associated with pulmonary eosinophilic granuloma. *Arch Pathol Lab Med* 115:499, 1991.

196. Troussard X, et al. Pulmonary veno-occlusive disease after bone marrow transplantation. *Thorax* 39:956, 1984.

197. Tsoi MS. Immunological mechanisms of graft-versus-host disease in man. *Transplantation* 33:459, 1982.

198. Tsunematsu Y, et al. A clinicopathological study of histiocytosis X. *Jpn J Clin Oncol* 14:633, 1984.

199. Ward HN. Pulmonary infiltrates associated with leukoagglutinin transfusion reactions. *Ann Intern Med* 73:689, 1970.

200. Wardman AG, Cooke NJ. Pulmonary infiltrates

in adult acute leukemia: Empirical treatment or lung biopsy. *Thorax* 39:647, 1984.

201. Weiner RS, et al. Interstitial pneumonitis following bone marrow transplantation: Assessment of risk factors. *Ann Intern Med* 104:168, 1986.

202. Weiss W, Waife SO. Tuberculosis and sickle-cell anemia. *Am Rev Tuberc* 65:735, 1952.

203. Whitcomb ME, et al. Hodgkin's disease of the lung. *Am Rev Respir Dis* 106:79, 1972.

204. Wick MR, et al. Immunologic, clinical, and pathologic aspects of human graft-versus-host disease. *Mayo Clin Proc* 58:603, 1983.

205. Wilimas JA, et al. Hemothorax and hemomediastinum in patients with hemophilia. *Acta Haematol (Basel)* 73:176, 1985.

206. Winterbauer RH, et al. Pleuropulmonary manifestations of Waldenstrom's macroglobulinemia. *Chest* 66:368, 1974.

207. The Writing Group of the Histiocyte Society. Histiocytosis syndromes in children. *Lancet* 1: 208, 1987.

208. Xaubet A, et al. Characteristics and prognostic value of pleural effusions in non-Hodgkin's lymphomas. *Eur J Respir Dis* 66:135, 1985.

209. Yellin A, Benfield JR. Pneumothorax associated with lymphoma. *Am Rev Respir Dis* 134:590, 1986.

210. Yousem SA, Weiss LM, Colby TV. Primary pulmonary Hodgkin's disease: A clinicopathologic study of 15 cases. *Cancer* 57:1212, 1986.

61

Renal Diseases

Udaya B. S. Prakash

The respiratory and renal systems are the two most important organ systems responsible for the maintenance of normal acid-base equilibrium. Failure of one system promptly elicits a compensatory response from the other. This close relationship is maintained not only in health but also in certain pathologic states. For example, the disease entities commonly referred to as pulmonary-renal syndromes affect both the kidney and the lung by diverse and, in many instances, unknown mechanisms. Some of the serious respiratory complications of kidney diseases described in the past are now uncommon because of the early diagnosis and treatment of renal disorders. However, successful treatment of renal failure by hemodialysis, peritoneal dialysis, and renal transplantation has led to some unusual complications related to the treatment itself. Elucidation of the basis for the pulmonary pathology in chronic hemodialysis has led to an understanding of some of the factors responsible for certain types of acute respiratory distress syndrome. Pulmonary complications after renal transplantation are well recognized. This chapter will address the pleuropulmonary manifestations of kidney diseases (Table 61-1), renal transplantation, and pulmonary alveolar hemorrhage syndromes.

Renal Failure

Pulmonary Edema

Pulmonary changes may be associated with either acute or chronic renal failure [208]. Pulmonary edema is the most serious complication of renal failure. The roentgenographic manifestations—variously referred to as *uremic lung, uremic pneumonia,* and *butterfly shadows* or *bat-wing shadows*—are manifestations of pulmonary edema. Similar features can occur in patients with congestive heart failure from various causes. Even when physical signs in the lungs are scant in comparison with the roentgenographic evidence, correction of overhydration results in rapid improvement. Typically, the chest roentgenogram exhibits bilaterally symmetric densities extending laterally from the hilum, leaving clear apices and peripheral zones (Figs. 61-1, 61-2). The reason for the central concentration of the abnormal shadows is unclear, but the severity of the changes increases with the degree of azotemia and acidosis, and it has been suggested that these conditions may increase capillary permeability [46]. In acute glomerulonephritis, children may die so rapidly from pulmonary edema that the diagnosis may be made only at necropsy [135].

In chronic renal failure, pulmonary edema may develop without uremia, probably in part from sodium retention and increased blood volume. Uremic pneumonitis (Fig. 61-3) does not occur in every patient with uremia, and its occurrence cannot be correlated with the degree of azotemia or the severity of left ventricular failure. However, the clearing of chest roentgenographic abnormalities is paralleled by a reduction in total body fluid.

The pathogenesis of pulmonary edema in renal failure is unknown. Fluid overload, left ventricular failure, and increased capillary permeability from uremia are some of the possibilities. Increased endothelial permeability to sodium and water [46] and increased alveolar permeability to technetium 99m–labeled compounds [14] before and during hemodialysis have been shown. Edema fluid sampled by endotracheal aspiration has shown an elevated protein content, suggesting increased vascular permeability to plasma proteins in renal failure [167]. A more recent study [177] reported that there was no evidence of increased pulmonary endothelial permeability to the plasma protein transferrin (75,000 daltons) in patients with pulmonary edema associated with renal failure.

Table 61-1. **Pulmonary complications in renal diseases**

Pulmonary manifestation	Renal etiology
Hypoxemia	Hemodialysis Pulmonary edema Pleural effusion Pulmonary infections Pulmonary calcification Pulmonary-renal syndromes (see Table 61-2)
Pulmonary edema	Renal failure (acute and chronic) Acute glomerulonephritis Nephrotic syndrome Hemodialysis Renal transplantation
Pleural effusion	Renal failure (acute and chronic) Nephrotic syndrome Acute glomerulonephritis Hemodialysis Peritoneal dialysis Ureteral obstruction Hydronephrosis Perinephric abscess Pulmonary embolism Pulmonary-renal syndromes Renal transplantation
Pleuritis	Uremia Hemodialysis
Pulmonary calcification	Hemodialysis Transplantation Chronic renal failure
Sleep apnea	Chronic renal failure
Infections	Hemodialysis Transplantation Renal failure
Lymphoma, lung cancer	Renal transplantation
Pulmonary-renal syndromes	See Table 61-2

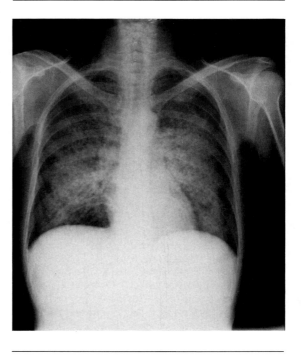

Fig. 61-1. Typical bat-wing (outer one-third of lungs) or butterfly (inner two-thirds of lungs) appearance in uremic pulmonary edema. Note sparing of both costophrenic angles.

Lung function studies in patients with severe renal failure have revealed a significant decrease in diffusing capacity, presumably from pulmonary edema [129]. Improvement in midexpiratory flow and reduction in air trapping after hemodialysis have been described, and it has been suggested that these changes could be attributed to alleviation of peribronchial edema [221]. The degree of restrictive dysfunction will depend on the chronicity and severity of the renal failure. Muscle weakness, myopathy, and reduced aerobic muscle function are common in chronic renal failure. Diaphragmatic involvement from a myopathic process contributes to dysfunction in patients with chronic renal failure [198]. Pulmonary function tests performed at least 12 hours after the preceding hemodialysis in one group of patients revealed significantly reduced diffusing capacity for carbon monoxide ($D_{L}CO$), even after correction for anemia [72]. There appeared to be no correlation between anemia and the severity of reduction in $D_{L}CO$.

The histopathologic findings in pulmonary edema include septal swelling and edema, proteinaceous fluid in alveoli and, in some cases, hyaline membrane formation. Two types of residual or chronic lesions consist of (1) round hyaline structures in alveolar septa that are well circumscribed and coated by a single layer of flat endothelial cells and (2) organized casts of alveoli, alveolar ducts, and bronchioles, many revealing marked cellularity [102]. Repeated episodes of

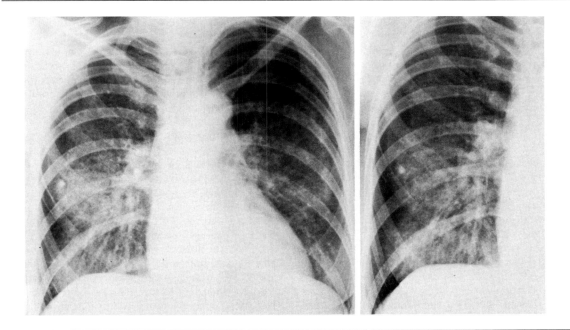

Fig. 61-2. Bilateral but asymmetric pulmonary edema in acute renal failure (left). Close-up shows clear demarcation of normal and abnormal lung.

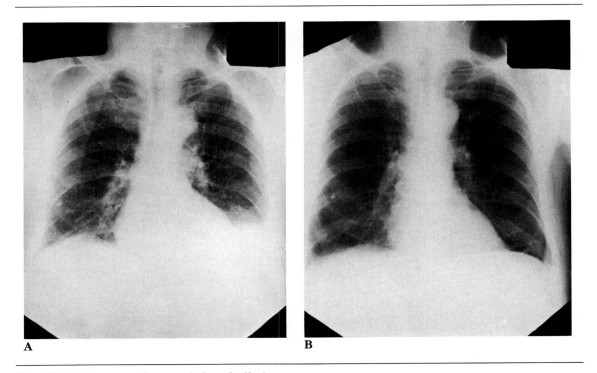

A

B

Fig. 61-3. Pulmonary edema and pleural effusion before (A) and after (B) hemodialysis for renal failure.

uremic pulmonary edema may result in interstitial fibrosis and deposition of hemosiderin in the alveoli.

Pleural Effusion

Pleural effusion is a common complication of renal diseases. Hemodialysis, peritoneal dialysis, and renal transplantation are also associated with this disorder. Various renal diseases that produce pleural effusion are listed in Table 61-1.

Pleural effusion occurs in nearly half the children who develop acute glomerulonephritis. The effusions probably are secondary to hypervolemia and raised capillary hydrostatic pressures, and they are usually transudative [183]. Many of these patients will exhibit edema and cardiomegaly.

Nephrotic syndrome is a common cause of pleural effusion in renal diseases. Pleural and pericardial effusions are seen in 20 to 25 percent of patients with the nephrotic syndrome, and subpulmonic effusions are not uncommon [183]. The pleural fluid is usually a transudate with a low protein content. The main factor leading to pleural transudation is the diminution of the plasma oncotic pressure, allowing easier transport of protein-poor fluid into the pleural space. Usually bilateral and sometimes massive, these effusions may produce significant respiratory distress. One of the peculiar features of subpulmonic effusion is its tendency not to obliterate the costophrenic angle (Fig. 61-4). It is likely that the pleuritis associated with uremia may cause areas of adhesion between the parietal diaphragmatic pleura and the visceral pleura, thereby preventing the fluid from pushing the lung upward. The chest roentgenogram may show only an elevated hemidiaphragm on the side of pleural effusion. A lateral decubitus chest roentgenogram frequently is necessary to demonstrate free layering of the fluid. The treatment of pleural effusion associated with the nephrotic syndrome should be aimed at decreasing the protein loss. Routine therapeutic thoracentesis is not recommended because of the additional loss of proteins. Fibrosing uremic pleuritis complicated by empyema has been described [140]. Tetracycline pleurodesis should be attempted for recurrent or symptomatic effusions [106].

Fig. 61-4. Subpulmonic left pleural effusion on chronic renal failure demonstrates (A) maintenance of sharp costophrenic angle on the left and (B) free layering of the pleural effusion in the lateral decubitus position.

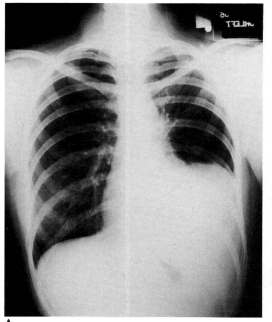

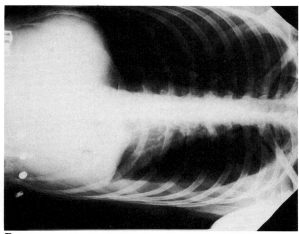

A   B

Fibrinous pleuritis is an uncommon but distinct entity and possibly a specific manifestation of uremia, although episodes of fibrinous pleuritis have been noted in patients on chronic hemodialysis [28]. Affected patients usually complain of recurrent episodes of pleuritic chest pain and dyspnea and low-grade fever. Pleural friction rubs are commonly heard on auscultation [153]. In some patients, the fluid is an exudate containing high levels of protein and lactate dehydrogenase, and a disruption of the pleural membrane has been blamed for this [28,78,178].

Patients undergoing chronic hemodialysis may develop pleural effusions. The fluid usually is serosanguineous as a result of heparinization during the procedure [15,75]. In one case, hemorrhagic effusion resulted in fibrinous pleuritis and pulmonary restriction requiring pulmonary decortication [75].

Ureteral obstruction from calculi, ureteral valves, malignancy, and gravid uterus may result in extravasation of urine into the pleural space and produce urinothorax or urinoma [170,196, 214]. Occasionally, retroperitoneal extravasation of urine as a result of hydronephrosis may lead to thoracic complications [41]. Intrapleural urinomas and mediastinal widening have been reported as a consequence of this phenomenon [11]. Perinephric abscess may be complicated by pleural effusions, which are sympathetic (similar to sterile parapneumonic effusions) and rarely become infected.

Fig. 61-5. Metastatic calcification associated with chronic renal failure or in patients on long-term hemodialysis. (A) Calcium is seen as deposits of dark and platelike material diffusely in alveolar walls. (B) A von Kossa stain for calcium shows diffuse black staining of calcium in alveolar walls.

The possibility that the pleural effusion is instigated by pulmonary embolism has to be considered even though the incidence of thromboembolic disease is reported to be low in patients with nephrotic syndrome. One study observed pulmonary embolism in 22 percent (8 patients) of 36 adult patients with nephrotic syndrome [133].

The hemolytic-uremic syndrome may involve the respiratory system, and a case of pleuritis and pericarditis associated with this syndrome has been described [205].

Although chylous ascites is known to be associated with nephrotic syndrome, chylous pleural effusion is rare. The edema of the intestines with resultant lacteal leakage or malabsorption may be responsible. Chylous pleural effusion has been described in a patient with nephrotic syndrome [149].

Pulmonary Calcification in Chronic Renal Failure

Soft-tissue calcification is divided into metastatic calcification, in which calcium salts are deposited in previously normal tissue, and dystrophic calcification, in which calcification occurs at pathologically altered sites [21,182]. The primary target of metastatic calcification is the lung [71,112,122]. Chronic renal failure may result in secondary hyperparathyroidism with hypercalcemia. Although pulmonary calcification is said to be a common occurrence with chronic renal diseases [69,147], it usually is sparse and identifiable only on histologic examination of the lungs (Fig. 61-5) [141]. The clinical manifestations are nonspecific. Chest roentgenograms show calci-

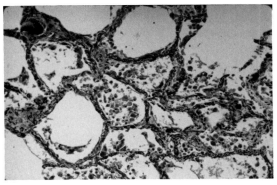

A

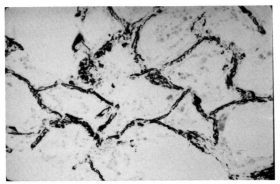

B

fications that are either localized or diffuse [36,141]. In most cases, they are identical to roentgenographic opacities produced by pneumonia or pulmonary edema [147], but sometimes definite punctate calcifications may be seen (Fig. 61-6). Upper lung zones are more commonly affected [71]. Even when pulmonary calcification cannot be demonstrated with certainty, the possibility should be considered in any case of renal failure if persistently unchanging pulmonary infiltrates develop. Physiologic studies have revealed the presence of a restrictive defect. Bone-seeking radionuclide (^{99m}Tc diphosphonate) lung scans have been used to establish an early diagnosis of pulmonary calcification (Fig. 61-7), especially in high-risk patients [52]. An unusual form of focal, nodular pulmonary calcification has been reported in a patient with renal failure resulting from polycystic kidney disease [194].

Although the pathogenesis of pulmonary calcification is unknown, Herbert and associates [94] suggested that the disorder occurs when the product of calcium and phosphate ions exceeds the solubility constant in the blood (the product of plasma calcium and phosphate being greater than 75 mg/100 ml). Others have suggested that the product of calcium and phosphorus is more relevant to the in vivo situation.

Crystallographic, spectroscopic, and chemical

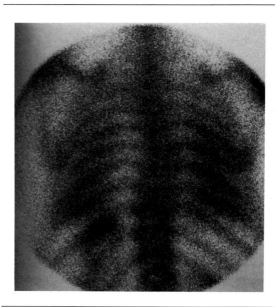

Fig. 61-7. A posterior view of ^{99m}Tc scan of lung in a patient with pulmonary calcification shows marked uptake of radionuclide by both lungs and the stomach (seen below the left lung).

studies have demonstrated two distinct types of calcium phosphate in tissues of patients with chronic renal failure. Calcifications found in the lungs are microcrystallites of magnesium, whitlockite, or an immediate precursor whose formation is promoted by the presence of magnesium [130]. Preferential calcification of the upper lung zones may be induced by the higher ventilation-perfusion ratio in the apical regions of lung relative to the basal regions, resulting in a lower alveolar carbon dioxide tension and higher tissue pH (blood pH at the apex is approximately 7.51, compared with 7.39 at the base). The resultant relative alkalinity favors precipitation of calcium phosphate [71].

Hemodialysis

Hypoxia

Hemodialysis-induced hypoxemia has been studied extensively. A fall in the partial pressure of arterial oxygen occurs during hemodialysis, and likely there are several mechanisms responsible for the hemodialysis-induced hypoxemia. Bischel and associates [18] concluded that it was due to

Fig. 61-6. Diffuse punctate calcification of pulmonary parenchyma in the right lower-lung zone in inadequately treated chronic renal failure.

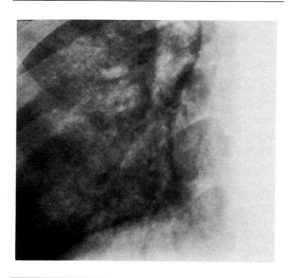

pulmonary arterial microembolization from the dialyzer membrane. Others demonstrated alveolar hypoventilation resulting from the substantial loss of carbon dioxide across the dialyzer membrane [7,189]. In addition, reversible lung damage due to intrapulmonary leukostasis as a consequence of the contact of blood with the dialyzer membrane may cause transient hypoxemia. Craddock and associates [44,45,192] demonstrated that complement- and leukocyte-mediated leukostasis is the underlying mechanism in hemodialysis-induced hypoxemia. Of 34 patients undergoing dialysis, 15 disclosed leukostasis or sequestration of leukocytes within the pulmonary vessels [44], leukopenia, and impaired pulmonary function. Histologic examination of animals undergoing hemodialysis revealed severe pulmonary vessel leukostasis and interstitial edema. This syndrome was prevented by preinactivation of complement but was reproduced by infusions of plasma in which complement was activated by zymosan. Hence, acute pulmonary dysfunction plays a significant role in the development of respiratory insufficiency during cellophane-membrane hemodialysis [35,44]. Observations by others suggest that activation of complement, leukopenia, and release of granulocyte-derived elastase are important interlinked pathophysiologic mechanisms for acute deterioration of pulmonary function during hemodialysis [120].

One study in hemodialysis patients has shown the occurrence of hypoxemia as a result of decreased minute ventilation without hypercapnia [159]. It is hypothesized that the diminished minute ventilation is unrelated to alterations in traditional chemoreceptor output, which depends on changing arterial oxygen tension. This theory suggests a carbon dioxide receptor somewhere in the central venous system. Blanchet and associates [20] found significant hypoxemia and diminished alveolar ventilation in acetate-treated patients. Whether acetate or bicarbonate is used in the dialysate does not seem to make a difference in dialysis-induced hypoxemia. Consumption of carbon dioxide in the metabolism of acetate has been suggested as the mechanism for hypoventilation and hypoxemia [155]. Some have suggested that hypoventilation, localized ventilation-perfusion abnormalities due to changes in the pulmonary vascular volume during dialysis, and increases in arterial pH contribute variably to dialysis-induced hypoxia [2,59]. However, the key factor seems to be hypoventilation [20,161]. Sorbent regenerative hemodialysis as a cause of acute hypercapnia has been observed [89].

Pulmonary Dysfunction

A decreased DLCO has been noted in both acetate-treated and bicarbonate-treated groups [20]. Leukocyte sequestration in the pulmonary capillary network may be the reason for this phenomenon. A study of 25 uremic patients observed hemodialysis-induced decreases in the DLCO in the majority of patients was due to reduced pulmonary capillary volume brought on by hemodialysis [60]. A significant fall in peak respiratory flow during the first 30 minutes of dialysis has been noted in 30 percent of patients [51]. The flow rates (forced expiratory flow in midcycle [FEF_{25-75}]) improve after hemodialysis, suggesting that peribronchial edema present before hemodialysis is responsible for the small airway dysfunction. Pulmonary dysfunction and eosinophilia have been noted in patients undergoing cuprophan dialysis [143].

Pulmonary Calcification

Metastatic calcification is more common in patients on long-term hemodialysis. Pulmonary calcification is more common with chronic hemodialysis than with peritoneal dialysis, and its extent usually reflects the duration of treatment (see Figs. 61-6, 61-7). In a prospective study of 31 patients, of whom 15 died, necropsy revealed pulmonary calcification in 9 [40]. Such calcification also occurs in patients with hyperphosphatemia who are being treated with a dialysate high in calcium [23].

A 1979 report noted that 7 of 13 patients with pulmonary calcification described in the literature died of respiratory failure [110]. In a group of 18 children on maintenance dialysis without evidence of pulmonary calcification on chest roentgenograms, 22 percent had positive technetium bone scans [58]. There were no significant differences between the groups with and without positive bone scans with respect to serum levels of calcium, phosphorus, bicarbonate, magnesium, and calcium-phosphorus product, as well as parathyroid hormone and vitamin D levels. Two factors that influenced the presence of pulmonary calcification were the long-term duration of dialysis and high serum aluminum levels. Biochemical analysis of pulmonary parenchyma in patients with pulmonary calcification has shown the presence of magnesium whitlockite [$(CaMg)_3(PO_4)_2$] as the main constituent. Ultrastructural studies of the lung parenchyma have shown linear or finely granular localization of the calcification along the alveolar septa [16].

Sleep Disorders

Sleep apnea seems to develop more commonly in patients with chronic renal failure. The association between end-stage renal failure and sleep apnea remains highly significant, though the cause for it remains unclear [54,119]. This association seems not to be altered acutely by conventional hemodialysis treatment [142]. In a report of 29 male patients maintained on outpatient hemodialysis, 12 had clinical features suggestive of sleep apnea. Polysomnography in eight of these patients documented obstructive sleep apnea in six. The role of testosterone was tested in these patients, but no relationship to sleep apnea was noted [145].

Progressive dialysis encephalopathy as well as spells of sudden respiratory arrest, in close association with the episodic electroencephalographic abnormalities characteristic of the syndrome, have been reported [76].

Hemodialysis-Induced Asthma

Asthmatic episodes have been observed during hemodialysis, and some believe that bronchial reactivity is more pronounced in this group of patients [61,211]. Hemodialysis-induced asthma has been attributed to the bronchospasm caused by acetate in the dialysate. Substitution of acetate with bicarbonate in the dialysate has resulted in resolution of this unusual problem. Others have inferred that hemodialysis does not commonly result in bronchial hyperactivity, their conclusion being based on a lack of airway hyperactivity to histamine challenge before and after hemodialysis [191]. Hemodialysis patients who are also asthmatics dependent on theophylline for maintenance of bronchodilatation need special care during dialysis. A shortened half-life of theophylline, from 5.7 hours to 1.6 hours, during hemodialysis has been described [32]. However, hemodialysis clearance of theophylline varies substantially and may be dependent on the dialysis system, different blood flow rates, and different dialyzers used. Hemodialysis patients who are receiving theophylline should be carefully monitored, via measurement of serum theophylline concentrations, for exacerbations of bronchospasm during and after the hemodialysis procedure [32].

Miscellaneous Problems in Dialysis

The risk of infections caused by *Legionella* species is increased in patients on chronic hemodialysis. In some cases, these infections were believed to result from infection of the dialysis fistula by *Legionella* species. Patients receiving hemodialysis and renal transplant recipients are at an increased risk of developing pneumonia caused by *Legionella pneumophila*. The hemodialysis fistula can become infected by such organisms and cause *Legionella* pneumonia [113].

Pleural effusion in hemodialysis and peritoneal dialysis were discussed earlier. Occasionally, a severe alkalemic shift is seen as a result of failure of dialysis to substitute for the kidney's normal response to simple respiratory alkalosis [118].

Postmortem studies in dialysis patients have shown a high incidence of pulmonary atherosclerosis, indicating chronic elevations in pulmonary artery pressure [66]. However, clinical pulmonary hypertension is uncommon in patients with chronic renal failure or those on chronic dialysis.

Tuberculosis

The risk of tuberculosis is increased in renal failure [193]. A British publication estimated the risk to be nearly 70 times higher in non-Europeans with chronic renal failure than in the native population [48]. The incidence of tuberculosis is higher in patients on maintenance dialysis. Active tuberculosis occurs in 3.7 to 6.0 percent of patients followed longitudinally while on dialysis, an infection rate that is 12 to 15 times higher than normal [63]. One study of 25 patients on dialysis detected tuberculosis in 28 percent; the majority were women, and extrapulmonary tuberculosis was common [146].

Peritoneal Dialysis

Many of the pulmonary complications associated with peritoneal dialysis are similar to those described for hemodialysis. However, several complications are peculiar to this group of patients. Patients on long-term peritoneal dialysis may develop extrapulmonary restrictive ventilatory defects. The filling of the peritoneal cavity with the dialysate induced, in both the supine and upright positions, significant reductions in the maximal inspiratory pressure and diminished lung volumes. The diaphragmatic dysfunction is most likely the result of physical alterations resulting from the dialysate infusion [83]. The D$_L$CO seems to diminish in patients who receive continuous ambulatory peritoneal dialysis [30,60].

Peritoneal dialysis is occasionally complicated by pleural effusion [151,180]. A review of the literature in 1990 noted 33 cases of pleural effusion associated with peritoneal dialysis; 28 of these cases occurred in women [203]. Detection occurred within 48 hours of acute peritoneal dialysis. All cases were unilateral, and all but one were right-sided. The mechanism of fluid accumulation is similar to that in ascites. Instillation of large volumes of fluid intraperitoneally will further stretch the diaphragmatic defects. The fluid can accumulate acutely and rapidly, within hours of initiating peritoneal dialysis, and produce respiratory distress [203]. The effusions tend to recur on reinstitution of peritoneal dialysis.

Disordered sleep occurs more frequently in patients on chronic peritoneal dialysis. In a prospective study of 11 patients on chronic peritoneal dialysis, six were found to have obstructive sleep apnea; the amount of dialysate drained in the morning was negatively correlated with the minimum arterial oxygen saturation during the night [209].

Severe shifts in systemic pH that occur in patients undergoing peritoneal dialysis are usually acidemic shifts resulting from inadequate replacement of the kidney's ability to excrete acid and regenerate bicarbonate. Hypercapnia and acute respiratory acidosis have resulted from an increased carbohydrate load associated with peritoneal dialysis; lipogenesis following a carbohydrate load in patients with renal failure is associated with a respiratory quotient of 8.0, reflecting the much greater production of carbon dioxide per unit of oxygen consumed [37,117].

Renal Transplantation and the Lung

Pulmonary problems in recipients of solid-organ transplants are a result of the transplant rejection process and immunosuppressive therapy. The reader is referred to Chapter 58 for more detailed discussions regarding the respiratory complications of organ transplantation. Pulmonary infections are common in renal transplant recipients and are, as a group, the major cause of death among them [96,173]. These infections may be caused by unusual bacteria or fungi, possibly favored by suppression of immune mechanisms by drugs and corticosteroids [97,172]. The incidence of cytomegalovirus infection in cadaveric renal transplant patients is reported to be as high as 43 to 92 percent [17,79]. Although many renal transplant patients remain asymptomatic during cytomegalovirus infection, pulmonary dysfunction is common. One report demonstrated that a decreased DLCO is common in virtually every patient with cytomegalovirus infection [207]. An interesting finding was activation of the complement system (C3d and C3a) in many of these patients, suggesting a causal relationship between complement activation and diminished DLCO. Earlier studies questioned whether cytomegalovirus played any role in the development of pneumonia among renal transplantation patients [81], but other reports show that cytomegalovirus pneumonia has become a leading cause of death in this patient group [162].

Study of pneumonia in renal transplant patients disclosed single-organism involvement by type 3 *Streptococcus pneumoniae, Staphylococcus aureus, Pseudomonas aeruginosa,* and *Escherichia coli* [27]. Nosocomial pneumonia caused by *Legionella pneumophila* has been described in this patient pool as well [131]. Systemic fungal infections with pulmonary involvement, particularly candidiasis and aspergillosis, are also common after renal transplantation [172]. *Pneumocystis carinii* infection is another opportunistic agent seen in renal transplant recipients [174]. Tuberculous infections have been reported, but the incidence is not high. In a series of 400 transplant patients, only 5 developed tuberculosis [43]. Several cases of pulmonary infection caused by *Mycobacterium xenopi* have been noted [212].

Pulmonary calcification, at times fatal, also is seen in renal transplant recipients [65,77,114, 121,144]. One patient developed extensive pulmonary calcification 6 days after renal transplantation and died from respiratory failure on the seventh day [77]. In a study of 17 pediatric patients, 4 developed pulmonary calcinosis and respiratory failure within 3 to 5 days of renal transplantation [144]. Common clinical features included poor allograft function with persistent uremia requiring dialysis, and evidence of moderate to severe hyperparathyroidism. Three patients had markedly elevated calcium-phosphorus product, to peak values of 122 to 147 mg/dl. This increase was noted at the time of onset of respiratory failure. All patients died of respiratory failure 5 to 58 days after transplantation [144].

Chronic immunosuppressive therapy in patients with renal transplants increases the risk of developing B-cell lymphoma and carcinoma of the lung [74]. Non-Hodgkin's lymphoma has been observed in up to 2.5 percent of renal transplant recipients [63]. The incidence of Kaposi's sarcoma in this patient population is estimated to be 400-to 500-fold more than the general population and may affect up to 4 percent of renal transplant recipients of Mediterranean or Jewish ancestry [86,92]. Although rare, pulmonary involvement from Kaposi's sarcoma has been described in recipients of renal transplants [86].

Abnormal pulmonary function, particularly a reduced DlCO, seems to persist even after renal transplantation. Subclinical pulmonary edema present in the pretransplantation period is presumed to progress to fibrosis before transplantation [30].

The incidence of pulmonary thromboembolism is markedly reduced in uremic patients [150]. However, renal transplant recipients exhibit a high occurrence of pulmonary embolism. Pulmonary embolism was the most frequent complication among 227 renal transplant recipients, being observed in 60 percent of those with a noninfectious process [168].

Pulmonary Alveolar Hemorrhage Syndromes

Pulmonary alveolar hemorrhage syndromes are discussed in this chapter because many belong to the group of diseases sometimes referred to as *pulmonary-renal syndromes*, to denote simultaneous occurrence of pulmonary and renal diseases, usually by the same pathologic process [67,127,128,139,169,220]. Because pulmonary alveolar hemorrhage is a common feature in most of these syndromes, the term *lung purpura* also has been used to describe these entities (Table 61-2). The mechanism of alveolar bleeding may vary from disease to disease. For instance, the bleeding in Goodpasture's syndrome is believed to be the result of pulmonary capillary wall damage caused by the destruction of type IV collagen by autoantibodies [215,216]. The alveolar hemorrhage in mitral stenosis is the result of stress failure of the capillary wall, caused by a tremendous increase in capillary pressure [216]. In vasculitic syndromes, capillaritis due to direct involvement by the vasculitic process leads to hemorrhage into the alveoli.

The common physiologic defect in these disorders is the diminished alveolar gas volumes evidenced by reduced total lung capacity and vital capacity. Airflow limitation is not a feature. Interestingly, DlCO can be elevated if fresh alveolar hemorrhage is present. Theoretically, DlCO may show a continual rise if measured repeatedly in a patient with continued alveolar hemorrhage, due to the increased uptake of carbon monoxide by the erythrocytes newly introduced into the alveoli. This test has been used in anecdotal cases and is reported to be a sensitive and useful indicator of the presence or absence of recurrent

Table 61-2. **Pulmonary-renal syndromes**

Goodpasture's syndrome
Churg-Strauss vasculitis
Wegener's granulomatosis
Polyarteritis nodosa
Systemic lupus erythematosus
Lymphomatoid granulomatosis
Henoch-Schönlein purpura
Hemolytic-uremic syndrome
Scleroderma
Rheumatoid arthritis
Mixed connective tissue disease
Drug-induced vasculitis
Granulomatous (giant-cell) arteritis
Hypocomplementemic urticarial vasculitis
Idiopathic rapidly progressive glomerulonephritis
Essential mixed cryoglobulinemia

intrapulmonary hemorrhage [3,12]. My own experience in several patients has shown that repeated measurement of DlCO for this purpose is unreliable. Furthermore, repeated testing is impractical because most patients with alveolar hemorrhage are markedly ill and may not be able to withstand the testing.

Quantitative measurement of macrophage hemosiderin content in the bronchoalveolar lavage effluent has been suggested as a useful test to determine the degree of alveolar hemorrhage [111]. The available data do not indicate that this is a dependable test. During bronchoalveolar lavage, incremental increase in the bloody discoloration of alveolar effluent is one strong indicator of alveolar hemorrhage. However, the possibility of bleeding induced by the procedure itself should be considered.

The antineutrophil cytoplasmic antibody (ANCA) test may aid in differentiating the various vasculitic syndromes (see Chapter 58). However, more recent data suggest that some patients with Goodpasture's syndrome may exhibit perinuclear ANCA [213].

Although the common feature of alveolar hemorrhage syndromes is the bleeding into alveolar spaces (Fig. 61-8), the disorders are diverse in etiology. However, many are immunologically mediated or belong to broad categories of vasculitides or collagenoses [3,128,163–165]. Differential diagnoses of alveolar hemorrhage syndrome (with or without renal involvement) are listed in Table 61-3.

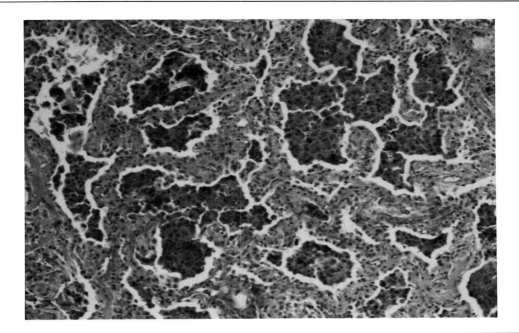

Fig. 61-8. Chronic pulmonary alveolar hemorrhage, regardless of cause, is seen as increased hemosiderin-filled alveolar macrophages associated with mild thickening and reactive changes in the surrounding alveolar walls.

Goodpasture's Syndrome

Of the four well-known basic immune reactions in the lung, the cytotoxic antibody-mediated reaction (type II) is responsible for Goodpasture's syndrome [70,84]. This syndrome is characterized by the presence of circulating antiglomerular basement membrane (anti-GBM) antibodies and characteristic linear deposits of IgG and complement along the basement membranes of alveoli and glomerular basement membrane. More recently, the autoantigen (Goodpasture's antigen) has been identified as the alpha$_3$ chain of type IV collagen (alpha$_3$(IV)NC$_1$), and its gene, COL4A3, maps to 2q36-2q37 [87,101,204]. Although the primary target of the antibodies is the kidney, the lungs are affected by cross-reactivity. The etiology is unknown, but influenza virus, hydrocarbon exposure, penicillamine, and unknown genetic factors are known to stimulate autoantibody production [134,160,185,197].

A recent review of the literature analyzed the data on 31 patients with hydrocarbon exposure and anti-GBM antibody–mediated nephritis and concluded that a causal relationship was present [22]. Further, inadvertent exposure to hydrocarbons has resulted in the exacerbation of Goodpasture's syndrome [118]. Goodpasture's syndrome has been described in identical twins [50]. It is noteworthy that anti-GBM antibody has been detected in systemic lupus erythematosus, polyarteritis nodosa, Henoch-Schönlein purpura, hydrocarbon exposure, and penicillamine sensitivity. Because of this, there is some confusion regarding the exact definition of Goodpasture's syndrome.

A study of 39 patients with anti-GBM antibody–mediated glomerulonephritis has suggested that HLA-B7-associated genes influence the severity of the renal disease but not that of the lung disease [171]. Short-term exposure to certain solvents, such as several halogenated hydrocarbons, petroleum distillates, ethylene glycol, ethylene glycol ethers, and diethylene glycol, may cause renal tubular necrosis, and tubular lesions with metabolic acidosis have been reported in addicts inhaling solvent vapor such as toluene [125]. Goodpasture's syndrome may be induced by acute or subacute exposure to solvents, but its incidence is rare. Although adequate proof is lacking to suggest that repeated exposure to nonsubstituted organic solvents may lead to the development of different types of chronic glomerulonephritis and, possibly, Goodpasture's syn-

***Table 61-3.* Causes of pulmonary alveolar hemorrhage**

Pulmonary hemosiderosis
    Childhood pulmonary hemosiderosis
    Chronic adult idiopathic pulmonary
       hemosiderosis
    Celiac sprue-associated hemosiderosis
Rapidly progressive glomerulonephritis
    With anti-GBM antibody (Goodpasture's
       syndrome)
    Without anti-GBM antibody
    Microscopic polyarteritis
    Systemic lupus erythematosus
    Wegener's granulomatosis
    Henoch-Schönlein purpura
Other collagenoses
    Mixed connective tissue disease
    Rheumatoid arthritis
    Scleroderma
Other vasculitides
    Churg-Strauss disease
    Behçet's disease
    Essential mixed cryoglobulinemia
Malignant disease of pulmonary parenchyma
    Leukemias
    Lymphomas
    Pulmonary Kaposi's sarcoma
    Metastatic malignancy
       Right atrial myxoma and other tumors
       Hematogenous metastasis
Bone marrow transplantation
Toxic alveolar hemorrhage
    D-Penicillamine
    Trimellitic anhydride
    Isocyanates
    Hydrocarbons
    Lymphangiographic dye
    Anticoagulants (superwarfarin)
Mitral stenosis
Miscellaneous diagnoses
    Pulmonary lymphangioleiomyomatosis
    Microangiopathic hemolytic anemia
    Pulmonary veno-occlusive disease
    Ventilator-associated pneumonia
    Immunocompromised patients with pneumonia
    IgA monoclonal gammopathy

anti-GBM = antiglomerular basement membrane.

drome, the available epidemiologic data suggest such an association [13]. Use of penicillamine and carbimazole for the treatment of rheumatoid arthritis and other diseases has been associated with Goodpasture's syndrome, circulating anti-GBM antibodies, focal necrotizing glomerulonephritis with crescents, and HLA typing of Dr3 and Dr4 being present [160].

The role of cigarette smoking in contributing to the pulmonary alveolar hemorrhage in Goodpasture's syndrome has been examined. In a study of 51 patients with glomerulonephritis due to anti-GBM antibody, 43 had pulmonary hemorrhage [55]; of these, 37 were smokers and all had pulmonary hemorrhage, as opposed to only 2 of 10 nonsmokers. There was no significant difference between the titers of circulating anti-GBM antibody in smokers and nonsmokers.

A review in 1985 observed that since 1919 nearly 400 cases of Goodpasture's syndrome have been published [115]. Patients with anti-GBM antibody–mediated nephritis demonstrate two principal patterns of disease—young men presenting in their twenties with Goodpasture's syndrome (glomerulonephritis and lung hemorrhage) and elderly patients, especially women, presenting in their sixties with glomerulonephritis alone. In the classic form of Goodpasture's syndrome, men are affected more often than women (male–female ratio 7 : 1), and the average age of onset is approximately 27 years. Recurrent hemoptysis, pulmonary insufficiency, renal involvement with hematuria and renal failure, and anemia are the classic features. Pulmonary hemorrhage almost always precedes renal manifestations. Chest roentgenograms typically reveal bilateral, diffuse, symmetric perihilar infiltrates with sparing of the costophrenic angles and apices (Fig. 61-9). The diagnosis is made by correlating the clinical features, chest roentgenographic abnormalities, and characteristic renal pathology. Lung biopsy also will demonstrate the characteristic linear deposition of immunofluorescent material along the

Fig. 61-9. Extensive dense alveolar infiltrates secondary to pulmonary alveolar hemorrhage in Goodpasture's syndrome. The costophrenic angles are spared.

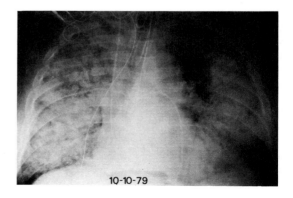

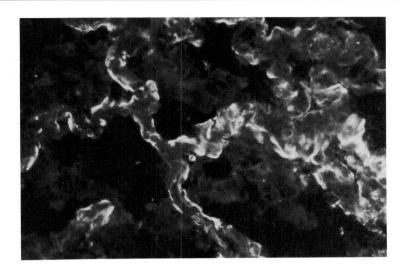

Fig. 61-10. Immunofluorescent staining of lung tissue in Goodpasture's syndrome reveals the characteristic linear deposits of IgG along alveolar basement membrane.

alveolar basement membrane (Fig. 61-10). Transbronchial lung biopsy has been used for diagnosis, but the diagnostic yield is approximately 30 percent [1,108].

The preceding description is that of the classic Goodpasture's syndrome. However, there is some confusion regarding the diagnosis because of inclusion of other alveolar hemorrhage syndromes under the eponym *Goodpasture's syndrome* [100]. An overall mortality of 58 percent was noted in 40 patients belonging to these groups, and most patients died of progressive disease or infection. Recurrent Goodpasture's syndrome has been described by several investigators [49]. A fatal relapse 3 years after plasmapheresis has been described in a smoker who had been exposed to hydrocarbon solvents and who had the HLA tissue antigens Dr2 and Mt3 [115]. More recent studies have recorded the presence of myeloperoxidase-ANCA in patients with Goodpasture's syndrome and other vasculitides (see Chapter 58), introducing further confusion into the understanding of Goodpasture's syndrome and other alveolar hemorrhage syndromes [6,176].

An interesting case was reported of a 19-year-old woman working as a hairdresser who developed severe anemia as a result of occult pulmonary hemorrhage followed by anti-GBM antibody–induced glomerulonephritis with normal renal function [88]. Withdrawal of the suspected toxic factor, products used for permanent waving, was followed by both clinical remission and disappearance of the linear deposits of immunoglobulin from the renal glomeruli. Anti-GBM antibodies were detected in the serum only after clinical healing. In patients with Goodpasture's syndrome, a careful search should be made to ascertain the possibility of toxin exposure [88].

One study looked into the factors that affected the clinical course of 22 patients with Goodpasture's syndrome with renal impairment and reported that the most important features associated with a bad prognosis were total anuria or a very high percentage of glomeruli showing crescents (>85 percent) in the initial renal biopsy [210]. Renal biopsies proved to be an extremely valuable guide for the progress and outcome of the disease.

Plasmapheresis is the treatment of choice in patients with Goodpasture's syndrome [9,116, 190,200]. It has been reported that since 1975, in nearly 100 patients with Goodpasture's syndrome treated with plasma exchange in addition to immunosuppression, remission was achieved in 50 percent, and in 7 percent a relapse was reported [115]. Long-term follow-up data on 29 patients disclosed that 31 percent recovered totally and remained symptom-free with normal renal function for a mean of 206 weeks [199]. Complete recovery has occurred in patients treated with systemic corticosteroids, immunosuppressive agents, or plasmapheresis [26,100,108].

A patient with autoantibody-mediated Goodpasture's syndrome was successfully treated with cytotoxic drugs, steroids, and plasma exchange. After an absence of 3 years, circulating anti-GBM antibodies reappeared, and linear IgG staining of the glomeruli was shown by immunofluorescence studies. Renal function did not change, and there was no evidence of pulmonary hemorrhage. Antibody levels then fell spontaneously over the succeeding 18 months [99].

Glomerulonephritis

Another major cause of alveolar hemorrhage is rapidly progressive glomerulonephritis. This disease is more common than reported, and more than 50 percent of cases are composed of Wegener's granulomatosis and microscopic polyarteritis [5]. Additionally, rapidly progressive glomerulonephritis can occur in patients with Goodpasture's syndrome (anti-GBM antibody disease), lupus nephritis (immune complex disease), and pauciimmune and other vasculitides or idiopathic nephritis. In a series of 1500 renal biopsies demonstrating glomerulonephritis with crescent formation, 44 percent had immune complex deposition, 5 percent had anti-GBM antibody, and 51 percent had a pauciimmune pattern [107]. In another review of alveolar hemorrhage syndrome associated with nephritis in 45 patients, the etiologies included anti-GBM disease (18 percent), a systemic vasculitis (56 percent), and idiopathic glomerulonephritis (27 percent), and a variety of acute pulmonary complications, the most common being acute respiratory failure (29 percent) [24]. Mortality directly due to pulmonary disease was uncommon, with 7 percent dying from fulminant lung hemorrhage. Follow-up studies in 22 patients 6 months after initial presentation indicated that although respiratory symptoms (14 percent) or pulmonary roentgenographic abnormalities (23 percent) were uncommon, the majority (73 percent) of patients had residual abnormalities on pulmonary function testing. Interstitial lung disease has occurred in association with glomerulonephritis caused by unusual vasculitic disorders such as Takayasu's arteritis [85]. Other vasculitic syndromes—for instance, giant cell arteritis—can produce pulmonary problems without alveolar hemorrhage [124]. Pulmonary hemorrhage is common in Behçet's disease.

Collagenoses and Vasculitides

The disorders classified as collagenoses and vasculitides are two of the most important causes of pulmonary alveolar hemorrhage syndrome [163–165]. In the former category, systemic lupus erythematosus is noteworthy, whereas in the latter, Wegener's granulomatosis and other vasculitic syndromes are significant. As a group, the vasculitic disorders are important in the etiology of alveolar hemorrhage syndrome. The clinical aspects of alveolar hemorrhage associated with these diseases are discussed in Chapters 58 and 59.

Idiopathic Pulmonary Hemosiderosis

It has become increasingly difficult to separate idiopathic pulmonary hemosiderosis from other causes of alveolar hemorrhage syndrome. The confusion stems from the inclusion of idiopathic pulmonary hemosiderosis with Goodpasture's syndrome and other causes of alveolar hemorrhage. Development of systemic vasculitis several years after the diagnosis of idiopathic pulmonary hemosiderosis has been described [126]. For instance, the alveolar hemorrhage caused by so-called microscopic polyarteritis (not to be confused with polyarteritis nodosa), associated with pauciimmune glomerulonephritis in combination with systemic small-vessel vasculitis but without granulomatous inflammation, has been labelled *idiopathic pulmonary hemosiderosis* [186]. Furthermore, Fraser and associates [73] regard *idiopathic pulmonary hemorrhage* as a preferable term to the more traditional *idiopathic pulmonary hemosiderosis*. Morgan and Turner-Warwick [148] have classified all pulmonary alveolar hemorrhage syndromes listed in Table 61-3 as variants of pulmonary hemosiderosis. Currently, idiopathic pulmonary hemosiderosis is a diagnosis of exclusion.

An uncommon disorder caused by recurrent intrapulmonary hemorrhage, idiopathic pulmonary hemosiderosis is characterized by the triad of hemoptysis, iron-deficiency anemia, and transient roentgenologic infiltrates. The etiology of this disorder remains unknown, even though its origin has been attributed to several mechanisms, including a heritable defect, an immunologic mechanism based on the presence of antibodies to cow's milk (Heiner's syndrome), cold agglutinins, and increased serum IgA, viral infections, a primary disorder of airway epithelial cells, and a structural defect of pulmonary capillaries [8,39,206]. Familial occurrence has been noted [25,202]. Idiopathic pulmonary hemosiderosis has been described in association with idiopathic thrombocytopenic purpura and autoimmune hemolytic anemia [29,148]. A significant number of patients with idiopathic pulmonary hemosiderosis and celiac disease have been described [123,148,156,187]. The implication of these associations is unclear, although an immunologically mediated mechanism seems most likely.

The clinical findings are extremely variable. Although most patients previously described have been children or young adults, the condition has been recognized in older adults [154]. Hemoptysis may be massive, with dyspnea, cough, and cyanosis, and recurrent bleeding may result in hypochromic anemia. Chest film abnormalities include poorly defined, coarse infiltrates, more common in the lower lobes bilaterally. Cessation of symptoms correlates with roentgenographic clearing. Intrathoracic lymphadenopathy is seen in up to 25 percent of cases. The clinical course is characterized by remissions and relapses, and a fatal end is common. Anemia is due to sequestration of iron in the lung parenchyma, often in alveolar macrophages. Since they cannot be mobilized for synthesis of hemoglobin, usable body iron stores become depleted, but they can be mobilized and excreted by the use of synthetic chelating agents [104]. Development of pulmonary fibrosis accounts for the chronic respiratory insufficiency evident in many patients with long-standing idiopathic pulmonary hemosiderosis.

Diagnosis is based on the clinical and roentgenographic features and the presence of hemosiderin-laden macrophages in the sputum. Microscopically, there is marked capillary dilatation with degeneration and hyperplasia of alveolar epithelial cells (see Fig. 61-8) [56]. Corticosteroid and immunosuppressive therapy have been utilized with varying results. Several cases of idiopathic pulmonary hemosiderosis that resolved with cyclophosphamide or chloroquine therapy have been reported [31,39]. Interestingly, resolution of idiopathic pulmonary hemosiderosis after institution of a gluten-free diet in patients with idiopathic pulmonary hemosiderosis and celiac disease has been reported [156].

Malignant Disease

Alveolar hemorrhage is an important complication of pulmonary malignancies, being more common in patients who develop hematogenous pulmonary metastasis or leukemic lung infiltrates. Autopsy studies in patients with leukemia frequently show alveolar hemorrhage that was occult during life [82,95,184,195]. Twelve percent of focal and 78 percent of diffuse pulmonary infiltrates have been attributed to alveolar hemorrhage in leukemic patients [201]. The alveolar hemorrhage is frequently related to other complications such as invasive aspergillosis or zygomycosis, which result from immunosuppression. Occasionally, nonfungal infections can also produce alveolar hemorrhage. In the majority of the documented cases, thrombocytopenia (platelet count of fewer than 20,000/µl) has been noted. Irrespective of the etiology, alveolar hemorrhage usually is not suspected or diagnosed before death; hemoptysis occurs in fewer than one-fourth of patients [95]. Many patients develop an immunocompromised state as a result of infections, neoplasms, cytotoxic chemotherapy, or for unknown reasons. The incidence of alveolar hemorrhage in this group of patients varies from 3 to 8 percent [95].

Pulmonary alveolar hemorrhage is also common in certain nonhematologic malignancies. In one study of 23 patients with bronchopulmonary Kaposi's sarcoma, occult alveolar hemorrhage was present in 16 (70 percent) [103]. Hematogenous malignancies with tumor emboli in the pulmonary vessels also cause alveolar hemorrhage (Fig. 61-11). Right atrial myxoma is reported to cause pulmonary hemorrhage [34].

Fig. 61-11. Diffuse alveolar-nodular infiltrates caused by hematogenous tumor emboli originating in a hypernephroma resulted in clinically significant alveolar hemorrhage.

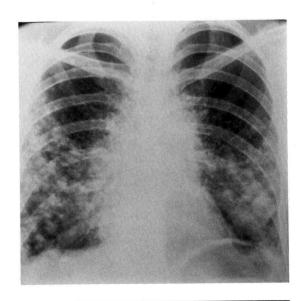

Bone Marrow Transplantation

Pulmonary alveolar hemorrhage is now recognized as a significant cause of pulmonary disease among marrow recipients, although the actual incidence is unknown [64,175]. A review of this complication found diffuse alveolar hemorrhage in 11 to 21 percent of patients, with a mortality ranging from 50 to 80 percent [64]. The use of dimethyl sulfoxide in the cryopreservation of the bone marrow of autologous transplants has been suggested as a possible cause of diffuse alveolar hemorrhage in these patients [33].

A high incidence of alveolar hemorrhage has been noted in patients with Hodgkin's and non-Hodgkin's lymphoma treated with high-dose radiation and chemotherapy and autologous bone marrow transplantation. Acute respiratory failure secondary to alveolar hemorrhage occurred within 2 weeks after bone marrow transplantation in 26 percent of 77 consecutive patients thus treated; the mortality was 100 percent [109]. Others have observed alveolar hemorrhage in 21 percent, with a mortality of 79 percent, in patients who received either allogeneic or autologous bone marrow transplant [175].

Hemoptysis is unusual in most cases of alveolar hemorrhage. The majority of patients exhibit clinical and roentgenologic signs of infection, including high fever, dyspnea, nonproductive cough, hypoxemia, and diffuse or focal alveolar infiltrates. The initial roentgenologic abnormalities develop within the first 2 weeks and precede the clinical diagnosis by an average of 3 days [217].

Mitral Stenosis

Although mitral valve disease is now an uncommon cause of alveolar hemorrhage in the developed countries, it remains an important etiology of hemoptysis and alveolar hemorrhage in developing countries. Earlier publications indicated that hemoptysis in mitral stenosis is caused by the rupture of dilated and varicose bronchial veins [53,152]. Hemoptysis from this mechanism usually occurs early in the course of mitral stenosis and may be the presenting symptom [188]. More recent studies suggest that the capillary wall stresses greatly increase when the capillary pressure is raised, and wall damage occurs at pressures of 40 mmHg and higher; alveolar hemorrhage in mitral stenosis is believed to be the result of stress failure of pulmonary capillaries [215,216]. Recurrent episodes of alveolar hemorrhage may result in pulmonary calcification and even true ossification. Pulmonary fibrosis may be seen in some patients.

Toxic Alveolar Hemorrhage

D-PENICILLAMINE

Alveolar hemorrhage is a rare manifestation of penicillamine toxicity. Several anecdotal case reports have suggested D-penicillamine as a cause of Goodpasture's syndrome [128,160,197]. The daily dose of the drug was high (0.75 to 2.0 gm) in almost all cases, and the duration of therapy prior to toxicity ranged from 10 months to 3 years. Uniformly severe alveolar hemorrhage occurred with glomerulonephritis, but other organs were not affected, and four deaths were recorded in a review of the subject in 1984 [128]. Immunopathologic features in these cases suggest immune-complex drug-induced disease with a granular pattern of immunofluorescence and with none of the hallmarks of Goodpasture's syndrome [148].

TRIMELLITIC ANHYDRIDE

Trimellitic anhydride is a component of epoxy resin used in the manufacture of epoxy resin coatings, plastics, and paints. Inhalation of fumes or powder can lead to several clinical syndromes, among which pulmonary alveolar hemorrhage is the most serious. Workers exposed to this chemical have developed allergic type of lung disease as well as alveolar hemorrhage. Presence of antibodies against haptenized erythrocytes and human serum albumin in these subjects suggests an immunologic basis [4]. The illness is characterized by cough, hemoptysis, dyspnea, weakness, and nausea or vomiting. Anemia is a common finding—hence the term *pulmonary disease–anemia syndrome*, sometimes used to describe this entity. A series of seven young men exposed to trimellitic anhydride developed typical symptoms, but all recovered quickly without treatment; light and electron microscopic studies of lung tissue showed extensive bleeding into alveoli, but no basement membrane deposits or anti-GBM antibodies were observed [93].

ISOCYANATES

Hemoptysis, dyspnea, and bilateral pulmonary opacities have been described in a 34-year-old man who was exposed to spray paint that contained hexamethylene diisocyanate and toluene diisocyanate; high levels of IgG and IgE antibodies were detected against these isocyanates [158].

ANTICOAGULANTS

A case of rodenticide-induced diffuse alveolar hemorrhage has been reported in a patient who consumed brodifacoum (D-Con), a derivative of warfarin [10]. Therapeutic use of anticoagulants is unlikely to cause alveolar hemorrhage unless the pulmonary parenchyma suffers trauma. Three cases were described in 1975, and the clinical features included dyspnea, unexplained acute anemia, and alveolar infiltrates, but hemoptysis was conspicuously absent; one patient died from massive pulmonary alveolar hemorrhage [68].

LYMPHANGIOGRAPHY

Lymphangiography has been complicated by pulmonary alveolar hemorrhage [80]. Hemoptysis has been estimated to occur in only 1 in 3000 cases and is limited to blood-tinged sputum [128]. A 1984 review of alveolar hemorrhage syndromes noted three reported cases of severe alveolar bleeding occurring 2, 5, and 10 days after the procedure, and one patient died [128].

Other Causes of Alveolar Hemorrhage

Immunocompromised patients develop a variety of infectious and noninfectious pulmonary complications, as discussed in Chapter 59. Among the noninfectious respiratory manifestations, alveolar hemorrhage is an important consideration. In a study of 51 immunocompromised patients, bronchoalveolar lavage studies documented severe alveolar hemorrhage in 27 percent of patients; thrombocytopenia and invasive fungal infections were significantly associated with this complication [111]. Clinical features include progressive dyspnea, cough, and hypoxemia. Hemoptysis is distinctly uncommon. Chest roentgenologic abnormalities vary considerably (Figs. 61-12, 61-13).

Ventilator-associated pneumonia is also known to produce alveolar hemorrhage. A study evaluated the roentgenologic aspects of autopsy-proved ventilator-associated pneumonia in 69 patients and observed alveolar hemorrhage in 38 percent of cases; the hemorrhage was associated with 29 percent of multiple air bronchograms and 30 percent of bilateral alveolar infiltrates in patients without pneumonia [218].

Pulmonary lymphangioleiomyomatosis is an uncommon cause of alveolar hemorrhage syndrome. Hemoptysis as a presenting symptom occurs in 7 percent of cases and in half the patients during the course of their illness [42]. The mechanism of alveolar hemorrhage is hypothesized to

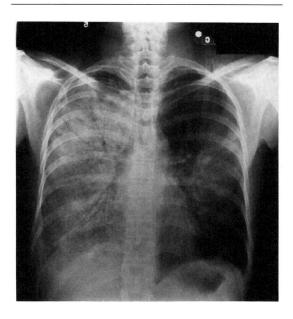

Fig. 61-12. Marked alveolar infiltrates in the right lung with only a patchy area of infiltrate in left midlung. Significant hemoptysis in this patient was caused by systemic lupus erythematosus complicated by renal failure. Not all cases of "diffuse" alveolar hemorrhage show bilaterally symmetric chest roentgenologic abnormalities.

be the venous obstruction and capillary hemorrhage caused by proliferation of muscle in the walls of the pulmonary veins [148].

Pulmonary veno-occlusive disease in a child is reported to have caused fatal alveolar hemorrhage [38]. Microangiopathic hemolytic anemia in association with alveolar hemorrhage syndrome has been described in several cases [148]. Anticardiolipin antibody syndrome (see Chapter 58) is another cause of alveolar hemorrhage [98].

Miscellaneous Renal Diseases

The risk of hemorrhage during surgical procedures is increased in renal failure because of platelet dysfunction caused by azotemia. Transbronchial lung biopsy in patients with serum creatinine levels in excess of 3.5 mg/dl carries a 40 percent risk of bleeding.

A study of 206 Taiwanese children with nephrotic syndrome revealed that boys had a three times higher incidence of bronchial asthma than the general population, whereas no difference

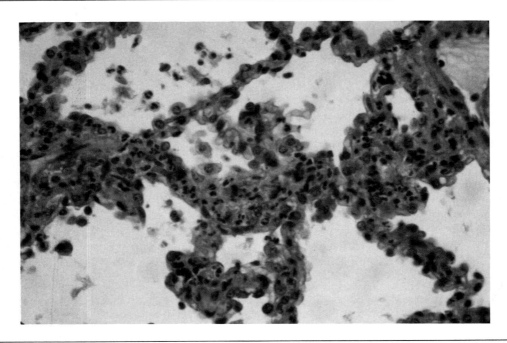

Fig. 61-13. Acute pulmonary alveolar hemorrhage showing infiltrates of neutrophils in the alveolar septa. The pattern here is nonspecific and could be seen in Goodpasture's syndrome, Wegener's granulomatosis, collagenoses, or vasculitis. In this particular case, a specific diagnosis could not be made.

was noted among girls. Both sexes had ten times more atopic dermatitis than the general population. The serum IgE level was elevated in most of the patients and seemed to serve as a prognostic factor in renal disease [132].

Nephrobronchial fistula is a rare sequel of perinephric abscess and other inflammatory renal diseases [57,179]. There are reports of nephrolithiasis complicated by obstruction leading to pyonephrosis, perinephric abscess, and nephrobronchial fistula that were treated successfully by nephrectomy [90]. Inflammatory renal diseases may involve the perirenal space and spread contiguously to other organs in the abdomen, as well as to the adjacent pleural space.

Acute respiratory distress has been described in a man undergoing nephrolithotripsy. Absorption of a large volume of irrigating fluid during the procedure was responsible for this complication [181]. Pyelonephritis in pregnancy also may be complicated by acute respiratory distress syndrome [47,62].

A unique case of biopsy-proved IgA nephropathy associated with IgA immune complex pneumonitis has been described in a 41-year-old man [91]. He developed dyspnea on exertion, restrictive ventilatory impairment, reduced DlCO, and hypoxemia. Transbronchoscopic lung biopsy re-

vealed interstitial pneumonitis and deposition of IgA and C3, closely resembling the pathologic findings in the renal mesangium.

Pulmonary alveolar microlithiasis is an uncommon disease of unknown etiology, characterized by deposition of tiny calcispherites in the alveolar spaces [166]. Although there is no relation between this disorder and nephrolithiasis, a case of pulmonary alveolar microlithiasis with pleural calcification and nephrolithiasis has been reported [157].

Renal cell carcinoma may produce hematogenous metastases, frequently referred to as *cannonball lesions*. Endobronchial metastases also are seen. Lobar or segmental atelectasis, hemoptysis, or expectoration of the metastatic tumor may be the presenting symptom [105].

Rounded atelectasis, also known as *folded-lung syndrome*, or atelectatic pseudotumor has been described in three patients with end-stage renal disease [219]. It is usually caused by chronic pleural effusion or pleural disease. Uremic pleurisy or recurrent small pleural effusion associated with chronic renal disease may well lead to rounded atelectasis.

Diagnostic and therapeutic procedures performed on the kidneys can lead to pulmonary complications. Life-threatening hypoxemia after lithotripsy due to shock wave–induced pulmonary contusion has been described in a patient [137]. Hemoptysis is another complication reported in a child who underwent extracorporeal shock-wave lithotripsy [136]. Hemothorax has occurred as a complication of percutaneous renal biopsy [19].

In a study of 19 patients with renal tubular acidosis, 4 were found to have pulmonary fibrosis with restricted pulmonary function and diminished DLCO [138].

References

1. Abboud RT, et al. Goodpasture's syndrome: Diagnosis by transbronchial lung biopsy. *Ann Intern Med* 89:635, 1978.
2. Abu-Hamdan DK, et al. Hypoxemia during hemodialysis using acetate versus bicarbonate dialysate. *Am J Nephrol* 4:248, 1984.
3. Addleman M, Logan AS, Grossman RF. Monitoring intrapulmonary hemorrhage in Goodpasture's syndrome. *Chest* 87:119, 1985.
4. Ahmad D, et al. Pulmonary haemorrhage and hemolytic anemia due to trimellitic anhydride. *Lancet* 2:328, 1979.
5. Andrassy K, et al. Rapidly progressive glomerulonephritis: Analysis of prevalence and clinical course. *Nephron* 59:206, 1991.
6. Arimura Y, et al. A case of Goodpasture's syndrome associated with anti-myeloperoxidase antibodies. *Ann Intern Med* 31:239, 1992.
7. Aurigemma NM, et al. Arterial oxygenation during hemodialysis. *N Engl J Med* 297:871, 1977.
8. Bailey P, Groden BM. Idiopathic pulmonary hemosiderosis: Report of two cases and review of the literature. *Postgrad Med J* 55:266, 1979.
9. Balow JE. Plasmapheresis: Development and application in treatment of renal disorders. *Artif Organs* 10:324, 1986.
10. Barnet TV, et al. Diffuse alveolar hemorrhage secondary to superwarfarin ingestion. *Chest* 102:1301, 1992.
11. Baron RL, et al. Intrathoracic extravasations of retroperitoneal urine collections. *AJR* 137:37, 1981.
12. Beechler CR, et al. Immunofluorescence of transbronchial biopsies in Goodpasture's syndrome. *Am Rev Respir Dis* 121:869, 1980.
13. Beirne GJ, Brennan JT. Glomerulonephritis associated with hydrocarbon solvents. *Arch Environ Health* 25:365, 1972.
14. Belcher NG, Rees PJ. Changes in pulmonary clearance of technetium labelled DTPA during hemodialysis. *Thorax* 41:381, 1986.
15. Berger HW, et al. Uremic pleural effusion: A study in 14 patients on chronic dialysis. *Ann Intern Med* 82:362, 1975.
16. Bestetti-Bosisio M, et al. Lung calcification in long-term dialysed patients: A light and electron microscopic study. *Histopathology* 8:69, 1984.
17. Betts RF. Cytomegalovirus infection in transplant patients. *Prog Med Virol* 28:44, 1982.
18. Bischel MD, Scoles BG, Mohler JG. Evidence for pulmonary microembolization during hemodialysis. *Chest* 67:335, 1975.
19. Bissler JJ, Warner BW, Welch TR. Hemothorax as a complication following percutaneous renal biopsy. *Am J Kidney Dis* 18:122, 1991.
20. Blanchet F, et al. Relative contribution of intrinsic lung dysfunction and hypoventilation to hypoxemia during hemodialysis. *Kidney Int* 26:430, 1984.
21. Bloodworth J, Tomashefski JF Jr. Localised pulmonary metastatic calcification associated pulmonary artery obstruction. *Thorax* 47:174, 1992.
22. Bombassei GJ, Kaplan AA. The association between hydrocarbon exposure and anti-glomerular basement membrane antibody-mediated disease (Goodpasture's syndrome). *Am J Ind Med* 21:141, 1992.
23. Boner G, et al. Diffuse calcification of lungs in a patient on maintenance hemodialysis. *Isr J Med Sci* 7:1182, 1971.
24. Boyce NW, Holdsworth SR. Pulmonary manifestations of the clinical syndrome of acute glomerulonephritis and lung hemorrhage. *Am J Kidney Dis* 8:31, 1986.
25. Breckenridge RL Jr, Ross JS. Idiopathic pulmonary hemosiderosis: A report of familial occurrence. *Chest* 75:636, 1979.
26. Briggs WA, et al. Antiglomerular basement-membrane antibody-mediated glomerulonephritis and Goodpasture's syndrome. *Medicine* 58:348, 1979.
27. Briggs WA, et al. Severe pneumonia in renal transplant patients. One year's experience. *Ann Intern Med* 75:887, 1971.
28. Brown CM, et al. Fibrosing uremic pleuritis during hemodialysis. *JAMA* 245:705, 1981.
29. Buchanan GR, Moore GC. Pulmonary hemosiderosis and immune thrombocytopenia: Initial manifestations of collagen-vascular disease. *JAMA* 246:861, 1981.
30. Bush A, Gabriel R. Pulmonary function in chronic renal failure: Effects of dialysis and transplantation. *Thorax* 46:424, 1991.
31. Bush A, Sheppard MN, Warner JO. Chloroquine

in idiopathic pulmonary haemosiderosis. *Arch Dis Child* 67:625, 1992.

32. Chang D-B, et al. Clearance of theophylline by hemodialysis in one patient with chronic renal failure. *Chest* 102:1621, 1992.

33. Chao NJ, et al. Corticosteroid therapy for diffuse alveolar hemorrhage in autologous bone marrow transplant recipients. *Ann Intern Med* 114:145, 1991.

34. Chaudhry AA, Dobson CM, Simpson FG. Pulmonary haemosiderosis associated with left atrial myxoma. *Thorax* 46:539, 1991.

35. Chervenick PA. Dialysis, neutropenia, lung dysfunction and complement (editorial). *N Engl J Med* 296:810, 1977.

36. Chinn DH, et al. Calcified pulmonary nodules in chronic renal failure. *AJR* 137:402, 1981.

37. Cohn J, Balk RA, Bone RC. Dialysis-induced respiratory acidosis. *Chest* 98:1285, 1990.

38. Cohn RC, et al. Death due to diffuse alveolar hemorrhage in a child with pulmonary veno-occlusive disease. *Chest* 100:1456, 1991.

39. Colombo JL, Stolz SM. Treatment of life-threatening primary pulmonary hemosiderosis with cyclophosphamide. *Chest* 102:959, 1992.

40. Conger JD, et al. Pulmonary calcification in chronic dialysis patients. Clinical and pathologic studies. *Ann Intern Med* 83:330, 1975.

41. Corriere JN Jr, Miller WT, Murphy JJ. Hydronephrosis as a cause of pleural effusion. *Radiology* 90:79, 1968.

42. Corrin B, Liebow AA, Friedman PJ. Lymphangioleiomyomatosis. A review. *Am J Pathol* 79:348, 1975.

43. Coutts II, Jegarajah S, Stark JE. Tuberculosis in renal transplant recipients. *Br J Dis Chest* 73:141, 1979.

44. Craddock PR, et al. Complement and leukocyte-mediated pulmonary dysfunction in hemodialysis. *N Engl J Med* 296:769, 1977.

45. Craddock PR, et al. Hemodialysis leukopenia: Pulmonary vascular leukostasis resulting from complement activation by dialyzer cellophane membranes. *J Clin Invest* 59:879, 1977.

46. Crosbie WA, Snowden S, Parsons V. Changes in lung capillary permeability in renal failure. *Br Med J* 4:388, 1972.

47. Cunningham FG, et al. Respiratory insufficiency associated with pyelonephritis during pregnancy. *Obstet Gynecol* 63:121, 1984.

48. Cuss FM, et al. Tuberculosis in renal failure: A high incidence in patients born in the third world. *Clin Nephrol* 25:129, 1986.

49. Dahlberg PJ, et al. Recurrent Goodpasture's syndrome. *Mayo Clin Proc* 53:533, 1978.

50. D'Apice AJF, Kincaid-Smith P, Becker GJ. Goodpasture's syndrome in identical twins. *Ann Intern Med* 88:61, 1978.

51. Davenport A, Williams AJ. Fall in peak expiratory flow during haemodialysis in patients with chronic renal failure. *Thorax* 43:693, 1988.

52. Devacaanthan K, et al. Pulmonary calcification in chronic renal failure: Use of diphosphonate scintiscan as a diagnostic tool. *Clin Nephrol* 6:488, 1976.

53. Diamond MA, Genovese PD. Life-threatening hemoptysis in mitral stenosis. Emergency mitral valve replacement resulting in rapid, sustained cessation of pulmonary bleeding. *JAMA* 215:441, 1971.

54. Dolan MJ, et al. Hypopnea associated with acetate hemodialysis: Carbon dioxide flow-dependent ventilation. *N Engl J Med* 305:72, 1981.

55. Donaghy M, Rees AJ. Cigarette smoking and lung haemorrhage in glomerulonephritis caused by autoantibodies to glomerular basement membrane. *Lancet* 2:1390, 1983.

56. Donlan CJ Jr, Srodes CH, Duffy FD. Idiopathic pulmonary hemosiderosis: Electron microscopic, immunofluorescent, and iron kinetic studies. *Chest* 68:577, 1975.

57. Doughney KB, Dineen MK, Venable DD. Nephrobronchial colonic fistula complicating perinephric abscess. *J Urol* 135:765, 1986.

58. Drachman R, et al. Pulmonary calcification in children on dialysis. *Nephron* 44:46, 1986.

59. Duarte R. Blood pressure, ventilation and lipid imbalance during hemodialysis: Effect of dialysate composition. *Blood Purif* 3:199, 1985.

60. Dujic Z, et al. The effects of hemodialysis and anemia on pulmonary diffusing capacity, membrane diffusing capacity and capillary blood volume in uremic patients. *Respiration* 58:277, 1991.

61. Ei K, et al. Hemodialysis-associated asthma in a renal failure patient. *Nephron* 25:247, 1980.

62. Elkington KW, Gelb LC. Adult respiratory distress syndrome as a complication of acute pyelonephritis during pregnancy: Case report and discussion. *Obstet Gynecol* 67(Suppl):18s, 1986.

63. Ettinger NA, Trulock EP. Pulmonary considerations of organ transplantation (part 1). *Am Rev Respir Dis* 143:1386, 1991.

64. Ettinger NA, Trulock EP. Pulmonary considerations of organ transplantation (part 2). *Am Rev Respir Dis* 144:213, 1991.

65. Evans TW, et al. Pulmonary calcification in a renal transplant recipient. *Br J Dis Chest* 77:202, 1983.

66. Fairshter RD, Vaziri ND, Mirahmadi MK. Lung pathology in chronic hemodialysis patients. *Int J Artif Organs* 5:97, 1982.

67. Feinstein EI, et al. Hemoptysis and acute renal failure in a young man (clinical conference). *Am J Nephrol* 5:64, 1985.

68. Finley TN, et al. Occult pulmonary hemorrhage in anticoagulated patients. *Am Rev Respir Dis* 112:23, 1975.

69. Firroznia H, et al. Diffuse interstitial calcification of the lungs in chronic renal failure mimicking pulmonary edema. *AJR* 129:1103, 1977.

70. Fish AJ, et al. Detection of Goodpasture antigen

in fractions prepared from collagenase digests of human glomerular basement membrane. *Clin Exp Immunol* 55:58, 1984.

71. Fogelfeld L, Gil I, Almong C. Pleurocolonic fistula secondary to calculous pyonephrosis. *Br J Urol* 55:125, 1983.

72. Forman JW, Ayres L, Miller WC. Pulmonary diffusing capacity in chronic renal failure. *Br J Dis Chest* 75:81, 1981.

73. Fraser RG, et al. Diseases of Altered Immunologic Activity. In RG Fraser et al (Eds.), *Diagnosis of Diseases of the Chest* (3rd ed). Philadelphia: Saunders, 1989. P 1177.

74. Fraumeni JF, Hoover R. Immunosurveillance cancers: Epidemiologic observations. *Natl Cancer Inst Monogr* 47:121, 1977.

75. Galen MA, et al. Hemorrhagic pleural effusion in patients undergoing chronic hemodialysis. *Ann Intern Med* 82:359, 1975.

76. Garcia-Bunuel L, Elliot DC, Blank NK. Apneic spells in progressive dialysis encephalopathy. *Arch Neurol* 37:594, 1980.

77. Giacobetti R, et al. Sudden fatal pulmonary calcification following renal transplantation. *Nephron* 19:295, 1977.

78. Gilbert L, et al. Fibrinous uremic pleuritis: A surgical entity. *Chest* 67:53, 1975.

79. Glenn J. Cytomegalovirus infection following renal transplantation. *Rev Infect Dis* 3:1151, 1981.

80. Glikson M, et al. Pulmonary complications of lymphangiography. *Harefuah* 117:14, 1989.

81. Gold E. Infections associated with immunologic deficiency diseases. *Med Clin North Am* 58:649, 1974.

82. Golde DW, et al. Occult pulmonary haemorrhage in leukaemia. *Br Med J* 2:166, 1975.

83. Gomez GME, et al. Respiratory muscle weakness in uremic patients under continuous ambulatory peritoneal dialysis. *Nephron* 36:21, 1984.

84. Goodpasture EW. The significance of certain pulmonary lesions in relation to the etiology of influenza. *Am J Med Sci* 158:863, 1919.

85. Green NB, Baughman RP, Kim CK. Takayasu's arteritis associated with interstitial lung disease and glomerulonephritis. *Chest* 289:605, 1986.

86. Gunawardena KA, et al. Pulmonary Kaposi's sarcoma in two recipients of renal transplants. *Thorax* 43:653, 1988.

87. Gunwar S, et al. Alveolar basement membrane: Molecular properties of the noncollagenous domain (hexamer) of collagen IV and its reactivity with Goodpasture autoantibodies. *Am J Respir Cell Mol Biol* 5:107, 1991.

88. Hamels J, et al. Remission of Goodpasture's syndrome after withdrawal of an unusual toxic. *Clin Nephrol* 23:312, 1985.

89. Hamm LL, Lawrence G, DuBose TD Jr. Sorbent regenerative hemodialysis as a potential cause of acute hypercapnia. *Kidney Int* 21:416, 1982.

90. Hampel N, Sidor TA, Persky L. Nephrobronchial fistula: Complication of perinephric abscess secondary to ureteral obstruction and pyonephrosis. *Urology* 16:608, 1980.

91. Harland RW, et al. Immunoglobulin A (IgA) immune complex pneumonitis in a patient with IgA nephropathy. *Ann Intern Med* 116:220, 1992.

92. Harwood AR, Osoba D, Hofstader SL. Kaposi's sarcoma in recipients of renal transplants. *Am J Med* 67:759, 1979.

93. Herbert FA, Orford R. Pulmonary hemorrhage and edema due to inhalation of resins containing trimellitic anhydride. *Chest* 76:546, 1979.

94. Herbert FK, Miller HG, Richardson GO. Chronic renal disease, secondary parathyroid hyperplasia, decalcification of bone and metastatic calcification. *J Pathol Bacteriol* 53:161, 1941.

95. Hildebrand FL Jr, et al. Pulmonary complications of leukemia. *Chest* 98:1233, 1990.

96. Hill RB Jr, et al. Death after transplantation: An analysis of sixty cases (editorial). *Am J Med* 42:327, 1967.

97. Hill RB Jr, Rowlands DT Jr, Rifkind D. Infectious pulmonary disease in patients receiving immunosuppressive therapy for organ transplantation. *N Engl J Med* 271:1021, 1964.

98. Hillerdal G, et al. Intra-alveolar haemorrhage in the anticardiolipin antibody syndrome. *Scand J Rheumatol* 20:58, 1991.

99. Hind CR, et al. Recurrence of circulating antiglomerular basement membrane antibody three years after immunosuppressive treatment and plasma exchange. *Clin Nephrol* 21:244, 1984.

100. Holdsworth S, et al. The clinical spectrum of acute glomerulonephritis and lung haemorrhage (Goodpasture's syndrome). *Q J Med* 55:75, 1985.

101. Hudson BG, et al. Goodpasture's syndrome: Molecular architecture and function of basement membrane antigen. *Lab Invest* 61:256, 1989.

102. Hughes RT. The pathology of butterfly densities in uraemia. *Thorax* 22:97, 1967.

103. Hughes-Davies L, et al. Occult alveolar haemorrhage in bronchopulmonary Kaposi's sarcoma. *J Clin Pathol* 45:536, 1992.

104. Hyatt RW, Adelstein ER, Halazun JF. Ultrastructure of the lung in idiopathic pulmonary hemosiderosis. *Am J Med* 52:822, 1972.

105. Jariwalla AG, et al. Intrabronchial metastases from renal cell carcinoma with recurrent tumor expectoration. *Thorax* 36:179, 1981.

106. Jenkins PG, Shelp W. Recurrent pleural transudate in the nephrotic syndrome: A new approach to treatment. *JAMA* 230:587, 1974.

107. Jennette JC, Wilkman AS, Falk RJ. Anti-neutrophil cytoplasmic autoantibody-associated glomerulonephritis and vasculitis. *Am J Pathol* 135:921, 1989.

108. Johnson JP, et al. Therapy of antiglomerular basement-membrane antibody disease: Analysis of prognostic significance of clinical, patho-

logic, and treatment factors. *Medicine* 64:219, 1985.

109. Jules-Elysee K, et al. Pulmonary complications in lymphoma patients treated with high-dose therapy and autologous bone marrow transplantation. *Am Rev Respir Dis* 146:485, 1992.

110. Justrabo E, Gonin R, Rifle G. Pulmonary metastatic calcification with respiratory insufficiency in patients on maintenance hemodialysis. *Thorax* 34:384, 1979.

111. Kahn FW, Jones JM, England DM. Diagnosis of pulmonary hemorrhage in the immunocompromised host. *Am Rev Respir Dis* 136:155, 1987.

112. Kaltreider HB, et al. So-called metastatic calcification of the lung. *Am J Med* 46:188, 1969.

113. Kalweit WH, et al. Hemodialysis fistula infection caused by *Legionella pneumophila*. *Ann Intern Med* 96:173, 1982.

114. Karasick SR. Case of the winter season: Metastatic pulmonary calcification in a renal transplant recipient. *Semin Roentgenol* 16:5, 1981.

115. Keller F, Nekarda H. Fatal relapse in Goodpasture's syndrome 3 years after plasma exchange. *Respiration* 48:62, 1985.

116. Keller F, et al. Membrane plasma exchange in Goodpasture's syndrome. *Am J Med Sci* 287:32, 1984.

117. Kenamond TG, et al. Severe recurrent alkalemia in a patient undergoing continuous cyclic peritoneal dialysis. *Am J Med* 81:548, 1986.

118. Keogh AM, et al. Exacerbation of Goodpasture's syndrome after inadvertent exposure to hydrocarbon fumes. *Br Med J* 288:188, 1984.

119. Kimmel PL, Miller G, Mendelson WB. Sleep apnea syndrome in chronic renal disease. *Am J Med* 86:308, 1989.

120. Knudson F, et al. Adult respiratory distress-like syndrome during hemodialysis: Relationship between activation of complement, leukopenia, and release of granulocyte elastase. *Int J Artif Organs* 8:187, 1985.

121. Kuhlman JE, et al. Fulminant pulmonary calcification complicating renal transplantation: CT demonstration. *Radiology* 173:459, 1989.

122. Kuzela DC, et al. Soft tissue calcification in chronic dialysis patients. *Am J Pathol* 86:403, 1977.

123. Lane DJ, Hamilton WS. Idiopathic steatorrhoea and idiopathic pulmonary haemosiderosis. *Br Med J* 2:89, 1971.

124. Larson TS, et al. Respiratory tract symptoms as a clue to giant cell arteritis. *Ann Intern Med* 101:594, 1984.

125. Lauweryns R, et al. Kidney disorders and hematotoxicity from organic solvent exposure. *Scand J Work Environ Health* 11(Suppl 1):83, 1985.

126. Leaker B, et al. Idiopathic pulmonary haemosiderosis: A form of microscopic polyarteritis. *Thorax* 47:988, 1992.

127. Leatherman JW. Immune alveolar hemorrhage. *Chest* 91:891, 1987.

128. Leatherman JW, Davies SF, Hoidal JR. Alveolar hemorrhage syndromes: Diffuse microvascular lung hemorrhage in immune and idiopathic disorders. *Medicine* 63:343, 1984.

129. Lee HY, Stretton TB, Barnes AM. The lungs in renal failure. *Thorax* 30:46, 1975.

130. LeGeros RZ, Contiguglia SR, Alfrey AC. Pathological calcifications associated with uremia: Two types of calcium phosphate deposits. *Calcif Tissue Res* 13:173, 1973.

131. Levin AS, et al. An outbreak of nosocomial Legionnaires' disease in a renal transplant unit in Sao Paulo, Brazil. Legionellosis Study Team. *J Hosp Infect* 18:243, 1991.

132. Lin C-Y, et al. A study of relationship between childhood nephrotic syndrome and allergic diseases. *Chest* 97:1408, 1990.

133. Llach F, Arieff AI, Massry SG. Renal vein thrombosis and nephrotic syndrome: A prospective study of 36 adult patients. *Ann Intern Med* 83:8, 1975.

134. Lockwood CM, et al. Autoimmunity and glomerulonephritis. *Adv Nephrol* 16:291, 1987.

135. Macpherson RI, Banerjee AK. Acute glomerulonephritis: A chest film diagnosis? *J Can Assoc Radiol* 25:58, 1974.

136. Malhotra V, Gomillion MC, Artusio JF Jr. Hemoptysis in a child during extracorporeal shock wave lithotripsy. *Anesth Analg* 69:526, 1989.

137. Malhotra V, Rosen RJ, Slepian RL. Life-threatening hypoxemia after lithotripsy in an adult due to shock-wave-induced pulmonary contusion. *Anesthesiology* 75:529, 1991.

138. Mason AMS, et al. Fibrosing alveolitis associated with renal tubular acidosis. *Br Med J* 4:596, 1970.

139. Matthay RA, Bromberg SI, Putman CE. Pulmonary-renal syndromes: A review. *Yale J Biol Med* 53:497, 1980.

140. McCabe TA, et al. Fibrosing uremic pleuritis complicated by empyema. *Arch Intern Med* 142:1369, 1982.

141. McLachlan MSF, Wallace M, Seneviratne C. Pulmonary calcification in renal failure: Report of three cases. *Br J Radiol* 41:99, 1968.

142. Mendelson WB, et al. Effects of hemodialysis on sleep apnea syndrome in end-stage renal disease. *Clin Nephrol* 33:247, 1990.

143. Michelson EA, et al. Eosinophilia and pulmonary dysfunction during Cuprophan hemodialysis. *Kidney Int* 24:246, 1983.

144. Milliner DS, Lieberman E, Landing BH. Pulmonary calcinosis after renal transplantation in pediatric patients. *Am J Kidney Dis* 7:495, 1986.

145. Millman RP, et al. Sleep apnea in hemodialysis patients: The lack of testosterone effect on its pathogenesis. *Nephron* 40:407, 1985.

146. Mitwalli A. Tuberculosis in patients on maintenance dialysis. *Am J Kidney Dis* 18:579, 1991.

147. Mootz JR, Sagel SS, Roberts TH. Roentgenographic manifestations of pulmonary calcifications: A rare cause of respiratory failure in chronic renal disease. *Radiology* 107:55, 1973.

148. Morgan PGM, Turner-Warwick M. Pulmonary haemosiderosis and pulmonary haemorrhage. *Br J Dis Chest* 75:225, 1981.

149. Moss R, Hinds S, Fedullo AJ. Chylothorax: A complication of nephrotic syndrome. *Am Rev Respir Dis* 140:1436, 1989.

150. Mossey RT, et al. Pulmonary embolism: Low incidence in chronic renal failure. *Arch Intern Med* 142:1646, 1982.

151. Nassberger L. Left-sided pleural effusion secondary to continuous ambulatory peritoneal dialysis. *Acta Med Scand* 211:219, 1982.

152. Nennhaus HP, Hunter JA. Massive hemorrhage from bronchial varices in mitral stenosis. *Surgery* 61:556, 1967.

153. Nidus BD, et al. Uremic pleuritis—a clinicopathological entity. *N Engl J Med* 281:255, 1969.

154. Ognibene AJ, Johnson DE. Idiopathic pulmonary hemosiderosis in adults: Report of case and review of literature. *Arch Intern Med* 111:503, 1963.

155. Oh MS, et al. Consumption of CO_2 in metabolism of acetate as an explanation for hypoventilation and hypoxemia during dialysis. *Proc Clin Dial Transplant Forum* 9:226, 1979.

156. Pacheco A, et al. Long-term clinical follow-up of adult idiopathic pulmonary hemosiderosis and celiac disease. *Chest* 99:1525, 1991.

157. Pant K, et al. Pulmonary alveolar microlithiasis with pleural calcification and nephrolithiasis. *Chest* 98:245, 1990.

158. Patterson R, et al. Immunologic hemorrhagic pneumonia caused by isocyanates. *Am Rev Respir Dis* 141:226, 1990.

159. Patterson RW, et al. Hypoxemia and pulmonary gas exchange during hemodialysis. *J Appl Physiol* 50:259, 1981.

160. Peces R, et al. Goodpasture's syndrome in a patient receiving penicillamine and carbimazole. *Nephron* 45:316, 1987.

161. Peces-Serrano R, Fernandez-Vega F, Alvarez-Grande J. Hypoxemia during hemodialysis in patients with impairment in pulmonary function. *Nephron* 42:14, 1986.

162. Peterson RW, Balfour H, Marker S. Cytomegalovirus disease in renal allograft recipients: A prospective study of the clinical features, risk factors, and impact on renal transplantation. *Medicine* 59:283, 1980.

163. Prakash UBS. Lungs in mixed connective tissue disease. *J Thorac Imaging* 7:1, 1992.

164. Prakash UBS. Rheumatological diseases. *Lung Biol Health Dis* 59:385, 1992.

165. Prakash UBS. Vasculitides. *Lung Biol Health Dis* 59:431, 1992.

166. Prakash UBS, et al. Pulmonary alveolar microlithiasis: A review including ultrastructural and pulmonary function studies. *Mayo Clin Proc* 58:290, 1983.

167. Rackow EC, et al. Uremic pulmonary edema. *Am J Med* 64:1084, 1978.

168. Ramsey PG, et al. The renal transplant patient with fever and pulmonary infiltrates: Etiology, clinical manifestations, and management. *Medicine* 59:206, 1980.

169. Rankin JA, Matthay RA. Pulmonary renal syndromes: II. Etiology and pathogenesis. *Yale J Biol Med* 55:11, 1982.

170. Redman JF, et al. Hypertension and urinothorax following an attempted percutaneous nephrostomy. *J Urol* 128:1307, 1982.

171. Rees AJ, et al. The influence of HLA-linked genes on the severity of anti-GBM antibody-mediated nephritis. *Kidney Int* 26:445, 1984.

172. Rifkind D, et al. Systemic fungal infections complicating renal transplantation and immunosuppressive therapy: Clinical, microbiologic, neurologic and pathologic features. *Am J Med* 43:28, 1967.

173. Rifkind D, et al. Infectious diseases associated with renal homotransplantation (parts 1 and 2). *JAMA* 189:397, 1964.

174. Rifkind D, Faris TD, Hill RB Jr. *Pneumocystis carinii* pneumonia: Studies on the diagnosis and treatment. *Ann Intern Med* 65:943, 1966.

175. Robbins RA, et al. Diffuse alveolar hemorrhage in autologous bone marrow transplant recipients. *Am J Med* 87:511, 1989.

176. Roberts DE, et al. Autoantibodies to native myeloperoxidase in patients with pulmonary hemorrhage and acute renal failure. *J Clin Immunol* 11:389, 1991.

177. Rocker GM, et al. Pulmonary vascular permeability to transferrin: The pulmonary edema of renal failure. *Thorax* 42:620, 1987.

178. Rodelas R, et al. Fibrosing uremic pleuritis during hemodialysis. *JAMA* 243:2424, 1980.

179. Rubin SA, Morettin LB. Nephrobronchial fistula: An uncommon manifestation of inflammatory renal disease. *J Urol* 127:103, 1982.

180. Rudnick MR, et al. Acute massive hydrothorax complicating peritoneal dialysis, report of 2 cases and a review of the literature. *Clin Nephrol* 12:38, 1979.

181. Rudy DC, et al. Adult respiratory syndrome complicating percutaneous nephrolithotripsy. *Urology* 23:376, 1984.

182. Russell RGG, et al. Calcium in mineralized tissues and pathological calcification. *Br Med Bull* 42:435, 1986.

183. Sahn SA, Miller KS. Obscure pleural effusion: Look to the kidney. *Chest* 90:631, 1986.

184. Saka H, et al. Diffuse pulmonary alveolar hemorrhage in acute promyelocytic leukemia. *Intern Med* 31:457, 1992.

185. Savage COS, et al. Antiglomerular basement membrane antibody-mediated disease in the British Isles 1980–1984. *Br Med J* 292:301, 1986.

186. Savage COS, et al. Microscopic polyarteritis: Presentation, pathology, and prognosis. *Q J Med* 56:467, 1985.

187. Savige JA, et al. Circulating anti-glomerular basement membrane antibodies in coeliac disease and epidermolysis bullosa acquisita. *Aust NZ J Med* 21:867, 1991.

188. Scarlat A, Bodner G, Liron M. Massive hemoptysis as the presenting symptom in mitral stenosis. *Thorax* 41:413, 1986.

189. Sherlock JE, et al. Respiratory gas exchange during hemodialysis. *Proc Clin Dial Transplant Forum* 2:171, 1972.

190. Shumak KH, Rock GA. Therapeutic plasma exchange. *N Engl J Med* 310:762, 1984.

191. Singh S, et al. Serial studies of pulmonary function in continuous ambulatory peritoneal dialysis: A prospective study. *Chest* 86:874, 1984.

192. Skubitz KM, Craddock PR. Reversal of hemodialysis granulocytopenia and pulmonary leukostasis: A clinical manifestation of selective down-regulation of granulocyte responses to $C5_{adesarg}$. *J Clin Invest* 67:1383, 1981.

193. Smith EC. Tuberculosis in dialysis patients. *Int J Artif Organs* 5:11, 1982.

194. Smith JC, et al. Nodular pulmonary calcification in renal failure: Report of a case. *Am Rev Respir Dis* 100:723, 1969.

195. Smith LJ, Katzenstein AL. Pathogenesis of massive pulmonary hemorrhage in acute leukemia. *Arch Intern Med* 142:2149, 1982.

196. Stark DD, et al. Biochemical features of urinothorax. *Arch Intern Med* 142:1509, 1982.

197. Sternlieb I, Bennett B, Scheinberg IH. d-Penicillamine-induced Goodpasture's syndrome in Wilson's disease. *Ann Intern Med* 82:673, 1975.

198. Tarasuik A, Heimer D, Bark H. Effect of renal failure in skeletal and diaphragmatic muscle contraction. *Am Rev Respir Dis* 146:1388, 1992.

199. Teaque CA, et al. Goodpasture's syndrome with normal renal function. *Kidney Int* 13:492, 1978.

200. Teichman S, et al. Goodpasture's syndrome: Two cases with contrasting early course and management. *Am Rev Respir Dis* 113:223, 1976.

201. Tenholder MF, Hooper RG. Pulmonary infiltrates in leukemia. *Chest* 78:468, 1980.

202. Thaell JF, et al. Idiopathic pulmonary hemosiderosis: Two cases in a family. *Mayo Clin Proc* 53:113, 1978.

203. Trust A, Rossoff LJ. Tension hydrothorax in a patient with renal failure. *Chest* 97:1254, 1990.

204. Turner N, et al. Molecular cloning of the human Goodpasture antigen demonstrates it to be the alpha 3 chain of type IV collagen. *J Clin Invest* 89:592, 1992.

205. Utting JA, Shreeve DR. Haemolytic-uraemic syndrome in an adult with pericarditis and pleurisy. *Br Med J* 2:591, 1973.

206. Valassi-Adam H, et al. Raised IgA in idiopathic pulmonary hemosiderosis. *Arch Dis Child* 50:320, 1975.

207. Van Son WJ, et al. Pulmonary dysfunction is common during a cytomegalovirus infection after renal transplantation even in asymptomatic patients. *Am Rev Respir Dis* 136:580, 1987.

208. Verberckmoes R, Bobbaers H. Pulmonary problems in renal patients. *Contrib Nephrol* 33:67, 1982.

209. Wadhwa NK, et al. Sleep related respiratory disorders in end-stage renal disease patients on peritoneal dialysis. *Perit Dial Int* 12:51, 1992.

210. Walker RG, et al. Clinical and morphological aspects of the management of crescentic anti-glomerular basement membrane antibody (anti-GBM) nephritis/Goodpasture's syndrome. *Q J Med* 54:75, 1985.

211. Walshaw MJ, et al. Bronchial reactivity in patients undergoing long-term haemodialysis for chronic renal failure. *Blood Purif* 9:70, 1991.

212. Weber J, et al. Pulmonary disease due to *Mycobacterium xenopi* in a renal allograft recipient: Report of a case and review. *Rev Infect Dis* 11:964, 1989.

213. Weber MF, et al. Antineutrophil-cytoplasmic antibodies and antiglomerular basement membrane antibodies in Goodpasture's syndrome and in Wegener's granulomatosis. *J Am Soc Nephrol* 2:1227, 1992.

214. Weiss Z, et al. Obstructive renal failure and pleural effusion caused by the gravid uterus. *Acta Obstet Gynecol Scand* 65:187, 1986.

215. West JB, Mathieu-Costello O. Strength of the pulmonary blood-gas barrier. *Respir Physiol* 88:141, 1992.

216. West JB, Mathieu-Costello O. Stress failure of pulmonary capillaries: Role in lung and heart disease. *Lancet* 340:762, 1992.

217. Witte RJ, et al. Diffuse pulmonary alveolar hemorrhage after bone marrow transplantation: Radiographic findings in 39 patients. *Am J Roentgenol* 157:461, 1991.

218. Wunderink RG, et al. The radiologic diagnosis of autopsy-proven ventilator-associated pneumonia. *Chest* 101:458, 1992.

219. Yao L, Killam DA. Rounded atelectasis associated with end-stage renal disease. *Chest* 96:441, 1989.

220. Young KR Jr. Pulmonary-renal syndromes. *Clin Chest Med* 10:655, 1989.

221. Zidulka A, et al. Pulmonary function with acute loss of excess lung water by hemodialysis in patients with chronic uremia. *Am J Med* 55:134, 1973.

62

Gastroenterologic Diseases

Udaya B. S. Prakash

The upper gastrointestinal tract and the tracheobronchial tree, as a result of their common embryologic origin, remain in close anatomic proximity throughout life. This predisposes diseases of the esophagus to affect the tracheobronchial tree and vice versa. The aspiration of gastric contents as a result of gastroesophageal reflux into the respiratory system is an excellent example. Malignant neoplasms originating in the esophagus frequently invade or compress the tracheobronchial tree, with resultant respiratory embarrassment. Congenital communications between the esophagus and the tracheobronchial tree are a relatively common finding in pediatric practice. Further, there is evidence to suggest the existence of local neuronal esophagolaryngotracheal reflexes in humans [23,121]. Pulmonary involvement in hepatic and pancreatic diseases is well-known. However, respiratory manifestations in other gastroenterologic diseases are fairly uncommon and hence are not very familiar to all. This chapter will discuss pulmonary manifestations in the common as well as several of the uncommon gastroenterologic diseases. The role of alcohol on lung function also is included.

Esophageal Disorders

Fistulas

Tracheoesophageal and bronchoesophageal fistulas may be congenital or acquired. Congenital fistulas are more commonly tracheal than bronchial. In 90 percent of congenital cases, there is a proximal blind-ending esophagus and usually a connection between the distal esophagus and the trachea (Fig. 62-1). In the remaining 10 percent of cases, an H type of fistula is seen. This latter congenital anomaly may remain undetected until adulthood, at which time resection of a chroni-

cally infected bronchiectatic segment of lung may disclose its presence. Sixty percent of acquired fistulas result from a malignancy in the mediastinum, the primary tumor originating either in the esophagus or in the tracheobronchial tree. The remainder are a consequence of infections and trauma. Instrumental perforation is an important cause of tracheoesophageal fistula and acute mediastinitis. Other causes of acquired tracheoesophageal fistula include mediastinal granulomas secondary to histoplasmosis, broncholithiasis, silicotic lymph nodes, and chemical corrosives [22,67,150,167]. Crohn's disease affects the esophagus in 0.3 percent of patients, but esophagography has demonstrated stricture in 38 percent and ulceration in 32 percent. Tracheoesophageal fistula is a potential complication and has been observed in 6 percent of patients with Crohn's disease [17,185].

Symptoms depend on the location and size of the fistula but, characteristically, there is coughing on swallowing liquids. Hemoptysis, recurrent pulmonary infection, wheezing, and bronchiectasis also are commonly seen. Diagnosis is accomplished by demonstrating, in the fistulous tract, contrast material introduced through the esophagus. The possibility of satisfactory surgical correction depends on the cause and location of the fistula.

Gastroenteric Cysts

Gastroenteric cysts develop from the foregut and represent a failure of the originally solid esophagus to become a hollow tube. The cysts occur in the paraspinal region of the posterior mediastinum and usually are round or oval and homogeneous in density (Fig. 62-2). Patients with gastroenterogenous cysts usually are asymptomatic.

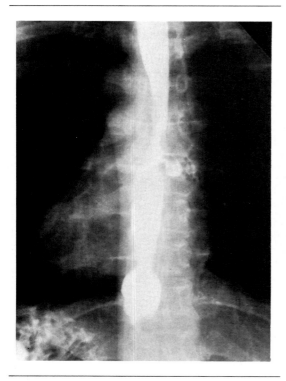

Fig. 62-1. Situs inversus and congenital fistula between esophagus and proximal left main stem bronchus, presenting in adulthood as asthma and cough induced by ingestion of liquids.

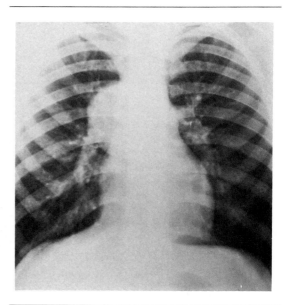

Fig. 62-2. A large gastroenteric cyst presenting as posterior mediastinal mass. This was asymptomatic and discovered during routine examination.

Zenker's Diverticulum

A pharyngoesophageal diverticulum of Zenker may be large enough to be identified as a superior mediastinal mass on chest roentgenograms. Symptoms included dysphagia, chronic cough due to aspiration, and recurrent aspiration pneumonia (Fig. 62-3).

Achalasia

Esophagomegaly (megaesophagus) secondary to achalasia can encroach on the upper airway and cause obstruction to airflow during the expiratory phase [27,70,202]. It is not unusual for the enlarged esophagus in achalasia to appear as mediastinal widening or density on routine chest roentgenograms (Fig. 62-4). Aspiration pneumonia is a serious complication of achalasia and may lead to acute respiratory distress syndrome [93]. Esophagobronchial fistula has been de-

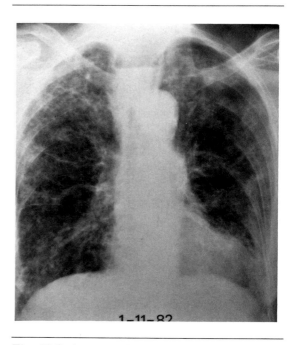

Fig. 62-3. Acute respiratory failure caused by aspiration from a large pharyngoesophageal diverticulum. Note the air-fluid level in upper esophagus just above the aortic arch.

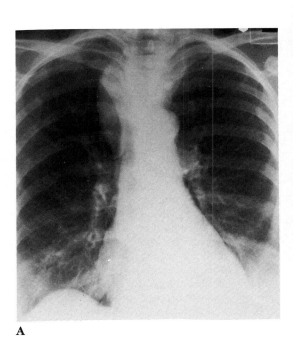

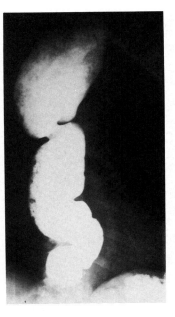

A   B

Fig. 62-4. Achalasia presenting as a superioposterior mediastinal mass. Posteroanterior chest roentgenogram (A) and barium contrast study (B) demonstrate the megaesophagus.

scribed in a patient with chronic achalasia [12]. Pulmonary infection caused by *Mycobacterium fortuitum* has been reported in a patient with achalasia [81].

Chagas' Disease

Chagas' disease, or American trypanosomiasis, is an infection caused by *Trypanosoma cruzi* and is characterized by an acute, often asymptomatic illness with a prolonged latent period and chronic cardiac and gastrointestinal sequelae. In patients with predominantly esophageal involvement (chagasic megaesophagus), the pleuropulmonary problems include pleural effusion in 36 percent, pulmonary embolism in 22 percent, pneumonia in 35 percent, and aspiration pneumonia in a small percentage. All these complications are more common in patients with chagasic megaesophagus and cardiomyopathy than in those without esophageal involvement [21].

Esophageal Perforation

Esophageal perforation is an uncommon entity. The majority of perforations are iatrogenic, and fewer than 15 percent are due to spontaneous rupture. Esophagoscopy, especially in the removal of foreign bodies, is the most common cause of iatrogenic perforation (Fig. 62-5). Other causes are the insertion of esophageal tubes, trauma, carcinomas of the esophagus or a Mallory-Weiss tear, Boerhaave's syndrome, mediastinal malignancy, radiation necrosis of the esophagus, foreign bodies, and external trauma [1,73].

The initial injury is acute mediastinitis. Approximately 60 percent of patients with esophageal perforation develop pleural effusion, and nearly 25 percent will exhibit a pneumothorax. Pleural effusion usually is left-sided, and analysis will reveal a high protein content, high amylase level, low pH, and the presence of squamous epithelial cells and, occasionally, food particles. The amylase is derived from the salivary juices leaking into the pleural space. The extremely low pH is due to the increased leukocytic and mesothelial metabolism. The diagnosis of esophageal per-

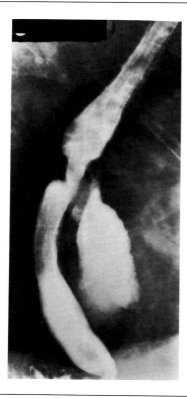

Fig. 62-5. Instrumental perforation of anterior midesophagus demonstrated by Gastrografin extravasation into the mediastinum.

foration is made by the clinical findings of chest pain, severe back pain, dysphagia, acute fever, and subcutaneous emphysema, and documentation of the tear by meglumine diatrizoate (Gastrografin) contrast studies of the esophagus [1]. Boerhaave's syndrome and Mallory-Weiss tear of the esophagus can lead to acute mediastinitis.

Sclerotherapy of Esophageal Varices

Sclerotherapy of the esophageal varices is one therapeutic method used to control variceal hemorrhage [193]. Either sodium morrhuate or ethanolamine oleate is used as the sclerosant and is injected into the varices under direct vision via the esophagoscope. Sclerotherapy for bleeding esophageal varices has not improved survival but has reduced the risk of rebleeding and the need for extensive bypass surgery. Within 6 hours of the injection, some patients develop mediastinal widening, presumably due to chemical mediasti-

nitis. The overall incidence of intrathoracic complications includes pleural effusion, 0 to 50 percent; mediastinitis, 63 percent; atelectasis, 16 percent; bronchitis, 8 percent; pneumonia, 0 to 5 percent; and esophagopleural fistula, 1 to 2 percent [50]. Other complications such as esophagobronchial fistula, empyema, acute respiratory distress syndrome, pulmonary infarction, and late expectoration of sclerosant are described but rare. Acute pulmonary edema leading to respiratory distress syndrome within 8 to 36 hours of sclerotherapy has been described [127]. A Mayo Clinic study of 223 patients who underwent 390 esophageal variceal sclerotherapy procedures with either ethanolamine oleate or tetradecyl sulfate evaluated the pulmonary complications and reported the following: retrocardiac or mediastinal widening in 35 percent, pleural effusion in 27 percent, atelectasis in 12 percent, and pulmonary infiltrates in 9 percent of procedures. Respiratory insufficiency was noted after 14 sclerotherapy procedures [212]. Most thoracic manifestations after variceal sclerotherapy are likely due to a local inflammatory response to the sclerosant.

Injection of sodium morrhuate in sheep causes marked but transient pulmonary hypertension and an increased flow of relatively protein-poor lymph. The constituent unsaturated fatty acids may be responsible for the pathogenesis of pulmonary edema. The edema from sodium morrhuate may be another example of hydrostatic (low lymph protein) pulmonary edema due to abrupt pulmonary hypertension without an increase in pulmonary capillary wedge pressure. Use of a Sengstaken tube immediately after sclerotherapy may increase the risk of pulmonary complications. On the other hand, acute respiratory failure resulting from sclerotherapy has resolved after aspiration of air via a Sengstaken tube [35].

Pleural effusion after endoscopic variceal sclerotherapy has been reported to occur in 50 percent of patients so treated. The incidence of pleural effusion is related to the amount of sclerosant injected [6]. The effusions are usually small, bilateral in a third, right-sided in a third, and left-sided in a third. They usually are exudative and transient. The pleural effusion is secsecondary to mediastinal pleuritis caused by the sclerosant. Chylothorax also has ensued after sclerotherapy [66,134].

Transmission of infection by gastrointestinal endoscopy can occur if endoscopy instruments are contaminated. Involved organisms have included *Salmonella* species, *Pseudomonas aeruginosa*, and *Helicobacter pylori*. A review of the literature disclosed 180 isolates causing disease in 67 cases and death in 2 as a result of infection transmitted by gastrointestinal endoscopy [172]. Pulmonary aspiration is a fairly common complication during emergency upper gastrointestinal endoscopy. In a study of 30 patients who underwent upper gastrointestinal endoscopy for diagnosis and treatment of acute bleeding, 6 (20 percent) developed new pulmonary infiltrates after the procedure and all but 1 exhibited fever, leukocytosis, and oxygen desaturation below 90 percent [115].

Gastroesophageal Reflux

Gastroesophageal reflux is an extremely common phenomenon, occurring on a daily basis in 10 percent and intermittently in 50 percent of healthy individuals [130]. Gastroesophageal reflux disease (GERD) is a syndrome that manifests as heartburn and the sequelae of esophagitis, ulceration, stricture, or Barrett's epithelium [31]. Gastroesophageal reflux and GERD have assumed importance in the pathogenesis of certain lung diseases, particularly laryngospasm, chronic cough, and bronchospasm. Mechanical reflux of gastric acid into the tracheobronchial tree is another mechanism responsible for the pulmonary complications. Reliable and practical techniques for ambulatory measurement and recording of gastroesophageal reflux and esophageal pH permit better understanding of these complications. This test is believed to be of diagnostic significance if intermittent symptoms can be shown to be regularly associated with a decrease in the intraesophageal pH to less than 4.0 during testing [23].

Vagally mediated local neuronal esophagolaryngotracheal reflexes have assumed an important role in the etiology of many respiratory complications associated with GERD [23,83,86,121]. Normal vagal reflexes in the respiratory tract include cough, laryngeal closure, forced inspiration, respiratory suppression, bronchoconstriction, and mucous secretion. Abnormal reflexes consist of laryngospasm, prolonged apnea, bronchospasm, and singultus (hiccup) [36]. There remains the question of whether gastroesophageal reflux is primary or secondary to the pulmonary disease. It is common knowledge that continuous coughing causes retching and vomiting. However, a study of 12 patients with chronic obstructive pulmonary disease used esophageal manometry, 24-hour pH monitoring, esophageal acid clearance, and pulmonary function tests to determine that these patients do not have a bronchoconstrictive reflex to distal esophageal acidification, and esophageal function in these patients is normal [136].

Reflux Laryngitis

The association of gastroesophageal reflux with chronic hoarseness and posterior laryngitis has been referred to as *reflux laryngitis* or *Cherry-Donner syndrome* [23]. Twenty-four-hour esophageal pH monitoring has revealed that as many as 75 percent of patients with chronic hoarseness will exhibit an abnormal amount of gastroesophageal reflux [99]. In a group of 33 patients referred for hoarseness, gastroesophageal reflux was found in almost 80 percent [199]. Abnormal laryngeal reflexes can be elicited by acidic (pH < 4.5) solutions [36]. GERD also contributes to the development of chronic throat clearing, cough, sore throat, contact ulcer and granuloma, globus pharyngeus, cervical dysphagia, subglottic stenosis, and cricoarytenoid arthritis [135].

Cough

Controlled studies have shown that chronic persistent cough that remains after a diagnostic evaluation is associated with increased episodes of otherwise asymptomatic gastroesophageal reflux. Indeed, cough may be the sole presenting manifestation of gastroesophageal reflux [88]. Prolonged exposure of esophageal mucosa to gastric acid may cause cough by stimulating esophagolaryngotracheal reflexes. It has been suggested that in those with gastroesophageal reflux, a self-perpetuating mechanism may exist whereby acid reflux causes cough via a local neuronal esophageal-tracheobronchial reflex, and the cough in turn amplifies reflux via increased transdiaphragmatic pressure or by inducing transient lower esophageal sphincter relaxation [84]. Impaired clearance of esophageal acid has been documented by 24-hour ambulatory monitoring of esophageal pH in patients with chronic cough [83]. Postnasal drip also may irritate the receptors located in the pharynx and larynx and contribute to cough; this phenomenon should be excluded in patients who have nocturnal cough and gastroesophageal reflux [87]. Cough caused by tobacco smoke may be aggravated by the lowered esophageal sphincter tone induced by the tobacco smoke [39].

Four to 21 percent of chronic cough is estimated to be secondary to gastroesophageal reflux [85,88,145]. Therefore, reflux should be considered an etiologic possibility in subjects with chronic persistent cough that remains unexplained after a standard diagnostic assessment [84].

Asthma

The association of asthma with GERD has been noted [47,72]. As many as 45 to 65 percent of adults with asthma have been estimated to have gastroesophageal reflux [3,47]. This reflux has been demonstrated to be the cause of nocturnal exacerbation of asthma in 27 percent of asthmatic children [207]. The mechanism of bronchospasm in the setting of gastroesophageal reflux is unclear. Although reflux of acid into the airways is well-known to produce bronchospasm, not all individuals with gastroesophageal reflux develop asthma. Asthma and gastroesophageal reflux are more common during sleep, but studies have shown that gastroesophageal reflux does not aggravate nocturnal asthma [56,181]. It has even been questioned whether esophageal reflux is caused by asthma because treatment of asthmatics with esophageal reflux has resulted in diminished reflux symptoms [139,168]. Nonetheless, compared to bronchitic patients with gastroesophageal reflux, asthmatics have exhibited more episodes and a shorter duration of gastroesophageal reflux [47]. It is important to recognize that asthmatic patients who take theophylline may develop gastroesophageal reflux because the drug is known to decrease lower esophageal sphincter tone and predispose to reflux. In addition, theophylline increases gastric acid secretion [62].

One study provided the results of long-term experience (average follow-up of 7.9 years) with a group of 44 asthmatic patients with gastroesophageal reflux who underwent Nissan fundoplication: The gastroesophageal reflux cleared in 42 patients (95 percent), asthma was markedly improved or cured in 18 (41 percent), and the reflux improved in 29 (66 percent) [143]. There was a significant association between cure of asthma after fundoplication and the presence of nocturnal attacks, nocturnal tracheitis, intrinsic tracheitis, intrinsic asthma, or a clear history of reflux symptoms preceding the onset of asthmatic symptoms. A clinically useful finding was that the positive response to a trial of medical treatment helped identify patients who would be cured. Another study of 15 asthmatics during sleep observed that gastroesophageal reflux did not contribute to nocturnal worsening of asthma [181]. Others have shown that esophageal acid stimulation is not a strong and immediate trigger of asthma [55].

An opposite view of the role of gastroesophageal reflux in asthmatics was presented in a report by Larrain and colleagues [112]. In 90 nonasthmatic patients with adult-onset wheezing, a 90 percent prevalence of gastroesophageal reflux was noted during a study in which the patients were assigned randomly to receive cimetidine or a placebo for a 6-month trial. Those assigned to cimetidine or surgical therapy of gastroesophageal reflux improved significantly. The intake of pulmonary medicine for wheezing decreased significantly [112]. Others have reported that antireflux treatment will provide only small improvements in asthma control in patients with a history of gastroesophageal reflux [54]. Unfortunately, there is no acceptable diagnostic method to confirm the presence of gastroesophageal reflux–induced asthma [171], and controversy about this issue is likely to continue.

A number of studies have documented excellent long-term results of surgical treatment for reflux-induced asthma. However, such therapy should be reserved for cases of severe asthma poorly controlled by medications and complicated by severe reflux that leads to ulcerative esophagitis [143].

Aspiration Pneumonia

Aspiration pneumonitis caused by gastroesophageal reflux is a serious acute medical problem and may lead to acute respiratory distress syndrome. The risk of developing significant aspiration pneumonia increases when the volume of gastric contents aspirated exceeds 50 ml and the pH of the aspirate is below 2.5. Although the initial pathologic features are directly related to the damaging effects of gastric acid, aspiration pneumonia frequently is complicated by bacterial pneumonitis. Community-acquired aspiration pneumonia is extremely uncommon except in alcoholics [194], those with poor dental hygiene, and debilitated individuals. Nosocomial aspiration pneumonia is more likely to be complicated by bacterial pneumonitis [24,186]. Debility and prolonged supine posture predispose to this complication. Elegant studies using technetium 99 sulfur colloid labeling of gastric contents and subsequent measurements of endobronchial secretions in patients on mechanical ventilation have shown that the supine position, and particularly the length of time the patient is kept in this position, are potential risk factors for aspiration of gastric contents [187]. The same microorganisms were isolated from stomach, pharynx, and endobronchial samples in 32 percent of studies done while patients were semirecumbent and in 68 percent of studies done while patients were in the supine position.

Alkalinization of gastric contents also can predispose to bacterial pneumonia, and gastric colonization by microorganisms is related to the degree of gastric alkalinization [34,162]. A gastric pH exceeding 4.0 seems to be the most important factor favoring gastric colonization [44,187]. Hospitalized patients, particularly those being mechanically ventilated, are systematically given antacids or histamine-2 (H2) blocking drugs, or both, to prevent the development of stress ulcers. Several studies have shown that the use of these drugs in critically ill patients is associated with a greater incidence of both nosocomial pneumonia and gastric and pharyngeal colonization [45,109, 189]. These studies also reported that the prophylactic use of a cytoprotective agent such as sucralfate does not alter gastric pH and thus prevents microbial colonization. Others have shown that treatment with cimetidine is an independent risk factor for developing pneumonia in mechanically ventilated patients [34]. Elevating the head of the bed to 45 degrees is reported to reduce the risk of aspiration pneumonia significantly [187].

Many subjects who remain asymptomatic despite frequent aspiration may develop pulmonary complications after chronic aspiration. Typical examples of insidious aspiration-induced lung disease include mild basal pulmonary fibrosis and patchy infiltrates. Ingestion of oil-based compounds for laxative purposes or other reasons may result in lipid pneumonia (Fig. 62-6).

Gastric pH and Nosocomial Pneumonia

Acid pH maintains the sterility of the stomach in the fasting state. Critically ill patients who receive ulcer prophylaxis with drugs to suppress or neutralize gastric acidity commonly demonstrate growth of intragastric gram-negative bacteria [38,45,46]. However, one study reported that the use of sucralfate was associated with a lower incidence of nosocomial pneumonia in comparison to agents that raise gastric pH [32]. Transmission of these bacteria from the stomach to the respiratory tract has been well documented [64]. In patients receiving stress ulcer prophylaxis, the stomach is a potential source of pathogenic bacteria that may colonize the respiratory tract [32]. Aspiration of these organisms is an important mechanism in the development of nosocomial pneumonia. The presence of an endotracheal tube does not afford complete protection from aspiration of the gastric bacteria.

Other Complications of GERD

Several other complications have been described in relation to gastroesophageal reflux. These include singultus (hiccup), bronchitis, bronchiectasis, atelectasis, hemoptysis, pulmonary fibrosis, apnea, and seizures related to hypoxia [86]. Many adults with obstructive sleep apnea suffer from gastroesophageal reflux. This may be related to lowered intrathoracic pressure caused by obstructive sleep apnea and increased arousal and repetitive body movement during sleep [95]. Treatment of obstructive sleep apnea with nasal continuous positive airway pressure has been shown to decrease thoracic gastroesophageal reflux in these patients [95]. The esophagus and central nervous system of asymptomatic volunteers have been shown to maintain an awareness for the presence and volume of intraesophageal acid, and the response time by the central nervous system is inversely related to acid volume [137]. The larger volumes of acid in the esophagus are reported to create an afferent warning signal to the central nervous system to produce rapid arousal from sleep along with a shortened interval to the first swallow [137].

Gastric Disorders

Hiatal Hernia

In esophageal hiatal hernia, chest roentgenograms often show the herniated portion of the stomach directly behind the heart, suggesting the possibility of a posterior mediastinal mass lesion. Presence of an air-fluid level and a barium contrast study usually confirm the diagnosis. Symptoms originating from hiatal hernia may resemble those of cardiopulmonary disease; however, careful attention to the clinical history often helps in making the distinction. Occasionally, a large hiatal hernia may compromise pulmonary function by occupying a large area of the chest cavity (Fig. 62-7).

One of the most serious respiratory complications of hiatal hernia is the occurrence of aspi-

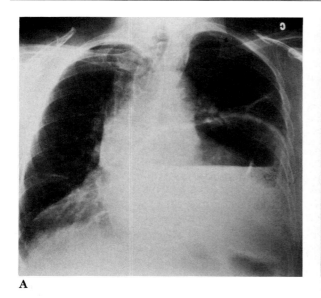

A

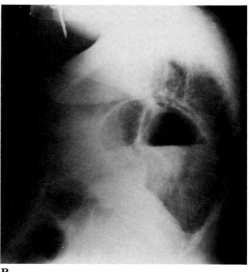

B

Fig. 62-6. (A) Chronic ingestion of mineral oil for laxative purposes resulted in an ill-defined mass in the right lower lobe. (B) Resection of lung revealed typical findings of lipid pneumonia.

ration pneumonia secondary to gastroesophageal reflux, as discussed previously. Roentgenologic and endoscopic investigations have reported that from 50 to 94 percent of patients with GERD have hiatal hernia [169]. A study of 34 patients with endoscopically documented hiatal hernia recorded that compared to normal volunteers, those with hiatal hernia had substantially higher reflux scores and reduced lower esophageal sphincter pressure [169].

Hernia Through the Foramina of Bochdalek and Morgagni

Hernia through the foramen of Bochdalek results from incomplete fusion of the posterolateral part of the diaphragm. Herniation is seen more frequently in children, and the abnormality is usually located on the left. Chest roentgenograms reveal a space-occupying mass lesion. Large herniations produce dyspnea, chest discomfort and, occasionally, respiratory failure. Sometimes these hernias mimic pleural effusion, with the lateral chest roentgenogram disclosing "free layering." Postmortem studies in infants with congenital diaphragmatic hernia have shown that the lungs are immature, especially the ipsilateral lungs. Additionally, intraalveolar hemorrhage is reported to be a common complication of congenital diaphragmatic hernia [65]. Hernia through the fora-

men of Morgagni tends to be on the right and anterior. Herniation of the liver may occur, though herniation of intestinal segments is more likely (Fig. 62-8).

Peptic Ulcer Disease

Peptic ulcer disease has been found in 10 to 35 percent of study groups with chronic obstructive lung disease, contrasting with 3 percent in control groups [211]. The increased incidence with such lung disease may be explained, at least partly, by gastric hypersecretion due to increased arterial carbon dioxide tension and decreased arterial oxygen tension. Peptic ulcers associated with chronic obstructive lung disease are more commonly duodenal than gastric. Often the peptic ulcer disease is not accompanied by pain and is recognized only after gastrointestinal hemorrhage calls attention to it. Perforation of a gastric ulcer occasionally may result in pleural effusion [16].

Effect of Gastrectomy on Tuberculosis

Gastrectomy has an adverse effect on preexisting, active pulmonary tuberculosis, and elective

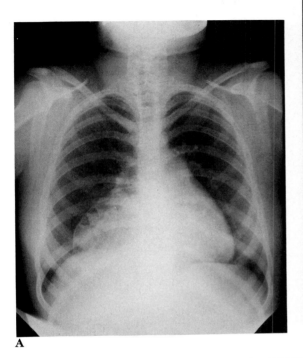

A

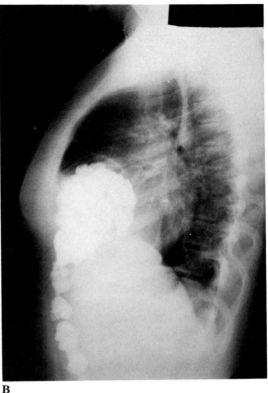

B

Fig. 62-7. A large hiatal hernia occupying most of the left chest cavity. (A) Anterior view. (B) Posterior view.

surgery is best postponed until a reasonable period of antituberculous therapy has been completed. An increased incidence of pulmonary tuberculosis after subtotal or total gastrectomy and jejunal or ileal bypass has been noted [10,18,198]. The incidence of tuberculosis after gastrectomy is estimated to be as high as 1 to 5 percent [170]. The prevalence of prior gastrectomy in patients with tuberculosis has ranged from 1.7 to 20 percent, the higher incidence being more common in elderly patients [4,170,201]. A poor response to treatment and an increased rate of reactivation has been noted in gastrectomy patients who develop infection caused by *Mycobacterium avium-intracellulare* [2]. The relationship between gastrectomy and tuberculosis that develops several years later is uncertain [29]. A plausible explanation for the increased incidence of tuberculosis in this group of patients is the decreased absorption of antituberculous drugs caused by gastrectomy. Pharmacokinetic studies have documented this phenomenon in anecdotal cases [201]. All this notwithstanding, fear of tuberculosis should not be a factor in deciding on elective gastrectomy.

Gastrobronchial Fistula

Gastrobronchial fistula is extremely rare. A review in 1985 found only 13 cases [126]. There are five causes for the development of these fistulas. The most common cause is the presence of a subphrenic abscess, which erodes through the diaphragm and leads to lung abscess. Traumatic rupture of the diaphragm, especially from penetrating injury, is the next most common cause. Perforated ulcer in an incarcerated hiatal hernia and necrosis of gastric tumors and areas of previous esophageal or gastric surgery are the other causes [5,126].

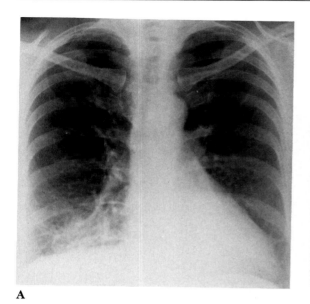

A

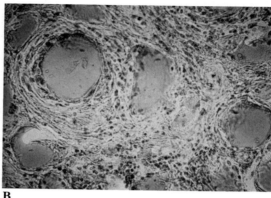

B

Fig. 62-8. (A) Foramen of Morgagni hernia presenting as an air-filled mass adjacent to right heart border. (B) Barium examination of the small intestine shows that much of the small bowel has herniated through the foramen of Morgagni.

Intestinal Diseases

Inflammatory Bowel Diseases

Both chronic ulcerative colitis and Crohn's disease (regional enteritis) are well-known for their propensity to produce various extraintestinal manifestations. Pulmonary involvement is now a documented but uncommon extraintestinal manifestation of inflammatory bowel diseases (Table 62-1). A variety of respiratory problems, including pulmonary vasculitis, apical fibrosis, chronic suppurative bronchitis, and bronchiectasis, have been reported (Fig. 62-9) [19,68,100]. However, in a series of 1400 patients with inflammatory bowel disease evaluated retrospectively, only 3 were found to have unexplained bronchopulmonary disease [100]. In a separate review of clinical material on 1400 patients with inflammatory bowel diseases whose diagnoses were recorded in a computerized registry between 1930 and 1970, there were only 6 unexplained pulmonary diseases [158]. However, in several publications on this subject, pulmonary function abnormalities in Crohn's disease have been reported with a prevalence rate ranging from 36 to 68 percent [132].

The pathogenesis of pulmonary disease secondary to inflammatory bowel diseases is not known. An unidentified systemic mechanism affecting both the bronchial and colonic epithelium may be responsible. Among 10 nonsmokers with chronic ulcerative colitis, 4 had exertional dyspnea, 4 exhibited abnormal chest roentgenograms, and 3 had obstructive changes in their pulmonary function tests [79]. Bronchial biopsies in 4 patients showed basal cell hyperplasia, submucosal inflammation, and thickening of the basement membrane, similar to the pathologic changes in the colonic mucosa. Several case reports are discussed here to provide some understanding of these uncommon pulmonary manifestations of the inflammatory bowel diseases.

In a study of 18 patients with Crohn's disease and no pulmonary symptoms, bronchoalveolar lavage has revealed lymphocytic alveolitis in 61 percent, with lymphocyte counts ranging from 18 to 79 percent [196]. There was no apparent correlation between lymphocyte count in the lavage effluent and the pulmonary dysfunction observed in 11 patients. These studies suggest that most patients with Crohn's disease have a latent pulmonary involvement. In one study, 71 percent of patients with Crohn's disease demonstrated increased superoxide production, but the significance of this in the pathogenesis of lung disease is unclear [14]. Pulmonary manifestations of both chronic ulcerative colitis and Crohn's disease can be considered under the broad headings of airways disease, pulmonary parenchymal disease, and other complications.

AIRWAYS DISEASE

In one study, pulmonary function was assessed in patients with ulcerative colitis and Crohn's disease and compared with that of a healthy population, and no statistically significant differences were found in the measurements observed among the three groups [91]. However, in a prospective study of 58 patients with Crohn's disease and 44 patients with chronic ulcerative colitis, a high incidence of respiratory abnormalities was identified in both groups [77]. Pulmonary function tests were abnormal in 50 percent of patients, with diminished flow rates (less than 50 percent of predicted forced expiratory volume in the first second [FEV_1]) in 31 percent and decreased diffusing capacity (less than 75 percent predicted) in 26 percent. Abnormally low diffusing capacity was the only abnormality in 16 patients (8 with Crohn's). Four patients with Crohn's and two with colitis had interstitial processes on the chest roentgenograms.

Another study assessed pulmonary function in 36 outpatients with inflammatory bowel diseases and reported that the diffusing capacity for carbon monoxide (DLCO) was significantly reduced in patients as compared with matched controls ($p < .01$) [48]. The reason for this reduction was not clear, though it was considered unlikely to be due to sulfasalazine (salazosulfapyridine). A further study of the lung function of 10 patients with Crohn's disease during and after an attack of the disease revealed that pulmonary volumes and DLCO were not impaired but functional residual capacity (FRC) was greater during the attack than during remission [140]; it was also greater than in normal subjects. FRC values, disease activity, and finger clubbing decreased concomitantly during remission. Another study disclosed that the prevalence of hay fever and asthma was raised among 242 patients with chronic ulcerative colitis and slightly higher among 45 patients with Crohn's disease [75]. A report on 29 patients with Crohn's disease noted that the lungs are rel-

Table 62-1. **Pulmonary abnormalities associated with intestinal diseases**

Intestinal disease	Pulmonary abnormality
Inflammatory bowel diseases*	Apical pulmonary fibrosis Bronchiectasis Bronchiolitis Bullous lung disease Chronic bronchitis Desquamative interstitial pneumonitis Increased incidence of asthma Lymphocytic alveolitis Pleural effusion Pulmonary edema Tracheoesophageal fistula Airflow obstruction Decreased DLCO Sulfasalazine-induced lung disease
Whipple's disease	Cough Pleuritic chest pain Pleural effusion Hilar lymphadenopathy Pulmonary parenchymal infiltrates Restrictive pulmonary dysfunction
Nontropical sprue (celiac disease)	Interstitial pneumonitis and fibrosis Hypersensitivity pneumonitis Chronic cough Increased incidence of asthma Peribronchial fibrosis Pulmonary hemosiderosis
Intestinal parasitic diseases	Asthma Pulmonary infiltrates with eosinophilia Pulmonary parasitic infiltrates
Intestinal lymphangiectasia	Pleural effusion (chylous)

*Includes chronic ulcerative colitis and Crohn's disease.

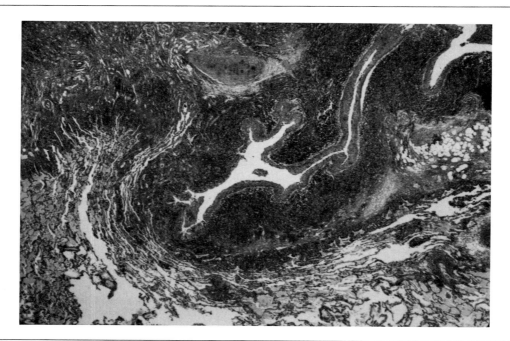

Fig. 62-9. Chronic bronchiectasis that was symptomatically steroid-responsive in this patient with ulcerative colitis. Dense infiltration of chronic inflammatory cells involving a small bronchus is shown.

atively unaffected by Crohn's disease [132]. Bronchiolitis with organizing pneumonitis, sclerosing peribronchiolitis, and diffuse panbronchiolitis are other abnormalities described in ulcerative colitis [40,178,203].

PULMONARY PARENCHYMAL DISEASE

Although the association of apical fibrosis and ankylosing spondylitis is widely recognized, only one case has been reported in which fibrosis was associated with both spondylitis and ulcerative colitis [124]. Dense basal pulmonary infiltrates responsive to steroid therapy have been reported in two patients: Lung biopsy in one revealed changes similar to those in idiopathic pulmonary fibrosis, and the second had nondiagnostic findings [166]. Pulmonary bullous lesions are also described in chronic ulcerative colitis [165]. Hypoproteinemia is common in Crohn's disease. A case has been described of a 29-year-old man who presented with recurrent pulmonary edema and hypoalbuminemia [15]. The diagnosis of Crohn's disease was made only after several episodes of pulmonary edema.

An 11-year-old child who presented with terminal ileitis associated with pulmonary lesions showing periodic progression was described [78].

The initial thoracic disorder developed 2 years before roentgenographic evidence of the ileitis, the second episode coinciding with the diagnosis of the ileal lesion. Pulmonary lesions progressed simultaneously with the clinical signs of digestive tract disturbances, which eventually stabilized.

In patients with inflammatory bowel disease, biopsy of the affected segment of intestine may show granulomatous changes. Noncaseous and nonconfluent granulomas are found in 30 percent of patients with Crohn's disease [42]. Interestingly, a report described three patients with classic chronic ulcerative colitis who developed histologically proved type III sarcoidosis during the course of their disease [161]. A case of acute segmental inflammation of the terminal ileum in a female patient who presented with signs and symptoms of acute appendicitis is reported [37]. The patient had associated bilateral pulmonary tuberculosis. The role of *M. tuberculosis* in the etiology of the segmental ileal disease is well-known, but the relationship between tuberculosis and inflammatory bowel disease is not clear.

Those with jejunal or ileal bypass exhibit an increased incidence of tuberculosis [18].

OTHER PULMONARY COMPLICATIONS
Pleuropericarditis may complicate ulcerative colitis and Crohn's disease. A review of the literature reveals approximately a dozen patients with ulcerative colitis and Crohn's disease who developed pleural effusions, bilateral in a third and left-sided in the rest. Many of these were associated with pericardial effusion. The pleuropericardial complications of inflammatory bowel disease may run an independent course and may be present at the time of inactive bowel disease [142,159].

Crohn's disease is complicated by esophageal stricture in 38 percent and ulcerations in 32 percent. The most common presenting symptom in Crohn's disease of the esophagus is dysphagia, seen in more than two-thirds of patients. Cough and repeated bouts of pneumonia occur in a small number of patients. Regurgitation and aspiration pneumonia are responsible for these symptoms. Esophagotracheal fistula has been described in 6 percent of patients. Histologic studies of these areas have shown submucosal fibrosis, lymphocytic infiltration, noncaseous granulomas, and hypertrophy of muscle [17,185]. Colobronchial fistula also has been described in a patient with Crohn's disease [42].

Sulfasalazine, used in the treatment of inflammatory bowel diseases, is known to produce pulmonary infiltrates and dyspnea [123,206]. However, most studies reporting on the pulmonary manifestations of inflammatory bowel disease have excluded this possibility and have concluded that the respiratory involvement was independent of sulfasalazine-induced lung disease [78,140]. A patient with ulcerative colitis receiving sulfasalazine therapy who developed interstitial pneumonitis and bronchiolitis has been described [206]. Open-lung biopsy in a patient with chronic ulcerative colitis showed severe interstitial fibrosis and bronchiectasis [123]. The pulmonary fibrosis progressed despite cessation of sulfasalazine therapy and a total colectomy. A child with chronic ulcerative colitis and hepatic cirrhosis developed progressive respiratory distress from desquamative interstitial pneumonitis despite cessation of sulfasalazine and institution of systemic corticosteroid therapy [183]. Bilateral interstitial infiltrates and gas exchange abnormalities were described in a patient who developed the pulmonary complication insidiously after 2 years of treatment with mesalamine (5-aminosalicylic acid), which is another drug used in the treatment of chronic ulcerative colitis [148].

Nontropical Sprue

Nontropical sprue (celiac disease) has been reported to exist with diffuse pulmonary fibrosis. Although each of those disorders may be associated with abnormal immunologic phenomena, the pathogenesis remains unclear [80]. However, other studies of patients with this combination of diseases have indicated that avian protein precipitins were present in sera [11,110]. The influence of extrinsic factors seems to be prominent in these cases of pulmonary fibrosis; in two other patients with the combination of nontropical sprue and pulmonary fibrosis, the presence of farmer's lung precipitins (*Micropolyspora faeni*) was noted [152].

Lung function studies and chest roentgenograms have shown features of interstitial lung disease in patients with nontropical sprue. It has been suggested that both nontropical sprue and extrinsic allergic alveolitis may be caused by a common immunologic mechanism, because extrinsic allergic alveolitis and nontropical sprue are both associated with HLA-D3, and an association has been reported between nontropical sprue and hypersensitivity pneumonitis from the European literature [98]. However, a study of 18 North American patients with nontropical sprue failed to corroborate this association [182]. Nonetheless, a history of asthma or chronic cough was present in a higher proportion of the celiac than the control subjects, and the patients with nontropical sprue showed objective evidence of obstructive lung disease.

A case is reported of a 62-year-old woman who had celiac sprue and developed lymphocytic interstitial pneumonia followed by abdominal lymphoma [131]. The patient presented with dyspnea, cough, weight loss, and bibasilar pulmonary infiltrates. Systemic corticosteroids resulted in improvement lasting 1 year. Whereas lymphocytic lymphomas are a well-known complication of sprue, lymphocytic interstitial pneumonitis is not. Postmortem examination of the respiratory system in a patient with nontropical sprue has revealed partial fibrous obliteration of small airways and dilatation of larger airways [52].

A more interesting relationship is between celiac disease and idiopathic pulmonary hemosiderosis. The coexistence has been reported in many cases. A study of seven patients with idiopathic pulmonary hemosiderosis revealed nontropical sprue in three patients and limitation to airflow and decreased DLCO in five [209]. Clinical documentation that treatment of celiac disease could lead to remission of idiopathic pulmonary hemosiderosis is worth noting. In the cases reported in the literature, 6 of 10 patients who were followed showed improvement in both diseases with a gluten-free diet, although histopathologic improvement in the intestinal lesion was shown in only 2 patients [138]. Despite these reports, there is some doubt regarding the relationship between nontropical sprue and idiopathic pulmonary hemosiderosis [138,209,210]. Nevertheless, it is worthwhile to look for the presence of celiac disease in patients who develop clinical features of idiopathic pulmonary hemosiderosis because both diseases may improve on a gluten-free diet. In patients with celiac disease, antibodies to reticulin and gliadin are found in 78 and 95 percent, respectively [92]. A positive serology for either reticulin or gliadin in a patient with idiopathic pulmonary hemosiderosis should lead to consideration of a gluten-free diet.

Whipple's Disease

Whipple's disease is a multisystem disorder with predominantly intestinal manifestations in the form of malabsorption syndrome. Descriptions of Whipple's disease normally place emphasis on the intestinal and joint manifestations. However, a significant number of patients with this disorder develop pleuropulmonary complications, which may include pleuritic pain, pleural effusion, dyspnea, cough, lung infiltrates, and restrictive lung dysfunction. Respiratory involvement without other symptoms such as arthralgias and fever has occurred. Cough is noted in nearly half of these cases [146]. Although intestinal and joint manifestations are attributed to intracellular infection, the pulmonary manifestations may be the result of an inflammatory reaction to locally deposited immune complexes containing bacterial antigens [179]. Whipple's disease is known to simulate pulmonary sarcoidosis [28,154]. One patient who developed chest roentgenographic features of sarcoidosis had noncaseous granulomas in the peripheral lymph nodes, pleura, and lung parenchyma. The pleuropulmonary disease resolved with appropriate treatment of Whipple's disease [154].

Whipple's disease presented as pleuropericarditis in a 48-year-old woman [141]. Peribronchiolar and perivascular histiocytic infiltrates in a patchy distribution have been described in this disease, with characteristic cytoplasmic bacilliform inclusions present in these cells [208]. Also, pulmonary fibrosis in a patient who had eosinophilic gastroenteritis with malabsorption has been reported [184].

Other Malabsorption Syndromes

Protein-losing enteropathy may predispose patients to developing pleural effusions, both transudative and chylous [10]. Primary intestinal lymphangiectasia is a rare condition of uncertain etiology characterized by dilated small-bowel lymphatics and often complicated by anomalous lymphatics elsewhere, typically in the limbs. Protein-losing enteropathy secondary to intestinal lymphangiectasia has been reported to produce chylothorax [8].

The combination of yellow nails, lymphedema, and pleural effusions is known as the yellow-nail syndrome. Lymphedema can occur as a distinct entity or as a result of lymphatic obstruction or loss of chyle from various mechanisms. More than 20 percent of patients with primary lymphedema have a protein-losing enteropathy resulting from lymphangiectasia of the small bowel. With significant loss of protein, these patients develop hypoproteinemia as well as hypogammaglobulinemia. Persistent pleural effusions and recurrent pulmonary infections may ensue in this setting [10,60].

Hepatic Diseases

Diseases of the liver produce or are associated with multiple pulmonary problems [13,103]. Hepatic cirrhosis is the most prevalent type of chronic liver disease in the United States. Approximately 15 to 45 percent of patients with cirrhosis demonstrate one or more of the following: arterial hypoxemia in conjunction with hemoglobin desaturation, clubbing, pleural effusions secondary to ascites, hyperventilation, and platypnea-orthodeoxia [103]. In a prospective study of 170 patients with various types of chronic hepatic diseases, mottled pulmonary parenchymal infiltrates were noted in 6 percent. Decreased DLCO was observed in 20 percent [177]. Clubbing of nails seemed to occur with a higher frequency in those with liver disease and abnormal chest roentgenograms. Various respiratory complications seen in hepatic diseases are listed in Table 62-2.

Pleural Effusion

Pleural effusion, usually right-sided and occasionally massive and symptomatic, may occur in cirrhosis or peritonitis. Pleural effusion is found in 6 percent of patients who have hepatic cirrhosis associated with ascites. The fluid is usually a transudate, and its chemical characteristics are similar to those of ascitic fluid. There are three

possible mechanisms for the development of pleural effusion in hepatic cirrhosis: hypoproteinemia, azygos hypertension, and transfer of peritoneal fluid to the pleural cavity via congenital defects in the diaphragm. Intraperitoneal injection of the radioisotope ^{99m}Tc sulfur colloid has demonstrated the one-way transdiaphragmatic flow of fluid from the peritoneal to the pleural space, and thoracotomy has allowed identification of the diaphragmatic defects, which were repaired [160]. In patients with massive pleural effusion secondary to ascites, drainage of pleural fluid for therapeutic purposes is usually futile because as long as the peritoneal cavity contains

Table 62-2. **Intrathoracic abnormalities in hepatic diseases**

Hepatic disorder	Intrathoracic complication	Hepatic disorder	Intrathoracic complication
Cirrhosis*	Intrapulmonary shunting Pleural shunting (pleural spider nevi) Portopulmonary shunting Pleural effusion (without ascites) Defective hypoxic vasoconstriction Ventilation-perfusion mismatch Diffusion abnormalities Pulmonary hypertension Rightward shift of oxyhemoglobin dissociation curve	Primary sclerosing cholangitis	Bronchiectasis Recurrent bronchitis
		Hepatic abscess	Pleurisy or pleural effusion Empyema Lung abscess
		Hepatic amebiasis	Pleurisy or pleural effusion Amebic empyema Hepatobronchial fistula
		Hepatic hydatid disease	Pleurisy or pleural effusion
		Hepatic or biliary surgery	Diaphragmatic elevation Pleurisy or pleural effusion Pulmonary bile embolism
Ascites	Diaphragmatic elevation Pleural effusion Empyema Decreased lung volumes	Hepatic malignancy	Pleural effusion Pulmonary nodules Diffuse lymphangitic infiltration
Hepatitis†	Pleuritis or pleural effusion Interstitial pneumonitis	Liver transplantation	Pleural effusion Opportunistic infections Atelectasis of right lower lobe Diaphragmatic dysfunction
Primary biliary cirrhosis	Lymphocytic alveolitis (subclinical) Lymphocytic interstitial pneumonitis Interstitial pneumonitis (nonspecific) Desquamative interstitial pneumonitis Interstitial noncaseous granulomas Airways obstruction (with Sjögren's syndrome) Restrictive disease (thoracic deformity)	Alpha$_1$-antitrypsin deficiency	Panlobular emphysema Bullous lung disease Intrapulmonary shunting

*Alcoholic, cryptogenic, and postnecrotic cirrhosis.
†Viral, drug-induced, and chronic active hepatitis.

fluid, the pleural fluid will continue to reaccumulate. Treatment should be aimed at controlling the ascites [163]. Pleural effusions also are seen with viral hepatitis [74]. In a prospective Italian study of hepatitis, 70 percent of 156 patients had some fluid in the pleural space [175].

Ascites, if large in volume, can interfere with normal pulmonary function by interfering with normal diaphragmatic excursion. Ascites and abnormal distension restrict full inflation of the lungs and thus reduce lung volume. This effect of ascites on the pulmonary system is reported to be mediated by a hydrostatic pressure exerted from within the peritoneal cavity on the diaphragm [76]. However, this effect varies among patients and seems to be dependent on the intraabdominal hydrostatic pressure (thought of as a pressure in excess of the height of the anterior abdominal wall) [76].

Hepatopulmonary Syndrome

The term *hepatopulmonary syndrome* is used to reflect the arterial hypoxemia in patients with cirrhosis [90,96,102,155]. It may be seen in other chronic liver diseases, such as chronic active hepatitis and nonspecific hepatitis. Arterial hypoxemia is a well-known complication of hepatic cirrhosis and is present in 30 to 50 percent of patients [59]. There are several mechanisms of hypoxemia in liver disease. Hypoxemia results from venoarterial shunting in the basal regions of the lung. Intrapulmonary shunting in liver disease is due to the following mechanisms: venous blood flowing through nonventilated alveoli, anatomic communications between pulmonary arteries and veins with bypassing of the capillary-alveolar interphase, and dilated capillary and precapillary beds in which diffuse oxygen ineffectively reaches the midstream deoxygenated hemoglobin molecules. Shunts can reach considerable proportions (20 to 70 percent) of the cardiac output [103]. Blood gas analysis discloses moderate hypoxemia and respiratory alkalosis. There may be more than one mechanism for the hypoxemia associated with liver cirrhosis [49]. Injection of radioactive krypton into the spleen has shown definite portopulmonary anastomoses. In some instances, venous blood in the portal system may reach the left side of the heart through anastomotic channels with pulmonary veins.

Anatomic shunting cannot be implicated as the sole reason for the severe hypoxemia in these patients because calculated shunts, determined while patients were breathing 100% O_2, ranged from 4 to 31 percent in one study [105]. One report suggests that the hypoxemia noted in patients with hepatic cirrhosis is not due to hypoxic pulmonary vasoconstriction [128], although in another study of patients with chronic hepatic cirrhosis, the most significant finding was the hypoxic pulmonary vasoconstriction and inadequate pulmonary vascular tone [157]. Yet another study concluded that the hypoxia of liver disease was caused by ventilation-perfusion mismatching, which cannot be explained by an abnormal hypoxic pulmonary vasoconstriction [125]. An experimental study in rats has shown that hepatic cirrhosis induces reversible depression of hypoxic pulmonary vasoconstriction, and this may be a suitable animal model for studying hepatopulmonary syndrome [26]. The definitive mechanism for the hypoxemia of hepatic cirrhosis remains undetermined. Hypoxemia produced by the assumption of an erect position and relieved by a recumbent position (orthodeoxia) in patients with hepatic cirrhosis results from the effect of the gravitational forces that increase the blood flow through intrapulmonary venoarterial shunts. When orthodeoxia is severe, patients develop increasing dyspnea while standing (platypnea) [151]. Although hypoxemia in patients with liver disease is common and multifactorial, severe hypoxia is unusual. In a large series of cirrhotic patients, 7 percent had an arterial oxygen tension of less than 60 mmHg while breathing room air [129]. Another cause of hypoxia in these patients is the pulmonary edema associated with liver disease. There appears to be high incidence of low-pressure pulmonary edema and acute respiratory distress syndrome in patients with fulminant hepatic failure [188].

Diffuse Pulmonary Disease

Primary biliary cirrhosis is a granulomatous liver disease characterized by chronic intrahepatic cholestasis. The etiology is unknown, and it is associated with the presence of non-organ-specific antibodies to mitochondria in more than 95 percent of patients [176]. The frequency and nature of pleuropulmonary manifestations in primary biliary cirrhosis are poorly documented. Interstitial lung disease has been observed on rare occasions. Many of the cases of lung involvement in primary biliary cirrhosis have been characterized by lung parenchymal granuloma formation and mononuclear cell alveolitis mimicking pulmonary sarcoidosis [176]. One study using bronchoalveolar lavage has shown an increase in the number of alveolar CD4+ (helper-inducer) T lympho-cytes (22 versus 12 percent in alcoholic cirrhosis) and activated alveolar macrophages in 50 percent of patients [195]. These data suggest that subclinical alveolar inflammation, comprising T lymphocytes and activated alveolar macrophages and mimicking sarcoid alveolitis, is present in a high proportion of patients with primary biliary cirrhosis. Pulmonary nodules simulating pulmonary carcinomatosis and later documented to be lymphocytic interstitial pneumonitis was described in a 51-year-old woman [200]. These changes were unrelated to the activity of primary biliary cirrhosis and underwent spontaneous resolution. Since sicca complex often is associated with primary biliary cirrhosis, part of the respiratory dysfunction noted in primary biliary cirrhosis may be related to sicca complex rather than to the liver disease [156].

Patients with primary biliary cirrhosis and Sjogren's syndrome have a high frequency of respiratory complaints, particularly productive cough and dyspnea [156]. The respiratory symptoms are most likely related to Sjogren's syndrome rather than liver disease. Although obstructive or restrictive pulmonary dysfunction can be demonstrated, reduction in DLCO is the most common abnormality reported [156,192].

Turner-Warwick [190] reported eight cases of pulmonary fibrosis associated with chronic active hepatitis (five cases) and interlobular hepatitis (three cases). Progression and regression of pulmonary and hepatic disease were parallel in seven of these patients. All had antibodies that were not organ-specific and one or more circulating immunoglobulins. Turner-Warwick [190] concluded that hepatic and pulmonary diseases in these patients may have several factors in common. An underlying systemic disorder, possibly autoimmune, may be responsible for some cases of cryptogenic fibrosing alveolitis, chronic active hepatitis, and autoimmune hemolytic anemia in the same patient [205]. In a study of 108 patients with chronic acute hepatitis, pulmonary function tests disclosed an abnormality in the DLCO in 26 percent [71].

Pulmonary Hypertension

The association of hepatic cirrhosis and pulmonary hypertension was first observed more than three decades ago. There has been some disagreement, however, regarding this. In a study of 2459 patients with biopsy-proved cirrhosis and 1241 patients with cirrhosis diagnosed at autopsy,

the incidences of idiopathic hypertensive pulmonary vascular disease were 0.6 and 0.73 percent, respectively, in contrast to 0.13 percent ($p < .001$) in all autopsies [122]. The data from this study suggest an association between cirrhosis and the development of pulmonary hypertension. Whereas the prevalence of cirrhosis alone was highest in the fifth decade, the average age of the cirrhotics with pulmonary hypertension was 35 years, and they tended to be women. The mechanisms responsible for the development of pulmonary hypertension in hepatic cirrhosis are unknown. Recurrent embolization from portal to pulmonary circulation, primary vasoconstriction, in situ thrombosis of pulmonary vessels, increased pulmonary vascular resistance from vasoactive peptides released as a result of portal hypertension, dietary alterations, and recurrent pulmonary emboli have been implicated.

Although most cases of pulmonary hypertension have been reported in patients with cirrhosis, hepatic parenchymal disease or failure is not necessary for its development. The strongest association appears to be with portal hypertension, and portal hypertension nearly always precedes by several years the diagnosis of pulmonary vacuolar disease [59]. Histologic features, including plexogenic arteriopathy, are similar to those in primary pulmonary hypertension [116]. Autopsy studies reveal a high incidence of intravascular thrombosis in association with plexiform lesions [51].

A prospective study of lung functions after liver transplantation in 95 patients before and 9 to 15 months following transplantation observed that the most common abnormality before transplantation was the impaired gas exchange as measured by DLCO. Obstructive airways disease, as measured by FEV_1 and FVC, was uncommon [106]. Arterial carbon dioxide tension and DLCO significantly improved after transplantation, the improvement in the former parameter indicating the resolution of pretransplant alkalosis.

Liver Transplant

Liver transplantation is a well-established treatment option for patients with end-stage liver diseases, with 1-year survival after transplant approaching 70 to 80 percent. It was reported that 2656 liver transplantations were performed in 1990 in the United States alone [59]. Pulmonary infections occur in 25 percent of transplant recipients [53]. The organisms responsible for pulmonary infections include gram-negative bacteria, cytomegalovirus, *Candida* species, *Aspergillus* species, and *Pneumocystis carinii*. The majority of the noninfectious complications are caused by prolonged general anesthesia, extensive upper abdominal surgery, and massive administration of blood products and colloids [104]. Noninfectious complications include atelectasis, pleural effusion, acute respiratory distress syndrome, and pulmonary calcification [59]. Although air embolism is common during liver transplantation, clinical sequelae are few [149].

Miscellaneous Hepatic Associations

Bile pulmonary embolism is a rare, occasionally fatal complication following biliary trauma. Communications between the biliary tract and hepatic veins after biliary surgery have been shown to result in bile emboli in small pulmonary arteries. Among the nine cases reported in the literature up to 1983, five had malignancies encroaching on the biliary tree and the rest had biliary trauma [144].

Drugs such as penicillamine, azathioprine, and sulfasalazine are used in various gastroenterologic diseases. These drugs have the potential to cause pulmonary toxicity, and this possibility should be considered in evaluating patients with gastroenterologic diseases and pulmonary problems. A case of azathioprine-associated alveolitis diagnosed by gallium 67 scanning and transbronchial biopsy is reported [101]. The patient denied respiratory symptoms, exhibited spiking fevers, and had normal chest roentgenograms. Allopurinol inhibition of azathioprine metabolism may have been a contributing factor [84].

Low levels of serum alpha$_1$-antitrypsin may be associated with cirrhosis of the liver in children and some adults. Chronic liver disease in patients with alpha$_1$-antitrypsin deficiency is associated with a high prevalence of liver infection by viruses. It has been suggested that the viral infection of the liver, rather than the alpha$_1$-antitrypsin deficiency alone, may be the cause of the liver disease in such patients [147]. Hepatocellular carcinoma is another complication. Individuals homozygous for alpha$_1$-antitrypsin deficiency may develop cirrhosis in infancy and emphysema in adulthood.

Pleuropulmonary complications in amebiasis are seen only if the liver is affected by this parasitic infection and occur in 7 to 20 percent of patients with amebic liver abscesses and in 2 to 3 percent of those with invasive disease [94]. The intrathoracic manifestations include sympathetic effusion over the infradiaphragmatic area of inflammation, rupture of the amebic abscess and amebic empyema, and rupture directly into the bronchial tree to produce hepatobronchial fistula [82,108] (Fig. 62-10).

Alcohol and the Lung

It is well documented that chronic alcohol consumption increases the risk of developing pulmonary tuberculosis, chronic bronchitis, aspiration pneumonitis, lung abscess, pulmonary complications of alcoholic cirrhosis, and pulmonary problems from alcoholic cardiomyopathy. The reported effects of alcohol on the respiratory system include diminished ciliary motion, decreased migration of alveolar macrophages, interference with surfactant production, and increased prevalence of oropharyngeal gram-negative bacilli. However, the effect of alcohol and alcoholism on respiratory function is still controversial [7,30,57,113,173].

Several studies in the 1970s led to the widely held belief that alcohol consumption caused airways obstruction and a reduction in diffusing ca-

Fig. 62-10. Right-sided pleuropulmonary involvement by amebic abscess.

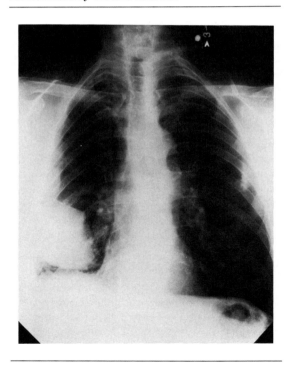

pacity. However, in the early 1980s, three large epidemiologic studies critically analyzed the effect of alcohol on respiratory function and found that alcohol has little, if any, effect on pulmonary function. The pulmonary functional abnormalities noted in earlier studies were apparently related to smoking, a common habit among subjects who consume alcohol. More recently, the effect of alcohol consumption on pulmonary function was evaluated in a population-based study of more than 8750 persons over a period of 5 years, among whom 301 men and 32 women (78 nonsmokers) with an alcohol consumption of 350 gm/wk or more were the study group. The results showed that alcohol consumption significantly accelerated the loss of FEV_1 and forced vital capacity, and the effects were comparable to the effect of smoking 15 gm tobacco daily [111]. An earlier study of 27 alcoholic subjects in the United Kingdom concluded that the high prevalence of respiratory disease in alcoholics is largely attributable to their smoking habits and that there was no evidence of a specific pulmonary toxic effect of ethanol on the lungs [119]. Still other reports have noted that short-term cessation of alcohol intake had no effect on pulmonary function parameters in cigarette-smoking alcoholics [7,30,57,113,173].

Impaired glottic reflex and cough reflex, aspiration pneumonias, aggravation of sleep apnea, respiratory failure from oversedation, and tuberculosis are some of the complications of alcohol ingestion. The effect of moderate amounts of alcohol (e.g., 120 ml scotch whiskey, with 40 percent alcohol) on nocturnal esophageal reflux was studied in healthy volunteers [194]. Monitoring of esophageal pH in ambulatory and supine postures revealed prolonged supine reflux episodes in 41 percent, whereas none in the control group had reflux. This study also found that there was a significant exposure of the distal esophagus to acid and that the normal acid clearance of the esophagus in the supine position was impaired after only moderate amounts of alcohol. A small number of persons of Asian and Native American extraction are reported to experience chest tightness and wheezing after alcohol ingestion, and this has been termed *alcohol asthma* [107].

Alcoholism is closely associated with tuberculosis, the prevalence of alcoholism being 49 percent in newly diagnosed tuberculous disease [61]. Among 970 subjects in New York City with alcohol and drug addiction, the prevalence of tuberculosis was 0.91 percent, which was 28 times the age-matched rate for the city and the screening;

only those with a positive tuberculin test and cough substantially increased the yield of active tuberculosis to 7.2 percent, or 225 times the rate for the city [63]. In view of the rising incidence of tuberculosis in the 1990s, screening for tuberculosis in the alcoholic population is highly recommended. A review of 23 patients with primary pulmonary sporotrichosis, presumably acquired by inhalation, revealed that this form of the disease affects middle-aged men with a history of alcoholism or chronic lung disease. Clinically and roentgenographically, the disease mimics chronic cavitary tuberculosis and histoplasmosis [58].

Deficiency of IgG subclass has been reported in 70 percent of patients with alcoholic liver disease, and the deficiency was reported to be closely correlated with the number and type of bacterial respiratory infections [174].

Pancreatic Diseases

Pleural Effusion

Acute, chronic, or relapsing pancreatitis is sometimes associated with pleuropulmonary complications. Pleural effusion has a reported incidence of 4 to 17 percent [20]. Roentgenographic abnormalities include pleural effusion, elevation of a hemidiaphragm, and basilar atelectasis. The effusions are predominantly left-sided. Characteristically, the fluid has increased protein content and an elevated amylase level, with hemorrhagic effusion in 30 percent of instances. Massive pleural effusions can occur in association with asymptomatic pancreatic disease [33]. The most common underlying cause of pancreatic pleural effusion is alcoholic pancreatitis [191].

Pleuropancreatic fistula may produce chronic massive pleural effusions [33,153]. Chronic massive pancreatic pleural effusion also may develop weeks, months, or years after an episode of acute pancreatitis and, in most of these patients, there is no history of pancreatitis [41]. Patients may present with dyspnea, cough, and chest pain. The pleural fluid amylase content is always markedly elevated. The fluid is an exudate with elevated concentrations of lactate dehydrogenase and protein. Chronic massive pancreatic pleural effusion is due to posterior disruption of the pancreatic duct into the retroperitoneal space, with tracking of secretions from the pancreas along the esophagus or aorta upward into the mediastinum [41]. The fluid can occasionally collect in the mediastinum and produce a mediastinal pseudocyst [41,89]. Pericardial effusion and tamponade has been described [164]. Very high levels of pleural fluid amylase also can be seen in pleural effusion secondary to esophageal perforation.

Acute Respiratory Distress Syndrome

Acute respiratory distress syndrome is the most serious complication of pancreatitis and is reported to occur in 20 to 50 percent of patients [197]. The mechanism of injury is unknown, but it is believed to be related to defective surfactant production. Lecithin is a main constituent of the pulmonary surfactant dipalmitoyl lecithin. The surfactant is split by a lecithinase, which is increased in acute pancreatitis. An experimental study suggests that pancreatic elastase plays a major role, by direct deleterious action on the pulmonary vasculature, in the development of pulmonary vascular injury after acute pancreatitis [118]. In another experimental model of pancreatitis, induced by injection of trypsin and sodium taurocholate into the pancreas, pulmonary injury was prevented by pretreatment of animals with trasylol, an antiprotease drug active toward trypsin and elastase [180]. Acute hemorrhagic pancreatitis frequently is associated with acute respiratory failure with pulmonary edema, which is generally believed to be due to increased alveolar membrane permeability [120]. Hypoalbuminemia seen in pancreatitis may aggravate the tendency to develop pulmonary edema.

Large intrathoracic fluid collections often complicate pancreatic pseudocysts [69]. Most, but not all, chronic or persistent pleural effusions are associated with, and caused by, a fistulous tract between the pseudocyst and the pleural space. Computed tomography is helpful in detecting the fistulous communication [117]. Subdiaphragmatic collection of fluid is common and may play a role in the accumulation of pleural effusion; ultrasonography or computed tomography is necessary to exclude such fluid collections [204]. Other pulmonary complications of chronic pancreatitis include bibasilar atelectasis, diaphragmatic elevation due to pleural effusion or atelectasis, and pleural calcification [20]. Mediastinal fat necrosis is another complication described [164].

Other Gastroenterologic Diseases

Subphrenic Abscess

With intraabdominal problems such as a rupture or perforation of a viscus and after intraabdom-

inal surgery, subphrenic abscess is a common complication. The incidence of involvement of either side is approximately equal, as is involvement of the anterior and posterior subphrenic spaces. Roentgenographically, evidence of subphrenic abscess appears within the lung, in the pleural space, and in the subphrenic space. Blunting of the costophrenic angle is seen in nearly 90 percent of patients. Retroperitoneal abscess also can cause pleural effusion [133].

Abdominal Surgery

Changes in respiratory function after abdominal surgery have been well documented. Intraoperative testing of lung function has shown both diminished vital capacity and diminished residual capacity [43]. Microatelectasis, seen commonly in postoperative states, is believed to be a major cause of persistent hypoxemia. Several mechanisms have been hypothesized to explain this, including diminished product of surfactant resulting from inhalation of high oxygen concentrations or from altered ventilatory patterns [9]; alveolar collapse due to complete resorption of alveolar gas following inhalation of 100% O_2; and peripheral airways obstruction by bronchoconstriction due to hypocapnia. In another study, mucociliary clearance (of tantalum introduced into the tracheobronchial tree for measurement of clearance) was grossly abnormal, with segmental atelectasis, after abdominal surgery but was normal after peripheral surgery.

Development of small pleural effusions is common after abdominal procedures. In one study, pleural fluid could be detected in 49 percent of 200 patients 48 to 72 hours after operation. The incidence was higher after upper abdominal surgery and in patients with atelectasis on the same side as the operation. Thoracentesis in 20 patients revealed that the fluid was an exudate in 16 of them. Almost all the effusions resolved spontaneously [114].

Abnormalities of the abdominal wall may interfere with normal pulmonary function. Large defects such as ventral hernia may produce respiratory embarrassment and therefore require surgical correction, especially in those with chronic obstructive lung disease [25].

Acute pulmonary embolism can be triggered by the act of defecation in patients with deep vein thrombosis. One retrospective chart review estimated that defecation-induced pulmonary embolism occurred in 6.8 percent of all patients with the discharge diagnosis of pulmonary embolism, and, of the nine patients with this combination, six died [97]. Increased intraabdominal pressure (due to Valsalva maneuver) during defecation followed by a sudden decrease in the pressure ("vacuum effect") is hypothesized to dislodge clots from deep veins [97]. We recommend that pulmonary embolism be considered in the differential diagnosis of patients with defecation syncope and defecation-associated sudden death.

References

1. Abbott OA, Mansour KA, Logan WD Jr. Atraumatic so-called "spontaneous" rupture of the esophagus: A review of 47 personal cases with comments on a new method of surgical therapy. *J Thorac Cardiovasc Surg* 59:67, 1970.
2. Ahn CH, et al. A four drug regimen for initial treatment of cavitary disease caused by *Mycobacterium avium* complex. *Am Rev Respir Dis* 134:438, 1986.
3. Allen CJ, Newhouse MT. Gastroesophageal reflux and chronic respiratory disease. *Am Rev Respir Dis* 129:645, 1985.
4. Alvarez S, Shell C, Berk SL. Pulmonary tuberculosis in elderly men. *Am J Med* 82:602, 1987.
5. Angelillo VA, et al. Gastrobronchial fistula secondary to a subphrenic abscess. *Chest* 84:85, 1983.
6. Bacon BR, Bailey-Newton RS, Connors AF Jr. Pleural effusions after endoscopic variceal sclerotherapy. *Gastroenterology* 88:1910, 1985.
7. Banner AS. Pulmonary function in chronic alcoholism. *Am Rev Respir Dis* 108:851, 1973.
8. Barrett DS, Large SR, Rees GM. Pleurectomy for chylothorax associated with intestinal lymphangiectasia. *Thorax* 42:557, 1987.
9. Bartlett RH, Gazzaniga AB, Geraghty TR. Respiratory maneuvers to prevent postoperative pulmonary complications: A critical review. *JAMA* 224:1017, 1973.
10. Battaglia A, et al. Pleural effusion and recurrent bronchopneumonia with lymphedema, yellow nails, and protein-losing enteropathy. *Eur J Respir Dis* 66:65, 1985.
11. Berrill WT, et al. Bird-fancier's lung and jejunal villous atrophy. *Lancet* 2:1006, 1975.
12. Berstein CN, Snape WJ Jr. Achalasia and development of benign esophagobronchial fistula. *Dig Dis Sci* 37:609, 1992.
13. Bihari DJ, Gimson AE, Williams R. Cardiovascular pulmonary and renal complications of fulminant hepatic failure. *Semin Liver Dis* 6:119, 1986.
14. Bonniere P, et al. Latent pulmonary involvement in Crohn's disease: Biological, functional, bronchoalveolar lavage and scintigraphic studies. *Gut* 27:919, 1986.
15. Bradshaw MJ, Harvey RF, Burns-Cox CJ. Crohn's disease presenting as recurrent pulmonary oedema. *Br Med J* 283:1437, 1981.
16. Brandstetter RD, et al. Pleural effusion due to communicating gastric ulcer. *NY State J Med* 85:706, 1985.
17. Britton CA, Jarmolowski CR, Winzelberg GG. A 34-year-old woman with persistent cough and diarrhea. *JAMA* 255:2785, 1986.
18. Bruce RM, Wise L. Tuberculosis after jejunojejunal bypass for obesity. *Ann Intern Med* 87:574, 1977.
19. Butland RJA, et al. Chronic bronchial suppuration and inflammatory bowel disease. *Q J Med* 197:63, 1981.
20. Bydder GM, Kreel L. Pleural calcification in pancreatitis demonstrated by computed tomography. *J Comput Assist Tomogr* 5:161, 1981.
21. Camara EJN, et al. Pulmonary findings in patients with chagasic megaesophagus. *Chest* 83:87, 1983.
22. Carasso B, Couropmitree C, Heredia R. Eggshell silicotic calcification causing bronchoesophageal fistula. *Am Rev Respir Dis* 108:1384, 1973.
23. Castell DO. Asthma and gastroesophageal reflux. *Chest* 96:2, 1989.
24. Celis R, et al. Nosocomial pneumonia. A multivariate analysis of risk and prognosis. *Chest* 93:318, 1988.
25. Celli BR, et al. Respiratory consequences of abdominal hernia in a patient with severe chronic obstructive pulmonary disease. *Am Rev Respir Dis* 131:178, 1985.
26. Chang S-W, Ohara N. Pulmonary circulatory dysfunction in rats with biliary cirrhosis. *Am Rev Respir Dis* 145:798, 1992.
27. Chijimatsu Y, et al. Airway obstruction in achalasia. *Chest* 78:348, 1980.
28. Cho C, et al. Sarcoid-like granulomas as an early manifestation of Whipple's disease. *Gastroenterology* 87:941, 1984.
29. Chofnas I, Love RW Jr. Postgastrectomy state and tuberculosis. *Arch Surg* 92:704, 1966.
30. Cohen BH, et al. Alcohol consumption and airway obstruction. *Am Rev Respir Dis* 21:205, 1980.
31. Cohen S. The pathogenesis of gastroesophageal reflux disease: A challenge in clinical physiology (editorial). *Ann Intern Med* 117:1051, 1992.
32. Cook DJ, et al. Nosocomial pneumonia and the role of gastric pH. A meta analysis. *Chest* 100:7, 1991.
33. Cooper CB, et al. Pleural effusions and pancreatico-pleural fistulae with asymptomatic pancreatic disease. *Br J Dis Chest* 82:315, 1988.
34. Craven DE, et al. Risk factors for pneumonia and fatality in patients receiving continuous mechanical ventilation. *Am Rev Respir Dis* 133:792, 1986.

35. Crawford DC, Ryan DW. Acute respiratory insufficiency after endoscopy for bleeding oesophageal varices. *Br Med J* 288:1639, 1984.

36. Cunningham ET, et al. Vagal reflexes referred from the upper aerodigestive tract: An infrequently recognized cause of common cardiorespiratory responses. *Ann Intern Med* 116:575, 1992.

37. Das CH, Raju MP. Acute regional ileitis with concomitant pulmonary tuberculosis. *Int Surg* 67:377, 1982.

38. Daschenr F, et al. Stress ulcer prophylaxis and ventilation pneumonia: Prevention by antibacterial cytoprotective agents. *Infect Control Hosp Epidemiol* 9:59, 1988.

39. Dennish GW, Castell DO. Inhibitory effect of smoking on the lower esophageal sphincter. *N Engl J Med* 284:1136, 1971.

40. Desai SJ, Gephardt GN, Stoller JK. Diffuse panbronchiolitis preceding ulcerative colitis. *Chest* 45:1342, 1989.

41. Dewan NA, Kinney WW, O'Donohue WJ Jr. Chronic massive pancreatic pleural effusion. *Chest* 85:497, 1984.

42. Domej W, et al. Colobronchial fistula: A rare complication of Crohn's colitis. *Am Rev Respir Dis* 142:1225, 1990.

43. Don HF, Wahba WM, Craig DB. Airway closure, gas trapping, and the functional residual capacity during anesthesia. *Anesthesiology* 36:533, 1972.

44. Donowitz LG, et al. Alteration of normal gastric flora in critical care patients receiving antacid and cimetidine therapy. *Infect Control* 7:23, 1986.

45. Driks MR, et al. Nosocomial pneumonia in intubated patients given sucralfate as compared with antacids or histamine type 2 blockers. The role of gastric colonization. *N Engl J Med* 317:1376, 1987.

46. du Moulin GC, et al. Aspiration of gastric bacteria in antacid-treated patients: A frequent cause of postoperative colonization of the airway. *Lancet* 2:242, 1982.

47. Ducolone A, et al. Gastroesophageal reflux in patients with asthma and chronic bronchitis. *Am Rev Respir Dis* 135:327, 1987.

48. Eade OE, et al. Pulmonary function in patients with inflammatory bowel disease. *Am J Gastroenterol* 73:154, 1980.

49. Edell ES, et al. Severe hypoxemia and liver disease. *Am Rev Respir Dis* 140:1631, 1989.

50. Edling JE, Bacon BR. Pleuropulmonary complications of endoscopic variceal sclerotherapy. *Chest* 99:1252, 1991.

51. Edwards BS, et al. Coexistent pulmonary and portal hypertension: Morphologic and clinical features. *J Am Coll Cardiol* 10:1233, 1987.

52. Edwards C, Williams A, Asquith P. Bronchopulmonary disease in coeliac patients. *J Clin Pathol* 38:361, 1985.

53. Ekberg H, et al. Major liver resection: Perioperative course and management. *Surgery* 100:1, 1986.

54. Ekstrom T, Lindgren BR, Tibbling L. Effects of ranitidine treatment on patients with asthma and history of gastro-oesophageal reflux: A double blind crossover study. *Thorax* 44:19, 1989.

55. Ekstrom T, Tibbling L. Esophageal acid perfusion, airway function, and symptoms in asthmatic patients with marked bronchial hyperreactivity. *Chest* 96:995, 1989.

56. Ekstrom T, Tibbling L. Gastroesophageal reflux and triggering of bronchial asthma: A negative report. *Eur J Respir Dis* 71:177, 1987.

57. Emirgil C, et al. Pulmonary function in alcoholics. *Am J Med* 57:69, 1974.

58. England DM, Hochholzer L. Primary pulmonary sporotrichosis: Report of eight cases with clinicopathologic review. *Am J Surg Pathol* 9:193, 1985.

59. Ettinger NA, Trulock EP. Pulmonary considerations of organ transplantation. *Am Rev Respir Dis* 143:1386, 1991.

60. Eustace PW, Gaunt JI, Croft DN. Incidence of protein-losing enteropathy in primary lymphedema using chromium 51 chloride technique. *Br Med J* 4:737, 1975.

61. Feingold AO. Association of tuberculosis with alcoholism. *South Med J* 69:1336, 1976.

62. Foster LJ, Trudeau WL, Goldman AL. Bronchodilator effects on gastric acid secretion. *JAMA* 241:2613, 1979.

63. Freidman LN, et al. Tuberculosis screening in alcoholics and drug addicts. *Am Rev Respir Dis* 136:1188, 1987.

64. Garvey BM, McCambley JA, Tuxen DV. Effects of gastric alkalinization on bacterial colonization in critically ill patients. *Crit Care Med* 17:211, 1989.

65. George DK, et al. Hypoplasia and immaturity of the terminal lung unit (acinus) in congenital diaphragmatic hernia. *Am Rev Respir Dis* 136:947, 1987.

66. Gertsch P, Mosimann R. Chylothorax complicating sclerotherapy for bleeding oesophageal varices. *Br J Surg* 70:562, 1983.

67. Gerzic Z, Rakic S, Randjelovic T. Acquired benign esophagorespiratory fistula: Report of 16 consecutive cases. *Ann Thorac Surg* 50:724, 1990.

68. Gibb WRG, et al. Bronchiectasis with ulcerative colitis and myelopathy. *Thorax* 42:155, 1987.

69. Girbes ARJ, et al. Massive pleural effusion due to pancreatic pseudocyst. *Thorax* 45:563, 1990.

70. Givan DC, et al. Achalasia and tracheal obstruction in a child. *Eur J Respir Dis* 66:70, 1985.

71. Golding PL, Smith M, William R. Multisystem involvement in chronic liver disease. *Am J Med* 55:772, 1973.
72. Goodall MJR, et al. Relationship between asthma and gastroesophageal reflux. *Thorax* 36:116, 1981.
73. Graeber GM, et al. A comparison of patients with endoscopic esophageal perforations and patients with Boerhaave's syndrome. *Chest* 92:995, 1987.
74. Gross PA, Gerding DN. Pleural effusion associated with viral hepatitis. *Gastroenterology* 60:898, 1971.
75. Hammer B, Ashurst P, Naish J. Diseases associated with ulcerative colitis and Crohn's disease. *Gut* 9:17, 1968.
76. Hanson CA, et al. Ascites: Its effect upon static inflation of the respiratory system. *Am Rev Respir Dis* 142:39, 1990.
77. Heatley RV, et al. Pulmonary function abnormalities in patients with inflammatory bowel disease. *Q J Med* 51:241, 1982.
78. Henrion F, et al. Pulmonary and cutaneous lesions and terminal ileitis in an 11-year-old child: An exceptional case. *J Radiol* 63:123, 1982.
79. Higenbottam T, et al. Bronchial disease in ulcerative colitis. *Thorax* 35:581, 1980.
80. Hood J, Mason AMS. Diffuse pulmonary disease with transfer defect occurring with coeliac disease. *Lancet* 1:445, 1970.
81. Howard RS II, et al. *Mycobacterium fortuitum* pulmonary infection complicating achalasia. *South Med J* 84:1391, 1991.
82. Ibarra-Perez C. Thoracic complication of the amebic abscess of the liver: Report of 501 cases. *Chest* 79:672, 1981.
83. Ing AJ, Ngu MC, Breslin ABX. Chronic persistent cough and clearance of esophageal acid. *Chest* 102:1668, 1992.
84. Ing AJ, Ngu MC, Breslin ABX. Chronic persistent cough and gastro-oesophageal reflux. *Thorax* 46:479, 1991.
85. Irwin RS, Curley FJ, French CL. Chronic cough: The spectrum and frequency of causes, key components of the diagnostic evaluation, and outcome of specific therapy. *Am Rev Respir Dis* 141:640, 1990.
86. Irwin RS, et al. Evaluation of technetium pertechnate as a radionuclide marker of pulmonary aspiration of gastric contents in rabbits. *Chest* 93:1270, 1988.
87. Irwin RS, et al. Postnasal drip causes cough and is associated with reversible upper airway obstruction. *Chest* 85:346, 1984.
88. Irwin RS, et al. Chronic cough as the sole presenting manifestation of gastro-esophageal reflux. *Am Rev Respir Dis* 140:1294, 1989.
89. Jaffe BM, et al. Mediastinal pancreatic pseudocysts. *Am J Surg* 124:600, 1972.
90. Johnson DA. Hepatopulmonary syndrome: Qualification of the defect. *Am J Gastroenterol* 87:401, 1992.
91. Johnson NM, et al. Pulmonary function in inflammatory bowel disease. *Digestion* 18:416, 1978.
92. Kelly J, et al. Humoral response to alpha-gliadin as serological screening test for coeliac disease. *Arch Dis Child* 62:469, 1987.
93. Kendall AP, Lin E. Respiratory failure as presentation of achalasia of the esophagus. *Anaesthesia* 46:1039, 1991.
94. Kennedy D, Sharma OP. Hemoptysis in a 49-year-old man. An unusual presentation of a sporadic disease. *Chest* 98:1275, 1990.
95. Kerr P, et al. Nasal CPAP reduces gastroesophageal reflux in obstructive sleep apnea syndrome. *Chest* 101:1539, 1992.
96. Kim S. Pulmonary dysfunction in advanced liver disease. *Dis Colon Rectum* 35:189, 1992.
97. Kollef MH, Schachter DT. Acute pulmonary embolism triggered by the act of defecation. *Chest* 99:373, 1991.
98. Konig G, et al. Extrinsic allergic alveolitis combined with celiac disease sprue in childhood. *Respiration* 43:444, 1982.
99. Koufman J, et al. Reflex laryngitis and its sequelae: The diagnostic role of ambulatory 24 hour pH monitoring. *J Voice* 2:78, 1988.
100. Kraft SC, et al. Unexplained bronchopulmonary disease with inflammatory bowel disease. *Arch Intern Med* 136:454, 1976.
101. Krowka MJ, Breuer RI, Kehoe TJ. Azathioprine-associated pulmonary dysfunction. *Chest* 83:696, 1983.
102. Krowka MJ, Cortese DA. Hepatopulmonary syndrome: An evolving perspective in the era of liver transplantation [comment]. *Hepatology* 11:138, 1990.
103. Krowka MJ, Cortese DA. Pulmonary aspects of chronic liver disease and liver transplantation. *Mayo Clin Proc* 60:407, 1985.
104. Krowka MJ, Cortese DA. Pulmonary aspects of liver disease and liver transplantation. *Clin Chest Med* 10:593, 1989.
105. Krowka MJ, Cortese DA. Severe hypoxemia associated with liver disease: Mayo Clinic experience and the experimental use of almitrine bismesylate. *Mayo Clin Proc* 62:164, 1987.
106. Krowka MJ, et al. A prospective study of pulmonary function and gas exchange following liver transplantation. *Chest* 102:1161, 1992.
107. Krumpe PE, Cummiskey JM, Lillington GA. Alcohol and the respiratory tract. *Med Clin North Am* 68:201, 1984.
108. Kubitscheck KR, Peters J, Nickeson D. Amebiasis presenting as pleuropulmonary disease. *West J Med* 142:203, 1985.
109. Laggner AN, et al. Prevention of upper gastroin-

testinal bleeding in long-term ventilated patients. Sucralfate versus ranitidine. *Am J Med* 86(Suppl):81, 1989.

110. Lancaster Smith MJ, Benson MK, Strickland ID. Coeliac disease and diffuse interstitial lung disease. *Lancet* 1:473, 1971.

111. Lange P, et al. Pulmonary function is influenced by heavy alcohol consumption. *Am Rev Respir Dis* 137:1119, 1988.

112. Larrain A, et al. Medical and surgical treatment of nonallergic asthma associated with gastroesophageal reflux. *Chest* 99:1330, 1991.

113. Liebowitz MD. Respiratory symptoms and disease related to alcohol consumption. *Am Rev Respir Dis* 123:16, 1981.

114. Light RW, George RB. Incidence and significance of pleural effusion after abdominal surgery. *Chest* 69:621, 1976.

115. Lipper B, Simon D, Cerrone F. Pulmonary aspiration during emergency endoscopy in patients with upper gastrointestinal hemorrhage. *Crit Care Med* 19:330, 1991.

116. Lockhart A. Pulmonary arterial hypertension in portal hypertension. *Clin Gastroenterol* 14:123, 1985.

117. Louie S, et al. Pancreatic pleuropericardial effusions: Fistulous tracts demonstrated by computed tomography. *Arch Intern Med* 145:1231, 1985.

118. Lungarella G, et al. Pulmonary vascular injury in pancreatitis: Evidence for a major role played by pancreatic elastase. *Exp Mol Pathol* 42:44, 1985.

119. Lyons DJ, et al. Contribution of ethanol and cigarette smoking to pulmonary dysfunction in chronic alcoholics. *Thorax* 41:197, 1986.

120. Malik AB. Pulmonary edema after pancreatitis: Role of humoral factors. *Circ Shock* 10:71, 1983.

121. Mansfield L, Stein MR. Gastro-esophageal reflux: A possible reflex mechanism. *Ann Allergy* 41:224, 1978.

122. McDonnell PJ, Toye PA, Hutchins GM. Primary pulmonary hypertension and cirrhosis: Are they related? *Am Rev Respir Dis* 127:437, 1983.

123. McKee AL. Severe interstitial pulmonary fibrosis in a patient with chronic ulcerative colitis. *Am J Gastroenterol* 78:86, 1983.

124. Meadway J. Ulcerative colitis, colitic spondylitis and associated apical pulmonary fibrosis. *Proc R Soc Med* 67:324, 1974.

125. Melot C, et al. Pulmonary and extrapulmonary contributors to hypoxemia in liver cirrhosis. *Am Rev Respir Dis* 139:632, 1989.

126. Moeller DD, Carpenter PR. Gastrobronchial fistula: Case report and review of the English literature. *Am J Gastroenterol* 80:538, 1985.

127. Monroe P, et al. Acute respiratory failure after sodium morrhuate esophageal sclerotherapy. *Gastroenterology* 85:693, 1983.

128. Naeije R, et al. Hypoxic pulmonary vasoconstriction in liver cirrhosis. *Chest* 80:570, 1981.

129. Naeije R, et al. Pulmonary hemodynamics in liver cirrhosis. *Semin Respir Med* 7:164, 1985.

130. Nebel OT, Fornes MF, Castell DO. Symptomatic gastroesophageal reflux: Incidence and precipitating factors. *Dig Dis Sci* 21:955, 1976.

131. Neil GA, et al. Lymphocytic interstitial pneumonia and abdominal lymphoma complicating celiac sprue. *J Clin Gastroenterol* 8:282, 1986.

132. Neilly JB, et al. Pulmonary abnormalities in Crohn's disease. *Respir Med* 83:487, 1989.

133. Nijhuis-Heddes JMA, Pannekoek BJM. The cause of pleural effusion diagnosed by a fixed gas bubble. *Chest* 94:851, 1988.

134. Nygaard SD, Berger HA, Fick RB. Chylothorax as a complication of oesophageal sclerotherapy. *Thorax* 47:134, 1992.

135. Olson NR. Laryngopharyngeal manifestations of gastroesophageal reflux disease. *Otolaryngol Clin North Am* 24:1201, 1991.

136. Orr WC, et al. Esophageal function and gastroesophageal reflux during sleep and waking in patients with chronic obstructive pulmonary disease. *Chest* 101:1521, 1992.

137. Orr WC, Robinson MG, Johnson LF. The effect of esophageal acid volume on arousals from sleep and acid clearance. *Chest* 99:351, 1991.

138. Pacheco A, et al. Long-term clinical follow-up of adult idiopathic pulmonary hemosiderosis and celiac disease. *Chest* 99:1525, 1991.

139. Pack AI. Acid: A nocturnal bronchoconstrictor (editorial)? *Am Rev Respir Dis* 141:1391, 1990.

140. Pasquis P, et al. Transient pulmonary impairment during attacks of Crohn's disease. *Respiration* 41:56, 1981.

141. Pastor BM, Geerken RG. Whipple's disease presenting as pleuropericarditis. *Am J Med* 55:827, 1973.

142. Patwardhan RV, et al. Pleuropericarditis: An extraintestinal complication of inflammatory bowel disease. Report of three cases and review of literature. *Arch Intern Med* 143:94, 1983.

143. Perrin-Fayolle M, et al. Long-term results of surgical treatment for gastroesophageal reflux in asthmatic patients. *Chest* 96:40, 1989.

144. Peven DR, Yokoo H, Bile pulmonary embolism: Report of a case and a review of the literature. *Am J Gastroenterol* 78:830, 1983.

145. Poe RH, et al. Chronic persistent cough: Experience in diagnosis and outcome using anatomic diagnostic protocol. *Chest* 95:723, 1989.

146. Pollock JJ. Pleuropulmonary Whipple's disease. *South Med J* 78:216, 1985.

147. Propst T, et al. High prevalence of viral infection in adults with homozygous and heterozygous alpha$_1$-antitrypsin deficiency and chronic liver disease. *Ann Intern Med* 117:641, 1992.

148. Reinoso MA, Schroeder KW, Pisani RJ. Lung

disease associated with orally administered mesalamine for ulcerative colitis. *Chest* 101: 1469, 1992.

149. Rettke S, et al. Anesthesia approach to hepatic transplantation. *Mayo Clin Proc* 64:224, 1989.

150. Richardson AJ, Tait N, O'Rourke IO. Gastrobronchial fistula owing to non-malignant causes. *Br J Surg* 79:331, 1992.

151. Robin ED, et al. Platypnea related to orthodeoxia caused by true vascular lung shunts. *N Engl J Med* 294:941, 1976.

152. Robinson TJ. Coeliac disease with farmer's lung. *Br Med J* 1:745, 1976.

153. Rockey DC, Cello JP. Pancreaticopleural fistula. Report of 7 patients and review of the literature. *Medicine* 69:332, 1990.

154. Rodarte JR, Garrison HO, Holley KE. Whipple's disease simulating sarcoidosis. *Arch Intern Med* 129:479, 1972.

155. Rodriguez-Roisin R, Agusti A, Roca J. The hepatopulmonary syndrome: New name, old complexities. *Thorax* 47:897, 1992.

156. Rodriguez-Roisin R, et al. Pulmonary involvement in primary biliary cirrhosis. *Thorax* 36: 208, 1981.

157. Rodriguez-Roisin R, et al. Gas exchange and pulmonary vascular reactivity in patients with liver cirrhosis. *Am Rev Respir Dis* 135:1085, 1987.

158. Rogers BHG, Clark LM, Kirsner JB. The epidemiologic and demographic characteristics of inflammatory bowel disease: An analysis of computerized file of 1400 patients. *J Chronic Dis* 24:743, 1971.

159. Rosenbaum AJ, Murphy PJ, Engel JJ. Pleurisy during the course of ulcerative colitis. *J Clin Gastroenterol* 5:517, 1983.

160. Rubinstein D, McInnes IE, Dudley FJ. Hepatic hydrothorax in the absence of clinical ascites: Diagnosis and management. *Gastroenterology* 88:188, 1985.

161. Rubinstein I, Baum GL. Association of ulcerative colitis and sarcoidosis? *Chest* 89:618, 1986.

162. Ruddell WS, et al. Effect of cimetidine on the gastric bacterial flora. *Lancet* 1:672, 1980.

163. Runyon BA, Greenblatt M, Ming RH. Hepatic hydrothorax is a relative contraindication to chest tube insertion. *Am J Gastroenterol* 81:566, 1986.

164. Shewring DJ, Naerger HG, Steer HW. Rare intrathoracic complications in acute pancreatitis. *Thorax* 46:399, 1991.

165. Shneerson JM. Lung bullae, bronchiectasis, and Hashimoto's disease associated with ulcerative colitis treated by colectomy. *Thorax* 36:313, 1981.

166. Shneerson JM. Steroid-responsive alveolitis associated with ulcerative colitis. *Chest* 101:585, 1992.

167. Singh AK, Kothawla LK, Karlson KE. Tracheo-

168. Singh V, Jain NK. Asthma as a cause for, rather than a result of, gastroesophageal reflux. *J Asthma* 20:241, 1983.

169. Sloan S, Rademaker AW, Kaharilas PJ. Determinants of gastroesophageal junction incompetence: Hiatal hernia, lower esophageal sphincter, or both? *Ann Intern Med* 117:977, 1992.

170. Snider DE. Tuberculosis and gastrectomy (editorial). *Chest* 87:414, 1985.

171. Sontag SJ. Gut feelings about asthma. The burp and the wheeze. *Chest* 99:1321, 1991.

172. Spach DH, Silverstein FE, Stamm WE. Transmission of infection by gastrointestinal endoscopy and bronchoscopy. *Ann Intern Med* 118: 117, 1993.

173. Sparrow D, et al. Alcohol consumption and pulmonary function. *Am Rev Respir Dis* 127:735, 1983.

174. Spinozzi F, et al. IgG subclass deficiency and sinopulmonary bacterial infections in patients with alcoholic liver disease. *Arch Intern Med* 152:99, 1992.

175. Sposito M, Petroni VA, Valeri L (cited by RL Owen, H Shapiro). Pleural effusion, rash, and anergy in icteric hepatitis. *N Engl J Med* 291:963, 1974.

176. Stanley NN, et al. Primary biliary cirrhosis or sarcoidosis—or both. *N Engl J Med* 287:1282, 1972.

177. Stanley NN, Woodgate DJ. Mottled chest radiograph and gas transfer defect in chronic liver disease. *Thorax* 27:315, 1972.

178. Swinburn CR, et al. Bronchiolitis organizing pneumonia in a patient with ulcerative colitis. *Thorax* 43:735, 1988.

179. Symmons DP, et al. Pulmonary manifestations of Whipple's disease. *Q J Med* 56:497, 1985.

180. Tahamont MV, et al. Increased lung vascular permeability after pancreatitis and trypsin infusion. *Am J Pathol* 109:15, 1982.

181. Tan WC, et al. Effects of spontaneous and simulated gastroesophageal reflux on sleeping asthmatics. *Am Rev Respir Dis* 141:1394, 1990.

182. Tarlo SM, et al. Association between celiac disease and lung disease. *Chest* 80:715, 1981.

183. Teague WG, Sutphen JL, Fechner RE. Desquamative interstitial pneumonitis complicating inflammatory bowel disease of childhood. *J Pediatr Gastroenterol Nutr* 4:663, 1985.

184. Thomas E, et al. Eosinophilic gastroenteritis with malabsorption, extensive villous atrophy, recurrent hemorrhage and chronic pulmonary fibrosis. *Am J Med Sci* 269:259, 1975.

185. Tishler JM, Helman CA. Crohn's disease of the esophagus. *J Can Assoc Radiol* 35:28, 1984.

esophageal and aortoesophageal fistulae complicating corrosive esophagitis. *Chest* 70:549, 1976.

186. Torres A, et al. Incidence, risk, and prognosis factors of nosocomial pneumonias in mechanically ventilated patients. *Am Rev Respir Dis* 142:523, 1990.

187. Torres A, et al. Pulmonary aspiration of gastric contents in patients receiving mechanical ventilation: The effect of body position. *Ann Intern Med* 116:540, 1992.

188. Trewby P, et al. The incidence and pathophysiology of pulmonary edema in patients with fulminant hepatic failure. *Gastroenterology* 74:859, 1978.

189. Tryba M. Risk of acute stress bleeding and nosocomial pneumonia in ventilated intensive care unit patients: Sucralfate versus antacids. *Am J Med* 83(Suppl):117, 1987.

190. Turner-Warwick M. Fibrosing alveolitis and chronic liver disease. *Q J Med* 37:133, 1968.

191. Uchiyama T, et al. Pancreatic pleural effusion: Case report and review of 113 cases in Japan. *Am J Gastroenterol* 87:387, 1992.

192. Uddenfelt P, et al. Lung function abnormalities in patients with primary biliary cirrhosis. *Acta Med Scand* 223:549, 1988.

193. Van Ruiswyk J, Byrd JC. Efficacy of prophylactic sclerotherapy for prevention of a first variceal hemorrhage. *Gastroenterology* 102:587, 1992.

194. Vitale GC, et al. The effect of alcohol on nocturnal gastroesophageal reflux. *JAMA* 258:2077, 1987.

195. Wallaert B, et al. Primary biliary cirrhosis: Subclinical inflammatory alveolitis in patients with normal chest roentgenograms. *Chest* 90:842, 1986.

196. Wallaert B, et al. Evidence of lymphocytic alveolitis in Crohn's disease. *Chest* 87:363, 1985.

197. Warshaw AL, et al. The pathogenesis of pulmonary edema in acute pancreatitis. *Ann Surg* 182:505, 1975.

198. Warthin TA. Reactivation of pulmonary tuberculosis in relation to subtotal gastrectomy for peptic ulcer. *Am J Med Sci* 225:421, 1953.

199. Weiner GJ, et al. Chronic hoarseness secondary to gastroesophageal reflux disease: Documentation with 24-h ambulatory pH monitoring. *Am J Gastroenterol* 84:1503, 1989.

200. Weissman E, Becker NH. Interstitial lung disease in primary biliary cirrhosis. *Am J Med Sci* 285:21, 1983.

201. Welsh CH. Drug-resistant tuberculosis after gastrectomy. Double jeopardy? *Chest* 99:245, 1991.

202. Westbrook JL. Oesophageal achalasia causing respiratory obstruction. *Anaesthesia* 47:38, 1992.

203. Wilcox P, et al. Airway involvement in ulcerative colitis. *Chest* 92:18, 1987.

204. Wilkinson MJ, Robson DK, Basran G. Pleural complications of acute pancreatitis—an autopsy study. *Respir Med* 83:259, 1989.

205. Williams AJ, Marsh J, Stableforth DE. Cryptogenic fibrosing alveolitis, chronic active hepatitis, and autoimmune hemolytic anemia in the same patient. *Br J Dis Chest* 79:200, 1985.

206. Williams T, Eidus L, Thomas P. Fibrosing alveolitis, bronchiolitis obliterans, and sulfasalazine therapy. *Chest* 81:766, 1982.

207. Wilson NM, et al. Gastrooesophageal reflux and childhood asthma: The acid test. *Thorax* 40:592, 1985.

208. Winberg C, Rose M, Rappaport H. Whipple's disease of the lung. *Am J Med* 65:873, 1978.

209. Wright PH, et al. Adult idiopathic pulmonary hemosiderosis: A comparison of lung function changes and the distribution of pulmonary disease in patients with and without coeliac disease. *Br J Dis Chest* 77:282, 1983.

210. Wright PH, et al. Adult idiopathic pulmonary hemosiderosis and coeliac disease. *Q J Med* 50:95, 1981.

211. Zasly L, Baum GL, Rumball JM. The incidence of peptic ulceration in chronic obstructive pulmonary emphysema: A statistical study. *Dis Chest* 37:400, 1960.

212. Zeller FA, Cannan CR, Prakash UBS. Thoracic manifestations after esophageal variceal sclerotherapy. *Mayo Clin Proc* 66:727, 1991.

63

Endocrine and Metabolic Diseases

Udaya B. S. Prakash

The lung, under certain conditions, may secrete or release various humoral substances that can produce specific endocrine syndromes or otherwise influence the functions of many organ systems. Ectopic endocrine syndromes, most often occurring with pulmonary malignancies, are the best known and most dramatic. It is not commonly recognized in clinical practice that the respiratory system can be involved in many of the endocrinologic diseases. In addition to the well-known respiratory compensatory mechanisms in metabolic acidosis and alkalosis, the pulmonary system may become involved in both common and uncommon metabolic disorders. This chapter deals with the pulmonary problems resulting from or associated with various endocrine and metabolic diseases. Several of the gonadal disorders usually are managed by the endocrinologist as well, and these entities are discussed in Chapter 67.

Pituitary Disorders

Pneumomegaly

The lungs are involved in the general visceromegaly of acromegaly and, if an excess of growth hormone is present in adult life, the lungs are capable of additional growth. Total lung capacity in acromegaly is significantly increased from predicted values measured by body plethysmography [163]. Large lungs, defined as a vital capacity greater than 120 percent of predicted normal, were noted in 34 percent of 35 patients with acromegaly [180]. Studies of pulmonary function in 10 male patients with acromegaly and 1 male pituitary giant revealed tremendous increases in all lung volumes. There was no evidence of airflow obstruction or air trapping; lung compliance was increased, but lung elastic recoil was normal [15]. Despite the large lung volumes, diffusing capacity

of carbon monoxide (DlCO) was normal, suggesting that the lung growth resulted from an increase in the size of alveoli rather than from an increase in their number. However, others have reported DlCO greater than 120 percent of normal in 22 percent of patients with acromegaly [180]. Pneumomegaly is believed by some [104] to be an uncommon cause of increased lung volumes, although others [35] have indicated that the increased lung size in acromegaly is due to pneumomegaly and not hyperinflation. That lung size has been shown to regress in adults with growth hormone deficiency lends support to this hypothesis [35]. There is disagreement among reports as to whether abnormal lung growth occurs in women with acromegaly [178]. In children with hypopituitarism, the mechanical properties of the lung are consistent with the height-related rather than age-related variations [110].

Airways Obstruction

Extrathoracic airway narrowing, presumably from vascular obstruction, has been noted in acromegalics [60]. Even though the pulmonary function tests are normal in most, reduced airflow due to upper airway involvement has been noted in 50 percent of patients [180]. Hypoxemia, believed to be a result of ventilation-perfusion mismatch [104], seems to be related to the duration of acromegaly. The role of growth hormone in causing hypoxemia is unclear. Pulmonary function testing and roentgenographic assessment of the larynx and trachea in a group of 26 acromegalics demonstrated upper airway obstruction in 23 percent, whereas laryngeal tomography revealed marked narrowing of the true and false vocal cords in 54 percent. These findings suggest that attention to laryngeal anatomy is important, especially in acromegalics scheduled for tracheal intubation and anesthesia [122].

Sleep Apnea

Obstructive sleep apnea is now a well-recognized complication in acromegaly [19,51,60,62,104, 116,132,139]. In one series of 11 patients, 5 had obstructive sleep apnea [132]. The large tongue and thickened tissues in the upper airways of acromegalic patients have been shown to reduce the ratio of airway space to tissue mass and thus to increase airways resistance at that level [87]. However, bronchoscopic examination in patients with sleep apnea due to acromegaly has shown that, on inspiration, the soft tissue of the posterior and lateral hypopharynx invaginates into the lateral vestibule before any posterior movement of the tongue. Enlargement of the tongue did not appear to be a primary factor in causing sleep apnea, but some reports have observed obstruction of the airways by the enlarged tongue [19,116]. Also, thickening of laryngeal mucosa can lead to stridor and progressive dyspnea in acromegalic patients.

The incidence of central sleep apnea is high in patients with acromegaly. In a study of 53 patients with acromegaly, central sleep apnea was the predominant type of apnea in 33 percent of patients [54]. Biochemical evidence of increased disease activity was associated with the presence of central apnea rather than with the degree of sleep apnea. An earlier study of 21 patients with sleep apnea and acromegaly has suggested that the central sleep apnea in acromegaly may result from defective respiratory drive caused by the elevated growth hormone level [62]. The resolution of sleep apnea after treatment of acromegaly indicates that it may clear after a normal level of growth hormone is restored. However, the hypercapnic ventilatory response was normal and unaffected by the growth hormone level.

Cardiopulmonary complications are responsible for significant mortality in acromegalic patients. In one series of 194 patients with acromegaly, there were 55 deaths, and nearly half of these were due to cardiopulmonary complications [196].

Thyroid Disorders

Goiter

Respiratory symptoms can result from both extrathoracic and intrathoracic goiters (Table 63-1). Intrathoracic goiter may be defined as any thyroid enlargement that has its greater mass inferior to the thoracic inlet [81]. Although extension

Table 63-1. Pulmonary complications in thyroid diseases

Goiter
  Cough
  Mediastinal mass
  Tracheal obstruction
  Superior vena caval syndrome
  Recurrent laryngeal nerve paralysis
  Chylothorax
Hyperthyroidism
  Thyrotoxic dyspnea
    Thyrotoxic myopathy
    Increased work of breathing
    Increased oxygen consumption
    Decreased compliance
  Exacerbation of asthma
    Thyrotoxic dyspnea
    ?Diminished cyclic adenosine monophosphate
    ?Diminished adrenergic responsiveness
    ?Decreased catecholamines
    ?Increased metabolism of bronchodilators
  Anterior mediastinal mass
    Benign thymic hyperplasia
  Aspiration pneumonia in thyrotoxic bulbar paralysis
Hypothyroidism
  Depressed respiratory center
    Decreased response to hypercapnia
    Decreased hypoxic drive
    Central sleep apnea
  Hypoventilation
    Myxedema coma
    Central hypoventilation
    Muscle weakness
  Decreased bronchospasm in asthma
  Pleural effusion
  Pulmonary edema (in myxedema heart)
  Leftward shift of oxyhemoglobin dissociation curve
  Myxedematous pulmonary infiltrates
  Aspiration pneumonia (in myxedema coma)
Riedel's thyroiditis
  Cough
  Tracheal obstruction
  Massive upper-lobe pulmonary fibrosis

of goiter into the thorax is seen in only 1 to 3 percent of thyroidectomy patients, thyroid masses constitute a considerable percentage of anterior mediastinal tumors. In most of these, there is a direct connection between the retrosternal mass and a palpable thyroid gland in the neck. The tumors usually are nodular colloid goiters and, although thyrotoxicosis is seen in some cases, malignant changes are uncommon. Up to 80 percent of these intrathoracic goiters arise from the isthmus or lower pole and extend into the anterior mediastinum in front of the trachea. The rest arise from the posterior aspect of the thyroid gland and extend into the posterior mediastinum, behind the trachea and almost always on the right [159].

Most patients with intrathoracic goiters are women and, in many, a previous history of thyroid surgery is present. From 50 to 96 percent of such patients have symptoms [159]. The most common symptoms associated with intrathoracic goiters are dyspnea, stridor, dysphagia, hoarseness, coughing, wheezing, and cervical mass. A small percentage of intrathoracic goiters produce stridor and respiratory embarrassment [3,74]. In a study of 273 patients with benign goiters, 33 percent had signs of tracheal compression, mostly from colloid goiters [3]. Another study of 132 patients used flow-volume loop to evaluate upper airways and reported upper airway obstruction in 31 percent of those with goiters [74]. The incidence of tracheoesophageal compression was higher (67 percent) in those with thyroiditis. Acute or subacute tracheal obstruction necessitated tracheostomy in 3 percent of these. Severe expiratory flow obstruction necessitating surgical removal of goiter has been described [79]. Acute life-threatening tracheal obstruction has been noted in patients with intrathoracic goiter. Histologic studies have shown that the acute problem is very likely related to the multiple foci of hemorrhage in the goiter [179].

Goiters may present with superior vena caval obstruction. Among 32 patients with superior vena caval syndrome, four had thyroid goiters [65]. Recurrent laryngeal nerve paralysis is uncommon in benign goiters, having been discovered in fewer than 1 percent of 3279 goiters [146]. A retrosternal goiter can compress the thoracic duct and brachiocephalic vessels and cause chylothorax [42]. Intrathoracic goiter with hyperthyroidism, tracheal compression, superior vena cava syndrome, and Horner's syndrome has been described [23].

In the evaluation of chronic cough, thyroid disease usually is ignored as a cause. The close proximity of the thyroid gland to the laryngotracheal structures is occasionally responsible for distressing chronic cough [71]. In the presence of goiter, the cough usually disappears after the goiter is removed. Thyroiditis also may present with chronic cough.

Chest roentgenograms reveal a sharply defined, lobulated or smooth mass of homogeneous density displacing the trachea posteriorly and laterally if the goiter is located in the anterior mediastinum (Fig. 63-1). Calcification is very common (Fig. 63-2). The majority of intrathoracic goiters produce no symptoms and are discovered incidentally on a routine chest roentgenogram. A small percentage of patients have symptoms: inspiratory and expiratory stridor, hoarseness and, rarely, respiratory distress. Radioisotopic studies (^{131}I thyroid scans) are diagnostic when positive, but these goiters are rarely, if ever, functioning. To evaluate the degree of tracheal obstruction

Fig. 63-1. Intrathoracic extension of thyroid goiter.

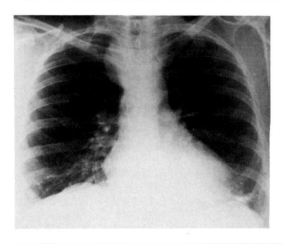

Fig. 63-2. Close-up view of upper-middle chest demonstrating calcification within the intrathoracic goiter.

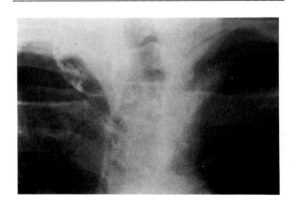

caused by thyroid goiter or masses, flow-volume loops may be superior to conventional roentgenologic methods [49,117].

Hyperthyroidism

Dyspnea at rest (thyrotoxic dyspnea) is a common symptom in thyrotoxicosis. There are several causes for this, but a reversible proximal myopathy may play a major role [6]. Skeletal muscle weakness has been reported in as many as 82 percent of thyrotoxic patients, and there is electromyographic evidence of myopathy in 93 percent [114,141]. Significant decreases in both inspiratory and expiratory maximal pressures have been demonstrated [161]. Respiratory muscle strength is proportional to the degree of thyroid dysfunction, and this muscle weakness is reversible with medical treatment [114,161]. Reduced vital capacity, diminished maximum inspiratory and expiratory pressures, and decreased compliance may occur. More recent studies show that hyperthyroid patients have higher ventilation than normal subjects during exercise [167]. The increased ventilation is secondary to increased central drive, which is correlated to circulating thyroid hormone level, and this abnormal drive can be normalized by beta blockade. These findings suggest that the inappropriately increased ventilatory drive may be the result of enhanced adrenergic stimulation. Diffusing capacity of the lung is reported to be normal. Dyspnea, in addition to myopathy, is related to a number of factors: decreased compliance, increased dead-space ventilation, and increased work of breathing required by greater oxygen uptake by the hypermetabolic body tissues.

Hyperthyroidism occasionally may cause, by unknown mechanisms, benign thymic hyperplasia. In most instances, the thymic enlargement is minimal and not noticed. On rare occasions, thymic hyperplasia may present as an anterior mediastinal mass [10,191]. The thymic enlargement associated with hyperthyroidism occasionally may produce dyspnea from extrinsic compression of the trachea, but usually the thymic hyperplasia is detected on computed tomographic scans performed for other reasons [46]. Treatment of hyperthyroidism is followed promptly by regression of thymic hyperplasia. Bulbar palsy is a well-known complication of thyrotoxicosis. Aspiration pneumonia and respiratory failure have been described in this setting [38].

Hypothyroidism

Hypothyroidism is associated with several respiratory problems owing to a combination of factors, including hypoactive respiratory center, disturbed neuronal and neuromuscular transmission (hypothyroid neuropathy), respiratory muscle weakness, and changes in pulmonary alveolar capillary membranes [90].

HYPOVENTILATION

Alveolar hypoventilation is known to occur in myxedema. Nearly 10 percent of patients with myxedema demonstrate diminished hypoxic drive [200]. One study demonstrated normal minute ventilation and oxygen and carbon dioxide tension in arterial blood in myxedema but a decreased response to breathing higher concentrations of carbon dioxide. The hypoventilation is believed to be related to the depressed hypoxic ventilatory drive that is responsive to thyroid replacement therapy [200]. A lesser-known mechanism is the myopathy, which occurs in 30 to 40 percent of all hypothyroid patients. Dysfunction of diaphragm, in addition to weakness of other inspiratory and expiratory muscles, also occurs in these patients [113]. Indeed, hypothyroidism can present as dyspnea secondary to reversible phrenic nerve neuropathy [97]. Diminished muscle strength, as indicated by diminished maximum voluntary ventilation, has been observed in patients with hypothyroidism. Rapid resolution of hypercapnia with thyroid replacement despite persistent muscle weakness in some patients suggests that thyroid hormone deficiency is hierarchically more important than myopathy [188]. However, more recent studies have shown that the significantly diminished inspiratory and expiratory maximal strengths return to normal with thyroid replacement therapy [162]. Prolonged hypothyroidism with gradual onset of respiratory failure and predominant hypercapnia has been described [198]. Coma is not uncommon in myxedema, occurring usually in elderly, obese women. Hypoventilation appeared to be responsible for the coma in a third of the patients.

SLEEP APNEA

Obstructive sleep apnea and oxygen desaturation have been observed increasingly in patients with hypothyroidism. However, in a study of 65 patients with proved obstructive sleep apnea, only 2 (3.1 percent) had hypothyroidism and, among

20 patients with hypothyroidism, 2 showed moderate to severe obstructive sleep apnea [102]. All hypothyroid patients in this study were snorers. Whereas obstructive sleep apnea without hypothyroidism is more common in men, obstructive sleep apnea associated *with* hypothyroidism is more common in women. Hypothyroidism can produce obstructive sleep apnea from the macroglossia and narrowing of the upper airways secondary to submucosal deposition of mucopolysaccharides and protein extravasation [166]. Central sleep apnea results from abnormalities in ventilatory control [118]. Episodes of sleep apnea occur more frequently in hypothyroid patients who are obese than in the nonobese. The impaired respiratory drive is corrected by thyroid hormone replacement therapy [102]. Thyroxine replacement therapy decreases apnea frequency, even without a change in body weight. Increases in the loaded respiratory effort and ventilation during thyroxine therapy have been demonstrated [139]. Restoration of euthyroid status usually results in complete resolution of obstructive sleep apnea [131,166].

PLEURAL EFFUSION

Myxedema is an uncommon cause of pleural effusions, and the incidence of this complication in hypothyroidism is unknown. A review of the literature in 1983 revealed 13 cases, of which 11 were in women whose mean age was 52 years [16]. The pleural effusions frequently were associated with ascites. Congestive heart failure also was noted in many patients. Usually, myxedematous patients with pleural effusion have a concomitant pericardial effusion. The pleural effusion associated with pericardial effusion is a transudate (Fig. 63-3) [168]. Another report in 1990 reviewed the record of 60 patients with hypothyroidism and noted pleural effusion in 15 (25 percent), but the effusions in the majority of patients were due to other diseases or hypothyroidism-related nonpulmonary complications [52]. Combining this with another group of 13 for a total of 28 patients with pleural effusions associated with hypothyroidism, Gotthrer and colleagues [52] found that only 5 patients (18 percent) had pleural effusions that could be ascribed to hypothyroidism; pleural fluid protein levels in 4 patients varied from 1.1 to 3.2 gm/dl. Usually, effusions are evident only on roentgenographic examination, but rarely is one sufficiently large to cause symptoms. The observation that the pleural effusion disappears after treat-

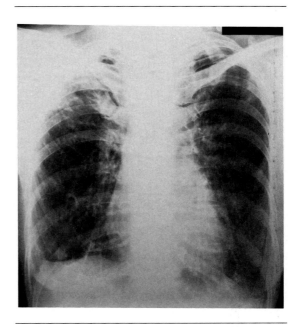

Fig. 63-3. Right-sided pleural effusion and pulmonary edema in a patient with severe myxedema. These findings resolved with thyroid replacement therapy.

ment of myxedema supports an etiologic relationship with myxedema. Increased pulmonary or pleural capillary permeability may play a role in the collection of fluid in the pleural space.

OTHER COMPLICATIONS

A decrease in vital capacity in the absence of heart failure also has been noted in myxedema. Hypothyroidism is a good example of the leftward shift of the oxyhemoglobin dissociation curve; hence, the tissue supply of oxygen is worse than is indicated by hypoxia alone [156]. Soft, patchy, nodular infiltrates (myxedematous lesions) are reported to occur in myxedema. Roentgenographic clearing of these infiltrates has been reported following replacement therapy with thyroid hormone [150]. The pathogenesis of these lesions is unknown, but studies have shown that thyroidectomized rats develop atelectasis due to decreased surfactant, and thyroxine therapy stimulates surfactant synthesis [144]. Thyroxine is reported to promote lung maturation in fetal rabbit lungs [197].

Asthma and the Thyroid Gland

The relationship between thyroid function and bronchial asthma has very interesting clinical implications. However, the coexistence of asthma and thyroid diseases has been reported only sporadically. A retrospective cohort mortality study of 3696 women treated for thyrotoxicosis at the Mayo Clinic from 1946 to 1964 showed that asthma was the underlying cause of death in 7 patients, compared with 2.6 expected deaths in the normal population [66]. Another retrospective study of 1107 patients found only 12 with coexistent hypothyroidism and asthma [38]. Treatment of hypothyroidism in three of these patients led to the worsening of their asthma. A similar experience has been described following administration of triiodothyronine for hypothyroidism [18,103]. In contrast, some patients with coexistent intractable asthma and hyperthyroidism have exhibited prompt and striking improvement in asthma when their hyperthyroidism was treated [158]. The positive therapeutic response to treatment of hyperthyroidism in asthmatic patients is not always uniform [126]. Interestingly, acute hypothyroidism is reported to increase nonspecific bronchial reactivity in nonasthmatic subjects [192].

A report on 11 hyperthyroid nonasthmatic patients concluded that hyperthyroidism actually reduced the severity of carbachol-induced changes in airways reactivity as measured by SGaw [72]. One proposed mechanism for the worsening asthma in hyperthyroidism is increased airways reactivity [27]. Reduced beta-adrenergic responsiveness and reduced beta receptors (downregulation of beta receptors) in asthma may contribute to the worsening of bronchospasm. A study of the effect of thyroid function on airways' beta-adrenergic responsiveness indicates that there is an inverse relationship between such responsiveness and the level of thyroid function and that changes distal to the beta adrenoreceptor are the most likely explanation for these findings [61]. An ingenious study induced thyrotoxicosis by administering triiodothyronine (T_3) to subjects with mild asthma and concluded that T_3-induced thyrotoxicosis of 4 weeks' duration had no effect on lung function, airway responsiveness, or exercise capacity in subjects with mild asthma [68].

It should be recognized that hyperthyroidism may worsen asthma by accelerating the metabolism of bronchodilators. Additionally, beta-adrenergic blocking drugs such as propranolol used in thyrotoxicosis may exacerbate asthma [44]. An asthmatic who develops hyperthyroidism should be closely monitored for deterioration of asthma. In contrast, even a slow and cautious restoration of the euthyroid state in hypothyroid patients may lead to increasing problems with asthma [115].

Iodide-induced thyrotoxicosis is a recognized complication after long-term administration of iodine or iodide-containing compounds to patients with preexisting thyroid disorders, particularly goiter. Interestingly, the saturated solution of potassium iodide (SSKI) was used in the past as an expectorant in asthmatic patients. Its use has resulted in hyperthyroidism, which in turn has aggravated the asthmatic condition [92]. Currently, iodinated glycerol (Organidin) is used as a mucolytic agent in the treatment of chronic obstructive pulmonary disease [134], although Organidin-induced thyrotoxicosis has been described in a patient with this disease [70].

Riedel's Thyroiditis

Riedel's thyroiditis is a rare disease characterized by extensive dense fibrosis of the thyroid gland, often extending into the strap muscles and adjacent structures in the neck. The condition is rare, 20 cases being discovered among 42,000 patients at the Mayo Clinic [195]. Respiratory symptoms are those from tracheal compression and the massive fibrotic process in both upper lobes of the lungs [186]. Severe upper airway obstruction has been described in a patient with Hashimoto's thyroiditis [182]. Lymphocytic interstitial pneumonitis has been described in four patients with autoimmune thyroiditis [85]. The association of idiopathic pulmonary hemosiderosis and autoimmune thyroiditis has been noted [7].

Parathyroid Disorders

Parathyroid tumors rarely present as anterior mediastinal masses and usually are small and encapsulated growths in the upper mediastinum. They may become large enough to widen the mediastinum, usually unilaterally [9]. Because most of these tumors are functioning, patients present with clinical hyperparathyroidism which, along with hypercalcemic crises, has been reported to produce pulmonary edema [69] and metastatic pulmonary calcification [28]. A review of more than 7000 autopsies disclosed 13 cases of "metastatic" pulmonary calcification. Chronic renal disease and parathyroid abnormalities accounted for seven of them, and the remainder were associated with malignancies [78].

Hypercalcemic states are well-known to produce calcifications of visceral organs, the so-called metastatic calcification. In the lungs, calcium deposits are found in bronchi, alveoli, and venous channels. Roentgenograms reveal premature calcification of the bronchi and an amorphous, diffuse, and finely dispersed calcification of the lungs radiating from the hilar regions. Although primary hyperparathyroidism, malignancies, and chronic renal failure are the more common causes of the hypercalcemic state, metastatic calcification is seen also in hypervitaminosis D, sarcoidosis, and milk alkali syndrome, as well as following intravenous calcium infusion.

Adrenal Disorders and Corticosteroids

Cushing's syndrome and long-term corticosteroid therapy can result in abnormal accumulation of fat in the upper mediastinum and both pleuroperi-

Fig. 63-4. (A) Cushing's syndrome with mediastinal widening. (B) Computed tomography in mediastinal lipomatosis reveals typical lipid density in the anterior mediastinum.

cardial angles. Roentgenograms reveal a smooth, symmetric widening of the upper mediastinum (Fig. 63-4A) extending from the thoracic inlet to both hilar areas. Computed tomography (Fig. 63-4B) is diagnostic because of its ability to demonstrate the lipid density in the mediastinum. It is well-known that long-term corticosteroid therapy suppresses some of the immune defense mechanisms of the body and predisposes the host to a number of unusual and opportunistic infections. Tuberculosis occurs with greater frequency in patients receiving long-term corticosteroid therapy; for younger tuberculin reactors in this situation, prophylactic isoniazid therapy is considered appropriate. Endogenous Cushing's syndrome has been complicated by cryptococcosis [93]. This syndrome, secondary to a hormonally active thymic carcinoid, was noted to exist with *Pneumocystis carinii* infection [5,48]. Patients with endogenous Cushing's syndrome who develop pulmonary infiltrates should be carefully evaluated to exclude the possibility of opportunistic infections.

Acute respiratory distress syndrome (ARDS) has been observed in a patient with pheochromocytoma [40]. A surge of catecholamines from pheochromocytoma may provoke pulmonary edema in a manner similar to that in neurogenic

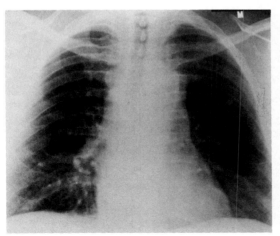

A

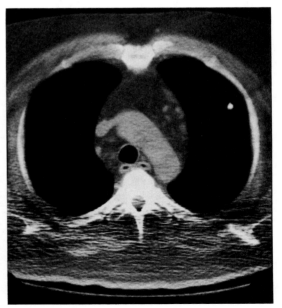

B

pulmonary edema [34]. Hemoptysis during paroxysms of hypertension caused by pheochromocytoma, cured by surgical resection of the tumor, has been reported [47].

Paragangliomas (chemodectomas) are tumors of the extraadrenal paraganglion system. The most common paragangliomas are carotid body chemodectomas, the glomus jugulare tumors,

Fig. 63-5. Paraganglioma located in the lower anterior mediastinum.

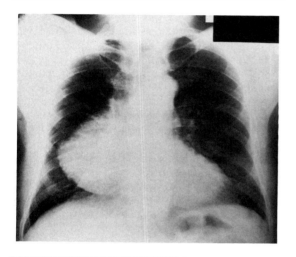

and globus tympanicum [32,95,130]. In the thorax, these are usually located above the aortic arch near the subclavian arteries. The reports of mediastinal paragangliomas have observed that most of these are located in the anterior mediastinum (Fig. 63-5). Female preponderance, an average age at the time of diagnosis of 49 years, and an average tumor size of 7.5 cm are reported from a review of 40 patients [130]. Nearly 50 percent of these patients are asymptomatic; the reported symptoms include hoarseness, cough, dysphagia, and chest pain. Distant metastasis may be noted in 23 percent of the 40 cases reported in 1979 [95]. Surgical resection is recommended for these tumors.

Carney's triad is a syndrome of pulmonary chondroma, multicentric gastric epithelioid leiomyosarcoma, and extraadrenal paraganglioma. This triad has been described in 28 patients since 1977 [20,21,88,111]. Several clinically important features of this unusual syndrome include the multicentricity of both the paragangliomas and the epithelioid leiomyosarcomas, the often indolent progression of metastatic leiomyosarcoma, the potential for late recurrences, and the importance of distinguishing intraadrenal from periad-

Fig. 63-6. Multiple pulmonary chondromas in the triad of multicentric gastric epithelioid leiomyosarcoma, functioning extraadrenal paraganglioma, and pulmonary chondroma.

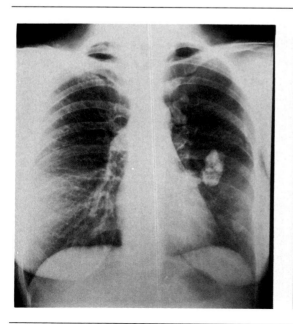
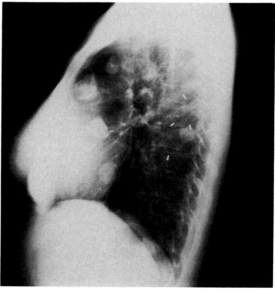

renal catecholamine-producing tumors (paragangliomas) [111]. Twenty-six patients were female, and the average age was 16.5 years. The most common clinical features were hematemesis and anemia due to the gastric lesion. Hypertension was the next most common finding. Multiple pulmonary tumors (two-thirds were uncalcified) and mediastinal widening were the chest roentgenographic abnormalities (Fig. 63-6). None of the patients had symptoms from the pulmonary lesions. If a new catecholamine-producing tumor is suspected, urine biochemical assays and computed tomography of the chest and abdomen are the first-choice localization procedures [111].

Metabolic Disorders

Diabetes Mellitus

Diabetes mellitus is a common disease that may be complicated by the involvement of other organs. Pulmonary complications may manifest clinically in different ways [56]. Table 63-2 lists the reported complications in diabetes mellitus.

PULMONARY INFECTIONS
It is generally agreed that hyperglycemic patients have a higher incidence of pulmonary infections. Diabetics are particularly prone to develop tuber-

culosis, frequently to an advanced stage. Among 106 patients in whom both diseases occurred, the diabetes came first in 48, the tuberculosis was first in 40, and the two were diagnosed simultaneously in 18 [67]. The increased incidence of tuberculosis in patients with diabetes mellitus is paralleled by the incidence of diabetes in those with tuberculosis [199]. Tuberculous infection in diabetics shows a predilection for the lower lobes of the lungs (Fig. 63-7). A study of 20 patients with both pulmonary tuberculosis and diabetes mellitus showed lower-lobe involvement in 10 percent of patients [123].

Diabetics also have been found to be more susceptible to mucormycosis. This is particularly true of patients with poorly controlled diabetes mellitus who have multiple complications [12,31, 56,98] (Fig. 63-8). It is apparent that diabetics with pulmonary mucormycosis have a striking tendency to develop major airways lesions. Because of the propensity of the *Mucor* species of fungi to invade vascular structures, the endobronchial lesion can invade the airway walls and the hilar vessels and produce pulmonary infarction or massive hemoptysis. Diagnostic features of major airways involvement include hoarseness, gross hemoptysis, or mediastinal widening on chest roentgenograms. Sudden, massive he-

Table 63-2. Pulmonary complications in diabetes mellitus

Reduced elastic lung recoil

Reduced diffusing capacity for carbon monoxide

Viral and bacterial infections

Tuberculosis

Mucormycosis

Pneumomediastinum

Pneumothorax

Acute pleuritic pain (in ketoacidosis)

Pulmonary fibrosis

Pulmonary edema (in ketoacidosis)

Mucous plugging of major airways (in ketoacidosis)

Central hypoventilation (in autonomic neuropathy)

Sleep apnea (with autonomic neuropathy)

Aspiration pneumonia (in diabetic gastroparesis)

Pulmonary xanthogranulomatosis

Respiratory alkalosis (in ketoacidosis)

Increased endogenous production of carbon dioxide

Fig. 63-7. Localized lesion secondary to *Mycobacterium tuberculosis* in a young patient with type I diabetes mellitus. The pulmonary lesion is located in the superior segment of left lower lobe.

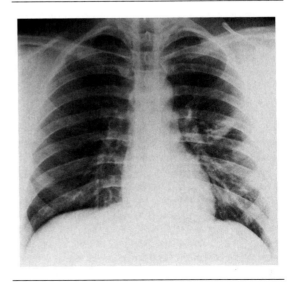

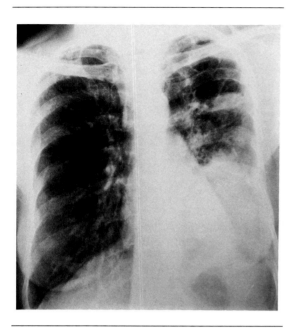

Fig. 63-8. Pneumonia of left lower lobe secondary to *Mucor* species in a patient with poorly controlled diabetes mellitus.

moptysis is a common fatal complication of endobronchial mucormycosis [36].

Carrier rates for aerobic gram-negative rods in pharyngeal secretions have been found to be higher for diabetics and alcoholics [108]. Bacterial pneumonias are by far the most common type of respiratory infections in patients with diabetes mellitus. The causative agents include gram-negative organisms (*Escherichia coli, Klebsiella pneumoniae*) and gram-positive bacteria (*Staphylococcus aureus*).

PULMONARY DYSFUNCTION

Diabetics are reported to develop pulmonary dysfunction, and the severity of diabetes mellitus may influence the degree of lung function impairment [140]. A study of 284 diabetics reported that, on average, forced vital capacity (FVC) and 1-second forced expiratory volume (FEV_1) were reduced by 334 ml and 239 ml, respectively, in insulin-treated diabetics, and by 184 ml and 117 ml, respectively, in diabetics treated with oral hypoglycemic agents [96]. An earlier study of 31,691 patients with diabetes mellitus observed pulmonary emphysema in 4.2 percent, asthma in 0.9 percent, and pulmonary fibrosis in 0.8 percent. Al-

though the incidence of asthma and emphysema among diabetics was the same as in the total hospital population, the incidence of fibrosis was reported to be moderately elevated [1]. Pulmonary function tests of 36 patients with insulin-dependent diabetes mellitus were compared with those of 40 nondiabetic controls, and the inspiratory vital capacity in the former group was found to be significantly reduced [185]. The authors concluded that this abnormality may have been caused partly by the reduced capacity of the inspiratory muscles. Diminished total lung capacity and DLCO in insulin-dependent diabetics has been ascribed to limited expansion of the rib cage and diabetes-related changes in pulmonary vasculature [29]. More recent studies show that insulin-dependent diabetes mellitus does not affect pulmonary function [106].

Diabetics with autonomic neuropathy have a higher threshold for the cough response to nebulized citric acid, thereby suggesting that vagal innervation of the bronchial tree is damaged by diabetic autonomic neuropathy [183]. This is further supported by the observation that bronchoconstrictive response to cold air and methacholine is impaired in patients with diabetic autonomic neuropathy [11,63]. Further studies in patients with diabetic autonomic neuropathy have demonstrated reduction in parasympathetic bronchomotor tone resulting in increased basal airway caliber [154]. These results raise the question: Is asthma uncommon in patients with diabetic autonomic neuropathy or, if an asthmatic patient develops this disorder, does the asthma either resolve or improve? The available clinical data are insufficient to respond reliably to this question.

Physiologic studies in juvenile diabetics have shown that the elastic lung recoil is significantly less than in normal individuals, and total lung capacity also is diminished. It is postulated that the disordered lung mechanics are manifestations of elastin and collagen abnormalities [157]. In a study involving 40 adult insulin-dependent diabetics, all lifelong nonsmokers without evidence of lung disease and compared to a matched group of healthy controls, detailed pulmonary function tests demonstrated that the diabetics had mild abnormalities of lung elastic recoil and DLCO, as well as a reduction in pulmonary capillary blood volume [152]. The degree of lung dysfunction was related directly to the duration of insulin-dependent diabetes mellitus. Similar findings have been reported in younger insulin-dependent diabetics [153]. The lean type I diabetic patients are reported to have a higher incidence of breathing abnormalities [121]. Histopathologic studies of streptozotocin-induced diabetes in rats have shown ultrastructural alterations in the granular pneumocytes in the alveolar septum [135], nonciliated bronchiolar epithelial (Clara) cells [136], and collagen and elastin in the alveolar wall [86]. Postmortem studies of diabetics also have documented thickening of epithelial and capillary basal laminae of alveoli [184], centrilobular emphysema, and diabetic microangiopathy in the capillaries of alveolar septa and the alveolar and pleural arterioles [89]. Clinical knowledge suggests that the pulmonary parenchymal defects and pulmonary dysfunctions in insulin-dependent diabetics are insufficient to cause significant respiratory embarrassment [153]. Reports have shown that DlCO is significantly lower in diabetic patients with microangiopathy, and this may reflect microangiopathy in the pulmonary circulation [189].

Despite these extensive studies on pulmonary dysfunction in patients with diabetes mellitus, routine pulmonary function testing is not indicated in the absence of pulmonary symptoms or a history of smoking.

PULMONARY EDEMA

Pulmonary edema is rare in diabetic ketoacidosis. Diabetic ketoacidosis is reported to produce noncardiogenic pulmonary edema, and it is suggested that altered pulmonary capillary permeability is the cause of the extravascular leakage of fluids [137]. The patient with diabetic ketoacidosis usually is administered large quantities of intravenous crystalloids over a short period. These solutions tend to elevate the hydrostatic pressure and diminish oncotic pressure, thereby facilitating the development of pulmonary edema [99,172]. Pulmonary vascular diabetic angiopathy may predispose some diabetics to pulmonary edema [17]. Additionally, endogenous fluid shifts due to severe hyperglycemia may contribute to pulmonary edema [77]. Recurrent episodes of acute alveolar and interstitial pulmonary edema have been noted on chest roentgenograms in anephric diabetics during periods of severe hyperglycemia. Clinical and chest roentgenographic resolution occurs immediately after insulin therapy and restoration of normoglycemia.

DISORDERED SLEEP

Sleep-related breathing abnormalities occur with greater frequency in diabetic patients with auto-nomic neuropathy. The ventilatory and heart rate response to hypoxia are impaired in diabetics, whereas the ventilatory response to hypercapnia is well preserved [129]. Although a diminished hypercapnic ventilatory response to progesterone therapy is described in a patient with diabetic autonomic neuropathy [164], detailed studies of the effect of this neuropathy on the respiratory system have shown that there is no difference in the ventilatory responses to hypoxemia and hypercapnia in patients with and without autonomic neuropathy [169]. Diabetic microangiopathy of muscles, resulting in a myopathic process and muscle weakness and central hypoventilation, may cause hypercapnia and respiratory failure. Another explanation for the diminished ventilatory response to hypoxia is that medullary depression of ventilation by hypoxia is greater in diabetic patients than in control subjects [129]. Others have reported normal breathing patterns in diabetics with severe autonomic neuropathy [22]. A relationship has been shown between neuropathy and sleep-related breathing abnormalities in type I insulin-dependent diabetics [121]. Sudden, unexplained deaths are relatively common in diabetic autonomic neuropathy.

OTHER COMPLICATIONS

In diabetic ketoacidosis, the oxygen tension in arterial blood is high due to hyperventilation secondary to acidosis and the increased glucose load. Additionally, the production of endogenous carbon dioxide from the metabolic acidosis causes a higher respiratory quotient and thus a higher-than-expected increase in oxygen tension in arterial blood [13,83]. Rarely, hypokalemic hypoventilation may complicate severe diabetic ketoacidosis [176].

Pleural effusion is reported to occur more commonly in diabetic patients, particularly in those with left ventricular failure. In a study of 40 patients with similar degrees of left ventricular dysfunction, pleural effusions were more common in diabetic patients and, indeed, 4 of 5 diabetic patients who had persistent pleural effusions had no evidence of either cardiomegaly or congestive cardiac failure [24]. Although several mechanisms, including those discussed under Pulmonary Edema above, were postulated to be responsible, the exact mechanism remains unclear.

The coexistence of diabetic ketoacidosis and pneumomediastinum has been reported in several instances [50,149,177]. The cause remains obscure, although ketoacidosis is believed to change the pressure gradient within the lungs by the hyperpnea induced by acidosis, by severe vomiting, or by a combination of both. The prognosis is excellent [50], and the pneumomediastinum regresses promptly after correction of the ketoacidosis.

Mucous plugging of major airways has been described as a specific complication of diabetic ketoacidosis. Lethargy, altered vagal tone, and autonomic neuropathy are proposed as contributing factors responsible for occult mucous plugging [13,37]. It has been demonstrated that there is reduced airway vagal tone and diminished cold responsiveness in nonsmoking, nonasthmatic diabetic patients with autonomic neuropathy [37,190].

Vomiting of gastric contents may lead to aspiration pneumonia in diabetic patients with unsuspected gastroparesis. This is of greater importance during anesthetic procedures [124]. Perivascular xanthogranulomatosis has been demonstrated in the lungs of 6 percent of diabetic patients (versus 2 percent in nondiabetics), but the effect on pulmonary function is unknown [145].

Hypoglycemic coma resulting in acute pulmonary edema in patients receiving insulin shock therapy for schizophrenia was noted several times in the 1930s [128]. In one series of seven patients treated with insulin shock, acute pulmonary edema ranked second to irreversible coma as the cause of death [109]. Most of the patients were otherwise healthy and were younger than 35 years. Animal studies support the hypothesis that the pulmonary edema seen in hypoglycemic coma results from neurogenic causes [107].

Obesity

PULMONARY DYSFUNCTION
Obesity, even when mild, is reported to impair lung function significantly [76]. Among 144 men with mild obesity (mean weight ± SD, 81.1 ± 9.0 kg), 63 percent exhibited diminished functional residual capacity (FRC), expiratory reserve volume, and arterial oxygen tension compared to 28 subjects of normal weight [76]. Spirometric evaluation of lung functions in morbidly obese patients before severe weight loss programs has shown no significant abnormalities and no significant improvement in their lung functions after considerable weight loss [31]. Several studies have reported decreases in FRC and forced expiratory flow in midcycle (FEF_{25-75}) and mildly

decreased arterial oxygen tension [25,39,58, 73,165]. These findings have been interpreted to show disease of the small airways [58,165]. The overall incidence of postoperative pulmonary complications in a large group of obese patients undergoing abdominal surgery (ileojejunal bypass) was 25 percent [181]. Altered respiratory function in obesity may result from a combination of mechanical impedance to breathing exerted by thoracic and abdominal fat and a ventilation-perfusion mismatch [91]. Studies suggest greater diaphragmatic efficiency in the upright than in the supine position in a majority of obese subjects, a reversal of the normal response. Diaphragmatic overstretching may be an important mechanism in the development of hypoventilation in the morbidly obese [160]. Ventilatory studies in obese patients show diminished tidal volume, vital capacity, and functional residual capacity, but normal diffusing capacity. Increased work of breathing and decreased efficiency of the respiratory system are also seen. Another study has shown an increase in DLCO in patients with weight-to-height ratios exceeding 0.6 [143]. It is postulated that the increase in DLCO is the result of increased pulmonary blood volume, which accompanies the elevated cardiac output noted in obesity. These findings suggest that the diminished DLCO in morbidly obese subjects indicates intrinsic pulmonary pathology. Abnormal ventilation-perfusion ratios have been demonstrated in the lung bases of obese patients with hypoxemia and low or normal carbon dioxide tension in arterial blood.

HYPOVENTILATION
The hypoventilation seen in obese patients with both hypoxemia and hypercapnia may result from one or more of the following proposed mechanisms: increased fat deposits around the chest wall and resultant increase in the work of breathing; extremely low ventilation-perfusion ratio at lung bases, promoted by lower expiratory reserve volume [91]; upper airways obstruction; or a disturbance in the respiratory center itself, making it insensitive to carbon dioxide. Considerable weight loss may reverse the symptoms in many cases [57]. However, in some instances, low arterial oxygen tension may persist, whereas in others there has been a significant reduction in the number of episodes of sleep-disordered breathing and nocturnal desaturation, lending support to the concept that obesity is the cause and not an effect of the sleep apnea syndrome in these patients [59].

PICKWICKIAN SYNDROME

The pickwickian syndrome consists of extreme obesity, alveolar hypoventilation, somnolence, twitching, cyanosis, periodic breathing, secondary polycythemia, and right-sided heart failure. Details of the etiology and pathogenesis of this obesity-hypoventilation syndrome are unknown, as is its true incidence. Studies show that the syndrome can exist in nonobese patients as well [55]. Among patients weighing 45 kg more than their ideal weights, hypoxemia has been observed in 40 to 50 percent, and hypoventilation, as manifested by hypercapnia, is seen in the same proportion. Studies of patients with the pickwickian syndrome suggest that two mechanisms may be responsible for the chronic hypercapnia in these patients: (1) a critical balance between the ventilation during the time spent awake and hypoventilation due to apneas, a mechanism resolved by treatment of obstructive sleep apnea, and (2) a sustained hypoventilation independent of the apnea mechanism and therefore not correctable. The true pickwickians may represent the second mechanism [142].

OTHER COMPLICATIONS

Detailed discussions of obstructive and central sleep apneas can be found in Chapter 43. Even though nonobese patients demonstrate obstructive sleep apnea, the external and internal neck circumferences and the degrees of obesity are important predictors of sleep apnea [82]. Patients with severe obesity and obstructive sleep apneas are known to have abnormal pulmonary function tests. Obesity may produce different degrees of sleep-related abnormalities depending on the sex of the patient [58]. Hormonal factors may play a significant role because progesterone is a known respiratory stimulant and is clinically useful in the treatment of pickwickian syndrome [175]. An alternative possibility is that testosterone or the androgen-estrogen ratio is an important factor in male subjects [58]. An obese man treated with testosterone for hypogonadism developed a blunted response to carbon dioxide, which was reversible with discontinuation of testosterone therapy, and recurrence of hypoventilation was noted when testosterone was resumed [173].

In summary, the major respiratory complications of obesity, with or without hypoventilation, include heightened demand for ventilation, elevated work of breathing, respiratory muscle insufficiency, decreased Ccw and Cl, diminished FRC and expiratory reserve volume, and a high CV-to-FRC ratio, which is associated with closure of peripheral lung units, ventilation-perfusion abnormalities, and hypoxemia, especially in the supine position [105]. In addition, the DlCO is elevated, and the reason is believed to be the increased pulmonary capillary blood volume [143]. Overweight children have been shown to have an increased incidence of respiratory symptoms [170].

Malnutrition

Clinically significant malnutrition is a common complication of long-term mechanical ventilation and in patients with severe emphysematous obstructive lung disease. These forms of malnutrition, as well as the malnutrition caused by starvation, affect the respiratory system [147]. Prolonged starvation significantly alters the structure and function of the lung. Morphometric and ultrastructural changes similar to those observed in elastase-induced emphysema have been noted in hamsters subjected to starvation [151]. Pulmonary defense mechanisms, as those of other organ systems, depend on optimal nutritional status. Diminished respiratory clearance of microbial organisms, decreased number of pulmonary alveolar macrophages, and marked decreases in secretory IgA and other immunoglobulins (as a result of hypoproteinemia) may predispose these patients to infections caused by various organisms [147]. Malnourished subjects also demonstrate reduced ventilatory drive from the effects of nutritional depletion on both the central nervous system and respiratory muscles. Diaphragmatic muscle mass is reduced in malnourished subjects.

In rachitic lung, the pulmonary changes seen include such roentgenographic abnormalities as lobar or segmental atelectasis, compression atelectasis, and interstitial pneumonitis [84]. These changes are attributed to hypoventilation in a distorted, small chest, along with chronic and recurrent pulmonary infections. Hypoventilatory failure has been described in these patients [119]. In a study of a large group of children with vitamin A deficiency, the incidence of respiratory disease was twice that of normal children, and the risk of respiratory disease was more closely associated with vitamin A status than with general nutritional status [171].

Gaucher's Disease

Gaucher's disease is an autosomal recessive error of metabolism due to a deficiency of glucosidase, the enzyme that catalyzes glucosylceramide. It is seen predominantly in Jewish women and occurs in a neurologic form, a visceral form, and an osseous form. Accumulation of glucosylceramide in cells of the reticuloendothelial system changes them to Gaucher's cells, which accumulate both there and in the lungs and other organs. Whereas pulmonary involvement and symptoms are not unusual in the infantile form of Gaucher's disease, it is distinctly uncommon in the adult form [43,155,194]. There is an increased incidence of pulmonary infections in these patients. Wolson's [194] review of the literature found 10 cases involving the lung. Roentgenograms of the lung reveal a diffuse reticulonodular or miliary pattern [194]. Microscopic examination indicates impressive consolidation of lung parenchyma by Gaucher's cells. Elevated levels of serum angiotensin-converting enzyme have been noted in this disease [101].

Niemann-Pick Disease

Niemann-Pick disease is characterized by an absolute or relative deficiency of the enzyme sphingomyelinase. Severe nodular pulmonary disease leading to cor pulmonale has been noted [100]. Association of widespread pulmonary nodules, linear strands, and honeycombing has been reported [94]. Large, multivacuolated "foam" cells can be found in pulmonary alveoli.

Angiokeratoma Corporis Diffusum (Fabry's Disease)

An X-linked sphingolipid storage disorder due to the lack of alpha-galactosidase, Fabry's disease is reported to be associated with multiple angiomas of the tracheobronchial tree and bullous emphysema leading to hyperinflation of the lungs. Recurrent pulmonary infections and hemoptysis may indicate respiratory involvement. Bronchial inclusion bodies and alveoli filled with ceramide hexosidase have been observed in patients with obstructive lung disease secondary to Fabry's disease [8,80,156]. The deposition of ceramide hexosidase in the bronchial tree may contribute to the intrinsic airways disease and functional airways obstruction [148].

Mucopolysaccharidosis

Lung involvement can be seen in other metabolic storage diseases. Deposition of mucopolysaccharides in the tracheal wall of 56 patients with mu-

copolysaccharidosis (including Hurler's disease, mucopolysaccharidosis type I) was noted to result in tracheal narrowing and airways compromise in 9 patients [133]. Airway obstruction is a frequent problem in these patients [125]. Morquio's disease, another type of mucopolysaccharidosis, is distinguished by the presence of a distinctive bony dystrophy (spondyloepiphyseal dysplasia). Marked hypoplasia of the odontoid process can cause cervical dislocation and spinal cord compression. Pulmonary function studies in these patients have noted the restrictive nature of the ventilatory defects. Upper airways collapse during head flexion may be an important cause of pulmonary disability in Morquio's disease [138]. Rapidly progressive respiratory failure in an 8-week-old boy with Krabbe's leukodystrophy has been described [26]. Ultrastructural examination of lungs revealed the presence of numerous intraalveolar macrophages.

Lipoid Proteinosis

A rare hereditary disorder of the autosomal recessive type, lipoid proteinosis involves multiple organs by deposition of an amorphous eosinophilic glycoprotein. Pulmonary abnormalities consist of infiltration of this anomalous glycoprotein into capillary walls. Roentgenograms reveal a diffuse reticulonodular pattern throughout both lungs [187].

Acute Intermittent Porphyria

Acute intermittent porphyria results from an inborn error of metabolism. Occasionally, this entity may present as acute respiratory insufficiency or with neurologic, psychiatric, or gastrointestinal manifestations. With respiratory involvement, the mortality may be high. The pulmonary features usually are like those of Guillain-Barré syndrome, in which the disease process involves the respiratory muscles and produces alveolar hypoventilation. Acute intermittent porphyria should be considered in the differential diagnosis of respiratory failure [53].

Carcinoid Syndrome

Carcinoid tumors of the lung are discussed fully in Chapter 54. The following is a review of pulmonary manifestations of the carcinoid syndrome, the classic form of which is caused by a hormonally active carcinoid tumor located most frequently in the terminal ileum. The tumor arises from the Kulchitzky (argentaffin) cells, which contain neurosecretory granules filled with serotonin (5-hydroxytryptamine). This hormone is responsible for most of the clinical features, which include episodic flushing, purplish cyanosis, diarrhea, bronchospasm, and valvular disease of the right side of the heart.

Among the 3718 cases of abdominal carcinoid tumors reported by Wilson [193], 3.7 percent had symptomatic endocrine activity. In a Mayo Clinic series [45], the carcinoid syndrome was observed with 7 percent of gastrointestinal carcinoids and 2 percent of bronchial carcinoids.

Pulmonary manifestations of the syndrome may include hyperventilation and wheezing. Most frequently, however, patients do not have symptoms referable to the chest, and evidence of bronchoconstriction is found only during flushing attacks. The most prominent cardiac symptoms arise from stenosis of the pulmonic and tricuspid valves, and these lesions can lead to intractable right heart failure. Elevation of urinary 5-hydroxyindoleacetic acid is helpful in establishing the diagnosis.

Miscellaneous Metabolic Disorders

Volume contraction is a common clinical problem, and its effects on pulmonary functions have been studied [75]. During hypohydration induced by diuretics in normal volunteers, lung volumes increased significantly. In addition, peak expiratory flow rate, FEV_1, maximal voluntary ventilation, and flow rates at low lung volumes also increased but returned to normal on rehydration. DLCO was unchanged. The mechanism is probably related to the loss of water in the airway walls or peribronchial space. The clinical significance of this finding is unclear.

Hypokalemia is a commonly encountered clinical problem. Respiratory muscle weakness may result from severe hypokalemia. Hypokalemic periodic paralysis has been described with hypoventilation [4]. Severe diarrhea, dehydration, and marked hypokalemia in a pediatric patient was followed by fatal respiratory failure due to respiratory muscle paralysis [33].

Hypophosphatemic states are known to produce respiratory failure secondary to muscle weakness [127]. A decrease in the body phosphate level diminishes adenosine triphosphate and results in muscle weakness. Phosphate replacement therapy in such cases dramatically improves muscle function and reverses respiratory failure. Chronic hypophosphatemia produces a decrease in 2,3-diphosphoglycerate, which increases the affinity of oxygen to hemoglobin, thereby decreasing the delivery of oxygen to the tissues.

Hypomagnesemia may contribute to respiratory muscle weakness [120]. Next to potassium, magnesium is the most abundant intracellular cation in the human body. It is required as a cofactor by many enzymes and is a cofactor in all transphosphorylation reactions. The incidence of hypomagnesemia varies from 30 percent in alcoholics to 2 percent in normal individuals. In patients with respiratory muscle weakness, hypomagnesemia should be sought as an etiologic factor because magnesium replacement therapy has been shown to improve all the indices of muscle power measured after treatment. Hypermagnesemia as a result of excessive ingestion of antacids, bowel obstruction, and renal failure may be followed by respiratory depression and coma. These features can be reversed by lowering the magnesium level [41].

Metabolic alkalosis is a common acid-base disorder in hospitalized patients. The compensatory hypoventilation may lead to atelectasis, deterioration in the ventilation-perfusion relationship, and an increased alveolar-arterial oxygen tension difference. The resultant hypoxia can be corrected significantly by reversing alkalosis with administration of hydrochloric acid [14].

Acute respiratory failure may ensue in patients receiving very high carbohydrate loads. This is a potential problem in those receiving total parenteral nutrition. The infused glucose is used as the primary energy source, which leads to substantial increases in carbon dioxide production and respiratory quotient. Respiratory failure is more likely to occur in patients with limited pulmonary reserve [30].

Total parenteral nutrition increases carbon dioxide production in patients on ventilation who cannot match their carbon dioxide excretion to the carbon dioxide load, leading to increased arterial carbon dioxide tension. This risk can be minimized by increasing minute ventilation before total parenteral nutrition is begun [64]. Hyperlipidemia is reported [174] to produce falsely low DLCO measurements as a result of interference with a hemoglobin-combining coefficient. This is of no clinical significance in healthy subjects.

Glycogen storage diseases predispose patients to bacterial infections. Staphylococcal infections may produce lung abscesses and pneumatoceles (Fig. 63-9).

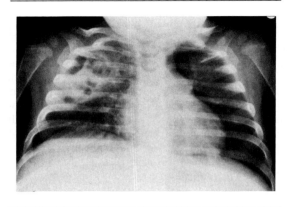

Fig. 63-9. Glycogen storage disease in an infant, complicated by *Staphylococcus aureus*–induced abscesses in the right upper lobe.

Acid-base abnormalities in asthma are discussed elsewhere. One point of interest is the highly variable acid-base relationships in acute asthma. In one large study of 109 adult asthmatics, arterial pH was lower than expected for the measured arterial carbon dioxide tension in 17 percent, suggesting metabolic acidosis and indicating that metabolic acidosis can confuse the diagnosis in asthmatic patients [2].

Gouty tophi of the larynx and vocal cords have been described, with accompanying stridor, hoarseness, and signs of extensive gouty disease [112].

References

1. Abramowitz S, Leiner GC, Small MJ. Chronic respiratory diseases and diabetes. *Rev Allergy* 23:972, 1969.
2. Alberts WM, Williams JH, Ramsdell JW. Metabolic acidosis as a presenting feature in acute asthma. *Ann Allergy* 57:107, 1986.
3. Alfonso A, et al. Tracheal or esophageal compression due to benign thyroid disease. *Am J Surg* 142:350, 1981.
4. Ali K. Hypokalemic periodic paralysis complicating thyrotoxicosis. *Br Med J* 4:503, 1975.
5. Anthony LB, Greco FA. *Pneumocystis carinii* pneumonia: A complication of Cushing's syndrome. *Ann Intern Med* 94:488, 1981.
6. Ayres J, et al. Thyrotoxicosis and dyspnoea. *Clin Endocrinol* (Oxf) 16:65, 1982.
7. Bain SC, Bryan RL, Hawkins JB. Idiopathic pulmonary hemosiderosis and autoimmune thyrotoxicosis. *Respir Med* 83:447, 1989.
8. Bartimno EE Jr, Guisan M, Moser KM. Pulmonary involvement in Fabry's disease: A reappraisal. *Am J Med* 53:755, 1972.
9. Becker FO, Tausk K. Radiologically evident functioning mediastinal parathyroid adenoma. *Chest* 58:79, 1970.
10. Bergman TA, Mariash CN, Oppenheimer JH. Anterior mediastinal mass in a patient with Graves' diseases. *J Clin Endocrinol Metab* 55:587, 1982.
11. Bertherat J, et al. Decreased bronchial response to methacholine in IDDM patients with autonomic neuropathy. *Diabetes* 40:1100, 1991.
12. Bigny TD, et al. Clinical spectrum of pulmonary mucormycosis. *Chest* 89:435, 1986.
13. Brandstetter RD, et al. Occult mucous airway obstruction in diabetic ketoacidosis. *Chest* 91:575, 1987.
14. Brimioulle S, Kahn RJ. Effects of metabolic alkalosis on pulmonary gas exchange. *Am Rev Respir Dis* 141:1185, 1990.
15. Brody JS, et al. Acromegalic pneumonomegaly: Lung growth in the adult. *J Clin Invest* 49:1051, 1970.
16. Brown SD, Brashear RE, Schnute RB. Pleural effusion in a young woman with myxedema. *Arch Intern Med* 143:1458, 1983.
17. Brun-Buisson CJ, et al. Recurrent high-permeability pulmonary edema associated with diabetic ketoacidosis. *Crit Care Med* 13:55, 1985.
18. Bush RK, Ehrlich EN, Reed CE. Thyroid disease and asthma. *J Allergy Clin Immunol* 59:398, 1977.
19. Cadieux RJ, et al. Endoscopic findings in sleep apnea associated with acromegaly. *J Clin Endocrinol Metab* 55:18, 1982.
20. Carney JA. The triad of gastric leiomyosarcoma, functioning extra-adrenal paraganglioma, and pulmonary chondroma: A 5-year review. *Medicine* 62:159, 1983.
21. Carney JA, et al. The triad of gastric leiomyosarcoma, functioning extra-adrenal paraganglioma, and pulmonary chondroma. *N Engl J Med* 296:1517, 1977.
22. Catterall JR, et al. Breathing, sleep, and diabetic autonomic neuropathy. *Diabetes* 33:1025, 1984.
23. Cengiz K, et al. Intrathoracic goiter with hyperthyroidism, tracheal compression, superior vena cava syndrome, and Horner's syndrome. *Chest* 97:1005, 1990.
24. Chertow BS, Kadzielawa R, Burger AJ. Benign pleural effusions in long-standing diabetes mellitus. *Chest* 99:1108, 1991.
25. Chodoff PM, et al. Massive weight loss following jejunoileal bypass: I. Effects on pulmonary function. *Surgery* 81:399, 1977.
26. Clarke JT, Ozere RL, Krause VW. Early infantile variant of Krabbe globoid cell leukodystrophy with lung involvement. *Arch Dis Child* 56:640, 1981.

27. Cockcroft DW, Silverberg JDH, Dosman JA. Decrease in nonspecific bronchial reactivity in an asthmatic following treatment of hyperthyroidism. *Ann Allergy* 41:160, 1978.

28. Cohen AM, et al. Metastatic pulmonary calcification in primary hyperparathyroidism. *Arch Intern Med* 137:520, 1977.

29. Cooper BG, et al. Lung function in patients with diabetes mellitus. *Respir Med* 84:235, 1990.

30. Covelli HD, et al. Respiratory failure precipitated by high carbohydrate loads. *Ann Intern Med* 95:579, 1981.

31. Crapo RO, et al. Spirometry as a preoperative screening test in morbidly obese patients. *Surgery* 99:763, 1986.

32. D'Altorio RA, Rishi US, Bhagwanani DG. Arteriographic findings in mediastinal chemodectoma. *J Thorac Cardiovasc Surg* 67:963, 1974.

33. da Silva OA, et al. Hypokalemic respiratory muscle paralysis following *Strongyloides stercoralis* hyperinfection. *Am J Trop Med Hyg* 30:69, 1981.

34. de Leeuw PW, Waltman FL, Birkenhager WH. Noncardiogenic pulmonary edema as the sole manifestation of pheochromocytoma. *Hypertension* 8:810, 1986.

35. De Troyer A, Desir D, Copinschi G. Regression of lung size in adults with growth hormone deficiency. *Q J Med* 195:329, 1980.

36. Donohue JF. Endobronchial mucormycosis. *Chest* 83:585, 1983.

37. Douglas NJ, et al. Reduced airway vagal tone in diabetic patients with autonomic neuropathy. *Clin Sci* 61:581, 1981.

38. Edelman J, Stewart-Wynne EG. Respiratory and bulbar paralysis with relapsing hyperthyroidism. *Br Med J* 283:275, 1981.

39. Emirgil E, Sobol B. The effects of weight reduction on pulmonary function and the sensitivity of the respiratory center in obesity. *Am Rev Respir Dis* 108:831, 1973.

40. Feldman JM. Adult respiratory syndrome in a patient with a pheochromocytoma. *J Surg Oncol* 29:5, 1985.

41. Ferdinandus J, Pederson JA, Whang R. Hypermagnesemia as a cause of refractory hypotension, respiratory depression, and coma. *Arch Intern Med* 141:669, 1981.

42. Fernandez-Cruz L, Serra-Batlles J, Picado C. Retrosternal goiter and chylothorax: Case report. *Respiration* 50:70, 1986.

43. Fisher MR, Sider L. Diffuse reticulonodular infiltrate associated with splenomegaly. *Chest* 84:609, 1983.

44. Fitzpatrick WJ, et al. Hyperthyroidism and acute bronchial asthma. *Br Med J* 288:314, 1984.

45. Fontana RS, et al. Serotonin and the carcinoid syndrome in patients with bronchial tumors. *Ann Otol Rhinol Laryngol* 72:1024, 1963.

46. Ford HC, Svage T, Delahunt JW. Anterior mediastinal mass and Graves' disease. *Thorax* 40:469, 1985.

47. Frymoyer PA, Anderson GH Jr, Blair DC. Hemoptysis as a presenting symptom of pheochromocytoma. *J Clin Hypertension* 2:65, 1986.

48. Fulkerson WJ, Newman JH. Endogenous Cushing's syndrome complicated by *Pneumocystis carinii* pneumonia. *Am Rev Respir Dis* 129:188, 1984.

49. Geraghty JG, et al. Flow volume loop in patients with goiters. *Ann Surg* 215:83, 1992.

50. Girard DE, et al. Pneumomediastinum in diabetic ketoacidosis: Comments on mechanism, incidence, and management. *Chest* 60:455, 1971.

51. Goldhill DR, Dalgleish JG, Lake RH. Respiratory problems and acromegaly: An acromegalic with hypersomnia, acute upper airway obstruction and pulmonary edema. *Anaesthesia* 37:1200, 1982.

52. Gotthrer A, et al. Hypothyroidism and pleural effusions. *Chest* 98:1130, 1990.

53. Greenspan GH, Block AJ. Respiratory insufficiency associated with acute intermittent porphyria. *South Med J* 74:954, 1981.

54. Grunstein RR, Ho KY, Sullivan CE. Sleep apnea in acromegaly. *Ann Intern Med* 115:527, 1991.

55. Guilleminault C, et al. Sleep apnea syndrome due to upper airway obstruction: A review of 25 cases. *Arch Intern Med* 137:296, 1977.

56. Hansen LA, Prakash UBS, Colby TV. Pulmonary complications of diabetes mellitus. *Mayo Clin Proc* 64:791, 1989.

57. Harman EM, Block AJ. Why does weight loss improve the respiratory insufficiency of obesity? *Chest* 90:153, 1986.

58. Harman E, et al. Sleep-disordered breathing and oxygen desaturation in obese patients. *Chest* 79:256, 1981.

59. Harman EM, Wynne JW, Block AJ. The effect of weight loss on sleep-disordered breathing and oxygen desaturation in morbidly obese men. *Chest* 83:291, 1982.

60. Harrison BDW, et al. Lung function in acromegaly. *Q J Med* 47:517, 1978.

61. Harrison RN, Tattersfield AE. Airway response to inhaled salbutamol in hyperthyroid and hypothyroid patients before and after treatment. *Thorax* 39:34, 1984.

62. Hart TB, et al. Sleep apnea in active acromegaly. *Arch Intern Med* 145:865, 1985.

63. Heaton RW, et al. Diminished bronchial reactivity to cold air in diabetic patients with autonomic neuropathy. *Br Med J* 289:149, 1984.

64. Herve P, et al. Hypercapnic acidosis induced by nutrition in mechanically ventilated patients: Glucose versus fat. *Crit Care Med* 13:537, 1985.

65. Hillerdahl G, et al. Intrathoracic goiter with the superior vena cava syndrome, hoarseness, and acute stridor. *Otol Rhinol Laryngol* 40:340, 1978.

66. Hoffman DA, McConahey WM. Thyrotoxicosis and asthma. *Lancet* 1:808, 1982.
67. Holden HM, Hiltz JE. The tuberculous diabetic. *Can Med Assoc J* 87:797, 1962.
68. Hollingsworth HM, et al. Effect of triiodothyronine-induced thyrotoxicosis on airway hyperresponsiveness. *J Appl Physiol* 71:438, 1991.
69. Holmes F, et al. Pulmonary oedema in hypercalcaemic crisis (letter). *Lancet* 1:311, 1974.
70. Huseby JS, Bennet SW, Hagensee ME. Hyperthyroidism induced by iodinated glycerol. *Am Rev Respir Dis* 144:1403, 1991.
71. Irwin RS, Pratter MR, Hamolsky MW. Chronic persistent cough: An uncommon presenting complaint of thyroiditis. *Chest* 81:386, 1982.
72. Israel RH, et al. Hyperthyroidism protects against carbachol-induced bronchospasm. *Chest* 91:242, 1987.
73. Jacobson E, Dano P, Skovsted P. Respiratory function before and after weight loss following intestinal shunt operation for obesity. *Scand J Respir Dis* 55:332, 1974.
74. Jauregui R, Lilker ES, Bayley A. Upper airway obstruction in euthyroid goiter. *JAMA* 238:163, 1977.
75. Javaheri S, et al. Effects of hypohydration on lung functions in humans. *Am Rev Respir Dis* 135:597, 1987.
76. Jenkins SC, Moxham J. The effects of mild obesity on lung function. *Respir Med* 85:309, 1991.
77. Kaldany A, et al. Reversible acute pulmonary edema due to uncontrolled hyperglycemia in diabetic individuals with renal failure. *Diabetes Care* 5:506, 1982.
78. Kaltreider HB, et al. So-called "metastatic" calcification of the lung. *Am J Med* 46:188, 1969.
79. Karbowitz SR, et al. Spectrum of advanced upper airway obstruction due to goiters. *Chest* 87:18, 1985.
80. Kariman K, Singletary WV Jr, Sieker HO. Pulmonary involvement in Fabry's disease. *Am J Med* 64:911, 1978.
81. Katlic MR, Wang CA, Grillo HC. Substernal goiter. *Ann Thorac Surg* 39:391, 1985.
82. Katz I, et al. Do patients with obstructive sleep apnea have thick necks? *Am Rev Respir Dis* 141:1228, 1990.
83. Keton JG, Collins FF. Exceptionally high arterial oxygen tension in diabetic ketoacidosis. *South Med J* 72:1127, 1979.
84. Khajavi A, Amirhakimi GH. The rachitic lung: Pulmonary findings in 30 infants and children with malnutritional rickets. *Clin Pediatr* 16:36, 1977.
85. Khardori R, et al. Lymphocytic interstitial pneumonitis in autoimmune thyroid disorders. *Am J Med* 90:649, 1991.
86. Kida K, et al. Changes in lung morphologic features and elasticity caused by streptozotocin-induced diabetes mellitus in growing rats. *Am Rev Respir Dis* 128:125, 1983.
87. Kitahata LM. Airway difficulties associated with anaesthesia in acromegaly: Three case reports. *Br J Anaesth* 43:1187, 1971.
88. Knake JE, Gross MD. Extra-adrenal paraganglionoma, pulmonary chondroma, and gastric leiomyoblastoma: Triad in young females. *AJR* 132:448, 1979.
89. Kodolova IM, Lysenko IV, Saltykov BB. Changes in the lungs in diabetes mellitus. *Arkh Patol* 44:35, 1982.
90. Koenig MP, Scherrer M. Respiratory functional abnormalities in hypothyroidism. *Excerpta Med* 378:527, 1975.
91. Kopelman PG. Clinical complications of obesity. *Clin Endocrinol Metab* 13:613, 1984.
92. Korsager S, Ostergard-Kristensen HP. Iodine-induced hypothyroidism and its effect on the severity of asthma. *Acta Med Scand* 205:115, 1979.
93. Kramer M, et al. Pulmonary cryptococcosis and Cushing's syndrome. *Arch Intern Med* 143:2179, 1983.
94. Lachman R, et al. Radiological findings in Niemann-Pick disease. *Radiology* 108:659, 1973.
95. Lack EE, et al. Aortico-pulmonary paragangliomas: Report of a case with ultrastructural study and review of the literature. *Cancer* 43:269, 1979.
96. Lange P, et al. Diabetes mellitus, plasma glucose and lung function in a cross-sectional population study. *Eur Respir J* 2:14, 1989.
97. Laroche CM, et al. Hypothyroidism presenting with respiratory muscle weakness. *Am Rev Respir Dis* 138:472, 1988.
98. Lehrer RI, et al. Mucormycosis. *Ann Intern Med* 93:93, 1980.
99. Leonard RC, et al. Acute respiratory distress in diabetic ketoacidosis: Possible contribution of low colloid osmotic pressure. *Br Med J* 286:760, 1983.
100. Lever AML, Ryder JB. Cor pulmonale in an adult secondary to Niemann-Pick disease. *Thorax* 38:873, 1983.
101. Lieberman J, Beutler E. Elevation of serum angiotensin-converting enzyme in Gaucher's disease. *N Engl J Med* 294:1442, 1976.
102. Lin C-C, Tsan K-W, Chen P-J. The relationship between sleep apnea syndrome and hypothyroidism. *Chest* 102:163, 1992.
103. Lipworth BJ, et al. Problems with asthma following treatment of thyrotoxicosis. *Br J Dis Chest* 82:310, 1988.
104. Luboshitzky R, Barzilai D. Hypoxemia and pulmonary function in acromegaly. *Am Rev Respir Dis* 121:471, 1980.
105. Luce JM. Respiratory complications of obesity. *Chest* 78:626, 1980.
106. Maccioni FJ, Colebatch HJH. *Am Rev Respir Dis* 143:1253, 1991.

107. MacKay EM, Pecka EF Jr. Experimental pulmonary edema: III. Hypoglycemia, a cause of pulmonary edema. *Proc Soc Exp Biol Med* 73:568, 1950.
108. Mackowiak PA, Martin RM, Smith JW. The role of bacterial interference in the increased prevalence of oropharyngeal gram-negative bacilli among alcoholics and diabetics. *Am Rev Respir Dis* 120:589, 1979.
109. Maclay WS. Death due to treatment: President's address. *Proc R Soc Med* 46:13, 1953.
110. Mansell AL, Levison H, Bailey JD. Maturation of lung function in children with hypopituitarism. *Am Rev Respir Dis* 127:166, 1983.
111. Margulies KB, Sheps SG. Carney's triad: Guidelines for management. *Mayo Clin Proc* 63:496, 1988.
112. Marion RB, Alperin JE, Maloney WH. Gouty tophus of the true vocal cord. *Arch Otolaryngol* 96:161, 1972.
113. Martinez FJ, Bermudez-Gomez M, Celli BR. Hypothyroidism. A reversible cause of diaphragmatic dysfunction. *Chest* 96:1059, 1989.
114. McElvaney GN, et al. Respiratory muscle weakness and dyspnea in thyrotoxic patients. *Am Rev Respir Dis* 141:1221, 1990.
115. McKechnie HL. Hypothyroidism with coexistent asthma: Problems in management. *South Med J* 77:401, 1984.
116. Mezon BJ, et al. Sleep apnea in acromegaly. *Am J Med* 69:615, 1980.
117. Miller MR, et al. Upper airway obstruction due to goitre: Detection, prevalence, and results of surgical management. *Q J Med* 74:177, 1990.
118. Millman RO, et al. Central sleep apnea in hypothyroidism. *Am Rev Respir Dis* 127:504, 1983.
119. Mogle P, et al. Respiratory failure and multiple fractures in vitamin D–dependent rickets. *Acta Paediatr Scand* 74:300, 1985.
120. Molloy DW, et al. Hypomagnesemia and respiratory muscle power. *Am Rev Respir Dis* 129:497, 1984.
121. Mondini S, Guilleminault C. Abnormal breathing patterns during sleep in diabetes. *Ann Neurol* 17:391, 1985.
122. Morewood DJ, et al. The extrathoracic airway in acromegaly. *Clin Radiol* 37:243, 1986.
123. Morris JT, Seaworth BJ, McAllister CK. Pulmonary tuberculosis in diabetics. *Chest* 102:539, 1992.
124. Mulhall BP, O'Fearghail M. The diabetic gastroparesis: Case report and review of the literature. *Anaesthesia* 39:468, 1984.
125. Myer CM III. Airway obstruction in Hurler's syndrome—radiographic features. *Int J Pediatr Otorhinolaryngol* 22:91, 1991.
126. Nakazawa T, Kobayashi S. Influence of antithyroidal therapy on asthma symptoms in the patients with both bronchial asthma and hyperthyroidism. *J Asthma* 28:109, 1991.
127. Newman JH, Neff TA, Ziporin P. Acute respiratory failure associated with hypophosphatemia. *N Engl J Med* 296:1101, 1977.
128. Nielsen JM, Ingham SD, Von Hagen KO. Pulmonary edema and embolism as complications of insulin shock in the treatment of schizophrenia. *JAMA* 111:2455, 1938.
129. Nishimura M, et al. Ventilatory and heart rate response to hypoxia and hypercapnia in patients with diabetes mellitus. *Thorax* 44:251, 1989.
130. Olson JL, Salyer WR. Mediastinal paragangliomas (aortic body tumor): A report of 4 cases and a review of the literature. *Cancer* 41:2405, 1978.
131. Orr WC, Males JL, Imes NK. Myxedema and obstructive sleep apnea. *Am J Med* 70:1061, 1981.
132. Perks WH, et al. Sleep apnea in acromegaly. *Br Med J* 280:894, 1980.
133. Peters ME, et al. Narrow trachea in mucopolysaccharidoses. *Pediatr Radiol* 15:225, 1985.
134. Petty TL. The national mucolytic study: Results of a randomized, double-blind, placebo-controlled study of iodinated glycerol in chronic obstructive bronchitis. *Chest* 97:75, 1990.
135. Plopper CG, Morishige WK. Alterations in granular (type II) pneumocyte ultrastructure by streptozotocin-induced diabetes in the rat. *Lab Invest* 38:143, 1978.
136. Plopper CG, Morishige WK. Alterations in the ultrastructure of nonciliated bronchiolar epithelial (Clara) cells by streptozotocin-induced diabetes in rats. *Am Rev Respir Dis* 120:1137, 1979.
137. Powner D, Snyder JV, Grenvik A. Altered pulmonary capillary permeability complicating recovery from diabetic ketoacidosis. *Chest* 68:253, 1975.
138. Pritzker MR, King RA, Kronenberg RS. Upper airway obstruction during head flexion in Morquio's disease. *Am J Med* 69:615, 1980.
139. Rajagopal KR, et al. Obstructive sleep apnea in hypothyroidism. *Ann Intern Med* 101:491, 1984.
140. Ramirez LC, et al. Relationship between diabetes control and pulmonary function in insulin-dependent diabetes mellitus. *Am J Med* 91:371, 1991.
141. Ramsay I. Thyrotoxic muscle disease. *Postgrad Med J* 44:385, 1968.
142. Rapoport DM, et al. Hypercapnia in the obstructive sleep apnea syndrome. A reevaluation of the "pickwickian syndrome." *Chest* 89:627, 1986.
143. Ray CS, et al. Effect of obesity on respiratory function. *Am Rev Respir Dis* 128:501, 1983.
144. Redding RA, Douglas WHJ, Stein M. Thyroid hormone influence upon lung surfactant metabolism. *Science* 175:994, 1975.
145. Reinila A. Perivascular xanthogranulomatosis

in the lungs of diabetic patients. *Arch Pathol Lab Med* 100:542, 1976.

146. Reuger RG. Benign disease of the thyroid gland and vocal cord paralysis. *Laryngoscope* 84:897, 1974.

147. Rochester DF, Esau SA. Malnutrition and the respiratory system. *Chest* 85:411, 1984.

148. Rosenberg DM, et al. Chronic airflow obstruction in Fabry's disease. *Am J Med* 68:898, 1980.

149. Ruttley M, Mills RA. Subcutaneous emphysema and pneumomediastinum in diabetic keto-acidosis. *Br J Radiol* 44:672, 1971.

150. Sadiq MA, Davies JG. Unusual lung manifestations of myxedema. *Br J Clin Pract* 31:224, 1977.

151. Sahebjami H, Macgee J. Changes in connective-tissue composition of the lung in starvation and refeeding. *Am Rev Respir Dis* 128:644, 1983.

152. Sandler M, Bunn AE, Stewart RI. Cross-sectional study of pulmonary function in patients with insulin-dependent diabetes mellitus. *Am Rev Respir Dis* 135:223, 1987.

153. Sandler M, Bunn AE, Stewart RI. Pulmonary function changes in young insulin-dependent diabetic subjects. *Chest* 90:670, 1986.

154. Santos-e-Fonseca CM, et al. Cholinergic bronchomotor tone and airway caliber in insulin-dependent diabetes mellitus. *Chest* 101:1038, 1992.

155. Schneider EL, et al. Severe pulmonary involvement in adult Gaucher's disease. *Am J Med* 63:475, 1977.

156. Schussler GC, Ranney HM. Thyroid hormone and the oxygen affinity of hemoglobin. *Ann Intern Med* 74:632, 1971.

157. Schuyler MR, et al. Abnormal lung elasticity in juvenile diabetes mellitus. *Am Rev Respir Dis* 113:37, 1976.

158. Settipane GA, Schoenfeld E, Hamolsky MW. Asthma and hyperthyroidism. *J Allergy Clin Immunol* 49:348, 1972.

159. Shahian D, Rossi RL. Posterior mediastinal goiter. *Chest* 94:599, 1988.

160. Sharp JT, Druz WS, Kondragunta VR. Diaphragmatic responses to body position changes in obese patients with obstructive sleep apnea. *Am Rev Respir Dis* 133:32, 1986.

161. Siafakas NM, et al. Respiratory muscle strength in hyperthyroidism before and after treatment. *Am Rev Respir Dis* 146:1025, 1992.

162. Siafakas NM, et al. Respiratory muscle strength in hyperthyroidism before and after treatment. *Chest* 102:189, 1992.

163. Siafakas NM, et al. Radiographic determination of total lung capacity in patients with acromegaly. *Br J Dis Chest* 81:280, 1987.

164. Silverstein D, et al. Right ventricular failure in a patient with diabetic neuropathy (myopathy) and central alveolar hypoventilation. *Respiration* 44:460, 1983.

165. Sixt S, Kral T. Closing volume and gas exchange in obese patients before and after intestinal bypass operation. *Scand J Respir Dis* [Suppl] 95:65, 1976.

166. Skatrud J, et al. Disordered breathing during sleep in hypothyroidism. *Am Rev Respir Dis* 124:325, 1981.

167. Small D, et al. Exertional dyspnea and ventilation in hyperthyroidism. *Chest* 101:1268, 1992.

168. Smolar EN, et al. Cardiac tamponade in primary myxedema and review of the literature. *Am J Med Sci* 272:345, 1976.

169. Soler NG, Eagleton LE. Autonomic neuropathy and the ventilatory responses of diabetics to progressive hypoxemia and hypercarbia. *Diabetes* 31:609, 1982.

170. Somerville SM, Rona RJ, Chinn S. Obesity and respiratory symptoms in primary school. *Arch Dis Child* 59:940, 1984.

171. Sommer A, Katz J, Tarwotjo I. Increased risk of respiratory disease and diarrhea in children with preexisting mild vitamin A deficiency. *Am J Clin Nutr* 40:1090, 1984.

172. Sprung CL, Rackow EC, Fein IA. Pulmonary edema: A complication of diabetic ketoacidosis. *Chest* 77:687, 1980.

173. Strumf IJ, et al. A possible relationship between testosterone, central control of ventilation and the pickwickian syndrome. *Am Rev Respir Dis* 117:183, 1978.

174. Sundstrom G, Zauner CW, Arborelius M Jr. Decrease in pulmonary diffusing capacity during lipid infusion in healthy men. *J Appl Physiol* 34:816, 1973.

175. Sutton FD, et al. Progesterone for outpatient treatment of pickwickian syndrome. *Ann Intern Med* 83:476, 1975.

176. Tillman CR. Hypokalemic hypoventilation complicating severe diabetic ketoacidosis. *South Med J* 73:231, 1980.

177. Toomey FB, Chinnock RF. Subcutaneous emphysema, pneumomediastinum, and pneumothorax in diabetic ketoacidosis. *Radiology* 116:543, 1975.

178. Toppell KL, Atkinson R, Whitcomb ME. Lung growth in acromegaly. *Am Rev Respir Dis* 108:1254, 1973.

179. Torres A, et al. Acute respiratory failure and tracheal obstruction patients with intrathoracic goiter. *Crit Care Med* 11:265, 1983.

180. Trotman-Dickenson B, Weetman AP, Hughes JM. Upper airflow obstruction and pulmonary function in acromegaly: Relationship to disease activity. *Q J Med* 79:527, 1991.

181. Tseuda K, et al. Pulmonary complications in the morbidly obese following jejunoileal bypass surgery under narcotic anesthesia. *Int Surg* 65:123, 1980.

182. Tsunoda T, et al. Hashimoto's thyroiditis pre-

senting with severe pressure symptoms—a case report. *Jpn J Surg* 21:450, 1991.

183. Vianna LG, et al. Cough threshold to citric acid in diabetic patients with and without autonomic neuropathy. *Thorax* 43:569, 1988.

184. Vracko R, Thorning D, Huang TW. Basal lamina of alveolar epithelium and capillaries: Quantitative changes with aging and in diabetes mellitus. *Am Rev Respir Dis* 120:973, 1979.

185. Wanke T, et al. Inspiratory muscle performance and pulmonary function changes in insulin-dependent diabetes mellitus. *Am Rev Respir Dis* 143:97, 1991.

186. Ward MJ, Davies D. Riedel's thyroiditis with invasion of the lungs. *Thorax* 36:956, 1981.

187. Weidner WA, Wenzl JE, Swischuk LE. Roentgenographic findings in lipoid proteinosis: A case report. *AJR* 110:457, 1970.

188. Weiner M, Chausow A, Szidon P. Reversible respiratory muscle weakness in hypothyroidism. *Br J Dis Chest* 80:391, 1986.

189. Weir DC, et al. Transfer factor for carbon monoxide in patients with diabetes mellitus with and without microangiopathy. *Thorax* 43:725, 1988.

190. Wheaton RW, et al. Diminished bronchial reactivity to cold air in diabetic patients with autonomic neuropathy. *Br Med J* 289:149, 1984.

191. White SR, Hall JB, Little A. An approach to mediastinal masses associated with hyperthyroidism. *Chest* 90:691, 1986.

192. Wieshammer S, et al. Effects of hypothyroidism on bronchial reactivity in non-asthmatic subjects. *Thorax* 45:947, 1990.

193. Wilson H. Carcinoid syndrome. *Curr Probl Surg*, Nov: 36,1970.

194. Wolson AH. Pulmonary findings in Gaucher's disease. *AJR* 123:712, 1975.

195. Woolner LB, McConahey WC, Beahrs OH. Thyroiditis. *J Clin Endocrinol* 17:201, 1957.

196. Wright AD, et al. Mortality in acromegaly. *Q J Med* 39:1, 1970.

197. Wu B, et al. Accelerated maturation of fetal rabbit lungs by thyroxine. *Physiologist* 14:253, 1971.

198. Yamamoto T. Delayed respiratory failure during treatment of myxedema coma. *Endocrinol Jpn* 31:769, 1984.

199. Zack MB, Fulkerson LL, Stein E. Glucose intolerance in pulmonary tuberculosis. *Am Rev Respir Dis* 108:1164, 1973.

200. Zwillich CW, et al. Ventilatory control in myxedema and hypothyroidism. *N Engl J Med* 292:662, 1975.

64

Neurologic Diseases

Udaya B. S. Prakash

The central and peripheral nervous systems play significant roles in the normal functioning of the respiratory system. The central component of the respiratory system resides mainly in the respiratory centers located in the medulla oblongata. Internuncial pathways connect these centers with higher brain centers, which also play a role in the normal breathing mechanism. The peripheral nervous system is responsible for normal functioning of the respiratory musculature. Depending on the type and extent of injury to either the central or peripheral nervous system, the respiratory apparatus may exhibit various abnormalities [104]. In this chapter, respiratory manifestations as they relate to disease processes at various levels of the nervous system will be discussed.

Neurogenic Breathing Disorders

The most common respiratory feature noted in intracranial disorders is a change in the breathing pattern. When damage is limited to one hemisphere, breathing is often normal, and hence respiratory abnormalities in a patient with an acute neurologic problem may indicate bilateral hemispheric injury. Abnormal breathing patterns have been related to prognosis after brain damage. Abnormalities of breathing are equally common in each of three large groups of patients: those with head injury, intracranial tumor, and subarachnoid hemorrhage [161]. In one report of 100 consecutive patients with severe head injuries who arrived at a major trauma center, hypoxia was noted in 30 percent and hypercapnia in 4 percent [144]. Elevation of intracranial pressure is the main pathologic event causing these breathing abnormalities. Abnormalities in the rate and depth of respiration occur in approximately 40 percent of cases of cerebral hemorrhage. Extensive lesions such as massive cerebral hemorrhage, major cerebral embolism, and the results

of severe head trauma are accompanied by a higher incidence of breathing-pattern abnormalities. Several types of abnormalities, including periodic breathing, irregular breathing, and tachypnea, have been described in patients with central nervous system trauma, tumor, or cerebrovascular accidents. In one report of 227 patients with these types of abnormalities, 60 percent demonstrated some type of abnormal breathing [161]. All patients with medullary lesions demonstrated respiratory abnormalities, whereas pontine lesions were associated with respiratory abnormalities in 60 to 70 percent of patients. Poor prognosis was associated with respiration exceeding 25 breaths per minute and an arterial carbon dioxide tension ($PaCO_2$) of less than 30 mmHg. Different breathing patterns observed with cerebrovascular diseases are shown in Figure 64-1.

Cheyne-Stokes Breathing

Cheyne-Stokes breathing is characterized by regularly alternating phases of hyperventilation and apnea and usually persists for long periods [32,174]. It occurs in approximately 25 percent of cases of cerebral embolism and in nearly 10 percent of cases of cerebral infarction. This respiratory dysrhythmia is also seen in other clinical situations, including lactic acidosis, diabetic ketoacidosis, and uremic coma. The mechanism of this respiratory pattern is not entirely clear. Instability of the ventilatory control system, with associated problems of controller sensitivity and the damping characteristics of carbon dioxide stores, may play a part in producing it [30]. Another possible cause is abnormal sensitivity of respiratory neurons to carbon dioxide, which results in hyperventilation that is unduly prolonged by impairment of forebrain ventilatory inhibition. Patients with Cheyne-Stokes respiration exhibit

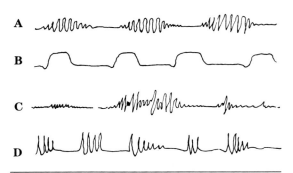

Fig. 64-1. Abnormal neurogenic breathing patterns. (A) Cheyne-Stokes respiration. (B) Apneustic breathing. (C) Biot's breathing. (D) Cluster breathing.

progressively increased tidal volume during the hyperpneic phase, with subsequent decreases without change in respiratory rate [150]. Arterial blood gas studies indicate that the hyperventilation phase is associated with decreased arterial oxygen tension (PaO_2) and pH and increased $PaCO_2$, whereas during the apneic phase, PaO_2 and pH are increased and $PaCO_2$ is decreased [66]. Patients with Cheyne-Stokes breathing who develop respiratory alkalosis have a higher mortality. Cardiac and pulmonary monitoring in 44 patients admitted within 48 hours of onset of stroke disclosed that the presence of intermittent Cheyne-Stokes breathing or tachypnea, seen in 88 percent, was associated with increased mortality [84]. In one study reporting on 11 patients with a $PaCO_2$ of less than 35 mmHg and a pH of more than 7.46, only 1 patient survived [186].

Ataxic Breathing

Plum and Brown [174] coined the term *ataxic breathing* to describe these various patterns: periodic hypoventilation, slow regular breathing, Biot's respiration, apneustic-like inspiratory pauses, and inspiratory gasps. Ataxic breathing is seen in lower pontine and medullary disorders, morphine poisoning, hypercapnic stupor, brain stem infarcts, meningitis, and tumors of the central nervous system. The term *chaotic breathing* is used also to describe ataxic breathing.

BIOT'S BREATHING

Biot's respiration is another term used in the past to describe some abnormal breathing patterns [13]. Many use the terms *ataxic* and *Biot's breathing* synonymously. Clinically, the breathing

pattern consists of irregular cycles of uniformly deep or shallow breaths separated by apnea. Biot's breathing can be seen in patients with lower pontine and medullary disorders, meningitis, lesions in the posterior fossa, morphine poisoning, and hypercapnic stupor.

APNEUSTIC BREATHING

Apneustic breathing refers to prolonged inspiratory "cramps" with cessation of breathing in the inspiratory position (*apneusis* is derived from the Greek term meaning "breathholding"). It is an extremely rare clinical entity, with only nine cases reported in the English literature [126]. The mechanism of this abnormality is unknown, but it is believed to be due to the dissociation of cerebral pathways. A report on five patients with achondroplasia, all of whom demonstrated apneustic breathing, speculated that compression of the lower medullary respiratory centers and afferent pathways in the spinal cord were responsible in these patients [126]. Apneustic breathing can be seen in patients with lower pontine and medullary disorders, brain stem infarction, hypercapnic stupor, meningitis, and hypoglycemia. A classic example of apneustic breathing has been described in a patient with Dandy-Walker syndrome, in which hydrocephalus associated with a cystic fourth ventricle, hypoplasia or agenesis of the cerebellar vermis, and atresia of the foramina of Luschka and Magendie are noted [110]. Typical apneustic breathing and other respiratory abnormalities have occurred in infants with this syndrome. Although the breathing pattern may revert to normal after a shunt procedure, respiratory failure is the major complication leading to death in infants with this syndrome.

Cluster Breathing

Clusters of normal breaths separated by irregular pauses constitute this abnormal breathing pattern, which can be seen in patients with high medullary or low pontine lesions.

Neurogenic Hyperventilation

A rare phenomenon, neurogenic hyperventilation is characterized by very regular, rapid breathing (24 to 38 breaths per minute) that keeps ventilation in a range of three to six times normal for hours or days at a time [175]. Lee and associates [121] suggested that for diagnosis of central hyperventilation, the PaO_2 should be normal (>80 mmHg) and the volume of breathing should be increased beyond body needs. Lesions in the region of the midbrain and upper pontine tegmentum—as seen in brain stem infarctions, acute encephalitis, hypoglycemia, severe sustained anoxia, trauma, and carbon monoxide poisoning—may cause central neurogenic hyperventilation. Several studies have shown that when central neurogenic hyperventilation or Cheyne-Stokes breathing is associated with respiratory alkalosis, the mortality is very high [186].

The mechanism underlying respiratory alkalosis in central neurogenic hyperventilation is not well understood, although lessened sensitivity of peripheral chemoreceptors to hypoxia may allow the PaO_2 to fall below 45 mmHg, at which point central hypoxic drive produces hyperventilation and augmentation of respiratory alkalosis. Although tachypnea and hyperventilation are observed in patients with various neurologic diseases, hyperventilation itself can be used as a diagnostic aid in patients with partial complex seizures. In a report that studied a large number of patients with partial complex seizures, hyperventilatory maneuvers evoked abnormal electroencephalographic discharges and clinical seizures in 11 percent of patients [143]. Central neurogenic hyperventilation has never been induced experimentally, and it is rare even in patients with severe neurologic problems [173].

Neurogenic Hypoventilation

Hypoventilation is characterized by elevated $PaCO_2$. The cause of neurogenic hypoventilation can be either central or peripheral. Hypoventilation associated with obesity (pickwickian syndrome) was described in Chapter 63. Hypoventilation may result from upper airways obstruction or central neurogenic failure. The direct depressant effects of overdosage with narcotic medication are a well-known cause of centrally induced hypoventilation. Cerebral trauma, vascular accidents, and infections also may result in alveolar hyperventilation, which has been found as a result of microinfarctions of basal ganglia in familial hemiplegic migraine as well [156].

True central alveolar hypoventilation (i.e., hypoventilation without any neurologic, cardiopulmonary, or metabolic disorder) is very rare, and only a few cases have been reported since it was first described in 1955 [155]. However, if disorders such as syringomyelia [183], Parkinson's disease [141], schizophrenia [183], and mental retardation [192] are included, approximately 45 cases of true central alveolar hypoventilation can be found in the literature up to 1978 [96]. Clinical features included cyanosis in 100 percent, poly-

cythemia in 33 percent, somnolence in 33 percent, and headache in 25 percent. Frequent findings were pulmonary hypertension in 80 percent and congestive cardiac failure in 50 percent [96].

An increasing number of newborn infants are now being seen who have central hypoventilation of congenital origin, and bilateral phrenic nerve pacing has been tried with varying success in these neonates [95]. Several pharmacologic agents, including medroxyprogesterone acetate and nocturnal administration of oxygen, have been used therapeutically for primary hypoventilation. Patients with severe cerebrovascular disease show a reduced steady-state ventilatory response to hypercapnia. The mechanism for this phenomenon is unknown.

Respiratory inhibitory apraxia is a breathing abnormality in which one is unable to stop breathing voluntarily. However, voluntary spontaneous respiration is unaffected. This type of breathing problem is often associated with other forms of apraxia or motor impersistence. Respiratory inhibitory apraxia is believed to be due to a minor hemisphere lesion, usually deep-seated [3]. Lesions in descending motor pathways in the internal capsule and middle cerebral artery branch territory may produce this abnormality.

Neurogenic Pulmonary Edema

Acute pulmonary edema resulting from elevated intracranial pressure is a well-recognized but relatively uncommon clinical phenomenon. In a publication on more than 2100 patients with serious head injuries and 132 serious cervical spinal cord or spinal column injuries, there were only 2 clear examples of pulmonary edema [72]. However, an autopsy study of 100 soldiers dying from combat wounds in Vietnam revealed pulmonary edema and alveolar hemorrhage in 89 percent, most commonly in those who died within 1 week of injury [131]. Respiratory disease was discovered most frequently, whether or not thoracic injury was present. The edematous changes are seen commonly in postmortem examination of the lungs of patients with bulbar poliomyelitis, hydrocephalus, tumors of the central nervous system, intracerebral hematomas, intraventricular and subarachnoid hemorrhages, and especially trauma to the central nervous system. The mechanism of neurogenic pulmonary edema is not thoroughly understood, although increases in microvascular pressure attributed to changes in the distribution of lung perfusion are believed to be of major importance in its pathogenesis (Fig. 64-2). These hemodynamic events occur within

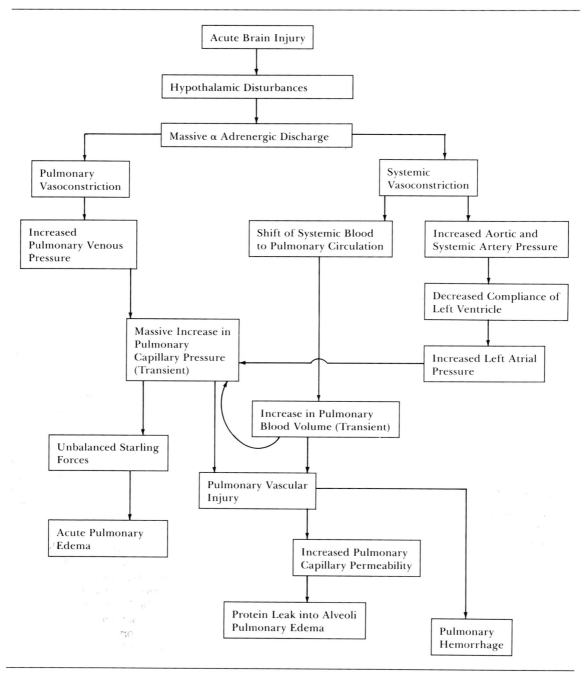

Fig. 64-2. Mechanism of neurogenic pulmonary edema. (Modified from TJ Robin [Ed], Speculations on neurogenic pulmonary edema [NPE]. *Am Rev Respir Dis* 113:405, 1976.)

seconds after injury to the central nervous system. They result from massive alpha-adrenergic sympathetic discharge brought about by stimulation of hypothalamic centers and hence are similar to the effects produced by large infusions of epinephrine. Elevations of both systemic and pulmonary arterial pressures reflect increased vascular resistance in both circulations due to vasoconstriction. The left ventricle is stiffened (so-called stone heart) as a result of overstimulation by the sympathetic nervous system and excessive release of catecholamine. Pulmonary edema develops during these hemodynamic alterations and persists after the vascular pressures return to normal. Presumably, the persistence of edema is due to pulmonary capillary endothelial damage caused by the abrupt changes in pressure and volume within the pulmonary vasculature [108, 202,203]. Protein also leaks into the alveoli, as has been shown in humans and animals [82]. There is some evidence that damage to the hypothalamus initiates the response just discussed and, in particular, the postchiasmatic area has been referred to as the *edemagenic center* [127].

In a study of dogs, sustained elevation of intracranial pressure at a level below mean arterial pressure induced action of the alpha-adrenergic mechanisms that resulted in pulmonary vasoconstriction [129]. This neurogenic pulmonary vasoconstriction resulted in increases in lung water, physiologic shunt, and alveolar dead space, as well as worsening of hypoxemia. The action of the vagus nerve in neurogenic pulmonary edema is not clear. In experiments on rats and rabbits, such edema did not occur if the vagi were sectioned before the brain was injured [26]. However, studies in dogs and monkeys have failed to corroborate these findings [44]. Although the hemodynamic changes, as hypothesized by Theodore and Robin [202,203], are believed to be responsible for the neurogenic pulmonary edema, measurements in humans after the onset of pulmonary edema have usually demonstrated normal pressures.

Head trauma is one of the most common causes of severe but nonfatal neurogenic pulmonary edema. In a retrospective clinical and pathologic analysis of 78 cases of fatal subarachnoid hemorrhage [211], a pathologic diagnosis of pulmonary edema was made in 71 percent, and 31 percent of this group had a clinical diagnosis of pulmonary edema. Neurogenic pulmonary edema after subarachnoid hemorrhage carries a poor prognosis, and postmortem studies indicate that between 33 and 71 percent of patients with fatal subarachnoid hemorrhage will have pulmonary edema [211].

Any situation that leads to severe cerebral hypoxia has the potential to produce pulmonary edema. The overall frequency of postictal edema is low; the literature yields approximately 100 cases. Postictal pulmonary edema can recur in the same patient [39,75]. Postictal pulmonary edema shows a predilection for young epileptic patients. It may develop immediately after an epileptic seizure or several hours later. Electric shock therapy for seizure disorder has resulted in fatal pulmonary edema [23]. Guillain-Barré syndrome, old poliomyelitis, and meningitis have caused neurogenic pulmonary edema [54,81]. A report on the pathologic findings in 200 cases of fatal meningococcal meningitis observed pulmonary edema in 60 percent [83]. Neurogenic pulmonary edema has followed trigeminal blockade [216].

The clinical features of neurogenic pulmonary edema include the obvious evidence of damage to the central nervous system, progressive respiratory distress, and chest roentgenographic dis-

Fig. 64-3. Neurogenic pulmonary edema. Bilateral alveolar infiltrates with air bronchograms are noted.

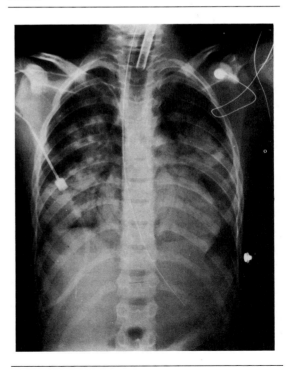

tribution of asymmetric alveolar type infiltrates [52] (Fig. 64-3), although a generalized pattern has been observed in most cases. Delayed onset of edema is unusual, but it has been observed in a number of cases [51].

Abnormal States of Consciousness

Unconsciousness and Coma

Unconsciousness and coma are conditions favorable to the development of aspiration pneumonitis, nosocomial pneumonia, hypoventilatory respiratory failure, and pulmonary thromboembolism. Aspiration pneumonia and nosocomial pneumonia from gram-positive, gram-negative, and anaerobic organisms are the major causes of morbidity and mortality in this group of patients. Neurogenic pulmonary edema also is seen in these patients. Although abnormal breathing patterns are common in these patients, especially at the lowest level of consciousness, no significant association has been found between any particular abnormal pattern and level of consciousness [161]. The unconscious patient breathes more rapidly and regularly than conscious patients. Increasing regularity of respiration seems to correlate well with deepening coma and accurately reflects ultimate outcome even when other clinical signs remain unchanged. Attention to prevention of these serious pulmonary problems will reduce the mortality among this highly susceptible group of patients.

Hypoxic pulmonary disorders and head injuries associated with raised intracranial pressure frequently coexist. Positive end-expiratory pressure breathing in patients with brain injuries has been shown to improve arterial oxygenation without increasing the intracranial pressure and, consequently, may be a form of treatment for the comatose patient with pneumonia or pulmonary edema [57].

Head Trauma

Neurogenic pulmonary edema and other complications discussed in this chapter can also result from closed head injury. The pulmonary complications depend on the degree of trauma, level of consciousness, and involvement of other organs. Closed head injury is a common condition requiring endotracheal intubation and mechanical ventilation. A study of 109 initially comatose patients with isolated closed head injuries who were ventilated for 24 hours or more concluded the fol-

lowing: Closed head injury is associated with a high incidence of pneumonia; pneumonia occurs earlier in closed head injury than in other patient groups, it does not tend to occur after the first week of hospitalization, and it prolongs stay in the intensive care unit [94].

Barbiturates are commonly used in patients with cerebral edema. A prospective study assessed the effect of barbiturates in mechanically ventilated patients with brain edema and discovered that the rate of nosocomial pneumonia was significantly higher in patients receiving barbiturates than in the control group, those receiving higher doses being at greater risk of developing pneumonia [46]. The colonization of the respiratory tract was observed in all barbiturate-treated patients, and 70 percent of the control group was colonized by organisms.

Epilepsy

Alterations in respiratory function associated with epileptic discharges have been described in the past. In petit mal seizure, short periods of apnea are almost always discovered. Whether the respiratory arrest occurs in expiration or inspiration depends on the phase of the respiratory cycle during which the epileptic discharge arises. Similar respiratory abnormalities have been observed in focal epilepsy, especially temporal lobe type. However, it should be noted that respiratory changes only rarely appear to be the principal and important components of the seizure, though such cases have been described. Several cases of respiratory failure as a seizure phenomenon have been reported [128,157]. The sudden death of an epileptic, unexplained by autopsy, is reported to be relatively frequent [128]. Such deaths have been attributed to acute functional disturbances in cardiorespiratory centers as a result of seizure discharges [90]. It is theorized that acute respiratory failure develops as a consequence of propagation of seizure discharges leading to dysfunction of brain stem respiratory centers. Fortunately, this complication of seizure disorders seems to be uncommon.

Breathing difficulties, including the presenting symptom of laryngospasm, have been noted in patients with temporal lobe seizures [176]. Severe hypoxia and acidosis after local anesthetic-induced convulsions have been reported; in these cases, convulsions were induced following local anesthesia with bupivacaine [148]. Neurogenic pulmonary edema is one of the complications associated with epileptic seizures. Prolonged apnea also has been noted in epileptic patients [50]. Prolonged spasm of the respiratory muscles leading to ventilatory problems has been reported in patients with status epilepticus [160].

Phenytoin-treated epileptic patients have been noted to have more frequent symptoms of respiratory diseases than controls. The high frequency of respiratory diseases in phenytoin-treated epileptic patients is probably related in part to immunoglobulin A deficiency. However, additional drug effects may be important. Phenytoin is reported to have a depressant effect on the immune system, and this effect may have clinical significance by causing frequent respiratory diseases in epileptic patients taking the drug [63].

Exaggerated vagal attack has been described in 58 children in whom reflex anoxic seizures secondary to provoked cardioinhibition (also known as *white breath-holding attacks*) were diagnosed. The seizures were diagnosed initially as epileptic in nature; however, detailed studies and reviews of the literature support the concept that these seizures result from vagally mediated reflex cardiac arrest, which can be prevented by atropine therapy [201].

Spinal Cord Disorders

Damage to the cervical spinal cord can interfere with both afferent and efferent spinal pathways concerned with respiratory function. Transection or other severe injury to the cervical spinal cord at a high level causes weakness of the respiratory muscles and may result in ventilatory failure. Transection of the cord below the fifth cervical vertebral level results in intercostal muscle paralysis. In such an instance, although the accessory neck muscles of respiration are affected, diaphragmatic function is preserved, and so hypoventilation does not occur. However, the work done by the diaphragm is many times normal, and therefore most patients with transection of the spinal cord experience dyspnea.

Quadriplegia (Tetraplegia)

Hemiplegia denotes loss of neuromuscular function on one side of the body, usually owing to a cerebrovascular accident on the contralateral side. The functional classification of spinal cord injuries includes pentaplegia, quadriplegia (tetraplegia), and paraplegia. In quadriplegia, C4 to C8 levels are involved, with motor and sensory loss in the arms and legs. In respiratory quadriplegia, the spinal cord is involved at the second through third cervical vertebral levels, and findings include motor and sensory loss of the arms, legs, and diaphragm. Pentaplegia results when the lesion is located in the brain stem to the first cervical vertebral level, with resultant motor and sensory loss of the neck, arms, legs, and diaphragm. In paraplegia, sensory and motor loss is noted in the legs as a result of involvement of the spinal cord between the levels of the first thoracic and first sacral vertebrae [200].

Hemingway and coworkers [85], in a comprehensive paper on pulmonary function in quadriplegic patients, reported that the vital capacity was approximately two-thirds normal and the maximum breathing capacity half normal. A mean decrease in vital capacity to 42 percent of the predicted value has been reported [58]. The impaired ventilatory function in quadriplegic patients is caused by the elimination of supraspinal control of respiratory muscles innervated from spinal segments below the level of the lesion. The spastic paralysis results in decreased compliance of the chest wall and reduction of both inspiratory and expiratory reserve volumes. The decrease in vital capacity is also due to altered body posture [58]. Duration of quadriplegia does not seem to alter pulmonary function testing response [130]. However, rib cage distortion is less severe in chronic than in acute quadriplegia [188]. Electromyographic studies of the intercostal muscles in quadriplegic patients show that once the stage of spinal shock subsides and full reflex activity of the isolated cord develops, the increase in electrical response of the intercostal muscles to the act of breathing is very conspicuous. In the early stages of quadriplegia, the intensity of the compensatory respiratory function of the sternomastoid muscle varies, and its development to full strength as an auxiliary force in the act of breathing may require some time and the use of systematic exercises. These studies also show that unilateral paralysis of the diaphragm greatly reduces, but does not abolish, reflex function of the intercostal muscles.

Studies of the motion of the abdomen and the rib cage in quadriplegic patients during breathing in supine and sitting postures have shown that in the former the rib cage moves paradoxically inward, with resultant functional deformity of the chest wall and increased work with breathing. In addition to the recoil of the whole respiratory system, there is also recoil of the deformed chest wall toward its passive configuration, with an expansion of the rib cage above its resting position during the first part of expiration and an alteration of the expiratory profile. In the sitting posture, the paradoxical inward motion disappears in the lower rib cage, whereas it is decreased but still present in the higher rib cage [151].

Further studies in quadriplegic patients have demonstrated postural hypoxemia, especially during the posture after the onset of quadriplegia. The postural hypoxemia probably results from relative hypoventilation of the upper lung fields caused by flaccid paralysis of the intercostal muscles. With time, the change from flaccid to spastic paralysis of the intercostal muscles is the most likely explanation for the disappearance of hypoxemia after 1 year [65]. The disappearance of paradoxical motion of the upper rib cage with time in quadriplegics has been attributed to the development of spasticity of the intercostal muscles, with better support of the rib cage preventing its in-drawing with inspiration [10]. The partial hypoxemia was noted in the head-down position in these quadriplegic patients [65]. The most conspicuous feature of the respiratory mechanics of the supine quadriplegic patient is the paradoxical inward movement of the rib cage during inspiration [152].

Most deaths that follow soon after acute quadriplegia are due to pulmonary complications. Respiratory problems include hypoventilation, recurrent infections due to aspiration and ineffective cough, pulmonary edema in the acute quadriplegic state, and an increased incidence of thromboembolic phenomena. Bergofsky [10] demonstrated that the work done by the diaphragm in quadriplegic patients is nine times greater than that in the normal individual. He postulated that this increased work of breathing is associated with dyspnea, which is minimized by a decrease in the respiratory rate to an inadequate level, and this is the basis for the chronic alveolar hypoventilation seen in such cases. A 20-year analysis of 54 quadriplegic patients showed that pulmonary complications were fairly common. Tracheostomy in these individuals was associated with a higher mortality [8]. Radiofrequency electrophrenic respiratory pacing has been used to support quadriplegic patients dependent on mechanical ventilatory assistance [64].

In a prospective study of 22 consecutive patients with quadriplegia reported from the Mayo Clinic, a high mortality was noted during the first months and 15 to 40 percent mortality was seen in the first year [133]. Most deaths were related to respiratory failure. However, with aggressive respiratory care, mortality was decreased. A retrospective analysis of 22 similar patients showed a 41 percent mortality within 5 years after quadriplegia. With time, lung functions improved, especially the diaphragmatic function. In another study of 10 quadriplegic patients, it was shown that diminished outward recoil of the rib cage was a prominent feature. Rib cage muscles seemed to recover and stabilize the chest wall with time. Sometimes electromyography may help in diagnosing the abnormal recoil and thereby assist in determining the necessary actions to decrease the incidence of respiratory failure [43].

Bronchorrhea or bronchial mucus hypersecretion is reported to occur in 20 percent of quadriplegic patients [11]. This occurs in the absence of well-known mechanisms such as smoking and respiratory infection, and the quantity of mucus produced may exceed 1.0 liter/day. The sudden onset and spontaneous recovery has led investigators to believe that quadriplegic bronchorrhea is due to disturbed neuronal control of bronchial mucous gland secretion rather than mucous gland hypertrophy and perhaps is related to initial disappearance and later reappearance of peripheral sympathetic nervous system tone [11].

Cervical cordotomy to relieve intractable pain may lead to respiratory dysfunction and result in sleep-induced apnea and even sudden death. It is believed that respiratory complications are related to dissection of efferent pathways to the phrenic nuclei, as well as distal respiratory control mechanisms, as a result of ablation of reticular formation spinal tracts.

Hemiplegia

In hemiplegia, spastic paralysis or weakness of the affected side of the body may include the diaphragm and intercostal muscles. However, respiratory complications ordinarily are not regarded as a complication of hemiplegia. Ipsilateral diaphragmatic dysfunction occurs frequently. The left diaphragm is more commonly involved in left hemiplegia than is the right hemidiaphragm in right hemiplegia, though the reason for this discrepancy is unclear. Forced vital capacity (FVC) and forced expiratory volume may be decreased to 60 percent of normal in these patients [163]. Ventilatory failure becomes imminent when the vital capacity is reduced to 25 percent or less of the predicted normal value. Spirometry in hemiplegic patients has shown reduction of both forced vital capacity and forced expiratory volume in 1 second (FEV$_1$) to approximately 60 and 70 percent, respectively, of the predicted values.

A restrictive type of pulmonary dysfunction in clinical patients with hemiplegia shows only mild signs of impaired ventilatory function. Furthermore, the lack of clinical symptoms may be due to the fact that patients with hemiplegia are less active than their normal counterparts. Therefore, the restrictive ventilatory defect in hemiplegic patients will be of more clinical importance in terms of exercise tolerance for strenuous exercise done in ordinary daily activities [182].

Paraplegia

Paraplegia is accompanied by a slight ventilatory restriction [106]. Studies in paraplegic patients have shown both normal vital capacity and maximal breathing capacity as well as diminished vital capacity to 60 percent in patients with high thoracic transections and to 78 percent in patients with low thoracic lesions [85].

Diaphragmatic Paralysis

The diaphragm is the most important muscle of respiration and, therefore, diaphragmatic paralysis can cause significant respiratory abnormalities. The paralysis can be unilateral or bilateral and transient or permanent. It may result from interruption of the nerve supply, from muscular atrophy, or transiently from diaphragmatic pleurisy. Acute unilateral diaphragmatic paralysis usually is due to interruption of the phrenic nerve by bronchogenic carcinoma or another tumor in the mediastinum, whereas chronic unilateral paralysis is idiopathic. Unilateral or bilateral paralysis can be caused by motor neuron disease, paralytic poliomyelitis, high cervical cord injuries, infectious polyneuritis of Landry-Guillain-Barré, or peripheral neuritis associated with measles, tetanus, typhoid, or diphtheria. Diaphragmatic involvement is often a late manifestation of a generalized neuromuscular disease. Diaphragmatic weakness has also been noted in patients with Charcot-Marie-Tooth disease [117].

Unilateral phrenic nerve paralysis followed 1.7 percent of 1891 consecutive cardiac surgical procedures during an 8-year period [137]. This complication was most frequently associated with Blalock-Taussig shunts. These procedures represented 22 percent of the series reported, and unilateral phrenic nerve paralysis complicated 7 percent of all Blalock-Taussig shunts [137]. Hypothermic cardioplegia, induced by placing ice around the heart prior to open heart surgery, is complicated by transient unilateral phrenic nerve

palsy ("frost-bitten phrenic") that lasts for 6 to 8 weeks. During a 1-year period, 2 cases of bilateral diaphragmatic paralysis were found among 360 prospectively studied patients; both patients had insulin-dependent diabetes mellitus [47]. Phrenic nerve isolation and protection from hypothermia during surgery resulted in no case of phrenic paralysis in a group of 76 control patients, compared to an 18 percent incidence in 76 patients whose phrenic nerves were exposed to cold [120]. Diaphragmatic paralysis has been associated with Erb's palsy, which is a well-circumscribed complication of birth trauma to the shoulder and neck, thoracotomy, and as a complication of central venous alimentation [12, 73,113]. The diseases associated with diaphragmatic paralysis are listed in Table 64-1.

In more than two-thirds of cases, the cause of diaphragmatic paralysis remains undetermined. The majority of patients studied were asymptomatic and remained so on follow-up examination. Approximately 25 percent of them regained diaphragmatic function after a period of several months to 3 years. In another study of 247 patients with diaphragmatic paralysis reported

Table 64-1. Causes of diaphragmatic paralysis

Cerebral hemispheric stroke

Spinal cord disorders
    Trauma to the cervical spinal cord
    Syringomyelia
    Poliomyelitis
    Motor neuron diseases

Peripheral neuropathies
    Trauma to the phrenic nerve (surgery, radiation, tumor)
    Phrenic nerve compression by tumor
    Landry-Guillain-Barré syndrome
    Brachial plexus neuritis
    Nutritional or alcoholic neuropathy
    Lead neuropathy
    Postinfectious neuropathies
        Diphtheria
        Tetanus
        Typhoid
        Measles

Myasthenia gravis

Muscular disorders
    Myotonic dystrophies
    Duchenne's muscular dystrophy
    Metabolic myopathies
    Polymyositis

Idiopathic

from the Mayo Clinic, 42.5 percent were found to have a cause for the diaphragmatic paralysis, whereas there was no identified reason for the paralysis in the remaining 57.5 percent (142 patients) [172]. Among this group, left-sided paralysis was seen in 58 percent, right-sided involvement in 41 percent, and bilateral involvement in 1 percent. Intrathoracic malignant lesions were subsequently diagnosed in 3.5 percent, and progressive neurogenic atrophy was seen in one patient.

Unilateral Diaphragmatic Paralysis

A diagnosis of unilateral diaphragmatic paralysis often is difficult to establish with certainty. Study of the motion of the abdominal wall and the rib cage with magnetometry in the supine position has failed to show paradoxical movements of the abdomen in unilateral paralysis [86]. This is in contrast to the findings in bilateral diaphragmatic paralysis, in which the anterior abdominal wall moves inward paradoxically with inspiration [193]. Measurement of transdiaphragmatic pressure using two balloon catheters has shown that at rest and expiration when the diaphragm is relaxed, the transdiaphragmatic pressure is zero

[159]. During maximal inspiration, the change in pressure exceeds 25 cmH$_2$O in normal individuals, whereas in patients with weakness of the diaphragm, this pressure is less than 6 cmH$_2$O [159].

Symptoms of unilateral phrenic paralysis are orthopnea and difficulty in inspiration. Significant arterial oxygen desaturation can occur in the supine position, but carbon dioxide retention is unusual. Roentgenographic findings include elevation of the diaphragm; diminished, absent, or paradoxical movements on inspiration; mediastinal shift on inspiration; and paradoxical movements of the diaphragm under conditions of augmented load such as sniffing. Paradoxical motion of the affected diaphragm during a "sniff test" under fluoroscopic guidance is a widely accepted test to establish the diagnosis (Fig. 64-4). However, it should be noted that nearly 6 percent of normal people may demonstrate paradoxical movement of one diaphragm or the other. If paradoxical excursion during sniffing exceeds 2 cm and involves the whole leaf of the diaphragm as

Fig. 64-4. Diaphragmatic motion in diaphragmatic paralysis. (A) Paradoxical upward motion of the paralyzed right diaphragm during sudden inspiratory breathing. (B) Paradoxical downward motion during expiration.

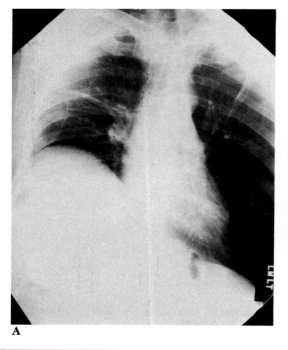
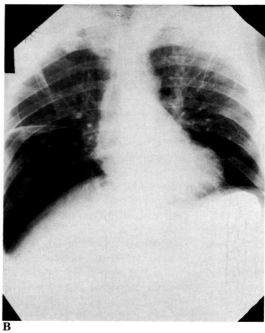

A   B

seen on the oblique view, it probably is pathologic, provided that the abdominal muscles are relaxed during the test. Perhaps the most scientific means of identifying weakness or paralysis of the diaphragm is the measurement of transdiaphragmatic pressure. This is accomplished by recording pressures in balloons placed in both the esophagus and the stomach [159]. Diaphragmatic electromyography is occasionally required to document the diagnosis.

Pulmonary function studies in patients with unilateral diaphragmatic paralysis have shown total lung capacity to be decreased by 37 percent and vital capacity (VC) and maximal voluntary ventilation (MVV) to be decreased by 20 percent, whereas bilateral paralysis diminishes vital capacity by 50 percent in the upright posture and by 60 to 75 percent in the supine position [178]. The effects of posture on lung volume, airway closure, and gas exchange studied in eight patients with hemidiaphragmatic paralysis showed the mean vital capacity in the sitting position to be 81 percent of predicted normal and in the supine posture to decrease by a further 19 percent in right-sided paralysis but only 10 percent in left-sided paralysis. Diffusing capacity for carbon monoxide (DLCO) was normal in all cases [34]. Overall pulmonary function in the sitting position in 17 subjects with hemidiaphragmatic paralysis revealed VC, MVV, and FEV_1 to be reduced by an average of approximately 25 percent.

Experimentally induced unilateral phrenic paralysis in eight subjects reduced the mean VC to 86 percent of the previous value and the total lung capacity to 91 percent; supine posture further reduced these capacities to 71 and 80 percent, respectively [67]. Regional lung function data in the same position showed a considerable decrease in perfusion (19 percent), ventilation (20 percent), and lung volume (7 percent) of the diseased side as compared to reference values obtained in healthy volunteers. PaO_2 was significantly below normal in the supine position and in the normal range in the sitting position and increased further during exercise [2]. Radioactive xenon 133 was used to study regional lung function in five patients with unilateral diaphragmatic paralysis not associated with intrathoracic disease. The results showed that both ventilation and perfusion were preferentially distributed to the middle and upper lung zones [178]. The quantity of ^{133}Xe inhaled was decreased on the paralyzed side [178].

Ipsilateral diaphragmatic dysfunction occurs frequently in hemiplegia. As stated previously, the left diaphragm is more commonly involved in left hemiplegia than is the right hemidiaphragm in right hemiplegia. The reason for this discrepancy is not clear. FVC and FEV may be decreased to 60 percent of normal in these patients [163]. Ventilatory failure becomes imminent when the vital capacity is reduced to 25 percent or less of the predicted normal value. Routine pulmonary function tests may suggest the possibility of respiratory neuromuscular disease when the lung parenchyma is normal with a decrease in total capacity or an increase in residual volume. Maximal inspiratory and expiratory pressures are very helpful in assessing respiratory muscle strength. Serial measurements aid in recognizing respiratory muscle fatigue or recovery of muscle strength [15,178]. Unilateral diaphragmatic paralysis is associated with an abnormal pattern of use of the respiratory muscles during quiet breathing, characterized by the use of intercostal and accessory inspiratory muscles or compensatory use of abdominal expiratory muscles [123]. A detailed physiologic study in one patient with right hemidiaphragmatic paralysis has suggested that to compensate for paralysis of a hemidiaphragm, a new pattern of inspiratory muscle recruitment develops, involving more rapid contraction of the remaining inspiratory muscles [45].

Bilateral Diaphragmatic Paralysis

Bilateral diaphragmatic paralysis is not as common as unilateral paralysis, but it can be life-threatening in acute cases. Nonetheless, reports suggest that bilateral paralysis or severe weakness of the diaphragm alone does not lead to respiratory failure unless weakness of other respiratory muscles is present [116]. The most striking clinical feature is severe orthopnea in the absence of heart and lung disease. The vital capacity is reduced to 50 percent of the predicted normal value; in the supine position there is further decrease, accompanied by orthopnea. In addition to the diminished lung volumes, especially in the supine posture, lung compliance is reduced, perhaps because of widespread atelectasis [61]. Although the $PaCO_2$ is usually normal in the erect position, in some cases an elevated $PaCO_2$ in the supine position as well as during sleep has been observed [159].

Further examples of disturbances of ventilation and perfusion in the lungs of patients with bilateral diaphragmatic paralysis have been reported. These patients demonstrate an increased alveolar-arterial oxygen tension difference $[P(A-a)O_2]$ on assuming the supine posture, and studies in the lateral decubitus posture using radioisotopes illustrate further mismatch of ventilation-perfusion relationships. Bilateral diaphragmatic paralysis leads to chronic respiratory failure with the worsening of hypoxemia and hypercapnia during sleep. The increased incidence of respiratory infection may be caused by chronic atelectasis and impaired mucociliary clearance [140]. Radiofrequency electrophrenic pacing has been used successfully in some patients with this problem [134]. Nocturnal ventilatory support, as well as treatment with nasal continuous positive airway pressure, has been suggested as a therapeutic alternative [124,218]. The chest cuirass also has been used in patients with bilateral diaphragmatic paralysis [93].

Myoneural and Muscular Disorders

Among these disorders are various neuromyopathies, demyelinating disease, motor neuron disease, and dystrophic muscle disorders. Although the etiology, pathogenesis, and nonrespiratory manifestations greatly vary in these diverse diseases, the main pulmonary problem relates to respiratory muscle weakness and chronic hypoventilation. In fact, respiratory failure may be the presenting symptom in many of these diseases. In the later stages of many of these diseases, respiratory failure is common and frequently is the cause of death.

Myasthenia Gravis

Involvement of respiratory muscles occurs in approximately 10 percent of myasthenics; the resultant respiratory failure may require prolonged ventilatory assistance [104]. The risk of respiratory insufficiency may be increased by surgery, infectious diseases, and the administration of corticosteroids or antimicrobial drugs. Untreated myasthenic patients show decreases in vital capacity, total lung capacity, dynamic lung volumes, and functional residual capacity, as well as maximal inspiratory and expiratory forces [15,180, 199]. Patients with myasthenia gravis may have severe respiratory muscle involvement even when peripheral muscle weakness is mild [142]. Repetitive surface electrode stimulation of phrenic nerves is reported to be a useful and noninvasive method for identifying patients with myasthenia gravis in whom weakness of the diaphragm is suspected [139].

The patient with myasthenia gravis undergoing thymectomy presents special problems during and after anesthesia. In a study of 24 myasthenic patients who underwent thymectomy, four risk factors—duration of myasthenia, respiratory disease, pyridostigmine dosage, and vital capacity—allowed prediction of which patients would need postoperative mechanical ventilation and which could readily have their tracheas extubated [122]. In addition, bulbar symptomatology, pyridostigmine dosage, and history of respiratory failure should be considered along with vital capacity in identifying those patients who need mechanical ventilation. Previous reports advocated tracheostomy in all instances to deal with complications in postoperative myasthenic patients [166]. Others recommended that tracheostomy be performed if bulbar weakness, previous history of respiratory and myasthenic crises, or a vital capacity of less than 2 liters was present [153]. In the previously cited study, vital capacity of less than 22.9 liters, pyridostigmine dosage of more than 750 mg/day, and myasthenia of more than 6 years' duration were considered risk factors [122]. The anesthetic management of patients with myasthenia gravis is complicated by the increased sensitivity to nondepolarizing myoneural blocking drugs and a resistance to depolarizing neuromuscular blocking drugs. Consequently, it is common practice to leave the endotracheal tube in place for 24 to 48 hours after the operation, and usually the patient's response to doses of anticholinesterase drugs is used as a guide to the progress of myasthenia after surgery [87]. The major problems in myasthenic patients undergoing general anesthesia involve maintenance of adequate ventilation with the provision of adequate relaxation and clearance of secretions.

Studies on the effect of administration of an anticholinesterase agent (pyridostigmine) on lung mechanics in eight patients with myasthenia gravis demonstrated impairment of the respiratory muscles, showing average vital capacity to increase by 14 percent without a change in residual volume [41]. Pyridostigmine did not seem to modify specific airway conductance or the relationship between static lung recoil pressure and maximal expiratory flow; by contrast, it increased markedly the peak expiratory flow and maximal inspiratory flow. The authors concluded that an increase in respiratory muscle force did not affect the elastic properties of the lungs and airways and was associated with an increased tendency of the chest wall to recoil outward. This study suggested that the changes observed in patients were related solely to the increase in respiratory muscle force, and the major effect of the drug was an increase in the ability to inflate the lungs [41]. Further studies using edrophonium chloride (Tensilon) have shown this drug to reduce the vital capacity as well as the maximal inspiratory flows. Hence, the use of Tensilon may be limited in patients with myasthenic crisis, especially in those complicated by obstructive lung disease. The increased airways resistance signals the limits of drug quantity that can be administered, especially in myasthenic patients suffering also from obstructive lung disease.

Antibodies directed against the acetylcholine receptor are present in the sera of most myasthenia gravis patients. Use of plasmapheresis, immunosuppressive therapy, and thymectomy may prove effective in improving respiratory function of some patients with myasthenia gravis. In a Mayo Clinic study of 22 patients who required prolonged mechanical ventilation because of respiratory failure secondary to myasthenia gravis, the most frequent cause of respiratory failure was surgery, and the most common type of procedure was thymectomy [68]. All but one of the patients were weaned from the ventilator after 1 to 32 days of respiratory support [68]. The only factor useful for predicting the probable need for prolonged postoperative mechanical ventilation is reported to be the degree of bulbar involvement [69].

Myasthenic Syndrome

Also known as Eaton-Lambert syndrome, myasthenic syndrome is a disorder of neuromuscular transmission in which IgG antibodies to presynaptic calcium channels lead to their downregulation, thereby reducing calcium-dependent, nerve impulse–evoked acetylcholine release. Nearly 70 percent of patients with this syndrome have an underlying small-cell carcinoma of lung [171]. In approximately half of all cases of myasthenic syndrome, a tumor is not detectable. The syndrome is characterized by proximal muscle weakness, easy tendency to fatigue, and progressive respiratory failure [71,118].

Myotonic and Progressive Muscular Dystrophy

Myotonic dystrophy and progressive muscular dystrophy can lead to insidious, chronic respiratory failure. Approximately 10 percent of patients with myotonic dystrophy develop this complica-

tion. Myotonic patients demonstrate a decreased minute ventilation, hypoxemia, hypercapnia, and pulmonary hypertension, whereas the patient with nonmyotonic dystrophy exhibits a greater decrease in vital capacity and maximal breathing capacity. FVC and MVV were decreased to 67 percent of predicted values, and peak expiratory flow rate was reduced to 72 percent in 14 men with pseudohypertrophic muscular dystrophy [24]. Children with nonmyotonic muscular dystrophy of the Duchenne type normally have well-preserved diaphragmatic function, but they commonly die of respiratory failure or pulmonary infection [97]. Blunted respiratory drive is occasionally seen in congenital myopathies [179]. Chronic alveolar hypoventilation has been reported in all major forms of muscular dystrophy. Studies of lung mechanics in patients with severe respiratory muscle weakness have shown that both maximal transpulmonary pressure and static expiratory compliance are low [61]. The low compliance, it was suggested, results from either microatelectasis or a generalized alteration of alveolar elastic properties [61].

Patients with muscular dystrophies face the same problems as those with other neuromyopathic diseases—namely, aspiration pneumonia, hypoventilation and, in patients with dystrophic myocardial involvement, cardiomyopathy and pulmonary edema [194]. The vital capacity improves following vigorous respiratory therapy, including breathing exercises and intermittent positive-pressure therapy. Daytime hypersomnolence is frequently reported by patients with myotonic dystrophy. Detailed sleep studies in six young male patients with mild myotonic dystrophy and a complaint of excessive daytime sleepiness showed evidence of sleep apnea syndrome with high apnea indices. There is no relation between hypoxic and hypercapnic ventilatory responses during wakefulness and sleep apnea indices. Both hypoxemia and hypercapnia worsened considerably during rapid-eye-movement (REM) sleep. Increased pulmonary and systemic arterial pressures also were noted during sleep in these patients [79]. These patients may demonstrate central apnea, an obstructive type of apnea, or a combination of the two [36,79].

A study of seven patients with mild myotonic dystrophy showed consistently decreased hypoxic ventilatory response with varying hypercapnic response [29]. The high incidence of respiratory failure in such patients is most likely related to the decreased hypoxic ventilatory response, occurring because of an underlying neurogenic deficit [29]. Ventilatory aids and mechanical respiratory assistance have been used in a domiciliary setting to support the respiratory function of such patients. It has been reported that these patients can have a meaningful life even though they require continuous mechanical ventilatory aids [1,5,88,146].

Friedreich's Ataxia

Friedreich's ataxia is characterized by cardiac myopathy with decreased ventricular compliance and varying degrees of hypertrophy and, less frequently, obstruction to ventricular outflow. Cardiopulmonary dysfunction is a primary cause of death in patients suffering from Friedreich's ataxia that occurs at a young age, averaging 28 years. Progression of the neuromuscular disease in these patients leads to total respiratory failure. Three mechanisms contribute to the eventual fatal outcome: (1) The severe scoliosis found in these patients leads to respiratory failure; (2) the neuromuscular dysfunction decreases the efficiency of the respiratory muscles; and (3) pulmonary edema occurs secondary to cardiomyopathy. Pulmonary function in patients with Friedreich's ataxia shows decreases in total lung capacity and VC with elevation of the residual volume and functional residual capacity (FRC). Scoliosis itself may cause most of the respiratory difficulty in patients with Friedreich's ataxia [25].

Further follow-up and a repeat study 3 years later in the 15 patients suffering from classic Friedreich's ataxia showed striking decreases in residual volume and FRC [25]. These changes could not be attributed entirely to progression of the scoliosis, since residual volume has been shown to be independent of the degree of scoliosis. Hence, it was concluded that the deterioration of cardiopulmonary function in Friedreich's ataxia was multifactorial, and the neuromyopathy appeared to be the main contributing factor to deterioration of cardiopulmonary function, which is exacerbated by the scoliosis and varying severity of the cardiomyopathy. Another surprising finding was the low incidence of pulmonary infections in these patients [37].

Steinert's Myotonic Dystrophy

Steinert's myotonic dystrophy is a genetically transmitted (autosomal dominant) neuromuscular disease that is known to lead to premature death from cardiopulmonary complications.

These patients develop both acute and chronic respiratory failure. The acute respiratory insufficiency is first diagnosed by the failure to generate the first postnatal breath, leading to ventilatory support in the neonatal period [195]. In adults with Steinert's dystrophy, acute respiratory disease can be precipitated during recovery from general anesthesia. In chronic respiratory complications of Steinert's dystrophy, pneumonia, weakness of the respiratory muscles with hypoventilation, increased work of breathing, and altered central control of respiration contribute to respiratory failure. Both the blunted chemical drive of breathing and the respiratory muscle weakness have been cited in the pathophysiology of premature death in these patients. However, refined studies have shown that the chemosensitivity of the respiratory centers is well preserved in Steinert's muscular dystrophy, but the output to breathing is modulated by the impaired ventilatory mechanics, which causes tachypnea, even in the absence of restricted lung volume [7].

Demyelinating Diseases

In patients with demyelinating diseases such as multiple sclerosis, respiratory complications are uncommon and, if present, only mild. In a report on the natural history of multiple sclerosis in 840 patients, it was noted that involvement of the vital centers of the central nervous system was rare and was confined to patients with acute disease who died within a few months of onset. This series included three deaths from respiratory failure, one of which was within 3 months of onset [132]. Studies on the natural cause of multiple sclerosis have observed a 1 to 2 percent instance of death due to bulbar dysfunction, often within months of disease onset.

In a report on four cases of respiratory failure in multiple sclerosis, the presence of quadriparesis and high segmental sensory levels was emphasized [80]. In these patients, the respiratory failure was believed to be secondary to demyelinating lesions involving the bulbar area (especially the area of the respiratory center) and pyramidal tracts bilaterally and possibly the anterior horns [20]. Severe spinal cord involvement by the demyelinating process may be accompanied by respiratory failure. Hyperventilation, decreased response to carbon dioxide, irregular breathing, and sleep-induced apnea have been noted in such patients, presumably caused by destruction of cervical spinal pathways [112,165,182]. Three cases of spontaneous pneumothorax have been described in patients with multiple sclerosis. These were found among 141 patients identified as incidence cases of spontaneous pneumothorax in an epidemiologic study [136]. This occurrence was reported to be unlikely on the basis of chance alone. A statistically low incidence (less than expected) of pulmonary embolism has been noted in multiple sclerosis [103]. A recent study of 40 patients concluded that descriptive clinical indices and clinical assessment were superior to spirometry as predictors of clinical illness; however, MVV uncovered subtle respiratory muscle weakness [198].

Other Neuropathies

Charcot-Marie-Tooth disease encompasses a collection of chronic degenerative neuropathic conditions and includes cases of hereditary motor and sensory neuropathies. The major clinical feature is the slowly progressive and predominantly distal and lower-limb effects of the disease. Diaphragmatic dysfunction has been described in several patients with this disease [117]. Neuropathic changes characteristic of the disease have been observed in phrenic nerves [62].

Other Myopathies

METABOLIC MYOPATHIES

Acid maltase deficiency is one of the metabolic myopathies known to cause respiratory failure. It is a type II glycogen storage disease, known also as *Pompe's disease*. Because of the deficiency of the enzyme acid maltase, engorgement of cellular vacuoles with glycogen occurs [107]. Acid maltase deficiency presenting with respiratory failure has been reported [159,184]. These patients can develop proximal myopathy and weakness as well as diaphragmatic dysfunction. Isolated diaphragmatic paralysis also has been noted [196]. Acid maltase deficiency classically affects infants and children, with a few sporadic cases occurring in adults.

Respiratory involvement, including ventilatory failure and diaphragmatic paralysis, has been described in various types of myopathies, including centronuclear myopathies (congenital myotubular myopathy), progressive congenital myopathy with type I fiber atrophy, Isaac's syndrome (myokymia, generalized muscular stiffness, and decreased tendon reflexes), and Kearns-Sayre syndrome (also known as *oculocraniosomatic neuromuscular disease*, characterized by a combination of all or some of the following: ptosis,

external ophthalmoplegia, retinal degeneration, axial muscle weakness, deafness, ataxia, pyramidal tract abnormalities, small stature, mental retardation, endocrine abnormalities, and cardiac conduction defects) [99,102,177]. Chronic respiratory failure requiring mechanical ventilation has been described in two patients with an adult-onset form of mitochondrial myopathy [38].

Hereditary porphyrias (acute intermittent porphyria, porphyria variegata, and hereditary coproporphyria) are disorders of porphyrin metabolism. Each of these may be associated with ascending paralysis and respiratory failure. The neuropathy in these diseases probably is caused by the toxic effect of the accumulated porphyrin precursors aminolevulinic acid and porphobilinogen.

Muscular weakness and respiratory failure have been noted in rhabdomyolysis (myoglobinuria) [9], hypophosphatemia [158], hypokalemia [51], polymyositis-dermatomyositis [101], and familial periodic paralysis [76].

TOXIC MYOPATHIES

Organophosphate and carbonate poisoning are a common occurrence in certain regions of the world where these compounds are used as agricultural insecticides. Accidental or suicidal ingestion can lead to serious respiratory problems as a result of muscarinic and nicotinic effects. They cause muscle paralysis by inhibiting acetylcholinesterase. The pulmonary features include rhinorrhea, excessive bronchial secretions, pulmonary edema, laryngospasm, bronchospasm, respiratory muscle paralysis, and paralysis of respiratory medulla. In a report on 107 subjects in Taiwan exposed to organophosphate or carbonate, 40 percent developed respiratory failure and 51 percent died [204]. The use of pralidoxime did not reduce the incidence of respiratory failure. Importantly, aggressive treatment within the first 96 hours resulted in prevention of respiratory failure [204].

Botulism is a disorder of the neuromuscular junction caused by the binding of one of eight neurotoxins (labeled *A* through *G*) elaborated by the bacterium *Clostridium botulinum*. Botulism characteristically causes multiple cranial motor neuropathies. Clinical findings include blurred vision, paralysis of pupillary muscles, ileus, dry mouth, and descending paralysis involving extraocular and bulbar muscles, with frequent progression to respiratory muscle weakness. Muscle weakness of upper airways may result in dysphonia and nasal regurgitation. A study of six patients with botulism observed weakness of ventilatory muscles early in the course of poisoning in all patients, but recovery was the rule, though it took several months [214]. Long-term follow-up in 13 patients revealed that residual symptoms including dyspnea and fatigue were common at 2 years after intoxication, even though lung functions had returned to normal in all [213].

Summary of the Respiratory Problems in Myoneuronal and Muscular Disorders

The main respiratory problems in neuropathies and dystrophic muscular diseases include hypoventilation with progressive respiratory failure, a restrictive type of pulmonary dysfunction, aspiration pneumonia, repeated infections, and cardiopulmonary problems in patients with cardiomyopathy associated with certain muscular dystrophies. Depending on the severity of the underlying disease, patients may complain of anxiety, lethargy, headaches, dyspnea and, occasionally, a sensation of suffocation. Severe hypoventilation will lead to confusion, coma, cyanosis, severe hypoxemia, hypercapnia, and death. In addition to the hypoventilation, these patients develop alveolar collapse, which produces low pulmonary compliance. It has been shown in patients with severe long-standing respiratory muscle weakness that marked alterations in the static mechanical properties of the lungs are noted. One study has revealed that these alterations cannot be reversed by a 15-minute period of intermittent positive-pressure breathing treatment [42]. Positive end-expiratory pressure treatment in patients with lobar atelectasis in amyotrophic lateral sclerosis has been reported to be useful [105]. Spirometric evaluation of lung function and assessment of respiratory muscles by performing inspiratory and expiratory pressures should aid in gauging the severity of the respiratory involvement in these patients [77]. The role of tracheostomy and chronic ventilatory assistance in these patients, especially those with amyotrophic lateral sclerosis, is questionable.

Diseases of Peripheral Nerves and Anterior Horn Cells

Poliomyelitis

Poliomyelitis is a typical example of an anterior horn cell disease that can lead to respiratory failure. Unless arterial blood gas analyses are performed in these patients, respiratory involvement from poliomyelitis may go undetected. Many of these patients remain in a state of chronic hypoventilation. Pulmonary function studies in patients who have recovered from poliomyelitis but who have residual muscle weakness have demonstrated that the majority experience exertional dyspnea and recurrent respiratory tract infections [40]. Late onset of respiratory failure and polycythemia have been described in a significant number of patients with previous poliomyelitis [114]. Kyphoscoliosis and diaphragmatic paralysis in these patients aggravate the respiratory problems and produce ventilation-perfusion imbalance, which eventually results in respiratory failure [114]. In a study of 55 patients with previous poliomyelitis, VC was almost immediately reduced to approximately 20 to 40 percent of the predicted normal values, often on the order of 1 liter or less. Total lung capacity was correspondingly reduced in the majority of patients, but residual volume was within normal limits. The PaO_2 was generally surprisingly normal despite severe restriction of the VC. However, at VCs below 50 percent of the predicted value, 60 percent of patients had a PaO_2 of less than 80 mmHg. Hypercapnia was seen at some stage in 35 percent of these patients [114]. The decreased VC may be due to diminished compliance of the chest wall and the lung parenchyma.

In patients with previous poliomyelitis and severe respiratory failure, long-term ventilatory assistance is required. Four years after the epidemic of poliomyelitis in Copenhagen in 1952, in which 264 patients were submitted to tracheostomy and 232 were treated with positive-pressure ventilation, 24 of 138 survivors were considered to be chronic respirator-dependent patients. Nine of these died during the next 17 years. Among the 24 chronic patients, 13 were alive in 1975 and were still receiving constant ventilatory assistance [33].

Landry-Guillain-Barré Syndrome

Landry-Guillain-Barré syndrome (acute polyneuritis) is probably the most common neuromuscular cause of acute respiratory failure [164]. It is a demyelinating disease of motor neurons and, clinically, it manifests as symmetric ascending paralysis and a lack of cellular response in the cerebrospinal fluid despite an increase in protein concentration. A typical patient is younger than 26 years or between 45 and 60 years of age. Seasonal clustering (late summer and autumn) is one of the features of this disease. However, atypical clinical features may make it difficult to diagnose and, therefore, a process of exclusion is necessary. The clinical course of Landry-Guillain-Barré syndrome is variable, but complete recovery can be expected in most patients, though the mortality without ventilatory support in the past has averaged from 20 to more than 60 percent. Most deaths occur from cardiopulmonary complications. Nearly half the patients with Landry-Guillain-Barré syndrome develop respiratory complications. Intercostal muscular and diaphragmatic paralysis produce progressive alveolar hypoventilation. The patient frequently is not disturbed by this weakness because of the gradual onset and slow progression. Significant respiratory muscle insufficiency can be present without being detected clinically. Hence, frequent bedside monitoring of basic respiratory parameters is extremely important. Paralysis of the ninth and tenth cranial nerves may lead to dysphagia, laryngeal paralysis, and aspiration. Although systemic corticosteroids have been used in these patients, because of the extremely variable course of the disease it is difficult to evaluate the role of this medication. In patients presenting with unexplained respiratory deficiency, careful evaluation should be performed to exclude an underlying variant of Landry-Guillain-Barré syndrome [190]. Neurogenic pulmonary edema has occurred in patients with Landry-Guillain-Barré syndrome.

Respiratory failure from Landry-Guillain-Barré syndrome often requires mechanical ventilatory support and precautions to prevent such complications as aspiration pneumonia and secondary infections [70]. The Mayo Clinic experience with 79 patients with acute Landry-Guillain-Barré syndrome seen during a 6-year period revealed that 27 percent required admittance to the respiratory intensive care unit for 14 to 105 days. Nasotracheal intubation followed by tracheostomy and mechanical ventilation were required in 18 percent. The mortality due to complications of the disease or its treatment was 3.8 percent [70]. Repeated VC measurements have been used as predictive parameters for the need for mechanical ventilation and weaning success [31].

Amyotrophic Lateral Sclerosis

Amyotrophic lateral sclerosis is the most common motor neuron disease in the United States [215]. Most patients with amyotrophic lateral sclerosis have progressive neurologic deterioration without remission, with an average life expectancy after the onset of symptoms of 3.6 years [154]. Destruction of the anterior horn cells in the spinal cord leads to atrophic muscle weakness.

Neuropathologic studies of this disease have shown that the anterior horn cell loss is most marked in the cervical, lumbosacral, and lower thoracic spinal segments, with relative sparing of upper and midthoracic areas. Some degree of respiratory muscle involvement can be detected in most patients before respiratory symptoms begin [138]. Occasionally, amyotrophic lateral sclerosis may present with respiratory failure as the initial manifestation [56]. Irreversible hypoventilation leading to fatal respiratory failure is common in the later stages of the disease [56]. Sleep hypopnea as the presenting symptom has been described [28]. The second major problem is aspiration pneumonia, as 25 percent of patients with amyotrophic lateral sclerosis have bulbar paralysis, which aggravates the problem of aspiration [56] (Fig. 64-5). Respiratory insufficiency in patients with amyotrophic lateral sclerosis also may be due to unilateral or bilateral diaphragmatic paralysis [170,197].

In a study of 218 patients with amyotrophic lateral sclerosis, 204 were found to have abnormal lung functions. Significantly, abnormal functions included decreased MVV and FVC [49]. Pulmonary function tests in patients with this disease normally show severe diminution of maximal inspiratory and expiratory pressures as well as severe reductions in VC, maximal midexpiratory flow, and maximal breathing capacity [15], but the majority of patients have been reported to

Fig. 64-5. Recurrent episodes of aspiration pneumonia secondary to bulbar involvement in amyotrophic lateral sclerosis.

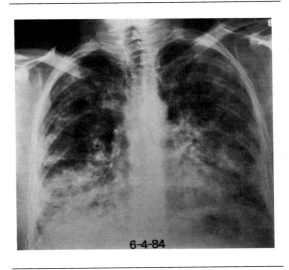

have abnormally low total lung capacity, VC, and MVV, an abnormally high residual volume and total lung capacity, and an unaltered residual volume and FRC. Although clinically it is not well recognized, obstructive pulmonary disease has been noted in up to 19 percent of patients with amyotrophic lateral sclerosis [49]. The etiology is likely related to bulbar incoordination leading to a repetitive aspiration and obstruction of the upper airways. Other studies have shown that total lung capacity is well preserved even in an advanced stage of the disease, provided that diaphragmatic function is not grossly compromised and elevation of residual volume is well correlated with severity of muscle weakness [109]. It has been shown that maximal expiratory flow-volume relationships serve to identify patients with more severe expiratory muscle weakness who may be predicted to have a marked decrease in VC and flow with small changes in resistance and thus may be at risk for developing respiratory failure during relatively minor respiratory illnesses [109,187]. In addition to the abnormally low MVV, the easiest test to measure respiratory muscle weakness is maximal inspiratory and expiratory pressures using the simple "bugle" spirometer [15]. Spirometry also can help in the continued evaluation of the status of respiratory failure.

The prognosis in the motor neuron diseases depends on the rapidity with which the underlying disorder progresses and the degree of respiratory muscle involvement [89]. Aggressive chronic ventilatory assistance and tracheostomy are not usually recommended in these patients because of the slow but relentless progression of the disease. Measures to prevent aspiration pneumonia and nonaggressive palliative therapy are the prudent goals.

An unusual type of motor neuron disease with peculiar flaccid paralysis has been recognized in some children recovering from episodes of asthma. Clinical features have included seizures and semiconsciousness. In addition, paralysis similar to poliomyelitis following severe episodes of asthma has been reported in at least 18 children, occurring between 1968 and 1976. It has been hypothesized that this syndrome may be due to subtle immunologic abnormalities [6].

Dyskinetic Disorders

Extrapyramidal diseases such as parkinsonian syndrome may produce severe, prolonged spasm of the respiratory musculature and consequent respiratory insufficiency. Respiratory abnormalities described in extrapyramidal diseases are now believed to involve the nigrostriatal dopaminergic system. In addition, these patients had episodes of respiratory spasms or tics associated with grunting, snorting, or puffing. It was postulated that the respiratory dyskinesias were related to destruction of mesoencephalopontine respiratory centers governing the lower bulbar regions.

Parkinson's Disease

Parkinson's disease is a common dyskinetic disorder and, although pulmonary involvement is frequent and considered to be the common cause of death, it rarely is recognized clinically. Parkinson's disease is associated with pathologic changes in the reticular formation of the brain stem, and hence the afferent or efferent pathways involved in the control of respiration may be affected. Studies have shown that more than 85 percent of patients have impaired ventilatory function, which appears to relate to the severity of the disease rather than to underlying lung disease [162,206]. Erratic breathing, also known as *chaotic breathing*, is a common finding in patients with Parkinson's disease. The ventilatory defect appears to be due to the rigidity and weakness of respiratory muscles, which are ameliorated with treatment, similar to the response of optimally treated skeletal muscles elsewhere [135].

Upper airways obstruction is relatively common in Parkinson's patients [17,208]. In a report on the detailed pulmonary function of 31 patients with Parkinson's disease, obstructive type of pulmonary functions were identified in one-third of the patients, and these had a history of chronic bronchitis and demonstrated no functional improvement with L-dopa (levodopa) therapy. However, significant improvement of symptoms from Parkinson's disease was noted, and hence it was concluded that the obstructive pulmonary disease did not result from the Parkinson's disease [162]. In contrast, another study of 10 patients exhibited a significant improvement in MVV following therapy with L-dopa, but there was no correlation between clinical and pulmonary functional improvement [115]. It has been postulated that the obstructive lung disease in Parkinson's disease may be related to increased parasympathetic tone and infections [4]. Levodopa therapy may reverse the upper airways obstruction in these patients [207].

Levodopa is a commonly used drug in Parkinson's disease. Patients with neuroleptic-induced tardive dyskinesia or with levodopa-induced dyskinesia may have acute dyspnea and chest pain secondary to severe, involuntary muscle incoordination [210]. Bromocriptine has been used in the treatment of Parkinson's disease [181]. In a review of 123 patients in whom this medication was used, 6 were found to have pleurisy accompanied by effusion, pleural thickening, and pulmonary infiltrates. The daily dose of bromocriptine ranged from 20 to 90 mg, and the duration of treatment ranged from 6 to 27 months. Three of the patients also were taking levodopa with benserazide, from 400 to 800 mg/day [181]. The pleural pulmonary complications are believed to be from bromocriptine rather than levodopa. Similar complications have been noted in a patient receiving cabergoline [55]. Bromocriptine is reported to cause coronary vasospasm and lead to myocardial infarction; 24 such cases were identified in the literature [119]. The bromocriptine-induced myocardial infarction and secondary pulmonary edema should be considered in any patient using this drug.

Respiratory Dyskinesia

Extrapyramidal dysfunction not related to Parkinson's disease has been shown to be associated with dyspnea, and the term *respiratory dyskinesia* has been used to describe this. Respiratory dyskinesia probably is related to destruction of mesoencephalopontine respiratory centers governing the lower bulbar regions and the abnormal, irregular respiratory movements resulting from a release of formerly inhibited brain stem areas. It may mimic chronic psychogenic hyperventilation syndrome, and so it has been called *pseudopsychogenic hyperventilation*. In both respiratory dyskinesia and chronic hyperventilation syndrome, abnormal respiratory movements worsen with stress and disappear with sleep. In patients with respiratory dyskinesia, speech is interrupted by involuntary sounds or grunts, respirations are awkward, and the patient appears distressed and anxious even when pain or dyspnea is denied [74]. Episodes of respiratory spasms or tics associated with grunting, snorting, or puffing may be seen.

In a report of four patients who suffered from severe involuntary respiratory dyskinesia, respiratory findings included irregular respiratory rate, shortness of breath, and discomfort in the chest [210]. The respiratory dyskinesia occurred as one aspect of more generalized choreiform movement disorders. Three of these patients had neuroleptic-induced tardive dyskinesias, and one had levodopa-induced dyskinesia. It is interesting to note that because of the nature of the complaints, some of these patients initially are believed to have cardiopulmonary disorders. Their respirations were irregular in rate and depth and associated with involuntary grunting and gasping noises. Dopaminergic manipulation was successful in correcting the subjective discomfort and the respiratory abnormalities in all these patients. Reserpine was used in three patients, and the levodopa dosage was lowered in another [210].

Tardive Dyskinesia

Tardive dyskinesia is a syndrome of involuntary movement with characteristic facial involvement and temporal association with neuroleptic drug ingestion. Control studies of patients with tardive dyskinesia have disclosed that respiratory dyskinesia may well be a part of tardive dyskinesia syndrome [100]. It is recommended that examinations of patients with subjective tardive dyskinesia should include an assessment of respiratory function [100]. Stiff-man syndrome is reported to be associated with progressive respiratory failure [27].

In a large group of chronically hospitalized patients with psychiatric illness, clinical evidence of irregular respiration (respiratory tardive dyskinesia) was observed in 2 percent. In patients with tardive dyskinesia, the respiratory abnormalities were noted in 7 percent. The prevalence of respiratory irregularities was significantly greater (11 percent) in patients with an organic mental disorder compared to those without. None had respiratory symptoms [217].

Cerebellar Disorders

Arnold-Chiari Malformation

Arnold-Chiari malformation is a congenital anomaly consisting of caudal displacement of the inferior cerebellar vermis, kinking of the medulla oblongata, a small posterior fossa, a low tentorium cerebelli, and displacement of the fourth ventricle into the spinal canal. Coexistence of spina bifida, hydrocephalus, and other anomalies of the neural axis is common. The most common respiratory problem is dramatic onset of laryngeal stridor. The stridor appears precipitously and is closely correlated with increased intracranial pressure. The cause remains controversial. Three mechanisms have been postulated, and all implied involvement of vagus nerves: brain stem disease, compression of the vagus nerves at the level of the foramen magnum, and traction of the vagus nerves by caudal displacement of the brain stem. In addition to the laryngeal stridor, studies in these patients have shown depressed ventilatory response to CO_2 [111]. In a series of 21 infants with this problem, respiratory obstruction and apnea with bilateral abductor vocal cord paralysis were described [92].

Arnold-Chiari malformation and syringomyelia both may produce respiratory problems by impairing the functions of the ninth, tenth, and twelfth cranial nerves, and have been described with total absence of a normal ventilatory response to hypoxia, presumably because of the destruction of afferent pathways in the ninth cranial nerve [18]. Respiratory abnormalities such as respiratory distress, apnea, vocal cord paralysis, and inability to swallow are known complications of the Arnold-Chiari malformation. Hemorrhages in the medulla oblongata and compression or traction of the vagus and other lower cranial nerves may cause these symptoms, but anatomic confirmation of the mechanism is sketchy. In a study of 14 children with Arnold-Chiari malformation, vascular lesions resulting in hemorrhage, hemorrhagic necrosis, or bland infarcts in the tegmentum of the medulla oblongata were found in 12 children with clinical abnormalities of respiratory function and dysfunction of the lower cranial nerves [169]. Respiratory problems frequently cause death or markedly shorten the life expectancy of affected children. Surgical decompression of the posterior fossa has been shown to relieve respiratory symptoms in some cases [91]. Respiratory dysfunction, dysphagia, and aspiration pneumonia often are temporarily related to increased intracranial pressure. Physiologic studies have shown that patients with uncomplicated Arnold-Chiari malformation have normal respiratory function [111].

Joubert's Syndrome

Joubert's syndrome is characterized by agenesis of the cerebellar vermis with abnormal eye movements, ataxia, retardation, and episodic hyperpnea. An abnormal respiratory pattern—namely, persistent tachypnea from birth—is the clinical hallmark of Joubert's syndrome and may be detectable in utero, thus permitting prenatal diagnosis. Peak respiratory rates in excess of 200

breaths per minute while awake and 150 breaths per minute with tachypneic episodes lasting up to 150 seconds have been described in these patients [19]. Apneic episodes in non-REM sleep lasting 10 to 20 seconds, with a maximum duration of 45 seconds, have been observed [19].

Ataxia-Telangiectasia

Also known as *Louis-Bar syndrome*, ataxia-telangiectasia is characterized by a progressive cerebellar ataxia, oculocutaneous telangiectasia, and recurrent sinopulmonary infections. This disorder is associated with deficiency of IgA and IgE and the development of lymphoreticular malignancies. In addition, granulocytopenia, noted in many of these patients, is a factor in frequent infections. Repeated sinopulmonary infections are noted in three-fourths of patients with ataxia-telangiectasia, usually starting at approximately 4 to 6 years of age. Infection in nonrespiratory organs is uncommon. Severe neurologic impairment, bronchiectasis, and pulmonary fibrosis are usually progressive, leading to death by the time of adolescence. Roentgenologically, abnormalities are similar to those in cystic fibrosis, and both diseases also manifest chronic paranasal sinusitis [167]. Upper airway dysfunction, identified by abnormal maximum inspiratory and expiratory flow-volume loops, has been described in patients with olivopontocerebellar atrophy [189].

Autonomic Nervous System and Peripheral Chemoreceptors

Carotid Body Resection

Respiratory hypoxic drive is controlled primarily by peripheral chemoreceptors situated in the carotid bodies. Therapeutic carotid body resection has been advocated for bronchial asthma, but beneficial effects have not been proved. Bilateral carotid endarterectomy in such patients may abolish compensatory hyperventilation, and these patients become hypoxemic [125]. Bilateral carotid body resection may preclude compensatory ventilation when hypoxemia develops [209]. In a report on patients who underwent bilateral carotid body resection for asthma, the ventilatory response to increased $PaCO_2$ was reduced, but hypoventilation did not occur. Although the carotid bodies are believed to initiate the hyperpneic response to hypoxia, they have no part in ventilatory control in normal persons at sea level, either at rest or after exercise [125,209]. A patient has been described who developed cough syncope and was found to have carotid sinus hypersensitivity with mixed cardioinhibitory and vasodepressive responses. Cough syncope was ameliorated by denervation of the more hypersensitive carotid sinus [212].

Sympathectomy

Dorsal sympathectomy is performed for a wide spectrum of diseases with abnormal sympathetic function. Most patients complain of some shortness of breath during the first days after the operation. Pulmonary function tests were performed in a group of 15 patients before and 1 to 3 months after upper dorsal sympathectomy [147]. Significant decreases in all compartments of lung volume and maximal expiratory flows were discovered. The reasons for these include a loss of diaphragmatic tone as a result of the surgical procedure, surgical transection of the scalenus anticus muscle leading to impairment of maximal inspiration and decreases in total lung capacity and vital capacity, and pneumoconstriction due to sympathetic denervation [147].

Familial Dysautonomia

Familial dysautonomia (Riley-Day syndrome) is a mendelian recessive disease that is associated with a relative familial unresponsiveness to hypoxia and hypercapnia [22]. This incapacity is believed to result from a defect in the carotid body. Breath-holding attacks have been seen in 66 percent of 210 children with familial dysautonomia [22], and fleeting episodes of hyperventilation followed by profound hypoxia have been observed. Hyperventilation followed by hypoxia, attributed to incoordinate central depression consequent to reduced cerebral blood flow, has been reported in these patients [149].

Acquired Dysautonomias

Both central and obstructive sleep apnea occur in patients with autonomic nervous system dysfunction. Dysautonomias as a result of diabetic autonomic neuropathy [168], amyloidosis [48], Shy-Drager syndrome [78], and Arnold-Chiari malformation and syringomyelia [18] can be associated with respiratory failure due to the inability of the chemoreceptors to respond to hypoxia. Presumably, this blunting of carotid body response is caused by destruction of the ninth cranial nerve. In a study of 13 patients with familial dysautonomia, polysomnographic recordings revealed abnormal sleep patterns with decreased amounts of REM sleep and increased REM latencies in all patients [59]. The average number of apneic spells was 73 per night. A detailed report of a 6-year-old girl who developed sleep-induced hypoventilation and apnea with diffused dysautonomic changes has been published. This patient died 2 years later during sleep. Detailed pathologic examination revealed a ganglioneuroma originating in the sympathetic ganglia. This type of acquired progressive dysautonomia is rare. Other causes of dysautonomia include botulism, generalized neuropathy, neoplasms, Parkinson's disease, bilateral cervical cordotomy, and bulbar poliomyelitis [53].

Miscellaneous Neurologic Disorders

Cerebral Palsy

Youngsters with cerebral palsy may be prone to respiratory infections because of alterations in the ventilatory capacity. These alterations are a result of involvement of the neuromotor control; hence, the muscles used for breathing may be affected, which results in decreased efficiency and poor coordination of the breathing mechanism. In one study of dynamic and static lung volumes in children with cerebral palsy, total capacity was significantly reduced, averaging 85 percent of the predicted normal values [14]: A 50 percent decrease in VC occurred for subjects with dyskinesia, and a 67 percent decrease in patients with spasticity also was noted. These children behaved like patients with chronic obstructive pulmonary disease [14]. Breathing exercises in a study of 10 children with spastic cerebral palsy showed a mean increase in VC to 30 percent more than the pretest values, and this increase in VC nearly matched the normal predicted levels [185]. Another study has shown that the chronic cerebellar stimulation in a patient with cerebral palsy improves respiratory muscle coordination [145].

Migraine

In patients with migraine headaches, severe hyperventilation leading to diagnostic difficulties has been described. In the reported cases, hyperventilation occurred at the height of the migraine, making the attack seem worse to the patient. It is speculated that the migraine was exacerbated by the vasoconstrictor effect of hyperventilation

[16]. The term *pulmonary migraine* was suggested to describe a localized atelectasis of the lung associated with migraine headaches in a 14-year-old girl [205]. Neuropathologic findings included deep microinfarctions in the basal ganglia and a remarkable sparing of brain stem nuclei associated with the function of respiration [156].

Reye's Syndrome

Reye's syndrome is characterized by encephalopathy and fatty accumulation in visceral organs in children. This disorder has been shown to be associated with hypoxemia, hypocapnia, and tachypnea, as well as interstitial pneumonitis, thickening of the alveolar walls, and intraalveolar foamy histiocytes. Excessive lipolysis and mobilization of fat occur in Reye's syndrome, and it is possible that the lungs and, in particular, the alveoli and the alveolar interstitial spaces would be confronted with excessive amounts of fatty acids, especially since there is evidence to suggest that fatty acids are sometimes excreted through respiration [21].

Krabbe's Globoid Cell Leukodystrophy

Krabbe's globoid cell leukodystrophy is a hereditary degenerative brain disease caused by lack of the enzyme galactosylceramide galactosidase. The disease is characterized by the progressive development of retardation, failure to thrive, seizures, spasticity, and blindness, culminating in death by age 2 to 3 years. Symptoms begin at 4 to 8 months of age. A report of an 8-week-old boy presenting with rapidly progressive respiratory failure and death, with lung biopsy showing presence of numerous intraalveolar and a few interstitial macrophages, has been published [35]. Cultures of the lung were negative for infection, and numerous intraalveolar macrophages were identified containing intracellular structures that stained positively for periodic acid–Schiff.

Electroconvulsive Therapy

Electroconvulsive therapy is used in the treatment of major depressive disorders, schizophrenia, mania, and other conditions. Aspiration may occur, especially in elderly patients. Neurogenic pulmonary edema is another complication observed in these patients [39,60,191].

Ventriculoatrial and ventriculoperitoneal shunts are placed to treat high-pressure hydrocephalus. The catheter tips occasionally become blocked or infected. Recurrent discharge of the proteinaceous debris from the catheter tip into the pulmonary circulation can produce recurrent embolic phenomena and secondary pulmonary hypertension. The onset of pulmonary hypertension in these patients is insidious and invariably leads to right ventricular failure. Empyema has been described as a complication of ventriculoperitoneal shunt [98].

References

1. Alexander MA, et al. Mechanical ventilation of patients with late-stage Duchenne muscular dystrophy: Management in the home. *Arch Phys Med Rehabil* 60:289, 1979.
2. Arborelius M Jr, Lilja B, Senyk J. Regional and total lung function studies in patients with hemidiaphragmatic paralysis. *Respiration* 32:253, 1975.
3. Atack EA, Suranyi L. Respiratory inhibitory apraxia. *Can J Neurol Sci* 2:37, 1975.
4. Bateman DN, et al. Levodopa dosage and ventilatory function in pulmonary disease. *Br Med J* 283:190, 1981.
5. Baydur A, et al. Decline in respiratory function and experience with long-term assisted ventilation in advanced Duchenne's muscular dystrophy. *Chest* 97:884, 1990.
6. Beede HE, Newcomb RW. Lower motor neuron paralysis in association with asthma. *Johns Hopkins Med J* 147:186, 1980.
7. Begin R, et al. Control and modulation of respiration in Steinert's myotonic dystrophy. *Am Rev Respir Dis* 121:281, 1980.
8. Bellamy R, Pitts FW, Stauffer ES. Respiratory complications in traumatic quadriplegia: Analysis of 20 years' experience. *J Neurosurg* 39:596, 1973.
9. Berenson M, Yarvote P, Grace WJ. Idiopathic myoglobinuria with respiratory paralysis. *Am Rev Respir Dis* 94:956, 1966.
10. Bergofsky EH. Mechanism for respiratory insufficiency after cervical cord injury: A source of alveolar hypoventilation. *Ann Intern Med* 61:435, 1964.
11. Bhaskar KR, et al. Bronchial mucus hypersecretion in acute quadriplegia. *Am Rev Respir Dis* 143:640, 1991.
12. Biberstein MP, Eisenberg H. Unilateral diaphragmatic paralysis in association with Erb's palsy. *Chest* 75:209, 1979.
13. Biot MC. Contribution a l'etude du phenomene respiratoire de Cheyne-Stokes. *Lyon Med* 23:517, 1876.
14. Bjure J, Berg K. Dynamic and static lung volumes of school children with cerebral palsy. *Acta Paediatr Scand Suppl* 204:35, 1971.

15. Black LF, Hyatt RE. Maximal static respiratory pressures in generalized neuromuscular disease. *Am Rev Respir Dis* 103:641, 1971.

16. Blau JN, Dexter SL. Hyperventilation during migraine attack. *Br Med J* 280:1254, 1980.

17. Bogaard JM, et al. Maximal expiratory and inspiratory flow-volume curves in Parkinson's disease. *Am Rev Respir Dis* 139:610, 1989.

18. Bokinsky GE, Hudson LD, Weil JV. Impaired peripheral chemosensitivity and acute respiratory failure in Arnold-Chiari malformations and syringomyelia. *N Engl J Med* 288:947, 1973.

19. Bolthauser E, et al. Joubert syndrome: Clinical and polygraphic observation in a further case. *Neuropediatrics* 12:181, 1981.

20. Boor JW, et al. Reversible paralysis of automatic respiration in multiple sclerosis. *Arch Neurol* 34:686, 1977.

21. Brown RE, Madge GE. Pulmonary findings in Reye's syndrome. *Arch Pathol* 92:475, 1971.

22. Brunt PW, McKusick VA. Familial dysautonomia: A report of genetic and clinical studies, with a review of the literature. *Medicine* 49:343, 1970.

23. Buisseret P. Acute pulmonary edema following grand mal epilepsy and as a complication of electric shock therapy. *Br J Dis Chest* 76:194, 1982.

24. Burke SS, et al. Respiratory aspects of pseudohypertrophic muscular dystrophy. *Am J Dis Child* 121:230, 1971.

25. Burreau MA, et al. Pulmonary function studies in Friedreich's ataxia. *Can J Neurol Sci* 3:343, 1976.

26. Cameron GR, De SN. Experimental pulmonary oedema of nervous origin. *J Pathol Bacteriol* 61:375, 1949.

27. Campbell JR. Stiff-man syndrome and emphysema. *Arch Neurol* 36:387, 1979.

28. Carre PC, et al. Amyotrophic lateral sclerosis presenting with sleep hypopnea syndrome. *Chest* 93:1309, 1988.

29. Carroll JE, Zwillich CW, Weil JV. Ventilatory response in myotonic dystrophy. *Neurology* 27:1125, 1977.

30. Cherniack NS, Longobardo GS. Cheyne-Stokes breathing: An instability in physiologic control. *N Engl J Med* 288:952, 1973.

31. Chevrolet J-C, Deleamont P. Repeated vital capacity measurements as predictive parameters for mechanical ventilation need and weaning success in the Guillain-Barré syndrome. *Am Rev Respir Dis* 144:814, 1991.

32. Cheyne J. A case of apoplexy in which the fleshy part of the heart was converted into fat. *Dublin Hosp Rec* 2:211, 1918.

33. Christensen MS, Kristensen HS, Hansen EL. Artificial hyperventilation during 21 years in three cases of complete respiratory paralysis. *Acta Med Scand* 198:409, 1975.

34. Clague HW, Hall DR. Effect of posture on lung volume: Airway closure and gas exchange in hemidiaphragmatic paralysis. *Thorax* 34:523, 1979.

35. Clarke JTR, Ozere RL, Krause VW. Early infantile variant of Krabbe globoid cell leukodystrophy with lung involvement. *Arch Dis Child* 56:640, 1981.

36. Coccagna G, et al. Alveolar hypoventilation and hypersomnia in myotonic dystrophy. *J Neurol Neurosurg Psychiatry* 38:977, 1975.

37. Cote M, LaRose A, Lamieux B. Evolution of cardiopulmonary involvement in Friedreich's ataxia. *Can J Neurol Sci* 6:151, 1979.

38. Cros D, et al. Respiratory failure revealing mitochondrial myopathy in adults. *Chest* 101:824, 1992.

39. Darnell JC, Jay SJ. Recurrent postictal pulmonary edema: A case report and review of the literature. *Epilepsia* 23:71, 1982.

40. Dean E, et al. Pulmonary function in individuals with a history of poliomyelitis. *Chest* 100:118, 1991.

41. De Troyer A, Borenstein S. Acute changes in respiratory mechanics after pyridostigmine injection in patients with myasthenia gravis. *Am Rev Respir Dis* 121:629, 1980.

42. De Troyer A, Deisser P. The effects of intermittent positive-pressure breathing on patients with respiratory muscle weakness. *Am Rev Respir Dis* 12:132, 1981.

43. De Troyer A, Heilporn HP. Respiratory mechanics in quadriplegia: The respiratory function of the intercostal muscles. *Am Rev Respir Dis* 122:591, 1980.

44. Ducker TB, Simmons RL. Increased intracranial pressure and pulmonary edema: II. The hemodynamic response of dogs and monkeys to increased intracranial pressure. *J Neurosurg* 28:118, 1968.

45. Easton PA, et al. Respiratory function after paralysis of the right hemidiaphragm. *Am Rev Respir Dis* 127:125, 1983.

46. Eberhardt KE, et al. Dose-dependent rate of nosocomial pulmonary infection in mechanically ventilated patients with brain oedema receiving barbiturates: A prospective case study. *Infection* 20:12, 1992.

47. Efthimiou J, et al. Bilateral diaphragm paralysis after cardiac surgery with topical hypothermia. *Thorax* 46:351, 1991.

48. Eisele JH, et al. Abnormal respiratory control in acquired dysautonomia. *N Engl J Med* 285:366, 1971.

49. Fallat RJ, et al. Spirometry in amyotrophic lateral sclerosis. *Arch Neurol* 36:74, 1979.

50. Feuerstein J, et al. EEG and massive digitalis intoxication: A case of epilepsy with respiratory manifestations and prolonged apnea. *Electroencephalogr Clin Neurophysiol* 34:313, 1973.

51. Fischer DS, Nichol BA. Intraventricular conduction defect and respiratory tract paralysis in diabetic ketoacidosis. *Am J Med* 35:123, 1963.

52. Fisher A, Aboul-Nasr HT. Delayed nonfatal pulmonary edema following subarachnoid hemorrhage. *J Neurosurg* 51:856, 1979.

53. Frank Y, et al. Sleep apnea and hypoventilation syndrome associated with acquired nonprogressive dysautonomia: Clinical and pathological studies in a child. *Ann Neurol* 10:18, 1981.

54. Frankel RJ, Bennett ED, Borland CD. Pulmonary edema in meningococcal meningitis. *Postgrad Med J* 52:529, 1976.

55. Frans E, Dom R, Demedts M. Pleuropulmonary changes during treatment of Parkinson's disease with a long-acting ergot derivative, cabergoline. *Eur Respir J* 5:263, 1992.

56. Fromm GB, Wisdom PJ, Block AJ. Amyotrophic lateral sclerosis presenting with respiratory failure: Diaphragmatic paralysis and dependence on mechanical ventilation in two patients. *Chest* 71:612, 1977.

57. Frost EAM. Effects of positive end-expiratory pressure and compliance in brain-injured patients. *J Neurosurg* 47:195, 1977.

58. Fugl-Meyer AR, Grimby G. Ventilatory function in tetraplegic patients. *Scand J Rehabil Med* 3:151, 1971.

59. Gadoth N, Sokol J, Lavie P. Sleep structure and nocturnal disordered breathing in familial dysautonomia. *J Neurol Sci* 60:117, 1983.

60. Gaspar D, Samarasinghe CA. Electroconvulsive therapy in psychogeriatric practice: A study of risk factors, indications, and outcome. *Compr Psychiatry* 23:170, 1982.

61. Gibson GJ, et al. Pulmonary mechanics in patients with respiratory muscle weakness. *Am Rev Respir Dis* 115:389, 1977.

62. Gilchrist D, Chan CK, Deck JHN. Phrenic involvement in Charcot-Marie-Tooth disease. A pathologic documentation. *Chest* 96:1197, 1989.

63. Gilhus NE, Aarli JA. Respiratory disease and nasal immunoglobulin concentrations in phenytoin-treated epileptic patients. *Acta Neurol Scand* 63:34, 1981.

64. Glenn WWL, et al. Characteristics and surgical management of respiratory complications accompanying pathologic lesions of the brain stem. *Ann Surg* 191:655, 1980.

65. Goldman AL, George J. Postural hypoxemia in quadriplegic patients. *Neurology* 26:815, 1976.

66. Gotoh F, Meyer JS, Takagi Y. Cerebral venous and arterial blood gases during Cheyne-Stokes respiration. *Am J Med* 47:534, 1969.

67. Gould L, et al. A method for the production of hemidiaphragmatic paralysis: Its application to the study of lung function in normal man. *Am Rev Respir Dis* 96:812, 1967.

68. Gracey DR, Divertie MB, Howard FM Jr. Mechanical ventilation for respiratory failure in myasthenia gravis. *Mayo Clin Proc* 58:597, 1983.

69. Gracey DR, et al. Postoperative respiratory care after transsternal thymectomy in myasthenia gravis. *Chest* 86:67, 1984.

70. Gracey DR, et al. Respiratory failure in Guillain-Barré syndrome: A 6-year experience. *Mayo Clin Proc* 57:742, 1982.

71. Gracey DR, Southorn PA. Respiratory failure in Lambert-Eaton myasthenic syndrome. *Chest* 91:716, 1987.

72. Graf CJ, Rossi NP. Pulmonary edema and the central nervous system: A clinicopathological study. *Surg Neurol* 4:319, 1975.

73. Green W, L'Heureux P, Hune CE. Paralysis of the diaphragm. *Am J Dis Child* 129:1402, 1975.

74. Greenberg DB, Murray GB. Hyperventilation as a variant of tardive dyskinesia. *J Clin Psychiatry* 42:401, 1981.

75. Greene R, Platt R, Matz R. Postictal pulmonary edema. *NY State J Med* 75:1257, 1975.

76. Griggs RC, Engel WK, Resnick JS. Acetazolamide treatment of hypokalemic periodic paralysis: Prevention of attacks and improvement of persistent weakness. *Ann Intern Med* 73:39, 1970.

77. Griggs RC, et al. Evaluation of pulmonary function in neuromuscular disease. *Arch Neurol* 38:9, 1981.

78. Guilleminault C, et al. The impact of autonomic nervous system dysfunction on breathing during sleep. *Sleep* 4:263, 1981.

79. Guilleminault C, et al. Respiratory and hemodynamic study during wakefulness and sleep in myotonic dystrophy. *Sleep* 1:19, 1978.

80. Guthrie TC, Berlin L. Acute respiratory failure in multiple sclerosis and its management. *Ann Intern Med* 37:1197, 1952.

81. Hajiroussou V, Joshi RC. Unilateral pulmonary edema associated with old poliomyelitis. *Thorax* 34:690, 1979.

82. Harari A, et al. Normal pulmonary-capillary pressures in the late phase of neurogenic pulmonary oedema (letter). *Lancet* 1:494, 1976.

83. Hardman JM, Earle KM. Meningococcal infections: A review of 200 fatal cases. *J Neuropathol Exp Neurol* 26:119, 1967.

84. Heaney LM. Cardiac and respiratory monitoring of acute stroke victim. *Heart Lung* 6:469, 1977.

85. Hemingway A, Bors E, Hobby RP. An investigation of the pulmonary function of paraplegics. *J Clin Invest* 37:773, 1958.

86. Higenbottom T, et al. Abdominal wall movement in normals and patients with hemidiaphragmatic and bilateral diaphragmatic palsy. *Thorax* 32:589, 1977.

87. Higgs BD, Bevan JC. Use of mandatory minute volume ventilation in the perioperative management of a patient with myasthenia. *Br J Anaesth* 51:1181, 1979.

88. Hill NS, et al. Sleep-disordered breathing in patients with Duchenne muscular dystrophy using negative pressure ventilators. *Chest* 102:1656, 1992.

89. Hill R, Martin J, Hakim A. Acute respiratory failure in motor neuron disease. *Arch Neurol* 40:30, 1983.

90. Hirsch CS, Martin DL. Unexpected death in young epileptics. *Neurology* 21:682, 1971.

91. Hoffman JH, Hendrick EB, Humphreys RP. Manifestations and management of Arnold-Chiari malformation in patients with myelomeningocele. *Child Brain* 1:255, 1979.

92. Holinger PC, et al. Respiratory obstruction and apnea in infants with bilateral abductor vocal cord paralysis, meningomyelocele, hydrocephalus, and Arnold-Chiari malformation. *J Pediatr* 92:368, 1978.

93. Holtackers TR, Loosbrock LM, Gracey DR. The use of chest cuirass in respiratory failure of neurologic origin. *Respir Care* 27:271, 1982.

94. Hseih AH-H, et al. Pneumonia following closed head injury. *Am Rev Respir Dis* 146:290, 1992.

95. Hunt CE, et al. Central hypoventilation syndrome: Experience with bilateral phrenic nerve pacing in 3 neonates. *Am Rev Respir Dis* 118:23, 1978.

96. Hyland RH, et al. Primary alveolar hypoventilation treated with nocturnal electrophrenic respiration. *Am Rev Respir Dis* 117:165, 1978.

97. Inkley SR, Oldenburg FC, Vignos PJ Jr. Pulmonary function in Duchenne muscular dystrophy related to stage of disease. *Am J Med* 56:297, 1974.

98. Iosif G, Fleischman J, Chitkara R. Empyema due to ventriculoperitoneal shunt. *Chest* 99:1538, 1991.

99. Jackson DL, et al. Isaacs syndrome with laryngeal involvement: An unusual presentation of myokymia. *Neurology* 29:1612, 1979.

100. Jackson IV, et al. The respiratory components of tardive dyskinesia. *Biol Psychol* 15:485, 1980.

101. James JL, Park HWJ. Respiratory failure due to polymyositis treated by intermittent positive-pressure respiration. *Lancet* 2:1281, 1961.

102. Jerusalem F, et al. Cytoplasmic body neuromyopathy presenting as respiratory failure and weight loss. *J Neurol Sci* 41:1, 1979.

103. Kaufman J, Khatri BO, Riendl P. Are patients with multiple sclerosis protected from thrombophlebitis and pulmonary embolism? *Chest* 94:998, 1988.

104. Kelly BJ, Luce JM. The diagnosis and management of neuromuscular diseases causing respiratory failure. *Chest* 99:1485, 1991.

105. Kiss GT, Rao K. Treatment of refractory lobar atelectasis in amyotrophic lateral sclerosis with positive end-expiratory pressure. *Chest* 78:353, 1980.

106. Kokkola K, Moller K, Lehtonen T. Pulmonary function in tetraplegic and paraplegic patients. *Ann Clin Res* 7:76, 1975.

107. Kolodny EH. Current concepts: Lysosomal storage diseases. *N Engl J Med* 294:1217, 1976.

108. Kosnik EJ, et al. Central neurogenic pulmonary edema: With a review of its pathogenesis and treatment. *Child Brain* 3:37, 1977.

109. Kreitzer SM, et al. Respiratory muscle function in amyotrophic lateral sclerosis. *Am Rev Respir Dis* 117:437, 1978.

110. Krieger AJ, Detwiler JS, Trooskin SZ. Respiration in an infant with Dandy-Walker syndrome. *Neurology* 24:1064, 1974.

111. Krieger AJ, Detwiler JS, Trooskin SZ. Respiratory function in infants with Arnold-Chiari malformation. *Laryngoscope* 86:718, 1976.

112. Kuperman AS, Krieger AJ, Rosomoff HL. Respiratory function after cervical cordotomy. *Chest* 59:128, 1971.

113. Lam D, et al. Paralysis of diaphragm complicating central venous alimentation. *Am J Dis Child* 135:382, 1981.

114. Lane DJ, Hazleman B, Nichols PJR. Late-onset respiratory failure in patients with previous poliomyelitis. *Q J Med* 43:551, 1974.

115. Langer H, Woolf CR. Changes in pulmonary function in Parkinson's syndrome after treatment with l-dopa. *Am Rev Respir Dis* 104:440, 1971.

116. Laroche CM, et al. Clinical significance of severe isolated diaphragm weakness. *Am Rev Respir Dis* 138:862, 1988.

117. Laroche CM, et al. Diaphragm weakness in Charcot-Marie-Tooth disease. *Thorax* 43:478, 1988.

118. Laroche CM, et al. Respiratory muscle weakness in the Lambert-Eaton myasthenic syndrome. *Thorax* 44:913, 1989.

119. Larrazet F, et al. Possible bromocriptine-induced myocardial infarction. *Ann Intern Med* 118:199, 1993.

120. Laub GW, et al. Phrenic nerve injury. A prospective study. *Chest* 100:376, 1991.

121. Lee MC, Klassen AC, Resch JA. Respiratory pattern disturbances in ischemic cerebral vascular disease. *Stroke* 5:612, 1974.

122. Leventhal SR, Orkin FK, Hirsh RA. Prediction for the need for postoperative mechanical ventilation in myasthenia gravis. *Anesthesiology* 53:26, 1980.

123. Lisboa C, et al. Inspiratory muscle function in unilateral diaphragmatic paralysis. *Am Rev Respir Dis* 134:488, 1986.

124. Loh L, Hughes JMB, Newsom-Davis J. Gas-exchange problems in bilateral diaphragmatic paralysis. *Bull Eur Physiopathol Respir* 15:137, 1979.

125. Lugliani R, et al. Effect of bilateral carotid-body resection on ventilatory control at rest and dur-

ing exercise in man. *N Engl J Med* 285:1105, 1971.

126. Mador MJ, Tobin MJ. Apneustic breathing. A characteristic feature of brainstem compression in achondroplasia. *Chest* 97:877, 1990.

127. Maire FW, Patton HD. Role of splanchnic nerve and adrenal medulla in the genesis of "preoptic pulmonary edema." *Am J Physiol* 184:351, 1956.

128. Malatinsky J, Prochazka J, Samel M. Respiratory failure as a seizure phenomenon: A case report. *Br J Anaesth* 47:1019, 1975.

129. Malik AB. Pulmonary vascular response to increase in intracranial pressure: Role of sympathetic mechanisms. *J Appl Physiol* 42:335, 1977.

130. Maloney FP. Pulmonary function in quadriplegia. *Arch Phys Med Rehabil* 60:261, 1979.

131. Martin AM Jr, Simmons RL, Heisterkamp CA III. Respiratory insufficiency in combat casualities: I. Pathologic changes in the lungs of patients dying of wounds. *Ann Surg* 170:30, 1969.

132. McAlpine D, Comston N. Some aspects of the natural history of disseminated sclerosis. *Q J Med* 21:135, 1952.

133. McMichan J, Michel L, Westbrook PR. Pulmonary dysfunction following traumatic quadriplegia. *JAMA* 243:528, 1980.

134. McMichan JC, et al. Electrophrenic respiration: Report of six cases. *Mayo Clin Proc* 54:662, 1979.

135. Mehta AD, Wright WB, Kirby BJ. Ventilatory function in Parkinson's disease. *Br Med J* 1:1456, 1978.

136. Melton LJ, Bartleson JD. Spontaneous pneumothorax in multiple sclerosis. *Ann Neurol* 7:492, 1980.

137. Mickell JJ, et al. Clinical implications of postoperative unilateral phrenic nerve paralysis. *J Thorac Cardiovasc Surg* 76:297, 1978.

138. Mier A. Respiratory muscle weakness. *Respir Med* 84:351, 1990.

139. Mier A, et al. Repetitive stimulation of phrenic nerves in myasthenia gravis. *Thorax* 47:640, 1992.

140. Mier A, et al. Tracheobronchial clearance in patients with bilateral diaphragmatic weakness. *Am Rev Respir Dis* 142:545, 1990.

141. Mier M. Mechanisms leading to hypoventilation in extrapyramidal disorders, with special reference to Parkinson's disease. *J Am Geriatr Soc* 15:230, 1967.

142. Mier-Jedrzejowicz AK, Brophy C, Green M. Respiratory muscle function in myasthenia gravis. *Am Rev Respir Dis* 138:867, 1988.

143. Miley CE, Forster FM. Activation of partial complex seizures by hyperventilation. *Arch Neurol* 34:371, 1977.

144. Miller JD, et al. Early insults to the injured brain. *JAMA* 240:439, 1978.

145. Miyasaka K, Hoffman HJ, Froese AB. The influence of cerebellar stimulation on respiratory muscle coordination in a patient with cerebral palsy. *Neurosurgery* 2:262, 1978.

146. Mohr CH, Hill NS. Long-term follow-up of nocturnal ventilatory assistance in patients with respiratory failure due to Duchenne-type muscular dystrophy. *Chest* 97:91, 1990.

147. Molho M, et al. Pulmonary functional abnormalities after upper dorsal sympathectomy. *Am Rev Respir Dis* 116:879, 1977.

148. Moore DC, Crawford RD, Scurlock JE. Severe hypoxia and acidosis following anesthetic-induced convulsions. *Anesthesiology* 53:259, 1980.

149. Moore GC, Zwillich CW, Battaglia JD. Respiratory failure associated with familial depression of ventilatory response to hypoxia and hypercapnia. *N Engl J Med* 295:861, 1976.

150. Morse SR, Chandrasekhar AJ, Cugell DW. Cheyne-Stokes respiration redefined. *Chest* 66:345, 1974.

151. Mortola JP, Sant'Ambrogio G. Mechanisms of breathing in tetraplegics. *Am Rev Respir Dis* 119(Suppl):131, 1979.

152. Mortola JP, Sant'Ambrogio G. Motion of the rib cage and the abdomen in tetraplegic patients. *Clin Sci Mol Med* 54:25, 1978.

153. Mulder DG, Herrmann CV, Buckberg GD. Effect of thymectomy in patients with myasthenia gravis. *Am J Surg* 128:202, 1974.

154. Nakano KK, et al. Amyotrophic lateral sclerosis: A study of pulmonary function. *Dis Nerv System* 37:32, 1976.

155. Naughton J, Block R, Welch M. Central alveolar hypoventilation: A case report. *Am Rev Respir Dis* 103:557, 1971.

156. Neligan P, Harriman DGF, Pearce J. Respiratory arrest in familial hemiplegic migraine: A clinical and neuropathological study. *Br Med J* 2:732, 1977.

157. Nelson DA, Ray CD. Respiratory arrest from seizure discharges in limbic system. *Arch Neurol* 19:199, 1968.

158. Newman JH, Neff TA, Ziporin P. Acute respiratory failure associated with hypophosphatemia. *N Engl J Med* 296:1101, 1977.

159. Newsom-Davis J, et al. Diaphragm function and alveolar hypoventilation. *Q J Med* 45:87, 1976.

160. Nisbet HIA. Status epilepticus treated with d-tubocurarine and controlled respiration. *Br Med J* 1:95, 1959.

161. North JB, Jennett S. Abnormal breathing patterns associated with acute brain damage. *Arch Neurol* 31:338, 1974.

162. Obenour WH, et al. The causes of abnormal function in Parkinson's disease. *Am Rev Respir Dis* 105:382, 1972.

163. Odia GI. Spirometry in convalescent hemiplegic patients. *Arch Phys Med Rehabil* 59:319, 1978.

164. O'Donohue WJ Jr, et al. Respiratory failure in neuromuscular disease: Management in a re-

spiratory intensive care unit. *JAMA* 235:733, 1976.

165. Oligiati R, Jacquet J, Di Prampero PE. Energy cost of walking and exertional dyspnea in multiple sclerosis. *Am Rev Respir Dis* 134:1005, 1986.

166. Osserman KE, Genkins GC. Myasthenia gravis: A review of twenty-years experience in over 1200 patients. *Mt Sinai J Med* 38:497, 1971.

167. Ozonoff MB. Ataxia-telangiectasia: Chronic pneumonia-sinusitis and adenoidal hyperplasia. *AJR* 120:297, 1974.

168. Page MMcB, Watkins PJ. Cardiorespiratory arrest and diabetic autonomic neuropathy. *Lancet* 1:14, 1978.

169. Papasozomenos S, Roessmann U. Respiratory distress and Arnold-Chiari malformation. *Neurology* 31:97, 1981.

170. Parhad IM, et al. Diaphragmatic paralysis in motor neuron disease. *Neurology* 28:18, 1978.

171. Patel AM, Davila DG, Peters SG. Paraneoplastic syndromes associated with lung cancer. *Mayo Clin Proc* 68:278, 1993.

172. Piehler JM, et al. Unexplained diaphragmatic paralysis: A harbinger of malignant disease? *J Thorac Cardiovasc Surg* 84:861, 1982.

173. Plum F. Hyperpnea, hyperventilation, and brain dysfunction (editorial). *Ann Intern Med* 76:328, 1972.

174. Plum F, Brown HW. The effect on respiration of central nervous system disease. *Ann NY Acad Sci* 109:915, 1963.

175. Plum F, Swanson AG. Central neurogenic hyperventilation in man. *Arch Neurol Psychiatry* 81:535, 1959.

176. Ravindran M. Temporal lobe seizure presenting as "laryngospasm." *Clin Electroencephalogr* 12:139, 1981.

177. Reitter B, Mortier W, Wille L. Neonatal respiratory insufficiency due to centronuclear myopathy. *Acta Pediatr Scand* 68:773, 1979.

178. Ridyard JB, Stewart RM. Regional lung function in unilateral diaphragmatic paralysis. *Thorax* 31:438, 1976.

179. Riley DJ, et al. Blunted respiratory drive in congenital myopathy. *Am J Med* 63:459, 1977.

180. Ringqvist I, Ringqvist T. Respiratory mechanics in untreated myasthenia gravis with special reference to the respiratory forces. *Acta Med Scand* 190:499, 1971.

181. Rinne UK. Pleuropulmonary changes during long-term bromocriptine treatment for Parkinson's disease. *Lancet* 1:44, 1981.

182. Rizvi SS, et al. Defect in automatic respiration in a case of multiple sclerosis. *Am J Med* 56:433, 1974.

183. Rodman T, et al. Alveolar hypoventilation due to involvement of the respiratory center by obscure disease of the central nervous system. *Am J Med* 32:208, 1962.

184. Rosenow EC III, Engel AG. Acid maltase deficiency in adults presenting as respiratory failure. *Am J Med* 64:485, 1978.

185. Rothman JG. Effects of respiratory exercises on the vital capacity and forced expiratory volume in children with cerebral palsy. *Phys Ther* 58:421, 1978.

186. Rout MW, Lane DJ, Wollner L. Prognosis in acute cerebrovascular accidents in relation to respiratory pattern and blood gas tensions. *Br Med J* 3:7, 1971.

187. Saunders NA, Kreitzer SM. Diaphragmatic function in amyotrophic lateral sclerosis. *Am Rev Respir Dis* 119:127, 1979.

188. Scanlon PD, et al. Respiratory mechanics in acute quadriplegia. *Am Rev Respir Dis* 139:615, 1989.

189. Schiffman PL, Golbe LI. Upper airway dysfunction in olivopontocerebellar atrophy. *Chest* 102:1291, 1992.

190. Schmalstieg EJ, et al. Neuropathy presenting as prolonged dyspnea. *Arch Neurol* 34:473, 1977.

191. Selvin BL. Electroconvulsive therapy, 1987. *Anesthesiology* 67:367, 1987.

192. Seriff NS. Alveolar hypoventilation with normal lungs: The syndrome of primary or central alveolar hypoventilation. *Ann NY Acad Sci* 121:691, 1965.

193. Shim C. Motor disturbances of the diaphragm. *Clin Chest Med* 1:125, 1980.

194. Siegel IM. Pulmonary problems in Duchenne muscular dystrophy. *Phys Ther* 55:160, 1975.

195. Simpson K. Neonatal respiratory failure due to myotonic dystrophy. *Arch Dis Child* 50:569, 1975.

196. Sirak ED, et al. Adult-onset acid maltase deficiency presenting as diaphragm paralysis. *Ann Neurol* 9:613, 1981.

197. Sivak ED, Streib EW. Management of hypoventilation in motor neuron disease presenting with respiratory insufficiency. *Ann Neurol* 7:188, 1980.

198. Smeltzer SC, et al. Respiratory function in multiple sclerosis. Utility of clinical assessment of respiratory muscle function. *Chest* 101:479, 1992.

199. Spinelli A, et al. Control of breathing in patients with myasthenia gravis. *Am Rev Respir Dis* 145:1359, 1992.

200. Stauffer ES, Bell GD. Traumatic respiratory quadriplegia and pentaplegia. *Orthop Clin North Am* 9:1081, 1978.

201. Stephenson JB. Reflex anoxic seizures ("white breath holding"): Nonepileptic vagal attacks. *Arch Dis Child* 53:193, 1978.

202. Theodore J, Robin ED. Pathogenesis of neurogenic pulmonary oedema. *Lancet* 2:749, 1975.

203. Theodore J, Robin ED. Speculations on neurogenic pulmonary edema (NPE). *Am Rev Respir Dis* 113:405, 1976.

204. Tsao TC-Y, et al. Respiratory failure of acute or-ganophosphate and carbonate poisoning. *Chest* 98:631, 1990.

205. Tucker GF Jr. Pulmonary migraine. *Ann Otol Rhinol Laryngol* 86:671, 1977.

206. Tzelepis GE, et al. Respiratory muscle dysfunction in Parkinson's disease. *Am Rev Respir Dis* 138:266, 1988.

207. Vincken WG, Darauay CM, Coisio MG. Reversibility of upper airway obstruction after levo-dopa therapy in Parkinson's disease. *Chest* 96:210, 1989.

208. Vincken WG, et al. Involvement of upper airway muscles in extrapyramidal disorders: A case of airflow obstruction. *N Engl J Med* 311:438, 1984.

209. Wade JG, et al. Effect of carotid endarterectomy on carotid chemoreceptor and baroreceptor function in man. *N Engl J Med* 282:823, 1970.

210. Weiner WJ, et al. Respiratory dyskinesias: Extrapyramidal dysfunction and dyspnea. *Ann Intern Med* 88:327, 1978.

211. Weir BK. Pulmonary edema following fatal aneurysm rupture. *J Neurosurg* 49:502, 1978.

212. Wenger TL, et al. Hypersensitive carotid sinus syndrome manifested as cough syncope. *PACE* 3:332, 1980.

213. Wilcox PG, et al. Long term follow-up of symptoms, pulmonary function, respiratory muscle strength, and exercise performance after botulism. *Am Rev Respir Dis* 139:157, 1989.

214. Wilcox PG, Morrison NJ, Pardy RL. Recovery of the ventilatory and upper airway muscles and exercise performance after type A botulism. *Chest* 98:620, 1990.

215. Williams DB, Windebank AJ. Motor neuron disease (amyotrophic lateral sclerosis). *Mayo Clin Proc* 66:54, 1991.

216. Wright RS, Feuerman T, Brown J. Neurogenic pulmonary edema after trigeminal nerve blockade. *Chest* 96:436, 1989.

217. Yassa R, Lai S. Respiratory irregularity and tardive dyskinesia: A prevalence study. *Acta Psychiatr Scand* 73:506, 1986.

218. Zajkowski EJ, Kravath RE. Bilateral diaphragmatic paralysis in the newborn infant. *Chest* 75:392, 1979.

65

Skeletal Diseases

Udaya B. S. Prakash

The skeletal thorax is as much a part of the respiratory system as are the lungs and hence plays a major role in normal pulmonary function. Instability of the chest wall can lead to respiratory failure, as exemplified by the ventilatory failure in patients with flail chest. Congenital and acquired defects and diseases of the thoracic cage may interfere with the normal respiratory mechanics. Occasionally, diseases of the nonthoracic skeleton may be associated with lung problems. An excellent example of this is the pulmonary parenchymal process in patients with ankylosing spondylitis. Many of the musculoskeletal diseases in which the respiratory system is involved are discussed in Chapter 57 and elsewhere in this book. In this chapter, we will discuss some of the common and uncommon skeletal diseases in which the respiratory system is involved. Certain disease entities such as Marfan's syndrome are also covered here, although they are not primary skeletal diseases, because of the obviously evident skeletal abnormalities in these patients. The major spinal deformities are scoliosis, kyphosis, pectus excavatum, pectus carinatum, and straight-back syndrome. Respiratory complications in ankylosing spondylitis and several other skeletal disorders are also included.

Kyphoscoliosis

Scoliosis is deformity of the spine by marked lateral curvature, and *kyphosis* is abnormally accentuated posterior curvature of the spine. A combination of these deformities results in *kyphoscoliosis*, a lateral bending and rotation of the vertebral column. Pulmonary problems occur in both scoliosis and kyphoscoliosis.

Scoliosis is by far the most common spinal deformity. An incidence of 4 per 1000 population was found by a roentgenographic survey [120]. Scoliosis is classified etiologically into five varieties: idiopathic, congenital, neuropathic (poliomyelitis, cerebral palsy, and syringomyelia), myopathic (muscular dystrophy, amyotonia, and Friedreich's ataxia), and traumatic [80]. Scoliosis is also seen in mesenchymal disorders and in association with neurofibromatosis [154]. In practice, 80 percent of scolioses are idiopathic. Among infants, the male-to-female ratio is 6 : 4, but among cases that begin in adolescence—the largest group—the ratio is 1 : 9, and overall it is 2 : 8. It has been claimed that infantile scoliosis usually involves a leftward curvature, whereas scoliosis in adolescent girls is usually toward the right [68]. A familial basis for idiopathic scoliosis has been shown. Among first-, second-, and third-degree relatives of children with idiopathic scoliosis, examination showed spinal curvature 20 times as often as in a comparable group of the general population [152]. In congenital scoliosis of early onset, there is failure of alveolar multiplication [15], whereas in idiopathic scoliosis, the alveoli do not enlarge normally [99].

Idiopathic scoliosis in adolescent girls usually involves 7 to 10 vertebrae. The curvature or angulation of a scoliotic spine is best measured by the Cobb method [26] (Fig. 65-1). Pulmonary symptoms are not seen until the curvature exceeds 70 degrees, but 25 percent of patients have an angulation of more than 100 degrees and nearly 65 percent have an angulation greater than 70 degrees at the time body growth is complete [72]. Adolescent idiopathic thoracic curves of 60 to 80 degrees have been observed to increase by an average of 30 degrees over a period of 25 years after completion of growth [28]. Symptoms and signs of respiratory failure usually do not appear until the fourth or fifth decade [51]. A retrospective survey of approximately 800 scoliotic subjects attending a chest clinic over a 25-year period revealed 54 subjects who had unfused scoliosis [16]. Cardiorespiratory failure attributable

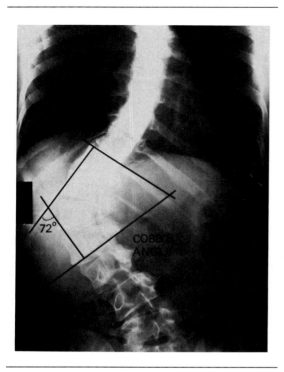

Fig. 65-1. The Cobb angle is determined by lines drawn perpendicular to the tangents from the end plates of the most tilted superior and inferior vertebrae.

to the scoliosis was the cause of death in 11 patients, and in 10 of these the scoliotic curve had first been observed at less than 5 years of age, whereas the onset was during early adolescence (11 years) in only 1.

Pulmonary Function Abnormalities

The most common abnormality of pulmonary function is a reduction in static lung volumes, including vital capacity and total lung capacity, in the absence of obstruction to expiratory outflow [11,22]. It is generally accepted that an inverse relationship exists between the angle of scoliotic curvature and the value (as a percentage of predictions) for vital capacity [11,12,22], total lung capacity, functional residual capacity, residual volume, and static compliance of the total respiratory system [79]. The ventilatory function may be impaired even in mild forms of scoliosis. One study suggested that the force developed by the respiratory muscles is a more important deter-

minant of ventilatory defect than the degree of spinal curvature [126]. The decreased lung compliance is most pronounced in scoliotics with muscle weakness, and the compliance can be increased by positive-pressure ventilation [125]. Flow rates are reduced only in proportion to the decrease in vital capacity, and direct measurement of airways resistance produces normal values. Cardiorespiratory failure is likely to occur when the vital capacity is less than 40 percent of the predicted normal value [57]. Total lung capacity usually is severely reduced in patients who develop cor pulmonale [18]. In kyphoscoliosis, prediction of lung volume from body height results in significant underestimation, but arm span serves satisfactorily for this purpose [64]. A method has been evolved by which the theoretic height of these patients is predicted from the angle of scoliosis, length of spine, and actual height [12,13].

Studies of respiratory function in children with idiopathic scoliosis have shown diminished vital capacity, one-second forced expiratory volume, gas transfer, and maximal static expiratory airways pressure, but no significant diminution in total lung capacity and maximal inspiratory pressure [29,76]. The characteristic deformity seen in scoliosis causes one hemithorax to become relatively smaller than the other. This inherent mechanical inefficiency of ventilation is the major factor in causing respiratory embarrassment. With scoliosis, arterial blood gas abnormalities occur in many adults and some younger patients [122,145]. Although hypoxemia often is present and has been attributed to alveolar hypoventilation resulting from small tidal volumes [11,48], arterial CO_2 tension ($PaCO_2$) usually is normal [11,18,78,81]. In advanced cases, however, increased $PaCO_2$ is common and signifies the onset of respiratory failure [11,18,81]. Increased ratios of physiologic dead space to tidal volume (V_D/V_T) and elevated alveolar-arterial oxygen tension gradients [$P(A-a)O_2$] have been demonstrated [78,81,145]. The gas exchange abnormality in idiopathic scoliosis is believed to be due primarily to ventilation-perfusion maldistribution resulting from deformity of the rib cage [80], and this has been confirmed by studies with ^{133}Xe [5]. The proportion of ventilation, oxygen consumption, and volume on the side of convexity is reported to be less than on the side of concavity [80]. However, a study with radionuclide methods did not find consistent differences in perfusion between the convex and concave sides of the curvature [5]. Although the adolescents with mild, asymptomatic scoliosis (thoracic curvature of less than 35 degrees) demonstrate little or no impairment of lung volumes at rest, abnormal ventilatory patterns do develop during exercise, hypoxia, or hypercapnia [127].

The severity of the scoliotic curvature is easily measured by the Cobb angle, but the rotation, which is probably more important, is not, and this has been a problem in comparative studies among patients [109] (Fig. 65-2). However, the scoliotic angle is an important predictor of respiratory failure. In a long-term study of 24 patients with unfused scoliosis, pulmonary function tests were performed 20 years apart, and respiratory failure occurred only in patients who had a vital capacity of less than 45 percent of that predicted during the initial testing and an angle greater than 110 degrees; the initial vital capacity was the strongest predictor of the development of respiratory failure, followed by scoliotic angle [103]. Cooper and associates [29] studied 29 patients with thoracic adolescent idiopathic scoliosis of less than 60 degrees and reported that maximal inspiratory pressure was reduced but maximal expiratory pressure was normal. They

concluded that if the expiratory muscles are normal, the inspiratory muscles probably are normal as well. The low maximal inspiratory pressure was attributed to the mechanical disadvantage resulting from the chest deformity.

Several types of breathing abnormalities have been documented during sleep in subjects with severe kyphoscoliosis (so-called Quasimodo syndrome), including severe obstructive sleep apnea and hypopnea [59]. Derangements in breathing pattern and arterial oxygen saturation had no apparent relation to the degree of thoracic deformity, the pulmonary function, PaCO$_2$, or chemical drives to breathe [96]. Patients with kyphoscoliosis hypoventilate during sleep, particularly in rapid eye movement sleep, resulting in hypoxia and hypercapnia [116]. The rate of rise in pulmonary artery pressure during and after exercise in scoliotics is more closely related to total lung capacity, vital capacity, or functional residual capacity [123,124]. Hypoventilation secondary to reduced chest wall movements is the main mechanism responsible for hypoxemia during sleep [97]. Obstructive sleep apnea caused by spinal deformity alone is uncommon [116].

Fig. 65-2. Severe thoracic kyphoscoliosis. (A) Posteroanterior view. (B) Lateral view.

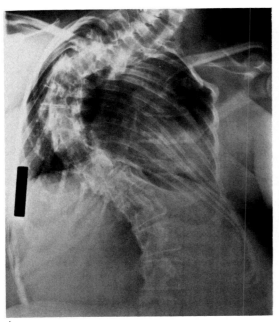

A

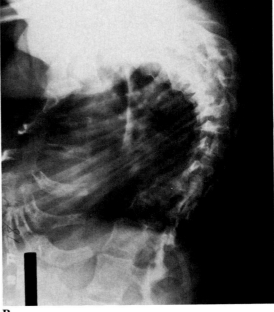

B

Treatment of Kyphoscoliosis

The treatment of scoliosis may be nonsurgical management with a Milwaukee brace [14] or surgical correction by spinal fusion and reduction of the deformity by the posterior placement of Harrington's distraction strut bars [63]. Many studies have shown no appreciable difference in lung function between patients with the Milwaukee brace and those with surgical correction [56,118]. In severe respiratory failure from kyphoscoliosis, cuirass respirators have been used with varying success [147]. Acute respiratory failure in adults with severe thoracic spinal deformity is associated with a higher mortality, but successful management of acute respiratory failure is possible in the majority of patients. These patients tend to be middle-aged, and their pulmonary function deteriorates at a slower rate after acute respiratory failure than in patients who develop acute respiratory failure as a result of chronic obstructive respiratory disease [88]. Nighttime ventilatory support, using continuous positive airway pressure, improves respiratory failure in secondary scoliosis [40,67,150]. Hypercapnia, a sign of worsening respiratory status in patients with severe kyphoscoliosis, is not a contraindication for long-term well-controlled domiciliary oxygen therapy [136].

Postoperative Respiratory Complications

After spinal fusion, postoperative respiratory complications are more common in those with nonidiopathic scoliosis who are 20 years or older and have mental retardation, anterior spinal fusion, relative arterial hypoxemia, or obstructive pulmonary function than in those with idiopathic scoliosis [3]. The long-term results of corrective surgery of spinal deformity are not well studied, but lung function measurements in anesthetized young patients undergoing spinal correction have shown immediate and short-term deterioration of respiratory mechanics [6]. However, one study assessed the effects of spinal fusion on pulmonary function tests in a homogeneous population of 42 women with idiopathic scoliosis by measuring lung functions before and a minimum of 3 years (mean 7.7 years) after surgery and found that the only significant preoperative abnormality was vital capacity reduced to 81 percent of predicted. A scoliotic angle exceeding 50 degrees was associated with significantly lower vital capacity. Postoperative evaluations showed that vi-

tal capacity increased significantly by 12 percent [55]. An interesting observation has been the significant association between scoliosis and pulmonary infection with *Mycobacterium avium* complex. Iseman and colleagues [70] evaluated 67 patients with pulmonary disease due to *M. avium* complex and discovered that 52 percent of patients had scoliosis and that this skeletal abnormality was significantly more common among all *M. avium* complex patients than among patients with *M. tuberculosis* or the general population [70]. This increased risk of infection among scoliotics is most likely related to structural bronchopulmonary abnormalities rather than immunologic or other well-known risk factors. Atelectasis of a lobe as a result of scoliosis-related bronchial stenosis has been described [138]. Subclinical lung damage by this mechanism may predispose to secondary infections.

Pectus Deformities

Pectus Excavatum

The congenital deformity pectus excavatum (also called *funnel chest*) is characterized by a depressed sternum (usually above the xiphisternal junction) with symmetric or asymmetric prominence of the ribs on either side. The origin of pectus excavatum is unknown, but it is believed to be due to excessive diaphragmatic traction on the lower sternum or displacement of the heart into the left hemithorax. A report on 10 cases of pectus excavatum noted pulmonary sequestration and other pulmonary abnormalities in 9 patients and suggested that there may be a connection between pulmonary sequestration and the formation of this abnormality [71]. Considering the common occurrence of pectus excavatum in clinical practice, however, this incidence seems unusually high. Pectus excavatum generally occurs sporadically, although a dominant pattern of inheritance has been described [60]. It is not infrequently associated with Marfan's syndrome and other connective tissue diseases. The majority of patients are asymptomatic, but some experience exertional dyspnea, precordial pain, palpitation, and a dizzy sensation [45]. Pulmonary function is usually normal but, with very severe deformity, the vital capacity, total lung capacity, and maximal breathing capacity may be decreased.

Chest roentgenograms may reveal displacement of the heart to the left [4]. The right parasternal soft tissues of the anterior chest wall give rise to the appearance of right middle-lobe disease on posteroanterior roentgenograms (Fig. 65-3A). Sternal depression is best appreciated on lateral views (Fig. 65-3B). Paradoxical increase in cardiac size on inspiration has been described [8].

In the study mentioned earlier [70], 27 percent of 67 patients with *M. avium* complex infection were found to have pectus excavatum deformity. By comparison, only 5 percent with *M. tuberculosis* had this skeletal abnormality. The prevalence of pectus excavatum among women with *M. avium* complex was significantly different from that among either the general population or patients infected with *M. tuberculosis*, whereas the prevalence of male pectus excavatum patients with *M. avium* infection was significantly different from that in the general population but not from that in patients infected with *M. tuberculosis*. Possible mechanisms for this putative association include bronchopulmonary structural abnormalities secondary to pectus excavatum, impaired mucociliary function, impaired pulmonary lymphatic drainage, and altered alveolar macrophage function. It is unlikely that the skeletal abnormalities occurred as a result of mycobacterial infection because there were no indications of chronic or past tuberculous infections. High-resolution computed tomography of the chest may provide more information regarding pulmonary parenchymal changes.

An earlier study reported that among a series of U.S. Air Force recruits with pectus excavatum, there was an apparent increase in infections of the lower respiratory tract [146].

Pectus Carinatum

Pectus carinatum is a congenital or acquired deformity of the chest cage characterized by protrusion of the sternum. It is a relatively rare chest deformity with an occurrence rate of 1 to 2 per 1000 population. Type 1 pectus carinatum, or "pigeon breast," is caused by an overgrowth of rib cartilages, resulting in forward buckling of the sternum [112]. Pectus carinatum type 2, or "pouter pigeon breast" (Currarino-Silverman syndrome) is characterized by premature fusion of the manubriosternal joint and sternal segments, resulting in high carinate chest deformity [24, 112,119]. Both types of pectus carinatum deformities are frequently associated with congenital heart disease [26,119]. The common cardiac anomalies in type 1 deformity are congenital atrial or ventricular septal defects. Conversely,

Fig. 65-3. Pectus excavatum. (A) Right heart border is obliterated, and there is appearance of an infiltrate in the right middle lobe. The ribs on the right appear crowded. (B) Lateral view shows sternal depression.

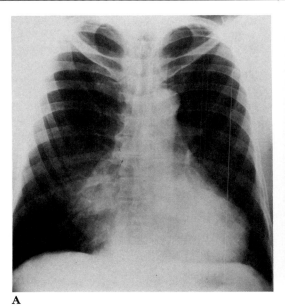

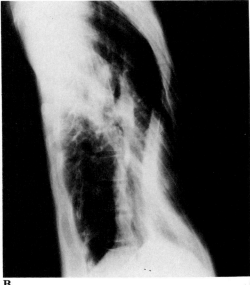

A   B

nearly 50 percent of patients with those forms of heart disease have pectus carinatum [34]. Prolonged asthmatic attacks are reported to produce this deformity [154]. Most patients with pectus carinatum are asymptomatic, but it has been suggested that they are subject to recurrent respiratory infections [87].

Pectus Deformatum

Pectus deformatum is the term used to describe an axially rotated sternum with an S-shaped frontal or sagittal plane. Among 80 patients with various abnormalities of the thoracic cage, pectus deformatum was noted in 13 (16 percent), and the incidence was identical to that of pectus carinatum [36]. Pulmonary function abnormalities are usually mild, somewhat similar to those in pectus excavatum and pectus carinatum.

Surgical Correction of Pectus Deformities

Pectus deformities are surgically corrected for cosmetic reasons, to alleviate cardiopulmonary dysfunctions, and to prevent progressive postural deformities. In a study of 88 patients who underwent surgical correction of any of the pectus deformities just discussed, the operation appeared to have a favorable effect on chest roentgenologic indices but resulted in undercorrection in pectus excavatum and overcorrection in pectus carinatum [36]. Furthermore, the study revealed that those with preoperative lung function values of less than 75 percent of those predicted experienced a functional improvement after corrective surgery. Interestingly, the pulmonary dysfunction worsened if lung function values were more than 75 percent of predicted. Another pulmonary function study of 138 patients before and after surgical correction of pectus excavatum reported that although the corrective procedures resulted in excellent cosmetic result, there was no beneficial effect on the pulmonary functions [77]. Similar conclusions have been reached by others [151].

Ankylosing Spondylitis

Ankylosing spondylitis, also known by many other names including *rheumatoid spondylitis* and *Marie-Strumpell disease*, is a chronic disorder characterized by progressive inflammation of the spine and the adjacent soft tissues. The sacroiliac, hip, and shoulder joints are commonly af-

fected. The disease affects men (male-to-female ratio 10 : 1) 16 to 40 years of age but begins most often in the third decade. The cause is unknown. Ankylosing spondylitis may be inherited by a single autosomal dominant factor, with a 70 percent penetrance in men and a 10 percent penetrance in women. A high association exists between ankylosing spondylitis and the histocompatibility antigen HLA-B27. Extraskeletal manifestations are numerous and include incompetence of aortic valve, varying degrees of heart block, acute anterior uveitis, fever, anemia, fatigue, and weight loss.

Although pulmonary involvement has been reported in 2 to 70 percent of these patients in the clinical setting, a small percentage (< 5 percent) demonstrate pulmonary problems [10,32,54,114, 117,141]. In a Mayo Clinic review of 2080 patients with ankylosing spondylitis, pleuropulmonary manifestations were noted in only 28 (1.3 percent) [114]. The most common chest roentgenologic finding was fibrobullous apical lesions in 26 patients. Other pleuropulmonary features included aspergilloma in 5 and pleural effusion with nonspecific pleuritis in 3 patients. A peculiar type of upper-lobe fibrotic process characterized by nodular and linear lesions has been observed in 14 to 30 percent of patients [23,31]. The process initially appears as linear strands in the upper lobes beginning medially and radiating laterally. When the spine resembles bamboo, these linear strands give rise to a telephone-pole appearance. Occasionally, the linear strands are replaced by small nodules that cavitate or appear cystic (Fig. 65-4). Computed tomography may reveal bullous changes, mycetomas, parenchymal fibrosis, pleural thickening, and bronchiectasis [115]. The cystic spaces and cavities occasionally become infected by *Aspergillus* species, *M. avium* complex, or *M. kansasii* [114,130]. Interstitial pneumonitis and fibrosis are uncommon findings [27]. Bilateral pleural effusion has been described in a patient with quiescent ankylosing spondylitis [83].

Upper airway involvement in the form of cricoarytenoid fixation occurs in some patients. Respiratory failure from cricoarytenoid ankylosis has necessitated therapeutic tracheostomy in 4 patients [9,88,148]. Calcification and ossification of cartilaginous structures may occur in the large airways. Obstruction by ossified arytenoid cartilage has been treated by endoscopic arytenoidectomy [89]. Carcinoma of the upper lobes of lungs is another unusual long-term complication [2,121]. Pathologic analysis of lung tissue in

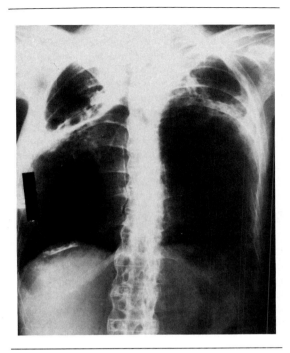

Fig. 65-4. Ankylosing spondylitis demonstrates "bamboo spine," bilateral apical fibrocavitary process, and right diaphragmatic calcification.

ankylosing spondylitis has exhibited nonspecific fibrosis with lymphocytic infiltrates, dilated bronchi, and thin-walled bullae and cavities. Diaphragmatic calcification is seen in a small number of patients with ankylosing spondylitis.

Furthermore, ankylosing spondylitis alters the lung function by modifying the mechanical properties of the thoracic cage. The ankylosis of the costovertebral joints rarely produces symptoms even though the pulmonary function tests are abnormal. Pulmonary function tests in patients with ankylosing spondylitis have revealed diminished total lung capacity, vital capacity, and diffusing capacity for carbon monoxide. Increases in residual volume and functional residual capacity are the other findings, although in some studies the functional residual capacity has been found to be decreased [31,129]. Lung function studies in 16 patients with ankylosing spondylitis recorded a mean total lung capacity of 83 percent of predicted and normal total respiratory resistance [142]. Ventilation studies using ^{133}Xe have shown decreases in ventilation and volumes in the upper lobes [129]. Another study has concluded that patients with ankylosing spondylitis do not underventilate the upper zones of the lungs except in the presence of radiographically visible fibrosis [100]. In another study of 32 patients with ankylosing spondylitis, pulmonary function tests were compared with those for a control population [44]. The patients had no lung symptoms, and their chest roentgenograms were normal. The main findings were reduced lung volumes, a raised closing volume–vital capacity ratio, and decreased airways conductance. The lung volume reduction correlated with disease duration, thoracic mobility, and degree of acute-phase reaction. The stiff spondylitic thorax probably was the main contribution to the impairment of lung function in these patients, but the findings in this study also suggest involvement of the small airways [44].

Pulmonary function tests before and after treatment with either diflunisal or phenylbutazone in 33 men with acute ankylosing spondylitis showed that vital capacity was not an appropriate variable for the evaluation of short-term therapy in ankylosing spondylitis [50]. The study was double-blinded and randomized and was conducted for 12 weeks, followed by an open extension period of 36 weeks. Spirometric studies were performed at baseline, week 12, and week 48. Despite abnormal pulmonary function tests, the majority of patients with ankylosing spondylitis are able to perform normal physical activities [47].

Cervical Hyperostosis

Cervical hyperostosis of the spine is anatomically manifested by bony outgrowths arising from the anterior aspects of the vertebral bodies and extending over the disc spaces. Also known as *diffuse idiopathic skeletal hyperostosis* (DISH), the condition was observed in 12 percent of 215 routine autopsies [108]. The pharyngeal masses formed by the bony outgrowths can be extensive and may occasionally be visualized or palpated at the time of physical examination. These hyperostotic spurs are known to cause dysphagia, foreign-body sensation, aspiration, respiratory distress, and dysphonia [82,144]. Bilateral vocal cord paralysis with airways obstruction has been described in these patients. The pathogenesis is the infection superimposed on ulceration of the cricoid produced by laryngeal movement over a large, sharp osteophyte [63]. Dysphagia and aspiration are the results of mechanical compression [144]. Nonsteroidal antiinflammatory drugs and antireflux precautions should be suggested for patients who complain of dysphagia. Surgical removal of the hyperostotic process is required in severe cases.

Cervical spondylosis can be associated with pressure symptoms in the neck area. Dyspnea and paretic left hemidiaphragm relieved by laminectomy are described [20].

Osteoporosis

Compression fractures of multiple thoracic vertebral bodies as a result of osteoporosis produce an anatomic anomaly akin to kyphosis. With severe compression fracture, some patients develop a gentle (nonacute angle) thoracic gibbus or hyperkyphosis. Furthermore, a markedly shortened thoracic vertebral column leads to reduced lung volumes. These mechanical factors and the pain secondary to compression fracture have the potential to cause respiratory dysfunction. The pulmonary effects of significant osteoporosis are similar to those observed in scoliosis. A study of 74 white women referred for evaluation of osteoporosis were subjected to pulmonary function testing, and those with thoracic wedge compression fractures secondary to osteoporosis had a significantly lower predicted forced vital capacity than did those without fractures. The degree of hyperkyphosis as measured by Cobb's angle had an appreciable effect on this parameter [86]. The authors of the study assess that, as a general rule, approximately a 9 percent fall in the predicted forced vital capacity might be expected for each thoracic vertebral fracture.

Sternotomy

Median sternotomy is a common surgical procedure in industrialized countries. Most such procedures are performed to correct coronary artery disease. A restrictive ventilatory defect follows median sternotomy [17,42,131]. Vital capacity, one-second forced expiratory volume, and functional residual capacity may decline to as little as 40 percent of preoperative values 1 to 3 days after coronary artery bypass grafting [73]. These changes are more pronounced after the use of internal mammary artery than after saphenous vein grafting [19,74], which may be related to disruption of the internal mammary artery–derived vascular supply of phrenic nerves [1]. The diminished lung function begins to reverse by the end of the first postoperative week, and recovery is almost total at 3 months [104]. The causes of the lung dysfunction include pain, atelecta-

sis, pulmonary edema, pulmonary embolism, hemothorax, diaphragmatic paralysis ("frost-bitten phrenic"), pleurotomy, and chest wall instability. A study of rib cage mechanics in 16 men before and 1 week and 3 months after median sternotomy for coronary artery grafting revealed that reduced and uncoordinated rib cage expansion contributed to the restrictive ventilatory defect [91]. Preexisting cardiopulmonary disease will influence the reduction in lung volumes. Obviously, resection of pulmonary parenchyma will result in permanent loss of lung function contributed by the resected segment or lobe.

Marfan's Syndrome

A heritable generalized disorder of connective tissue, Marfan's syndrome is manifested clinically by abnormalities of the skeletal system (excessive length of long bones), eyes (ectopia lentis), and cardiovascular system (aneurysm of the thoracic aorta, septal and valvular cardiac anomalies) [105]. Pulmonary abnormalities are observed in approximately 10 percent of Marfan's patients [49] and include emphysema [110], generalized honeycombing of the lungs [90], spontaneous pneumothorax [140], and bronchiectasis [137] (Fig. 65-5). Of these, spontaneous pneumothorax is the most common and is seen in nearly 5 percent of adolescents and adults [38,61,90, 140,149]. Spontaneous pneumothorax and bullae are causally related to Marfan's syndrome [149]. Necropsy studies of 4 infants with this syndrome and pulmonary emphysema showed that the elastic fibers in alveolar ducts and sacs were irregularly thickened, wavy, fragmented, and clumped [110]. Diffuse honeycombing of the lungs and spontaneous pneumothorax were reported as the presenting features of Marfan's syndrome in a boy [90]. In 2 cases, bilateral bullous disease with spontaneous pneumothorax has been reported [140]. Upper-lobe fibrosis is also reported in Marfan's syndrome [33,149]. A report described 3 members of 1 family—a father and 2 sons—all afflicted with Marfan's syndrome, who suffered multiple bilateral episodes of pneumothoraces that required repeated drainage procedures [153].

Structural abnormalities of the right middle lobe have been described [110]. Ciliary dyskinesia also has been observed in a patient with Marfan's syndrome [106]. Additionally, deformities of the thoracic cage by abnormalities of the vertebral column, ribs, and sternum are common in this syndrome and may occur in any combination and degree of severity [140]. Both scoliosis and

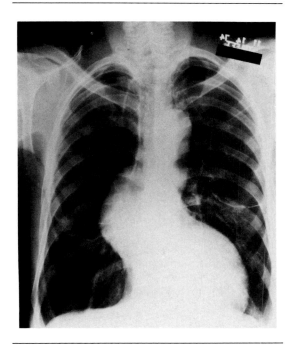

Fig. 65-5. Marfan's syndrome with hyperinflation, bullous changes, dilated tortuous aorta, and "tall" lungs.

pectus excavatum occur and may cause pulmonary dysfunction [143]. Tracheal weakness, presumably due to structural deficiency of the cartilages, may deteriorate, as has been reported in a patient who underwent posterior spinal fusion for ankylosing spondylitis [95].

Several extensive reviews have described the pulmonary manifestations in Marfan's syndrome. A review of published reports disclosed nearly 50 patients with bullous lesions, lung cysts, or emphysema, 22 of whom were younger than 20 years and two-thirds of whom were male [149]. In the same review, of an additional 100 patients with Marfan's syndrome, 11 had spontaneous pneumothorax, with recurrence in 10 and bilateral appearance in 6, pneumonia or recurrent respiratory infections in 8, and bronchiectasis in 2 [149]. Chest roentgenograms revealed emphysematous bullae in 5, upper-lobe fibrosis in 4, and aspergilloma in 2. Another review of 249 patients older than 12 years reported the frequency of pneumothorax to be 4.4 percent, with recurrent or bilateral pneumothorax in 3 percent [61]. This study suggests that definitive surgical therapy should be considered at the first occurrence of pneumothorax because of the high rate of recurrence after treatment with a chest tube.

Pulmonary dysfunction is present in the absence of thoracic cage abnormality. An important aspect of interpreting the pulmonary function test results is the recognition that the values are based on age, sex, and standing height. Thus the unusually longer length of the leg in Marfan's syndrome contributes disproportionately to these calculations [105,135]. Studies of pulmonary function in patients with Marfan's syndrome have revealed diminished total lung capacity and vital capacity and mildly lowered flow rates at low lung volumes, with decreased diffusing capacity and elastic lung recoil [25,53,140], whereas in some cases, only minimal abnormalities of pulmonary function have been noted [25]. A study involving 79 Marfan's patients concluded that persons with this syndrome who have, at most, mild thoracic deformity do not have significant abnormalities of static pulmonary function [135], and thus the connective tissue defects in the lungs seem to have minimal clinical impact beyond the risk of pneumothorax. However, tests of dynamic lung function were not done in this group of subjects. Another report on 11 children with Marfan's syndrome observed airway reactivity, as measured by methacholine challenge, in all children even though only 1 patient had a diagnosis of asthma [84]. An unusual case of Marfan's syndrome with hypercoagulability complicated by multiple pulmonary emboli has been described [69].

Achondroplasia

Achondroplasia is the most common skeletal dysplasia resulting in short-limbed dwarfism [111]. The disorder results from abnormal endochondral bone formation. Pulmonary complications are common in achondroplastic infants and children younger than 2 years. Factors that influence respiratory manifestations include associated deformities of the chest wall and involvement of respiratory centers at the level of the brain stem and upper cervical cord [107]. The thoracic skeletal abnormalities include reduced chest cage measurements, pectus excavatum, accentuated thoracic kyphosis, or thoracic lordosis [107,133]. Detailed physiologic abnormalities in 12 healthy subjects with achondroplasia showed that the reduction in vital capacity was out of proportion to what would be expected if these subjects had normal limb size; the other pulmonary function parameters were normal [132]. Another study of

58 female and 44 male achondroplastic subjects between 7 and 60 years of age showed vital capacity of 68 percent and 72 percent of that predicted for normally proportioned men and women, respectively [134].

Upper airway involvement, nasal obstruction, hypoxemia, and obstructive sleep apnea are more common in younger achondroplastic subjects. Sleep apnea with death due to acute or chronic compression of the lower brain stem or cervical spinal cord has been noted in infants with achondroplasia. Obstructive sleep apnea has been reported in older subjects as well [139]. Resolution of sleep apnea by tracheostomy in achondroplastic dwarfs has resulted in normalization of growth hormone release and normal growth [58]. Apneustic breathing is a rare neurogenic breathing characteristic (see Chapter 64). A report on 5 patients with achondroplasia, all of whom demonstrated apneustic breathing, speculated that compression of the lower medullary respiratory centers and afferent pathways in the spinal cord were responsible for the abnormal breathing pattern in these patients [93].

Rigid Spine Syndrome

Rigid spine syndrome consists of a rigid spine associated with a myopathy predominantly affecting proximal limb muscles [39]. Although this syndrome is more common in children, respiratory failure secondary to respiratory muscle weakness has been described in an adult [39]. The cause of respiratory failure is secondary to extreme flattening of the chest and fixation of the thorax as a result of contracture of costovertebral joints. In almost all reported cases of rigid spine syndrome, the patients have died from respiratory failure. Nocturnal ventilator assistance has been employed to assist 2 patients, both of whom had a vital capacity of less than 30 percent of that predicted [98].

Craniofacial Deformities

Several types of craniofacial deformities have been described in the literature, and these structural aberrations frequently are associated with upper airway problems. Severe sleep apnea, sometimes necessitating tracheostomy, is now a recognized complication of various craniofacial structural abnormalities. Different grades of respiratory distress from obstructive sleep apnea have been described in adults with craniofacial dysostosis [65], achondroplasia [58,101], meta-

tropic dwarfism [7], Hallerman-Streiff syndrome [52], and Treacher Collins syndrome [75,85]. Sleep apnea is a well-recognized aspect of micrognathia and Pierre Robin syndrome [128]. Tracheostomy is recommended in pediatric craniofacial abnormalities with sleep apnea before reconstructive surgery is undertaken [85].

Pierre Robin syndrome is characterized by mandibular hypoplasia (micrognathia) and glossoptosis, often associated with a cleft palate [74,113]. Upper respiratory obstruction is commonly present in this disorder. The tongue is posteriorly displaced (glossoptosis) because of micrognathia and anterior insertion of the tongue to the mandible [35]. Severe airways obstruction may persist for months but may improve with time [74,94].

Because of micrognathia, patients with Treacher Collins syndrome are at greater risk for developing obstructive sleep apnea. Surgical correction of the micrognathia may relieve sleep apnea [75].

Gorham's Disease

Gorham's disease (disappearing or vanishing bone disease) is characterized by massive osteolysis. It generally appears in the second and third decades of life with an equal sex distribution. Although any skeletal bone can be affected, the commonly involved bones are the innominate bones, thorax, and spine. Clinically, patients present with dull aching and weakness in an affected extremity. Pain is usually caused by pathologic fractures, which are a prominent feature of this disease. Histologically, lymphangiomatous tissue is observed in the affected skeletal structures. The predominant feature is the lymphatic dysplasia in skeletal structures as well as thorax.

Pleuropulmonary manifestations include pleural effusion and development of lymphangiomatous tissue in the mediastinum [102]. Massive pleural effusions, sometimes chylous, with high mortality have been described in these patients [37,43]. Pneumothorax may be associated with chylothorax and may be seen in conjunction with chylous pleural effusion [46]. Pulmonary lymphangiectasia, described in patients with some of these skeletal abnormalities, may be responsible for the chylous pleural effusion.

Adult Still's Disease

Adult Still's disease is characterized by high fever, arthritis, evanescent rash, serositis, lymphadenopathy, splenomegaly, leukocytosis, and absence of rheumatoid factor and antinuclear antibodies [21,41]. Pleuropulmonary complications such as pleuritis and pneumonitis may occur frequently. The incidence of pleuropulmonary complications is reported to be approximately 30 percent, but estimates of up to 60 percent are recorded [92]. The most common symptom is pleurisy with or without effusion. Persistent or severe pulmonary parenchymal infiltrates are uncommon [30]. Fatal adult respiratory distress syndrome complicated by opportunistic pulmonary infections has been described in a 65-year-old Japanese woman [66].

References

1. Abd AG, et al. Diaphragmatic dysfunction after open heart surgery: Treatment with a rocking bed. *Ann Intern Med* 111:881, 1989.
2. Ahern MJ, et al. Ankylosing spondylitis and adenocarcinoma of the lung. *Ann Rheum Dis* 41:292, 1982.
3. Anderson PR, et al. Postoperative respiratory complications in nonidiopathic scoliosis. *Acta Anaesthesiol Scand* 29:186, 1985.
4. Backer OG, Brunner S, Larsen V. Radiologic evaluation of funnel chest. *Acta Radiol* 55:249, 1961.
5. Bake B, et al. Regional pulmonary ventilation and perfusion distribution in patients with untreated idiopathic scoliosis. *Thorax* 27:703, 1972.
6. Baydur A, et al. Respiratory mechanics in anesthetized young patients with kyphoscoliosis. Immediate and delayed effects of corrective spinal surgery. *Chest* 97:1157, 1990.
7. Belik J, et al. Respiratory complications of metatropic dwarfism. *Clin Pediatr* (Phila.) 24:504, 1985.
8. Ben-Menachem Y, O'Hara AE, Kane HA. Paradoxical cardiac enlargement during inspiration in children with pectus excavatum: A new observation. *Br J Radiol* 46:38, 1973.
9. Berendes J, Miehkle A. A rare ankylosis of the cricoarytenoid joints. *Arch Otolaryngol* 98:63, 1973.
10. Bergofsky EH. Respiratory failure in disorders of the thoracic cage. *Am Rev Respir Dis* 119:643, 1979.
11. Bergofsky EH, Turino GM, Fishman AP. Cardiorespiratory failure in kyphoscoliosis. *Medicine* 38:263, 1959.
12. Bjure J, et al. Respiratory impairment and airway closure in patients with untreated scoliosis. *Thorax* 25:451, 1970.
13. Bjure J, Grimby G, Nachemson A. Correction of body height in predicting spirometric values in scoliotic patients. *Scand J Clin Lab Invest* 21:190, 1968.
14. Blount WP, Moe JH. *The Milwaukee Brace.* Baltimore: Williams & Wilkins, 1973.
15. Boffa P, Stovin P, Shneerson J. Lung development abnormalities in severe scoliosis. *Thorax* 39:681, 1984.
16. Branthwaite MA. Cardiorespiratory consequences of unfused idiopathic scoliosis. *Br J Dis Chest* 80:360, 1986.
17. Braun SR, Birnbaum ML, Chopra PS. Pre- and post-operative pulmonary function abnormalities in coronary artery revascularisation surgery. *Chest* 73:316, 1978.
18. Bruderman I, Stein M. Physiologic evaluation and treatment of kyphoscoliotic patients. *Ann Intern Med* 55:94, 1961.
19. Burgess GE, et al. Pulmonary effect of pleurotomy during and after coronary artery surgery with internal mammary artery versus saphenous vein grafts. *J Thorac Cardiovasc Surg* 76:230, 1978.
20. Buszek MC, et al. Hemidiaphragmatic paralysis: An unusual complication of cervical spondylosis. *Arch Phys Med Rehabil* 64:601, 1983.
21. Bywaters EGL. Still's disease in the adult. *Ann Rheum Dis* 30:121, 1971.
22. Caro CG, DuBois AB. Pulmonary function in kyphoscoliosis. *Thorax* 16:282, 1961.
23. Chakera TM, et al. The chest radiograph in ankylosing spondylitis. *Clin Radiol* 26:455, 1975.
24. Chidambaram B, Mehta AV. Currarino-Silverman syndrome (pectus carinatum type 2 deformity) and mitral valve disease. *Chest* 102:780, 1992.
25. Chishold JC, Cherniack NS, Carton RW. Results of pulmonary function testing in 5 persons with the Marfan syndrome. *J Lab Clin Med* 71:25, 1968.
26. Cobb JR. Outline for the study of scoliosis (Instructional Course Lectures). *Am Acad Orthop Surg* 5:261, 1948.
27. Cohen AA, Natelson EA, Fechner RE. Fibrosing interstitial pneumonitis in ankylosing spondylitis. *Chest* 59:369, 1971.
28. Collis DK, Ponseti IV. Long-term follow-up of patients with idiopathic scoliosis not treated surgically. *J Bone Joint Surg* 51A:425, 1969.
29. Cooper DM, et al. Respiratory mechanics in adolescents with idiopathic scoliosis. *Am Rev Respir Dis* 130:16, 1984.
30. Corbett AJ, Zizic TM, Stevens MB. Adult-onset Still's disease with an associated severe restrictive pulmonary defect: A case report. *Ann Rheum Dis* 42:452, 1983.
31. Cruickshank B. Pathology of ankylosing spondylitis. *Bull Rheum Dis* 10:211, 1960.
32. Davies D. Ankylosing spondylitis and lung fibrosis. *Q J Med* 41:395, 1972.
33. Davies D, Crowther JS, MacFarlane A. Idio-

pathic progressive pulmonary fibrosis. *Thorax* 30:316, 1975.

34. Davies H. Chest deformities in congenital heart disease. *Br J Dis Chest* 53:151, 1959.

35. Dennison WM. The Pierre Robin syndrome. *Pediatrics* 36:336, 1965.

36. Derveaux L, et al. Preoperative and postoperative abnormalities in chest x-ray indices and in lung function in pectus deformities. *Chest* 95:850, 1989.

37. Ducharme JC, et al. Chylothorax, chylopericardium with multiple lymphangioma of bone. *J Pediatr Surg* 17:365, 1982.

38. Dwyer EM, Troncale F. Spontaneous pneumothorax and pulmonary disease in the Marfan syndrome. *Ann Intern Med* 62:1285, 1965.

39. Efthimiou J, et al. Diaphragm paralysis causing ventilatory failure in an adult with the rigid spine syndrome. *Am Rev Respir Dis* 136:1483, 1987.

40. Ellis ER, et al. Noninvasive ventilatory support during sleep improves respiratory failure in kyphoscoliosis. *Chest* 94:811, 1988.

41. Esdaile JM, Tannenbaum HM, Hawkins D. Adult Still's disease. *Am J Med* 68:825, 1980.

42. Estenne M, et al. Phrenic and diaphragm function after bypass grafting. *Thorax* 40:293, 1985.

43. Feigl D, Seidel L, Marmor A. Gorham's disease of the clavicle with bilateral pleural effusions. *Chest* 79:242, 1981.

44. Feltelius N, et al. Pulmonary involvement in ankylosing spondylitis. *Ann Rheum Dis* 45:736, 1986.

45. Fink A, Rivin A, Murray JF. Pectus excavatum: An analysis of twenty-seven cases. *Arch Intern Med* 108:427, 1961.

46. Fisher E, et al. Spontaneous chylothorax in Noonan's syndrome. *Eur J Pediatr* 138:282, 1982.

47. Fisher LR, Cawley MI, Holgate ST. Relation between chest expansion, pulmonary function, and exercise tolerance in patients with ankylosing spondylitis. *Ann Rheum Dis* 49:921, 1990.

48. Fishman AP, Goldring RM, Turino GM. General alveolar hypoventilation: A syndrome of respiratory and cardiac failure in patients with normal lungs. *Q J Med* 35:261, 1966.

49. Foster ME, Foster DR. Bronchiectasis in Marfan's syndrome. *Postgrad Med J* 56:718, 1980.

50. Franssen MJ, et al. Lung function in patients with ankylosing spondylitis: A study of the influence of disease activity and treatment with nonsteroidal antiinflammatory drugs. *J Rheumatol* 13:936, 1986.

51. Freyschuss U, Nilsonne U, Lundgren KD. Idiopathic scoliosis in old age: I. Respiratory function. *Acta Med Scand* 184:365, 1968.

52. Friede H, et al. Cardiorespiratory disease associated with Hallerman-Streiff syndrome: Analysis of craniofacial morphology by cephalometric roentgenograms. *J Craniofac Genet Dev Biol* 1(Suppl):189, 1985.

53. Fuleihan FJ, Suh JK, Shephard RH. Some aspects of pulmonary function in the Marfan syndrome. *Bull Johns Hopkins Hosp* 113:320, 1963.

54. Gacad G, Hamosh P. The lung in ankylosing spondylitis. *Am Rev Respir Dis* 107:286, 1973.

55. Gagnon S, Jodoin A, Martin R. Pulmonary function test study and after spinal fusion in young idiopathic scoliosis. *Spine* 14:486, 1989.

56. Gazioglu K, et al. Pulmonary function in idiopathic scoliosis: Comparative evaluation before and after orthopaedic correction. *J Bone Joint Surg* 50A:1391, 1968.

57. Godfrey S. Respiratory and cardiovascular consequences of scoliosis. *Respiration* 27 (Suppl):67, 1970.

58. Goldstein SJ, et al. Achondroplasia and obstructive sleep apnea: Correction of apnea and abnormal sleep-entrained growth hormone release by tracheostomy. *Birth Defects* 21:93, 1985.

59. Guilleminault C, et al. Severe kyphoscoliosis, breathing, and sleep. The "Quasimodo" syndrome during sleep. *Chest* 79:626, 1981.

60. Guller B, Hable K. Cardiac findings in pectus excavatum in children: Review and differential diagnosis. *Chest* 66:165, 1974.

61. Hall JR, et al. Pneumothorax in the Marfan syndrome: Prevalence and therapy. *Ann Thorac Surg* 37:500, 1984.

62. Harrington PR. Treatment of scoliosis: Correction and internal fixation by spine instrumentation. *J Bone Joint Surg* 44A:591, 1962.

63. Hassard AD. Cervical ankylosing hyperostosis and airway obstruction. *Laryngoscope* 94:966, 1984.

64. Hepper NGG, Black LF, Fowler WS. Relationships of lung volume to height and arm span in normal subjects and in patients with spinal deformity. *Am Rev Respir Dis* 91:356, 1965.

65. Hess CW, Sauter K, Bonfils P. Severe adult hypersomnia–sleep apnea syndrome in craniofacial dysostosis. *Respiration* 50:147, 1986.

66. Hirohita S, et al. Adult Still's disease complicated with adult respiratory distress. *Arch Intern Med* 146:2409, 1986.

67. Hoeppner VH, et al. Nighttime ventilation improves respiratory failure in secondary scoliosis. *Am Rev Respir Dis* 129:240, 1984.

68. Howell JBL. Scoliosis. In PB Beeson, W McDermott (Eds), *Textbook of Medicine* (14th ed). Philadelphia: Saunders, 1975. Pp 817–820.

69. Humphries JE, et al. Hypercoagulability in a patient with Marfan syndrome. *J Med Genet* 28:349, 1991.

70. Iseman MD, Buschman DL, Ackerson LM. Pectus excavatum and scoliosis. Thoracic anomalies associated with pulmonary disease caused

by *Mycobacterium avium* complex. *Am Rev Respir Dis* 144:914, 1991.

71. Iwa T, Watanabe Y. Unusual combination of pulmonary sequestration and funnel chest. *Chest* 76:314, 1979.

72. James JIP. *Scoliosis.* Baltimore: Williams & Wilkins, 1967. P 43.

73. Jenkins SC, et al. Lung function after coronary artery surgery using the internal mammary artery and the saphenous veins. *Thorax* 44:209, 1989.

74. Jeresaty RM, Huszar RJ, Basu S. Pierre Robin syndrome: Cause of respiratory obstruction, cor pulmonale and pulmonary edema. *Am J Dis Child* 117:712, 1969.

75. Johnston C, et al. Obstructive sleep apnea in Treacher Collins syndrome. *Cleft Palate J* 18:39, 1981.

76. Jones RS, et al. Mechanical inefficiency of the thoracic cage in scoliosis. *Thorax* 36:456, 1981.

77. Kaguraoka H, et al. Degree of severity of pectus excavatum and pulmonary function in preoperative and postoperative periods. *J Thorac Cardiovasc Surg* 104:1483, 1992.

78. Kafer ER. Idiopathic scoliosis: Gas exchange and the age dependence of arterial blood gases. *J Clin Invest* 58:825, 1976.

79. Kafer ER. Idiopathic scoliosis: Mechanical properties of the respiratory system and the ventilatory response to carbon dioxide. *J Clin Invest* 55:1153, 1975.

80. Kafer ER. Respiratory and cardiovascular functions in scoliosis. *Bull Eur Physiopathol Respir* 13:299, 1977.

81. Kafer ER. Respiratory function in paralytic scoliosis. *Am Rev Respir Dis* 110:450, 1974.

82. Karlins NL, Yagan R. A complication of diffuse idiopathic skeletal hyperostosis. *Spine* 16:235, 1991.

83. Kinnear WJ, Shneerson JM. Acute pleural effusion in inactive ankylosing spondylitis. *Thorax* 40:150, 1985.

84. Konig P, et al. Bronchial hyperreactivity in children with Marfan syndrome. *Pediatr Pulmonol* 11:29, 1991.

85. Lauritzen C, Lilja J, Jaristad J. Airway obstruction and sleep apnea in children with craniofacial abnormalities. *Plast Reconstr Surg* 77:1, 1986.

86. Leech JA, et al. Relationship of lung function to severity of osteoporosis in women. *Am Rev Respir Dis* 141:68, 1990.

87. Lester CW. Pectus carinatum, pigeon breast and related deformities of the sternum and costal cartilages. *Arch Pediatr* 77:399, 1960.

88. Libby DM, et al. Acute respiratory failure in scoliosis or kyphosis: Prolonged survival and treatment. *Am J Med* 73:532, 1982.

89. Libby DM, Schley WS, Smith JP. Cricoarytenoid arthritis in ankylosing spondylitis: A cause of

acute respiratory failure and cor pulmonale. *Chest* 80:641, 1981.

90. Lipton RA, Greenwald RA, Seriff NS. Pneumothorax and bilateral honeycombed lung in Marfan syndrome: Report of a case and review of the pulmonary abnormalities in this disorder. *Am Rev Respir Dis* 104:924, 1971.

91. Locke TJ, et al. Rib cage mechanics after median sternotomy. *Thorax* 45:465, 1990.

92. Lundberg MS, Ward JR. Pulmonary manifestations of other rheumatic diseases. *Lung Biol Health Dis* 45:351, 1990.

93. Mador MJ, Tobin MJ. Apneustic breathing. A characteristic feature of brainstem compression in achondroplasia. *Chest* 97:877, 1990.

94. Mallory JB, Paradise JL. Glossoptosis revisited: On the development and resolution of airway obstruction in the Pierre Robin syndrome. *Pediatrics* 64:946, 1979.

95. Mesrobian RB, Epps JL. Midtracheal obstruction after Harrington rod placement in a patient with Marfan syndrome. *Anesth Analg* 65:411, 1986.

96. Mezon BL, et al. Sleep breathing abnormalities in kyphoscoliosis. *Am Rev Respir Dis* 122:617, 1980.

97. Midgren B, et al. Nocturnal hypoxaemia in severe scoliosis. *Br J Dis Chest* 82:226, 1988.

98. Morita H, et al. Rigid spine syndrome with respiratory failure. *J Neurol Neurosurg Psychiatr* 53:782, 1990.

99. Olgiati R, et al. Diffusing capacity in idiopathic scoliosis and its interpretation regarding alveolar development. *Am Rev Respir Dis* 126:229, 1982.

100. Parkin A, Robinson PJ, Hickling P. Regional lung ventilation in ankylosing spondylitis. *Br J Radiol* 55:833, 1982.

101. Pauli RM, et al. Apnea and sudden unexplained death in infants with achondroplasia. *J Pediatr* 104:342, 1984.

102. Pediceli G, et al. Gorham syndrome. *JAMA* 252:1449, 1984.

103. Pehrsson K, et al. Lung function in adult idiopathic scoliosis: A 20-year follow up. *Thorax* 46:474, 1991.

104. Peters RM. Pulmonary Function and Its Evaluation. In WWL Glenn et al (Eds), *Thoracic and Cardiovascular Surgery.* Norwalk, CT: Appleton-Century-Crofts, 1983.

105. Pyeritz RE, McKusick VA. The Marfan syndrome: Diagnosis and management. *N Engl J Med* 300:772, 1979.

106. Ras GJ, Van Wyk CJ. Primary ciliary dyskinesia in Marfan syndrome: A case report. *S Afr Med J* 64:212, 1983.

107. Reid CS, et al. Cervicomedullary compression in young patients with achondroplasia: Value of comprehensive neurologic and respiratory evaluation. *J Pediatr* 110:522, 1987.

108. Resnick D, et al. Diffuse idiopathic skeletal hyperostosis (DISH): Ankylosing hyperostosis of Forestier and Rotes-Querol. *Semin Arthritis Rheum* 7:153, 1978.

109. Respiratory function in scoliosis (editorial). *Lancet* 1:84, 1985.

110. Reye RDK, Bale PM. Elastic tissue in pulmonary emphysema in Marfan syndrome. *Arch Pathol* 96:427, 1973.

111. Rimoin DL. The chondrodystrophies. *Adv Hum Genet* 5:1, 1975.

112. Robicsek F, et al. Pectus carinatum. *J Thorac Cardiovasc Surg* 78:52, 1979.

113. Robin P. La chute de la base de la langue consideree comme une nouvelle cause de gene dans la respiration naso-pharyngienne. *Bull Acad Natl Med* 89:37, 1923.

114. Rosenow EC III, et al. Pleuropulmonary manifestations of ankylosing spondylitis. *Mayo Clin Proc* 52:641, 1977.

115. Rumancik WM, et al. Fibrobullous disease of the upper lobes: An extraskeletal manifestation of ankylosing spondylitis. *J Comput Assist Tomogr* 8:225, 1984.

116. Sawicka EH, Branthwaite MA. Respiration during sleep in kyphoscoliosis. *Thorax* 42:801, 1987.

117. Scobie BA. The lung in ankylosing spondylitis. *Br Med J* 4:560, 1971.

118. Sevastikoglou JA, Linderholm H, Lindgren U. Effect of the Milwaukee brace on vital and ventilatory capacity of scoliotic patients. *Acta Orthop Scand* 47:540, 1976.

119. Shamberger RC, Welch KJ. Surgical correction of chondromanubrial deformity (Currarino-Silverman syndrome). *J Pediatr Surg* 23:319, 1988.

120. Shands AR Jr, Eisberg HB. The incidence of scoliosis in the state of Delaware: A study of 50,000 minifilms of the chest made during a survey for tuberculosis. *J Bone Joint Surg* 37A:1243, 1955.

121. Shankar PS. Ankylosing spondylitis with fibrosis and carcinoma of the lung. *CA* 32:177, 1982.

122. Shaw DB, Read J. Hypoxia and thoracic scoliosis. *Br Med J* 2:1486, 1960.

123. Shneerson JM. The cardiorespiratory response to exercise in thoracic scoliosis. *Thorax* 33:457, 1978.

124. Shneerson JM. Pulmonary artery pressure in thoracic scoliosis during and after exercise while breathing air and pure oxygen. *Thorax* 33:747, 1978.

125. Sinha R, Bergofsky EH. Prolonged alteration in lung mechanics in kyphoscoliosis by positive pressure hyperinflation. *Am Rev Respir Dis* 106:47, 1972.

126. Smyth RJ, et al. Pulmonary function in adolescents with mild idiopathic scoliosis. *Thorax* 39:901, 1984.

127. Smyth RJ, et al. Ventilatory patterns during hypoxia, hypercapnia, and exercise in adolescents with mild scoliosis. *Pediatrics* 77:692, 1986.

128. Spier S, et al. Sleep in Pierre Robin syndrome. *Chest* 90:711, 1986.

129. Stewart RM, Ridyard JB, Pearson JD. Regional lung function in ankylosing spondylitis. *Thorax* 31:433, 1976.

130. Stiksa G, et al. Bilateral pulmonary aspergilloma in ankylosing spondylitis treated with transthoracic intracavitary instillations of antifungal agents. *Scand J Respir Dis* 57:163, 1976.

131. Stock MC, et al. Effect of pleurotomy on pulmonary function after median sternotomy. *Ann Thorac Surg* 42:441, 1986.

132. Stokes DC, et al. The lungs and airways in achondroplasia. Do little people have little lungs? *Chest* 98:145, 1990.

133. Stokes DC, et al. Respiratory complications of achondroplasia. *J Pediatr* 102:534, 1983.

134. Stokes DC, et al. Spirometry and chest wall dimensions in achondroplasia. *Chest* 93:364, 1988.

135. Streeten EA, Murphy EA, Pyeritz RE. Pulmonary function in the Marfan syndrome. *Chest* 91:408, 1987.

136. Strom K, et al. Survival of patients with severe thoracic spine deformities receiving domiciliary oxygen therapy. *Chest* 102:164, 1992.

137. Teoh PC. Bronchiectasis and spontaneous pneumothorax in Marfan's syndrome. *Chest* 72:672, 1977.

138. Ter-Wee PM, et al. Scoliosis as cause of pulmonary atelectasis. *Eur Respir J* 4:371, 1991.

139. Thomas JN. Partial upper airway obstruction and sleep apnea. *J Laryngol Otol* 92:41, 1978.

140. Turner JA McM, Stanley NN. Fragile lung in the Marfan syndrome. *Thorax* 31:771, 1976.

141. Vale JA, Pickering JG, Scott GW. Ankylosing spondylitis and upper lobe fibrosis and cavitation. *Guys Hosp Rec* 123:97, 1974.

142. van Noord JA, et al. Total respiratory resistance and reactance in ankylosing spondylitis and kyphoscoliosis. *Eur Respir J* 4:945, 1991.

143. Wanderman KL, Goldstein MS, Farber J. Cor pulmonale secondary to severe kyphoscoliosis in Marfan syndrome. *Chest* 67:250, 1975.

144. Warnick C, Sherman MS, Lesser RW. Aspiration pneumonia due to diffuse cervical hyperostosis. *Chest* 98:763, 1990.

145. Weber B, et al. Pulmonary function in asymptomatic adolescents with idiopathic scoliosis. *Am Rev Respir Dis* 111:389, 1975.

146. Weg JG, Krumholz RA, Harkleroad LE. Pulmonary dysfunction in pectus excavatum. *Am Rev Respir Dis* 96:936, 1967.

147. Wiers PWJ, et al. Cuirass respirator treatment of chronic respiratory failure in scoliotic patients. *Thorax* 32:221, 1977.

148. Wojtulewski JA, et al. Cricoarytenoid arthritis in ankylosing spondylitis. *Br J Med* 3:145, 1973.

149. Wood JR, et al. Pulmonary disease in patients with Marfan syndrome. *Thorax* 39:780, 1984.

150. Woolf CR. Kyphoscoliosis and respiratory failure. A patient treated with assisted ventilation for 27 years. *Chest* 98:1297, 1990.

151. Wynn SR, et al. Exercise cardiorespiratory function in adolescents with pectus excavatum. Observations before and after operation. *J Thorac Cardiovasc Surg* 99:41, 1990.

152. Wynne-Davies R. Familial (idiopathic) scoliosis: A family survey. *J Bone Joint Surg* 50B:24, 1968.

153. Yellin A, Shiner RJ, Lieberman Y. Familial multiple bilateral pneumothorax associated with Marfan syndrome. *Chest* 100:577, 1991.

154. Zorab PA. Chest deformities. *Br Med J* 1:1155, 1966.

66

Dermatologic Diseases

Udaya B. S. Prakash

Among the myriad dermatologic disorders are those that reflect diseases of other organs. Not uncommonly, the dermatologic sign is the initial signal of an internal illness. The cutaneous manifestations of both benign and malignant internal diseases are clinically well recognized. Among the malignant disorders, respiratory neoplasms are well known to cause paraneoplastic syndromes such as clubbing, dermatomyositis, acanthosis nigricans, and bullous pemphigoid. Many vasculitic syndromes and collagenoses produce significant cutaneous lesions. These diseases are discussed in Chapters 57 and 58. This chapter will address the respiratory manifestations of primary dermatologic diseases. However, many of these disorders cannot be classified as primary dermatoses, though their clinical presentations with cutaneous lesions warrant their inclusion here [153]. Because of the lack of connection between most of the diseases included here, which makes an appropriate classification difficult, the diseases are discussed in alphabetic order.

Acanthosis Nigricans and Other Paraneoplastic Dermatoses

Acanthosis nigricans is an uncommon cutaneous disorder characterized by hyperpigmentation and epidermal hypertrophy (Fig. 66-1) [27]. The paraneoplastic category of acanthosis nigricans is associated, in 90 percent of cases, with gastric adenocarcinoma and other intraabdominal malignancies [45]. Skin changes and an underlying neoplasm appear together in 60 percent of cases, whereas the cutaneous changes appear before clinical evidence of carcinoma in 20 percent of patients. Acanthosis nigricans may be the presenting clinical feature of lung cancer [99], adenocarcinoma of the lung being the most common type of pulmonary malignancy associated with

this skin disorder. Acanthosis nigricans has been observed also in a patient with bronchoalveolar cell carcinoma [126]. The prognosis in patients with acanthosis and associated cancer is dismal. Progressive skin changes signify a higher mortality.

Many lesser-known dermatoses are also associated with lung cancer. Bowen's disease is a chronic dermatosis characterized by the development of in situ epidermoid carcinoma of the skin [24]. This disease has been linked to arsenic exposure in some cases. An association between lung cancer and Bowen's disease has been described [73]. Other paraneoplastic cutaneous dermatoses associated with bronchogenic carcinoma include epidermolysis bullosa [2], pemphigoid [1], tylosis or hyperkeratosis palmaris et plantaris [46,151, 177], porphyria cutanea tarda [141], acquired hypertrichosis lanuginosa [181], and tripe palms [41]. Many of these dermatoses precede the onset of the malignancy.

Acute Febrile Neutrophilic Dermatosis

Acute febrile neutrophilic dermatitis (Sweet's syndrome) is an uncommon, recurrent, often dramatic cutaneous disease manifested by painful, plaque-forming inflammatory papules and usually associated with fever, arthralgia, and leukocytosis [191]. Approximately 20 percent of patients have associated malignancies, particularly hematologic neoplasms [195]. Chest roentgenograms have revealed patchy pulmonary parenchymal infiltrates. Histologic features in lung biopsies have included diffuse interstitial edema, neutrophilic interstitial and alveolar exudates, recent hemorrhages, and hyperplasia of type I and II cells [71,195]. Pulmonary pathologic findings in one patient consisted of marked intraalveolar

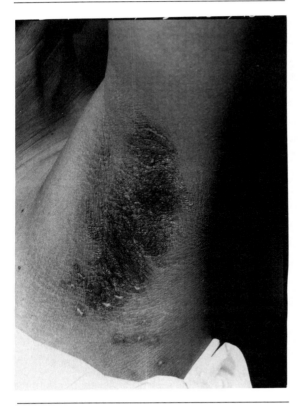

Fig. 66-1. Acanthosis nigricans involving left axilla in a patient with adenocarcinoma of lung. Marked hyperpigmentation and epidermal hypertrophy are the pathologic features.

neutrophilic infiltrate similar to skin biopsy findings, chronic interstitial pneumonitis, and minimal fibrosis; resolution was reported after corticosteroid therapy [103].

Anhidrotic Ectodermal Dysplasia

Anhidrotic ectodermal dysplasia is a hereditary, usually X-linked disorder characterized by insufficient sweating, sparse hair, and scanty teeth. Predisposition to severe bronchitis has been observed [15]. The common upper respiratory infections occur often in these patients and have been ascribed to scanty mucus and deficient cilia. Absence of mucous glands in the tracheobronchial tree and increased incidence of asthma are the other respiratory aspects of this disorder [32, 52,157].

Blue Rubber Bleb Nevus Syndrome

More than 40 cases of the blue rubber bleb nevus syndrome (Bean's syndrome), which is characterized by the presence of rubbery blue hemangiomas of the skin and gastrointestinal tract associated with gastrointestinal hemorrhage, have been reported in the literature [16]. The rubbery angiomas of skin are variable in size, compressible, and refill on release of pressure. Hemangiomas may occur in other organs, including the pleura. Those of the gastrointestinal tract cause profuse hemorrhage, whereas hemothorax has resulted from pleural hemangiomas [102]. Histologic assessment of pleural specimens has shown features similar to those in the skin.

Chest Wall Lesions

Confusion arises when chest roentgenograms reveal unusual abnormalities caused by lesions located in the chest wall. Initially diagnosed as pulmonary parenchymal lesions, many of these undergo extensive diagnostic testing. Good physical examination with a posteroanterior stereo chest roentgenogram and a lateral view will exclude an intrathoracic lesion. Unusual density, significant calcification, and association with skin lesions in areas other than the thoracic cage assist in excluding an intrathoracic lesion (Figs. 66-2, 66-3).

Fig. 66-2. Thick braid of hair masquerading as superior mediastinal mass in right paratracheal region.

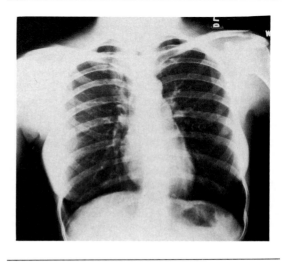

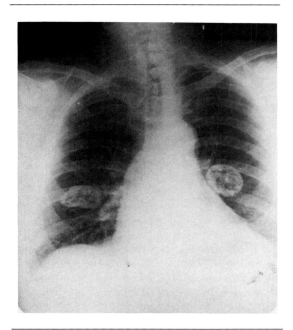

Fig. 66-3. Calcified skin lesions appearing as intrapulmonary lesions on a single posteroanterior view.

Chronic Mucocutaneous Candidiasis

Mucocutaneous candidiasis is an uncommon disorder associated with certain immunologic defects. Deficiency of the IgG_2/IgG_4 subclass and absence of antibodies against pneumococcal and *Hemophilus* polysaccharide have been observed in patients with this disorder. Detailed studies of a pediatric patient with mucocutaneous candidiasis and recurrent pulmonary infections revealed a severe defect in cell-mediated immunity, but humoral immune responses were normal [97]. The disease may be complicated by candidiasis involving the larynx, trachea, bronchi, and esophagus. Symptoms consist of hoarseness, hemoptysis, and dysphagia [100]. Bacterial pneumonia, bronchopneumonic infiltrates, and bronchiectasis are some of the pulmonary manifestations described [25].

Cutis Laxa

Cutis laxa (generalized elastolysis) is a rare systemic disorder of connective tissue in which the elastic fibers become fragmented, disorganized, and fewer in number. A congenital (X-linked re-

cessive) as well as an acquired variety have been described [20,30,78,156,204]. The acquired cases manifest in midlife and their origin, genetic or otherwise, is unknown. The dermatologic abnormalities in cutis laxa seem to result mainly from a developmental defect of the elastic network in the papillary dermis [104]. Both the congenital and acquired varieties exhibit identical clinical, physiologic, and pathologic abnormalities. Cutaneous pathologic findings are characterized by the disappearance of elastic fibers of the skin (Fig. 66-4). The skin changes lead to an appearance of early senility [65]. Because the disease affects connective tissues all over the body, the clinical manifestations can be varied. Cutis laxa (loose skin), emphysema, aortic aneurysms, diverticula of bowel, and hernias are some of the complications [81]. This disorder is distinct from Marfan's syndrome, Ehlers-Danlos syndrome, and pseudoxanthoma elasticum.

The respiratory system ranks only second to the skin as the most commonly affected organ [81]. The most frequent and serious pulmonary

Fig. 66-4. Cutis laxa (generalized elastolysis) shows loss of skin elasticity over lower trunk and external genitalia. This patient also had severe emphysema.

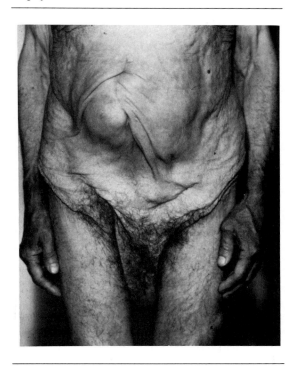

problem associated with cutis laxa is panlobular emphysema [202]. Markedly elevated activity of an elastase-like serum enzyme, observed in some patients with cutis laxa, may predispose to the development of emphysema [5]. Severe and rapidly progressive emphysema leads to early cor pulmonale, which is the most common cause of death among patients with the congenital variety. A review of the literature in 1989 noted 31 cases of congenital and 17 cases of acquired cutis laxa (UBS Prakash, EC Rosenow III, unpublished data). In each variety, the incidence of emphysema was 50 percent. Other observed respiratory complications include pneumothorax, pulmonary fibrosis, pulmonary artery stenosis, eventration of the diaphragm, recurrent pulmonary infections, bronchiectasis, tracheobronchomegaly, and thoracic-aortic aneurysms [85,213].

Ehlers-Danlos Syndrome

Ehlers-Danlos syndrome is a group of inherited disorders in which connective tissue diseases result from disorganization of collagen fibers [13]. Deficiency of type III collagen may be responsible for the respiratory complications. Ultrastructural and biochemical analysis of the lung tissue have revealed a marked decrease in type III collagen and the production of less type III procollagen relative to type I procollagen by fibroblasts cultured from the abnormal lung. Electron-microscopic examination of the lung tissue has shown dilated endoplasmic reticulum of the fibroblasts with normal collagen [14]. Of the six subtypes of Ehlers-Danlos syndrome, which generally are too difficult to distinguish from one another, only types 1 and 4 are reported to be associated with a substantial risk of arterial rupture [146]. The disorder is clinically characterized by abnormal skin flaccidity, hyperextensibility of the joints, bleeding tendencies, atrophic scars, easy skin bruising, and pseudotumors.

Pulmonary involvement in Ehlers-Danlos syndrome results from weakness of the collagen in the lung tissue. Respiratory complications recorded include pneumothorax and bullous lung disease [184]. Severe panacinar emphysema of lungs has been observed [36,44], and transient pulmonary cysts have been reported with this syndrome [14]. Bronchiectasis resulting from weakened bronchial walls also has been reported [68]. A dilated trachea, similar to that in Mounier-Kuhn syndrome, was noted in a patient with this disorder [36]. Weakness of the pulmonary arterial wall may result in rupture and hemoptysis [10].

Pulmonary artery regurgitation and pulmonary valvular stenosis are described as well [105, 106,120]. Spontaneous dissection of the aorta may occur [19].

Eosinophilic Fasciitis

The syndrome of eosinophilic fasciitis consists of symmetric thickening of the deep fascia between muscle and subcutis of the arms, legs, and torso. Skin biopsy reveals a normal epidermis and an inflammatory infiltrate in the deep fascia. More than 200 cases of this unusual syndrome have been reported [58]. Clinically, the affected skin is thickened and indurated. When the skin around the thoracic cage becomes involved, the work of breathing is increased due to the constricting effect of the thickened noncompliant skin ("hidebound chest"). This extrapulmonary thoracic restriction has led to progressive respiratory limitation, documented by pulmonary function tests [37]. Pulmonary parenchymal disease is not a feature, even though the diffusing capacity of carbon monoxide (D_LCO) in some patients with this disorder has been found to be reduced to a very low level.

Epidermolysis Bullosa Dystrophica

Epidermolysis bullosa dystrophica is an uncommon inherited skin disorder generally presenting in newborns and characterized by noninflammatory bullous lesions that may affect the tracheobronchial mucosa and cause respiratory distress [199]. Postmortem analysis of the airways in a 29-month-old boy who died from laryngeal obstruction secondary to this disorder showed intense mucosal inflammation and swelling of the seromucinous glands in the supraglottic airway [72]. Localized subglottic edema and the formation of an inflammatory membrane in the trachea has led to chronic subglottic stridor [178]. The laryngeal cysts are distinct from the cutaneous bullae or bullous pemphigoid. As noted earlier, bullous pemphigoid may be a paraneoplastic manifestation of bronchogenic carcinoma.

Erythema Multiforme

Erythema multiforme is a systemic disorder characterized by generalized eruptions of red or violaceous macules similar to urticaria, papules, vesicles, or bullae, involvement of various internal organs, and fever. The most characteristic skin lesion is known as a *target* or *bull's-eye*. A more severe form is generally described as Stevens-Johnson syndrome, in which mucocutaneous ulcerations are seen [189].

Although the association of erythema multiforme with respiratory infection caused by *Mycoplasma pneumoniae* is well-known [66], the most common association of this disorder is with bacterial pneumonias caused by streptococci, *Pseudomonas* species, pneumococci, *Legionella* species, and *Hemophilus influenzae* [176]. Erythema multiforme is also seen in association with histoplasmosis and blastomycosis [59,125]. Noninfectious causes of erythema multiforme include penicillin, antipyretics, barbiturates, and sulfonamides.

Reported respiratory complications include bronchopneumonic infiltrates, massive pneumonic consolidations, miliary lesions, hilar lymphadenopathy and, uncommonly, pleural effusions [18]. Clinically, the pulmonary manifestations are indicated by laryngotracheobronchitis, cough, hemoptysis, dyspnea, and cyanosis. In a 46-year-old woman with active systemic lupus erythematosus, severe Stevens-Johnson syndrome developed 8 hours after intravenous urography with the nonionic contrast medium iopamidol. The illness included erythema multiforme, intrahepatic cholestasis, pulmonary infiltrates, and acute renal failure, which led to her death [172]. Rapidly progressive and fatal bronchiolitis obliterans was observed in a middle-aged woman; an unusual feature of her disease was the membranous obliteration of larger cartilaginous bronchi [201].

The diagnosis and management of erythema multiforme and Stevens-Johnson syndrome are complex and controversial. Systemic corticosteroids have been used successfully in many instances [144].

Erythema Nodosum

Erythema nodosum is a self-limited cutaneous disorder characterized by inflammatory nodules in the dermis and subcutaneous tissues, commonly along the extensor aspects of the legs. This form of panniculitis is clinically characterized by pain in the anterior tibial area, followed by development of tender pink nodules on the shins. The lesions normally resolve spontaneously over a period of several weeks. The appearance is so characteristic that biopsy seldom is required. Erythema nodosum is most likely a hypersensitivity reaction to a broad variety of disorders, especially drug reactions and infection by viruses, bacteria, and fungi. The cause

is unknown in approximately half the patients [29].

Sarcoidosis is one of the common diseases associated with erythema nodosum. The skin lesion has been observed in 13 percent of two large series of patients with sarcoidosis [206,219]. Erythema nodosum can be the presenting manifestation of this disease [43]. The presence of erythema nodosum in sarcoidosis patients is associated with good prognosis [129]. Acute onset of sarcoidosis with erythema nodosum signifies a good prognosis and spontaneous resolution [179]. The generally good prognosis associated with erythema nodosum and bilateral hilar lymphadenopathy was confirmed in a retrospective study of 818 patients with sarcoidosis, even though 16 percent of patients presenting with erythema nodosum followed a chronic course [138]. Bronchoalveolar lavage in patients who had an acute inflammatory onset of sarcoidosis and erythema nodosum has demonstrated high CD4/CD8 lymphocyte ratios and a higher proportion of T lymphocytes than in patients presenting with respiratory complications after erythema nodosum has resolved [211]. Erythema nodosum in conjunction with non-Hodgkin's lymphoma that presents as a solitary pulmonary nodule has also been described [158].

In the United States, histoplasmosis and coccidioidomycosis are common causes of erythema nodosum [91,172]. Pulmonary blastomycosis associated with erythema nodosum has been described [128]. Another common association is tuberculosis, observed in 37 (12 percent) of 305 children with postprimary tuberculosis [54]. As in sarcoidosis, erythema nodosum in association with these infections denotes a good prognosis because such a combination confirms the development of hypersensitivity. Erythema nodosum was observed in 28 percent of 88 cases of tularemia in northern Finland, pulmonary tularemia being present in 27 percent of the patients [192]. Erythema nodosum was seen more often in patients with pulmonary tularemia than in other forms of the disease.

Familial Mediterranean Fever

Familial Mediterranean fever, also known as *periodic disease*, is an autosomal recessive inherited disorder characterized by recurrent episodes of fever accompanied by inflammation of the peritoneum, pleura, synovial membranes (recurrent polyserositis), and skin. The disorder predominantly affects persons of Mediterranean origin (Sephardic Jews, Armenians, and Arabs) and is very rare in other races. The most serious complication of the disease is amyloidosis, which is the cause of death in a substantial proportion of adult patients. Important clinical features include abdominal pain in more than 95 percent of patients, pleuritic chest pain in 35 to 85 percent, and acute arthritis in 17 to 75 percent [62,175,186]. Recurrent pleuritic chest pains are common and may be associated with small pleural effusions. Right-sided effusions are reported to be more common [62,63]. Pulmonary hypertension and pulmonary amyloidosis have been described in familial Mediterranean fever [92].

Hereditary Hemorrhagic Telangiectasia

Hereditary hemorrhagic telangiectasia (Osler-Weber-Rendu disease) is an autosomal dominantly inherited disorder characterized by telangiectasia of the skin and mucous membranes and intermittent bleeding from arteriovenous malformations and fistulas. The prevalence of simultaneous hereditary hemorrhagic telangiectasia and pulmonary arteriovenous malformation during a 10-year period in one Scandinavian county of more than 429,207 inhabitants was 2.6 per 100,000 [205]. The male-female ratio is 1 : 2 [47,168]. Telangiectasias of the skin and oral, nasal, and conjunctival mucosa manifest in the second and third decades of life. They appear bright red, punctate, or linear, and blanch under pressure. Gastrointestinal bleeding occurs in approximately 15 percent of patients [3].

Hereditary hemorrhagic telangiectasia is the most common cause of pulmonary arteriovenous fistula, and 15 to 20 percent of the patients with the disease have pulmonary arteriovenous fistulas [88,147,159]. The majority of the fistulas occur in the lower lobes of lungs and are multiple in nearly 35 percent of patients [74,169]. Typically, chest roentgenograms show the pulmonary arteriovenous fistulas as oval or round, homogenous nodular lesions that measure from a few millimeters to several centimeters in diameter. These fistulas tend to evolve and continue to enlarge over long periods, sometimes as long as 24 years [197,205]. A standard chest roentgenogram may show nodular shadow but can easily obscure small afferent and efferent vessels attached to the fistula (Fig. 66-5). The risk of relying solely on the standard chest roentgenogram becomes apparent when a transthoracic needle aspiration

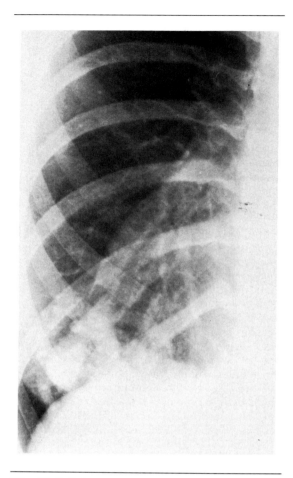

Fig. 66-5. Pulmonary arteriovenous malformation in right lower lobe of a patient with hereditary hemorrhagic telangiectasia reveals afferent and efferent vessels attached to the fistula.

is performed, with resultant serious hemorrhage. Therefore, anteroposterior tomography should be considered before invasive procedures such as transthoracic or bronchoscopic lung biopsy of such a nodule are attempted. Tomography generally discloses an artery entering the fistula and a vein leaving it (Fig. 66-6). Pulmonary angiography confirms the diagnosis in virtually all cases and is required before embolotherapy or surgical resection of a fistula is undertaken (Fig. 66-7). Cases of spontaneous pneumothorax and hemothorax secondary to intrapleural rupture of an arteriovenous fistula have been observed [96,180].

Dyspnea and hemoptysis are the two common symptoms. The degree of dyspnea depends on the degree of right-to-left shunting. The majority

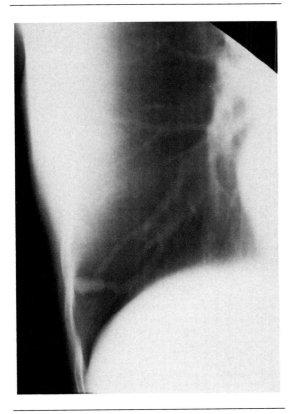

Fig. 66-6. Localized tomography sometimes is necessary to identify pulmonary arteriovenous malformation, especially when the fistula is small.

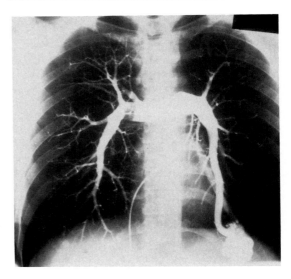

Fig. 66-7. Pulmonary angiogram in hereditary hemorrhagic telangiectasia shows a large arteriovenous malformation in left lower lobe.

of pulmonary fistulas are detected in the third and fourth decades of life. Although dyspnea is present in nearly 60 percent of patients, hemoptysis (occurring in 10 to 20 percent) is the most common presenting symptom [74]. This can be brisk but usually is not life-threatening. Clinical examination may reveal cyanosis, clubbing of fingers, and a bruit or a continuous bruit over the site of the fistula [74]. Endobronchial telangiectases are distinctly uncommon [111]. Pulmonary artery catheterization generally reveals diminished arterial oxygen tension and saturation but normal pulmonary artery pressure [169]. Echocardiography with dye studies is a less invasive method for detecting these extracardiac right-to-left shunts. After venous injection of indocyanine green dye, the characteristic contrast flow pattern consists of a markedly delayed appearance of echoes in the left ventricle [47,182]. However, this type of assessment does not calculate the degree of shunt. Using intravenously injected albu-

min microspheres labeled with technetium 99m at rest and during exercise has been reported to be an efficient and noninvasive method of measuring right-to-left shunt [217].

Brain abscess and abscesses in other organs, as the result of paradoxic embolism, are possible serious complications [70,131]. Various neurologic manifestations are reported in up to 30 percent of patients. Brain abscess, estimated to occur in approximately 1 percent of patients, can be the presenting feature of hereditary hemorrhagic telangiectasia [155,216]. Mental obtundation, headache, visual disturbances, hemiplegia, and seizures are the most common presenting features with neurologic involvement [155]. Leukocytosis and fever are not prominent features, and blood cultures are generally sterile. However, in patients with brain abscesses, anaerobic and microaerophilic streptococci are the most common pathogens isolated. In a series of 31 patients with hereditary hemorrhagic telangiectasia and neurologic involvement, 13 patients died and patients without abscess drainage or with delayed diagnosis had a higher mortality [155]. Another report observed that 4 of 5 patients with asymptomatic small or moderately sized pulmonary arteriovenous malformations presented with stroke caused by paradoxic embolism [86]. Among 67 patients with pulmonary arteriovenous malformations associated with hereditary hemorrhagic telangiectasia, strokes and transient ischemic attacks were recorded in 37 percent [216]. A review of the English literature in 1990 disclosed 52 cases of neurologic complications [131], but not all are caused by paradoxic emboli originating in pulmonary arteriovenous fistulas. Indeed, among a series of more than 200 reported patients with hereditary hemorrhagic telangiectasia and associated neurologic sequelae, 61 percent developed neurologic lesions secondary to pulmonary arteriovenous fistula whereas 36 percent of the patients with neurologic manifestations exhibited vascular malformations of the brain and spinal cord [162].

High-output congestive cardiac failure and portosystemic encephalopathy from hepatic arteriovenous malformations are among the unusual complications. Disseminated intravascular coagulation was observed in 51 percent of 47 patients with documented hereditary hemorrhagic telangiectasia [22].

The treatment of choice in current practice is pulmonary artery embolotherapy (therapeutic embolization) using coils and other intravascular devices [83]. As new fistulas evolve in the same patient over a period of time, repeated embolizations may be necessary (Figs. 66-8, 66-9). White and colleagues [216] reported their 10-year experience with embolotherapy of 276 pulmonary arteriovenous malformations in 76 patients, 67 (88 percent) of whom had hereditary hemorrhagic telangiectasia. Physiologic improvements remained stable for 5 years after embolotherapy, complications were minimal, and surgery was not required in any patient. Chilvers and associates [39] assessed the effects of embolotherapy (using steel coils) on pulmonary function and exercise capacity in 11 patients with pulmonary arteriovenous malformations secondary to hereditary hemorrhagic telangiectasia. Lung function tests before embolotherapy disclosed normal vital capacity and one-second forced expiratory volume–to–vital capacity ratios, reduced DLCO (mean, 71 percent of predicted; range, 36 to 123 percent), a resting supine arterial oxygen saturation of 86 percent (range, 67 to 95 percent), and mean shunt fraction of 33 percent (range, 15 to 47 percent). Exercise capacity was well preserved. Six months after therapy, the mean shunt fraction increased from 33 to 19 percent and resting arterial oxygen saturation from 86 to 92 percent. There was no change in vital capacity. A consistent improvement in DLCO was also seen.

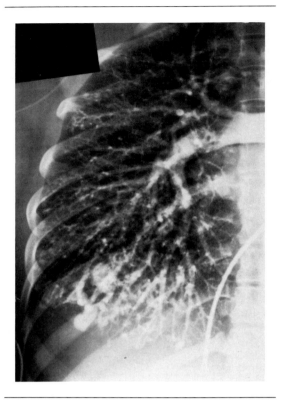

Fig. 66-8. Multiple arteriovenous malformations in right lower lobe. This patient had multiple bilateral arteriovenous malformations.

There were no long-term complications following embolotherapy. Others have documented the immediate improvement in respiratory symptoms, exercise capacity, and gas exchange at rest and during exercise as a result of the embolization-induced reduction in shunt [148].

Large arteriovenous fistulas (diameter of efferent vessel exceeding 10 mm) may require surgical resection [28,57]. The life expectancy of patients with hereditary hemorrhagic telangiectasia is not reduced provided treatable complications are diagnosed and treated promptly.

Hyperhidrosis

Hyperhidrosis, or abnormally excessive production of sweat, can signify an underlying malignancy. The association of intrathoracic malignancy with neurologic involvement, such as Horner's syndrome, is a well-acknowledged para-

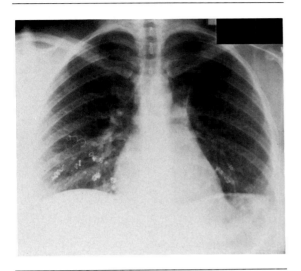

Fig. 66-9. Chest roentgenogram of patient shown in Figure 66-8 after multiple steel-coil embolizations. This patient has required several embolizations for recurrent arteriovenous malformations.

neoplastic feature. In most reported cases, hyperhidrosis has been limited to the same side as the tumor. It has been speculated that direct irritation of nerves may excite the autonomic efferent fibers. Unilateral hyperhidrosis of the chest cage has been described in patients with lung cancer [112]. The presence of hyperhidrosis indicates a poor prognosis. Resection of a cervical rib may abolish the hyperhidrosis.

Malignant Atrophic Papulosis

Malignant atrophic papulosis (Degos' disease) is a rare multisystemic disorder characterized by typical skin and gastrointestinal symptoms. Many patients demonstrate a rapidly fatal course. The presenting clinical feature is the appearance of crops of asymptomatic oval skin lesions, ranging from 2 to 8 mm in diameter. A review of 60 reported cases of Degos' disease found that 17 included intrathoracic abnormalities, most of which were found incidentally at postmortem [150]. The most common intrathoracic findings were pleuritis and pericarditis. Bilateral hemorrhagic pleural effusions, pleural plaques, pulmonary infarcts, and pulmonary abscess also were noted [150].

Mastocytosis

Systemic mastocytosis, or mast cell disease, is an uncommon disorder characterized by urticaria pigmentosa, hepatosplenomegaly, osteosclerotic bone lesions, and diarrhea, nausea, vomiting, and flushing. Respiratory manifestations include interstitial lung disease and extensive peribronchial and alveolar infiltration with mast cells [135,161].

Neurofibromatosis

Neurofibromatosis (von Recklinghausen's disease) is a common disease of variably expressive autosomal dominant inheritance characterized by café au lait spots, freckling, and neurofibromas of skin and internal organs. Its incidence is 1 per 3000; approximately half the cases occur sporadically. Cutaneous lesions are the result of the maldevelopment of neural crest cells. The number of dermal neurofibromas vary from individual to individual. Large plexiform neurofibromas develop along peripheral nerves and involve deeper tissues. Extracutaneous (visceral) involvement may not be apparent during life unless such lesions produce symptoms [149,203].

Respiratory involvement is reported in 10 to 15 percent of patients [50,122,160,212]. Although neurofibromatosis is a congenital disorder, the lung involvement does not become evident until adulthood. Approximately 20 percent of patients older than 35 years develop diffuse interstitial fibrosis [203]. With pulmonary involvement in a patient with cutaneous neurofibromatosis evaluated by radioisotope techniques, there is diminished perfusion and ventilation to apices of the lungs [154]. Bullous lung disease may occur alone or in combination with diffuse pulmonary fibrosis [79]. Pulmonary fibrosis usually is seen in the basal areas of the lungs, whereas the bullous lesions occur predominantly in the apical areas (Fig. 66-10) [98,212]. Cystic lung disease resembling honeycomb lung also has been described [121].

The pulmonary parenchymal disease is attributed to a mesenchymal defect resulting in primary deposition of collagen [8]. The histologic features mimic those of idiopathic pulmonary fibrosis [122]. Ultrastructural studies have shown fragmentation of collagen fibers in the lung [143]. The clinical manifestations are mild, usually consisting only of exertional dyspnea, but a restrictive pattern of pulmonary function and dimin-

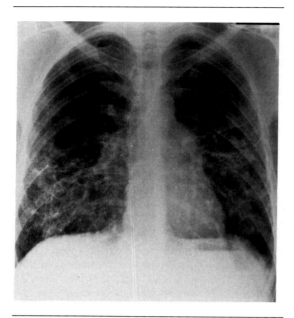

Fig. 66-10. Neurofibromatosis with pulmonary manifestations showing bullous changes in the upper lung zone and honeycomb changes in the lower lungs.

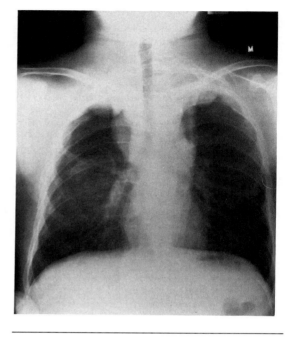

Fig. 66-11. Neurofibromatosis with intrathoracic neurofibromas.

ished diffusing capacity often are observed [212].

Intrathoracic neurofibromas and meningoceles may be associated with a dermal form of neurofibromatosis, but these usually remain undetected because they rarely are symptomatic (Fig. 66-11) [203]. An earlier review of the literature reported 27 cases of intrathoracic meningocele with neurofibromatosis [137]. Since then, more than a dozen such associations have been reported [170]. When these lesions are situated in the posterior mediastinum, as they commonly are, they may represent so-called dumbbell tumors with intraspinal extension [79]. Magnetic resonance imaging of the involved spinal area is helpful in assessing the anatomic extent of such tumors. Primary pulmonary parenchymal neurofibromas are rare [149,203]. Benign neurogenous tumors arising in the trachea are also uncommon. A report described a patient with neurofibromatosis who presented with dyspnea caused by endotracheal neurofibroma [114]. Hoarseness may result from recurrent laryngeal nerve involvement [8].

Primary or secondary malignancy in the lung has been overlooked in 2 patients with generalized neurofibromatosis owing to roentgeno-graphic confusion caused by overlying cutaneous lesions (see above regarding chest wall lesions) [173]. Neurofibromatosis is associated with an increased incidence of malignancy, ranging from malignant tumors of the central nervous system to Wilms' tumor, rhabdomyosarcoma, leukemia, and pheochromocytoma [8]. In 5 percent of patients, the neurofibromas in neurofibromatosis undergo transformation to malignant degeneration and commonly metastasize to the lungs [8]. "Scar" cancer of the lung has been reported as a complication of the chronic pulmonary process in neurofibromatosis [55].

Nonsuppurative Panniculitis

Sometimes referred to as *Weber-Christian disease*, nonsuppurative panniculitis is characterized by cutaneous nodular fat necrosis of the panniculus adiposum. Tender, erythematous subcutaneous nodules appear over the extremities and trunk.

A review in 1976 reported pulmonary involvement in only 5 cases [64]. Pulmonary manifestations include pulmonary fat emboli and infarcts, lipogranulomatous pneumonitis with nodules measuring 0.8 to 3 cm in diameter [174], and fluffy roentgenographic densities bilaterally [64]. Recurrent pneumonia and pleural effusion also occur [188]. Interestingly, alpha₁-antitrypsin deficiency has been found in some patients with acute panniculitis [163]. There is no report of emphysematous lung disease occurring as a result of this.

Cogan's Syndrome

Cogan's syndrome is a disease of unknown origin characterized by audiovestibular symptoms, nonsyphilitic interstitial keratitis, and systemic manifestations that include fever, anemia, elevated sedimentation rate, leukocytosis, and thrombocytosis. Complications are serious and may include deafness, blindness, vasculitis, aortic insufficiency, and death. An upper respiratory tract infection precedes onset of the syndrome in approximately 40 percent of patients. Respiratory involvement is present in approximately 20 percent of patients, and the pulmonary manifestations include mild, sometimes transient, chest roentgenologic abnormalities and pleuropericarditis. A review of 78 patients noted transient pulmonary infiltrates and pleuritis in 9 and 5 percent, respectively [208]. Recurrent lung infiltrates have been described.

Oculocutaneous Albinism

Sometimes called *pulmonary ceroidosis* or the *Hermansky-Pudlak syndrome*, oculocutaneous albinism is an autosomal recessive disorder characterized by oculocutaneous tyrosinase-positive albinism, platelet pool disease with moderate bleeding tendency, and ceroid-like inclusions in the reticuloendothelial system [49,53,69]. Ceroid is believed to be a product of oxidation and polymerization of unsaturated lipids. A review of the literature in 1989 recorded more than 200 cases of the Hermansky-Pudlak syndrome [53], the most striking feature of which is the presence of recognizable oculocutaneous albinism. However, the most frequent clinical complication is hemorrhage, and epistaxis is the most common hemorrhagic manifestation [53].

Respiratory involvement is a well-recognized complication in oculocutaneous albinism, with more than 20 patients with respiratory problems reported in the literature [69]. The disease affects men and women equally, but the incidence of lung disease is twice as high in women as in men. The lung disease is similar to idiopathic pulmonary fibrosis and usually begins in the third or fourth decade of life. Constant nonproductive cough and progressive dyspnea are the main symptoms. Dyspnea can develop suddenly over several weeks or gradually over years, and the lung disease can progress to end-stage fibrosis and death. The pulmonary pathology in oculocutaneous albinism is compatible with oxidant injury as it parallels pathologic alterations seen with pulmonary oxygen toxicity. Bronchoalveolar lavage may show alveolar macrophages containing typical ceroid-like material [215]. Increased levels of immunoglobulins, numbers of IgG- and IgA-secreting cells, and normal percentages of helper and suppressor T cells are observed. Brown-pigmented histiocytes have been demonstrated in the alveolar spaces [171]. The pulmonary fibrosis is an irreversible and progressive process. No specific therapy is available for the lung disease.

Pulmonary ceroidosis occurs in many of the approximately 30 disorders in which systemic or localized deposition of ceroid occurs [171]. Sea-blue histiocytosis syndrome is an example of ceroidosis, and lung involvement is present in 11 percent of these patients [193]. Idiopathic pulmonary ceroidosis may represent pulmonary alveolar deposition of ceroid-like material in the absence of clinical or biochemical data characteristic of any specific ceroid storage disease [171,194]. Interestingly, deposition of ceroid-like pigment in the alveolar macrophages has been reported in 8 patients with carcinoma of the stomach [116].

Pseudoxanthoma Elasticum

Pseudoxanthoma elasticum is a rare disorder characterized by fragmentation and calcification of elastic fibers in skin, blood vessels, and retina [4]. Both autosomal dominant and recessive forms have been described. The basic defect is unknown. One patient with pseudoxanthoma elasticum has been reported in whom the lung biopsy showed widespread deposition of calcium in the walls of some arteries, arterioles, and venules, with swollen, short, irregularly clumped elastic fibers and irregularity of the elastic laminae [90].

Pyoderma Gangrenosum

Pyoderma gangrenosum is a painful, chronic, destructive, and ulcerating skin disease of unknown origin. The occurrence of this disorder in intestinal diseases is well known. In a report on 86 patients with this disease, inflammatory bowel disease was present in 36 percent [152]. Asthma or chronic obstructive pulmonary disease was noted in 5 percent. Pulmonary abscess has been described in a patient with pyoderma gangrenosum [207], but the relationship between pyoderma gangrenosum and pulmonary disease remains unclear.

Tuberous Sclerosis

Tuberous sclerosis (Bourneville's disease) is an autosomal dominant disease of mesodermal development characterized clinically by epilepsy and mental retardation and pathologically by congenital tumors and malformations of the brain, skin, and viscera [23]. The classic clinical triad in tuberous sclerosis consists of adenoma sebaceum, mental retardation, and seizures. Skin lesions, in addition to adenoma sebaceum or dermal angiofibroma, include ash leaf spots (a hypopigmented skin lesion, the earliest to appear in tuberous sclerosis), shagreen patches (hamartomas of connective tissue seen in 50 percent of patients and located over the lumbosacral area), and periungual fibromas (benign pink fibrous neoplasms adjacent to the nails and seen in 15 to 20 percent of patients). Poliosis, or hypopigmentation of the scalp hair or eyelashes, also is seen [35,132]. Extracutaneous manifestations include seizure disorder, electroencephalographic abnormalities, or both in 80 to 90 percent, mental retardation of wide-ranging severity, a hamartomatous lesion of the central nervous system, retinal phakomas, angiomyolipomas of the kidney and renal and bone cysts, and cardiac rhabdomyomas [35,75,109,132]. Only 25 percent of affected children live beyond their twentieth year [80].

Respiratory disease is seen in fewer than 1% of patients. Pulmonary tuberous sclerosis usually involves other organs [80]. Patients with pulmonary involvement are generally women of childbearing age (between 18 and 34 years) [61,101, 109]. Lung disease has been observed in a mother and daughter from a family with tuberous sclerosis for four generations [183]. Men with tuberous sclerosis seldom develop lung disease [67]. Exertional dyspnea is the most common respiratory symptom and may progress to the point of disability. The diffuse pulmonary interstitial process may progress to honeycombing and cyst formation, spontaneous pneumothorax, and cor pulmonale (Fig. 66-12). A review of the literature revealed 19 cases of spontaneous pneumothorax

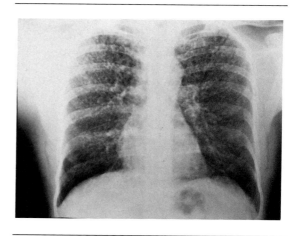

Fig. 66-12. Tuberous sclerosis with extensive reticulonodular infiltrates with some sparing of lower lung zones.

secondary to tuberous sclerosis, with 8 patients dying of this complication [8,12,108]. Chylous pleural effusion secondary to lymphatic obstruction from mediastinal lymphadenopathy can occur [67]. Significant pulmonary hypertension also has been reported [94,209]. Overall, respiratory disease is reported to be associated with a more benign course, compared to tuberous sclerosis without pulmonary manifestation [84].

Chest roentgenograms in tuberous sclerosis may show diffuse interstitial infiltrates in later stages of the disease. In the early stages, reticulonodular changes and pleural effusions are found. Spontaneous pneumothorax is common. Thin-section computed tomographic (CT) scans of lungs in tuberous sclerosis have shown thin-walled cysts less than 20 mm in diameter scattered randomly in all parts of the lungs, with normal-appearing lung tissue between cysts. The CT findings are identical in tuberous sclerosis and pulmonary lymphangioleiomyomatosis (Fig. 66-13). CT findings correlate better with DLCO than do chest roentgenograms [107].

Morphologic analysis of the lungs reveals multiple cysts measuring a few millimeters in diameter [127]. The cyst walls are formed of smooth-muscle cells identical to pulmonary lymphangioleiomyomatosis. Ultrastructural morphologic analysis of the lung in tuberous sclerosis has shown findings identical to those in lymphangioleiomyomatosis [33,34]. Cystic disease of the lung with focal adenomatoid proliferation is

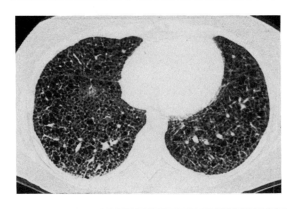

Fig. 66-13. Tuberous sclerosis of lung evaluated by high-resolution computed tomography, showing typically diffuse fine honeycombing.

among the least common pathologic feature of tuberous sclerosis. It tends to develop in adult life, occurs more commonly among female patients who do not have mental retardation and epileptic seizures, and may be rapidly fatal after the onset of respiratory symptoms [110]. Mesodermal tumors containing smooth muscle and other structures are seen frequently [80,190].

Pulmonary function tests generally demonstrate an obstructive airways disease despite the nodular interstitial appearance of lungs on the chest roentgenograms. Compression of the smaller airways by the smooth-muscle hyperplasia is one of the mechanisms for the development of obstructive airways disease. However, airspace lesions are reported to be more important than muscular proliferation in small airways in producing airflow limitation [185]. Interestingly, lung function studies have shown increased lung volumes [42]. Small airways collapse occurs because of the surrounding emphysema.

Some consider tuberous sclerosis and pulmonary lymphangioleiomyomatosis to be the same clinical entity [33,93,115]. However, the presence of hormonal (estrogen, progesterone) receptors in lymphangioleiomyomatosis may distinguish it from tuberous sclerosis, although not all patients with the former disease exhibit these receptors. Because some patients with lymphangioleiomyomatosis respond to hormones, tuberous sclerosis also has been treated with these agents [214].

Yellow Nail Syndrome

The term *yellow nail syndrome* was first employed in 1964 to describe yellow discoloration of the fingernails in association with lymphedema in 13 patients (Fig. 66-14) [167]. Further experience with more than 150 patients portrayed in the literature has demonstrated the association of yellow nails with pleural effusion, bronchiectasis, and lymphedema of the breasts [56,87]. Nails of both hands and feet are affected, becoming thickened, excessively curved along both axes, very slow growing, and of yellowish-gray hue; cuticle and lunula are usually absent, and onycholysis generally is evident. Lymphangiography of the lower extremities has shown hypoplasia or aplasia of the lymphatics, similar to that occurring in primary lymphedema [134,167].

The origin of yellow nail syndrome is unknown, although a few cases seemed to follow episodes of pneumonia. The mechanism of nail discoloration is undefined, and the nail changes are not present in all patients. Histopathologic changes in the nail matrix and bed demonstrate dense, fibrous tissue replacing subungual stroma with numerous ectatic, endothelium-lined vessels that mimic pleural alterations in this syndrome. Based on these findings, it is hypothesized that primary stromal sclerosis may lead to lymphatic obstruction [51]. Nail discoloration may precede or follow pleural effusion and lymphedema [17].

Among 97 patients with yellow nail syndrome, most developed the disease in early middle age, and the male-to-female ratio was 1:1.6 [139]. Yellow nail syndrome has been described in an 8-year-old [117]. Whereas more than half the pa-

Fig. 66-14. Yellow nail syndrome with characteristic yellow discoloration of nails.

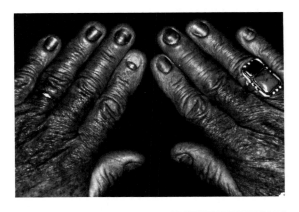

tients develop nail changes, the majority do not notice the nail discoloration because its onset is subtle.

The recurrent pleural effusions are most likely the result of lymphatic hypoplasia. Measurements of the rate of pleural fluid turnover have indicated that accumulation of pleural fluid in yellow nail syndrome is due to defective lymphatic drainage rather than excess production [119,164]. On histologic examination, the pleura is thickened with fibrosis, chronic inflammatory infiltration, and dilatation of lymphatic capillaries in the visceral pleura. Ectasia of lymphatic capillaries has been documented by electron microscopy [187]. The pathologic process affects not only the lymphatic system but also the pleural capillaries [21].

Pleural effusion may precede the onset of nail changes by several years [165]. The fluid may be an exudate or a transudate. In some patients, the pleural fluid glucose level may be reduced [6]. Pleural effusions range from small, unilateral, and asymptomatic to large, bilateral, recurrent, and debilitating [17]. The pulmonary symptoms depend on the size of the pleural effusion and the severity of associated bronchiectasis. Empyema thoracis has been reported as a complication of the yellow nail syndrome [113].

Bronchiectasis of lower lobes is now included in the definition of yellow nail syndrome. Additionally, many patients develop sinus infections [31,82,87,133,136]. Bronchiectasis limited to upper lung zones has been noted in a patient [124], but the mechanism responsible for its development is unknown. Ciliary beat frequency measured in 2 patients was within normal limits (12 Hz) [130].

A report of 8 patients with proved diagnoses of the acquired immunodeficiency syndrome (AIDS) and *Pneumocystis carinii* pneumonia observed yellow discoloration of the distal portions of the nails in 4 patients, with some showing ridging, loss or decrease in size of lunulae, and opaqueness [38]. Yellow nail syndrome has been described in association with rheumatoid arthritis in 3 patients [123], as well as in 2 mentally retarded siblings [95].

Nonpulmonary complications of yellow nail syndrome include keratosis obturans involving the external ear and excess cerumen [7,133], chylous ascites [60,196], hypoalbuminemia [166], chyluria [200], intestinal lymphangiectasia [60, 142], pericardial effusion [210], giant cell interstitial infiltrates [77], lymphedema of the eyelids [118], nephrotic syndrome [40], and Raynaud's phenomenon [9].

Even though several cases have been described in association with carcinomas of breast, lung, and larynx, there is no clear indication that yellow nail syndrome is a paraneoplastic process [76,77,119,198]. Nevertheless, it is of interest that the nail changes resolved after the malignancy was treated [76,77]. There has been one report of a case of yellow nail syndrome following penicillamine therapy that resolved after discontinuation of the drug [89].

Large, recurrent, or debilitating pleural effusions require repeated thoracentesis, pleuroperitoneal shunting, medical or surgical pleurodesis, or pleurectomy [17,26,48]. There are reports of successful treatment of the nail changes with topical vitamin E solution [11,140,218]. Treatment of pulmonary disease also may resolve the nail changes [145]. There is even a report of spontaneous resolution of nail discoloration without change in the patient's respiratory status [51]. Chylous effusions are more difficult to cure, although a report of successful therapy consisting of dietary restriction of fat and supplements of medium-chain triglycerides is noteworthy [196].

References

1. Abadir R. Pemphigoid, bronchial neoplasm and radiotherapy. *Proc R Soc Med* 60:1271, 1967.
2. Almeyda J. Epidermolysis bullosa associated with neoplasm of the bronchus. *Br J Dermatol* 87:70, 1972.
3. Alper J, Kegel M. Skin signs in pulmonary disease. *Clin Chest Med* 8:299, 1987.
4. Altman LK, et al. Pseudoxanthoma elasticum: An undiagnosed genetically heterogeneous disorder with protean manifestations. *Arch Intern Med* 134:1048, 1974.
5. Anderson CE, et al. Association of hemolytic anemia and early-onset pulmonary emphysema in three siblings. *J Pediatr* 105:247, 1984.
6. Angelillo VA, O'Donohue WJ Jr. Yellow nail syndrome with reduced glucose level in pleural fluid. *Chest* 75:83, 1979.
7. Armitage JM, et al. Ear involvement in the yellow nail syndrome. *Chest* 98:1534, 1990.
8. Aughenbaugh GL. Thoracic manifestations of neurocutaneous disease. *Radiol Clin North Am* 22:741, 1984.
9. Awerbuch MS. The yellow nail syndrome, bronchiectasis and Raynaud's disease—a relationship. *Med J Aust* 2:829, 1976.
10. Ayers J, Rees J, Cochrane GM. Haemoptysis and non-organic upper airways obstruction in a pa-

tient with previously undiagnosed Ehlers-Danlos syndrome. *Br J Dis Chest* 75:309, 1981.

11. Ayres S Jr, Mihan R. Yellow nail syndrome: Response to vitamin E. *Arch Dermatol* 108:267, 1973.

12. Babcock TL, Synder BA. Spontaneous pneumothorax associated with tuberous sclerosis. *J Thorac Cardiovasc Surg* 83:100, 1982.

13. Barabas AP. Heterogeneity of the Ehlers-Danlos syndrome: Description of three clinical types and a hypothesis to explain the basic defect(s). *Br Med J* 2:612, 1967.

14. Baumer JH, Hankey S. Transient pulmonary cysts in an infant with the Ehlers-Danlos syndrome. *Br J Radiol* 53:598, 1980.

15. Beahrs JO, et al. Anhidrotic ectodermal dysplasia: Predisposition to bronchial disease. *Ann Intern Med* 74:92, 1971.

16. Bean WB. *Vascular Spiders and Related Lesions of the Skin.* Springfield, IL: Thomas, 1958. P 178.

17. Beer DJ, Pereira W Jr, Snider GL. Pleural effusion associated with primary lymphedema: A perspective on the yellow nail syndrome. *Am Rev Respir Dis* 117:595, 1978.

18. Beerman H, Kirshbaum BA. Some associated pulmonary and cutaneous diseases: A review of recent literature. *Am J Med Sci* 242:494, 1961.

19. Beighton P. Lethal complications of the Ehlers-Danlos syndrome. *Br Med J* 3:656, 1968.

20. Beighton P. The dominant and recessive forms of cutis laxa. *J Med Genet* 9:216, 1972.

21. Ben-Yehuda A, Ben-Chetrit E, Eliakim M. Yellow nail syndrome: Case report and review of the literature. *Isr J Med Sci* 22:117, 1986.

22. Bick RL. Hereditary hemorrhagic telangiectasia and disseminated intravascular coagulation: A new clinical syndrome. *Ann NY Acad Sci* 370:851, 1981.

23. Bourneville DM. Sclerose tubereuse des circonvolutions cerebrales: Idiotie et epilepsie hemiplegique. *Arch Neurol* (Paris) 1:81, 1880.

24. Bowen JT. Precancerous dermatoses: A study of two cases of chronic atypical epithelial proliferation. *J Cutan Dis* 30:241, 1912.

25. Brägger C, et al. IgG2/IgG4 subclass deficiency in a patient with chronic mucocutaneous candidiasis and bronchiectases. *Eur J Pediatr* 149:168, 1989.

26. Brofman JD, et al. Yellow nails, lymphedema and pleural effusion: Treatment of chronic pleural effusion with pleuroperitoneal shunting. *Chest* 97:743–745, 1990.

27. Brown J, Winkelmann RK. Acanthosis nigricans: A study of 90 cases. *Medicine* 47:33, 1968.

28. Brown SE, et al. Staged bilateral thoracotomies for multiple pulmonary arteriovenous malformations complicating hereditary hemorrhagic telangiectasia. *J Thorac Cardiovasc Surg* 83:285, 1982.

29. Bullock WE. The clinical significance of erythema nodosum. *Hosp Pract* [Off], 15(21):102E, 1986.

30. Byers PH, et al. An X-linked form of cutis laxa due to deficiency of lysyl oxidase. *Birth Defects* 12:293, 1976.

31. Camilleri AE. Chronic sinusitis and the yellow nail syndrome. *J Laryngol Otol* 104:811, 1990.

32. Capitano MA, et al. Congenital anhidrotic ectodermal dysplasia. *Am J Roentgenol* 103:168, 1968.

33. Capron F, et al. Pulmonary lymphangioleiomyomatosis and Bourneville's tuberous sclerosis with pulmonary involvement: The same disease? *Cancer* 52:851, 1983.

34. Carrington CB, et al. Lymphangioleiomyomatosis: Physiologic, pathologic, radiologic correlations. *Am Rev Respir Dis* 116:977, 1977.

35. Cassidy SB. Tuberous sclerosis in children: Diagnosis and course. *Compr Ther* 10:43, 1984.

36. Cavanaugh MJ, Cooper DM. Chronic pulmonary disease in a child with the Ehlers-Danlos syndrome. *Acta Paediatr Scand* 65:679, 1976.

37. Chalker RB, et al. Extrapulmonary thoracic restriction (hidebound chest) complicating eosinophilic fasciitis. *Chest* 100:1453, 1991.

38. Chernosky ME, Finley VK. Yellow nail syndrome in patients with acquired immunodeficiency disease. *J Am Acad Dermatol* 13:731, 1985.

39. Chilvers ER, et al. Effect of percutaneous transcatheter embolization on pulmonary function, right-to-left shunt, and arterial oxygenation in patients with pulmonary arteriovenous malformations. *Am Rev Respir Dis* 142:420, 1990.

40. Cockram CS, Richards P. Yellow nails and nephrotic syndrome. *Br J Dermatol* 101:707, 1979.

41. Cohen PR, et al. Tripe palms and malignancy. *J Clin Oncol* 7:669, 1989.

42. Corrin B, Liebow AA, Friedman PJ. Pulmonary lymphangiomyomatosis. *Am J Pathol* 79:348, 1975.

43. Crawley FE. Erythema nodosum as initial manifestation of Boeck's sarcoidosis. *Br Med J* 2:1362, 1950.

44. Cupo LN, et al. Ehlers-Danlos syndrome with abnormal collagen fibrils, sinus of Valsalva aneurysms, myocardial infarction, panacinar emphysema and cerebral heterotopias. *Am J Med* 71:1051, 1981.

45. Curth HO, Hilberg AW, Machacek GF. The site and histology of the cancer associated with malignant acanthosis nigricans. *Cancer* 15:364, 1962.

46. Cuzick J, Harris R, Mortimer PS. Palmar keratoses and cancers of the bladder and lung. *Lancet* 1:530, 1984.

47. Dansky HM, Schwinger ME, Cohen MV. Using contrast material-enhanced echocardiography

to identify abnormal pulmonary arteriovenous connections in patients with hypoxemia. *Chest* 102:1690, 1992.

48. David I, et al. Thoracic surgical implications of the yellow nail syndrome. *J Thorac Cardiovasc Surg* 91:788, 1986.

49. Davies BH, Tuddenham EGD. Familial pulmonary fibrosis associated with oculocutaneous albinism and platelet function defect: A new syndrome. *Q J Med* 45:219, 1976.

50. Davies PDB. Diffuse pulmonary involvement in von Recklinghausen's disease: A new syndrome. *Thorax* 18:198, 1963.

51. De Coste SD, Imber MJ, Baden HP. Yellow nail syndrome. *J Am Acad Dermatol* 22:608, 1990.

52. De Jager H. Congenital anhidrotic ectodermal dysplasia: Case report. *J Pathol Bacteriol* 90:321, 1965.

53. Depinho RA, Kaplan KL. The Hermansky-Pudlak syndrome: Report of three cases and review of pathophysiology and management considerations. *Medicine* 64:192, 1985.

54. Derham RJ. Postprimary intrathoracic tuberculosis in childhood: With special reference to its sequelae. *Tex State J Med* 52:583, 1956.

55. De Scheerder I, et al. Desquamative interstitial pneumonia and scar cancer of the lung complicating generalised neurofibromatosis. *Eur J Respir Dis* 65:623, 1984.

56. Dilley JJ, et al. Primary lymphedema associated with yellow nails and pleural effusions. *JAMA* 204:670, 1968.

57. Dines DE, Seward JB, Bernatz PE. Pulmonary arteriovenous fistulas. *Mayo Clin Proc* 58:176, 1983.

58. Doyle JA, Ginsburg WWz. Eosinophilic fasciitis. *Med Clin North Am* 73:1157, 1989.

59. Drake RG Jr. North American blastomycosis: A review. *J Ky Med Assoc* 83:77, 1985.

60. Duhra PM, Quigley EMM, Marsh MN. Chylous ascites, intestinal lymphangiectasia and the 'yellow-nail' syndrome. *Gut* 26:1266, 1985.

61. Dwyer JM, Hickie JB, Garvan J. Pulmonary tuberous sclerosis: Report of three patients and a review of the literature. *Q J Med* 40:115, 1971.

62. Ehrenfeld EN, Eliakim M, Rachmilewitz M. Recurrent polyserositis familial Mediterranean fever (periodic disease): A report of fifty-five cases. *Am J Med* 31:107, 1961.

63. El-Kassimi F. Acute pleuritic chest pain with pleural effusion and plate atelectasis. *Chest* 91:265, 1987.

64. Federman Q, Abrams RM, Lee T. Pulmonary radiographic findings in a case of febrile, relapsing, nonsuppurative panniculitis (Weber-Christian disease). *Mt Sinai J Med* 43:174, 1976.

65. Ferreira MC, Spina V. A case of cutis laxa with abnormal copper metabolism. *Br J Plast Surg* 26:283, 1973.

66. Fleming PC, et al. Febrile mucocutaneous syndrome with respiratory involvement, associated with isolation of *Mycoplasma pneumoniae*. *Can Med Assoc J* 97:1458, 1967.

67. Foresti V, et al. Chylous pleural effusion in tuberous sclerosis. *Respiration* 57:398–401, 1990.

68. Fraser RG, et al. *Diagnosis of Diseases of the Chest* (3rd ed). Philadelphia: Saunders, 1991. Vol. 4, p. 2595.

69. Garay SM, et al. Hermansky-Pudlak syndrome: Pulmonary manifestations of a ceroid storage disorder. *Am J Med* 66:737, 1979.

70. Gelfand MS, et al. Brain abscess: Association with pulmonary arteriovenous fistula and hereditary hemorrhagic telangiectasia. Report of three cases. *Am J Med* 85:718, 1988.

71. Gibson LE, Dicken CH, Flach DB. Neutrophilic dermatoses and myeloproliferative disease: Report of two cases. *Mayo Clin Proc* 60:735, 1985.

72. Glossop LP, Michaels L, Bailey CM. Epidermolysis bullosa letalis in the larynx causing acute respiratory failure: A case presentation and review of the literature. *Int J Pediatr Otorhinolaryngol* 7:281, 1984.

73. Goldman AL. Lung cancer in Bowen's disease. *Am Rev Respir Dis* 108:1205, 1973.

74. Gomes MMR, Bernatz PE. Arteriovenous fistulas: A review and ten-year experience at the Mayo Clinic. *Mayo Clin Proc* 45:81, 1970.

75. Gomez MR, Kuntz NL, Westmoreland BF. Tuberous sclerosis, early onset of seizures, and mental subnormality: A study of discordant homozygous twins. *Neurology* 32:604, 1982.

76. Guin JD, Elleman JH. Yellow nail syndrome: Possible association with malignancy. *Arch Dermatol* 115:734, 1979.

77. Gupta AK, Davies GM, Haberman HF. Yellow nail syndrome. *Cutis* 37:371, 1986.

78. Hajjar BA, Joyner EN III. Congenital cutis laxa with advanced cardiopulmonary disease. *J Pediatr* 73:116, 1968.

79. Hardcastle SW, Hendricks ML. Neurofibromatosis (von Recklinghausen's disease)—an unusual cause of parenchymal lung disease. *S Afr Med J* 66:959, 1984.

80. Harris JO, Waltuck BL, Swenson EW. The pathophysiology of the lungs in tuberous sclerosis: A case report and literature review. *Am Rev Respir Dis* 100:379, 1969.

81. Harris RB, Heaphy MR, Perry HO. Generalized elastolysis (cutis laxa). *Am J Med* 65:815, 1978.

82. Hassard AD, Martin J, Ross JB. Yellow nail syndrome and chronic sinusitis. *J Otolaryngol* 13:318, 1984.

83. Hatfield DR, Fried AM. Therapeutic embolization of diffuse pulmonary arteriovenous malformations. *AJR* 137:861, 1981.

84. Hauck RW, et al. Tuberous sclerosis with pulmonary involvement. *Respiration* 57:289, 1990.

85. Hayden JG, Talner NS, Klaus SN. Cutis laxa as-

sociated with pulmonary artery stenosis. *J Pediatr* 72:506, 1968.

86. Hewes RC, Auster M, White RI Jr. Cerebral embolism—first manifestation of pulmonary arteriovenous malformation in patients with hereditary hemorrhagic telangiectasia. *Cardiovasc Intervent Radiol* 8:151, 1985.

87. Hiller E, Rosenow EC III, Olsen AM. Pulmonary manifestations of the yellow nail syndrome. *Chest* 61:452, 1972.

88. Hodgson CH, et al. Hereditary hemorrhagic telangiectasia and pulmonary arteriovenous fistula: Survey of a large family. *N Engl J Med* 261:625, 1959.

89. Ilchyshyn A, Vickers CFH. Yellow nail syndrome associated with penicillamine therapy. *Acta Derm Venereol (Stockh)* 63:554, 1983.

90. Jackson A, Loh CL. Pulmonary calcification and elastic tissue damage in pseudoxanthoma elasticum. *Histopathology* 4:607, 1980.

91. Joffe B. An epidemic of coccidioidomycosis probably related to soil. *N Engl J Med* 262:720, 1960.

92. Johnson WJ, Lie JT. Pulmonary hypertension and familial Mediterranean fever: A previously unrecognized association. *Mayo Clin Proc* 66:919, 1991.

93. Józwiak S. Pulmonary lymphangioleiomyomatosis: A "forme fruste" of tuberous sclerosis (letter)? *AJR* 155:419, 1990.

94. Józwiak S. Severe pulmonary hypertension with diffuse smooth muscle proliferation of the lungs (letter). *Chest* 98:250, 1990.

95. Kamatani M, et al. Yellow nail syndrome associated with mental retardation in two siblings. *Br J Dermatol* 99:329, 1978.

96. Kintzer JS, Jones FL, Pharr WF. Intrapleural haemorrhage complicating pulmonary arteriovenous fistula. *Br J Dis Chest* 72:155, 1978.

97. Kirkpatrick CH, et al. Reconstitution of defective cellular immunity with foetal thymus and dialysable transfer factor: Long-term studies in a patient with chronic mucocutaneous candidiasis. *Clin Exp Immunol* 23:414, 1976.

98. Klatte EC, Franken EA, Smith JA. The radiographic spectrum in neurofibromatosis. *Semin Roentgenol* 11:17, 1976.

99. Knowles JH, Smith LH Jr. Extrapulmonary manifestations of bronchogenic carcinoma. *N Engl J Med* 262:505, 1960.

100. Kobayashi RH, et al. *Candida* esophagitis and laryngitis in chronic mucocutaneous candidiasis. *Pediatrics* 66:380, 1980.

101. Lagos JC, Gomez MR. Tuberous sclerosis: Reappraisal of a clinical entity. *Mayo Clin Proc* 42:20, 1967.

102. Langleben D, et al. Hemothorax and hemopericardium in a patient with Bean's blue rubber bleb nevus syndrome. *Chest* 95:1352, 1989.

103. Lazarus AA, McMillan M, Miramadi A. Pulmonary involvement in Sweet's syndrome (acute febrile neutrophilic dermatosis): Preleukemic and leukemic phases of acute myelogenous leukemia. *Chest* 90:922, 1986.

104. Ledoux-Corbusier M. Cutis laxa, congenital form with pulmonary emphysema: An ultrastructural study. *J Cutan Pathol* 10:340, 1983.

105. Lees MH, et al. Ehlers-Danlos syndrome associated with multiple pulmonary artery stenoses and tortuous systemic arteries. *J Pediatr* 75:1031, 1969.

106. Leier CV, et al. The spectrum of cardiac defects in the Ehlers-Danlos syndrome, types I and III. *Ann Intern Med* 92:171, 1980.

107. Lenoir S, et al. Pulmonary lymphangiomyomatosis and tuberous sclerosis: Comparison of radiographic and thin-section CT findings. *Radiology* 175:329, 1990.

108. Liberman BA, Chamberlain DW, Goldstein RS. Tuberous sclerosis with pulmonary involvement. *Can Med Assoc J* 130:287, 1984.

109. Lie JT. Cardiac, pulmonary, and vascular involvements in tuberous sclerosis. *Ann NY Acad Sci* 615:58, 1991.

110. Lie JT, Miller RD, Williams DE. Cystic disease of the lungs in tuberous sclerosis: Clinicopathologic correlation, including body plethysmographic lung function tests. *Mayo Clin Proc* 55:547, 1980.

111. Lincoln MJ, Shigeoka JW. Pulmonary telangiectasia without hypoxemia. *Chest* 93:1097, 1988.

112. Lindsay DC, Freeman JG, Record CO. Unilateral hyperhidrosis associated with underlying intrathoracic neoplasia. *Thorax* 41:814, 1986.

113. Lodge JPA, Hunter AM, Saunders NR. Yellow nail syndrome associated with empyema. *Clin Exp Dermatol* 14:328, 1989.

114. Lossos IS, Breuer R, Lafair JS. Endotracheal neurofibroma in a patient with von Recklinghausen's disease. *Eur Respir J* 1:464, 1988.

115. Luna CM, et al. Pulmonary lymphangiomyomatosis associated with tuberous sclerosis: Treatment with tamoxifen and tetracycline-pleurodesis. *Chest* 88:473, 1985.

116. Maeda R. The origin and characteristics of ceroid. *Acta Pathol Jpn* 17:439, 1967.

117. Magid M, et al. The yellow nail syndrome in an 8-year-old girl. *Pediatr Dermatol* 4:90, 1987.

118. Maisels DO, Korachi AO. Lymphoedema of the eyelids in the yellow nail syndrome. *Br J Plast Surg* 38:93, 1985.

119. Mambretti-Zumwalt J, Seidman JM, Higano N. Yellow nail syndrome: Complete triad with pleural protein turnover studies. *South Med J* 73:995, 1980.

120. Marquez J, Juffé A, Rufilanchas JJ, Maitre M, Artaza M. Successful correction of valvular and fibromuscular subpulmonary ring stenosis in a patient with Ehlers-Danlos syndrome. *J Cardiovasc Surg* (Torino) 19:271, 1978.

121. Massaro D, et al. Von Recklinghausen's neurofibromatosis associated with cystic lung disease. *Am J Med* 38:233, 1965.

122. Massaro D, Katz S. Fibrosing alveolitis: Its occurrence, roentgenographic, and pathologic features in von Recklinghausen's neurofibromatosis. *Am Rev Respir Dis* 93:934, 1966.

123. Mattingly PC, Bossingham DH. Yellow nail syndrome in rheumatoid arthritis: Report of three cases. *Ann Rheum Dis* 38:475, 1979.

124. McNicholas WT, Quigley C, FitzGerald MX. Upper lobe bronchiectasis in the yellow nail syndrome: Report of a case. *Ir J Med Sci* 153:394, 1984.

125. Medeiros AA, et al. Erythema nodosum and erythema multiforme as clinical manifestations of histoplasmosis in a community outbreak. *N Engl J Med* 274:415, 1966.

126. Menzies DG, et al. Acanthosis nigricans associated with alveolar cell carcinoma. *Thorax* 43:414, 1988.

127. Milledge RD, Gerald BE, Carter WJ. Pulmonary manifestations of tuberous sclerosis. *Am J Roentgenol* 98:734, 1966.

128. Miller DD, Davies SF, Sarosi GA. Erythema nodosum and blastomycosis. *Arch Intern Med* 142:1839, 1982.

129. Milman N, Selroos O. Pulmonary sarcoidosis in the Nordic countries 1950–1982. Epidemiology and clinical picture. *Sarcoidosis* 7:50, 1990.

130. Miro AM, Vasudevan V, Shah H. Ciliary motility in two patients with yellow nail syndrome and recurrent sinopulmonary infections. *Am Rev Respir Dis* 142:890, 1990.

131. Momma F, et al. Brain abscess associated with congenital pulmonary arteriovenous fistula. *Surg Neurol* 34:439, 1990.

132. Monaghan HP, et al. Tuberous sclerosis complex in children. *Am J Dis Child* 135:912, 1981.

133. Moran MF, Larkworthy W. Upper respiratory problems in the yellow nail syndrome. *Clin Otolaryngol* 1:333, 1976.

134. Müller RP, et al. Roentgenographic and clinical signs in yellow nail syndrome. *Lymphology* 12:257, 1979.

135. Mutter RD, Tannenbaum M, Ultmann JE. Systemic mast cell disease. *Ann Intern Med* 59:887, 1963.

136. Nakielna EM, Wilson J, Ballon HS. Yellow-nail syndrome: Report of three cases. *Can Med Assoc J* 115:46, 1976.

137. Nanson EM. Thoracic meningocele associated with neurofibromatosis. *J Thorac Surg* 33:650, 1957.

138. Neville E, Walker AN, James DG. Prognostic factors predicting the outcome of sarcoidosis: An analysis of 818 patients. *Q J Med* 52:525, 1983.

139. Nordkild P, Kromann-Andersen H, Struve-Christensen E. Yellow nail syndrome—the triad of yellow nails, lymphedema and pleural effusions: A review of the literature and a case report. *Acta Med Scand* 219:221, 1986.

140. Norton L. Further observations on the yellow nail syndrome with therapeutic effects of oral alpha-tocopherol. *Cutis* 36:457, 1985.

141. Nyman CR. Porphyria cutanea tarda, carcinoma of bronchus, rheumatoid arthritis, right hydronephrosis. *Proc R Soc Med* 65:688, 1972.

142. Ocaña I, et al. Intestinal lymphangiectasia and the yellow nail syndrome (letter). *Gastroenterology* 94:858, 1988.

143. Patchefsky AS, et al. Interstitial pulmonary fibrosis and von Recklinghausen's disease. An ultrastructural and immunofluorescent study. *Chest* 64:459, 1973.

144. Patterson R, et al. Erythema multiforme and Stevens-Johnson syndrome. Descriptive and therapeutic controversy. *Chest* 98:331, 1990.

145. Pavlidakey GP, Hashimoto K, Blum D. Yellow nail syndrome. *J Am Acad Dermatol* 11:509, 1984.

146. Pearl W, Spicer M. Ehlers-Danlos syndrome. *South Med J* 74:80, 1981.

147. Peery WH. Clinical spectrum of hereditary hemorrhagic telangiectasia (Osler-Weber-Rendu disease). *Am J Med* 82:989, 1987.

148. Pennington DW, et al. Treatment of pulmonary arteriovenous malformations by therapeutic embolization. Rest and exercise physiology in eight patients. *Am Rev Respir Dis* 145:1047, 1992.

149. Petersen JM, Ferguson DR. Gastrointestinal neurofibromatosis. *J Clin Gastroenterol* 6:529, 1984.

150. Pierce RN, Smith GJW. Intrathoracic manifestations of Degos' disease (malignant atrophic papulosis). *Chest* 73:79, 1978.

151. Powell F, Mackey JP. Bronchial carcinoma and hyperkeratosis palmaris et plantaris. *Postgrad Med J* 57:57, 1981.

152. Powell FC, et al. Pyoderma gangrenosum: A review of 86 patients. *Q J Med* 55:173, 1985.

153. Prakash UBS. Dermatological diseases. *Lung Biol Health Dis* 59:471, 1992.

154. Prediletto R, Viegi G, Bernard P. Lung involvement in a patient with cutaneous neurofibromatosis evaluated by radioisotope techniques. *J Nucl Med Allied Sci* 31:249, 1987.

155. Press OW, Ramsey PG. Central nervous system infections associated with hereditary hemorrhagic telangiectasia. *Am J Med* 77:86, 1984.

156. Reed WB, Horowitz RE, Beighton P. Acquired cutis laxa: Primary generalized elastolysis. *Arch Dermatol* 103:661, 1971.

157. Reed WB, Lopez DA, Landing B. Clinical spectrum of anhidrotic ectodermal dysplasia. *Arch Dermatol* 102:134, 1970.

158. Reverter JC, et al. Erythema nodosum and pulmonary solitary nodule as the first manifesta-

tions of a non-Hodgkin's lymphoma. *Br J Dis Chest* 81:397, 1987.

159. Revill D, Matts SGF. Pulmonary arteriovenous aneurysm in hereditary telangiectasia. *Br J Tuber* 52:222, 1958.

160. Riccardi VM. Von Recklinghausen neurofibromatosis. *N Engl J Med* 305:1617, 1981.

161. Roberts PL, McDonald HB, Wells RF. Systemic mast cell disease in a patient with unusual gastrointestinal and pulmonary abnormalities. *Am J Med* 45:638, 1968.

162. Román G, et al. Neurological manifestations of hereditary hemorrhagic telangiectasia (Rendu-Osler-Weber disease): Report of 2 cases and review of the literature. *Ann Neurol* 4:130, 1978.

163. Rubinstein HM, et al. Alpha $_1$-antitrypsin deficiency with severe panniculitis: Report of two cases. *Ann Intern Med* 86:742, 1977.

164. Runyon BA, Forker EL, Sopko JA. Pleural-fluid kinetics in a patient with primary lymphedema, pleural effusions, and yellow nails. *Am Rev Respir Dis* 119:821, 1979.

165. Ryan CJ, et al. The outcome of patients with pleural effusion of indeterminate cause at thoracotomy. *Mayo Clin Proc* 56:145, 1981.

166. Sahi SP, Bansal SK. Yellow nail syndrome with persistent hypoalbuminaemia. *Br J Clin Pract* 42:36, 1988.

167. Samman PD, White WF. The "yellow nail" syndrome. *Br J Dermatol* 76:153, 1964.

168. Sammons BP. Arteriovenous fistula of the lung. *Radiology* 72:710, 1959.

169. Sanders JS, Martt JM. Multiple small pulmonary arteriovenous fistulas: Diagnosis by cardiac catheterization. *Circulation* 25:383, 1962.

170. Sarkar PK, Fagan AM. Intrathoracic meningocele in a patient with neurofibromatosis. *Respir Med* 85:163, 1991.

171. Sastre J, et al. Pulmonary ceroidosis. *Chest* 91:281, 1987.

172. Savill JS, et al. Fatal Stevens-Johnson syndrome following urography with iopamidol in systemic lupus erythematosus. *Postgrad Med J* 64:392, 1988.

173. Schabel SI, Schmidt GE, Vujic I. Overlooked pulmonary malignancy in neurofibromatosis. *J Can Assoc Radiol* 31:135, 1980.

174. Schoen I, Reingold IM, Meister L. Relapsing nodular nonsuppurative panniculitis with lung involvement: Clinical and autopsy findings, with notes on pathogenesis. *Ann Intern Med* 49:687, 1958.

175. Schwabe AD, Peters RS. Familial Mediterranean fever in Armenians: Analysis of 100 cases. *Medicine* 53:453, 1974.

176. Schwartz BK, Clendenning WE. Bullous erythema multiforme associated with *Hemophilus influenzae* pneumonia. *Cutis* 36:255, 1985.

177. Schwindt WD, Bernhardt LC, Johnson SAM. Ty-

losis and intrathoracic neoplasms. *Chest* 57:590, 1970.

178. Shackelford GD, et al. Upper airway and external genital involvement in epidermolysis bullosa dystrophica. *Radiology* 143:429, 1982.

179. Sharma OP. Sarcoidosis. *Dis Mon* 36:469, 1990.

180. Shashy SS, Jones BC, Kitchens CS. Spontaneous hemothorax in a patient with Osler-Weber-Rendu disease. *South Med J* 78:1393, 1985.

181. Shee CD, Graham VAL. Acquired hypertrichosis lanuginosa and carcinoma of the bronchus. *Thorax* 36:153, 1981.

182. Shub C, et al. Detecting intrapulmonary right-to-left shunt with contrast echocardiography: Observations in a patient with diffuse pulmonary arteriovenous fistulas. *Mayo Clin Proc* 51:81, 1976.

183. Slingerland JM, et al. Pulmonary manifestations of tuberous sclerosis in first degree relatives. *Thorax* 44:212, 1989.

184. Smit J, Alberts C, Balk AG. Pneumothorax in the Ehlers-Danlos syndrome: Consequence or coincidence. *Scand J Respir Dis* 59:239, 1978.

185. Sobonya RE, Quan SF, Fleishman JS. Pulmonary lymphangioleiomyomatosis: Quantitative analysis of lesions producing airflow limitation. *Hum Pathol* 16:1122, 1985.

186. Sohar E, et al. Familial Mediterranean fever: A survey of 470 cases and review of the literature. *Am J Med* 43:227, 1967.

187. Solal-Celigny P, Cormier Y, Fournier M. The yellow nail syndrome: Light and electron microscopic aspects of the pleura. *Arch Pathol Lab Med* 107:183, 1983.

188. Sorensen RU, Abramowsky CR, Stern RC. Ten-year course of early-onset Weber-Christian syndrome with recurrent pneumonia: A suggestion for pathogenesis. *Pediatrics* 78:115, 1986.

189. Stevens AM, Johnson FC. A new eruptive fever associated with stomatitis and ophthalmia: Report of two cases in children. *Am J Dis Child* 24:526, 1922.

190. Stovin PGI, et al. The lungs in lymphangiomyomatosis and in tuberous sclerosis. *Thorax* 30:497, 1975.

191. Sweet RD. An acute febrile neutrophilic dermatoses. *Br J Dermatol* 76:349, 1964.

192. Syrjälä H, Karvonen J, Salminen A. Skin manifestations of tularemia: A study of 88 cases in northern Finland during 16 years (1967–1983). *Acta Derm Venereol (Stockh)* 64:513, 1984.

193. Tachibana F, et al. Syndrome of the sea-blue histiocyte: The first case report in Japan and review of the literature. *Acta Pathol Jpn* 29:73, 1979.

194. Takahashi K, Hakozaki H, Kojima M. Idiopathic pulmonary ceroidosis. *Acta Pathol Jpn* 28:301, 1978.

195. Takimoto CH, Warnock M, Golden JA. Sweet's

syndrome with lung involvement. *Am Rev Respir Dis* 143:177, 1991.

196. Tan WC. Dietary treatment of chylous ascites in yellow nail syndrome. *Gut* 30:1622, 1989.

197. Teragaki M, et al. Hereditary hemorrhagic telangiectasia with growing pulmonary arteriovenous fistulas followed for 24 years. *Am J Med Sci* 295:545, 1988.

198. Thomas PS, Sidhu B. Yellow nail syndrome and bronchial carcinoma (letter). *Chest* 92:191, 1987.

199. Thompson JW, Ahmed AR, Dudley JP. Epidermolysis bullosa dystrophica of the larynx and trachea: Acute airway obstruction. *Ann Otol Rhinol Laryngol* 89:428, 1980.

200. Toal BJ, Doherty CC, Johnston SR. Chyluria and the yellow nail syndrome. *Br J Urol* 61:360, 1988.

201. Tsunoda N, et al. Rapidly progressive bronchiolitis obliterans associated with Stevens-Johnson syndrome. *Chest* 98:243, 1990.

202. Turner-Stokes L, et al. Emphysema and cutis laxa. *Thorax* 38:790, 1983.

203. Unger PD, Geller SA, Anderson PJ. Pulmonary lesions in a patient with neurofibromatosis. *Arch Pathol Lab Med* 108:654, 1984.

204. Van Maldergem L, et al. Severe congenital cutis laxa with pulmonary emphysema: A family with three affected sibs. *Am J Med Genet* 31:455, 1988.

205. Vase P, Holm M, Arendrup H. Pulmonary arteriovenous fistulas in hereditary hemorrhagic telangiectasia. *Acta Med Scand* 218:105, 1985.

206. Veien NK, Stahl D, Brodthagen H. Cutaneous sarcoidosis in Caucasians. *J Am Acad Dermatol* 16:534, 1987.

207. Vignon-Pennamen MD, et al. Pyoderma gangrenosum with pulmonary involvement. *Arch Dermatol* 125:1239, 1989.

208. Vollertson RS, et al. Cogan's syndrome: 18 cases and a review of the literature. *Mayo Clin Proc* 61:344, 1986.

209. Wagener OE, Roncoroni AJ, Barcat JA. Severe pulmonary hypertension with diffuse smooth muscle proliferation of the lungs: Pulmonary tuberous sclerosis? *Chest* 95:234, 1989.

210. Wakasa M, et al. Yellow nail syndrome associated with chronic pericardial effusion. *Chest* 92:366, 1987.

211. Ward K, et al. Prognostic value of bronchoalveolar lavage in sarcoidosis: The critical influence of disease presentation. *Thorax* 44:6, 1989.

212. Webb WR, Goodman PC. Fibrosing alveolitis in patients with neurofibromatosis. *Radiology* 122:289, 1977.

213. Weir EK, et al. Cardiovascular abnormalities in cutis laxa. *Eur J Cardiol* 5:255, 1997.

214. Westermann CJJ, et al. Pulmonary tuberous sclerosis treated with tamoxifen and progesterone. *Thorax* 41:892, 1986.

215. White DA, et al. Hermansky-Pudlak syndrome and interstitial lung disease: Report of a case with lavage findings. *Am Rev Respir Dis* 130:138, 1984.

216. White RI Jr, et al. Pulmonary arteriovenous malformations: Techniques and long-term outcome of embolotherapy. *Radiology* 169:663, 1988.

217. Whyte MKB, et al. Quantification of right to left shunt at rest and during exercise in patients with pulmonary arteriovenous malformations. *Thorax* 47:790, 1992.

218. Williams HC, Buffham R, du-Vivier A. Successful use of topical vitamin E solution in the treatment of nail changes in yellow nail syndrome. *Arch Dermatol* 127:1023, 1991.

219. Winterbauer RH, Belic N, Moores KD. A clinical interpretation of bilateral hilar adenopathy. *Ann Intern Med* 78:65, 1973.

67

Obstetric, Gynecologic, and Gonadal Disorders

Udaya B. S. Prakash

Pulmonary involvement in obstetrics is peculiar in that the respiratory symptoms and signs, although common, are not viewed as abnormalities because pregnancy, parturition, and the attendant alterations in bodily systems' function are considered normal physiologic events. Nonetheless, the pulmonary system can be involved by pathologic processes exclusive to pregnancy, gynecologic diseases, and diseases of the gonads. Additionally, in pregnancy, the clinical course of primary pulmonary diseases such as asthma, sarcoidosis, and certain infectious processes may vary from that in the nonpregnant patient. Similarly, the treatment of pulmonary disease in the pregnant patient may differ because some of the drugs normally used may interfere with pregnancy or cross the placental barrier and adversely affect the fetus [170,197]. The pulmonary complications described in pregnancy and the postpartum period are listed in Table 67-1. In this chapter, the physiologic changes noted in normal pregnancy, lung involvement by obstetric and gynecologic pathology, and pulmonary manifestations in the disorders of the gonads in both sexes are discussed.

Pregnancy

Dyspnea

Dyspnea due to mechanical, biochemical, and hemodynamic factors during pregnancy is a common occurrence [187]. By the twelfth week of pregnancy, more than 20 percent of women experience dyspnea at rest, whereas nearly two-thirds are dyspneic on exertion [102]. The incidence of dyspnea increases from 15 percent in the first trimester to 50 percent by the nineteenth week and 75 percent by the thirty-first week of gestation [121]. Upward displacement of the diaphragm by the enlarging uterus results in slightly diminished lung volumes in the second half of pregnancy [197]. Diaphragmatic fatigue following prolonged contractions, particularly before and during labor, may contribute to the occurrence of dyspnea [131]. A consistent decrease in expiratory reserve volume, a mild decrease in functional residual capacity, and a slightly reduced total lung capacity are common findings during late pregnancy. Airway closure is too insignificant to cause clinical problems. Diffusing capacity during early pregnancy is unchanged or slightly increased over nonpregnant values in the same patient and then diminishes to a plateau during the latter half of pregnancy [120,197]. Severe hyperventilation in labor has resulted in tetany [5].

Resting ventilation and, to a lesser extent, oxygen consumption are increased at rest and during exercise in pregnancy as well as during labor [45,197]. Hyperventilation is a common feature of pregnancy, but the overall pH remains relatively intact because of increased renal excretion of bicarbonate [107]. Arterial oxygen tension (PaO_2) is elevated because of the hyperventilation [4,186]. However, an abnormally high alveolar-arterial oxygen tension difference near term, possibly due to small airways closure, partially offsets the high PaO_2 [197]. Changes in concentrations of progesterone are instrumental in producing the ventilatory changes in pregnancy.

Smoking in Pregnancy

Studies in older children have demonstrated a clear association between passive exposure to maternal smoking and frequency of acute respiratory illness and chronic pulmonary conditions such as wheezing or asthma [129]. In an excellent

Table 67-1. **Pulmonary complications in pregnancy**

Pulmonary complications	Obstetric causes and effects
Dyspnea of pregnancy	Mechanical Hormonal (biochemical) Hemodynamic changes Pulmonary disease (see below)
Pneumothorax and pneumomediastinum	Valsalva maneuver (second stage of labor)
Pulmonary edema	Aspiration pneumonia Eclampsia Tocolytic therapy Pulmonary embolism Amniotic fluid embolism Disseminated intravascular coagulation Trophoblastic embolism Transfusion reactions Sepsis (septic abortion)
Pleural effusion	Postpartum Eclampsia Pulmonary edema (see above) Pulmonary embolism Amniotic fluid embolism Metastatic choriocarcinoma
Pulmonary embolism	Thromboembolism Amniotic fluid embolism Septic embolism (septic abortion)
Pulmonary hypertension	Unknown Recurrent pulmonary embolism Trophoblastic emboli

Note: Sarcoidosis, rhinitis, asthma, coccidioidomycosis, tuberculosis, and cystic fibrosis, though not complications due to pregnancy, may be present in conjunction with, and thereby affect, pregnancy, and vice versa.

study in which healthy infants born to women who smoked during pregnancy were compared to infants born to women who did not smoke during pregnancy, the researchers observed that maternal smoking was associated with significant reductions in forced expiratory flow in their young offspring. The authors inferred that maternal smoking during pregnancy may impair in utero airway development or alter lung elastic properties and that these effects may be important factors predisposing infants to the occurrence of wheezing illness later in childhood [71].

Barotrauma

Spontaneous pneumothorax and pneumomediastinum may appear during pregnancy, but these are more likely to occur during the second stage of labor. Repeated Valsalva maneuvers are the most frequent cause of these problems [128]. Pneumomediastinum is a rare complication of

pregnancy, and symptoms are not noted until after delivery [100].

Pulmonary Edema

Obstetric causes of pulmonary edema include aspiration pneumonia, sepsis, transfusion reactions, allergic reactions, disseminated intravascular coagulation, amniotic fluid embolism, toxemia of pregnancy, tocolytic therapy, and eclampsia, the latter being the most common cause of pulmonary edema in pregnancy [132]. In a recent report on 32 obstetric patients who required admission to a critical care unit, preeclampsia was the most common reason (22 percent) [91]. Eclampsia is the leading cause of maternal mortality in developing countries. A study of 126 patients with eclampsia showed acute respiratory insufficiency in 24 percent and a mortality of 6 percent [132]. Microscopic examination of the lungs reveals intravascular coagulation, fibrin deposition, and intraalveolar hemorrhage. Focal areas of bronchopneumonia may occur in this situation. Invasive hemodynamic monitoring of these patients revealed reductions in colloid osmotic pressure, pulmonary capillary leak, and left ventricular failure [14]. Impedance plethysmography in pregnant women with iatrogenic pulmonary edema has suggested that decreased venous tone and venous resistance are the cause [60]. Surgical procedures and infections, particularly pyelonephritis, during pregnancy may be accompanied by an increased risk for the development of pulmonary edema and acute respiratory distress syndrome [30,47,48].

As mentioned, the use of tocolytic agents, usually beta agonists such as terbutaline to arrest uterine contractions, is associated with the development of pulmonary edema. The frequency of this phenomenon is not certain, but estimates of occurrence vary from 0 to 4.4 percent. A literature review of tocolytic therapy–induced pulmonary edema from 1966 to 1988 revealed 58 cases reported [140]. Women with twin gestations were more likely to develop this complication, and the syndrome occurred within 12 hours in postpartum cases. Among these cases, terbutaline (41 percent) was the most commonly used tocolytic agent, following by isoxsuprine (33 percent), ritodrine (17 percent), and salbutamol (10 percent). The mean duration of tocolytic therapy was 54 hours. Symptoms included dyspnea (76 percent), chest pain (24 percent), and cough (17 percent), and these occurred before delivery in 70 percent of cases. The mean PaO_2 was 50 mmHg. Chest roentgenograms showed bilateral alveolar infiltrates and a normal-sized heart. The response to diuresis was rapid, with full recovery over a period of 24 hours, but there were 2 deaths (3 percent).

The mechanism of tocolytic therapy–induced pulmonary edema remains unknown. However, a combination of volume overload, decreased colloid oncotic pressure, and the physiologic alterations caused by pregnancy and tocolysis produce pulmonary edema that is more likely due to increased hydrostatic pressure than to increased permeability [140].

Pleural Effusion

Pleural effusions occur with toxemia of pregnancy, preeclampsia, pulmonary edema, pulmonary embolism, choriocarcinoma, and amniotic fluid embolism [74]. Surprisingly, a large number of pregnant women have asymptomatic pleural effusions during the postpartum period. In a retrospective study of 112 pregnant women who underwent normal delivery, pleural effusion was noted in 46 percent, and a prospective study of 30 normal pregnancies revealed pleural effusion in 67 percent. These effusions were noted within 24 hours of delivery, and all were asymptomatic and small [84]. The increased blood volume and decreased colloid osmotic pressure normally seen in pregnancy and the impaired lymphatic drainage secondary to elevated systemic venous pressure from Valsalva maneuvers during the second stage of labor are believed to be responsible for the accumulation of fluid in the pleural space. Acute renal failure due to ureteral obstruction by the gravid uterus is an uncommon complication of pregnancy. Pleural effusion is also an uncommon complication of ureteral obstruction by the gravid uterus and has been described in a patient [198]. Several cases of transudative pleural effusion in connection with severe preeclampsia are reported [180].

Pulmonary Embolism

Pulmonary embolism is a rare complication of pregnancy, but it is second only to abortion as a cause of maternal death [39,75]. It occurs with higher frequency during the postpartum period [1], especially after a difficult labor and an abnormal postpartum hemorrhage. A review of several series in 1965 showed the incidence of deep vein thrombosis to be 0.29 per 100 deliveries [195]. Among the 32,337 pregnancies reviewed at the Mayo Clinic, superficial phlebitis was seen in 12 per 1000 patients and deep phlebitis was seen in 2 per 1000 pregnancies. The prepartum and postpartum incidences of thrombophlebitis were 1 in 1902 patients and 1 in 622 patients, respectively. More than 75 percent of phlebitic episodes occurred during the first month after delivery, especially within the first 3 days postpartum. Calf veins were involved in 50 percent. Pulmonary embolism was noted to have an incidence of 0.4 per 1000 persons (13 of 32,337 pregnancies), and 10 of these occurred during the first postpartum month [2]. The incidence of pulmonary embolism is increased even during the first trimester [75].

Coumarin drugs, unlike heparin, cross the placenta and may cause fetal hemorrhage and congenital malformations, with a perinatal mortality of 18 percent [195,197]. Treatment of antepartum thrombophlebitis or pulmonary embolism should start with intravenous heparin, followed by coumarin after the first trimester. Coumarin should be replaced by intravenous heparin at the thirty-seventh week of gestation. All anticoagulants are withheld from the time of labor to 6 hours after delivery. Then heparin and coumarin should be resumed as in conventional patients [195,197].

Pulmonary Hypertension

The incidence of primary pulmonary hypertension in pregnancy is higher than that in nonpregnant nubile women. Wagenvoort and Wagenvoort [196] reviewed 602 cases of primary pulmonary hypertension from 51 medical centers and found that 4.5 percent were associated with pregnancy. A more recent analysis at Stanford University, during a 12-month period, of 73 women with primary pulmonary hypertension showed that 8 percent of cases were related to pregnancy [36]. A rigorous screening of these patients (all of whom were referred for heart-lung transplantation) for an underlying reason for the pulmonary hypertension failed to disclose evidence of thromboembolic disease. Recurrent noncardiogenic pulmonary edema has been described in patients with pregnancy-induced hypertension [63]. The reason for the increased incidence of primary pulmonary hypertension in pregnancy remains unknown.

Amniotic Fluid Embolism

Amniotic fluid embolism is an uncommon consequence of parturition [114]. In the United States, the incidence is in the range of 1 in 20,000 to 30,000 deliveries [171]. Amniotic fluid embolism carries an exceedingly high mortality, with a fatal outcome in 86 percent of cases [125]. Nearly 10 percent of maternal deaths in 1967 were attributed to this lesion [139]. As the frequency of other causes of mortality in pregnancy has diminished, the percentage of deaths due to amniotic fluid embolism has risen, and it is second only to pulmonary thromboembolism in most recent studies [83].

The average age at occurrence of amniotic fluid embolism is 32 years, and the risk factors include multiparity, very strong (tetanic) uterine contractions during labor, a large fetus, a dead fetus, and large quantities of particulate matter, including meconium. In one study of 40 cases of amniotic fluid embolism, the occurrence of abruptio placentae and placenta previa was noted in 45 percent [138]. Rupture of the cervix

(in 54 to 60 percent of cases), amniocentesis, and legal abortions also have caused amniotic fluid embolism [171].

Originally, the pathogenesis was attributed to an anaphylactoid reaction, but there has been no proof of this [171]. The pathogenesis probably comprises a combination of three factors: (1) pulmonary microvascular obstruction with subsequent systemic hypotension, (2) pulmonary hypertension with acute cor pulmonale, and (3) ventilation-perfusion inequality. Recent studies have shown that left ventricular failure is the only consistent abnormality [27].

Clinically, the patient develops, during labor or immediately postpartum, chills, shivering, cough, cyanosis, convulsions, and profound shock. The survivors almost always develop disseminated intravascular coagulopathy, with bleeding from the uterus. The diagnosis is made on a clinical basis presumptively and definitively at postmortem. The diagnosis also can be made by identifying mucin and squamous cells in a blood smear taken from a central venous line such as Swan-Ganz catheter [144,177].

Pathologic examination of the lungs will show that the pulmonary arteries are overwhelmingly obstructed by amniotic fluid contents—namely, mucin, fetal squamous cells, vernix fat globules, meconium, and lanugo hairs (Fig. 67-1). Mucin is almost always present, and the cellular elements are seen 80 percent of the time, with special stains and immunoperoxidase [142,171,191]. Treatment is supportive, as the use of corticosteroids and anticoagulants has not changed the course of the disease [171].

Asthma

Asthma is encountered in pregnancy with an estimated frequency of 0.4 to 1.3 percent and is reported to complicate gestation in approximately 1 percent of pregnant women [66,121]. Various reports note improvement in asthma during pregnancy in approximately 5 to 46 percent, with a similar range for worsening [197]. A study of 31 asthmatic women reported that mild to moderately severe asthmatics exhibit an improvement in asthma in the last trimester, but in more than one-third there may be a postnatal deterioration [199]. A prospective Finnish study of 198 pregnancies among 181 asthmatics reported that asthma caused no emergencies during labor and there was no difference between asthmatic and control subjects with regard to length of gestation, birth weight, incidence of perinatal deaths,

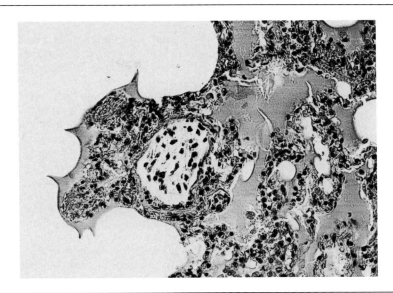

Fig. 67-1. Amniotic fluid embolism. Pulmonary arteriole occluded by fetal cells, vernix, and mucin.

low Apgar scores, neonatal respiratory difficulties, hyperbilirubinemia, or malformations [174]. However, the study observed that severe asthma or systemic corticosteroid treatment (or both) during pregnancy increased the incidence of preeclampsia in the mother and hypoglycemia in the infant. Another significant finding was that among the asthmatic women, 28 percent of births were by cesarean section, compared with 17 percent in the control group. Another study analyzed the hormonal factors and clinical and physiologic parameters during the preconception period (in 20 asthmatic women) and after conception and delivery (in 16 of 20 women), and noted that both airway responsiveness and asthma severity show statistically and clinically significant improvements during pregnancy and return toward preconception levels postpartum [89].

The mechanisms responsible for the improvement in asthma during pregnancy may include progesterone- and other substance-induced reduction in the contractility of airway smooth muscle, as yet unknown pregnancy-related circulating antiinflammatory factors, increased free serum cortisol, and the steroid's prolonged duration of action. The latter possibilities are supported by the observation that other inflammatory conditions, such as rheumatoid arthritis and ankylosing spondylitis, also improve during pregnancy [89]. The effect of mechanical factors responsible for dyspnea in nonasthmatic pregnant, discussed above, is also important in the deterioration of asthma during pregnancy.

Management of asthma during pregnancy is similar to that in the nonpregnant patient [66]. In a prospective study of 181 asthmatic women with 198 pregnancies, 40 percent of the patients were managed during pregnancy with the same antiasthmatic medications as before pregnancy, 18 percent required less medication, and 42 percent needed more. Theophylline therapy at term did not influence labor or delivery. Methylxanthines appear to present no danger to the fetus, and there is no teratogenic effect in humans. Beta agonists are also safe, but an increased risk of fetal malformation has been mentioned with the use of epinephrine [197]. Catecholamines inhibit uterine contractions. Corticosteroids may cause fetal adrenal insufficiency, but this risk is believed to be negligible. Hypoglycemia in the infant is a complication of maternal corticosteroid therapy, and therefore plasma glucose must be carefully monitored in the newborn [174]. Status asthmaticus unresponsive to medical therapy during pregnancy may necessitate termination of the pregnancy [57]. Respiratory distress can complicate pregnancy in women with severe obstructive pulmonary disease. Endotracheal intubation and mechanical ventilation in the postpartum period may be necessary in some to support the pulmonary system [99]. Bronchiectasis, if mild, does not seem to pose special problems for the pregnant patient [81].

Tuberculosis

The annual incidence of tuberculosis among pregnant women has varied depending on the period during which the data were collected [68]. A report in 1972 recorded an incidence of tuberculosis among pregnant women in New Orleans of 4.8 percent [8]. The rate of tuberculosis among American women of childbearing age (15 to 45 years) declined from 3.8 per 100,000 in 1977 to 2.35 per 100,000 in 1987, then increased to 2.5 per 100,000 in 1989 among Hispanic white women [191]. A recent increase in the rate of tuberculosis in the United States suggests that pregnant women will also be at greater risk of developing this disease.

Pregnancy neither predisposes to the development or progression of tuberculosis nor alters the clinical presentation of the disease [38,149,201]. A study of 1565 pregnancies during which tuberculosis was active showed no evidence of a negative consequence of pregnancy on tuberculosis during gestation, although most of the relapses developed in the postpartum period [149]. A corollary to this is that tuberculosis neither affects nor complicates the course of pregnancy or the type of delivery [68,149]. However, mother-to-fetus or -newborn transmission of tuberculosis is an important clinical consideration in managing the pregnant tuberculous patient. The modes of spread of tubercle bacilli from mother to fetus or newborn include hematogenous or lymphogenous spread, transmission through placenta, and tuberculous endometritis during pregnancy. In a detailed review of the topic, Hamadeh and Glassroth [68] conclude that despite the potential for transmission in utero, the newborn is at greater risk of acquiring tuberculosis postpartum than congenitally, particularly if born to a mother whose sputum contains tubercle bacilli and whose condition remains undiagnosed and untreated.

Radiation hazard from repeated chest roentgenography should be minimized in pregnant women. In those suspected of having tuberculosis, a chest roentgenogram should be obtained after the twelfth week of gestation with proper shielding of the abdomen, and it should be performed only when a positive result of a tuberculin skin test requires exclusion of active pulmonary tuberculosis [68]. However, it may be necessary sooner if the patient has symptoms

that are highly suggestive of pulmonary tuberculosis. Tuberculin skin testing is not contraindicated in pregnancy as it does not affect pregnancy or the fetus. The tuberculin response in pregnancy is no different from that in nonpregnancy [141]. Induced sputum and gastric washings on a repeated basis are valuable.

Active pulmonary tuberculosis diagnosed during pregnancy should be treated promptly, the initial drug combination being isoniazid (300 mg/day) and rifampin (600 mg/day) for at least 9 months. Ethambutol may be used if the clinical situation warrants addition of the third or an alternate drug. Because of their potential to cause fetal toxicity, pyrazinamide, streptomycin, and other aminoglycosides should be avoided [166]. Active disease detected at the time of delivery should be treated likewise [3]. During the postpartum period, antituberculous drugs are continued until the prescribed treatment period is completed. Antituberculous therapy is not a contraindication to breast-feeding [167]. Other precautions—namely, the isolation precautions, study of contacts, and preventive therapy for the infant and close contacts—is similar to the approach in nonpregnant tuberculous patients. Tuberculosis is not an indication for routine therapeutic interruption of pregnancy.

Sleep Apnea

Even though several cases of obstructive sleep apnea in pregnancy are reported, the prevalence of sleep apnea in pregnancy is unknown [24,28,87,97,152]. The effects of pregnancy on the severity of preexistent sleep apnea also are unknown. More important is the effect of obstructive sleep apnea–induced hypoxemia on fetal maturation. Chronic hypoxemia causes fetal polycythemia in an animal model, but the heart rate and respiratory movements return to baseline [16,95]. Intrauterine growth retardation in maternal obstructive sleep apnea has been reported [24,152] and may be present even if external cardiotocography shows normal fetal heart rate reactivity to fetal movements despite apneic episodes and periods of desaturation [24]. Early recognition and treatment of obstructive sleep apnea in pregnancy might prevent problems with fetal development. Nasal continuous positive airway pressure (CPAP) treatment and other nonhormonal therapies pose no threat to the development of the fetus, but careful monitoring of fetal status and maternal cardiopulmonary condition is imperative [24].

Molar Pregnancy

Thoracic complications can occur after removal of a benign hydatidiform mole. The incidence of trophoblastic pulmonary emboli varies between 2 and 11 percent [135]. Clinically, these patients manifest a wide spectrum of pulmonary findings, including the development of pulmonary hypertension and pulmonary edema [7,76,94,108,126, 189]. Among 128 patients with hydatidiform mole undergoing evacuation, 12 patients (9.4 percent) developed acute, severe respiratory distress, and trophoblastic embolism was identified in 7 patients [190]. The incidence of respiratory complications increased from 0 at less than 16 weeks' gestation to 27 percent when the uterus had developed beyond 16 weeks. In a recent review of 60 patients with benign trophoblastic disease, 5 developed pulmonary complications, with 2 progressing into acute respiratory distress syndrome from pulmonary edema. Possible etiologies include trophoblastic emboli, hypervolemia, and intravascular coagulation [82]. Chest roentgenograms in these patients may reveal rounded lesions [9,135].

Choriocarcinoma

Choriocarcinoma is most often preceded by molar pregnancy. It is a fetal neoplasm that invades maternal tissue and it occurs in 1 in 20,000 pregnancies. The interval between pregnancy and pulmonary metastases varies from 1 to 60 months. Pulmonary metastases have been reported in 68 percent of patients. The pulmonary lesions may be multiple, discrete, calcified, and associated with pleural effusion [49]. Hemoptysis is seen in patients with chest roentgenographic abnormalities [204]. In a series of 179 patients, 36 presented with pulmonary symptoms, and all but 1 had abnormal chest roentgenograms [113]. Tumor emboli and hemothorax also can occur [178]. Gestational choriocarcinoma has presented as endobronchial carcinoma [117].

Miscellaneous Obstetric Disorders

Sarcoidosis does not seem to have any adverse effects on the course of pregnancy [197], whereas pregnancy may influence sarcoidosis, which remains unchanged or improves during pregnancy [40,54,115,134]. Some observations have been made regarding the behavior of sarcoidosis during and after pregnancy [148]. In patients whose chest roentgenograms demonstrated disease resolution before pregnancy, a normal chest roentgenogram is likely to persist through the prenatal period and gestation. Patients with active sarcoidosis usually experience partial or complete resolution of chest roentgenographic abnormalities during pregnancy, although many in this group will experience exacerbation of sarcoid within 3 to 6 months after delivery. Those with a fibrotic process secondary to sarcoidosis are likely to show no changes in their chest roentgenograms [148]. One possible explanation for the frequent ameliorating effect of pregnancy on sarcoidosis is the increased concentration of circulating corticosteroids [115]. Occasional relapse during the postpartum period has been noted [115]. There is no indication for termination of pregnancy in sarcoidosis.

Rhinitis occurs frequently during pregnancy, and although many causes, including altered vagal function, hormonal imbalance, and others, have been proposed, the rhinitis of pregnancy may not be a distinct entity [111]. Varicella pneumonia seems to occur more commonly in pregnant women. A review of the literature in 1980 noted that approximately 10 percent of all reported cases of varicella pneumonia were in pregnant women, and the maternal mortality rate was approximately 45 percent [197].

Coccidioidomycosis has a propensity to disseminate during pregnancy. One report observed 50 percent dissemination among 50 pregnant women [72]. The risk of dissemination was higher in those who contracted the infection during pregnancy, particularly in the second and third trimesters. Amphotericin B, the drug of choice in disseminated coccidioidomycosis, has no detrimental effects on pregnancy and poses minimal risk to the fetus [118].

As more patients with cystic fibrosis reach adulthood, the occurrence of pregnancy among such patients will increase [96]. In a study of 11 pregnancies among 8 women with cystic fibrosis, the maternal condition deteriorated during and after pregnancy and did not return to the pregravid state [136]. Quantitative evaluation of pregravid nutritional and pulmonary status is useful in counseling women with cystic fibrosis about the risk of pregnancy.

Systemic lupus erythematosus may be exacerbated during pregnancy. Several cases of lupus pneumonitis developing during the postpartum period have been described [103,130].

Pregnant patients with pulmonary arteriovenous malformations from hereditary hemorrhagic telangiectasia face the risk of increased hypoxemia due to elevation of the intrapulmonary shunt fraction. In a report of a case, the pregnancy was terminated at 35 weeks' gestation because of life-threatening hypoxemia; the increased shunting was the result of the physiologic increase in blood volume during pregnancy [181]. There is some indication that these fistulas enlarge during pregnancy and cause serious complications such as massive hemothorax and increasing hypoxia.

Diaphragmatic rupture leading to respiratory failure is another rare but potentially lethal complication of pregnancy [203].

Gynecologic Disorders

Several gynecologic diseases produce pulmonary complications. Some of these represent a peculiar association of pulmonary and gynecologic disorders rather than complications. Table 67-2 lists the pulmonary complications of the gynecologic diseases described in the literature.

Catamenial Pneumothorax

Catamenial pneumothorax is a syndrome of spontaneous recurrent pneumothorax occurring within 48 to 73 hours of the onset of menses [12,23,106,122]. Until pneumothorax recurs, it is impossible to determine clinical coincidence from the specific syndrome of catamenial pneumothorax [23]. This is the most common thoracic complication of endometriosis [35,78,106,122, 160]. By 1974, 30 cases of catamenial pneumothorax were reported in the literature [160], and another dozen cases were added by 1976 [168]. A review in 1990 noted that there were approximately 100 cases in the literature [23]. Among 196 cases of spontaneous pneumothoraces in women younger than 50 years, 5.6 percent were catamenial [160]. Usually seen in women between the ages of 30 and 35 years, catamenial pneumothorax is almost always (90 to 95 percent) right-sided and small. The majority of patients present with chest pain or mild dyspnea, though the syndrome can be asymptomatic.

Pneumothorax is believed by some to be caused by pleural endometriosis [35] (Fig. 67-2). However, clinical and pathologic evidence of pelvic endometriosis is demonstrated in only 22 to 37 percent of cases [151]. Pleural or diaphragmatic endometrial implants have been visualized at thoracotomy in 23 to 35 percent of patients [12,151]. Air originating in the genital tract is believed to make its way through defects in the diaphragm. Examination at the time of thoracotomy for treatment of catamenial pneumothorax has revealed defects in the diaphragm, and closure of these defects has resulted in the absence of recurrent pneumothorax [175]. However, such diaphragmatic defects or fenestrations have been found in only 19 to 33 percent of the cases explored [151]. The diaphragmatic defects have been observed with thoracoscopy using a bronchoscope [56].

Ovulation-suppressing agents such as danazol sometimes are helpful in preventing recurrent pneumothorax [179]. Recently, a case of catamenial pneumomediastinum that responded to danazol was described [159]. Spontaneous pneumothorax has also been described in a patient with carcinoma of the cervix [184].

Table 67-2. **Pulmonary complications in gynecologic diseases**

Pulmonary complication	Gynecologic origin
Pneumothorax, pneumomediastinum (catamenial)	Pleural endometriosis Air entry via genital tract into pleural space
Hemoptysis	Endobronchial endometriosis
Pulmonary nodules or atelectasis	Endobronchial endometriosis Benign metastasizing leiomyoma Pulmonary lymphangioleiomyomatosis
Pleural effusion	Ovarian neoplasm (Meigs-Salmon syndrome) Pulmonary lymphangioleiomyomatosis Uterine fibroids Pleural endometriosis
Premenstrual exacerbation of asthma	Hormonal imbalance (?)

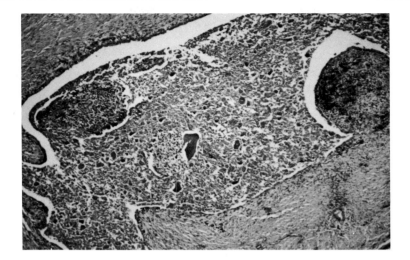

Fig. 67-2. Pleural endometriosis causing pneumothorax.

Premenstrual Exacerbation of Asthma

Premenstrual worsening of asthma (so-called premenstrual asthma) has been observed by many practitioners [33,70,143]. In a recent study involving 126 consecutive women aged 14 to 46 years who attended an outpatient asthma clinic, a detailed questionnaire and twice-daily peak expiratory flow measurements revealed premenstrual deterioration of asthma in 40 percent [59]. The falls in peak flow were modest and of a degree that would not be expected to result in increased dyspnea. No correlations were found between premenstrual exacerbation of asthma and symptoms of premenstrual tension, consumption of aspirin, use of the contraceptive pill, cycle length, or behavior of asthma during pregnancy. Severe asthmatics are reported to be more prone to premenstrual deterioration [59]. Even mild asthmatics who were previously unaware of premenstrual asthma have been shown to observe a premenstrual deterioration of asthmatic symptoms and peak expiratory flow rate without showing any significant changes in spirometry or airway reactivity [137].

The mechanism of premenstrual exacerbation of asthma is unclear. Progesterone level reaches a peak approximately 7 days before menstruation and rapidly falls almost to zero at the onset of the period [20]. It is known that progesterone is a smooth-muscle relaxant in the gastrointestinal tract, genitourinary system, and vascular tree [19], and the fall in progesterone concentration in the late luteal phase might be associated with the withdrawal of a relaxant effect on bronchial smooth muscle [59]. There are earlier reports on treatment of "ovarian asthma" by irradiation of the ovaries and progesterone preparations [13,32,53]. Progesterone is a well-known respiratory stimulant and is known to cause hyperventilation, which may heighten the sensation of breathlessness. However, the peak serum concentrations of progesterone are reached several days before symptomatic deterioration of asthma, and therefore, progesterone-induced hyperventilation is an unlikely explanation for premenstrual exacerbation of asthma [59].

Effect of Menses on Respiration

In addition to the menses-exacerbated asthma just discussed, the menses also affect normal respiration in nonasthmatic women. The respiratory-stimulating effect of progesterone has been mentioned already. The level of progesterone varies during the menstrual cycle in adult women. In a study of 30 healthy female adults, respiratory muscle function, measured by maximal static inspiratory and expiratory pressures, was assessed during the midfollicular and midluteal phases of the menstrual cycle; the results showed that inspiratory muscle endurance was 26 percent higher in the midluteal phase than in the mid-follicular phase, whereas the respiratory muscle strength and pulmonary function were unchanged [25]. Other studies have shown that resting ventilation, ventilatory response to hypoxia or hypercapnia, and resistance to genioglossal activity are elevated during the luteal phase [44,104,150,183]. These findings imply that the high inspiratory muscle endurance in the midluteal phase may be related, at least in part, to high plasma progesterone levels [25]. Transforming this information into variations in athletic performance is purely speculative.

Pulmonary Endometriosis

Endometriosis of the lung is rare. The presence of endometrial tissue in the lung is presumed to originate from hematogenous spread or celomic metaplasia [122]. Pleural endometriosis is believed to spread from pelvic or peritoneal deposits [41]. Another possibility is the hematogenous metastasis of viable endometrial tissue after uterine surgery or cesarean section [145]. This argument is supported by the finding that pulmonary endometriosis is almost always detected in the lower lung, which receives a higher blood supply. Pathologic analysis of pleuropulmonary tissue generally shows changes typical of endometriosis [101]. Endobronchial endometriosis has been reported to cause catamenial hemoptysis and airways obstruction with segmental atelectasis [51,145]. Other symptoms include chest pain, dyspnea, or pleural effusion. Asymptomatic pulmonary density is another manifestation. Chest roentgenograms have revealed solitary pulmonary nodules in parenchymal endometriosis [122].

A review of the literature in 1981 revealed 65 cases of pulmonary endometriosis, 11 cases of which were parenchymal and 54 cases that were pleural [51]. A half-dozen cases were reported by 1989 [41]. The review by Foster and associates [51] noted that pleural disease is more common in the younger age group (mean age, 33.6 years), is associated more frequently with pelvic endometriosis, usually occurs on the right, and more often is associated with pneumothorax. Pulmonary parenchymal endometriosis, on the other hand, appears later (mean age, 39 years) and is associated with pelvic endometriosis in only 10 percent of cases, catamenial hemoptysis in 82 percent, and catamenial pain and dyspnea in 18 percent.

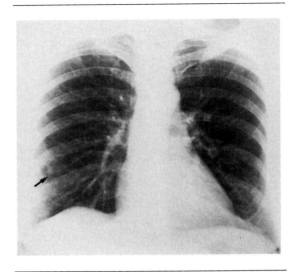

Fig. 67-3. Benign metastasizing leiomyoma in the lungs. *Arrows* point to small nodules in the lungs.

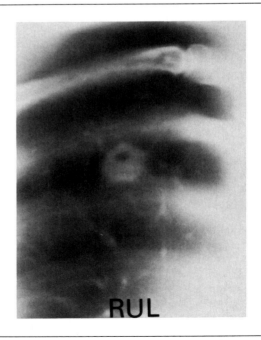

Fig. 67-4. Benign metastasizing leiomyoma in right upper lobe (*RUL*); cavitation as a result of secondary infection is demonstrated.

Metastasizing Benign Leiomyoma

Metastasizing benign leiomyoma is an oddity in pulmonary diseases. Uterine fibroleiomyomas (also called *well-differentiated leiomyosarcoma*) are known to be associated with multiple pulmonary fibroleiomyomas [6,26,173]. Although slow-growing, these are believed to be pulmonary metastases—hence the term *metastasizing benign leiomyoma*. A review of 23 reported cases revealed the following: The age span among patients studied was 30 to 74 years (mean, 47 years), three-fourths had uterine leiomyomas, and all but 2 were white [80]. Most cases were discovered during routine chest roentgenographic examination. The lesions were nodular, bilateral in 15, recurrent in 3, and increased in size in 7 patients. Roentgenographically, these nodular densities may range from 0.5 to 4.5 cm in diameter (Figs. 67-3, 67-4) and, occasionally, pleural effusion is also seen. Nodules may grow in premenopausal women and remain stationary in postmenopausal women [80,147].

Gonadal Disorders

Diseases of the gonads occasionally are associated with pulmonary problems. The main entities included in this discussion are Meigs-Salmon syndrome, Klinefelter's syndrome, Turner's syndrome, and Young's syndrome. Lymphangioleiomyomatosis is also included here because recent knowledge of this unusual disorder suggests that although it is not a primary gonadal disease, it responds to ovarian hormones.

Meigs-Salmon Syndrome

Meigs-Salmon syndrome is a clinical entity characterized by the coexistence of ovarian fibroma or other solid ovarian tumors, ascites, and pleural effusion [119]. Pleural effusions are observed in 3 percent of patients with ovarian neoplasms that measure more than 6 cm in diameter [43]. A variant of this syndrome is described in which the clinical features were highly suggestive of Meigs-Salmon syndrome but the ovary showed degenerative changes without tumor [188]. The effusions and ascites usually disappear with removal of the ovarian tumor. The pleural effusions in this syndrome are more common on the right, are transudative chemically, and may become voluminous. The transportation of fluid from the peritoneum to the pleural space is via the diaphrag-

matic lymphatics. Massive edema of the ovary without neoplastic changes has been reported to cause hydrothorax and ascites [55]. Very large ovarian tumors are capable of producing respiratory failure by upward push on the diaphragm [73].

At least a dozen patients have been reported to have developed pleural effusion in association with uterine fibroids [58]. These patients were between the ages of 30 and 45 years and presented with abdominal distension and mass. There were no menstrual abnormalities. The pleural effusions were right-sided in 75 percent and hemorrhagic in 1 patient [58]. Both transudates [200] and exudates [169] have been described. The pathogenesis of the pleural effusion in these patients and in Meigs-Salmon syndrome is unknown, although there exists the possibility of active secretion by the tumors or inflamed peritoneum and lymphatic or venous obstruction.

Lymphangioleiomyomatosis

Lymphangioleiomyomatosis is a rare disorder that affects women of childbearing age and is characterized by progressive dyspnea, spontaneous pneumothorax, chylothorax, and hemoptysis caused by diffuse cystic changes in the pulmonary parenchyma and marked proliferation of peribronchial smooth muscle in a lymphatic distribution. Lymphangioleiomyomatosis is an uncommon pulmonary condition of unknown origin and pathogenesis [22,29,52,93,185]. However, this disorder should be considered primarily an ovarian one with predominantly respiratory manifestations. The rationale for this assumption is as follows: First, the disease generally presents in women during their childbearing years. Second, there is exacerbation of the disease during menses and pregnancy [22,29,65]. Third, estrogen and progesterone receptors are present in lung tissue [18]. Fourth, clinical improvement has been documented following treatment with progesterone or oophorectomy [10,42,46,116]. There have been reports of only 6 women older than 55 years developing symptomatic lymphangioleiomyomatosis [17,162,163].

Lymphangioleiomyomatosis is sometimes discussed with tuberous sclerosis because of the similarities noted in the pulmonary pathologic specimens [86,88,98,116,123,165,193]. Further, lymphangioleiomyomatosis and tuberous sclerosis have been reported to coexist in a patient [110]. Nevertheless, the usual presence of clinical features such as mental retardation, development of angiomyolipomas, adenoma sebaceum, subungual fibromas, and various other skin lesions in patients with tuberous sclerosis distinguish these two entities (see Chapter 66).

Clinical features include progressive dyspnea resembling that of ordinary chronic obstructive lung disease, recurrent pneumothorax (in more than 60 percent), unilateral or bilateral chylous pleural effusions (in 25 percent), and hemoptysis (in 50 percent) in nubile women. The abnormal proliferation of smooth muscles around the distal airways causes venular congestion and disruption, resulting in hemoptysis and alveolar hemosiderosis [79]. Abdominal and thoracic lymphatics as well as lymph nodes may become involved [15,110,162]. Chylous ascites and a "doughy" abdomen are sometimes the presenting features.

Chest roentgenograms show diffuse reticulonodular infiltrates in 50 to 80 percent of patients (Fig. 67-5). Lung hyperinflation is observed in up to 25 percent. Cystic spaces measuring 0.5 to 1.5 cm in diameter and bullous changes are seen in 12 to 40 percent of patients. Pneumothorax (50 to 80 percent) and pleural effusion (30 to 40 percent) may be present. The smooth-muscle proliferation around the distal airways leads to alveolar destruction and development of cystic changes and pneumothorax. Likewise, the

Fig. 67-5. Lymphangioleiomyomatosis of lungs. Diffuse nodular infiltrates, relative sparing of lower lung zones, and hyperinflation of lungs can be seen.

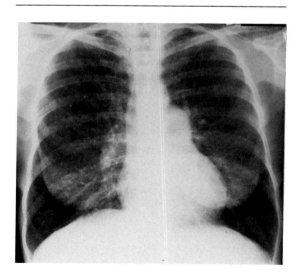

smooth-muscle proliferation around the pulmonary lymphatics produces lymphatic obstruction and development of chylothorax. Despite the presence of the above-noted typical clinical and roentgenologic features, the diagnosis was delayed by an average of 44 months (range, 1 to 219 months) in a series of 32 patients with lymphangioleiomyomatosis [185]. Bronchoscopic lung biopsy may be adequate, or an open-lung biopsy may be required for the diagnosis. However, typical clinical features combined with characteristic findings depicted by high-resolution computed tomography may establish the diagnosis (Fig. 67-6). Histopathologic features of lung parenchyma include accumulation of smooth-muscle bundles in the alveolar walls, especially around bronchioles and venules (Fig. 67-7). Ultrastructural and immunofluorescent examination of these smooth-muscle bundles has shown higher glycogen content of muscle cells [90] and smooth-muscle antigens [172].

The abnormal smooth-muscle proliferation occurs around the smaller airways. Compression of the airways by the smooth muscles is responsible for the severe obstructive pulmonary dysfunction in these patients. Studies of pulmonary mechanics in 8 women with lymphangioleiomyomatosis showed increased total lung capacity (114 ± 7 percent of predicted) and residual volume (207 ± 24 percent of predicted), reduced ratios of 1-second forced expiratory volume to forced vital capacity (61 ± 6 percent), moderately reduced retractive force at total lung capacity (67 ± 10 percent of predicted), increased static compliance (128 ± 19 percent of predicted), and markedly elevated pulmonary flow resistance (266 ± 46 percent) [21]. Maximal flow-static recoil

Fig. 67-6. Lymphangioleiomyomatosis of lungs imaged with high-resolution computed tomography showing typical cystic spaces.

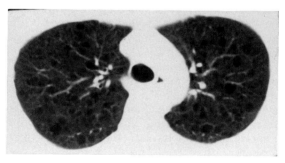

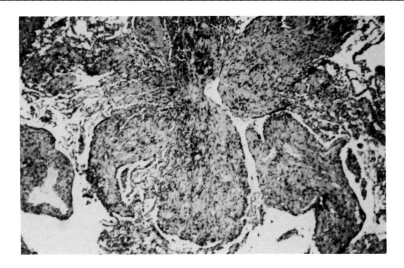

Fig. 67-7. Lymphangioleiomyomatosis in the lung tissue showing hypertrophy of bronchial smooth-muscle bundles.

curves also were evident in patients with airway obstruction, the cause being predominantly airway narrowing rather than loss of lung elastic forces [21]. Lymphangioleiomyomatosis is one of the rare diseases in which even though the chest roentgenogram suggests a restrictive type of process (nodular or interstitial), the pulmonary function tests reveal characteristics of obstructive pulmonary disease [161,176].

Treatment should be initiated as soon as the diagnosis is established because of the progressive nature of the disease. Patients should be advised against pregnancy and the use of estrogen preparations. Treatment options for lymphangioleiomyomatosis continue to evolve. A meta-analysis of 30 cases reported in the literature noted that although eight treatment regimens were used, progesterone or oophorectomy or both were the most effective treatments, resulting in improvement or stabilization of the disease in the majority of cases [46]. A more recent report on 8 women with lymphangioleiomyomatosis treated by various antiestrogen therapies concluded that without a control group, it was difficult to ascertain whether the treatments were responsible for the apparent improvement of the disease [192]. Medroxyprogesterone is given in doses equivalent to at least 10 mg/day on either a daily or monthly basis. Rapidly progressive cases should be considered for both progesterone ther-

apy and oophorectomy. Tamoxifen therapy and tetracycline pleurodesis have been used successfully to control recurrent chylothorax [10,110,202]. However, tamoxifen therapy is reported not only to lack evidence of proved effectiveness but also to be closely associated with the recurrence of pneumothoraces and exacerbation of the disease [79]. Persistent chylothorax may require surgical pleurodesis or placement of a pleuroperitoneal shunt. Single or double lung transplantation has become a therapeutic option for refractory cases [109,164], which develop progressive respiratory distress and lead to death within 10 years [22,161].

Klinefelter's Syndrome

Klinefelter's syndrome is the most common example of male hypogonadism in phenotypic men, characterized by the presence of two or more X chromosomes, the most common karyotype being XXY. It is morphologically manifested by varying degrees of seminiferous tubular failure and decreased Leydig cell function. Clinical features include small and firm testes, infertility, decreased testosterone level, gynecomastia and, frequently, eunuchoid features and mild mental retardation. Respiratory disease is known to be more prevalent in these patients than in the population at large [34,146]. Pulmonary manifestations described have included asthmatic bronchitis, recurrent pulmonary infections, bronchiectasis, pectus excavatum, kyphoscoliosis, pulmonary cysts, respiratory infections, and emphysema [64]. Restrictive lung dysfunction is attributed to chest wall abnormalities, even though pulmonary restriction has been demonstrated in the absence of parenchymal or musculoskeletal abnormalities [85,194]. A detailed physiologic study of 13 patients with Klinefelter's syndrome reported that none exhibited chest wall restriction, but 4 patients demonstrated significantly reduced lung compliance [124]. The authors concluded that the likely cause of pulmonary restriction, noted in 8 patients (62 percent), was a decrease in the compliance of the lung matrix, probably related to the absence of testosterone.

Turner's Syndrome

Turner's syndrome is a disorder of sex differentiation. Its clinical features include an XO sex chromosome constitution, dwarfism, sexual infantilism, webbing of the neck, and cubitus valgus. Thoracic manifestations consist of square and shieldlike chest, pleural effusions, coarctation of the aorta, and rib notching [61].

Young's Syndrome

Young's syndrome, or obstructive azoospermia, denotes primary infertility in men who have normal spermatozoa in the epididymides but none in the ejaculate [77,205]. This entity differs from the well-known links between infertility and lung diseases noted in ciliary dysmotility syndromes and cystic fibrosis. Unlike the immotile cilia syndrome, Young's syndrome demonstrates an absence of ultrastructural ciliary disorders and, unlike cystic fibrosis, normal sweat and pancreatic functions are present [77]. Electron microscopy of nasal cilia in 12 patients with Young's syndrome has confirmed normal ciliary ultrastructure [67]. Handelsman and associates [69] suggest that this disorder has a prevalence rate comparable to that of Klinefelter's syndrome and higher than that of either cystic fibrosis or the immotile cilia syndrome.

The underlying abnormality in Young's syndrome is unknown, although it is presumed to be a mucous defect [31]. Mucociliary clearance, as determined by nasal ciliary beat frequency, is shown to be abnormal in Young's syndrome [67]. It is not clear whether this is the cause or effect of sinusitis. The relative disorientation of distal ciliary axoneme in patients with Young's syndrome may be due to a structural defect but is more likely a consequence of abnormal mucus

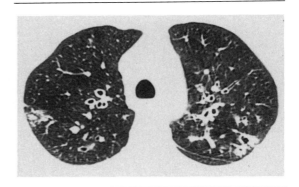

Fig. 67-8. Young's syndrome with bronchiectasis documented by high-resolution computed tomography showing bilateral bronchiectasis.

[37]. However, use of mucoregulatory agents in these patients has not been helpful [31].

More than half the patients in the original series had severe chest disease in childhood [205]. In a recent study of 34 infertile men with obstructive azoospermia and normal controls, the following abnormalities were noted in those with Young's syndrome: grossly abnormal sinus roentgenograms (59 percent), sinusitis (56 percent), repeated otitis media (32 percent), chronic bronchitis (35 percent), abnormal chest roentgenograms (53 percent), and bronchiectasis (29 percent) [133] (Fig. 67-8). Airflow obstruction was observed in 15 patients. Although this controlled study confirmed that a significant excess of sinopulmonary disease exists in this group, the reason for the relationship between obstructive azoospermia and lung disease remains undefined [133]. Interestingly, hypoxemia causes disturbances in the function of the hypothalamic-pituitary-gonadal axis in men [153–156]. Hypoxemia as a consequence of respiratory diseases has been shown to result in depression of serum concentrations of testosterone and atrophy of Leydig cells in the testes of men with bronchitis and emphysema [62].

Sexual Activity and the Lung

The coital act is physically strenuous even in healthy humans. The presence of chronic respiratory disease affects this function in many patients in the form of functional impotence or lack of libido [105]. Although a considerable number of patients with respiratory diseases are concerned about their inability to have normal sexual intercourse, very few mention this aspect of their health to their physicians. Part of the reason is the patients' embarrassment in bringing up this "medically irrelevant" topic, and part is due to physicians' failure to inquire about it. It is well recognized that several medications, particularly beta-blocking agents, used to treat cardiac diseases and hypertension cause impotence. However, none of the drugs used in chronic obstructive pulmonary disease or other common lung diseases is known to affect sexual function. Medroxyprogesterone used in some patients with central sleep apnea may result in impotence after long-term therapy. In hypoxemic patients, supplemental oxygen therapy during sexual intercourse is helpful.

Hemoptysis during sexual intercourse has been described in a patient with coronary artery disease [11]. Despite recurrent episodes of hemoptysis that necessitated several visits to his physician, the patient did not provide the history of sexual activity in relation to hemoptysis. Increased cardiovascular demands and left ventricular dysfunction brought on by sexual activity were concluded to be physiologic reasons for the hemoptysis. Postcoital catamenial pneumothorax not associated with endometriosis has also been reported [127].

Asthma (postcoital asthma) and rhinitis (honeymoon rhinitis) brought on by sexual activity have been described by several practitioners [50,112,158,182]. A study of 3 men and 1 woman with postcoital asthma or rhinitis observed clinically significant attacks of asthma or rhinorrhea during and immediately after sexual intercourse; indeed, 1 man required several visits to the emergency department and hospitalization on one occasion [158]. All had a previous history of asthma, and anxiety was noted to be a predominant feature in the patients and their sexual partners. Sexual excitement, rather than exercise, may have caused asthma in one of the patients who developed asthmatic symptoms before sexual intercourse. Allergy to human seminal plasma in female subjects has also been reported to cause postcoital asthma [157]. Exaggerated autonomic imbalance and coitus-induced exercise are likely the responsible factors.

Reflux dyspareunia denotes heartburn occurring during sexual intercourse. In a prospective study of 100 women with known gastroesophageal reflux, 77 percent suffered from reflux symptoms (severe in 6, moderate in 22, and mild in 49) during sexual intercourse [92]. The supine position and increased intraabdominal pressure may account for the reflux symptoms during sexual intercourse. Although the number of women with hiatal hernia was not mentioned, such herniation is as important as other factors in causing reflux dyspareunia. No mention was made in the literature of reflux dyspareunia–related aspiration.

References

1. Aaro LA, Juergens JL. Thrombophlebitis and pulmonary embolism as complications of pregnancy. *Med Clin North Am* 58:829, 1974.
2. Aaro LA, Juergens JL. Thrombophlebitis associated with pregnancy. *Am J Obstet Gynecol* 109:1128, 1971.
3. American Thoracic Society. Treatment of tuberculosis and tuberculosis infection in adults and children. *Am Rev Respir Dis* 134:355, 1986.
4. Anderson GJ, et al. The maternal oxygen tension and acid-base status during pregnancy. *J Obstet Gynaecol* 76:16, 1969.
5. Argent VP. Treatment of severe tetany due to hyperventilation during labour with a mixture of nitrous oxide, oxygen, and carbon dioxide. *Br Med J* 285:117, 1982.
6. Bachman D, Wolff M. Pulmonary metastases from benign-appearing smooth muscle tumors of the uterus. *AJR* 127:441, 1976.
7. Bagshawe KD, Noble MIM. Cardiorespiratory aspects of trophoblastic tumors. *Q J Med* 137:39, 1966.
8. Bailey WC, Thompson DH, Greenberg HB. Indigent pregnant women of New Orleans require tuberculosis control measures. *Hum Serv Report* 87:737, 1972.
9. Band PR, et al. Hydatidiform mole metastasizing to the lung. *Can Med Assoc J* 114:813, 1976.
10. Banner AS, et al. Efficacy of oophorectomy in lymphangioleiomyomatosis and benign metastasizing leiomyoma. *N Engl J Med* 305:204, 1981.
11. Bansal S, Day JA Jr, Braman SS. Hemoptysis during sexual intercourse. Unusual manifestation of coronary artery disease. *Chest* 93:891, 1988.
12. Barrocas A. Catamenial pneumothorax: Case report and a review of the literature. *Am Surg* 45:340, 1979.
13. Beaumont GE. Ovarian Asthma. In *The Clinical Approach to Medical Practice*. London: Churchill, 1956.
14. Benedetti TJ, Kates R, Williams V. Hemodynamic observations in preeclampsia complicated by pulmonary edema. *Am J Obstet Gynecol* 152:330, 1985.
15. Berberich FR, et al. Lymphangiomyomatosis with chylothorax. *J Pediatr* 87:941, 1975.
16. Boddy K, et al. Foetal respiratory movements, electrocordal and cardiovascular responses to

hypoxemia and hypercapnia in sheep. *J Physiol* 243:599, 1974.

17. Bradley SL, et al. Pulmonary lymphangioleiomyomatosis. *Lung* 158:69, 1980.

18. Brentani MM, et al. Steroid receptors in pulmonary lymphangioleiomyomatosis. *Chest* 85:96, 1984.

19. Briggs MH, Brotherton J. *Steroid Chemistry and Pharmacology.* New York: Academic, 1970.

20. Brush MC. Endocrine and other biochemical factors in the aetiology of the premenstrual syndrome. *Curr Med Res Opin* 6(Suppl 5):19, 1979.

21. Burger CD, Hyatt RE, Staats BA. Pulmonary mechanics in lymphangioleiomyomatosis. *Am Rev Respir Dis* 143:1030, 1991.

22. Carrington CB, et al. Lymphangioleiomyomatosis. *Am Rev Respir Dis* 116:977, 1977.

23. Carter EJ, Ettensohn DB. Catamenial pneumothorax. *Chest* 98:713, 1990.

24. Charbonneau M, et al. Obstructive sleep apnea during pregnancy. Therapy and implications for fetal health. *Am Rev Respir Dis* 144:461, 1991.

25. Chen H-I, Tang Y-R. Effects of the menstrual cycle on respiratory muscle function. *Am Rev Respir Dis* 140:1359, 1989.

26. Clark DH, Weed JC. Metastasizing leiomyoma: A case report. *Am J Obstet Gynecol* 127:672, 1977.

27. Clark SL, Montz FJ, Phelan JP. Hemodynamic alterations associated with amniotic fluid embolism: A reappraisal. *Am J Obstet Gynecol* 151:617, 1985.

28. Conti M, et al. Sleep apnea syndrome in pregnancy: A case report. *Eur J Anesthesiol* 5:151, 1988.

29. Corrin B, Liebow AA, Friedman PJ. Pulmonary lymphangioleiomyomatosis. *Am J Pathol* 79:347, 1975.

30. Cunningham FG, et al. Respiratory insufficiency associated with pyelonephritis during pregnancy. *Obstet Gynecol* 63:121, 1984.

31. Currie DC, et al. Efficacy of "mucoregulatory" agents in Young's syndrome. *Thorax* 43:480, 1988.

32. Dalton K. Menstruation and accidents. *Br Med J* 11:1425, 1960.

33. Dalton K. *The Premenstrual Syndrome and Progesterone Therapy.* London: Heinemann, 1977.

34. Daly JJ, Hunter H, Rickards DF. Klinefelter's syndrome and pulmonary disease. *Am Rev Respir Dis* 98:717, 1968.

35. Davies R. Recurring spontaneous pneumothorax concomitant with menstruation. *Thorax* 23:370, 1968.

36. Dawkins KD, et al. Primary pulmonary hypertension and pregnancy. *Chest* 89:383, 1986.

37. de Iongh R, Ing A, Rutland J. Mucociliary function, ciliary ultrastructure, and ciliary orientation in Young's syndrome. *Thorax* 47:184, 1992.

38. DeMarch P. Tuberculosis and pregnancy. 68:800, 1975.

39. Demers C, Ginsburg JS. Deep venous thrombosis and pulmonary embolism in pregnancy. *Clin Chest Med* 13:645, 1992.

40. Dines DE, Banner E. Sarcoidosis during pregnancy: Improvement in pulmonary function. *JAMA* 200:726, 1967.

41. Di Palo S, et al. Endometriosis of the lung. *Respir Med* 83:255, 1989.

42. Dishner W, et al. Pulmonary lymphangioleiomyomatosis. *Chest* 85:796, 1984.

43. Dockerty MB. Ovarian neoplasms: A collective review of the recent literature. *Int Abstr Surg* 81:179, 1945.

44. Dombovy ML, et al. Exercise performance and ventilatory response in the menstrual cycle. *Med Sci Sports Exerc* 19:111, 1987.

45. Eliasson AH, et al. Oxygen consumption and ventilation during normal labor. *Chest* 102:467, 1992.

46. Eliasson AH, Phillips YY, Tenholder MF. Treatment of lymphangioleiomyomatosis. A meta-analysis. *Chest* 196:1352, 1989.

47. Elkington KW, Gelb LC. Adult respiratory distress syndrome as a complication of acute pyelonephritis during pregnancy: Case report and discussion. *Obstet Gynecol* 67(Suppl):18s, 1986.

48. Erling MA, Schmidt WA, Katz AR. Fatal fulminant postoperative pulmonary edema: An unusual cause of second trimester maternal mortality. *Diagn Gynecol Obstet* 2:209, 1980.

49. Evans KT, Cockshott WP, Hendrickse PdeV. Pulmonary changes in malignant trophoblastic disease. *Br J Radiol* 38:161, 1965.

50. Falliers CJ. Sexercise-induced asthma. *Lancet* 2:1078, 1976.

51. Foster DC, et al. Pleural and parenchymal pulmonary endometriosis. *Obstet Gynecol* 58:552, 1981.

52. Frank MD, Simon L, Dawson BH. The lymphangiomyomatosis syndrome. *Cancer* 72:428, 1968.

53. Frank RT. The hormonal causes of pre-menstrual tension. *Arch Neurol Psychol* 26:1053, 1931.

54. Fried KH. Sarcoidosis and pregnancy. *Acta Med Scand* 176(Suppl 425):260, 1964.

55. Fukuda O, et al. Massive edema of the ovary associated with hydrothorax and ascites. *Gynecol Oncol* 17:231, 1984.

56. Furman WR, et al. Catamenial pneumothorax: Evaluation by fiberoptic pleuroscopy. *Am Rev Respir Dis* 121:137, 1980.

57. Gelber M, et al. Uncontrollable life-threatening status asthmaticus: An indicator for termination of pregnancy by caesarian section. *Respiration* 46:320, 1984.

58. Gianoutsos P, Laverty CR. Uterine fibroid: An unusual cause of recurrent hemorrhagic pleural effusion. *Med J Aust* 2:600, 1975.

59. Gibbs CJ, et al. Premenstrual exacerbation of asthma. *Thorax* 39:833, 1984.

60. Goodlin RC. Leg static pressure values in pregnant women with iatrogenic pulmonary edema. *Am J Obstet Gynecol* 154:634, 1986.

61. Gordon RR, O'Neill EM. Turner's infantile phenotype. *Br Med J* 1:483, 1969.

62. Gosney JR. Atrophy of Leydig cells in the testes of men with longstanding chronic bronchitis and emphysema. *Thorax* 42:615, 1987.

63. Gottlieb JE, et al. Recurrent noncardiac pulmonary edema accompanying pregnancy-induced hypertension. *Chest* 100:1730, 1991.

64. Grand RJ, et al. Unusual case of XXY Klinefelter's syndrome with pancreatic insufficiency, hypothyroidism, deafness, chronic lung disease, dwarfism, and microcephaly. *Am J Med* 41:478, 1966.

65. Gray SR, Carrington CB, Corong JL. Lymphangioleiomyomatosis: Report of a case with urethral involvement and chyluria. *Cancer* 35:490, 1975.

66. Greenberger PA. Asthma in pregnancy. *Clin Perinatol* 12:571, 1985.

67. Greenstone MA, et al. Ciliary function in Young's syndrome. *Thorax* 43:153, 1988.

68. Hamadeh MA, Glassroth J. Tuberculosis and pregnancy. *Chest* 101:1114, 1992.

69. Handelsman DJ, et al. Obstructive azoospermia and chronic sinopulmonary infections. *N Engl J Med* 310:3, 1984.

70. Hanley SP. Asthma variation with menstruation. *Br J Dis Chest* 75:306, 1981.

71. Hanrahan JP, et al. The effect of maternal smoking during pregnancy on early infant lung function. *Am Rev Respir Dis* 145:1129, 1992.

72. Harris RE. Coccidioidomycosis complicating pregnancy. *Obstet Gynecol* 28:401, 1966.

73. Harrison AR, Purcell GRG. Ovarian cyst: An unusual case of respiratory arrest. *Anaesthesia* 33:617, 1978.

74. Heffner JE, Sahn SA. Pleural disease in pregnancy. *Clin Chest Med* 13:667, 1992.

75. Henderson SR, Lund CJ, Creasman WT. Antepartum pulmonary embolism. *Am J Obstet Gynecol* 112:476, 1972.

76. Hendrickse JP, Willis AJ, Evans KT. Acute dyspnea with trophoblastic tumors. *Br J Obstet Gynecol* 72:376, 1965.

77. Hendry WF, et al. Obstructive azoospermia: Respiratory function tests, electron microscopy and the results of surgery. *Br J Urol* 50:598, 1978.

78. Hibbard LT, Schumann WR, Goldstein GE. Thoracic endometriosis: A review and report of two cases. *Am J Obstet Gynecol* 140:227, 1981.

79. Hofford JM. Lymphangioleiomyomatosis. *Chest* 98:1043, 1990.

80. Horstmann JP, et al. Spontaneous regression of pulmonary leiomyomatosis during pregnancy. *Cancer* 39:314, 1977.

81. Howie AD, Milne JA. Pregnancy in patients with bronchiectasis. *Br J Obstet Gynecol* 85:197, 1978.

82. Huberman RP, Fon GT, Bein ME. Benign molar pregnancies: Pulmonary complications. *AJR* 138:71, 1982.

83. Hughes EC, Cochrane NE, Czyz PL. Maternal mortality study 1970–1975. *NY State J Med* 76:2206, 1976.

84. Hughson WG, et al. Postpartum pleural effusion: A common radiologic finding. *Ann Intern Med* 97:856, 1982.

85. Huseby JS, Peterson D. Pulmonary function in Klinefelter's syndrome. *Chest* 80:31, 1981.

86. Jao J, Gilbert S, Messer R. Lymphangiomyoma and tuberous sclerosis. *Cancer* 29:1188, 1972.

87. Joel-Cohen SJ, Schoenfeld A. Fetal response to periodic sleep apnea: A new syndrome in obstetrics. *Eur J Gynecol Reprod Biol* 8:77, 1978.

88. Joliat G, Stadler H, Kapanci Y. Lymphangiomyomatosis: A clinicoanatomical entity. *Cancer* 31:455, 1973.

89. Juniper EF, et al. Improvement in airway responsiveness and asthma during pregnancy. A prospective study. *Am Rev Respir Dis* 140:924, 1989.

90. Kane PB, et al. Ultrastructure of the proliferating cells in pulmonary lymphangiomyomatosis. *Arch Pathol Lab Med* 102:618, 1978.

91. Kilpatrick SJ, Matthay MA. Obstetric patients requiring critical care. A five-year review. *Chest* 101:1407, 1992.

92. Kirk AJB. Reflux dyspareunia. *Thorax* 41:215, 216.

93. Kitzsteiner KA, Mallen RG. Pulmonary lymphangioleiomyomatosis: Treatment with castration. *Cancer* 46:2248, 1980.

94. Kohorn EI, et al. Pulmonary embolization of trophoblastic tissue in molar pregnancy. *Obstet Gynecol* 51(Suppl):16s, 1978.

95. Koos BJ, et al. Fetal breathing adaptation to prolonged hypoxemia in sheep. *J Dev Physiol* 10:161, 1988.

96. Kotloff RM, FitzSimmons SC, Fiel SB. Fertility and pregnancy in patients with cystic fibrosis. *Clin Chest Med* 13:613, 1992.

97. Kowall J, et al. Precipitation of obstructive sleep apnea during pregnancy. *Obstet Gynecol* 74:453, 1989.

98. Kreisman H, et al. Lymphangiomyomatosis syndrome with hyperparathyroidism: A case report. *Cancer* 42:364, 1972.

99. Lalli CM, Raju L. Pregnancy and chronic ob-

structive pulmonary disease. *Chest* 80:759, 1981.

100. Larson EM, Saltzman D, Davis MR. Pneumomediastinum in pregnancy: Two case reports and a review of the literature. *Obstet Gynecol* 64(Suppl):39s, 1984.

101. Lattes R, et al. A clinical and pathologic study of endometriosis of the lung. *Surg Gynecol Obstet* 103:552, 1956.

102. Lehmann V. Dyspnea in pregnancy. *J Perinat Med* 3:154, 1975.

103. Leikin JB, Arof HM, Pearlman LM. Acute lupus pneumonitis in the postpartum period: A case history and review of the literature. *Obstet Gynecol* 68(Suppl):29s, 1986.

104. Leither JC, et al. Respiratory activity of genioglossus. Interaction between alcohol and the menstrual cycle. *Am Rev Respir Dis* 135:383, 1987.

105. Levine SB, Stern RC. Sexual function in cystic fibrosis: Relationship to overall health status and pulmonary disease severity in 30 married people. *Chest* 81:422, 1982.

106. Lillington GA, Mitchell SP, Wood GA. Catamenial pneumothorax. *JAMA* 219:1328, 1972.

107. Lim VS, Katz AI, Lindheimer MD. Acid-base regulation in pregnancy. *Am J Physiol* 231:1764, 1976.

108. Lipp RG, Kindschi JD, Schmitz R. Death from pulmonary embolism associated with hydatidiform mole. *Am J Obstet Gynecol* 83:1644, 1962.

109. Lizotte PE, et al. Lymphangioleiomyomatosis. *Chest* 98:1045, 1990.

110. Luna CM, et al. Pulmonary lymphangioleiomyomatosis associated with tuberous sclerosis. *Chest* 88:473, 1985.

111. Mabry RL. Rhinitis of pregnancy. *South Med J* 79:965, 1986.

112. Mackay IS. Rhinitis and sinusitis. *Br J Dis Chest* 82:1, 1988.

113. Magrath IT, Golding PR, Bagshaw KD. Medical presentation of choriocarcinoma. *Br Med J* 2:633, 1971.

114. Masson RG. Amniotic fluid embolism. *Clin Chest Med* 13:657, 1992.

115. Mayock RL, Sullivan RD, Greening RS Jr. Sarcoidosis and pregnancy. *JAMA* 164:158, 1957.

116. McCarty KS, et al. Pulmonary lymphangioleiomyomatosis responsive to progesterone. *N Engl J Med* 303:1461, 1980.

117. McCleod DT. Gestational choriocarcinoma presenting as endobronchial carcinoma. *Thorax* 43:410, 1988.

118. McCoy MJ, Ellenberg JF, Killam AP. Coccidioidomycosis complicating pregnancy. *Am J Obstet Gynecol* 137:739, 1980.

119. Meigs JV. Pelvic tumors other than fibromas of the ovary with ascites and hydrothorax. *Obstet Gynecol* 3:471, 1954.

120. Milne JA, et al. Large airways function during normal pregnancy. *Br J Obstet Gynaecol* 84:448, 1977.

121. Milne JA, Howle AD, Pack AI. Dyspnea during normal pregnancy. *Br J Obstet Gynaecol* 85:260, 1978.

122. Mobbs GA, Pfanner DW. Endometriosis of the lung. *Lancet* 1:472, 1963.

123. Monteforte WJ Jr, Kohnen PW. Angiomyolipomas in a case of lymphangiomyomatosis syndrome: Relationships to tuberous sclerosis. *Cancer* 34:317, 1974.

124. Morales P, et al. Pathogenesis of the lung in restrictive defects of Klinefelter's syndrome. *Chest* 102:1550, 1992.

125. Morgan M. Amniotic fluid embolism. *Anaesthesia* 34:20, 1979.

126. Morrow CP, et al. Clinical and laboratory correlates of molar pregnancy and trophoblastic disease. *Am J Obstet Gynecol* 128:424, 1977.

127. Muller NL, Nelems B. Postcoital catamenial pneumothorax: Report of a case not associated with endometriosis and successfully treated with tubal ligation. *Am Rev Respir Dis* 134:803, 1986.

128. Munsell WP. Pneumomediastinum: A report of 28 cases and review of the literature. *JAMA* 202:689, 1967.

129. Murray AB, Morrison BJ. The effect of cigarette smoke from the mother on bronchial responsiveness and severity of symptoms in children with asthma. *J Allergy Clin Immunol* 77:575, 1986.

130. Myers SA, Podczaski E, Freese U. Acute lupus pneumonitis in the puerperium: A case report and literature review. *J Reprod Med* 25:285, 1980.

131. Nava S, et al. Evidence of acute diaphragmatic fatigue in a "natural" condition. The diaphragm during labor. *Am Rev Respir Dis* 146:1226, 1992.

132. Negovsky VA, Manevich LE, Kassil VL. Anaesthesia and intensive care in eclampsia. *Resuscitation* 3:157, 1974.

133. Neville E, et al. Respiratory tract disease and obstructive azoospermia. *Thorax* 38:929, 1983.

134. O'Leary JA. Ten-year study of sarcoidosis and pregnancy. *Am J Obstet Gynecol* 84:462, 1962.

135. Orr JW Jr, et al. Acute pulmonary edema associated with molar pregnancies: A high risk factor for development of persistent trophoblastic disease. *Am J Obstet Gynecol* 136:412, 1980.

136. Palmer J, et al. Pregnancy in patients with cystic fibrosis. *Ann Intern Med* 99:596, 1983.

137. Pauli BD, et al. Influence of the menstrual cycle on airway function in asthmatic and normal subjects. *Am Rev Respir Dis* 140:358, 1989.

138. Peterson M, Taylor H. Amniotic fluid embolism: An analysis of 40 cases. *Obstet Gynecol* 35:787, 1970.

139. Philip RS. Amniotic fluid embolism. *NY State J Med* 67:2085, 1967.

140. Pisani RJ, Rosenow EC III. Pulmonary edema associated with tocolytic therapy. *Ann Intern Med* 110:714, 1989.

141. Present PA, Comstock GW. Tuberculin sensitivity in pregnancy. *Am Rev Respir Dis* 112:413, 1975.

142. Price TM, Baker VV, Cefalo RC. Amniotic fluid embolism: Three case reports with a review of the literature. *Obstet Gynecol Surv* 40:462, 1985.

143. Rees L. An aetiological study of premenstrual asthma. *J Psychosom Res* 7:191, 1963.

144. Resnik R, Swartz WH, Plumer MH. Amniotic fluid embolism with survival. *Obstet Gynecol* 47:295, 1976.

145. Rodman MH, Jones CW. Catamenial hemoptysis due to bronchial endometriosis. *N Engl J Med* 266:805, 1962.

146. Rohde RA. Klinefelter's syndrome with pulmonary disease and other disorders. *Lancet* 2:149, 1964.

147. Sargent EN, Barnes RA, Schwinn CP. Multiple pulmonary fibroleiomyomatous hamartomas: Report of case and review of the literature. *AJR* 110:694, 1970.

148. Scadding JG. *Sarcoidosis*. London: Eyre and Spottiswood, 1967.

149. Schaefer G, Zervoudakis IA, Tucks FF. Pregnancy and pulmonary tuberculosis. *Obstet Gynecol* 46:706, 1975.

150. Schoene RB, et al. Respiratory drives and exercise in menstrual cycles of athletic and nonathletic women. *J Appl Physiol* 50:1300, 1981.

151. Schoenfeld A, et al. Catamenial pneumothorax: A literature review and report of an unusual case. *Obstet Gynecol Surv* 41:20, 1986.

152. Schoenfield A, Ovidia A, Freedman S. Obstructive sleep apnea (OSA): Implications in maternal-fetal medicine. A hypothesis. *Med Hypotheses* 30:51, 1989.

153. Semple Pd'A, Beastall GH, Hume R. Sexual dysfunction, low serum testosterone, and respiratory hypoxia. *Br J Sex Med* 7:48, 1980.

154. Semple Pd'A, et al. Hypothalamic-pituitary dysfunction in respiratory hypoxia. *Thorax* 36:605, 1981.

155. Semple Pd'A, et al. Serum testosterone suppression associated with hypoxia in respiratory failure. *Clin Sci* 58:105, 1980.

156. Semple Pd'A, et al. Hypoxia, depression of testosterone and impotence in pickwickian syndrome reversed by weight reduction. *Br Med J* 289:801, 1984.

157. Shah A, Agarwal MK. Human seminal plasma allergy as a cause of postcoital asthma. *Eur Respir J* 1:972, 1988.

158. Shah A, Sarkar M. Postcoital asthma and rhinitis. *Chest* 100:1039, 1991.

159. Shahar J, Angelillo VA. Catamenial mediastinum. *Chest* 90:776, 1986.

160. Shearin RPN, Hepper NGG, Payne WS. Recurrent pneumothorax concurrent with menses. *Mayo Clin Proc* 49:98, 1974.

161. Shuman RL, Engelman R, Kittle CF. Pulmonary lymphangioleiomyomatosis. *Ann Thorac Surg* 27:70, 1979.

162. Silverstein EF, et al. Pulmonary lymphangioleiomyomatosis. *AJR* 120:832, 1974.

163. Sinclair W, Wright JL, Churg A. Lymphangioleiomyomatosis presenting in a postmenopausal woman. *Thorax* 40:475, 1985.

164. Sleiman C, et al. Pulmonary lymphangioleiomyomatosis treated by single lung transplantation. *Am Rev Respir Dis* 145:964, 1992.

165. Slingerland JM, et al. Pulmonary manifestations of tuberous sclerosis in first degree relatives. *Thorax* 44:212, 1989.

166. Snider DE, et al. Treatment of tuberculosis during pregnancy. *Am Rev Respir Dis* 122:65, 1980.

167. Snider DE, Powell KE. Should women taking antituberculous drugs breast-feed? *Arch Intern Med* 14:589, 1984.

168. Soderberg CH Jr, Dahlquist EH Jr. Catamenial pneumothorax. *Surgery* 79:236, 1976.

169. Solomon S, Farber SJ, Caruso LJ. Fibromyomata of the uterus with hemothorax: Meig's syndrome? *Arch Intern Med* 127:307, 1971.

170. Spector SL. Reciprocal relationship between pregnancy and pulmonary disease. *Chest* 86 (Suppl):1s, 1984.

171. Sperry K. Amniotic fluid embolism: To understand an enigma. *JAMA* 255:2183, 1986.

172. Steffelaar JW, Nijkamp DA, Hilvering CV. Pulmonary lymphangiomyomatosis: Demonstration of smooth muscle antigens by immunofluorescence technique. *Scand J Respir Dis* 58: 103, 1977.

173. Steiner PE. Metastasizing fibroleiomyoma of the uterus. *Am J Pathol* 15:89, 1939.

174. Stenius-Aarniala B, Piirila P, Teramo K. Asthma and pregnancy: A prospective study of 198 pregnancies. *Thorax* 43:12, 1988.

175. Stern A, Toole AL, Merino M. Catamenial pneumothorax. *Chest* 78:480, 1980.

176. Stovin PGI, et al. The lungs in lymphangiomyomatosis and tuberous sclerosis. *Thorax* 30: 497, 1975.

177. Stromme WB, Fromke VL. Amniotic fluid embolism and disseminated intravascular coagulation after evacuation of missed abortion. *Obstet Gynecol* 52(Suppl):76s, 1978.

178. Sudduth CD, et al. Metastatic choriocarcinoma of the lung presenting as hemothorax. *Chest* 99:527, 1991.

179. Suginami H, Hamada K, Yano K. A case of endometriosis of the lung treated with danazol. *Obstet Gynecol* 66(Suppl):68s, 1985.

180. Suonio S, Saaranen M, Saarioski S. Left-sided hydrothorax in connection with severe eclampsia: Case reports. *Int J Gynecol Obstet* 22:357, 1984.

181. Swinburne AJ, et al. Hereditary telangiectasia and multiple pulmonary arteriovenous fistulas: Clinical deterioration during pregnancy. *Chest* 89:459, 1986.

182. Symington IS, Kerr JW. Sexercise-induced asthma. *Lancet* 2:693, 1976.

183. Takano N. Changes of ventilation and ventilatory response to hypoxia during menstrual cycle. *Pflugers Arch* 402:312, 1984.

184. Tawney S, Berger HW, Stauber SL. Spontaneous pneumothorax in metastatic carcinoma of the cervix. *Chest* 84:650, 1983.

185. Taylor JR, et al. Lymphangioleiomyomatosis. Clinical course in 32 patients. *N Engl J Med* 323:1254, 1990.

186. Templeton A, Kelman GR. Maternal blood gases (PaO$_2$-PaO$_2$), physiological shunt and Vd/Vt in normal pregnancy. *Br J Anaesth* 48:1001, 1976.

187. Tenholder MF, South-Paul JE. Dyspnea in pregnancy. *Chest* 96:381, 1989.

188. Teshima T, et al. A variant of Meig's syndrome without ovarian neoplasm. *Respir Med* 83:363, 1989.

189. Twiggs LB, Morrow CP, Schloerth JB. Acute pulmonary complication of molar pregnancy. *Am J Obstet Gynecol* 135:189, 1979.

190. Tuck CS. Amniotic fluid embolus. *Proc R Soc Med* 65:94, 1972.

191. United States Department of Health and Human Services. *1989: Tuberculosis Statistics in the United States* [HHS publication no. (CDC) 91-8322]. Atlanta: Centers for Disease Control, 1991.

192. Urban T, et al. Pulmonary lymphangioleiomyomatosis. Follow-up and long-term outcome with antiestrogen therapy: A report of eight cases. *Chest* 102:472, 1992.

193. Valenzi QJ. Pulmonary lymphangiomyoma: A probable "forme fruste" of tuberous sclerosis. A case report and survey of literature. *Am Rev Respir Dis* 108:1411, 1973.

194. Varkey B, Funahashi A. Restrictive defect in Klinefelter's syndrome. *Chest* 82:132, 1982.

195. Villasanta U. Thromboembolic disease in pregnancy. *Am J Obstet Gynecol* 93:142, 1965.

196. Wagenvoort CA, Wagenvoort N. Primary pulmonary hypertension: A pathologic study of lung vessels in 156 clinically diagnosed cases. *Circulation* 42:1163, 1970.

197. Weinberger SE, et al. Pregnancy and the lung. *Am Rev Respir Dis* 121:559, 1980.

198. Weiss Z, et al. Obstructive renal failure and pleural effusion cased by the gravid uterus. *Acta Obstet Gynecol Scand* 65:187, 1986.

199. White RJ, et al. A prospective study of asthma during pregnancy and the puerperium. *Respir Med* 83:103, 1989.

200. Williamson JG, Patel D, Menzies DN. Leiomyomata of the uterus associated with ascites and hydrothorax. *J Obstet Gynecol* 79:273, 1972.

201. Wilson EA, Thelin TJ, Dilts PV. Tuberculosis complicated by pregnancy. *Am J Obstet Gynecol* 115:526, 1973.

202. Winter JA. Oophorectomy in lymphangiomyomatosis and benign metastasizing leiomyoma. *N Engl J Med* 305:1416, 1981.

203. Wolfe CA, Peterson MW. An unusual case of massive pleural effusion in pregnancy. *Thorax* 43:484, 1988.

204. Wood T, Meltzer D, Carroll E. Hemoptysis and chest mass related to pregnancy. *Chest* 75:67, 1979.

205. Young D. Surgical treatment of male infertility. *J Reprod Fertil* 23:541, 1970.

X

Congenital, Developmental, and Genetic Diseases of the Lung

68

Developmental Anomalies of the Respiratory System

Robert Bilenker

Embryologic Review of the Respiratory System

In embryonic development, the larynx and trachea begin as a groove in the floor of the gut, running lengthwise. Furrows appear laterally and then fuse to separate the developing larynx and trachea from the esophagus. The external appearance of this structure is a ridge, rounded at its caudal end to form the lung bud.

The larynx develops from endoderm lining the cranial end of the laryngotracheal ridge. Supporting structures are derived from mesoderm of the fourth and fifth branchial arches. Arytenoid swellings form lateral to the opening in the trachea or glottis. These swellings move cranially and forward to fuse into the primitive epiglottis. Proliferating epithelium obliterates the larynx before 10 weeks [5]. After continuity is restored, the vocal folds appear below the lateral recesses of the ventricles. Innervation is provided by the vagus nerve, which supplies the structures derived from the fourth and fifth branchial arches [107].

The trachea develops from the midportion of the laryngotracheal tube and then elongates and descends into the thoracic cavity, as do the lungs. The muscles and cartilage-supporting structures derive from splanchnic mesoderm. The tracheal glands develop from the epithelial lining. The lung buds divide into right and left bronchopulmonary buds that later become the mainstem bronchi. These buds extend into the primitive pleural cavities, at this time the pericardioperitoneal canals. Secondary bronchi then form— two on the right, one on the left. These correspond to the eventual three-lobed right lung and two-lobed left lung. By 7 weeks' gestation, third-order bronchi appear and develop into the 18 bronchopulmonary segments—10 on the right, 8 on the left. Twenty-four generations of bronchi and bronchioles develop by 16 weeks' gestation.

The intrauterine development of the fetal lung has been divided into several stages by different workers. The following is based on Boyden's description [20]:

1. *Pseudoglandular period* (5 to 17 weeks), so named because cut sections of the lung appear as acinous glands. The elaborate branching of the airway and pulmonary vasculature dominates. The epithelium is cuboidal toward the periphery and pseudostratified near the hilum. By the end of this period, all prealveolar structures have developed.
2. *Canalicular period* (13 to 25 weeks). The bronchi and bronchiolar lumina enlarge during this period. At 24 to 25 weeks, each terminal bronchiole elongates and divides into two respiratory bronchioles. Vascularization has proceeded rapidly, and developing vessels thin the cuboidal lining of these respiratory bronchioles. This process prepares for the terminal sac and alveolar development that follows.
3. *Terminal sac period* (24 weeks to birth). During the final trimester, new respiratory bronchioles continue to appear buried within a thinned epithelium. Two types of pneumocytes, the epithelial lining cell, can be recognized. Surfactant, thought to be produced by the type II cells, can first be detected at this time. The developing pulmonary vasculature and thinned epithelial lining allow for extrauterine survival of increasing numbers of infants born preterm (<38 weeks' gestation).
4. *Alveolar period* (late fetal period to 8 years). Pulmonary alveoli reach adult numbers by the age of 8 years. The newborn has one-sixth to one-eighth as many alveoli as does the adult.

Developmental Anomalies Involving the Larynx and Trachea

Embryology of the Larynx and Trachea

The upper portion of the larynx develops the epiglottis anteriorly, which broadens and grows upward toward the posterior pharynx. The arytenoid swellings form the lateral boundaries of the glottal opening. Proliferation of this epithelium temporarily occludes the larynx, which lengthens and reopens at 10 weeks' gestation. The laryngeal ventricles are lateral outpouchings below the glottis opening. The vocal folds, eventually lined with stratified squamous epithelium, are just caudal. From this point down, the lining is pseudo-stratified columnar respiratory epithelium. The trachea lengthens considerably during development as the primary lung buds differentiate and move approximately eight segments downward into the pleural cavities [34]. Developmental anomalies of the larynx and trachea result from aberrations in normal differentiation [23,62,94, 115,119].

Developmental Anomalies

LARYNGOMALACIA

Sometimes called *congenital stridor*, laryngomalacia is caused by the flaccidity of a long epiglottis, short arytenoepiglottic folds, or bulky arytenoid swellings. These structures may prolapse upward on inspiration, causing stridor. Some patients may have a soft expiratory component as well. Stridor may present at birth or during an upper respiratory tract infection and subsequently recur with or without infection. The stridor increases with quiet breathing and may occur only during sleep [3]. Approximately half the affected infants have associated feeding difficulties, with vomiting or prolonged feeding time. The diagnosis is suspected clinically and confirmed with direct laryngoscopy. The problem tends not to persist, with most cases resolving by the age of 1 to 2 years. Findings on indirect laryngoscopy in 19 children done 7 to 12 years after diagnosis were normal [95]. Some children have experienced stridor under stress in later childhood [91]. No association with mental retardation was found.

SUBGLOTTIC STENOSIS

Congenital narrowing of the subglottic area may be caused by cricoid cartilage anomalies or increased soft-tissue mass surrounding the subglottis. The cause is said to be external compression by sixth branchial arches before 10 weeks' gestation. The affected infant has chronic stridor from birth [69]. Differentiation from laryngotracheobronchitis (croup) may be aided by roentgenographic findings. In both entities, the subglottic air column is narrowed on inspiration, with the hypopharynx distended with air. On expiration, however, the narrowing associated with subglottic stenosis appears fixed, while the narrowed lumen often widens on expiration in croup [56,131]. The roentgenographic attempt to determine if a lesion is "fixed" may expose the infant to more radiation than necessary, based on yield of positive diagnosis. Subglottic lesions causing only anterior or posterior indentation on the air column are unlikely to be croup. Infants with mild symptoms of subglottic stenosis may require no treatment; others require tracheostomy and other possible surgical interventions. The extreme form of subglottic stenosis is subglottic atresia. Prolonged endotracheal intubation for respiratory support has caused an increase in acquired laryngotracheal stenosis. Laryngotracheal reconstruction has been accomplished for those patients in whom other modalities have not succeeded [31].

LARYNGOTRACHEOESOPHAGEAL CLEFT

Laryngotracheoesophageal (LTE) cleft is a rare disorder associated with significant morbidity and mortality [10,48]. The disorder is separated into milder forms involving the posterior larynx but not extending through the cricoid cartilage, through the cartilage into the cervical tracheal rings, and complete LTE cleft involving the thoracic trachea [48,89]. LTE cleft is usually caused by a lack of rostral extension or failure in formation of the tracheoesophageal septum. Failure in fusion of the dorsal portion of the developing cricoid cartilage plays a contributory role [16]. These infants have increased oral secretions, cyanosis, and choking with all feedings. The presentation may simulate esophageal atresia (EA) or tracheoesophageal fistula (TEF), and in 20 percent of patients, the two anomalies—LTE cleft and EA or TEF—have been found to coexist. The diagnosis may be suspected from the anterior position of a nasogastric tube placed in the esophagus. On occasion, the diagnosis is delayed by a physiologic apposition of the edges of the cleft with inspiration. Cineesophagram shows high spillover into the larynx and trachea on swallowing [14]. Laryngoscopy is the preferred method for diagnosis and repair of supraglottic clefts [78]. LTE clefts extending to the carina or beyond to the mainstem bronchi present major challenges to successful surgical and postoperative management [43,118]. Postoperative management may entail nasotracheal intubation or prolonged tracheostomy.

TRACHEAL AGENESIS

Floyd and associates [50] divided tracheal agenesis into three types: (1) agenesis of the upper trachea with communication between the esophagus and the distal patent trachea; (2) the most common form, present in 70 percent of reported cases, in which there is agenesis of the entire trachea with a small fistulous connection between the esophagus and the carina (the bronchi form normally and are joined at the carina); and (3) complete agenesis of the trachea with the bronchi arising from the esophagus. There is very high incidence (70 percent) of major associated malformations in other organ systems, particularly cardiac, renal, and gastrointestinal [21,38,134,135]. Of the embryologic explanations offered, Bremer's theory of a marked ventral location of the developing LTE system appears most tenable [23].

COMPLETE TRACHEAL RINGS

The posterior membranous portion of the tracheal rings may rarely be replaced by cartilage [54]. The trachea is then poorly distensible, which causes respiratory distress that worsens markedly with infection. When the defect is limited, segmental resection may be attempted. The more general anomaly has not been successfully repaired thus far.

LARYNGEAL WEB

This is a rare anomaly of the larynx, with an estimated incidence of 1 in 10,000 births. The web is caused by partial or complete failure of the larynx to reopen at 10 weeks' gestation after closure caused by epithelialization. Seventy-five percent of laryngeal webs are membranes extending across the anterior one-half to two-thirds of the true vocal cords. The remainder are supraglottic (1.5 percent), subglottic (7.5 percent), or combined [92]. An absent or hoarse cry is usually present at birth. Respiratory distress may be a presenting sign. Diagnosis is made by direct laryngoscopy. The membrane may be quite dense, with muscle, fat, and cartilage present. Insertion of a Silastic or tantalum keel to prevent the incised edges from rejoining is needed in such cases [62]. Simple incision is insufficient for well-differentiated webs.

LARYNGOCELE

This rare anomaly presents as an air-filled cystic outpouching of the laryngeal wall [133]. It is most often palpated in the anterior triangle of the neck at the level of the thyrohyoid membrane. The cyst increases with Valsalva's maneuver and decreases with palpation [75]. These lesions may become infected, increase in size, and obstruct the airway. Surgical intervention is necessary; an external approach is preferred.

VASCULAR RINGS

Extrinsic compression of the trachea by anomalous vessels may cause respiratory difficulty during infancy. The anomalous vessels represent persistent branchial arch vessel(s), as in double aortic arch, the most common of the vascular compression syndromes. A lateral chest film may show tracheal compression. Diagnosis can be confirmed on esophagram, since contrast shows narrowing of the esophagus. Detailed discussion may be found in pediatric cardiology texts.

Esophageal Atresia and Tracheoesophageal Fistula

The anomalous development of the esophagus was first described by Gibson in 1696, with a report of proximal EA with distal TEF. As with anomalies in other body systems, many cases were cited before the first successful surgical correction. The first gastrostomy was done in 1888 by Steele, to measure the blind distal segment. In 1913, Richter made the first attempts at transpleural ligation of a distal fistula with establishment of a feeding gastrostomy. In the late 1930s, adoption of an extrapleural approach plus establishment of cervical esophagostomy foreshadowed the subsequent eventual primary repair. This was completed in 1939 by Leven in St. Paul [85] and Ladd in Boston [83]. Both children underwent gastrostomy, ligation of the distal fistula, cervical esophagostomy, and eventual anastomotic repair of the proximal and distal esophagus.

Several different categorizations have been proposed for these anomalies [75]. EA with distal TEF is by far the most common type (86.6 percent) [76]. Atresia without fistula (7.7 percent), TEF without EA or H-type TEF (4.2 percent), EA with proximal fistula (0.8 percent), and EA with

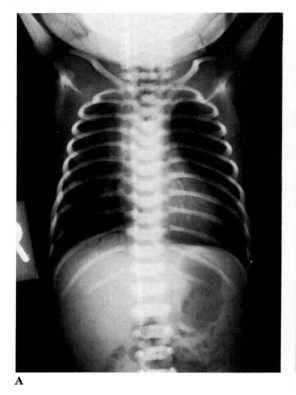

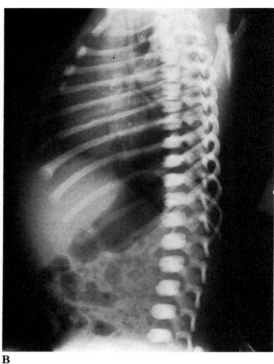

A   B

Fig. 68-1. Tracheoesophageal fistula. Note the curving nasogastric tube in the proximal esophagus. Presence of air throughout the remainder of the gastrointestinal tract results from the fistulous connection.

proximal and distal fistulas (0.7 percent) are much rarer in occurrence.

These entities occur with an incidence of 1 in 3000 live births. The occurrence is sporadic, with only a few examples of more than one case in a family reported [74]. When the proximal esophagus ends in a blind pouch, there is overflow of saliva and swallowed feeding into the trachea. Aspiration causes pneumonitis. The existence of a proximal TEF causes direct flow of proximal esophageal contents into the tracheobronchial structures. The occurrence of distal TEF causes regurgitation of stomach contents in a retrograde manner into the trachea. Crying causes acute gastric dilatation followed by flow of gastric acid into the lungs. Attempts at feeding such infants cause crying, choking, regurgitation, and cyanosis. Capacity of the proximal segment is limited at times to a few milliliters. Anteroposterior and lateral films should be obtained to confirm the diagnosis (Fig. 68-1). Absence of air in the gastrointestinal system probably means no asso-

ciated distal fistula, and a technically more difficult surgical repair can be anticipated.

There is a significant (50 percent) incidence of other anomalies in these patients [135]. Morbidity and mortality associated with repair vary with occurrence of these other anomalies, which are listed below [67]:[1]

Patients with no associated anomalies	553 (52%)
Patients with associated anomalies	505 (48%)
Congenital heart disease	201
Gastrointestinal anomalies	134
Genitourinary anomalies	109

[1]Table reprinted with permission from [67]. Copyright American Academy of Pediatrics, 1964.

Imperforate anus	99
Musculoskeletal anomalies	91
Central nervous system anomalies	63
Facial anomalies	53
Other	99
Total number of anomalies	849

More recent surveys delineated the associated cardiac, renal, and skeletal anomalies [7,13,28]. EA also has been associated with pulmonary agenesis [24].

Division of the TEF and primary anastomotic reconstruction of the esophagus are the procedures of choice in term infants. With sick, preterm, or small-for-gestational-age infants, staged repair has been advocated by some authors to decrease morbidity and mortality [33,68,79]. A gastrostomy is done, followed in a few days by retropleural division of the distal TEF. After controlling aspiration pneumonitis and feeding through gastrostomy, an end-to-end anastomosis can be undertaken. EA without TEF (approximately 7.7 percent of cases) and EA with proximal TEF (<1 percent of cases) are associated with the widest gaps between the proximal and distal segments. When primary repair is not possible, colonic interposition using an isoperistaltic segment of transverse colon has been the procedure of choice [8,121]. Postoperative complications have included stricture, leak at the anastomotic site, and pneumonia.

Long-term follow-up has shown an increased incidence of respiratory infection secondary to aspiration from reverse peristalsis [32,45] and mild restrictive deficits on a congenital or acquired basis. Such patients should continue to be fed and to sleep in a 60-degree upright position indefinitely.

Congenital Diaphragmatic Hernia

Congenital herniation of abdominal contents into the thoracic cavity was rarely recognized during life before roentgenography was available. Successful surgical correction began in the 1930s, and the techniques were well described by Ladd and Gross in 1940 [84]. Survival rates have not improved despite improved newborn care, anesthesia, and surgical management [39,40]. Advances in care have allowed patients with more severe abnormalities to survive until operation [18,60,112]. Mortality rates range from 30 to 80 percent and depend on (1) the severity of the de-

fect, (2) persistent fetal circulation with associated pulmonary hypertension, and (3) associated pulmonary hypoplasia—ipsilateral, contralateral, and bilateral [102].

The incidence of congenital diaphragmatic hernia (CDH) is often cited as 1 in 2200 births, based on the British Perinatal Mortality Survey [25]. There is no significant correlation with increased parity, advanced maternal age, or socioeconomic status. Males are twice as often affected as females. While CDH is almost always sporadic in occurrence, some families with near-total unilateral agenesis of the diaphragm inherited as an autosomal recessive trait have been described [109].

The diaphragm results from the embryonic fusion of four structures. The largest of these, the septum transversus, arises from the same cervical somites (C3–5) as the phrenic nerve that innervates it. The septum extends inward from the ventral surface to separate the pericardial and peritoneal cavities. The bilateral pleuropericardial and pleuroperitoneal folds arise from the body wall to surround and separate the embryonic lungs from the heart and abdominal viscera. The mediodorsal portion of the diaphragm is formed from the dorsal mesentery. The pleuroperitoneal folds join the septum transversus to form the diaphragm. Failure of this fusion allows herniation to occur through the patent pleuroperitoneal canals [39]. This accounts for the posterolateral herniation through the foramen of Bochdalek in 80 percent of all CDH patients. Retrosternal herniation through the foramen of Morgagni accounts for most remaining patients. Congenital eventration is caused by hypoplasia of the diaphragm muscle. Lung development at this gestational age (10 to 12 weeks) is at the stage of bronchi and bronchiolar differentiation [4]. Infants with CDH through the foramen of Bochdalek present in the first day(s) of life with dyspnea, tachypnea, and cyanosis. There may be dullness to percussion and decreased breath sounds on the affected side, prominence of the affected hemithorax, and a scaphoid abdomen due to displacement of abdominal contents into the thorax. The herniated contents consist of stomach, small intestine, and the descending colon. Herniation of some, but not all bowel would fail to produce a scaphoid abdomen. In Figure 68-2, note the presence of air in the descending colon. Herniation occurs through the left hemidiaphragm approximately five times as often as the right [15]. Accurate prenatal diagnosis can be made with ul-

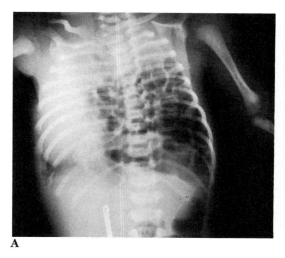 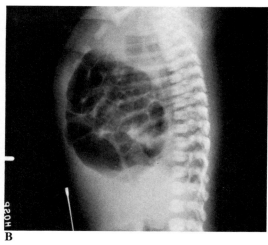

A   B

Fig. 68-2. Congenital diaphragmatic hernia. There is a herniation of small intestine, large intestine, and stomach (or parts thereof) into the left hemithorax. Note the air in the descending colon.

trasonography; polyhydramnios, shift of the mediastinum, and absence of an infraabdominal stomach bubble suggest the diagnosis [1]. Fetal abdominal organs are then located in the fetal chest. Diagnosis can be confirmed with a chest x-ray film showing the herniated contents and mediastinal shift toward the opposite side. Contrast studies are rarely needed [11].

Rapid surgical intervention is mandatory. Several authors advocate an abdominal approach because of easier reduction by traction and the high incidence of associated malrotation (30 percent) [2,125]. A transthoracic approach also has been used, with comparable survival rates [72]. Bowel reduction does not ensure the patient's survival. The associated pulmonary hypoplasia affects the ipsilateral and, in some cases, contralateral lung [4,12,29,35,103,113]. Even when unilateral, there is associated elevated pulmonary arterial pressure and vascular resistance [126]. Naeye and colleagues [102] observed increased pulmonary arterial muscle mass in children dying with CDH. These changes followed by decreased output from the right side of the heart may stimulate a return to fetal circulation after birth. In addition to pharmacologic management, extracorporeal membrane oxygenation (ECMO) was employed in the early 1980s [61,129,137]. Individual hospitals have shown the benefit for ECMO in improved survival rates following its introduction [6,64]. Comparisons in outcome among institutions are difficult and may be facilitated by using predictors of severity such as best postductal

PO_2. Values higher than 100 mmHg were associated with survival in 41 (91 percent) of 45 patients while only 1 (7 percent) of 14 patients survived with a best postductal PO_2 less than 100 mmHg [138]. High mortality rates continue to be shown for patients with CDH diagnosed in early gestation. This has occurred despite optimal postnatal therapy including ECMO [17]. Harrison's group reported successful correction of CDH in utero in fetuses between 22 and 30 weeks' gestation [63].

Congenital Cystic Diseases of the Lung

This group of entities is characterized by a cystic appearance of pulmonary tissue. While the exact embryogenesis of various forms is disputed, all result in aberrant differentiation of bronchi, bronchioles, alveoli, and pulmonary vasculature. Four distinct categories are discussed: bronchogenic cyst, pulmonary sequestration, congenital cystic adenomatoid malformation, and congenital lobar emphysema.

Bronchogenic Cyst

These cysts result from an abnormal diverticulum of the lung bud in the third to sixth week of fetal life. They are usually located adherent to the

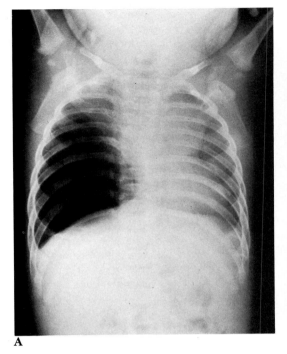
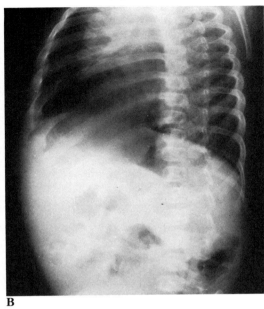

A

B

Fig. 68-3. Bronchogenic cyst. Hyperaeration with definable boundary within a lobe.

left mainstem bronchus or carina, are extrapulmonary in location, and so are within the middle mediastinum. Abnormal budding in the distal tracheobronchial tree causes intraparenchymal cysts [42]. The cyst wall contains all elements of the normal bronchus-columnar, mucus-secreting epithelium; smooth muscle; elastic tissue; and cartilage.

Most children with obstructing cysts who present in early infancy have moderate or severe respiratory distress and clinical signs of airway obstruction such as stridor, wheezing, and cyanosis. Chest x-ray films may not show a mass but do show emphysema or severe obstructive atelectasis with mediastinal shift. Bronchoscopy and bronchography are too dangerous and are not usually recommended. Chest x-ray films may show the lucent cystic area containing curvilinear shadows, demonstrating hyperaeration within a lobe (Fig. 68-3). Subcarinal bronchogenic cysts have been demonstrated using real-time ultrasonography with a parasternal approach [116]. Bronchogenic cysts shown by computed tomography (CT) may appear solid or cystic [96]. Mediastinal bronchogenic cyst was re-

cently diagnosed by magnetic resonance imaging [136].

Preoperative diagnosis can usually be confirmed by barium swallow or other contrast swallow examinations. The esophagus usually deviates backward and to the right, with the trachea pushed forward and narrowed. A communication between the cyst and the tracheobronchial tree is usually not demonstrated on x-ray films or at operation; these cysts range in size from 1.5 to 4.0 cm. After surgical removal, prognosis is almost always excellent [47,53,106]. All identified bronchogenic cysts should be surgically removed. Imaged thoracoscopic surgery has been successful in removing mediastinal cysts without a thoracotomy [87]. Two cases of embryonal rhabdomyosarcoma have been found within lung cysts [81].

Pulmonary Sequestration

These tissue masses are not connected with the tracheobronchial tree. They are generally divided into intralobar sequestration, which is part of a lobe, and extralobar sequestration or accessory

Table 68-1. **Pulmonary sequestration**

Distinguishing feature	Extralobar	Intralobar
Bronchopulmonary tissue	Found above or below the diaphragm	Confined to posterior basilar segments of lower lobe
Pleural covering	Separate from the rest of the lung	No pleural separation
Side affected	Left > 90%	Left 65%
Foregut communication present	Occasionally	Rarely
Associated anomalies	Frequent	Uncommon
Found in neonates	Often	Never
Age at diagnosis	<1 y in 60%	>20 y in 50%
Sex distribution	M/F = 4 : 1	M = F
Venous drainage	Systemic or portal	Pulmonary

Source: From P Hutchin. Congenital cystic disease of the lung. *Rev Surg* 28:82, 1971 [70].

lobe, which has its own pleural covering [37]. There are two main theories of embryogenesis: (1) accessory bronchial buds inside (intralobar) or outside (extralobar) the developing lung [71], and (2) persistence of a pulmonary branch of the dorsal aorta secondary to failure of the pulmonary artery to vascularize the periphery of the lower lobe [123]. Exposure to systemic pressure then causes cystic degeneration of the sequestered lobe. One review of 42,000 pediatric autopsies questions the designation of intralobar sequestration as a congenital malformation [128]. The clinical presentation varies in several ways, as summarized in Table 68-1. There are several reports of pulmonary sequestration presenting with congestive heart failure rather than the far more common respiratory symptoms [30,86].

Extralobar sequestration is associated with diaphragmatic hernia on the left in almost 60 percent of cases. Sequestration, as originally used, meant adherence of growing lung buds to the septum transversus as it developed into the diaphragm, which caused both anomalies. Intralobar sequestration presents as an inflammatory mass in the posterobasal segments of the lower lobes

Fig. 68-4. Intralobar sequestration in the right lower lobe. Retrograde arteriogram shows that the blood supply is from the aorta below the level of the diaphragm. Opaque material remains from the previous bronchogram.

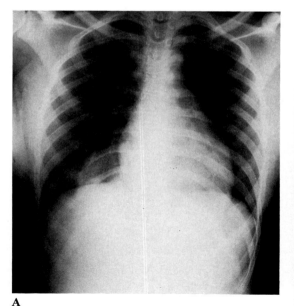

A

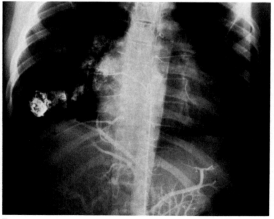

B

(Fig. 68-4). Preoperative contrast studies may demonstrate the occasional extralobar sequestration with a fistulous connection to the esophagus. Magnetic resonance angiography and ultrasonography have been useful in demonstrating the aberrant systemic blood supply [44,104]. Cure is effected by surgical removal [88]. A lobectomy or segmental resection is done, depending on the case.

Congenital Cystic Adenomatoid Malformation

Congenital cystic adenomatoid malformation (CCAM) is a rare form of congenital cystic disease of the lung, with less than 100 cases reported before 1978 [59,127]. The lesion is caused by an arrest in alveolar development with a proliferation of terminal bronchioles in the affected lobe. These bronchioles are lined by columnar or cuboidal epithelium and have soft walls. Air enters and then is trapped, causing cystic dilatation of the bronchioles. The entire malformation may cause mediastinal shift to the opposite side and compression atelectasis of otherwise normal adjacent lung tissue. Three morphologic types have been described. Type I has large cysts 3 to 10 cm in size. Type II lesions have numerous smaller cysts, each between 0.5 and 3.0 cm in size. Type III lesions have many small cysts, each less than 0.5 cm. The CCAM specimen shown in Figure 68-5 demonstrates radiolucent areas with curvilinear densities and scattered coalescent soft-tissue density, representing areas of atelectasis, which also may be seen with bronchogenic cysts.

CCAM has three distinct clinical presentations. About a third of patients present as stillborns with anasarca with or without a history of maternal polyhydramnios. Early detection of these patients by ultrasonography is now possible [82,92, 97]. The presenting indication for investigation is polyhydramnios. The CCAM in these cases is severe. The involved lobe hampers cardiac function and obstructs venous return, causing anasarca [73]. In type I lesions, in utero intervention with placement of a thoracoamniotic catheter allowed resolution of hydrops and mediastinal shift. The CCAM was then excised after delivery. A multicystic CCAM was removed during fetal life at 23 weeks' gestation [63]. A second presentation is in the newborn infant with tachypnea, dyspnea, and cyanosis. Roentgenographic diagnosis of the mass may be confusing. In particular, a large cyst in the mass may be confused with congenital lobar emphysema (CLE). Treatment is surgical. On occasion, an anomalous vessel may be found. Lobectomy rather than segmental resection is advocated. Preoperative bronchography or aortography is generally not advocated. These patients should do well postoperatively and on long-term follow-up [22,51,82]. Less commonly, patients with CCAM present in childhood with a history of recurrent pulmonary infection or when the mass ruptures into the pleural space.

Congenital Lobar Emphysema

CLE is a surgically correctable cause of severe respiratory distress in infancy [100,122]. Affected infants may present with respiratory distress that is mild or severe, precipitated by crying, feeding, or on occasion, respiratory infection [117]. Males are somewhat more often affected than females. When CLE involves a single lobe, the left upper lobe is most frequently involved, followed by the right middle lobe. Disease of the lower lobes and bilateral disease are rare (Fig. 68-6). CLE is almost always not of genetic origin. There have been reports of two affected sisters and an affected mother and daughter, however [132].

The pathology of CLE has often been attributed to deficient bronchial cartilage in the affected main bronchus. This may cause endobronchial proliferation of mucous membrane and subsequent obstruction. Deficient cartilage has been demonstrated in 25 percent of cases; endobronchial obstruction, in 13 percent; extrinsic compression of the bronchus (as by an anomalous vessel), in 1 percent; diffuse bronchial abnormality within a lobe, in 4 percent; and in 50 percent of cases no cause has been identified [65]. To explain CLE of unknown cause, an alveolar wall defect in the quantity, quality, or distribution of collagen or elastin has been postulated [17].

The clinical presentation is respiratory distress in a neonate or infant. Half the cases present in neonates and three-fourths in infants under the age of 6 months. The thoracic wall may be prominent over the involved lung, with hyperresonance on percussion and decreased breath sounds over the involved lobe. The apical beat may be shifted away from the involved side, and the diaphragm may be depressed on the affected side. Chest x-ray films show the hyperinflated lobe with a displaced mediastinum away from the affected lobe and in some cases herniation of the emphysematous lobe across the mediastinum. In several cases, retained fetal fluid initially causes the lung to have a more solid appearance [49].

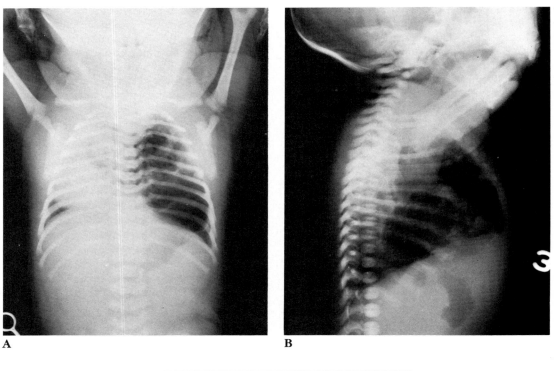

A

B

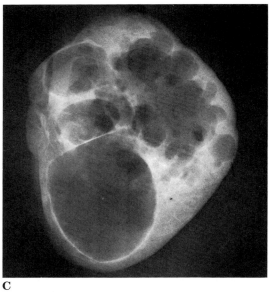

C

Fig. 68-5. *A, B.* Congenital cystic adenomatoid malformation of the lung. *C.* A roentgenogram of the surgically resected specimen.

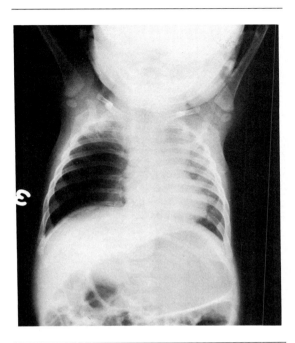

Fig. 68-6. Congenital lobar emphysema with hyperexpansion of the right middle lobe. The compressed lower lobe is visible as a triangular shadow in the cardiophrenic angle.

With clearing, a more typical radiolucent lobe is revealed. Differential diagnosis of CLE often includes pneumothorax, pneumatocele, and congenital cyst of the lung. CLE may be distinguished by the persistence of lung markings seen on x-ray films of the affected lobe. The other lesions cited have absent lung markings in involved areas [90]. In CLE, the vessels may be attenuated and abnormally separated within the emphysematous lobe. Lung scanning has provided helpful information on ventilation and perfusion in affected areas. Pneumothorax is rarely associated with CLE. There are associated cardiac defects in a much higher percentage of patients with CLE than with other congenital cystic diseases of the lungs. Most often these are ventricular septal defect or patent ductus arteriosus. Some authors have speculated that dilatation of the pulmonary artery is pathogenetically related to the evolution of CLE in some patients.

CLE may be treated surgically with excellent results. Lobectomy is generally advocated [36,99]. High-frequency jet ventilation has been used intraoperatively to maintain oxygenation and provide a near-motionless lung during surgery [52]. Segmental resection may be curative in some instances [46]. Conservative management is almost never indicated. There have been some reports of nonsurgical treatment when CLE presented with concurrent viral infection during infancy or when patients were older (7 and 10 years) at initial diagnosis [93,99].

Developmental Anomalies of Mediastinal Structures

The mediastinum contains all the viscera of the thorax, with the exception of the lungs and their surrounding pleurae. The developing pleural cavities define the mediastinum as well. Pleuropericardial folds appear longitudinally against the lateral body wall in the fourth week of gestation. These grow together in the midline and separate the developing heart from the lungs as they grow downward into the pleural canals. When the primary lung buds appear in the fifth week, the heart is a large structure. Over the next 2 weeks, the lungs undergo two subsequent divisions, and the bronchopulmonary segments are established. The lung enlarges, compared with the heart. The pleural membranes form the lateral boundaries of the mediastinum.

Clinical anatomic divisions of the mediastinum have usually been into superior and inferior compartments, with the inferior divided into anterior, middle, and posterior portions. Alternatively, the entire mediastinum may be divided into anterior, middle, and posterior segments. The latter classification is used in the following description [48].

The anterior mediastinum contains the thymus and the anterior portion of the pericardium and the heart. There are a few anterior mediastinal lymph nodes and a rare substernal extension of the thyroid. The most common anterior mediastinal mass in infancy is a hyperplastic thymus gland (Fig. 68-7) [57]. Regardless of the size of the thymus, it does not cause tracheal compression or displacement. If compression of the anterior tracheal wall is noted, an esophagram is indicated. Findings positive for a mass exclude enlarged thymus from the differential diagnosis. Surgical intervention should not be required because the thymus undergoes involution. Thymomas can occur but are rare. The occurrence of a thymoma is frequently associated with immunodeficiency. Thymomas presenting in adult life may be associated with myasthenia gravis, diabetes, chronic hepatitis, or arthritis.

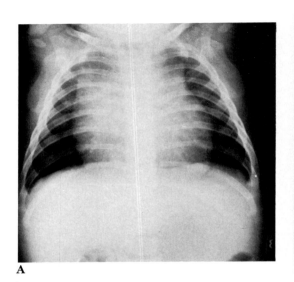

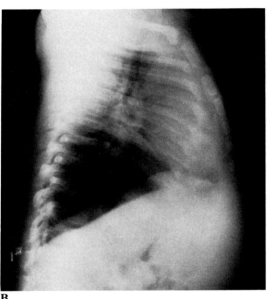

A   B

Fig. 68-7. Normal thymus. Note the absence of the retrosternal clear space and of tracheal compression.

Teratomas also can occur in the anterior mediastinum. These lesions contain all three germ layers (Fig. 68-8). Teratomas also may be specifically intrapericardial in origin (Fig. 68-9). When symptomatic, mediastinal teratomas produce respiratory compromise, and newborns may present with signs of cardiac tamponade or hydrops fetalis. Teratomas may be benign or malignant. Pericardial cysts may present on chest x-ray films at the right cardiophrenic angle. They are neither symptomatic nor premalignant [19,105,114].

Thoracic CT has markedly changed the evaluation of suspected mediastinal masses. CT differentiates among cystic, solid, vascular, and fatty lesions. Diagnostic thoracotomy or mediastinoscopy may be delayed in some patients showing benign fat deposition or asymptomatic cysts [77, 98,111,124].

Enterogenous Cysts (Duplications)

Foregut duplications may present in the mediastinum [41,55]. Occasionally, the presence of cervical vertebral anomalies such as hemivertebrae may suggest a foregut duplication. The endoderm of the foregut develops in close proximity to the notochord. A portion of endoderm may adhere to notochord as the latter is surrounded by paraxial mesoderm to form the vertebral bodies. Defects in these bodies are then formed. There may or

Fig. 68-8. Mediastinal teratoma. Air in the pleural space outlines the inferior margin of the teratoma. This particular lesion had no distinguishing characteristics such as teeth or bone. Obliteration of the upper portion of the heart border is a positive silhouette sign indicating anterior location of the mass.

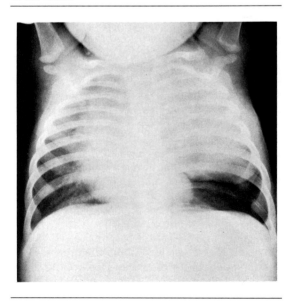

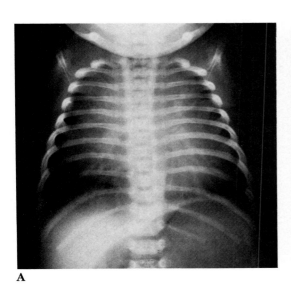
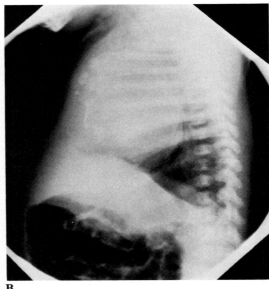

A   B

Fig. 68-9. Pericardial teratoma. Note the calcification within the pericardium on the lateral view.

may not be a fistulous connection to an enterogenous cyst, which forms at the cervical level and is then pulled into the thorax with the developing fetal lung. More commonly, duplications result from accessory foregut budding in early fetal life.

Enterogenous cysts present as rounded densities in a retropleural, paraesophageal position adherent to the esophageal wall (Fig. 68-10). They are lined by the columnar epithelium of the primitive esophagus. Other duplications may present in the mediastinum but are lined by gastric mucosa or other distal endodermal lining. In the latter cases, erosion with perforation into the right lower lobe may occur. These patients present with respiratory distress and hemoptysis from massive hemorrhage. Treatment is surgical when vertebral anomalies accompany the mediastinal cyst; a spinal cyst may be present as well. CT scanning with myelography should be done even when the patient is asymptomatic [130].

Anomalies of the Pleural Fissures

As noted previously, the visceral pleura constitutes the most distal layer of the visceral mesothelial tissues enveloping the lung, and the fissures may be regarded as inward plications of the pleura, separating the several pulmonary lobes.

There are some anomalies of these fissures or pleural extensions that, though seldom of clinical importance, deserve brief mention because they should be recognized, especially in differential diagnosis.

Absence or Incomplete Development of Fissures

One or more of the major interlobar fissures may be absent or incomplete. Such a defect may be suspected when an expected fissure marking is not visible in the posteroanterior or, more likely, lateral roentgenogram, but its existence can be proved only at thoracotomy. These defects are significant because absence of a natural barrier may permit direct extension of lesions, notably tuberculous lesions, from one lobe to another, and also because it may complicate operative procedures such as lobectomy.

Complete or Incomplete Accessory Fissures

Complete or incomplete accessory fissures are responsible for the formation of the following accessory lobes: (1) a dorsal lobe, set apart from the superior segment of one of the lower lobes; (2) a cardiac lobe, a bit of lung tissue cut off from the medial basal segment of one of the lower

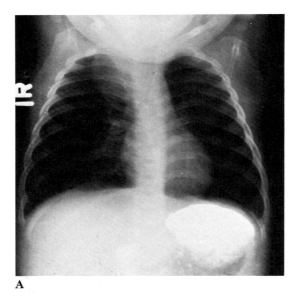

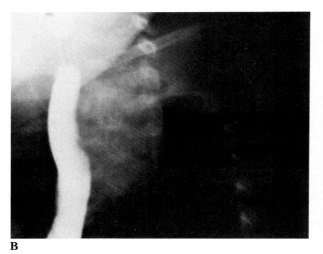

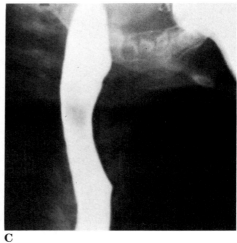

Fig. 68-10. Esophageal duplication. *A.* Anteroposterior chest x-ray film shows a rounded soft-tissue density of mediastinal origin. *B, C.* Spot films from esophagram show pressure on the esophageal wall from an extrinsic mass. The obtuse angle of the barium above and below the mass shows it to be submucosal in origin.

lobes; (3) an anterior basal lobe, a fragment separated from one of the anterior basal segments; and at times, (4) a true left middle or lingula lobe, the lingula fully separated from the rest of the left upper lobe by an accessory fissure.

These accessory fissures may be recognized in roentgenograms as linear densities at the locations indicated. They have no clinical importance unless they happen to act as barriers to the direct spread of disease.

AZYGOS LOBE

The azygos lobe is actually a portion of the right upper lobe. It is separated from the rest of that lobe by an abnormally laterally placed azygos vein, which is invaginated into the pleural covering of the lobe, producing a linear roentgenographic density that courses upward and outward from the upper pole of the right hilum to midclavicle or apex. This anomaly, of no practical significance, is said to occur in about 1 percent of individuals.

SUBCARDIAC LOBE

The so-called subcardiac lobe (lobus caval) is created when a part of the right lower lobe herniates into a pocket formed by the parietal pleura, in close relationship to the inferior vena cava. Like the azygos lobe, it has no clinical importance.

Anomalies of the Thoracic Cage

Pectus Deformities

Pectus excavatum and pectus carinatum are congenital abnormalities of the anterior chest wall. They are probably caused by abnormal growth rates in costal cartilages causing retrusion (excavatum) or protrusion (carinatum) of the sternum. Excavatum is seen 8 to 12 times as frequently as carinatum and occurs three times more often in males than females. Most cases are sporadic, although genetic transmission occurs.

The functional consequences of these deformities have been difficult to document. Some children complain of chest pain and reduced exercise tolerance. Studies of pulmonary function have shown mild restrictive deficits compared with normal controls, with decreases in vital capacity, total lung capacity, and maximal breathing capacity [27,108,110]. There were no differences when patients were studied both preoperatively and postoperatively. Surgeons have corrected these deformities with a number of different techniques. Reviews of surgical series report good cosmetic and psychological results [101]. Some patients have improved exercise tolerance after surgery [26]. Cardiac function has been studied in some patients [9]. Results of complete right-sided heart catheterization were normal, as was the response to supine exercise. Upright treadmill exercise showed decreased cardiac output compared with that of normal controls. Cardiac output was improved after surgery, although neither value was in the abnormal range. A recent review summarized cardiorespiratory studies in this patient group [120].

Many patients with pectus deformities require no surgical intervention. There is generally no progression of the deformity. Indications for correction include intervention in young children (ages 4 to 6 years) to prevent compressive thoracic deformity, to prevent pulmonary and cardiac dysfunction, and to improve cosmetic appearance [58]. Current surgical technique for excavatum, described by Haller and colleagues, includes subperichondrial removal of all abnormal cartilages preserving the perichondrium [58]. A sternal osteotomy is then done and the sternum is elevated and fixed in place with nonabsorbable sutures. In older children and adults, the correction is supported by a metal strut placed anterior to the rib cage and beneath the sternum in a perpendicular position. In patients with carinatum deformity, the lateral depression on either side of the deformity is surgically corrected.

Acknowledgement

The author thanks Norman Glazer, MD, late Clinical Professor of Radiology, Case Western Reserve University School of Medicine, who supplied and interpreted the roentgenograms accompanying this chapter.

References

1. Adzick NS, et al. Fetal diaphragmatic hernia: Ultrasound diagnosis and clinical outcome in 38 cases. *J Pediatr Surg* 24:654, 1989.
2. Allen MS, Thomson SA. CDH in children under one year of age: A 24-year review. *J Pediatr Surg* 1:157, 1966.
3. Apley I. Infant with stridor. *Arch Dis Child* 28:423, 1953.
4. Areechon W, Reid L. Hypoplasia of lung with CDH. *Br Med J* 1:230, 1963.
5. Arey LB, Rea RL. *Developmental Anatomy: A Textbook and Laboratory Manual of Embryology.* Philadelphia: Saunders, 1965.
6. Atkinson JB, et al. Impact of extracorporeal membrane support in the treatment of congenital diaphragmatic hernia. *J Pediatr Surg* 26:791, 1991.
7. Atwell JD, Beard RC. Congenital anomalies of upper urinary tract associated with esophageal atresia and tracheoesophageal fistula. *J Pediatr Surg* 9:825, 1974.
8. Azar H, Crispin AR, Waterston DJ. Esophageal replacement with transverse colon in infants and children. *J Pediatr Surg* 6:3, 1971.

9. Beiser GD, et al. Impairment of cardiac function, etc. *N Engl J Med* 287:267, 1972.

10. Bell DW, et al. Laryngotracheoesophageal cleft: The anterior approach. *Ann Otol Rhinol Laryngol* 86:616, 1977.

11. Bell MJ, Ternberg JL. Antenatal diagnosis of diaphragmatic hernia. *Pediatrics* 60:738, 1977.

12. Berdon WE, Baker DH, Amoury R. The role of pulmonary hypoplasia in the prognosis of newborn infants with diaphragmatic hernia and eventration. *AJR* 103:413, 1968.

13. Berkhoff WBC, et al. Urogenital tract abnormalities associated with esophageal atresia and tracheoesophageal fistula. *J Urol* 141:362, 1989.

14. Berkovits RNP, et al. Congenital LTE cleft. *Arch Otolaryngol* 100:442, 1974.

15. Blank E, Campbell JR. Congenital posterolateral defect in right side of the diaphragm. *Pediatrics* 57:807, 1976.

16. Blumberg JB, et al. LTE cleft, the embryologic implications: Review of the literature. *Surgery* 57:559, 1965.

17. Bolande RB, Schneider AF, Boggs JD. Infantile lobar emphysema. *Arch Pathol* 61:289, 1956.

18. Boles ET, Schiller M, Weinberger M. Improved management of neonates with CDH. *Arch Surg* 103:344, 1971.

19. Bower RJ, Kiesewetter WB. Mediastinal masses in infants and children. *Arch Surg* 112:1003, 1977.

20. Boyden EA. Development of the Human Lung. In *Brennermann's Practice of Pediatrics*, vol 4 Hagerstown, MD: Harper & Row, 1972. Chap 64.

21. Bradenkamp JK, Maceri DR, Crockett DM. Tracheal agenesis: The importance of an endoscopic diagnosis. *Otolaryngol Head Neck Surg* 101:688, 1989.

22. Breckenridge RL, Rehermann RL, Gibson ET. Congenital cystic adenomatoid malformation of the lung. *J Pediatr* 67:863, 1965.

23. Bremer JL. *Congenital Anomalies of the Viscera: Their Embryologic Basis.* Cambridge, MA: Harvard University Press, 1957. Pp 27–31.

24. Brereton RJ, Rickwood AMK. Esophageal atresia with pulmonary agenesis. *J Pediatr Surg* 18:618, 1983.

25. Butler N, Claireaux AE. CDH as a cause of perinatal mortality. *Lancet* 1:659, 1962.

26. Cahill JL, Lees GM, Robertson HT. A summary of preoperative and postoperative cardiorespiratory performance in patients undergoing pectus excavatum and carinatum repair. *J Pediatr Surg* 19:430, 1984.

27. Castile RG, Staats BA, Westbrook PR. Symptomatic pectus deformities of the chest. *Am Rev Respir Dis* 126:564, 1982.

28. Chetcuti P, Dickens DRV, Phelan PD. Spinal deformity in patients born with oesophageal atresia and tracheo-oesophageal fistula. *Arch Dis Child* 64:1427, 1989.

29. Chinn DH, et al. Prenatal ultrasonographic diagnosis of congenital diaphragmatic hernia. *Radiology* 148:119, 1983.

30. Choplin RH, Siegel MJ. Pulmonary sequestration: Six unusual presentations. *AJR* 134:695, 1980.

31. Cotton RT. Pediatric laryngotracheal stenosis. *J Pediatr Surg* 19:699, 1984.

32. Couriel JM, et al. Long-term pulmonary consequences of esophageal atresia and tracheoesophageal fistula. *Acta Paediatr Scand* 71:973, 1982.

33. Cozzi R, Wilkinson AW. Low-birth-weight babies with esophageal atresia or tracheoesophageal fistula. *Arch Dis Child* 50:791, 1975.

34. Crelin ES. Development of the upper respiratory system. *Clin Symp* 28:3, 1976.

35. DeLorimier AA, Tierney DF, Parker HR. Hypoplastic lungs in fetal lambs with surgically produced CDH. *Surgery* 62:12, 1967.

36. DeMuth GR, Sloan H. Congenital lobar emphysema: Long-term effects and sequelae in treatment cases. *Surgery* 59:601, 1966.

37. DeParades CG, et al. Pulmonary sequestration in infants and children: A 20-year experience and review of the literature. *J Pediatr Surg* 5:136, 1970.

38. Diaz EM Jr, et al. Tracheal agenesis: A case report and literature review. *Arch Otolaryngol Head Neck Surg* 115:741, 1989.

39. Dibbins AW. Neonatal diaphragmatic hernia. *Am J Surg* 131:408, 1976.

40. Dibbins AW, Wiener ES. Mortality from neonatal CDH. *J Pediatr Surg* 9:653, 1974.

41. Dickson JA, Clajett T, McDonald JR. Intrathoracic gastric cyst. *J Thorac Surg* 15:318, 1946.

42. DiLorenzo M, et al. Bronchogenic cysts. *J Pediatr Surg* 24:988, 1989.

43. Donahoe PK, Gee GE. Complete laryngotracheoesophageal cleft: Management and repair. *J Pediatr Surg* 19:143, 1984.

44. Doyle AJ. Demonstration of blood supply to pulmonary sequestration by M R angiography. *Am J Radiol* 158:989, 1992.

45. Dudley NE, Phelan PD. Respiratory complications in long-term survivors of esophageal atresia. *Arch Dis Child* 51:279, 1976.

46. Eigen H, Lemen RJ, Weruig WW. Congenital lobar emphysema: Long-term evaluation of surgically conservatively treated children. *Am Rev Respir Dis* 113:823, 1976.

47. Eraklis AJ, Criscan NT, McGovern JB. Bronchogenic cysts of the mediastinum in infancy. *N Engl J Med* 281:1150, 1969.

48. Evans JNG. Management of the cleft larynx and tracheoesophageal clefts. *Ann Otol Rhinol Laryngol* 94:627, 1985.

49. Fagan CJ, Swischuk LD. The opaque lung in lobar emphysema. *Am J Roentgenol Radium Ther Nucl Med* 114:300, 1972.

50. Floyd J, Campbell DC, Dominy DE. Agenesis of trachea. *Am Rev Respir Dis* 86:557, 1962.
51. Frenchkner B, Freyschuss V. Pulmonary function after lobectomy for congenital lobar emphysema and congenital cystic adenomatoid malformation. *Scand J Cardiovasc Surg* 16:293, 1982.
52. Goto H, et al. High-frequency jet ventilation for resection of congenital lobar emphysema. *Anesth Analg* 66:684, 1987.
53. Grafe WR, Goldsmith EI, Redo SF. Bronchogenic cysts of the mediastinum in children. *J Pediatr Surg* 1:384, 1966.
54. Greene DA. Congenital complete tracheal rings. *Arch Otolaryngol* 102:241, 1976.
55. Grosfeld JL, O'Neill JA, Clathworthy HW. Enteric duplications in infancy and childhood. *Ann Surg* 172:83, 1970.
56. Grunebaum M. The roentgenologic investigation of congenital subglottic stenosis. *AJR* 125:877, 1975.
57. Haller JA, Mazur DO, Morgan WW. Masses in children. *J Thorac Cardiovasc Surg* 58:385, 1969.
58. Haller JA, et al. Evolving management of pectus excavatum based on a single institutional experience of 664 patients. *Ann Surg* 209:578, 1989.
59. Halloran LG, Silverberg SC, Salzberg AM. Congenital cystic adenomatoid malformation of the lung. *Arch Surg* 104:714, 1972.
60. Harberg FJ, Meaher D, Wetchlers Harris F. Congenital anomalies of the diaphragm: Personal experience with thirty-five consecutive cases. *Am J Surg* 132:748, 1976.
61. Hardesty RL, et al. Extracorporeal membrane oxygenation: Successful treatment of persistent fetal circulation following repair of congenital diaphragmatic hernia. *J Thorac Cardiovasc Surg* 81:556, 1981.
62. Hardingham M, Walsh-Warin GP. The treatment of a congenital laryngeal web. *J Laryngol Otol* 89:273, 1975.
63. Harrison MR, et al. Correction of congenital diaphragmatic hernia in utero. V. Initial clinical experience. *J Pediatr Surg* 25:47, 1990.
64. Heiss K, et al. Reversal of mortality for congenital diaphragmatic hernia with ECMO. *Ann Surg* 209:225, 1989.
65. Hendren WH, et al. Surgical management of pectus deformities. *Ann Thorac Surg* 23:417, 1977.
66. Holder TM, Ashcraft JW. Esophageal atresia and tracheoesophageal fistula. *Curr Probl Surg* 1966. Pp 1–68.
67. Holder TM, et al. Esophageal atresia and tracheoesophageal fistula: A survey of its members by the surgical section of the American Academy of Pediatrics. *Pediatrics* 34:542, 1964.
68. Holder TM, McDonald VG, Woolley MM. The premature or critically ill infant with esophageal atresia: Increased success with a staged approach. *J Thorac Cardiovasc Surg* 44:344, 1962.
69. Hollinger PH. Clinical aspects of congenital anomalies of the larynx, trachea, bronchi and esophagus. *J Laryngol Otol* 75:1, 1961.
70. Hutchin P. Congenital cystic disease of the lung. *Rev Surg* 28:79, 1971.
71. Ito T, Sugito T, Nagaya M. Delayed primary anastomosis in poor-risk patients with esophageal atresia associated with tracheoesophageal fistula. *J Pediatr Surg* 19:243, 1984.
72. Johnson DG, Deaner RM, Koop CE. Diaphragmatic hernia in infancy: Factors affecting the mortality rate. *Surgery* 62:1082, 1967.
73. Johnson JA, et al. Cystic adenomatoid malformations: Antenatal demonstration. *AJR* 142:483, 1984.
74. Kashuk JL, Lilly JR. Esophageal atresia in father and son. *J Pediatr Surg* 18:621, 1983.
75. Kattan KR, Zaheer MA. Laryngocele: Audiological diagnosis. *JAMA* 244:1617, 1980.
76. Keith JD, Rowe RD, Vlad R. *Heart Disease in Infancy and Childhood* (3rd ed). New York: Macmillan, 1978.
77. Kirschner PA. Cervicomediastinal cystic hygroma. *Surgery* 60:1104, 1966.
78. Koltai PJ, Morgan D, Evans JNG. Endoscopic repair of supraglottic laryngeal clefts. *Arch Otolaryngol Head Neck Surg* 117:273, 1991.
79. Koop CE, Hamilton JP. Atresia of the esophagus: Increased survival with staged procedures in the poor-risk infant. *Ann Surg* 162:389, 1965.
80. Koop CE, Schnaufer L, Broennie AM. Esophageal atresia and tracheoesophageal fistula: Supportive measures that affect survival. *Pediatrics* 54:558, 1974.
81. Krous HF, Sexauer CL. Embryonal rhabdomyosarcoma arising within a congenital bronchogenic cyst in a child. *J Pediatr Surg* 16:506, 1981.
82. Kwittken T, Reiner L. Congenital cystic adenomatoid malformation of the lung. *Pediatrics* 30:759, 1962.
83. Ladd WE. The surgical treatment of esophageal atresia and tracheoesophageal fistula. *N Engl J Med* 230:625, 1944.
84. Ladd WE, Gross RE. Congenital diaphragmatic hernia. *N Engl J Med* 233:917, 1940.
85. Leven NL. Congenital atresia of esophagus with tracheoesophageal fistula. *J Thorac Surg* 10:648, 1941.
86. Levine MM, et al. Pulmonary sequestration causing congestive heart failure in infancy: A report of two cases and review of the literature. *Ann Thorac Surg* 34:581, 1982.
87. Lewis RJ, Caccavale RJ, Sisler GE. Imaged thoracoscopic surgery: A new thoracic technique

for resection of mediastinal cysts. *Ann Thorac Surg* 53:318, 1992.

88. Lilly JR, Wesenberg RL, Shikes RH. Segmental lung resection in the first year of life. *Ann Thorac Surg* 22:16, 1976.

89. Lim TA, Spanier SS, Kohut RI. Laryngeal clefts: A histopathologic study and review. *Ann Otol Rhinol Laryngol* 88:837, 1979.

90. Lowery J, O'Bradovich H, Coates G. Ventilation scintigraphy with submicronic radioaerosol as an adjunct in the diagnosis of congenital lobar emphysema. *J Nucl Med* 28:1213, 1987.

91. MacFarlane PI, Olinsky A, Phelan PD. Proximal airway function 8 to 16 years after laryngomalacia: Follow-up using flow-volume loop studies. *J Pediatr* 107:216, 1985.

92. Madewell JE, Stocker JT, Korosower JM. Cystic adenomatoid malformation of the lung. *AJR* 124:436, 1975.

93. Man DWK, et al. Congenital lobar emphysema: Problems in diagnosis and management. *Arch Dis Child* 58:709, 1983.

94. McHugh HE, Loch WE. Congenital webs of the larynx. *Laryngoscope* 52:43, 1942.

95. McSwiney PF, Cavanagh NPC, Languth P. Outcome in congenital stridor (laryngomalacia). *Arch Dis Child* 52:215, 1977.

96. Mendelson DS, et al. Bronchogenic cysts with high CT numbers. *AJR* 140:463, 1983.

97. Mendoza A, et al. Prenatal ultrasonographic diagnosis of congenital adenomatoid malformation of the lung. *Arch Pathol Lab Med* 110:402, 1986.

98. Mills NL, Grosfeld JL. One-stage operation for cervicomediastinal cystic hygroma in infancy. *J Thorac Cardiovasc Surg* 65:608, 1973.

99. Morgan WJ, Lemen RJ, Rojas R. Acute worsening of congenital lobar emphysema with subsequent spontaneous improvement. *Pediatrics* 71:844, 1983.

100. Murray GF. Congenital lobar emphysema. *Surg Gynecol Obstet* 124:611, 1967.

101. Naef AP. Surgical treatment of pectus excavatum: An experience with 90 operations. *Ann Thorac Surg* 21:63, 1976.

102. Naeye RL, et al. Unsuspected pulmonary vascular abnormalities associated with diaphragmatic hernia. *Pediatrics* 58:902, 1976.

103. Nakayama DK, et al. Prenatal diagnosis and natural history of the fetus with a congenital diaphragmatic hernia: Initial clinical experience. *J Pediatr Surg* 20:118, 1985.

104. Newman B. Real-time ultrasound and color Doppler imaging in pulmonary sequestration. *Pediatrics* 86:620, 1990.

105. Oldham HN, Sabiston DC. Primary tumors and cysts of the mediastinum. *Arch Surg* 96:71, 1968.

106. Opsahl T, Bergman EJ. Bronchogenic medias-

tinal cysts in infants: Case report review of the literature. *Pediatrics* 30:372, 1962.

107. O'Rahilly R, Muller F. Respiratory and alimentary relations in staged human embryos. *Ann Otol Rhinol Laryngol* 93:421, 1984.

108. Orzalesi MM, Cook CD. Pulmonary function in children with pectus excavatum. *J Pediatr* 66:898, 1965.

109. Passarge E, Halsey H, German J. Unilateral agenesis of the diaphragm. *Humangenetik* 5:226, 1968.

110. Polgar G, Koop CE. Pulmonary function in pectus excavatum. *Pediatrics* 32:209, 1963.

111. Pugutch RD, et al. CT diagnosis of benign mediastinal abnormalities. *AJR* 134:685, 1980.

112. Raphaely RC, Downes JJ. CDH: Prediction of survival. *J Pediatr Surg* 8:815, 1973.

113. Reid IS, Hutcherson RJ. Long-term follow-up of patients with congenital diaphragmatic hernia. *J Pediatr Surg* 11:939, 1976.

114. Reynolds JL, Donahue JK, Pearce CW. Intrapericardial teratoma: A case of acute pericardial effusion in infancy. *Pediatrics* 43:71, 1969.

115. Richardson MA, Cotton RT. Anatomic abnormalities of the pediatric airway. *Pediatr Clin North Am* 31:821, 1984.

116. Ries T, et al. Real-time ultrasonography of subcarinal bronchogenic cysts in two children. *Radiology* 145:121, 1982.

117. Robertson R, James ES. Congenital lobar emphysema. *Pediatrics* 8:795, 1951.

118. Ryan DP, et al. Laryngotracheoesophageal cleft (type IV): Management and repair of lesions beyond the carina. *J Pediatr Surg* 26:962, 1991.

119. Schaffer AJ, Avery E. *Diseases of the Newborn* (4th ed). Philadelphia: Saunders, 1977.

120. Schamberger RC, Welch KJ. Surgical repair of pectus excavatum. *J Pediatr Surg* 23:615, 1988.

121. Schiller M, Frye TR, Boles ET Jr. Evaluation of colonic replacement of the esophagus in children. *J Pediatr Surg* 6:753, 1971.

122. Sloan H. Lobar emphysema in infancy treated by lobectomy. *J Thorac Surg* 26:1, 1953.

123. Smith RA. A theory of the origin of intralobar sequestration of lung. *Thorax* 11:10, 1956.

124. Snyder ME, et al. Diagnostic dilemmas of mediastinal cysts. *J Pediatr Surg* 20:810, 1985.

125. Snyder WH, Greaney EM Jr. CDH: 77 consecutive cases. *Surgery* 57:576, 1965.

126. Starrett RW, DeLorimier AA. CDH in lambs: Hemodynamic and ventilatory changes with breathing. *J Pediatr Surg* 10:575, 1975.

127. Stocker JT, Madewell JE, Drake RM. Congenital cystic adenomatoid malformation of the lung. *Hum Pathol* 8:155, 1977.

128. Stocker JT, Malczak HT. A study of pulmonary ligament arteries: Relationship to intralobar pulmonary sequestration. *Chest* 86:611, 1984.

129. Stolar CJH, Diaan PW, Stalcup SA. Extracorpo-

real membrane oxygenation and congenital diaphragmatic hernia: Modification of the pulmonary vasoactive profile. *J Pediatr Surg* 20:681, 1985.

130. Superina RA, Ein SH, Jumphreys RP. Cystic duplications of the esophagus and neurenteric cysts. *J Pediatr Surg* 19:527, 1984.

131. Swischuk LE, Smith PC, Fagan CJ. Abnormalities of pharynx and larynx in childhood. *Semin Roentgenol* 9:283, 1974.

132. Wall MA, Eisenberg JD, Campbell JR. Congenital lobar emphysema in a mother and daughter. *Pediatrics* 70:131, 1982.

133. Walpita PR. Laryngocele in an infant. *J Pediatr Surg* 10:843, 1975.

134. Warfel KA, Schulz DM. Agenesis of the trachea. *Arch Pathol Lab Med* 100:357, 1976.

135. Weigel W, Kaufman HJ. The frequency and types of other congenital anomalies in association with tracheoesophageal malformations. *Clin Pediatr* 15:819, 1976.

136. Wiatrak BJ, Myer CM III, Bratcher GO. Mediastinal bronchogenic cyst. *Ann Otol Rhinol Laryngol* 99:413, 1990.

137. Wiener ES. Congenital posterolateral diaphragmatic hernia: New dimensions in management. *Surgery* 92:670, 1982.

138. Wilson JM, et al. Congenital diaphragmatic hernia: Predictors of severity in the ECMO era. *J Pediatr Surg* 26:1028, 1991.

69

Genetic Diseases of the Tracheobronchial Tree

Robert E. Wood   Irwin A. Schafer

Virtually all pulmonary diseases may be viewed as having both genetic and nongenetic components in their causation. There are some conditions, inherited as Mendelian traits, in which the disease is primarily due to the effects of a single mutant gene, but which are influenced to different degrees by environmental factors. These entities are relatively few and usually represent systemic diseases in which pulmonary manifestations are prominent. At the opposite end of the spectrum are many common pulmonary disorders in which environmental factors predominate, but in which genetic factors may play some modulating role. The genetic component in this latter group may fit the model for polygenic or multifactorial inheritance, in which several genes, each with a small additive effect, place the individual at increased risk of developing disease when exposed to inciting environmental factors. The multifactorial inheritance model fits when applied to some congenital malformations, including spina bifida and cleft palate. Similar analysis for common pulmonary diseases has not been published. Disorders with a significant polygenic component would be expected to show familial aggregation and possibly differences among ethnic groups or races. The identification of the polygenic components of pulmonary disease would provide clinically useful data, since individuals at increased risk could be counseled and the patients' environment modified to prevent the disease or ameliorate its course.

In the following sections, several diseases in which a genetic cause is implied but not proved are described. It will become apparent that for many entities, detailed information is lacking on the mode of inheritance, the frequency of the mutant gene in populations, or the basic biochemical defect producing the disease. Cystic fibrosis (CF) is an exception to this, as the gene has recently been cloned.

Cystic Fibrosis

CF is the most common lethal genetic disease in white populations [107], and is the cause of much of the chronic progressive pulmonary disease encountered in children. With improving prognosis over the past several decades—the median survival age is now nearly 30 years—CF has also become a disease of young adults.

CF is characterized by the clinical triad of excessive concentrations of sodium and chloride in exocrine sweat, chronic obstructive pulmonary disease (typically with chronic bacterial infection with such species as *Staphylococcus aureus* and *Pseudomonas aeruginosa*), and exocrine pancreatic insufficiency. The severity of expression is variable, especially with regard to pancreatic function.

It has long been known that CF is an autosomal recessive disorder, involving approximately 1 in 2500 newborns in North America. Within the past several years, the gene for CF has been cloned and characterized, and our understanding of the pathophysiology of the disease has been greatly enhanced [123].

Genetics

CF results from a mutation in a gene located on the long arm of chromosome 7 (7q31.3). The most common mutation involves a 3 base-pair deletion, which results in the absence of a phenylalanine residue at amino acid position 508 of the gene product [63,92,95]. This mutation is referred to as the ΔF508 mutation. About two-thirds of all CF chromosomes examined to date carry this mutation. Several hundred other mutations, some of which are associated with relatively mild clinical involvement, have been documented in this same gene. Non-ΔF508 mutations are more common in southern European populations than in those of northern Europe [141].

Heterozygotes for the CF mutation are clinically normal. It is estimated that approximately 1 in 25 to 1 in 35 white individuals in North America is a heterozygote. Various theories have been proposed to explain a putative heterozygote advantage and the high gene frequency. In view of the current understanding of the gene and its function, the most attractive such hypothesis is that heterozygotes are relatively protected against the effects of chloride-secreting diarrhea in infancy [94].

The gene product, known as the *cystic fibrosis transmembrane regulator* (CFTR), is a large, glycosylated protein of approximately 1480 amino acids [41,92]. CFTR is presumed to act as at least part of a chloride-selective ion channel through the apical membrane of epithelial cells in the airways, sweat glands, and intestine [10,60]. Some regions of the protein apparently act as regulators of the ion channel, in response to changes in intracellular cyclic adenosine monophosphate (cAMP) [28a].

Incidence and Prevalence

The incidence of CF varies widely in different populations, being most common in southern Europe and least common in Asian and black African populations. Likewise, the incidence of specific mutations varies. The ΔF508 mutation is more common in northern European populations than in southern Europe. Reported incidence figures range from 1 : 620 live births in individuals of Dutch descent in southwest Africa [119] to 1 : 90,000 live births in Orientals. CF is predominately a disease of the white population; the incidence in US blacks has been estimated to be about 1 : 17,000 [72], as compared with an incidence of about 1 : 2500 in white births. The incidence of heterozygotes can be estimated from the latter figure to be approximately 3 to 4 percent.

The total number of patients with CF is unknown. The Patient Registry of the Cystic Fibrosis Foundation (Bethesda, MD) records data on each patient followed by care centers in the United States. At the end of 1991, approximately 19,000 patients were reported to the Registry (un-published data). Many patients are not seen in this center network (or are not diagnosed), and the total number is generally estimated to be about twice that of the Registry data.

Pathophysiology

The most important clinical feature of CF is chronic obstructive pulmonary disease, which is characterized by accumulation of thick airway secretions and chronic bacterial infection. Although ciliary structure and beat are apparently normal, mucociliary clearance is impaired, and mucous plugging of small airways can be detected in infants with no discernible pulmonary infection [137]. The current explanation for this involves the role of CFTR (and chloride permeability of respiratory epithelial cells) in the regulation of mucociliary transport.

Cilia beat in an aqueous medium with their tips touching the overlying layer of mucus. The depth of the periciliary fluid layer is of critical importance to integrated mucociliary function. If it is too deep, the cilia cannot touch (and thus propel) the mucous layer, while if it is too shallow (i.e., dehydrated) the cilia are "mired in clay." In CF, because of the dysfunctional gene product, the apical membrane of the respiratory epithelial cells is impermeable to chloride, and the normal flux of chloride to the luminal surface is thus reduced. At the same time, there is excessive active sodium reabsorption. These phenomena are reflected in the bioelectric properties of the airway epithelium [65]. The resting transepithelial electrical potential is elevated, from the normal range of 25 to 35 mV to 55 to 90 mV. Selective inhibition of the sodium pump (i.e., by a drug such as amiloride) reduces the transepithelial potential to nearly 0 mV. In normal subjects, amiloride does not reduce the potential nearly as much, as continued flux of chloride maintains a potential of 10 to 15 mV (lumen-negative). Furthermore, chloride flux is normally increased by beta agonists such as isoproterenol, but this response is absent in CF. These electrophysiologic phenomena have been utilized to facilitate the diagnosis in patients with equivocal sweat test results or atypical clinical manifestations. The best evidence today suggests that CFTR is itself the chloride channel (or at least is capable of functioning as a chloride channel) [10].

Although definitive proof is yet lacking, it is widely assumed that failure of normal regulation of the periciliary fluid results in impaired clearance of pulmonary secretions, thus leading to the obstructive pulmonary disease. However, failure of mucociliary transport alone cannot be the whole story, as patients with congenitally absent ciliary function (immotile cilia syndrome, primary ciliary dyskinesia) do not have the same degree of viscous changes in their pulmonary secretions, nor are they characteristically infected with *P. aeruginosa*. The role of CFTR in other cellular membranes (such as the Golgi apparatus) is not yet understood, but it is possible that alterations in the function of such membranes could play a role in other CF-specific phenomena, such as the marked susceptibility to infection with *P. aeruginosa* and the increased sulfation of mucus glycoproteins [20].

The abnormalities of chloride permeability are also found in nonrespiratory epithelia, including the pancreatic and sweat ducts. In the pancreas, obstruction of small ducts, presumably due to decreased fluid secretion [75] (in turn, presumably due at least in part to failure of chloride permeability [29]), results in autodigestion of the exocrine pancreas. In the majority of patients, this process has progressed to the point of clinical pancreatic insufficiency by the time of birth. Ultimately, 85 to 90 percent of patients require enzyme replacement therapy. Deficiency of pancreatic enzyme secretion and the consequent maldigestion in turn lead to a myriad of secondary problems, including protein-calorie malnutrition and fat-soluble vitamin deficiencies.

The primary secretory product of sweat glands is isotonic with plasma, and the composition of sweat at the skin is regulated by the relative reabsorption of water and electrolytes by the sweat duct. The volume of sweat is regulated by blood flow into the gland and thus by the total volume of ultrafiltrate in the primary secretory coil. Normally, sodium and chloride are actively reabsorbed, leaving a hypotonic fluid to reach the surface. The concentration of chloride in normal sweat is on the order of 10 to 20 mEq/liter; in CF, the ductal epithelial cells are relatively impermeable to chloride, so that the concentration of chloride in the sweat at the skin exceeds 60 mEq/liter. If the rate of sweat formation is very low, there may be enough reabsorption of chloride to reach the normal range (<60 mEq/liter), so that for diagnostic purposes, it is important to measure sweat chloride concentrations on the output of maximally stimulated sweat glands (see below).

Diagnosis

The traditional diagnostic criteria for CF include a sweat chloride concentration exceeding 60 mEq/liter, and at least one of the following: chronic obstructive pulmonary disease (especially if associated with *P. aeruginosa*), exocrine pancreatic insufficiency, and confirmed family history (sibling, parent, child, or first cousin) of classic CF. Some authorities will accept a diagnosis of CF with normal sweat chloride values if there is typical, chronic pulmonary disease and well-documented pancreatic insufficiency. Such patients are unusual, most likely represent a specific mutation, and usually have sweat chloride concentrations in the range of 45 to 60 mEq/liter [109].

In practice, the most important aspect of diagnosis is the sweat test (Table 69-1). This test, while simple in concept, is difficult to perform accurately [28]. The sweat glands must be stimulated to produce maximal output (falsely low electrolyte values may be obtained at low sweat rates); this is accomplished by iontophoresis of pilocarpine. At least 100 mg of sweat should be collected to ensure an adequate sweat rate. The sweat is collected with great care to avoid evap-

Table 69-1. **Indications for sweat testing for cystic fibrosis**

Pulmonary
  Chronic cough
  Recurrent or chronic pneumonia
  Staphylococcal pneumonia
  Recurrent bronchiolitis
  Atelectasis
  Hemoptysis
  Mucoid *Pseudomonas* infection
Gastrointestinal
  Meconium ileus
  Steatorrhea
  Malabsorption
  Rectal prolapse
  Childhood cirrhosis (portal hypertension or
    bleeding esophageal varices)
  Hypoprothrombinemia (beyond the neonatal
    period)
Other
  Family history of cystic fibrosis
  Failure to thrive
  Salty sweat
  Nasal polyps
  Heat prostration
  Hyponatremia and hypochloremia, especially in
    infants
  Pansinusitis
  Aspermia

Source: From RE Wood, TF Boat, CF Doershuk. State of the art: Cystic fibrosis. *Am Rev Respir Dis* 113:833, 1976.

oration, and is analyzed titrimetrically for chloride. Alternative methods for sweat analysis involve pilocarpine iontophoresis, but quantify the chloride by ion-specific electrodes or by conductivity. These methods should be considered unreliable, even for screening purposes. Sweat osmolality has been used instead of electrolyte measurements [36,131], but may be less specific [120]. The use of nonstandard sweat test methods is at least partly responsible for the high rate of false-negative [73a] and false-positive results commonly seen in patients referred to major CF centers.

The normal value for sweat chloride is less than 60 mEq/liter, and in the majority of normal subjects is less than 40 mEq/liter [103]. There may be a slight increase in normal values with age, with an occasional normal adult having a sweat chloride concentration as high as 70 mEq/liter [26,44]. In patients with suggestive clinical presentations who consistently have sweat chloride values in the range of 50 to 60 mEq/liter, additional testing, including DNA studies, may be helpful. Physiologic studies may help clear the picture if the genetics are uncertain. Such studies include measurement of the transepithelial bioelectric potential in the nasal epithelium and the response to amiloride and isoproterenol [69] (the abnormal response will be an elevated basal potential, with marked response to amiloride but none to isoproterenol), and the response of sweat glands to intracutaneous injection of atropine and isoproterenol (the abnormal response is the lack of secretion) [99].

In a genetic disease with an identified mutation, such as CF, diagnostic tests based on DNA analysis can be very helpful. However, since several hundred different mutations have been reported in families with CF, it seems unlikely, from a purely practical standpoint, that DNA testing will completely replace sweat testing for clinical diagnosis. Even if the results of the DNA testing are unambiguous for known mutations that cause CF, most clinicians today would perform a sweat test for confirmation.

The most important and practical aspects of DNA-based diagnostic tests for CF involve prenatal diagnosis and the identification of family members who are heterozygous for the gene [8]. Within families, even though the affected individuals may have an unusual or as-yet-undefined mutation, it may be possible to identify heterozygotes with reasonable accuracy. DNA-based population screening (i.e., universal newborn screening), however, seems impractical with present technology.

Other methods have been advocated for population screening. Sweat testing would be extremely expensive and therefore impractical. Screening for pancreatic insufficiency in newborns has been done by detecting increased amounts of albumin in the meconium [38,108] or evidence of active pancreatic destruction (elevated serum levels of immunoreactive trypsin [24,93]). These tests will not necessarily detect those patients with normal pancreatic function, and are of somewhat limited value. A positive result from any screening test must be confirmed by definitive testing.

Diagnosis in Adults

The majority of patients are diagnosed in the first year of life [91], but many will escape recognition until adolescence or even adulthood [110]. Ten percent of patients reported to the Patient Registry of the Cystic Fibrosis Foundation [91] were diagnosed after the age of 10. These patients may have had milder or atypical forms of the disease, and thus escaped clinical suspicion. It is a mistake to think that a patient "looks too good to have CF" or is too old. Well-characterized patients have been diagnosed in the sixth decade of life [66]. CF should be suspected in patients with early onset of chronic bronchitis, especially if accompanied by chronic gastrointestinal symptoms of nearly any kind. Chronic sinusitis, male (or female) infertility, nasal polyps, a history of rectal prolapse or heat prostration, and pulmonary colonization with *Pseudomonas* species (especially if a mucoid strain) are all potential indications for further investigation. Many adult patients will successfully deny their gastrointestinal problems (malabsorption) and may hide their chronic cough behind a cloud of tobacco smoke.

Pathology

LUNG

The earliest manifestation of CF in the lung is dilation and hypertrophy of bronchial glands and goblet cell metaplasia. As obstruction proceeds, infection develops and a vicious cycle is established, the end result of which is bronchiectasis and decreased lung function. Early in the course of disease, the bronchioles are the principal focus of obstruction and inflammation, while peribronchial abscess formation and fibrosis develop late. The alveolar spaces are relatively spared [34,142], although interstitial disease has been reported [124].

The hypothesis that the primary event is hypersecretion or clearance failure has been challenged. Autopsy studies of young infants with CF suggested that in at least some patients, evidence of infection begins prior to evidence of airway obstruction [85]. In our own laboratory, however [137], we have performed bronchoalveolar lavage on young children with CF and found clear evidence of obstructive lung disease (mucous casts) without evidence of infection or inflammation. Destruction of the bronchial epithelium by infection or impairment of mucociliary transport by abnormally viscous secretions also contributes to widespread airway obstruction. Chronic inflammation itself may contribute substantially to the progressive bronchiolectasis and bronchiectasis that are so characteristic of CF. High concentrations of neutrophil elastase are found in the purulent airway secretions, which may overwhelm the indigenous antiprotease activity. For this reason, there has been interest in the use of antiinflammatory therapy as part of the comprehensive management of CF patients [13,71].

GASTROINTESTINAL TRACT
Exocrine pancreatic insufficiency, which occurs in more than 85 percent of patients, is due to inspissation of secretions in the pancreatic ducts. The consequent autolytic destruction of the exocrine portions of the organ gives the disorder its original name, *cystic fibrosis of the pancreas* [9]. The islet tissue is relatively spared despite near-total fibrofatty replacement of the remainder of the pancreas.

Intestinal mucous glands are hypertrophic, with extensive ductal obstruction, and goblet cells are prominent. Similar changes in mucus-secreting elements may be seen in salivary glands. Fatty changes occur in the liver of as many as 30 percent of patients, while biliary cirrhosis, due to inspissation of bile, may be found in 20 to 30 percent of older patients. Portal hypertension with esophageal varices occurs in 2 to 3 percent of patients [115].

GENITOURINARY
Male infertility is almost universal and is due to absence or atresia (perhaps due to in utero obstruction) of the vas deferens. Testicular function and spermatogenesis are normal [86]. There are no specific abnormalities of the female reproductive tract, although evidence of mucus hypersecretion and inspissation of gland ducts may be seen [87].

SWEAT GLANDS
The sweat glands are anatomically normal, despite their failure to reabsorb sodium and chloride.

Clinical Manifestations

The clinical manifestations of CF [84,138] are variable and are influenced by treatment and environmental (as well as genetic) variables. In the majority of patients, the pulmonary component predominates, but some patients have virtually no lung symptoms until the second or third decade of life. Patients with clinically normal pancreatic function tend to have a milder degree of pulmonary involvement [23].

PULMONARY
Cough is the earliest and most prominent clinical manifestation of pulmonary disease. It may begin as an infrequent and nonproductive cough, but progresses inexorably (usually over years) to become productive of thick sputum. The chest often remains clear on auscultation until the airways disease is relatively advanced; radiographic and physiologic (i.e., spirometric) evaluation is helpful in following the course. In infants or in older patients with acute exacerbations, wheezing may be prominent [74], but more often rales and rhonchi are heard. There is a distinct predilection for involvement of the right upper lobe, and many patients have worse disease in the right lung than the left. With progression, digital clubbing develops, the lungs become hyperinflated, physical findings become persistent, and the patient grows more symptomatic. Usually, however, patients do not exhibit cyanosis or marked decreases in exercise tolerance until relatively late in the course. In contrast with chronic obstructive lung disease in adults, the clinical course of CF is usually precipitous once overt respiratory failure develops.

The upper airway may also be involved. Pansinusitis is very common, and nasal polyps are present in 10 to 15 percent of patients [112].

Chronic pulmonary infection is a constant finding in CF patients [45,50,76,78]. Early in the course, *S. aureus, Hemophilus influenzae*, and a variety of other organisms may be found. Eventually, however, *P. aeruginosa* (or other *Pseudomonas* species) becomes the predominant or only organism in the majority of patients. Viral agents are often responsible for symptomatic exacerbations and may be implicated in the development of lung damage early in life. Fungi, especially *Aspergillus* species, also may be important. Recently in several CF centers, *Pseudomonas cepacia* became a major pulmonary pathogen [122]. Strains of atypical mycobacteria are also found in sputum specimens, and may be pathogenic.

Pulmonary complications include hemoptysis (which may be massive) [53,116], atelectasis [111], pneumothorax [117], and cor pulmonale [113].

GASTROINTESTINAL

Meconium ileus (neonatal intestinal obstruction) occurs in at least 10 percent of patients with CF [91]. In addition to the usual clinical findings of obstruction, there may be radiographic evidence of in utero perforation, with sterile peritonitis resulting in peritoneal calcifications [52]. Malrotation or volvulus may also occur in association with meconium ileus.

Approximately 85 percent of patients have clinically significant exocrine pancreatic insufficiency. In some, secretion of bicarbonate and total enzyme output may be decreased, while sufficient function remains to prevent steatorrhea. In these latter patients, episodes of acute pancreatitis may occur, especially at older ages [102]. The effects of pancreatic insufficiency include fat and protein maldigestion with consequent malabsorption and bulky, greasy, foul-smelling stools. Secondary caloric, protein, and vitamin deficiencies may develop in untreated or inadequately treated patients. Rectal prolapse is common in younger, untreated patients [114].

Late intestinal obstruction ("meconium ileus equivalent") may develop as a result of inspissation of bowel contents in the cecum or terminal ileum [55]. The colon tends to be distended because of the malabsorption, and intussusception (often relatively painless and sometimes without obstipation) is not uncommon.

GENITOURINARY

Almost all men with CF are sterile, but a semen analysis is required to be certain, as some patients have normal sperm counts [121]. Female fertility is reduced, both by chronic illness and by thick cervical mucus. However, a significant number of women with CF have conceived. Those with moderate to advanced disease who become pregnant are at risk of worsening their clinical condition. Infants born to these women are obligate heterozygotes; the incidence of CF is half that of the prevalence of the gene in the population, or 2.5 percent.

SWEAT GLANDS

Failure to reabsorb salt from the sweat ducts is almost universal in patients with CF, with sweat electrolyte concentrations above 60 mEq/liter. With adequate replacement of salt in the diet, there are usually no significant manifestations of the sweat defect other than the use of the sweat test for diagnosis. However, excessive loss of salt can lead to heat prostration, and in infants, metabolic alkalosis can develop, even in cold weather [83].

METABOLIC

Many patients develop glucose intolerance in the late second or third decade of life [14]. While ketoacidosis is unusual, many require insulin to control their glucosuria.

Treatment

While recent advances in understanding of the molecular basis of CF have been impressive, improvements in therapy have been somewhat slower to evolve. The most promising new developments include aerosol therapy with amiloride or DNase. Amiloride blocks the increased absorption of sodium from the airway lumen, thus (presumably) maintaining better hydration of the periciliary fluid and secretions. Results of pilot studies in adult patients have been encouraging [67]; larger-scale clinical trials are currently in progress. Nucleotide triphosphates (ATP, uridine triphosphate) appear to open the chloride channel in airway epithelial cells [68]; perhaps this may lead to more effective therapy in the future. Clinical trials are also underway with human recombinant DNase [100], as a method of reducing the viscosity of airway secretions. Ultimately, gene transfer seems the best hope for a cure. Successful experiments with in vitro gene transfer have been reported from several laboratories.

The treatment of CF is empirical, since the basic defect has not yet been reversed in vivo. There is considerable disagreement as to the most effective therapeutic regimen, and objective data in support of one or another method are scant. In general, it may be said that since CF is a complex disorder that involves multiple organ systems, its treatment is best handled in specialized centers where concentrated expertise and experience are available.

PULMONARY THERAPY

The main goal of pulmonary therapy is to reverse or prevent the progression of pulmonary disease.

This is approached in two ways: efforts to improve airway clearance, and efforts to reduce infection.

Physical measures to enhance clearance of pulmonary secretions include chest percussion, forced expiratory maneuvers, vigorous exercise, and cough. Airway obstruction begins at a very early age, and chest physiotherapy should be initiated at the time of diagnosis, even in patients who are asymptomatic. At times of symptomatic exacerbation, the frequency or the intensity, or both, of such therapy is increased.

Various forms of aerosol therapy, including mucolytic agents, bronchodilators, and antibiotics, have been used. There is little evidence, however, to support the use of mucolytic aerosols. Beta-adrenergic agents have been shown to increase mucociliary transport in patients with CF [139], but the clinical efficacy of such therapy is unknown. Some patients exhibit increased airway obstruction following bronchodilator therapy, and the response is not necessarily consistent over time [88]. Therefore, such treatment must be individualized. Aminoglycoside aerosols may be effective [106], either alone or in combination with parenteral therapy. In general, aerosolized agents may be expected to be more effective in the earlier stages of the pulmonary disease, since obstruction with thick secretions limits the penetration of aerosols.

Antibiotic therapy is important in reducing the pulmonary bacterial burden. The presence of large numbers of bacteria in the airways induces secondary inflammatory responses that may in themselves be harmful; reducing bacterial numbers is usually helpful. In addition, there is increasing evidence that at least in some patients, antiinflammatory agents may be effective. The role of such agents (prednisone, nonsteroidal antiinflammatory agents) is currently the subject of considerable investigation [12,71]; they should not be considered the standard of care at this time.

Early in the course of disease, patients may produce little or no sputum, and it may be difficult to determine the bacterial flora of the lower respiratory tract. In young children, infection with *H. influenzae, S. aureus*, and other common agents is more common than with *P. aeruginosa*, although this organism is also seen in infants and young children. Oral antibiotics may be efficacious for younger patients, but with *P. aeruginosa* infection, or in those with significant disease, parenteral therapy may be necessary. The choice of antibiotics should be guided by cultures of respiratory secretions. If sputum is not available, then induced sputum, swabs of the posterior pharynx after vigorous coughing, or even bronchoscopic specimens may be used.

Patients with CF require higher doses of virtually all antibiotics than do other patients; there is a larger volume of distribution and more rapid renal clearance of most drugs [54], and more rapid metabolism of others [56]. When drugs such as aminoglycosides are used, care must be taken to ensure that the doses are sufficient to produce effective levels while avoiding toxicity.

When the patient's disease cannot be controlled by oral or aerosolized antibiotic therapy, or when only parenteral drugs can be effectively used, hospitalization is indicated. Indications for intensified therapy or even hospitalization include weight loss; increased cough and sputum production lasting more than 2 weeks; worsening pulmonary function; and the development of complications such as pneumothorax, significant hemoptysis, or cor pulmonale. In selected patients, parenteral therapy can be continued at home. In the hospital, intensive chest physiotherapy, nutritional support, psychosocial support, and other therapeutic modalities are employed. In the majority of patients, clinical improvement will be evident after 5 to 7 days, but courses of therapy shorter than 2 weeks rarely result in a satisfactory clinical response. In many patients, longer (or even continuous) therapy is necessary. Monitoring of the patient for drug toxicity and for the development of resistant organisms is essential.

End-stage lung disease in CF patients is increasingly being managed by lung transplantation [31,126,135]. This procedure is expensive; is difficult for patient, family, and physician alike; and will not be appropriate for all patients. The indications for transplantation are not yet well defined. The long-term prognosis for patients who have undergone lung transplantation is as yet unclear, although many patients exhibit amazing improvement. One of our patients fell out of a boat 5 months after lung transplantation, and managed to swim for 2 hours before he was rescued.

GASTROINTESTINAL THERAPY

Nutrition plays a major role in the global well-being of CF patients [37]. Because of inefficient digestion and absorption, as well as other factors, CF patients require 125 to 150 percent of the usual daily requirement for calories and other nutrients. High-fat diets are important to provide sufficient calories. In addition, fat-soluble vitamins should be given in water-miscible form.

Pancreatic insufficiency is treated with pancreatic enzyme replacement. The enteric coated preparations are most effective, and the dosage should be spread throughout the meal to achieve optimal mixing. Dosage is totally empirical, and is adjusted according to the quantity and nature of the food ingested, as well as patterns of growth and stool character. Steatorrhea is almost never totally eliminated, despite adequate enzyme replacement.

Meconium ileus can sometimes be relieved nonoperatively by an enema of hygroscopic radiographic contrast material [77], but more often, surgery is necessary. Late intestinal obstruction can usually be relieved by enemas, as can intussusception, and such methods should be tried before resorting to surgery. Cleansing of the bowel with oral electrolyte solutions can also be effective if the obstruction is not complete.

Liver disease develops in a small percentage of patients, with symptomatic portal hypertension. Endoscopic sclerotherapy, vascular shunting, and even liver transplantation have been utilized for management. Hepatocellular damage may respond to treatment with ursodeoxycholic acid [22].

TREATMENT OF THE SWEAT DEFECT
Patients should be encouraged to maintain a high salt intake, especially in hot weather. No other treatment is necessary unless salt depletion has occurred. Some years ago, when low-sodium infant foods and formulas were introduced generally, the incidence of hypochloremic alkalosis in infants increased significantly [73].

PSYCHOSOCIAL THERAPY
CF is a chronic, progressive, and ultimately fatal disease. The importance of a positive attitude on the part of the patient, family, and the patient's physician and other caretakers cannot be overemphasized. A fatalistic attitude can literally be fatal. As more and more patients reach adulthood, problems with education, career planning, marriage and family, sterility, dependence-independence, fear of impending death or disability, and the cost of medical care assume major proportions and can be overwhelming. It may well be as important to pay attention to mental health as to physical health.

Prognosis
The outlook for patients with CF has improved dramatically over the past several decades. In 1966, the median survival age of patients reported to the Patient Registry of the Cystic Fibrosis Foundation was just over 10 years [136]. By 1991, the median survival age had increased to nearly 29 years (unpublished data). Females have a slightly worse prognosis than do males. The prognosis for individuals is difficult to predict [64].

The reasons for the improving prognosis are not fully understood. The mean age at diagnosis has not changed substantially over the past several decades, suggesting that neither earlier diagnosis nor diagnosis of older, more mildly affected patients makes the difference. Significant differences in survival patterns are reported by various centers, suggesting that differences in treatment may be of importance. Centers in Europe and Australia have reported survival experience similar to that of major North American centers.

What is clear is that further improvements in prognosis will depend on advances in therapy [17]. Several large centers that have traditionally had very high survival rates have not seen increases in survival rates over the past two decades, while survival rates in other centers have been "catching up." The rapid progress in the molecular biology of CF over the past several years promises dramatic changes in our approach to therapy and hopefully, improvements in prognosis. In anticipation of potentially curative therapy in the relatively near future, it is important to treat patients aggressively today, with current methods.

Immotile Cilia Syndrome (Primary Ciliary Dyskinesia)

The clinical triad of situs inversus, bronchiectasis, and pansinusitis was recognized as a distinct entity by Kartagener [59], who also noted the occurrence of the triad in siblings. Kartagener's syndrome remained a clinical oddity until Afzelius and colleagues [5] reported that sperm from these patients were immotile and that the ciliary ultrastructure was abnormal. Subsequently, the generalized nature of the ciliary abnormality was recognized [2,39,89]. Several kindreds have since been reported to have a variety of ultrastructural abnormalities and a common clinical picture of chronic sinus and bronchial disease, with or without situs inversus [4,127].

Pathophysiology

Normal mucociliary transport [129] requires normal ciliary structure (Fig. 69-1) and function. The ultrastructural detail of cilia is quite constant, with two central microtubules surrounded by nine outer microtubule doublets. The microtubules are composed of tubulin, a protein with no intrinsic contractile activity. Radial spokes extend from the central doublet to the outer tubules, which are also connected by a nexin link. Structures projecting from the outer doublets (dynein arms) have ATPase activity. Motion of the cilia is thought to occur by interaction of the dynein arms with the adjacent microtubule in a sliding mechanism similar to that of muscle contraction [98].

Mucociliary function depends on a number of factors, including the number, orientation, and beat frequency of cilia and the dimensions and viscoelastic properties of the mucus and the aqueous periciliary fluid layers.

Electron microscopy of cilia from sperm tails and from nasal and bronchial epithelium of patients with Kartagener's syndrome reveals the partial or complete absence of dynein arms [2]. Other kindreds have been reported in which the radial spokes are absent [127]. Several other ultrastructural patterns have also been reported [118]. Sperm from males with these conditions are biochemically normal but immotile. Thus, these patients are infertile [11]. When cough is suppressed, there is virtually no tracheobronchial clearance [18], which accounts for the eventual development of bronchiectasis and pansinusitis.

Not all patients with chronic sinopulmonary disease have immotile cilia, yet many of these patients do demonstrate abnormal ciliary ultrastructure [3,48]. Chronic infection or inflammation may itself produce abnormalities [19]. Furthermore, not all patients with clinically abnormal ciliary function have truly immotile cilia, even though the ciliary ultrastructure may be abnormal. The name *dyskinetic cilia syndrome* has been proposed for this group of disorders [96]. Clinical and ultrastructural data must be interpreted with caution, and it is difficult to assign a genetic basis to a given patient's problem unless the ultrastructure is classic (i.e., absence of dynein arms) or there is familial clustering. It also should be pointed out that fixation and staining

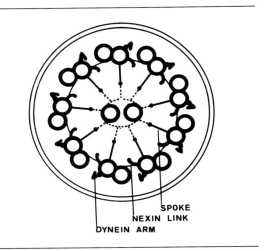

Fig. 69-1. Cross section of a cilium. (Reproduced from R Eliasson et al. The immotile-cilia syndrome, a congenital ciliary abnormality as an etiologic factor in chronic airway infections and male sterility. *N Engl J Med* 297:3, 1977.)

techniques may have a great impact on the ultrastructure visualized, and artifacts are common.

It has been postulated that ciliary beat is necessary for the normal embryonic rotation of the primitive foregut and that the situs inversus associated with immotile cilia (as in Kartagener's syndrome) results from an essentially *random* rotation [2]. While this hypothesis is unproved, it is clear that siblings of patients with Kartagener's syndrome often have pansinusitis and bronchiectasis without situs inversus. Many other patients with immotile cilia who do not have situs inversus have been reported [3,32]. In 65 patients with Polynesian bronchiectatic disease [49], there were none with situs inversus. These patients have been reported to have deficient dynein arms on their ciliary microtubules [128], but the relationship between the two syndromes remains unclear.

Patients with immotile cilia develop bronchial disease much more slowly than do those with CF and do not usually have the extensive mucous hypersecretion and airway plugging so characteristic of CF [70]. The very existence of the clinical syndrome emphasizes the physiologic importance of cilia in the respiratory tract, but it is clear that other factors are of importance in the pathogenesis of severe bronchopulmonary disease.

Incidence and Prevalence

Situs inversus occurs with an incidence of 1 in 8000 to 1 in 24,000 live births, and of these, only 12 to 25 percent have the complete triad of Kartagener's syndrome [21,125]. It is not clear whether situs inversus occurs with a 50 percent (i.e., random) incidence in all patients with immotile cilia. However, with a few assumptions it may be estimated that the incidence of immotile cilia syndrome may be as high as 1 in 20,000 live births.

Genetics

The familial pattern of Kartagener's syndrome is consistent with an autosomal recessive mode of inheritance [118]. The syndrome has been documented in siblings of both sexes but has not been seen in two consecutive generations [51]. Other variants of the immotile cilia syndrome have been observed in siblings [4,127]. From the estimated incidence figures above, it may be calculated that approximately 1 in 70 persons is heterozygous for one form or another of the disorder.

Pathology

Immotile cilia syndrome affects all ciliated epithelia, including those of the middle ear, eustachian tube, nose, paranasal sinuses, tracheobronchial tree, and perhaps other locations [3]. However, there is no distinctive histologic picture, and these patients cannot be distinguished from those with other forms of bronchiectasis or sinusitis on the basis of light microscopy.

Clinical Manifestations

The clinical manifestations of immotile cilia syndrome may begin early in life, or they may not develop until the second or third decades [3,39]. In infants and children, cough and recurrent otitis media may be the primary signs. Patients are often suspected of having CF, but sweat testing will definitively exclude this possibility. The usual signs and symptoms of sinusitis, bronchitis, and bronchiectasis are present in most patients; cough and sputum production, recurrent fevers, hemoptysis, digital clubbing, and eventually cyanosis also may be present. Recurrent otitis media and conductive hearing loss are common. Males are infertile, although sperm counts are normal, with immotile sperm.

Diagnosis

The diagnosis of immotile cilia syndrome may be suspected on the basis of the clinical picture, and it must be emphasized that situs inversus is *not* a necessary finding. A simple screening test may be performed by obtaining scrapings of nasal epithelium and immediately observing for ciliary beat through a microscope. If adequate specimens are obtained and the patient does not have an acute infection, the absence of ciliary beat on repeated testing is presumptive evidence of immotile cilia. (In adult men, sperm also may be examined.) In such a screening test, it is important to obtain sheets of ciliated epithelium rather than isolated cells and to compare the ciliary motility of the specimen with that of control material. Most isolated cells will not be viable and their cilia will not beat. Confirmation of the diagnosis depends on the demonstration of characteristic ciliary ultrastructural abnormalities. No other laboratory findings are diagnostic. Specimens for ultrastructural study may be obtained from the nose or a bronchus.

Patients may have defective mucociliary transport for reasons other than immotile cilia, and the demonstration of normal ciliary beat or normal ciliary ultrastructure does *not* mean that mucociliary function is normal [129].

Treatment

There is no specific treatment that will alter ciliary function in patients with immotile cilia. The bronchopulmonary disease is treated by chest physiotherapy, antibiotics, and bronchodilators as needed. Sinusitis should be treated with antibiotics and drainage if necessary. Attention to the management of upper respiratory tract infections and otitis media should help reduce the complications of conductive hearing loss. When bronchiectasis is localized and severe, excision of involved areas of the lung may be indicated if medical management is insufficient.

Prognosis

The complete spectrum of immotile cilia syndrome is not yet defined. What is clear is that the involvement and severity are quite variable. Patients with Kartagener's syndrome can reach advanced age, and many live a comparatively normal life [7]. The majority of patients appear to develop bronchitis in childhood and to demonstrate findings of airway obstruction after two to three decades. Infections may be most severe in childhood and adolescence, with a partial clinical remission in adult life [32].

Asthma

The familial disposition toward asthma has long been a part of conventional clinical wisdom, but no studies have succeeded in defining the precise role of genetic factors in its pathogenesis [80,104]. The imprecise nature of the definition of asthma emphasizes the diversity of predisposing factors and the difficulty of defining a genetic role. A study of 7000 Swedish twin pairs [30] found that while 4.8 percent of the dizygotic twin pairs were concordant for asthma, 19 percent of the monozygotic twin pairs were concordant. These figures, while helping to establish a genetic role in the pathogenesis of asthma, also indicate that factors other than genetics are probably more important. The genetic basis of asthma is most likely polygenic [40,105].

Cystic Lung Disease (Localized Saccular Bronchiectasis)

Cystic lung disease is a name given to a wide variety of conditions in which bronchiectasis is associated with fluid- or air-filled, sharply defined, round structures that have a definite wall. The cysts are discovered on chest roentgenograms or in anatomic specimens. In most patients, cysts found with the cylindrical variety of bronchiectasis have been related to the syndrome of infectious chronic bronchitis. Localized saccular bronchiectasis, which appears to be a distinct entity, has been described in Sephardic Jews immigrating to Israel [15] and in the Maoris, Polynesian natives of New Zealand [49]. Whether these are examples of genetic lung disease remains a somewhat open question. A recent report suggests that the Polynesian patients with bronchiectatic disease may have deficient dynein arms on their ciliary microtubules [128]. Thus, the disease in the Maoris may have the same basis as the immotile cilia syndrome. This observation lends further credence to the hypothesis that it is a genetic disorder. In the Jewish patients, the striking findings were cylindrical dilatations of the medium-size and small bronchi with cystlike cavities that were usually connected to the bronchi. The cylindrical nature of the bronchiectatic changes strongly suggests that these cases were not the classic, acquired forms of bronchiectasis.

Perhaps the most compelling evidence to support a genetic component in this form of bronchiectasis was the ethnic clustering. In Israel, 92 percent of the patients were found among immigrants from Yemen, Iraq, and Morocco, groups that have been isolated and highly inbred for 2000 years. Jews who emigrated from central and western Europe made up only 8 percent of the patient population. Similar clustering was observed in the Maoris as compared with the Anglo-Saxon immigrant populations of New Zealand. Higher frequencies of a disease in specific population groups suggest a genetic component in its cause if environmental conditions are held constant. Thus far, multiple cases in a family or transmission in two consecutive generations have not been reported. The hypothesis that saccular bronchiectasis has a genetic basis needs to be confirmed by additional studies.

Yellow Nail Syndrome

The association of primary lymphedema with yellow discoloration of the nails has been termed the *yellow nail syndrome* [97]. A third manifestation is unexplained recurrent pleural effusion. Patients studied by lymphangiography show lymphatic abnormalities consisting mostly of lymphatic hypoplasia. Of 12 patients described with this disorder, 5 had bronchiectasis [47]. The recurrent pleural effusions are most likely due to hypoplastic lymphatics. Chronic cough is present in all patients. Dyspnea may be present and is related to the extent of pleural effusion or to bronchiectasis. Lymphedema, pleural effusion, or bronchiectasis may not become evident for years after the nails become yellow. Lymphedema usually occurs before pleural effusions become manifest. The disorder appears to be congenital and may have a genetic component that has yet to be defined [132].

Tracheobronchiomegaly

Mounier-Kuhn [81] presented the first clinical description of tracheobronchiomegaly, a unique syndrome characterized by striking dilatation of the trachea and bronchi. The occurrence of two documented cases in a single family suggests a familial cause, but the genetic basis has not yet been firmly established [57]. Affected individuals show a distinctive clinical and roentgenographic picture consisting of marked dilatation of the trachea and major bronchi associated with chronic respiratory infection [61]. The symptoms of chronic respiratory disease in this condition do not differ from those of a great variety of other respiratory diseases. Patients may have cough, dyspnea, hoarseness, and copious production of purulent sputum. The course is often of long duration, with onset of symptoms in infancy or childhood.

The diagnosis is based on roentgenographic findings. Plain films of the chest may reveal the width of the tracheal air column to be equal to that of the vertebra. Bronchographic findings are pathognomonic, confirming the unusual width of the trachea and bronchi, with saclike recesses containing pools of contrast material. Computed tomography is a convenient and noninvasive method to confirm the diagnosis [140]. The size of the trachea and bronchi in adults deviates by more than 3 standard deviations from that in normal adults [57,90]. Similar data are now available for infants and young children [42,43]. Occasionally, cystic changes in the peripheral bronchi are noted on bronchograms.

The pathogenesis of tracheobronchiomegaly is not known, but it has been speculated that it is caused by a sparsity of elastic and muscular fibers in the airway walls. It is of interest that the syndrome has been reported in a patient with the Ehlers-Danlos syndrome [1]. Acquired forms of tracheobronchiomegaly may be related to prolonged respiratory support with positive pressure ventilation [58].

The incidence of tracheobronchiomegaly in the general population is unknown. Six cases were discovered in a series of 1200 adults undergoing bronchography for chronic pulmonary disease [35]. Treatment measures include chest physiotherapy to improve clearance of secretions and prompt treatment of infections. If pulmonary clearance of secretions can be maintained, the prognosis is relatively good, but if there are recurrent infections, the prognosis is poor [16,57].

Other Forms of Airways Disease with Possible Genetic Bases

Williams and Campbell [133] described a group of patients with bronchiectasis due to a generalized deficiency of bronchial cartilages. The clinical picture is characterized by persistent cough and wheezing, digital clubbing, chest deformities, and short stature. In the original reports [133,134], no familial pattern was seen, but more recently two siblings with this syndrome have been reported

[130]. Recurrent respiratory infections are the rule in these patients, and pulmonary function studies reveal marked air trapping and airway obstruction on expiration. Bronchographic studies demonstrate ballooning of the bronchi during inspiration and collapse during exhalation. Approximately 25 percent of the reported patients died before age 5, and most of the remainder have chronic pulmonary disease with persistent symptoms. Treatment is the same as for other forms of bronchiectasis.

At least one sibship has been reported in which four or five siblings had symptomatic bronchiectasis of the right middle lobe [25].

Generalized bronchomalacia without bronchiectasis has been reported on a familial basis [6]. Laryngomalacia also has been reported to have a familial pattern [101]. One family has been reported in which two siblings had severe tracheal obstruction due to an anomalous innominate artery, requiring emergency surgery [79]. Two sets of siblings with nasal polyps in infancy, aplasia of the nasal sinuses, and bronchiectasis have been described [62]. This condition has been termed *Woake's syndrome*.

There are a number of familial immunologic disorders that lead to sinopulmonary infection and bronchiectasis [27,46] (see Chap. 26). Esophageal atresia with associated tracheoesophageal fistula has been reported to occur in families, including two generations [33]. Infants with bronchopulmonary dysplasia may have a higher proportion of first-degree relatives with asthma than infants with normal lungs [82]. It is possible that infants with a genetic predisposition toward reactive airways may respond adversely to neonatal insults, with consequent development of permanent airways disease.

References

1. Aaby GC, Blake HA. Tracheobronchiomegaly. *Ann Thorac Surg* 2:64, 1966.
2. Afzelius BA. A human syndrome caused by immotile cilia. *Science* 193:317, 1976.
3. Afzelius BA. The immotile-cilia syndrome and other ciliary diseases. *Int Rev Exp Pathol* 19:1, 1979.
4. Afzelius BA, Eliasson R. Flagellar mutants in man: On the heterogeneity of the immotile-cilia syndrome. *J Ultrastruct Res* 69:43, 1979.
5. Afzelius BA, et al. Lack of dynein arms in immotile human spermatozoa. *J Cell Biol* 66:222, 1975.
6. Agosti E, et al. Generalized familial bronchomalacia. *Acta Pediatr Scand* 63:616, 1974.

7. Amjad H, Richburg F, Adler E. Kartagener syndrome: Case report in an elderly man. *JAMA* 227:1420, 1974.

8. Amos JA, Janes SR, Erbe RW. DNA analysis of cystic fibrosis genotypes in relatives with equivocal sweat test results. *Clin Invest Med* 13:1, 1990.

9. Andersen DH. Cystic fibrosis of the pancreas and its relation to celiac disease: A clinical and pathologic study. *Am J Dis Child* 56:344, 1938.

10. Anderson MP, et al. Demonstration that CFTR is a chloride channel by alteration of its anion selectivity. *Science* 253:202, 1991.

11. Arge E. Transposition of the viscera and sterility in men. *Lancet* 1:412, 1960.

12. Auerbach HS. The use of steroids in cystic fibrosis. *Antibiot Chemother* 42:254, 1989.

13. Auerbach HS, et al. Alternate-day prednisone reduces morbidity and improves pulmonary function in cystic fibrosis. *Lancet* 2:686, 1985.

14. Bardon A. Cystic fibrosis. Carbohydrate metabolism in CF and in animal models for CF. *Acta Paediatr Scand Suppl* 332:1, 1987.

15. Baum GL, et al. Cystic disease of the lung: Report of 88 cases, with ethnologic relationship. *Am J Med* 40:578, 1966.

16. Beachly MD, Ghahremani GD. Tracheobronchiomegaly (Mounier-Kuhn syndrome). *South Med J* 69:1228, 1976.

17. Boucher RC. Drug therapy in the 1990's. What can we expect for cystic fibrosis? *Drugs* 43:431, 1992.

18. Camner P, Mossberg B, Afzelius BA. Evidence for congenitally nonfunctioning cilia in the tracheobronchial tree in two subjects. *Am Rev Respir Dis* 112:807, 1975.

19. Carson JL, Collier AM, Hu SS. Acquired ciliary defects in nasal epithelium of children with acute viral upper respiratory infections. *N Engl J Med* 312:463, 1985.

20. Cheng PW, et al. Increased sulfation of glycoconjugates by cultured nasal epithelial cells from patients with cystic fibrosis. *J Clin Invest* 84:68, 1989.

21. Cockayne EA. The genetics of transposition of the viscera. *Q J Med* 7:479, 1938.

22. Colombo C, et al. Effects of ursodeoxycholic acid therapy for liver disease associated with cystic fibrosis. *J Pediatr* 117:482, 1990.

23. Corey M, et al. Improved prognosis in CF patients with normal fat absorption. *J Pediatr Gastroenterol Nutr* 3(Suppl 1):S99, 1984.

24. Crossley JR, Elliott RB, Smith PA. Dried-blood spot screening for cystic fibrosis in the newborn. *Lancet* 1:472, 1979.

25. Danielson GK, Hanson CW, Cooper EC. Middle lobe bronchiectasis. Report of an unusual familial occurrence. *JAMA* 201:111, 1967.

26. Davis PB, et al. Sweat chloride concentration in adults with pulmonary diseases. *Am Rev Respir Dis* 128:34, 1983.

27. Davis PB, et al. Familial bronchiectasis. *J Pediatr* 102:177, 1983.

28. Denning CR, et al. Cooperative study comparing three methods of performing sweat tests to diagnose cystic fibrosis. *Pediatrics* 66:752, 1980.

28a. Denning GM, et al. Localization of cystic fibrosis transmembrane conductance regulator in chloride secretory epithelia. *J Clin Invest* 89:339, 1992.

29. Durie PR. The pathophysiology of the pancreatic defect in cystic fibrosis. *Acta Paediatr Scand Suppl* 363:41, 1989.

30. Edfors-Lubs ML. Allergy in 7000 twin pairs. *Acta Allergol* 26:249, 1971.

31. Egan TM, et al. Isolated lung transplantation for end-stage lung disease: A viable therapy. *Ann Thorac Surg* 53:590, 1992.

32. Eliasson R, et al. The immotile-cilia syndrome, a congenital ciliary abnormality as an etiologic factor in chronic airway infections and male sterility. *N Engl J Med* 297:1, 1977.

33. Erichsen G, et al. Two-generation transmission of oesophageal atresia with tracheo-oesophageal fistula. *Acta Paediatr Scand* 70:253, 1981.

34. Esterly JR, Oppenheimer EH. Observations in cystic fibrosis of the pancreas. 3. Pulmonary lesions. *Johns Hopkins Med J* 122:94, 1968.

35. Fisher F, et al. Tracheobronchiomegaly. *Scand J Respir Dis* 50:147, 1969.

36. Franckx J, Shmerling DH. The use of sweat osmolality in the diagnosis of cystic fibrosis. *Helv Paediatr Acta* 39:347, 1984.

37. Gaskin KJ. The impact of nutrition in cystic fibrosis: A review. *J Pediatr Gastroenterol Nutr* 7(Suppl 1):S12, 1988.

38. Green MN, Shwachman H. Presumptive tests for cystic fibrosis based on serum protein in meconium. *Pediatrics* 41:989, 1968.

39. Greenstone M, et al. Primary ciliary dyskinesia: Cytological and clinical features. *Q J Med* 67:405, 1988.

40. Gregg I. Environmental Aspects of Asthma. In TJH Clark, S Godfrey (Eds), *Asthma*, (2nd ed). London: Chapman and Hall, 1980. P 242.

41. Gregory RJ, et al. Expression and characterization of the cystic fibrosis transmembrane conductance regulator. *Nature* 347:382, 1990.

42. Griscom NT. CT measurement of the tracheal lumen in children and adolescents. *AJR* 156:371, 1991.

43. Griscom NT, Wohl ME, Fenton T. Dimensions of the trachea to age 6 years related to height. *Pediatr Pulmonol* 6:186, 1989.

44. Hall SK, Stableforth DE, Green A. Sweat sodium and chloride concentrations—Essential criteria for the diagnosis of cystic fibrosis in adults. *Ann Clin Biochem* 27:318, 1990.

45. Hein J, Wiersbitzky S, Wunderlich P. [Broncho-pulmonary infections in mucoviscidosis]. *Z Erkr Atmungsorgane* 170:201, 1988.

46. Heiner DC, Myers A, Beck CS. Deficiency of IgG$_4$: A disorder associated with frequent infections and bronchiectasis that may be familial. *Clin Rev Allergy* 1:259, 1983.

47. Heller E, Rosenow EC, Olsen AM. Pulmonary manifestations of the yellow nail syndrome. *Chest* 61:452, 1972.

48. Herzon FS. Upper respiratory tract ciliary ultrastructural pathology. *Ann Otol Rhinol Laryngol Suppl* 83:1, 1981.

49. Hinds JR. Bronchiectasis in the Maori. *NZ Med J* 57:328, 1958.

50. Hoiby N. Epidemiological investigations of the respiratory tract bacteriology in patients with cystic fibrosis. *Acta Pathol Microbiol Scand [B]* 82:541, 1974.

51. Holmes LB, Blennerhassett JR, Austin KF. A reappraisal of Kartagener's syndrome. *Am J Med* 255:13, 1968.

52. Holsclaw DH, Eckstein HB, Nixon HH. Meconium ileus: A 20 year review of 109 cases. *Am J Dis Child* 109:101, 1965.

53. Holsclaw DS, Grand RJ, Shwachman H. Massive hemoptysis in cystic fibrosis. *J Pediatr* 76:829, 1970.

54. Horrevorts AM, et al. Pharmacokinetics of antimicrobial drugs in cystic fibrosis. Aminoglycoside antibiotics. *Chest* 94:120S, 1988.

55. Hunton DB, Long WK, Tsumagari HY. Meconium ileus equivalent: An adult complication of fibrocystic disease. *Gastroenterology* 50:99, 1966.

56. Hutabarat RM, et al. Disposition of drugs in cystic fibrosis. I. Sulfamethoxazole and trimethoprim. *Clin Pharmacol Ther* 49:402, 1991.

57. Johnston RF, Green RA. Tracheobronchiomegaly. Report of five cases and demonstration of familial occurrence. *Am Rev Respir Dis* 91:35, 1965.

58. Karsh S, Mahboubi S. Tracheomegaly in children. *Clin Imaging* 13:77, 1989.

59. Kartagener M. Bronchiektasien bei situs inversus. *Beitr Klin Erforsch Tuberk* 83:489, 1933.

60. Kartner N, et al. Expression of the cystic fibrosis gene in non-epithelial invertebrate cells produces a regulated anion conductance. *Cell* 64:681, 1991.

61. Katz I, LeVine M, Herman P. Tracheobronchiomegaly. The Mounier-Kuhn syndrome. *AJR* 88:1084, 1963.

62. Kellerhals B, Uthemann B. Woakes' syndrome: The problems of infantile nasal polyps. *Int J Pediatr Otorhinolaryngol* 1:79, 1979.

63. Kerem B, et al. Identification of the cystic fibrosis gene: Genetic analysis. *Science* 245:1073, 1989.

64. Kerem E, et al. Prediction of mortality in patients with cystic fibrosis. *N Engl J Med* 326:1187, 1992.

65. Knowles M, Gatzy J, Boucher R. Increased bioelectric potential difference across respiratory epithelia in cystic fibrosis. *N Engl J Med* 305:1489, 1981.

66. Knowles MR, et al. Mild cystic fibrosis in a consanguineous family. *Ann Intern Med* 110:599, 1989.

67. Knowles MR, et al. A pilot study of aerosolized amiloride for the treatment of lung disease in cystic fibrosis. *N Engl J Med* 322:1189, 1990.

68. Knowles MR, Clarke LL, Boucher RC. Activation by extracellular nucleotides of chloride secretion in the airway epithelia of patients with cystic fibrosis. *N Engl J Med* 325:533, 1991.

69. Knowles MR, et al. Abnormal respiratory epithelial ion transport in cystic fibrosis. *Clin Chest Med* 7:285, 1986.

70. Kollberg H, et al. Cystic fibrosis compared with the immotile-cilia syndrome: A study of mucociliary clearance, ciliary ultrastructure, clinical picture and ventilatory function. *Scand J Respir Dis* 59:297, 1978.

71. Konstan MW, Vargo KM, Davis PB. Ibuprofen attenuates the inflammatory response to *Pseudomonas aeruginosa* in a rat model of chronic pulmonary infection. Implications for antiinflammatory therapy in cystic fibrosis. *Am Rev Respir Dis* 141:186, 1990.

72. Kulczycki LL, Schauf V. Cystic fibrosis in blacks in Washington, DC: Incidence and characteristics. *Am J Dis Child* 127:64, 1974.

73. Laughlin JJ, Brady MS, Eigen H. Changing feeding trends as a cause of electrolyte depletion in infants with cystic fibrosis. *Pediatrics* 68:203, 1981.

73a. LeGrys VA, Wood RE. Incidence and implications of false-negative sweat test reports in patients with cystic fibrosis. *Pediatr Pulmonol* 4:169, 1988.

74. Lloyd Still JD, Khaw KT, Shwachman H. Severe respiratory disease in infants with cystic fibrosis. *Pediatrics* 53:678, 1974.

75. Marino CR, et al. Localization of the cystic fibrosis transmembrane conductance regulator in pancreas. *J Clin Invest* 88:712, 1991.

76. May JR, Herrick NC, Thompson D. Bacterial infection in cystic fibrosis. *Arch Dis Child* 47:908, 1972.

77. McPartlin JF, Dickson JA, Swain VA. The use of Gastrografin in the relief of residual and late bowel obstruction in cystic fibrosis. *Br J Surg* 60:707, 1973.

78. Mearns MB, Hunt GH, Rushworth R. Bacterial flora of respiratory tract in patients with cystic fibrosis, 1950–71. *Arch Dis Child* 47:902, 1972.

79. Mok JY, Simpson H. Tracheal compression by

an anomalous innominate artery: Report of two cases in a family. *Arch Dis Child* 56:791, 1981.

80. Morrison J, Higenbottam T. The molecular genetics of atopy. *Ann Med* 23:21, 1991.
81. Mounier-Kuhn P. Dilatation de al trachee: Constations radiographiques et bronchoscopiques. *Lyon Med* 150:106, 1932.
82. Nickerson BG, Taussig LM. Family history of asthma in infants with bronchopulmonary dysplasia. *Pediatrics* 65:1140, 1980.
83. Nussbaum E, et al. Cystic fibrosis with acute hypoelectrolytemia and metabolic alkalosis in infancy. *Am J Dis Child* 133:965, 1979.
84. O'Mahony MS, FitzGerald MX. Cystic fibrosis and seizures. *Lancet* 338:259, 1991.
85. Oppenheimer EH. Similarity of the tracheobronchial mucous glands and epithelium in infants with and without cystic fibrosis. *Hum Pathol* 12:36, 1981.
86. Oppenheimer EH, Esterly JR. Observations on cystic fibrosis of the pancreas. V. Developmental changes in the male genital system. *J Pediatr* 75:806, 1969.
87. Oppenheimer EH, Esterly JR. Observations on cystic fibrosis of the pancreas. VI. The uterine cervix. *J Pediatr* 77:991, 1970.
88. Pattishall EN. Longitudinal response of pulmonary function to bronchodilators in cystic fibrosis. *Pediatr Pulmonol* 9:80, 1990.
89. Pederson H, Mygind N. Absence of axonemal arms in nasal cilia in Kartagener's syndrome. *Nature* 262:494, 1976.
90. Rahbar M, Tabatabai D. Tracheobronchiomegaly. *Br J Dis Chest* 65:66, 1971.
91. *Report of the Patient Registry, 1978*. Rockville, MD: Cystic Fibrosis Foundation, 1980.
92. Riordan JR, et al. Identification of the cystic fibrosis gene: Cloning and characterization of complementary DNA. *Science* 245:1066, 1989.
93. Rock MJ, et al. Newborn screening for cystic fibrosis is complicated by age-related decline in immunoreactive trypsinogen levels. *Pediatrics* 85:1001, 1990.
94. Romeo G, Devoto M, Galietta LJ. Why is the cystic fibrosis gene so frequent? *Hum Genet* 84:1, 1989.
95. Rommens JM, et al. Identification of the cystic fibrosis gene: Chromosome walking and jumping. *Science* 245:1059, 1989.
96. Rossman CM, et al. The dyskinetic cilia syndrome: Ciliary motility in the immotile cilia syndrome. *Chest* 78:580, 1980.
97. Sammon PD, White WF. The yellow nail syndrome. *BR J Dermatol* 76:153, 1964.
98. Satir P. How cilia move. *Sci Am* 231:44, 1974.
99. Sato K, Sato F. Defective beta adrenergic response of cystic fibrosis sweat glands in vivo and in vitro. *J Clin Invest* 73:1763, 1984.
100. Shak S, et al. Recombinant human DNase I reduces the viscosity of cystic fibrosis sputum. *Proc Natl Acad Sci USA* 87:9188, 1990.
101. Shulman JB, et al. Familial laryngomalacia: A case report. *Laryngoscope* 86:84, 1976.
102. Shwachman H, Lebenthal E, Khaw KT. Recurrent acute pancreatitis in patients with cystic fibrosis with normal pancreatic enzymes. *Pediatrics* 55:86, 1975.
103. Shwachman H, Mahmoodian A, Neff RK. The sweat test: Sodium and chloride values. *J Pediatr* 98:576, 1981.
104. Sibbald B, et al. Genetics of asthma and atopy: An overview. *Clin Exp Allergy* 21:178, 1991.
105. Sibbald B, et al. Genetic factors in childhood asthma. *Thorax* 35:671, 1980.
106. Smith AL, et al. Safety of aerosol tobramycin administration for 3 months to patients with cystic fibrosis. *Pediatr Pulmonol* 7:265, 1989.
107. Steinberg AG, Brown DC. On the incidence of cystic fibrosis of the pancreas. *Am J Hum Genet* 12:416, 1960.
108. Stephan U, et al. Cystic fibrosis detection by means of a test-strip. *Pediatrics* 55:35, 1975.
109. Stern RC, et al. Intermediate range sweat chloride concentration and pseudomonas bronchitis. A cystic fibrosis variant with preservation of exocrine pancreatic function. *JAMA* 239:2676, 1978.
110. Stern RC, et al. Cystic fibrosis diagnosed after age 13. Twenty-five teenage and adult patients including three asymptomatic men. *Ann Intern Med* 87:188, 1977.
111. Stern RC, et al. Treatment and prognosis of lobar and segmental atelectasis in cystic fibrosis. *Am Rev Respir Dis* 118:821, 1978.
112. Stern RC, et al. Treatment and prognosis of nasal polyps in cystic fibrosis. *Am J Dis Child* 136:1067, 1982.
113. Stern RC, et al. Heart failure in cystic fibrosis. Treatment and prognosis of cor pulmonale with failure of the right side of the heart. *Am J Dis Child* 134:267, 1980.
114. Stern RC, et al. Treatment and prognosis of rectal prolapse in cystic fibrosis. *Gastroenterology* 82:707, 1982.
115. Stern RC, et al. Symptomatic hepatic disease in cystic fibrosis: Incidence, course, and outcome of portal systemic hunting. *Gastroenterology* 70:645, 1976.
116. Stern RC, et al. Treatment and prognosis of massive hemoptysis in cystic fibrosis. *Am Rev Respir Dis* 117:825, 1978.
117. Stowe SM, et al. Open thoracotomy for pneumothorax in cystic fibrosis. *Am Rev Respir Dis* 111:611, 1975.
118. Sturgess JM, et al. Genetic aspects of immotile cilia syndrome. *Am J Med Genet* 25:149, 1986.
119. Super M. Cystic fibrosis in the South West African Afrikaner. An example of population drift,

possibly with heterozygote advantage. *S Afr Med J* 49:818, 1975.

120. Symon DN, Stewart L, Russell G. Abnormally high sweat osmolality in children with Down's syndrome. *J Ment Defic Res* 29:257, 1985.

121. Taussig LM, et al. Fertility in males with cystic fibrosis. *N Engl J Med* 287:586, 1972.

122. Thomassen MJ, et al. *Pseudomonas cepacia* colonization among patients with cystic fibrosis. A new opportunist. *Am Rev Respir Dis* 131:791, 1985.

123. Tizzano EF, Buchwald M. Cystic fibrosis: Beyond the gene to therapy. *J Pediatr* 120:337, 1992.

124. Tomashefski JFJ, et al. The pathologic characteristics of interstitial pneumonia cystic fibrosis. A retrospective autopsy study. *Am J Clin Pathol* 91:522, 1989.

125. Torgersen J. Transposition of the viscera, bronchiectasis and nasal polyps. *Acta Radiol* 28:17, 1947.

126. Trulock EP, et al. The Washington University-Barnes Hospital experience with lung transplantation. Washington University Lung Transplantation Group. *JAMA* 266:1943, 1991.

127. Turner JAP, et al. Clinical expressions of immotile cilia syndrome. *Pediatrics* 67:805, 1981.

128. Waite D, et al. Cilia and sperm tail abnormalities in Polynesian bronchiectatics. *Lancet* 2:132, 1978.

129. Wanner A. State of the art: Clinical aspects of mucociliary transport. *Am Rev Respir Dis* 116:73, 1977.

130. Wayne KS, Taussig LM. Probable familial congenital bronchiectasis due to cartilage deficiency (Williams-Campbell syndrome). *Am Rev Respir Dis* 114:15, 1976.

131. Webster HL. Laboratory diagnosis of cystic fibrosis. *CRC Crit Rev Clin Lab Sci* 18:313, 1983.

132. Wells GC. Yellow nail syndrome with familial primary hypoplasia of lymphatics, manifest late in life. *Proc R Soc Med* 59:447, 1966.

133. Williams HE, Campbell P. Generalized bronchiectasis associated with deficiency of cartilage in the bronchial tree. *Arch Dis Child* 35:182, 1960.

134. Williams HE, Landau LI, Phelan PD. Generalized bronchiectasis due to extensive deficiency of bronchial cartilage. *Arch Dis Child* 47:423, 1972.

135. Wood A, et al. Airway mucosal bioelectric potential difference in cystic fibrosis after lung transplantation. *Am Rev Respir Dis* 140:1645, 1989.

136. Wood RE. Prognosis. In LM Taussig (Ed), *Cystic Fibrosis*. New York: Thieme-Stratton, 1984. Pp 434–460.

137. Wood RE. Treatment of CF lung disease in the first two years. *Pediatr Pulmonol Suppl* 4:68, 1989.

138. Wood RE, Boat TF, Doershuk CF. Cystic fibrosis. *Am Rev Respir Dis* 113:833, 1976.

139. Wood RE, et al. Tracheal mucociliary transport in patients with cystic fibrosis and its stimulation by terbutaline. *Am Rev Respir Dis* 111:733, 1975.

140. Woodring JH, Howard RS II, Rehm SR. Congenital tracheobronchomegaly (Mounier-Kuhn syndrome): A report of 10 cases and review of the literature. *J Thorac Imaging* 6:1, 1991.

141. Worldwide survey of the delta F508 mutation—Report from the Cystic Fibrosis Genetic Analysis Consortium. *Am J Hum Genet* 47:354, 1990.

142. Zuelzer WW, Newton WA. The pathogenesis of fibrocystic disease of the pancreas: A study of 36 cases with special reference to the pulmonary lesions. *Pediatrics* 4:53, 1949.

70

Genetic Diseases of the Pulmonary Parenchyma

Arthur B. Zinn

This chapter presents a discussion of a heterogeneous group of genetic disorders that cause parenchymal pulmonary disease. Alpha$_1$-antitrypsin deficiency receives the most attention because of its relative significance as a cause of pulmonary disease and because of the relative amount of information available about it. Familial pulmonary fibrosis, familial alveolar microlithiasis, familial spontaneous pneumothorax, Hermansky-Pudlak syndrome, and two phakomatoses, neurofibromatosis and tuberous sclerosis, are also discussed.

Alpha$_1$-Antitrypsin Deficiency

In 1963, Laurell and Eriksson [105] reported an association between the development of a severe form of emphysema and deficiency of serum alpha$_1$-antitrypsin. Eriksson [50,51] went on to establish that alpha$_1$-antitrypsin deficiency is genetically determined and causally related to the development of emphysema. Subsequent work has shown that alpha$_1$-antitrypsin deficiency is an important clinical disorder, responsible for perhaps as many as 100,000 cases of emphysema in the United States. This represents about 2 percent of the total number of patients with emphysema in this country. The molecular basis and pathophysiology of this disorder have been identified, and recent clinical trials have suggested that it may be possible to treat this disease by alpha$_1$-antitrypsin replacement. In broader terms, alpha$_1$-antitrypsin deficiency is important because it provides insight into the pathogenesis of other forms of emphysema. Several excellent reviews of alpha$_1$-antitrypsin deficiency have appeared in recent years [19,33,38,39,52,56,111,128].

Molecular Basis

Alpha$_1$-antitrypsin is a glycoprotein that derives its name from the fact that it migrates as an alpha$_1$ globulin in the electrophoretic analysis of serum proteins and is an inhibitor of the proteolytic activity of trypsin. Subsequent studies demonstrated that alpha$_1$-antitrypsin inhibits a broad range of serine proteases and could more correctly be termed *alpha$_1$-antiprotease*. However, historical precedent has prevailed over biochemical accuracy and the original name has persisted. About 90 percent of the alpha$_1$-globulin fraction is alpha$_1$-antitrypsin.

Alpha$_1$-antitrypsin is produced primarily by hepatocytes, but small amounts are also produced by macrophages and neutrophils. The primary role of the liver in alpha$_1$-antitrypsin production has been demonstrated in a variety of ways. The most dramatic demonstration has been provided by the transition of alpha$_1$-antitrypsin phenotype in patients with alpha$_1$-antitrypsin deficiency who have undergone liver transplantation. The physiologic role of alpha$_1$-antitrypsin produced by other cells is uncertain.

The gene encoding for alpha$_1$-antitrypsin has been mapped to band q32.1 on the long arm of chromosome 14 [33,41]. The alpha$_1$-antitrypsin–coding region is 10.2 kb in length and contains four exons [33,38,103]. There appears to be a different pattern of transcription in liver compared to macrophages and neutrophils [33,39]. A homologous gene encoding for the related protease inhibitor, alpha$_1$-antichymotrypsin, is located close to the alpha$_1$-antitrypsin gene on chromosome 14; the physiologic role of alpha$_1$-antichymotrypsin has not been established.

The alpha$_1$-antitrypsin gene encodes for a

418–amino acid residue polypeptide [33,39]. The amino terminus of the polypeptide contains a 24-residue sequence which serves as a signal sequence that directs its transport through the rough endoplasmic reticulum. The signal sequence is cleaved during the recognition and transport process, producing a mature protein with 394 amino acid residues [33,39]. Three carbohydrate side chains are attached during passage through the endoplasmic reticulum. The mature protein has a molecular mass of about 52,000 daltons and contains 12% carbohydrate. The half-life of circulating alpha$_1$-antitrypsin is 4 to 5 days.

Alpha$_1$-antitrypsin is a highly polymorphic protein, for which more than 75 variants have been described [33,38,56,111]. These variants have been resolved by a variety of electrophoretic systems and named according to their relative mobilities in these electrophoretic systems. The different electrophoretic variants are referred to as *protease inhibitor* (designated as *Pi* or *PI*) types. Faster migrating variants (i.e., more anodal) are designated with letters nearer the beginning of the alphabet than are variants that move more slowly. There are two systems of nomenclature currently in use for designating the genotype and phenotype of alpha$_1$-antitrypsin variants.

The first system was introduced about 20 years ago. In this system, the allele encoding for each variant is designated as "Pi" with the appropriate alphabetic superscript. For example, the allele that encodes for the most common *M* variant is designated Pi^M. Since alpha$_1$-antitrypsin alleles are codominantly expressed, Pi genotypes must include designations for both parental alleles. For example, the genotype of an individual who is homozygous for the Pi^M allele is designated Pi^M/Pi^M. Phenotype is designated as "Pi" followed by capital letters corresponding to the appropriate genotype. Accordingly, the phenotype of an individual homozygous for the *M* allele is Pi MM. There are rare alleles for which no protein can be found in serum; these alleles are designated as *null* alleles, designated Pi^{null}. Subtypes of electrophoretically indistinguishable variants are designated by the electrophoretic variant followed by a subscript indicating the geographic origin of the first patient identified with that mutation (e.g., M$_{mineral springs}$ or null$_{bellingham}$).

The more recently introduced system of nomenclature [33] refers to the various alpha$_1$-antitrypsin variants as the PI locus. Each allele is designated by the symbol "PI*" followed by a capital letter referring to the electrophoretic mobility (e.g., PI*M). Phenotypes are designated as in the first system except that "PI" is substituted for "Pi" (e.g., PI MM). *Null* mutations are designated as QO alleles, with the individual mutation shown as a subscript (e.g., genotype, PI*QO$_{bellingham}$; phenotype, PI QO$_{bellingham}$). The first system of nomenclature appears to be used more commonly than the second, and is adopted for use in this text.

The Pi MM phenotype is the most common pattern found in different populations; it has been observed in more than 90 percent of individuals from all ethnic groups examined [56,111]. About 92 percent of Caucasians in the United States are Pi MM. There are four "normal" subtypes of Pi^M that do not produce a deficiency state. These variants are designated as M1(val^{213}), M1(ala^{213}), M2, and M3, where "val^{213}" and "ala^{213}" designate the amino acid difference between the M1 variants. There are other *M* variants (e.g., M$_{malton}$) that are associated with clinically significant deficiencies.

The most common abnormal variants are encoded by the *S* and *Z* alleles. The *S* allele is found most commonly in southern European populations. In Spain and Portugal, for example, the gene frequencies are 0.112 and 0.141, respectively, compared to 0.023 in Norwegians [56,111]. The *S* allele is less common in blacks and Orientals. Approximately 8 percent of Caucasian Americans carry the *S* allele. The *Z* allele is most frequent in individuals from Scandinavian backgrounds, less frequent in individuals from southern European backgrounds, and rare in African blacks, Orientals, and Native Americans. The gene frequency of the *Z* allele in the Norwegian population, for example, is approximately 0.016 [56,111]. These observations suggest a single site of origin for the *Z* allele, with subsequent geographic migration. The molecular biologic studies of Cox and colleagues [37] support this suggestion. Approximately 3 percent of Caucasian Americans are heterozygous for the *Z* allele. *Null* alleles account for less than 1 percent of all abnormal alleles, with individual gene frequencies on the order of 1 in 10,000. Based on these gene frequencies, about 1 in 3500 white Americans are homozygous for the *Z* allele (Pi ZZ) and 1 in 800 have a Pi SZ phenotype.

Primary-sequence studies of the peptide component of the normal *M* alleles and the most common abnormal variants, *S* and *Z*, have shown that the variants differ from one of the *M* variants by a single amino acid substitution. The *S* protein contains valine in place of glutamic acid at residue 264 [136,190], whereas the *Z* protein contains lysine in place of glutamic acid at residue 342 [137,191]. The biochemical basis of many other abnormal variants has been defined in recent years. These too, for the most part, are caused by single amino acid substitutions. Some of the rare Pi[null] alleles are caused by other mechanisms, which have been explained only since the advent of advances in genetic analysis of the Pi locus.

Within the past several years, the molecular basis of alpha$_1$-antitrypsin deficiency has been defined at the genomic level. All of the normal *M* variants and most of the abnormal variants identified to date are the result of point mutations. The *S* and *Z* alleles are associated with single base pair missense mutations, which produce single amino acid substitutions. The *S* and *Z* alleles result from G → A and A → T substitutions, respectively [33,39,103]. The *S* protein is derived from the M1(val^{213}) variant; the *Z* protein is derived from M1(ala^{213}) variant [33,39]. The *null* mutations are caused either by point mutations leading to severe alterations in translation (e.g., premature stop codons) or by gene deletions/insertions [33,39]. Thus, there is now abundant evidence that alpha$_1$-antitrypsin deficiency is a genetically heterogeneous disorder.

Table 70-1 lists a summary of the six pathogenetic mechanisms that have been shown to produce clinically significant alpha$_1$-antitrypsin deficiency. In mechanism one, severe deficiency is caused by large deletions of the alpha$_1$-antitrypsin gene. The null$_{isola\ di\ procida}$ allele is an example of this type of mutation [38]. In mechanism two, the mutation (e.g., null$_{bellingham}$) permits transcription to occur, but the transcript is unstable and is degraded before significant amounts of protein can be produced. In mechanism three, the mutations permit normal transcription and translation, but yield a protein that is not secreted from the liver. The most common example of this class of mutation is the *Z* allele; the M$_{duarte}$ and M$_{malton}$ alleles are less common examples. In the case of the *Z* allele, the amino acid substitution alters posttranslational modification and interferes with secretion, resulting in accumulation of the protein in intracellular globules within the liver and reduction in its serum concentration [91,154,193]. In mechanism four, a mutant protein that has a decreased half-life is produced. The *S* variant is thought to have reduced protein stability and an increased rate of degradation. In mechanism five, the mutation leads to production of a protein with reduced catalytic activity (e.g., M$_{mineral\ springs}$). Lastly, in mechanism six, the abnormal protein has an altered substrate specificity. The only known example of this mechanism is Pi Pittsburgh, in which there is an enhanced substrate specificity for thrombin producing a clinical disorder characterized by an increased bleeding tendency rather than pulmonary or hepatic disease [136].

Thus, alpha$_1$-antitrypsin deficiency can result from a variety of genetic mechanisms. Except in the rare case of a protein with altered substrate specificity, the mutation results in a deficiency of alpha$_1$-antitrypsin in the lungs, leading to emphysema. Rare mutations result in the accumulation of alpha$_1$-antitrypsin in liver as well as a paucity of alpha$_1$-antitrypsin in the lungs; patients with these mutations have an increased predisposition for hepatic disease and emphysema.

Pathogenesis

Alpha$_1$-antitrypsin is a broadly specific inhibitor of serine proteases, including trypsin, chymotrypsin, plasmin, thrombin, various bacterial and plant proteases, kallikrein, and the neutrophil proteases elastase and collagenase [87,173]. Given this range of activity, alpha$_1$-antitrypsin might be more aptly named *alpha$_1$-antiprotease*. However, its physiologic role appears to be more circumscribed. Alpha$_1$-antitrypsin serves primarily as an inhibitor of neutrophil elastase. Neutrophil proteases digest the debris of cellular and inflammatory exudates within the pulmonary parenchyma. Alpha$_1$-antitrypsin protects the lung parenchyma from uncontrolled proteolytic activity by these proteases. Hence, there is a balance between protease and antiprotease activity. In alpha$_1$-antitrypsin deficiency, the protease-anti-

Table 70-1. Genetic mechanisms that can produce clinically significant alpha$_1$-antitrypsin deficiency

Pathogenetic mechanism	Example
Major gene deletion	Null$_{isola\ di\ procida}$
Increased rate of mRNA degradation	Null$_{bellingham}$
Protein is not secreted from liver	*Z*
Increased intracellular protein degradation	*S*
Protein has reduced catalytic activity	M$_{mineral\ springs}$
Protein has altered substrate specificity	Pittsburgh

protease balance (or, more correctly, the elastase-antielastase balance) is disturbed, leading to excessive proteolytic activity and alveolar damage.

The protease-antiprotease theory for the pathogenesis of alpha$_1$-antitrypsin deficiency is supported by several lines of work [33,87,111]. First, alpha$_1$-antitrypsin is a highly effective inhibitor of neutrophil elastase and other proteases [173]. Second, elastin is destroyed in the alveolar wall of patients with alpha$_1$-antitrypsin deficiency. Third, leukocytic proteases extracted from purulent sputum digest both human and hamster lung tissue, and human serum strongly inhibits these proteases [86,112]. Fourth, elastase produces emphysema when administered intratracheally to animals, whereas concurrent administration of alpha$_1$-antitrypsin prevents the development of emphysema [95]. Fifth, serum levels of alpha$_1$-antitrypsin provide an accurate reflection of protein levels within the lungs of normal and deficient patients. The concentration of alpha$_1$-antitrypsin in the epithelial lining fluid of the lung is approximately 10 to 15 percent of the serum concentration [183]. Finally, other proteases with which alpha$_1$-antitrypsin interacts, such as those of the blood clotting system, are not deranged in patients with alpha$_1$-antitrypsin deficiency.

The protease-antiprotease theory also provides the basis for understanding the pathogenesis of other forms of emphysema, including the most common form associated with cigarette smoking. Other forms of emphysema may be associated with disturbances on either side of the balance. In alpha$_1$-antitrypsin deficiency, it is the antiprotease component of the balance that is compromised. Cigarette smoking appears to be associated with disturbances of both sides, thereby explaining its role as a cause of emphysema and why it serves to hasten the deterioration of patients with alpha$_1$-antitrypsin deficiency. Cigarette smoking increases the levels of protease activity in the alveoli by causing alveolar macrophages to release neutrophil chemoattractants and by stimulating the release of proteases by the neutrophil [15,87]. On the other side of the balance, the neutrophil also releases oxidants that oxidize the methionine in the active site of alpha$_1$-antitrypsin, thereby destroying its ability to serve as an antielastolytic agent. Thus, the deleterious effects of cigarette smoking are not simply additive with those of alpha$_1$-antitrypsin deficiency, but are synergistic.

It is also possible to explain the pattern of emphysema seen in patients with alpha$_1$-antitrypsin deficiency. These patients have more pronounced emphysema in the lung bases than in the apices [8]. This phenomenon may be related to the fact that the lungs serve as a repository for circulating leukocytes [10] and blood flow is much greater through the bases of the lungs than through the apices. Leukocytes may therefore be sequestered primarily within the lower parts of the lung, leading to a more unfavorable balance between protease and antiprotease activities and severe emphysema in this region of the lung.

How much antiprotease is needed to maintain a "healthy" protease-antiprotease balance? The answer to this question has been provided by correlating the alpha$_1$-antitrypsin phenotype, serum alpha$_1$-antitrypsin concentration, and clinical phenotype of patients with alpha$_1$-antitrypsin deficiency [19,39,56]. A summary of these correlations is presented in Table 70-2. Levels below 35 percent of that found in Pi MM individuals are

Table 70-2. **Relationship between alpha$_1$-antitrypsin phenotype, serum alpha$_1$-antitrypsin concentration, and clinical phenotype**

Phenotype	Serum concentration (as % of Pi MM)	Clinical phenotype	
		Lung disease	Liver disease
Pi MM	100	–	–
Pi MS	80	–	–
Pi MZ	60	–	–
Pi SS	50–60	–	–
Pi SZ	30–40	+	–
Pi ZZ	10–15	+	+
Pi null-null	0	+	–

generally associated with the development of pulmonary disease. In absolute amounts, the clinical threshold is thought to be 11 μM. The patients who are principally at risk are individuals homozygous for the *Z* allele (10 to 15 percent) or the null allele (0 percent). Patients who are compound heterozygotes for the *null* allele and either the *S* or *Z* allele would also be at increased risk (i.e., patients with the Pi S-null or Pi Z-null phenotype). Most Pi SZ patients have a serum alpha$_1$-antitrypsin concentration greater than the 35 percent threshold, but those who do not are at increased risk. Intermediate levels of alpha$_1$-antitrypsin are found in Pi SS homozygotes (50 to 60 percent) and in Pi MS (80 percent) and Pi MZ (60 percent) heterozygotes, and these patients generally do not have a clinically significant deficiency.

Two additional points can be made about the information in Table 70-2. First, the lower the serum alpha$_1$-antitrypsin concentration the greater the relative risk of developing emphysema. The phenotypes associated with a relative risk for developing disease are, in descending order, Pi null-null, Pi ZZ, and Pi SZ. The Pi null-null phenotype is associated with the highest relative risk for developing disease, the earliest age of onset, and the most rapidly progressive course. Second, the development of liver disease is not simply a function of the serum concentration of alpha$_1$-antitrypsin, but is only associated with specific Pi phenotypes in which there is abnormal alpha$_1$-antitrypsin accumulation in liver.

There has been controversy regarding the normal serum concentration of alpha$_1$-antitrypsin. For many years the concentration of alpha$_1$-antitrypsin in sera of individuals with the Pi MM phenotype was thought to be 180 to 240 mg/dl. Clinically significant deficiency was not found in patients who had concentrations greater than 80 mg/dl. Normal serum levels have been reassessed in recent years using a more purified protein as a standard, and were found to be about 35 percent lower [173]. To indicate that a more refined protein is being used as a standard, current practice is to state the units of concentration in terms of micromoles per liter rather than as milligrams per deciliter. According to this current convention, the range of normal is 21 to 34 μM [19] and clinically significant deficiency is associated with concentrations less than 11 μM [38,183]. Pi SZ individuals have serum alpha$_1$-antitrypsin concentrations ranging between 8 and 19 μM, thereby explaining why some of these individuals develop lung disease and others do not.

Clinical Manifestations

Alpha$_1$-antitrypsin deficiency primarily causes two distinct disorders: emphysematous pulmonary disease and hepatic disease. The pulmonary manifestations are more prevalent than the hepatic ones, and are the focus of this discussion. Our understanding of the pulmonary disease caused by alpha$_1$-antitrypsin deficiency is a paradigm of the successful interaction of clinical and laboratory investigations [52]. In the 25 years since its discovery, the molecular basis, pathogenesis, and a rationale basis for treatment of emphysema caused by alpha$_1$-antitrypsin deficiency have been established.

PULMONARY DISEASE

Eriksson's 1965 [51] summary of the clinical pulmonary manifestations of alpha$_1$-antitrypsin deficiency associated with the Pi ZZ phenotype remains an excellent description of this disease. Of the 37 patients described, 23 (62 percent) had chronic obstructive pulmonary disease. The sex distribution of the entire group of 37 patients was equal, but 15 (65 percent) of the 23 patients with obstructive pulmonary disease were men and only 8 (35 percent) were women. The distribution of age of onset in the patients in Eriksson's series was shifted toward a younger age than that seen in patients with obstructive lung disease not associated with alpha$_1$-antitrypsin deficiency. Onset was generally in the fourth decade of life. The main symptom was dyspnea; cough and increased sputum production were present in less than half the group. Weight loss was common. Hyperresonance, diminished breath sounds, and an increase in the anteroposterior diameter of the chest were common physical findings. Heart sounds were diminished in intensity, but physical signs of heart failure were not usually seen. More recent studies substantiated these findings in a variety of populations [74,104,171,172].

Radiographic findings include enlarged and hyperlucent lungs [8] (Fig. 70-1). Lower lung involvement predominates in essentially all patients with radiographic evidence of disease and is confined to the lower lung fields in about two-thirds of such patients. In keeping with these observations, ventilation to the bases is commonly found to be reduced when assessed with radioactive xenon scanning [57]. Shunting of blood to the upper lung fields and enlargement of the proximal pulmonary artery shadows in patients with heart failure also have been noted.

Pulmonary function testing demonstrates typi-

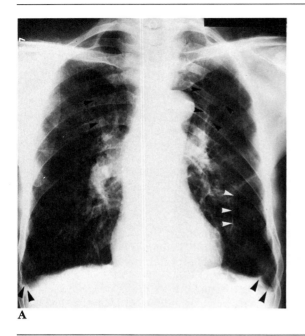

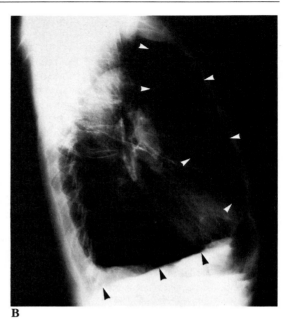

A

B

Fig. 70-1. *A.* Posteroanterior teleroentgenogram of the chest showing the major features of alpha$_1$-antitrypsin deficiency emphysema. Note the relatively flattened diaphragms, with blunting of the costophrenic angle and tenting from pleural scarring (*large black arrows*). The lung bases are hyperlucent with loss of normal vascular markings; occasional septa demarcate a bulla (*white arrows*). In contrast, blood flow is redistributed to the apices, so that vascularity is prominent there (*small black arrows*). *B.* Lateral chest teleroentgenogram of the same patient illustrating the low, flattened diaphragms (*black arrows*). The diaphragms have lost their normal convex appearance. In some patients, the diaphragms will assume a concave silhouette. This patient also shows the increased retrosternal airspace (*white arrows*) frequently seen in emphysema patients. Note also that the anteroposterior chest diameter is slightly increased in this patient.

cal findings of emphysema. There is evidence of airway obstruction and a striking increase in lung volume [51,74,171]. Airway resistance is increased, with reductions in forced expiratory flow rates (i.e., a decreased forced expiratory volume [FEV$_1$] and FEV$_1$/forced vital capacity [FVC]) and specific conductance. Marked increases in residual volume (RV), functional residual capacity (FRC), and total lung capacity (TLC) also have been noted. Diffusion capacity is commonly diminished, and hypoxemia is present in patients with end-stage disease. This pattern of laboratory impairment is similar to the pattern observed in patients with emphysema who do not have alpha$_1$-antitrypsin deficiency, but the course of disease is accelerated. Patients with alpha$_1$-antitrypsin deficiency do not usually show any improvement with aerosolized bronchodilator therapy [94]. Heart failure or cor pulmonale may be manifestations of this disease; there are no characteristic electrocardiographic (ECG) changes associated with these manifestations.

Patients with alpha$_1$-antitrypsin deficiency may present with bronchiectasis rather than emphysema. For example, Jones and associates [92] described three women with the Pi ZZ phenotype who presented with bronchiectasis, chronic cough, purulent sputum production, and bronchograms demonstrating saccular and tubular

bronchiectasis. Symptoms appeared relatively late in life (ages 53 to 69 years) in these patients, although all three women had progressive clinical and radiographic deterioration following diagnosis. Two of these patients, however, had no clinical or radiographic evidence of emphysema. Although it is impossible to prove that bronchiectasis was related to alpha$_1$-antitrypsin deficiency in these patients, only one of the patients gave a history of a preceding illness (i.e., whooping cough) known to cause bronchiectasis. Further studies are required before an etiologic role of alpha₁-antitrypsin in bronchiectasis can be assumed.

The most characteristic histologic finding in patients with alpha₁-antitrypsin deficiency is the destruction of acinar lung units distal to terminal bronchioles. In a study of 38 patients with alpha₁-antitrypsin deficiency, examination of autopsy and thoracotomy specimens showed that most patients had predominantly panlobular emphysema [135]. Several patients had a mild, "insignificant degree" of centrilobular emphysema, and one patient had predominantly centrilobular emphysema. Chronic bronchitic changes were found in 11 of 17 patients, with the extent and severity of the changes appearing unrelated to the degree of emphysema. Right ventricular hypertrophy was reported in 12 of the 38 patients but was absent in 3 with very severe emphysema. Vascular lesions (panarteritis) were observed in 1 patient in conjunction with proliferative glomerulonephritis. No extrapulmonary lesions were reported.

Patients who have deficiency associated with phenotypes other than Pi ZZ have the same basic clinical, radiologic, and histologic findings as those with Pi ZZ, except that the course of the disease is more or less severe. Patients with Pi null-null disease, for example, have onset of disease in their second or third decade of life and progress rapidly whether they smoke or not [34,65,167].

Risk Factors and Natural History. Patients who are homozygous for the *Z* allele have significantly reduced levels of alpha₁-antitrypsin and clearly have an increased risk of developing premature emphysema. It was initially thought that a very high proportion of these patients developed pulmonary disease. This is no longer thought to be so. There is now considerable evidence that the natural history of homozygous alpha₁-antitrypsin deficiency is highly variable and that other genetic or environmental factors influence the development of emphysema in these patients.

In one of the first studies to use subject groups that were carefully matched for identifiable environmental factors, Kueppers and Black [14,101] examined a group of 18 patients with homozygous Pi ZZ alpha₁-antitrypsin deficiency who had lived in rural communities most of their lives, had little or no known exposure to occupational air pollutants, and had never smoked. Only 7 (39 per-

cent) of these patients had classic roentgenographic evidence of emphysema in the lower lung fields, whereas 8 (44 percent) had no roentgenographic evidence of emphysema and 3 had atypical roentgenographic findings. This contrasted sharply with observations in a comparable group of 36 homozygous patients who were cigarette smokers. Twenty-six (72 percent) of these patients had classic roentgenographic findings of emphysema in the lower lung fields, 8 patients (22 percent) had atypical roentgenographic findings, and only 2 patients (6 percent) had normal-appearing chest roentgenograms. Black and Kueppers [14] found that cigarette smoking also had a deleterious effect on lung function, as well as on the radiographic appearance of the lungs. On the whole, patients who smoked developed impaired lung function earlier in life than did patients who did not smoke.

Several more recent studies confirmed these observations [88,104,156,171]. Larsson [104] studied 248 adults with homozygous alpha₁-antitrypsin deficiency (Pi ZZ) and found that patients who smoked as well as those who did not had a life expectancy shorter than that for the general population; however, patients who smoked had a significantly shorter life expectancy than did nonsmokers. This study also found that about one-third of patients identified through family studies had normal lung function. Janus and coauthors [88] reported on the progression of pulmonary function in a group of 69 Pi ZZ patients. Thirty-three of the patients had developed emphysema. The mean age of onset of symptoms (dyspnea) was 32 years in the group of patients who smoked, compared to 51 years for the group who did not smoke. Nonsmokers did not develop disabling symptoms until the ages of 60 to 65 years. Smokers died earlier (48 years) than nonsmokers (67 years). The FEV_1 was smaller at the time of initial examination and declined more rapidly in smokers compared to nonsmokers. In nonsmokers, the FEV_1 was initially 77 percent of predicted and declined at 80 ml/year, whereas in smokers the FEV_1 was initially 38 percent of predicted and declined at 317 ml/year. The rate of decline correlated with the degree of cigarette smoking in pack-years for the group of patients who smoked. Clearly, patients with the Pi ZZ phenotype should not smoke.

What about patients with heterozygous deficiencies? The relative risk of heterozygotes developing emphysema is less clear and an area of some controversy [102]. In brief, it appears that the prognosis for heterozygotes depends foremost on their relative level of deficiency, but that other factors may influence their risks. Patients with relatively minor degrees of deficiency (i.e., Pi MZ and Pi MS heterozygotes with 60 and 80 percent, respectively, of normal serum levels) are probably not at increased risk of developing clinically significant emphysema, although there is some evidence that they may have subclinical alterations in pulmonary function [18,21,88,110,113, 122,125]. The Pi SZ phenotype is associated with a greater level of deficiency (about 35 percent) and places the patient at an increased risk [38,85]. The assertion has been made [38] that the only Pi SZ patients at increased risk are those who have serum alpha$_1$-antitrypsin concentrations less than 11 μM. While this assertion provides a useful conceptual guide, it is almost certainly simplistic because it ignores the potential influence on phenotypic expression of both environmental factors, such as smoking, and other genetic factors. The arguments against cigarette smoking are valid for patients with heterozygous deficiencies as well as those with homozygous disease, although perhaps not as compelling.

Other factors, both genetic and environmental, may influence the development of emphysema in patients with alpha$_1$-antitrypsin deficiency. Possible genetic factors include variations in elastolytic activity in circulating leukocytes and the composition of the alveolar wall. Environmental factors may include respiratory irritants other than cigarette smoking. Identifying and modifying these factors may permit alteration of the natural history of alpha$_1$-antitrypsin deficiency, and may be useful in developing guidelines for choosing patients for different treatment protocols.

LIVER DISEASE

Alpha$_1$-antitrypsin deficiency is also a cause of liver disease in children [127,142,154,164] and adults [33,54,104]. Less is known about the epidemiology and pathogenesis of the hepatic manifestations than the pulmonary manifestations. The development of liver disease appears to be limited to those patients who are homozygous for the Z allele or other, rarer alleles (e.g., M$_{malton}$ and M$_{duarte}$) [33,39]. These alleles appear to cause hepatic disease by virtue of producing an abnormal protein that accumulates in the endoplasmic reticulum of the hepatocyte. Liver disease does not develop in patients who merely have very low serum levels of alpha$_1$-antitrypsin. For example, patients who are homozygous for the Pi^{null} allele have serum levels that are lower than those

found in Pi ZZ homozygotes, but they do not develop liver disease.

Approximately 15 percent of patients with the Pi ZZ phenotype develop cholestatic jaundice in the neonatal period, and about 50 percent have laboratory evidence of abnormal liver function [142,164]. One-third of patients with neonatal jaundice go on to develop chronic hepatitis or die from fulminant hepatic insufficiency, whereas the majority have regression of their liver disease [127,142,165].

The proportion of patients who do not have significant liver disease in the newborn period but develop hepatic disease in later life is uncertain. There is evidence that adults with the homozygous Pi ZZ phenotype are at increased risk for developing cirrhosis and primary liver carcinoma [36,53,54,104]. In a retrospective, population-based autopsy study, Eriksson and colleagues [53] demonstrated that men with alpha$_1$-antitrypsin deficiency have a significantly increased relative risk for developing cirrhosis or primary liver cancer. The relative risk for women was also increased, but not to a statistically significant degree. No explanation for the difference between homozygous men and women is available, although it certainly suggests that other genetic or environmental factors play a role in the development of liver disease in these patients. There is no compelling evidence that Pi SZ and Pi MZ heterozygotes are at increased risk for developing cirrhosis or primary liver carcinoma.

It remains unclear why some patients develop pulmonary disease and others develop hepatic disease, even within the same family. Glasgow and colleagues [69], for example, described a family in which one child with the Pi ZZ phenotype had liver disease, while a sibling with the same genotype was clinically unaffected. In families in which more than one sibling has liver disease, the severity of the liver disease is similar in about two-thirds and dissimilar in the remaining one-third [142]. This variability in phenotypic expression may be due to environmental agents or the actions of other genetic loci that affect expression of liver and/or lung disease.

Finally, it is important to note that a significant fraction of Pi ZZ patients never develop clinically significant disease. Eriksson's studies [53], for example, found that about one-third of patients with the Pi ZZ phenotype developed neither emphysema nor liver disease during their lives. This observation is important because it points out the need to determine the nature and role of other factors that influence expression of the deficiency state. It is also important in terms of designing and evaluating potential therapies for this disease. The relative risks for patients who have other genotypes are less clearly established.

Diagnosis

The diagnosis of alpha$_1$-antitrypsin deficiency should be suspected in young adults with severe emphysema or cholestatic liver disease at any age [19,33]. Focusing on the pulmonary presentation, the criteria suggested by Talamo and associates [166] include a family history of emphysema; the onset of symptoms of obstructive airway disease early in life, that is, in the third or fourth decade; the early development of dyspnea; and generally, the absence of significant cough and sputum.

When the deficiency is suspected, patients should have serum protein electrophoresis performed for estimating alpha$_1$-antitrypsin levels. Since alpha$_1$-antitrypsin makes up about 90 percent of the alpha$_1$-globulin fraction, a reduction in the size of this fraction suggests the possibility of alpha$_1$-antitrypsin deficiency and should lead to more specific testing. Because of the small size of the alpha$_1$-globulin peak and the fact that this protein is an acute-phase reactant, serum protein electrophoresis patterns may sometimes be misinterpreted by automated detectors and should be examined visually when there is a question [118].

A number of specific enzymatic assays are available for determining alpha$_1$-antitrypsin activity. The serum inhibitory capacity can be measured for either trypsin or elastase. When measured against trypsin, the activity is termed the *serum trypsin inhibitory capacity* (STIC). The STIC is equal to or greater than 0.95 units/ml in normal individuals, between 0.5 and 0.95 units/ml in patients with intermediate deficiency, and less than 0.5 units/ml in patients with severe deficiency [111,113]. Other inhibitors of trypsin may be present in serum and can yield false-negative results.

The preferred approach to measuring the concentration of alpha$_1$-antitrypsin is to use an immunologic assay, such as radial immunodiffusion [56,111]. With this technique, the concentration in serum was traditionally reported in milligrams per deciliter. For many years the concentration of alpha$_1$-antitrypsin in sera of individuals with the Pi MM phenotype was thought to be 180 to 240 mg/dl [33]. With more purified protein as a standard, normal serum levels have been reassessed and found to be somewhat lower. The normal serum alpha$_1$-antitrypsin concentration, expressed in the now standard units of micromoles per liter, is now stated to range between 21 and 34 μM [19]. The minimal alpha$_1$-antitrypsin threshold is thought to be 11 μM [20].

A low alpha$_1$-antitrypsin level establishes the diagnosis of alpha$_1$-antitrypsin deficiency. However, a normal level does not rule out the heterozygous state, since alpha$_1$-antitrypsin is an acute-phase reactant and may increase twofold to fourfold in response to an inflammatory process, rising to the normal range. The serum alpha$_1$-antitrypsin level of homozygotes increases only slightly during stress or infection, making it unlikely that a false-negative value will be observed in these patients.

Following determination of alpha$_1$-antitrypsin deficiency, the Pi phenotype should be established either by acid-starch gel electrophoresis, alone or combined with cross-immunoelectrophoresis, or by the more sensitive polyacrylamide gel isoelectric focusing technique [56,111]. With the recognition of an ever-increasing number of mutant alleles, newly diagnosed patients with unusual clinical phenotypes or clinical phenotypes that appear "inconsistent" with the Pi phenotype should have their genotype determined. For example, take the case of an unusually young patient with unusually severe emphysema who is found to have a Pi MZ phenotype. The initial response may be to assume that the patient's disease is not related to the Pi phenotype. It may be the case, however, that the *M* allele is in fact an abnormal *M* variant (e.g., M$_{duarte}$). Thus, genotyping permits making a specific diagnosis and more accurate predictions about prognosis. Specific genotyping can be accomplished using the polymerase chain reaction followed by recognition with allele-specific oligonucleotides or by allele-specific gene amplification using the polymerase chain reaction [133].

Treatment

Following diagnosis, a number of baseline studies are recommended, and include chest roentgenograms (posteroanterior and left lateral), pulmonary function tests (spirometry before and after inhaling a bronchodilator, lung volumes, and diffusion capacity), arterial blood gas measurement, and liver function tests [20]. Symptomatic patients should receive conventional forms of therapy for emphysema. If there is a reversible component to airways obstruction, this should be treated with bronchodilators. In addition, antibiotics should be used to treat serious parenchymal infections. Cor pulmonale and polycythemia should be treated, when present. In addition, oxygen therapy, respiratory muscle conditioning, and influenza and pneumococcal vaccinations should be employed when appropriate. Most important, patients should not smoke.

Within the last several years, considerable effort has been spent to develop more specific, active interventions for these patients. These efforts have been along four lines: (1) stimulation of endogenous production of alpha$_1$-antitrypsin, (2) development of a synthetic antielastolytic agent, (3) replacement therapy with purified alpha$_1$-antitrypsin, and (4) organ transplantation. Currently, the third approach appears most promising for patients with pulmonary disease caused by alpha$_1$-antitrypsin deficiency.

Efforts to increase endogenous production of alpha$_1$-antitrypsin were tried using estrogen, since estrogen increases the serum levels of this protein in Pi MM individuals. It was found that estrogen did not increase the levels of protein in patients with the Pi ZZ phenotype. A number of other steroidal hormones were tried, and Gadek and coworkers [62] found that danazol, an impeded androgen, increased alpha$_1$-antitrypsin levels in five of six patients with the Pi ZZ phenotype. Despite its apparent success initially, enthusiasm for danazol therapy waned because it induces a relatively small increase in serum levels (about 40 percent) and because of its potential for causing liver damage.

A series of synthetic elastase inhibitors was developed with the general structural classification of peptidyl chloromethyl ketones. These inhibitors appeared to serve effectively in animal studies, but their clinical use in humans was abandoned when it was found that they produced severe myocardial, hepatic, and renal side effects [99]. The search for a safe inhibitor is still underway.

Replacement therapy is being explored using purified human alpha$_1$-antitrypsin. In a key observation, Gadek and coworkers [63] showed that parenteral replacement therapy with an alpha$_1$-antitrypsin concentrate of normal plasma produces an increase in serum levels sufficient to establish effective levels of antielastase activity in alveolar fluid obtained by bronchoalveolar lavage. This study was important because it demonstrated that replacement therapy might be both technically possible and a physiologically useful approach to therapy. In a follow-up of these studies, Wewers and colleagues [183] reported the results of a clinical trial in which they administered 60 mg of purified alpha$_1$-antitrypsin per kilogram of body weight once a week for up to 6 months to 21 patients with Pi ZZ disease. They found clear evidence of biochemical improvement: increased alpha$_1$-antitrypsin levels and increased antineutrophil elastase capacities in serum and the epithelial lining of the lung (as measured in bronchoalveolar lavage fluid). They were unable to identify any associated improvement in clinical status during the relatively short time frame of their study. Infusion therapy was well tolerated, and the only side effect noted was transient fever following three infusions of inhibitor (out of a total of 360 infusions in the study). These studies suggest that it may be possible to restore the elastase-antielastase balance within the lung of genetically deficient individuals, thereby preventing further progression of their disease.

Purified alpha$_1$-antitrypsin is now commercially available for clinical use for patients with severe deficiency. It is estimated that over 1000 patients are currently receiving this form of therapy. There have been no serious side effects observed to date [20,38,80]. The National Institutes of Health has established a registry for monitoring augmentation therapy; however, this registry is not part of a systematic prospective study, which has been judged to be unfeasible. About two dozen regional treatment centers have been designated as part of this registry.

The American Thoracic Society recently issued a position statement entitled "Guidelines for the approach to the patient with severe hereditary alpha-1-antitrypsin deficiency" [20]. These guidelines include several recommendations for patient selection for augmentation therapy (also see [19]). These recommendations are summarized in Table 70-3. The first recommendation is that augmentation therapy only be offered to patients who are at significant risk for developing emphysema (i.e., they have a serum alpha$_1$-antitrypsin concentration < 11 μM). This recommendation would have the effect of limiting treatment to Pi ZZ, Pi Z-null, Pi S-null, and Pi null-null patients and a small fraction of Pi SZ patients. Treatment is not advocated for patients with the Pi SS, Pi MS, or Pi MZ phenotype. Two recommendations—a minimum age requirement of 18 years and the presence of abnormal pulmonary

Table 70-3. **Recommendations from the American Thoracic Society for selection of patients who should receive alpha$_1$-antitrypsin augmentation therapy [20], as modified by Buist [19]**

Treatment reserved for patients with severe deficiency (serum alpha$_1$-antitrypsin < 11 μM)

Age > 18 y

Lung function studies abnormal

No history of smoking for a minimum of 3 mo

Condition stabilized by maximum supportive care

function—are proposed to ensure that potentially asymptomatic patients are not treated prematurely (i.e., patients who have low levels of alpha$_1$-antitrypsin but will never manifest disease). Conversely, treatment would ideally be instituted as early as possible because augmentation therapy will not reverse existing lung damage, but offers only the promise of preventing further progression of disease. A fourth recommendation is designed to exclude patients who are unlikely to benefit from treatment (e.g., patients who continue to smoke should not be treated). Last, all patients should receive maximal conventional therapy before being evaluated as to their need for augmentation therapy.

These recommendations have not been met with universal approval [58,159]. The Canadian Thoracic Society, for example, argued that the potential clinical benefits of augmentation therapy had not been established, the potential complications have not been determined, the criteria for patient selection were too broad and potentially very costly, and the cost-benefit ratio of alternative treatment protocols had not been established [58]. The estimated cost of treating an adult male in the United States is $25,000 per year [159]. Although the cost considerations of augmentation therapy may soon decrease in importance with the availability of recombinant protein, direct answers to these reservations are needed and unfortunately, may not be forthcoming in the near future.

One potential problem with replacement therapy is the large quantity of plasma required to obtain sufficient inhibitor for treating all affected individuals. Casolaro and coworkers [26] examined the feasibility of employing alpha$_1$-antitrypsin produced by recombinant DNA technology. A nonglycosylated form of alpha$_1$-antitrypsin was produced using yeast engineered to contain a full-length segment of human DNA encoding for alpha$_1$-antitrypsin. The plasma half-life of this nonglycosylated protein was extremely short, but sufficient amounts were transferred to the lung to provide significant increases in alveolar antielastase activity.

Other efforts have been directed toward correcting alpha$_1$-antitrypsin deficiency by providing the protein as an aerosol. Hubbard and coworkers demonstrated that it was possible to prepare an aerosol of purified plasma [81] or recombinant [82] alpha$_1$-antitrypsin that effectively reached distal alveoli. They showed that the aerosolized alpha$_1$-antitrypsin could be recovered from pulmonary lavage fluid, lung lymph fluid, and blood. However, they found that they did not increase the levels of alpha$_1$-antitrypsin in the interstitial space above the minimal threshold considered necessary. This limitation notwithstanding, this mode of therapy appears very promising, especially in light of the possibility that it can be augmented using an engineered recombinant form of alpha$_1$-antitrypsin that will function as a "superinhibitor" [33,38].

There are two approaches currently being explored for gene therapy of alpha$_1$-antitrypsin deficiency. The first approach is to incorporate the human alpha$_1$-antitrypsin gene into various cell types outside of the pulmonary tract, which will in turn provide increased serum concentrations of alpha$_1$-antitrypsin; the second approach is to incorporate the gene into the epithelial cells of the lower respiratory tract. Both approaches appear promising. For example, Garver and associates [66] incorporated the human alpha$_1$-antitrypsin gene into a modified retroviral vector, which was in turn inserted into murine fibroblasts. They showed that the modified fibroblasts produced functional human alpha$_1$-antitrypsin. The fibroblasts were then transplanted into the peritoneal space of nude mice, where they continued to produce human protein that was demonstrated in blood and lung of the murine subjects. Much attention is currently being directed at developing improved vectors for incorporating the alpha$_1$-antitrypsin gene into epithelial cells of the respiratory lining and into hepatocytes.

The last therapeutic approach is organ transplantation. Lung transplantation has been performed for relatively few patients who have advanced emphysema associated with alpha$_1$-antitrypsin deficiency. These patients were initially thought to require double-lung transplants because a single transplant would leave in place one abnormal, hyperinflatable lung, which would lead to ventilation-perfusion maldistribution between the two lungs. However, recent technical advances in the procedures for single-lung transplantation have significantly improved the results of this procedure (see Chap. 48). Both double-lung and single-lung transplantation are now used for treating patients with advanced alpha$_1$-antitrypsin deficiency disease [174]. Whereas the short-term outcome for these patients appears good, it is too early to provide specific information about their long-term outcome.

The only therapy available for patients with irreversible liver disease is liver transplantation [143,162]. Protein replacement therapy would not help these patients because their disease is secondary to the accumulation of nonsecreted alpha$_1$-antitrypsin in hepatocytes, not to the deficiency state itself. In the future, it may be possible to treat these patients by devising means of inhibiting endogenous alpha$_1$-antitrypsin synthesis using a molecular biologic tool such as antisense RNA [31]. Liver transplantation has not been explored as a treatment for patients who have only pulmonary disease. Although early transplantation would presumably provide effective prophylaxis for the lung disease, the risks associated with the transplantation procedure are currently considered too great to justify this approach.

Genetics

Alpha$_1$-antitrypsin alleles are expressed as co-dominant traits; that is, each allele produces a discrete phenotype. The disease state is associated with the homozygous state for two mutant alleles. Thus, alpha$_1$-antitrypsin deficiency *disease* is inherited as an autosomal recessive trait. Genetic counseling should be provided to affected patients and their families. Probands and their spouses should be counseled regarding reproductive planning and prenatal testing. Siblings of affected patients should be counseled about their own risk of developing disease and their reproductive risks. Counseling for families at risk for the hepatic form of alpha$_1$-antitrypsin has a special set of concerns [142].

Genetic counseling should only be provided after Pi typing has been performed, since counseling differs for the homozygote compared to the heterozygote. The homozygous Pi ZZ patient will transmit the *Z* allele to each of his or her offspring. If the patient's spouse also possesses a *Z* allele, then their offspring are at 50 percent risk for homozygous disease. If the patient's spouse does not have the *Z* allele, their children are at

100 percent risk for the heterozygous state, but are not at risk for the homozygous disease state. An asymptomatic sibling of a homozygous patient also may be homozygous and should have Pi typing. Following testing, siblings should be advised of appropriate prophylaxis depending on their genetic status.

Prenatal diagnosis of alpha$_1$-antitrypsin deficiency has been accomplished, but its use has been limited to families at risk for the forms of alpha$_1$-antitrypsin deficiency associated with childhood liver disease. Prenatal diagnosis was first accomplished by determining Pi status and alpha$_1$-antitrypsin levels of fetal blood obtained by fetoscopy [90]. Although reliable, this method is limited by the relatively high risk for fetal loss posed by the fetoscopic procedure (about 5 percent). A safer alternative was described by Kidd and coauthors [97], who determined Pi status using direct analysis of the mutation site in fetal DNA derived from amniocytes that were obtained by amniocentesis (fetal risk of ≤ 1 percent). These workers synthesized short oligonucleotide probes that were complementary to the gene sequence surrounding the mutation site of the *M* and *Z* alleles. These oligonucleotides differed in only a single base but were recognized with sufficient specificity that they did not cross-react; the *M*-specific probe did not recognize the *Z* allele and the *Z*-specific probe did not recognize the *M* allele. This approach has been applied successfully in a relatively large number of at-risk pregnancies and is now in routine clinical use.

Prenatal diagnosis can also be accomplished using restriction fragment polymorphisms of fetal DNA [33,35]. Extensive studies have demonstrated that a number of restriction site polymorphisms are in linkage disequilibrium with the *Z* allele; that is, they are found exclusively or almost exclusively in patients who carry the Pi^Z allele. These polymorphisms permit prenatal diagnosis to be accomplished without full knowledge of the parental and sibling haplotypes. Additionally, there are other polymorphisms that are not in disequilibrium but do co-segregate with the Pi allele. These polymorphisms permit prenatal diagnosis of all the mutant Pi alleles, but require prior or concurrent family studies to determine the pattern of linkage between the abnormal Pi allele and the polymorphic markers.

The methods used to accomplish prenatal diagnosis also can be applied to patients at risk for the adult-onset form of pulmonary disease, but the relative merits of doing so are problematic.

Familial Pulmonary Fibrosis

Familial pulmonary fibrosis (also termed *hereditary miliary bronchoalveolar cystic disease* or *familial fibrocystic pulmonary dysplasia*) is clinically, radiographically, physiologically, and morphologically indistinguishable from the more common, nonfamilial form of idiopathic interstitial pulmonary fibrosis. The familial form of this disease appears to be transmitted genetically as an autosomal dominant trait with incomplete penetrance.

Clinical Manifestations

Patients with familial pulmonary fibrosis present with progressive exertional dyspnea, cyanosis, cough, chest pain, and weight loss. The age of onset is variable, ranging from infancy to the sixth decade [83,100]. Symptoms generally begin in middle age. Cyanosis, clubbing, bibasilar rales, and cor pulmonale develop as the disease progresses. Diffuse reticulonodular infiltrates are seen on chest roentgenograms, along with linear and irregular pulmonary opacities that eventually obliterate normal markings. Honeycombing may be seen in advanced disease. Spontaneous pneumothorax has been reported, including three cases in one family [130]. Bronchogenic carcinoma may also develop.

Pulmonary function testing shows a reduced lung volume, a reduced diffusion capacity, and a widened alveolar-arterial oxygen gradient at rest, which widens further during exercise. Static recoil measurements show an increased maximal transpulmonary pressure.

Pathogenesis

The histologic findings in the familial disorder are identical to those found in idiopathic interstitial pulmonary fibrosis. There is thickening of the alveolar septa by fibroblast proliferation, edema, and collagen deposition. The septa contain variable numbers of inflammatory cells. The alveolar space may contain a granular exudate or an accumulation of mononuclear cells. The bronchiolar epithelium is cuboidal and arteriolar walls are thickened by muscular hyperplasia and subintimal fibrosis. At a more advanced stage, typical honeycombing may be seen, with numerous fibrous-walled cysts being present. The surface of the lung is nodular, with these nodules representing subpleural cystic spaces of 3 to 15 mm in size.

Fibrosis and honeycombing may coexist in adjacent zones. Parenchymal involvement may be localized or diffuse, which suggests the need for adequate tissue sampling to grade the disorder histologically.

The basic defect responsible for familial pulmonary fibrosis is unknown, but understanding of the familial disorder has improved as more has been learned about the nonfamilial form of idiopathic pulmonary fibrosis [12]. The evidence for a chronic inflammatory process in the latter is convincing: Findings on gallium scans of the lung are generally positive; bronchoalveolar lavage fluid from the lower respiratory tract contains an excess number of neutrophils [84]; and alveolar macrophages, which spontaneously release neutrophil chemotactic factors and mediators that stimulate fibroblast replication, fibronectin, and alveolar macrophage-derived growth factor, are present [11].

Early evidence suggesting that the familial disorder results from an abnormal immunologic or inflammatory process was provided by pedigrees in which there was an association between familial pulmonary fibrosis and other disorders thought to have an immunologic basis. Bonanni and colleagues [14] noted an association between dysglobulinemia and interstitial fibrosis in several members of one family. An association of a positive rheumatoid factor with pulmonary fibrosis, with or without clinical manifestations of rheumatoid arthritis, was observed in several pedigrees [67,72,79,175]. Hilton and Pitkeathly [79] reported an association between familial pulmonary fibrosis and rheumatoid arthritis in a family in which the father and two children had arthritis and roentgenographic evidence of fibrosis, while four siblings had abnormal pulmonary function despite normal-appearing roentgenograms and no clinical evidence of arthritis.

To evaluate further the hypothesis that chronic alveolar inflammation precedes pulmonary fibrosis, Bitterman and coworkers [13] examined asymptomatic members of three families who were at risk for developing the disorder. They examined 17 patients, all of whom had normal findings on pulmonary function tests and chest radiograms. There was evidence of alveolar inflammation on the gallium scans of four patients and in the bronchoalveolar lavage fluid from eight patients (increased numbers of neutrophils and activated macrophages, which released neutrophil chemotactic factor and one or more fibroblast growth factors). The frequency of patients with abnormal findings (8 of 17) is consistent with an autosomal dominant trait. It remains to be seen whether the patients who had evidence of alveolar inflammation will go on to develop clinically significant disease.

The basic defect responsible for the abnormal inflammatory response remains unknown. There is some evidence of an association between human leukocyte antigen (HLA) haplotype and familial pulmonary fibrosis in some families, but not all [61]. Musk and associates [130] reported on a family in which all six affected members shared the same immunoglobulin haplotype (Gml) and suggested that the gene defect responsible for familial interstitial fibrosis may be on chromosome 14, close to the loci encoding for immunoglobulin structure. Similarly, the reported association of alpha$_1$-antitrypsin type and the development of interstitial fibrosis within a given family [67] may be explained by a gene defect on chromosome 14, since the alpha$_1$-antitrypsin gene is also located on this chromosome. Alternatively, immunoglobulin or alpha$_1$-antitrypsin status may influence expression of the familial fibrosis gene.

Diagnosis

This diagnosis should be suspected when the typical clinical, radiologic, and physiologic derangements of idiopathic pulmonary fibrosis are present, plus a consistent family history. The presence of two or more affected family members, in two or more generations, should raise the possibility of this disorder.

Treatment

Therapy for these patients is the same as that used for treating sporadic cases of interstitial fibrosis and is generally unsuccessful [40] (also see Chap. 42). Steroids may be of benefit in some cases. The most dramatic advance in treating pulmonary fibrosis in recent years has been the use of lung transplantation. There are currently three general surgical approaches to lung transplantation: single-lung, double-lung, and combined heart-lung. The last approach is not required for familial pulmonary fibrosis because the heart is generally not involved in this disease. The relative advantages and disadvantages of single-lung versus double-lung transplantation for this disease are currently being assessed [73,174] (also see Chap. 48). Although the double-lung procedure was initially favored, it appears that the unilateral procedure may be satisfactory. Following single-lung transplantation, patients continue to have evidence of restrictive lung disease manifested from the native lung, but are able to maintain normal or near-normal oxygenation at rest and show improved exercise tolerance.

Genetics

The initial description of this disorder by Sandoz [147] in 1907 was of pulmonary disease in 18-year-old twin sisters. Pathologic descriptions of these two patients, in retrospect, did not clearly establish whether these patients had interstitial fibrosis or emphysema, since findings consistent with both were reported. Subsequently, numerous reports [13,47,49,116,139,192] established the familial association of this disorder. The report by Javaheri and coworkers [89] of interstitial fibrosis in monozygotic twins separated in childhood further supports a genetic rather than environmental cause for the familial clustering reported in other families. Several reports [100, 130,192] documented father-to-son transmission of this disorder, thereby excluding an X-linked inheritance pattern. The prevailing evidence, especially that provided by Bitterman and associates [13], strongly supports an autosomal dominant mode of inheritance.

Pulmonary Alveolar Microlithiasis

Harbitz [76] first described pulmonary alveolar microlithiasis in 1918 as a disorder characterized by the presence of laminated calcium hydroxyapatite spheres in the alveoli. Since his original description, approximately 200 cases have been reported and a worldwide distribution noted. Its cause remains unknown, and no effective treatment is available.

Clinical Manifestations

Pulmonary alveolar microlithiasis may present at any age, ranging from 29 weeks' gestation (twins) [23] to 80 years [152]. The average age of diagnosis is between 30 and 40 years [141,161]. Most patients are ascertained by a routine chest radiograph prior to the onset of symptoms. At presentation, symptoms are generally milder than would be anticipated from the strikingly abnormal roentgenographic findings [5,161]. Findings on physical examination may be normal until relatively late in the course of the disease.

The course of the disease is highly variable. There is often little progression of either clinical symptoms or radiologic signs for many years. For example, Prakash and colleagues [141] and Sosman and associates [161] reported on patients who remained asymptomatic for as long as 30 years. The proportion of patients in whom this disorder progresses to become clinically significant disease is unknown. In those patients in whom the disorder progresses, dyspnea generally develops, followed by respiratory insufficiency, cor pulmonale, and death. Spontaneous pneumothorax sometimes occurs [185]. In later stages of the disease, clubbing, cyanosis, and findings of right ventricular failure are observed.

The chest roentgenogram typically shows diffuse, multiple punctate calcium opacities over the entire lung fields [5,161]. The pattern resembles a snowstorm or sandstorm appearance, and literally obliterates the lung fields. The roentgenograms generally need to be overexposed in order to reveal the discrete nature of the calcifications. The calcifications are most prominent at the lung bases. There may be thickening of the minor fissure and pericardial calcifications; apical bullae may be seen. These roentgenographic findings superficially resemble those seen in stannous oxide exposure, hemosiderosis, and miliary tuberculosis, but the relative well-being of the patient coupled with the lack of exposure to industrial dusts should point to the diagnosis of pulmonary alveolar microlithiasis. Computed tomography (CT) examination also shows microliths diffusely distributed throughout the lung fields, and may be better than a standard chest radiograph at revealing small pleural blebs [29, 185]. Diffusely increased lung uptake of technetium diphosphonate tracer has been reported [17].

Pulmonary function may also be normal at the time of diagnosis, since many patients are asymptomatic at this time [134,141,170]. Although this disease is characterized by an intraalveolar accumulation of microliths, the clinical and functional abnormalities are characteristic of interstitial lung disease. With time, patients generally develop a restrictive defect with reduced vital capacity, reduced diffusion capacity, and hypoxemia that worsens with exercise [16,141].

Pathogenesis

The microcalculi observed in this disorder are composed primarily of calcium oxide and phosphate, small amounts of magnesium and aluminum, and trace amounts of silicon and iron; organic material makes up about 20 percent of the microlith [161]. Excised microliths are homogeneous, laminated eosinophilic spheres, which are 0.01 to 3.00 mm in diameter [141]. X-ray energy dispersive spectroscopic analysis of microliths has shown that they contain calcium and phosphorus in a $2:1$ ratio, consistent with a Ca_2PO_3 structure [7,141]. Microscopic infrared spectroscopic analysis recently showed that the microliths are composed of calcium carboxyapatite [7].

Microliths have been observed in expectorated sputum and on microscopic examination of sedimented bronchopulmonary lavage fluid [138]. In the early stages of this disease, microliths are generally contained entirely within the alveolar lumina. The microliths later coalesce and impinge on and through alveolar walls. In end-stage disease, the alveolar wall itself becomes thickened and fibrotic. Up to 75 percent of the alveoli may be involved by this process.

Several hypotheses have been advanced to explain the etiology of this entity, but none have been proved. Sosman and associates [161] noted the familial incidence of this disease and postulated that microlithiasis might be caused by an inborn error of metabolism. They proposed, for example, that there is an enzyme deficiency of the alveolar cells that results in an abnormally alkaline alveolar surface, leading to precipitation and deposition of calcium salts on that surface. This hypothesis cannot explain the observation that typical microliths have been found within bronchial walls [152] and in the lumbar sympathetic chain and testes [30] of patients with this disease. Such observations would suggest that there is a more generalized defect affecting many cell types and organs. To date, however, no systemic defect in calcium or phosphorus metabolism has been identified [134].

A second proposal is that this disorder results from a hyperimmune reaction by the alveolar wall to inhalant exposure [96]. According to this proposal, a hyperimmune inflammatory response produces a protein-rich exudate that then dehydrates and provides a medium for subsequent calcification. The presence of typical microlithiasis in young children and in premature infants would be difficult to explain by this mechanism.

Finally, Tao [168] observed that microliths are seen in 26 percent of sputum samples from patients with chronic obstructive lung disease, but not in sputum from patients with other types of respiratory or nonrespiratory diseases. He postulated that pulmonary alveolar microlithiasis represents an acceleration of the normal process of calcification associated with formation of

Curschmann's spirals. However, the absence of obstructive lung disease in most patients with microlithiasis makes it difficult to accept this hypothesis.

Diagnosis

Pulmonary alveolar microlithiasis is unique among respiratory disorders insofar as the degree of discordance observed between clinical and radiographic findings. Many patients have minimal or no clinical symptoms in the face of a strikingly abnormal chest radiograph. Pulmonary microlithiasis can almost always be diagnosed on the basis of the characteristic radiographic findings and clinical-radiographic discordance. The presence of microliths in open lung biopsy specimens, transbronchial biopsy specimens [24], or bronchopulmonary lavage fluid [138] may sometimes be required to confirm the diagnosis.

Treatment

Chelating agents and steroids are of no therapeutic value in this condition [141,170]. Bronchoalveolar lavage is also ineffective in producing clinical, roentgenographic, or laboratory improvement [138]. It is extremely difficult to remove microliths with lavage, probably because many are larger in diameter than the terminal bronchioles. In short, there is no effective treatment presently available.

Genetics

There have been numerous reports of familial cases of this disease [5,23,98,134,161,170,185]. Caffrey and Altman [23] reviewed 68 published cases of patients with pulmonary alveolar microlithiasis and found that half had a family history of the disease. Parental consanguinity has been reported for several affected families. The sex ratio is approximately equal. Most of the pedigrees that have been reported show patterns consistent with autosomal recessive inheritance. However, there are rare pedigrees in which a parent and child have been affected, suggesting autosomal dominant inheritance. These pedigrees may also reflect environmentally determined phenocopies of pulmonary alveolar microlithiasis. These observations suggest that this disorder may be causally heterogeneous.

Following diagnosis, all siblings should have chest radiographs made to determine if they are presymptomatic affected individuals. They

should also receive genetic counseling. It is unlikely that affected individuals will have affected children because the disorder is an autosomal recessive trait that presumably has a low carrier frequency. There is no method for carrier testing. Prenatal diagnosis is not available.

Familial Spontaneous Pneumothorax

Spontaneous pneumothorax occurs most commonly either as an isolated sporadic problem or in association with acquired pulmonary disease. Less commonly, it occurs as a component of a familial disorder. There are several genetic disorders that may cause spontaneous pneumothorax, including pleiotropic defects that affect connective tissue, for example, Marfan syndrome and Ehlers-Danlos syndrome (see Chap. 72), and pleiotropic defects that affect lung parenchyma directly, for example, tuberous sclerosis (see below). There also exists a familial form of isolated spontaneous pneumothorax that is not associated with other clinical problems. It is this disorder, generally referred to as *familial spontaneous pneumothorax*, that is discussed in this section.

Clinical Manifestations

Spontaneous familial pneumothorax may occur at any age, but most typically it presents in early adulthood. For example, Lenler-Petersen and coauthors [107] recently reported on a single, large pedigree in which 27 members were examined, 8 of whom were affected. The average age (± standard deviation) of onset of the first pneumothorax was 28 ± 9 years (range, 17 to 43 years). Clearly, the age of onset may be quite variable, even within a single pedigree. As an extreme example of this variability, Wilson and Aylsworth [184] described a family in which some individuals presented in infancy whereas others did not present until the fifth decade. The sex ratio (male-female) is about 2:1, which differs from the female preponderance seen in patients with nonfamilial spontaneous pneumothorax. This entity may [45] or may not [68] predominate in people of above-average height.

No clinical features distinguish a pneumothorax that develops in patients with familial spontaneous pneumothorax from a pneumothorax that develops in other contexts. Patients often have multiple recurrences. Some patients have presented with simultaneous bilateral pneumothoraces. Chest radiographs demonstrate localized, subpleural bullae and, during acute attacks, pneumothoraces. CT scanning detects many, but not all bullae found later at the time of surgery [132]. Pulmonary function is generally normal following the acute episode, but some patients have increased residual volumes and reduced diffusion capacity in the absence of acute symptoms [68].

Pathogenesis

The cause of familial spontaneous pneumothorax is unknown. For example, no relationship has been found between familial spontaneous pneumothorax and HLA haplotypes, alpha$_1$-antitrypsin phenotype, or dynamic lung measurements [107]. Several hypotheses have been put forward to explain the etiology of this disorder, and include the presence of hereditary lung cysts (subpleural blebs) that are predisposed to rupture, the presence of an unusually sharp inner margin of the first or second rib, and the presence of an as-yet-unappreciated defect in connective tissue. The most favored hypothesis is the first. Subpleural blebs have been demonstrated at the time of thoracoscopy in some patients, but not in others [68]. These hypotheses are not mutually exclusive, and different mechanisms may operate in different patients.

Diagnosis

The diagnosis can only be made in the presence of a family history of isolated spontaneous pneumothorax, and after exclusion of an acquired pulmonary disease, a relationship to menstrual cycle (catamenial pneumothorax), and a familial disorder known to be associated with spontaneous pneumothorax. There is no specific laboratory test to establish or confirm the diagnosis.

One disorder that must often be ruled out is Marfan syndrome. As a rule, patients with Marfan syndrome who present with pneumothorax have extensive pulmonary disease with generalized emphysema and honeycombing on radiographic examination, whereas patients with familial spontaneous pneumothorax have neither. The diagnosis of Marfan syndrome can generally be established on the basis of characteristic skeletal, cardiac, and ocular manifestations; body measurements; and a family history. However, some patients with Marfan syndrome who develop pneumothoraces have neither radiographic evidence of underlying lung disease nor the charac-

teristic manifestations of this disorder. A careful history and examination of family members may be required to identify whether these individuals have Marfan syndrome. The recent demonstration that the basic defect in Marfan syndrome involves fibrillin biosynthesis (see Chap. 72) should facilitate making the diagnosis in patients with a mild form of this disease and distinguishing them from patients with familial spontaneous pneumothorax.

Treatment

The chief danger to individuals with familial spontaneous pneumothorax is the occurrence of hypoventilation and death. Although patients with no respiratory or cardiac embarrassment may recover from small pneumothoraces with bed rest, tube thoracotomy is required for larger pneumothoraces. The incidence of recurrence is high, and the probability of recurrence increases with each successive pneumothorax. As a result, it is recommended that surgical procedures to obliterate the pleural space be done if pneumothoraces recur. (See Chap. 74 for a fuller discussion of the medical and surgical management of pneumothorax.) Some authors [132] advocate very aggressive surgical intervention following the first episode. In their view, a young patient who presents with spontaneous pneumothorax and an unambiguous family history should have surgical intervention following the first episode in the form of bilateral bullectomy and/or pleurectomy.

Genetics

A number of multigenerational pedigrees with familial spontaneous pneumothorax have been described [45,68,106,107,184]. These pedigrees have traditionally been described as consistent with an autosomal dominant pattern of inheritance with incomplete penetrance and variable expression.

Abolnik and colleagues [1] recently reported a detailed genetic study of 32 families with familial spontaneous pneumothorax. They personally examined 15 of these families, and ascertained the remainder from previously published cases that had included sufficiently detailed pedigree information. These authors proposed two alternate hypotheses to explain the segregation patterns they observed. The first hypothesis was that familial spontaneous pneumothorax was an autosomal dominant trait with incomplete penetrance; the penetrance differed for male (50 percent) and female (21 percent) heterozygotes. The second hypothesis was that familial spontaneous pneumothorax is a genetically heterogeneous disorder that is transmitted as an X-linked recessive trait in some families and as an autosomal dominant trait with incomplete penetrance (males, 50 percent; females, 35 percent) in others. The second hypothesis was proposed to explain the relative preponderance of unaffected female carriers. The second hypothesis is supported by the authors' finding that there were differences in the mean age of onset and severity of pneumothorax in families whose pedigrees were more consistent with X-linked recessive inheritance compared to those pedigrees more consistent with autosomal dominant inheritance. Further studies will be required to test these hypotheses.

Hermansky-Pudlak Syndrome

There are several lipid storage disorders that lead to interstitial pulmonary fibrosis. Two of these disorders, Gaucher disease and Niemann-Pick disease, are well-characterized sphingolipidoses that are discussed in detail in Chapter 72. A third disorder, Hermansky-Pudlak syndrome, is discussed here. This disorder is not a sphingolipidosis; its cause is unknown.

The Hermansky-Pudlak syndrome is an autosomal recessive disorder characterized by a highly distinctive phenotype comprised of three unusual clinical abnormalities: oculocutaneous albinism; a bleeding diathesis caused by platelet storage pool deficiency; and ceroid deposition in the reticuloendothelial system, oral and intestinal mucosa, kidneys, and lung parenchyma [46,187]. The Hermansky-Pudlak syndrome has been identified in many different ethnic groups, but its frequency is particularly high among Puerto Ricans, in whom the incidence is estimated to be about 1 in 2000 [187].

Clinical Manifestations

The Hermansky-Pudlak syndrome is characterized by a highly variable clinical phenotype, with most patients showing some expression of each component of the characteristic clinical triad [46,187]. Patients generally exhibit a degree of oculocutaneous albinism that is comparable to that seen in patients with tyrosinase-positive albinism; the degree of albinism is generally milder than that seen in patients with classic tyrosinase-negative albinism who have essentially complete absence of pigmentation. In all cases, there is a significant degree of ocular involvement. Patients invariably have photophobia, nystagmus, foveal hypoplasia, albinoid fundi, and decreased visual acuity. Visual evoked potentials show a characteristic abnormality consistent with a defect in decussation of the optic tracts [187].

The second feature of this syndrome, a bleeding diathesis, is almost always present, but may be quite variable in severity. The bleeding disorder is generally mild. Patients exhibit easy bruisability, epistaxis, and prolonged bleeding following routine surgical procedures (e.g., tooth extraction). In a few patients, the bleeding disorder has led to serious and even life-threatening consequences. Most women with this disease have minimal difficulty with childbirth, but some women have died because of massive intrapartum bleeding. Other patients have died from gastric hemorrhage, often associated with ill-advised use of acetylsalicylic acid. Acetylsalicylic acid exacerbates the platelet dysfunction that characterizes Hermansky-Pudlak syndrome, and should not be used by these patients [46,187]. Witkop and colleagues [187] found that the deaths of about 15 percent of patients were caused by uncontrollable bleeding.

Ceroid deposition in the oral and intestinal mucosa, kidneys, and lung parenchyma is associated with significant clinical manifestations. The ceroid deposition appears to be age-dependent; the onset of symptoms associated with aberrant ceroid deposition is generally in adulthood, although children with gastrointestinal manifestations have been reported [117]. Pulmonary fibrosis is the most frequent of the disorders caused by ceroid deposition, followed by gastrointestinal disease, kidney disease, and least frequently, cardiomyopathy. Patients may have more than one of these organs affected at the same time [46, 64,150,187].

The precise proportion of patients with Hermansky-Pudlak syndrome who develop diffuse interstitial pulmonary fibrosis is unknown [46, 64]. Recent estimates suggest that greater than one-half of patients have evidence of decreased pulmonary function, which is often evident before clinical or radiologic abnormalities can be documented [188]. Pulmonary function studies have revealed changes characteristic of interstitial lung disease beginning in the second decade of life, whereas clinically significant disease generally does not begin until the fourth decade. Hermansky-Pudlak syndrome produces interstitial lung disease with clinical, radiographic, and physiologic characteristics typical of sporadic interstitial pulmonary fibrosis. The pulmonary disorder is generally progressive, leading to severe respiratory insufficiency and often death in the fourth or fifth decade [42,46,64,187]. Pulmonary fibrosis accounts for about 60 percent of deaths among patients with Hermansky-Pudlak syndrome, making it the leading cause of their death [188].

Hermansky-Pudlak syndrome may lead to severe granulomatous bowel disease, and sometimes granulomatous gingival disease as well [150,187]. This clinical manifestation generally presents in the second or third decade, but may present in childhood [117]. Although the bowel disease closely resembles Crohn's disease in its clinical and pathologic presentation, it generally proves more refractory to standard medical management and is more likely to require surgical intervention. About 5 percent of Hermansky-Pudlak patients die from the complications of granulomatous bowel disease.

Ceroid deposition in the proximal tubular epithelium may lead to clinically significant kidney disease, including renal failure. Hermansky-Pudlak syndrome does not cause glomerular disease. Renal disease is an uncommon cause of death for these patients. Lastly, ceroid deposition in the myocardium is a rare cause of cardiomyopathy in these patients.

Pathogenesis

The underlying cause for this pleiotropic disorder remains unknown, although much has been learned about the pathogenesis of the various clinical manifestations. For example, there is convincing evidence that the oculocutaneous albinism seen in patients with Hermansky-Pudlak syndrome is not caused by a primary defect in tyrosinase, the enzyme that catalyzes the first step in the conversion of tyrosine to melanin. Ultrastructural studies have shown that reduced skin pigmentation is characterized by a defect in melanosome maturation. It appears that there is an inability to activate tyrosinase rather than a defect in the tyrosinase molecule itself. Current evidence suggests that the primary defect is in the thioredoxin–thioredoxin reductase pathway which is required for activating tyrosinase [149, 187]. Further proof is required to confirm this suggestion.

The most consistent morphologic finding in these patients is the absence of platelet dense bodies. Dense bodies store adenine nucleotides, serotonin, and calcium, all of which are required for the second wave of platelet aggregation. Absent these storage bodies, platelets from Hermansky-Pudlak syndrome patients demonstrate a normal first wave of aggregation, but do not undergo a normal second wave. The cause for the dense body deficiency is unknown. Witkop and colleagues [186] proposed that the absence of platelet dense bodies is the most specific and sensitive diagnostic indicator for Hermansky-Pudlak syndrome.

The ceroid material that accumulates morphologically resembles that seen in patients with neuronal ceroid lipofuscinosis, a group of rare autosomal recessive disorders associated with neurodevelopmental retardation. The storage material was thought previously to be composed of unsaturated fatty acids derived from phagocytized red blood cells, but this does not appear to be true. Current evidence shows that ceroid is composed of dolichols derived from incompletely processed lysosomal membranes; dolichols are very long (90 to 105 carbons/molecule) polyisoprenoid alcohols that are located in lysosomal membranes [187]. Ceroid cannot be degraded, but can only be removed from cells by exocytosis. Thus, once formed, ceroid tends to accumulate progressively with time if there is a defect in exocytosis. Witkop and coworkers [187] proposed that ceroid accumulation may be caused by a defect in the thioredoxin pathway, which affects a thioendoproteinase that is required for exocytosis.

The pathogenesis of the interstitial pulmonary disease in patients with Hermansky-Pudlak syndrome appears to be related to an interaction of ceroid with the pulmonary macrophage [188]. Examination of fibrotic and nonfibrotic sections of lung showed that ceroid deposition precedes fibrosis. Ultrastructural analysis showed ceroid accumulation in the alveolar space and the alveolar macrophage, as well as in alveolar macrophages obtained from pulmonary lavage fluid. It remains unknown whether the origin of the ceroid is exogenous (i.e., derived from endocytosis of ceroid-laden cells) or endogenous (i.e., derived from an intrinsic defect in macrophage metabolism). Analysis of the pulmonary lavage fluid also showed an increased concentration of platelet-derived growth factor (PDGF), which is a stimulant of mesenchymal cell proliferation and fibrosis. These observations suggest a key role for the pulmonary macrophage in the pathogenesis of pulmonary fibrosis in patients with Hermansky-Pudlak syndrome.

Diagnosis

Diagnosis has required demonstrating the features of the clinical triad that defines this disorder. This is generally not difficult once the diagnosis is considered, although it can be difficult in some patients because of the high variability of the disorder. More recently, Witkop and colleagues [186] described a new method for diagnosing Hermansky-Pudlak syndrome that utilizes morphometric analysis of platelet dense bodies. These authors proposed that the absence of platelet dense bodies was the most reliable diagnostic criterion for Hermansky-Pudlak syndrome.

Treatment

There is no specific therapy for the interstitial pulmonary disease of Hermansky-Pudlak syndrome [46,187]. Immunosuppressive drugs have been reported to have no effect, but well-controlled studies have not been performed. Vitamin E may ameliorate the bleeding diathesis of these patients, but has not been effective against the pulmonary manifestations.

Genetics

The disease is transmitted as an autosomal recessive trait. There is evidence that the basic defect may be in the activity of thioredoxin reductase. Schallreuter and coworkers [149] examined obligate heterozygotes (i.e., carriers) from several pedigrees and found that they had reduced thioredoxin activity. Further substantiation of this finding is required. Presymptomatic detection and prenatal diagnosis are not currently available.

Phakomatoses

The *phakomatoses* are a highly heterogeneous group of disorders that share the characteristic of patchy skin lesions. The phakomatoses include neurofibromatosis, tuberous sclerosis, von Hippel-Lindau disease, and Sturge-Weber syndrome. Pulmonary disease is generally not a component of the phakomatoses, but a small proportion of patients with neurofibromatosis and tuberous sclerosis manifest significant pulmonary disease. These disorders are therefore discussed in this chapter. In addition, lymphangioleiomyomatosis is discussed because there are significant similarities between lymphangioleiomyomatosis and

pulmonary tuberous sclerosis. Von Hippel-Lindau disease and Sturge-Weber syndrome (encephalotrigeminal angiomatosis) occasionally show pulmonary angiomatous tumors and hemangiomas, respectively, but these manifestations are rarely clinically significant; these disorders therefore are not discussed.

Neurofibromatosis

There has been recognition in recent years that there are several forms of neurofibromatosis. A National Institutes of Health Consensus Development Conference [131] proposed a classification scheme and diagnostic criteria for the different forms of neurofibromatosis. The most common form is von Recklinghausen's neurofibromatosis, which has been designated *neurofibromatosis type 1* or *NF-1*. NF-1 has an incidence of approximately 1 in 3000; about 80,000 Americans currently suffer from this disorder [114,131, 145]. The other well-characterized form of neurofibromatosis has been termed *NF-2;* NF-2 was known previously as the central or acoustic form of neurofibromatosis because it is characterized by the development of bilateral acoustic neuroma. NF-1 and NF-2 are genetically and clinically distinct disorders [114,129,131]. There are several other forms of neurofibromatosis that are poorly characterized. The remainder of this discussion deals only with NF-1 because it is the only form of neurofibromatosis that is associated with significant pulmonary disease.

CLINICAL MANIFESTATIONS

NF-1 is a highly pleiotropic disorder, and is highly variable in its severity of expression [114,131,145, 146]. Until recently, NF-1 was generally considered a uniformly severe disorder. It now appears that most patients manifest relatively mild disability, whereas only a minority are moderately or severely affected.

The clinical hallmarks of NF-1 are areas of skin pigmentation termed *café-au-lait spots* and multiple neurofibromas [131]. Diagnosis is based on the presence of these and other clinical findings; the specific diagnostic criteria are presented below. The size and number of café-au-lait spots and neurofibroma generally increase with age. NF-1 may affect almost any organ in the body [114,131,145,146]. Males and females are equally affected. Central nervous system involvement may include developmental delay or mental retardation, learning or behavioral disabilities, and tumors. Peripheral nervous system involvement may lead to the previously mentioned neurofibroma, which on occasion may become large, disfiguring plexiform lesions. Autonomic dysfunction may result from involvement of the autonomic nervous system. Malignant degeneration may develop in any part of the nervous system. Musculoskeletal deformities may develop, and a wide variety of endocrinopathies have been observed.

Pulmonary Disease. Thoracic manifestations are thought to occur in about 15 percent of patients with NF-1 [3]. However, their true frequency is unknown. Pulmonary disease may be produced either indirectly through extrapulmonary intrathoracic lesions or directly from intrinsic pulmonary disease. Extrapulmonary intrathoracic manifestations include thoracic skeletal deformities, paravertebral meningoceles, and tumors of the sympathetic chain and vagus, recurrent laryngeal, phrenic, and intercostal nerves [3,144,145]. In one study [55], over 80 percent of all intrathoracic meningoceles were found in association with NF-1. Kyphoscoliosis is found in 10 percent or less of patients. A characteristic pattern of rib notching and a "twisted ribbon" deformity are seen on chest roentgenograms. Paravertebral tumors may present as posterior mediastinal masses, appearing as dumbbell-shaped lesions on radiographic examination. Management of these extrapleural lesions in patients with NF-1 does not differ from their management when they occur in other circumstances.

Intrinsic parenchymal disease may develop in the form of interstitial pulmonary fibrosis either alone or in combination with bullae [43,77,120, 181]. Webb and Goodman [181] found clinical evidence of interstitial fibrosis in about 10 percent of the 70 patients they studied. However, Massaro and Katz [120] found evidence of interstitial fibrosis in lung biopsy specimens from patients who had normal-appearing chest radiographs, suggesting that the frequency of interstitial pulmonary disease may be greater than currently appreciated. Interstitial fibrosis is generally symmetric, affecting both lung bases, whereas bullae are generally asymmetric, affecting primarily the upper lobes. The onset of pulmonary parenchymal disease is generally in later life, with variable progression. Symptoms are usually mild, but the disease may progress to severe respiratory insufficiency, cor pulmonale, and death. Pulmonary hypertension may also develop [140]. CT examination may be useful in the diagnosis of patients who have normal-appearing chest x-ray films [9].

Pulmonary function testing has shown that these patients may have either obstructive or restrictive defects, or both, and decreased diffusion capacity. The histologic pattern seen in patients with interstitial infiltrates is similar to that seen in other conditions that lead to pulmonary fibrosis.

PATHOGENESIS
Dramatic progress has been made in understanding the molecular basis of NF-1 since publication of the last edition of this textbook. The NF-1 locus has been mapped to a specific region of chromosome 17; the gene itself has been identified, cloned, and sequenced; specific mutations responsible for producing disease have been identified; and epigenetic factors influencing expression of the disease have been identified.

Chromosomal mapping of the NF-1 gene to the pericentric region of chromosome 17 was accomplished by classic linkage studies [6,153]. The location of the gene was defined more narrowly to band 17q11.2 by high-resolution cytogenetic analysis of chromosomal rearrangements which were identified in two patients who had unusual clinical phenotypes [151]. The NF-1 gene was subsequently identified and cloned from this chromosome segment [28,177,179]. The NF-1 gene is a large gene (about 300 kb) with a complex structure. Although the full function of the NF-1 gene has not been elucidated, it has been established that the gene encodes for a guanosine diphosphatase-activating protein (GAP), which is involved in the control of cell proliferation through interaction with *ras* oncogenes [189]. The NF-1 gene also encodes, on the antisense strand, for three smaller genes: two ecotropic viral-insertion-site genes and an oligodendrocyte-myelin glycoprotein gene [28,179]. The relationship of these genes to the pathogenesis of NF-1 is unknown. The large size of the NF-1 gene may explain the high frequency of new mutations observed for this disorder (see below).

The mechanism(s) whereby the NF-1 gene produces the various clinical manifestations of the disease are still unknown. It appears that the oncogenic potential of the disease requires interaction with at least one other gene, a suppressor gene (p53) located on the short arm of chromosome 17 [123]. The rate of progress in deciphering the molecular pathogenesis of NF-1 is rapid, and there is considerable confidence that this progress will lead to improved methods for diagnosis and hopefully, for prevention and treatment.

DIAGNOSIS

Despite the significant advances that have been made in understanding the molecular basis of NF-1, diagnosis is still based on clinical criteria for most patients. The dependence on clinical diagnostic criteria remains absolute for sporadic cases and for patients with a family history of neurofibromatosis in whom genetic linkage has not been established. The diagnostic criteria, as recommended by the National Institutes of Health Consensus Development Conference [131], are shown in Table 70-4. There are seven diagnostic criteria. Diagnosis requires that at least two of these criteria be satisfied. For an individual with a proven family history (i.e., a first-degree relative who satisfies two of these criteria), only one other clinical criterion is required.

Patients who are suspected of having NF-1 should have careful physical examinations directed toward identifying these criteria. The search for café-au-lait spots should include examination with a Wood's lamp. Special attention should be directed to the axillary and inguinal folds and, in postpubertal women, to the areolar area of the breast. The search for iris Lisch nodules should be performed using a slit lamp. A recent, systematic study of 167 patients with NF-1 showed that the prevalence of Lisch nodules increases with age; Lisch nodules were invariably present by the age of 20 years [114,115].

Table 70-4.* Clinical criteria for the diagnosis of NF-1

*Diagnosis requires the presence of two or more of these criteria:

Six or more café-au-lait spots > 5 mm in greatest diameter in prepubertal individuals and > 15 mm in greatest diameter in postpubertal individuals

Two or more neurofibromas of any type or one plexiform neurofibroma

Freckling in the axillary or inguinal regions

Optic glioma

Two or more Lisch nodules (iris hamartoma)

A distinctive osseous lesion such as sphenoid dysplasia or thinning of long-bone cortex, with or without pseudarthrosis

A first-degree relative (parent, sibling, or offspring) with NF-1 by the above criteria

Source: From National Institutes of Health Consensus Development Conference. Neurofibromatosis. Conference statement. *Arch Neurol* 45:575, 1988.

Presymptomatic diagnosis can be accomplished for patients who have a positive family history using linkage analysis [180]. A number of flanking, tightly linked DNA markers are available for analyzing at-risk family members. Linkage analysis is highly accurate at this time. The results of linkage analysis will be very useful for directing medical surveillance of at-risk patients (i.e., patients who may have inherited the NF-1 gene). At-risk patients shown not to have inherited the NF-1 gene by linkage analysis will be spared the radiation exposure, inconvenience, cost, and anxiety of anticipatory medical surveillance, whereas those patients demonstrated to have inherited the NF-1 gene will be best served by rigorous surveillance.

TREATMENT

There is no specific treatment available for the clinical manifestations of NF-1, including the pulmonary manifestations. Treatment for the various tumors that involve the thorax and affect pulmonary function is discussed in Chapter 56. Treatment for the pulmonary fibrosis that may accompany NF-1 is nonspecific.

GENETICS

Neurofibromatosis is inherited as an autosomal dominant disorder, with almost complete penetrance and highly variable expressivity [131]. Thus, almost all patients who possess the NF-1 gene manifest some signs of the disorder, but the degree of involvement varies. There may be considerable intrafamilial variation in the severity of disease. No explanation for the variable expressivity of the disorder is available.

An unusually high proportion of patients has NF-1 as a consequence of a new mutation. About half the patients with NF-1 have a family history of the disorder and half do not. The mutation rate is estimated to be 1 in 10^4, which is about an order of magnitude greater than the rate for most other autosomal dominant disorders. The high mutation rate is associated with an advanced paternal age effect. There appears to be no difference in the degree or pattern of involvement of patients with a family history compared to those without. Similarly, there is no difference in the degree or pattern of disease between patients who inherited the NF-1 gene from their mother and patients who inherited the gene from their father.

Genetic counseling requires determining whether the affected individual is a sporadic or a familial case. This may not be possible in all cases. All first-degree relatives should have a careful examination, including a Wood's lamp inspection of the skin for café-au-lait spots and a slit-lamp examination of the eyes for Lisch nodules. Presymptomatic testing and prenatal diagnosis are possible by linkage analysis in those families in whom there are two or more affected individuals, and at least one affected individual is available for DNA analysis. Linkage analysis is not available for families in whom there is only one sporadic case.

Tuberous Sclerosis

Tuberous sclerosis is a relatively uncommon genetic disorder with an incidence of about 1 in 100,000 [70,71]. It was originally recognized as a triad of clinical findings: adenoma sebaceum (dermal angiofibroma), epilepsy, and mental retardation. Subsequently, tuberous sclerosis became recognized as a highly pleiotropic disorder associated with a wide variety of clinical problems including interstitial pulmonary fibrosis [70,71].

CLINICAL MANIFESTATIONS

Patients with tuberous sclerosis may present at any age. One-fourth of patients present in the first 2 years of life, one-half present by the end of the first decade, and three-fourths present by the end of the second decade; thus, about one-fourth of patients do not present until adulthood [70]. Males and females are affected with equal frequency and severity. Seizures are the most common cause for presentation, followed by developmental delay or mental retardation. The seizures may be generalized and/or partial; the most characteristic pattern is that of infantile spasms. Similarly, the degree of mental retardation is highly variable, ranging from mild to severe. Other manifestations include hamartoma of the brain and kidney, sclerotic bone lesions, and cardiac rhabdomyoma. There is considerable clinical variation among patients, even among affected individuals in the same family.

Physical examination of affected patients reveals a wide range of findings. Nearly all patients have one or more characteristic skin lesions including hypomelanotic macules (86 percent), facial angiofibroma (47 percent), ungual fibromas (20 percent), and shagreen patches (19 percent) [70]. About one-half of patients have retinal hamartoma. CT may be helpful in establishing the diagnosis by revealing intracranial, periventricular calcifications [119].

With increasing recognition of this disorder, a broader spectrum of involvement is being appreciated, and its diagnosis should be considered in the adult who presents with renal cyst disease (angiomyolipoma) or pulmonary interstitial disease. These manifestations are a significant cause of morbidity and mortality for patients with tuberous sclerosis. Shepherd and colleagues [155] summarized their experience with 355 patients and reported the causes of death for the 40 patients who had died. Renal disease was the leading cause of death (11 deaths); 4 patients died of lung disease.

Pulmonary Disease. Pulmonary disease is an uncommon problem for patients with tuberous sclerosis, affecting less than 3 percent of patients [48,70,78,155]. The average age of onset of pulmonary disease is in the fourth decade, and onset before the age of 20 years is rare [48]. The great majority of patients with pulmonary disease have been women, in contrast to the equal sex ratio found for patients with tuberous sclerosis as a whole. It also has been found that pulmonary symptoms generally occur in patients who do not have mental retardation or seizures, which is again in contrast to the experience with the entire group of patients with tuberous sclerosis. This observation may, however, represent as ascertainment bias.

Patients generally present with dyspnea, but they may present with spontaneous pneumothorax or hemoptysis [4,48]. Symptoms generally do not begin before the third decade. Findings on radiologic studies may be normal. Abnormal radiologic findings include a reticulated interstitial pattern followed by a cystic honeycomb appearance, which is often associated with bullae [3]. Thin-section CT examinations reveal numerous small, thin-walled cysts that are evenly distributed throughout the lung. The CT findings appear to be more sensitive and distinctive than those of chest radiographs, and correlate better with results of pulmonary function studies [108]. Lung volumes are either normal or increased. Pulmonary function studies demonstrate both obstructive and restrictive patterns. The diffusion capacity is commonly reduced, and severe hypoxemia may be present.

Microscopic examination of the lungs reveals that the pleura are thickened and have a nodular surface, with numerous cysts [44,48,109]. The cysts are lined by columnar epithelium, and their walls are composed of fibrous connective tissue, hypertrophic smooth muscle, and dilated thin-walled vessels. The microscopic picture closely resembles that of pulmonary lymphangioleiomyomatosis, that is, proliferation and hypertrophy of smooth muscle in bronchioles and alveoli and around lymphatics and arterioles. Nodular masses of smooth muscle may press on pulmonary veins. Erosion of veins by nodules may produce hemoptysis, and occlusion of bronchioles may result in airway obstruction. It is thought that rupture of subpleural cysts is the cause of spontaneous pneumothorax in these patients.

The prognosis for patients who develop lung disease is poor [44,48,155,158]. Pulmonary symptoms are generally progressive; the mean length of survival after diagnosis is less than 5 years. The severity of disease is often made worse by pregnancy. Death usually occurs because of progressive cor pulmonale, but it may result from tension pneumothorax. In a recent review of the causes of death for patients with tuberous sclerosis, Shepherd and colleagues [155] found that pulmonary disease was the cause of death for 10 percent of the patients who had died. All the patients who died because of lung disease did so after the age of 40 years.

Relationship Between Tuberous Sclerosis and Lymphangioleiomyomatosis. In 1968, Frank and colleagues [59] introduced the term *lymphangiomyomatosis* (now generally termed *lymphangioleiomyomatosis*) to describe a condition characterized by multifocal hyperplasia of smooth-muscle cells in the mediastinal and retroperitoneal lymph nodes, as well as in the peribronchial, perivascular, and perilymphatic regions of the lung. There is a striking similarity between the pulmonary manifestations of tuberous sclerosis and lymphangioleiomyomatosis.

There have been several excellent reviews on lymphangioleiomyomatosis [32,157,163,169]. This condition is thought to occur exclusively in women. Affected women generally present during their childbearing years, and symptoms often develop during pregnancy. As the disease progresses, there is occlusion of lymphatic drainage and bronchiolar cysts develop. Hence, patients present with progressive dyspnea, chylous pleural and peritoneal effusions (seen in over 80 percent of cases), spontaneous pneumothorax, and hemoptysis.

Progressive reticulonodular interstitial infiltrates, recurrent pneumothoraces, recurrent pleural effusions, or a combination of these findings are seen on chest roentgenograms. CT is of help in diagnosing this condition, and may offer significant advantages over the standard chest x-ray study [108,124,169]. Lymphangiography commonly demonstrates dilated lymphatic channels, aberrant fistulas, and enlarged lymph nodes along lymphatic channels [157]. Characteristically, obstructive defects or a combination of obstructive and restrictive defects are found on pulmonary function testing [163,169].

The histologic features of the pulmonary disease found in patients with lymphangiomyomatosis are generally thought to be the same as those found in patients with pulmonary manifestations of tuberous sclerosis, although some small differences may be present [25]. In addition, some patients with lymphangiomyomatosis have been found to have angiomyolipoma of the kidney, similar to patients with tuberous sclerosis [109,126]. Conversely, some patients with tuberous sclerosis develop chylothorax. It has been suggested, therefore, that lymphangiomyomatosis may be a limited form ("forme fruste") of tuberous sclerosis [176]. The main argument against this suggestion is that familial recurrence has not been found for lymphangiomyomatosis. The exact relationship between tuberous sclerosis and lymphangiomyomatosis remains unclear [25].

In lymphangiomyomatosis, as in tuberous sclerosis, no form of therapy for the lung disease has been tested systematically in large numbers of patients and there is no satisfactory therapy.

PATHOGENESIS

The underlying cause of tuberous sclerosis is unknown. Recent genetic evidence suggests that tuberous sclerosis is genetically heterogeneous [60,75]. There is a subset of families for which the disease locus has been mapped to chromosome segment 9q32-9q34. In other families, linkage to this locus has been disproved, and a second disease locus must exist elsewhere in the genome. A second locus has been mapped provisionally to the long arm of chromosome 11, but linkage with this locus has been disproved for some families. Thus, there is currently evidence for two or more loci for tuberous sclerosis. In the small number of families studied to date, no difference between the clinical features of patients having chromosome 9–linked disease and other patients has been found, but additional families will need to be examined before a definitive genotype-phenotype correlation can be established. None of the genes responsible for tuberous sclerosis has been identified, but progress has been very rapid and the tuberous sclerosis genes will almost certainly be cloned in the near future.

DIAGNOSIS

The diagnosis of tuberous sclerosis is generally based on clinical criteria. There is no laboratory test currently available for diagnosis, except for those few families in whom genetic linkage analysis has been established. The diagnostic criteria recommended by Gomez [70] are summarized in Table 70-5. Gomez [70] proposed two sets of criteria, one set that permits definitive diagnosis and a second set that permits presumptive diagnosis. Definitive diagnosis can be established by the presence of at least one of the "definitive" criteria; the diagnosis of tuberous sclerosis is presumed until proved otherwise for any patient who has two or more of the "presumptive" criteria. The presence of a proven family history (an affected first-degree relative) plus one of the presumptive criterion is sufficient for diagnosis.

A patient who is suspected of having tuberous sclerosis should have careful physical and radiologic examinations directed to identifying these criteria. The search for characteristic skin lesions should include examination with a Wood's lamp. A complete family history should be obtained and all first-degree relatives should be examined (see below).

TREATMENT

There is no consistently effective treatment for the pulmonary manifestation of tuberous sclerosis. Dietary manipulation, irradiation, thoracic duct ligation, and cyclophosphamide (Cytoxan) have failed to halt progression of the disease [48,78,169]. The most actively explored treatment approach has been hormonal ablation or supplementation therapy. The rationale for this approach is the evidence showing the clinical and pathologic similarities between pulmonary tuberous sclerosis and lymphangioleiomyomatosis. Both diseases occur predominantly or exclusively in premenopausal women, and are often exacerbated during pregnancy. Furthermore, estrogen and progesterone receptors have been demonstrated in affected lung tissue from patients with both diseases.

The variety of hormonal therapies that have been tried include oophorectomy, tamoxifen, progesterone, and different combinations of these individual therapies. A few remissions have been reported with oophorectomy plus tamoxifen, oophorectomy plus progesterone, or progesterone alone [2,121,148]. It is very difficult to draw any conclusions from these various studies because so many different protocols have been used and because patients were generally started on treatment relatively late in their course of disease [169]. Since hormonal therapy appears to stabilize rather than reverse the development of lung disease, early treatment may be required. Further studies, including consistent measurement of hormonal receptors in affected lung tissue, are needed to evaluate the efficacy of hor-

Table 70-5. **Clinical criteria for the diagnosis of tuberous sclerosis***

Definitive criteria	Presumptive criteria
Adenoma sebaceum (facial angiofibroma)	Hypomelanotic macules
Ungual fibroma	Shagreen patches
Retinal hamartoma	Peripapillary retinal hamartoma
Cortical tuber	Gingival fibromas
Subependymal glial nodule	Dental enamel pits
Renal angiomyolipoma	Single renal angiomyolipoma
	Multicystic kidneys
	Cardiac rhabdomyoma
	Pulmonary lymphangiomyomatosis
	Radiographic "honeycomb" lungs
	Infantile spasms
	Myoclonic, tonic, or atonic seizures
	First-degree relative (parent, sibling, or offspring) with tuberous sclerosis

*Definitive diagnosis requires the presence of at least one of the "definitive" criteria, whereas presumptive diagnosis requires the presence of at least two of the "presumptive" criteria.
Source: From MR Gomez. *Tuberous Sclerosis* (2nd ed). New York: Raven, 1988.

monal therapy in both lymphangiomyomatosis and pulmonary tuberous sclerosis. Heart-lung transplantation has been used for treating patients who have far-advanced lymphangioleiomyomatosis [182].

GENETICS

Tuberous sclerosis is an autosomal dominant trait with high penetrance and variable expressivity [22,70]. The major limitation in providing genetic counseling for this disorder is the ambiguity in establishing whether an affected individual is a sporadic or a familial case. Approximately 80 percent of patients have no family history of the disease and presumably represent new mutations. As opposed to the observations for many other autosomal dominant disorders, the frequency of new mutations does not correlate with advanced parental ages. There do not appear to be significant phenotypic differences between patients who have a family history of the disease and those who do not. However, the genetic implications for other family members depend on whether or not the proband represents a new mutation. Therefore, all first-degree relatives (parents, siblings, and children) of the proband should be examined to identify other affected individuals. The examination of these relatives should include careful ophthalmologic examination and skin inspection using a Wood's lamp, and probably echocardiography, renal ultrasonography, and cranial CT or magnetic resonance imaging [27,160].

Prenatal diagnosis is not generally possible because there is no biologic marker for the disease. Theoretically, linkage analysis should permit prenatal diagnosis, as well as presymptomatic diagnosis. However, this is generally not possible because (1) many cases are the result of new mutations, in which case linkage cannot be established, and (2) even for cases in which there is a family history of the disease, linkage analysis is limited by the genetic heterogeneity of tuberous sclerosis. As a result of these limitations, prenatal diagnosis is not generally available.

Prenatal diagnosis is available in the special circumstance when prenatal ultrasonography reveals evidence of fetal cardiac rhabdomyoma. Since cardiac rhabdomyomas are rare tumors that are associated with tuberous sclerosis at least 50 percent of the time [93,178], the demonstration of fetal cardiac rhabdomyoma suggests that the fetus is affected. This is particularly true in the setting of a pregnancy at risk for this disease.

References

1. Abolnik IZ, et al. On the inheritance of primary spontaneous pneumothorax. *Am J Med Genet* 40:155, 1991.
2. Adamson D, et al. Successful treatment of pulmonary lymphangiomyomatosis with oophorectomy and progesterone. *Am Rev Respir Dis* 132:916, 1985.
3. Aughenbaugh GL. Thoracic manifestations of neurocutaneous diseases. *Radiol Clin North Am* 22:741, 1984.
4. Babcock TL, Snyder BA. Spontaneous pneumothorax associated with tuberous sclerosis. *J Thorac Cardiovasc Surg* 83:100, 1982.
5. Balikian JP, Fuleihan FJD, Nucho CN. Pulmonary alveolar microlithiasis. Report of five cases with special reference to roentgen manifestations. *AJR* 103:509, 1968.
6. Barker D, et al. Gene for von Recklinghausen neurofibromatosis is in the pericentric region of chromosome 17. *Science* 236:1100, 1987.
7. Barnard NJ, et al. Pulmonary alveolar microlithiasis. A new analytical approach. *Histopathology* 11:639, 1987.
8. Bell RS. The radiographic manifestations of α_1-antitrypsin deficiency: An important recognizable pattern of chronic obstructive pulmonary disease (COPD). *Radiology* 95:19, 1970.
9. Bergin CJ, Muller NL. CT in the diagnosis of interstitial lung disease. *AJR* 145:505, 1985.
10. Bierman HR, Kelly KH, Cortus FL. The sequestration and visceral circulation of leukocytes in man. *Ann NY Acad Sci* 59:850, 1955.
11. Bitterman PB, Adelberg S, Crystal RG. Mechanisms of pulmonary fibrosis: Spontaneous release of the alveolar macrophage-derived growth factor in the interstitial lung disorders. *J Clin Invest* 72:1801, 1983.
12. Bitterman PB, Crystal RG. Is there a fibrotic gene? *Chest* 78:549, 1980.
13. Bitterman PB, et al. Familial idiopathic pulmonary fibrosis. Evidence of lung inflammation in unaffected family members. *N Engl J Med* 314:1343, 1986.
14. Black LF, Kueppers F. α_1-Antitrypsin deficiency in non-smokers. *Am Rev Respir Dis* 117:421, 1978.
15. Blue M-L, Janoff A. Possible mechanisms of emphysema in cigarette smokers: Release of elastase from human polymorphonuclear leukocytes by cigarette smoke condensate in vitro. *Am Rev Respir Dis* 117:317, 1978.
16. Brown J, Leon W, Felton C. Hemodynamic and pulmonary studies in pulmonary alveolar microlithiasis. *Am J Med* 77:176, 1984.
17. Brown ML, et al. Pulmonary uptake of ^{99m}Tc diphosphonate in alveolar microlithiasis. *AJR* 131:703, 1978.
18. Bruce RM, et al. Collaborative study to assess

risk of lung disease in PiMZ phenotype subjects. *Am Rev Respir Dis* 130:386, 1984.

19. Buist AS. α_1-Antitrypsin deficiency in lung and liver disease. *Hosp Pract* 24:51, 1989.

20. Buist AS, et al. Guidelines for the approach to the patient with severe hereditary alpha-1-antitrypsin deficiency. *Am Rev Respir Med* 140:1494, 1989.

21. Buist AS. Pulmonary function in heterozygotes for α_1-antitrypsin deficiency: A case-control study. *Am Rev Respir Dis* 120:759, 1979.

22. Bundey S, Evans K. Tuberous sclerosis: A genetic study. *J Neurol Neurosurg Psychiatry* 32:591, 1969.

23. Caffrey PR, Altman RS. Pulmonary alveolar microlithiasis occurring in premature twins. *J Pediatr* 66:758, 1965.

24. Cale WF, Petsonk EL, Boyd CB. Transbronchial biopsy of pulmonary alveolar microlithiasis. *Arch Intern Med* 143:358, 1983.

25. Capron F, et al. Pulmonary lymphangioleiomyomatosis and Bourneville's tuberous sclerosis with pulmonary involvement: The same disease? *Cancer* 52:851, 1983.

26. Casolaro A, et al. Augmentation of the lung antielastase defenses of primates with parental administration of recombinant DNA produced α_1-antitrypsin. *Am Rev Respir Dis* 133:A103, 1986.

27. Cassidy SB, et al. Family studies in tuberous sclerosis: Evaluation of apparently unaffected parents. *JAMA* 249:1302, 1983.

28. Cawthon RM, et al. A major segment of the neurofibromatosis type 1 gene: cDNA sequence, genomic structure, and point mutations. *Cell* 62:193, 1990.

29. Chalmers AG, Wyatt J, Robinson PJ. Computerized tomographic and pathological findings in pulmonary alveolar microlithiasis. *Br J Radiol* 59:408, 1986.

30. Coetzee T. Pulmonary alveolar microlithiasis with involvement of the sympathetic nervous system and gonads. *Thorax* 25:637, 1970.

31. Cohen AB. Unraveling the mysteries of alpha$_1$-antitrypsin deficiency (editorial). *N Engl J Med* 314:778, 1986.

32. Corrin B, Liebow AA, Friedman PJ. Pulmonary lymphangiomyomatosis: A review. *Am J Pathol* 79:348, 1975.

33. Cox DW. α_1-Antitrypsin Deficiency. In CS Scriver et al (Eds), *The Metabolic Basis of Inherited Disease* (6th ed). New York: McGraw-Hill, 1989. Pp 2409–2437.

34. Cox DW, Levison H. Emphysema of early onset associated with a complete deficiency of alpha-1-antitrypsin (null homozygotes). *Am Rev Respir Dis* 137:371, 1988.

35. Cox DW, Mansfield T. Prenatal diagnosis of α_1-antitrypsin deficiency and estimates of fetal risk for disease. *J Med Genet* 24:52, 1987.

36. Cox DW, Smyth S. Risk for liver disease in adults with alpha$_1$-antitrypsin deficiency. *Am J Med* 74:221, 1983.

37. Cox DW, Woo SLC, Mansfield T. DNA restriction fragments associated with α_1-antitrypsin indicate a single origin for deficiency allele PI Z. *Nature* 316:79, 1985.

38. Crystal RG. α_1-Antitrypsin deficiency, emphysema, and liver disease: Genetic basis and strategies for therapy. *J Clin Invest* 85:1343, 1990.

39. Crystal RG, et al. The α_1-antitrypsin gene and its mutations: Clinical consequences and strategies for therapy. *Chest* 95:197, 1989.

40. Crystal RG, et al. Interstitial lung disease: Current concepts of pathogenesis, staging, and therapy. *Am J Med* 70:542, 1981.

41. Darlington GJ, et al. Assignment of human α_1-antitrypsin in chromosome 14 by somatic cell hybrid analysis. *Proc Natl Acad Sci USA* 79:870, 1982.

42. Davies BH, Tuddenham EGD. Familial pulmonary fibrosis associated with oculocutaneous albinism and platelet function defect. A new syndrome. *Q J Med* 178:219, 1976.

43. Davies PDB. Diffuse pulmonary involvement in von Recklinghausen's disease: A new syndrome. *Thorax* 18:198, 1963.

44. Dawson J. Pulmonary tuberous sclerosis and its relationship to other forms of the disease. *Q J Med* 23:113, 1954.

45. Delaney JC, Gale A, Walker BA. Familial spontaneous pneumothorax. *Postgrad Med J* 50:648, 1974.

46. DePinho RA, Kaplan KL. The Hermansky-Pudlak syndrome: Report of three cases and review of pathophysiology and management considerations. *Medicine* 64:192, 1985.

47. Donohue WL, et al. Familial fibrocystic pulmonary dysplasia and its relation to the Hamman-Rich syndrome. *Pediatrics* 24:786, 1959.

48. Dwyer JM, Hickie JB, Garvan T. Pulmonary tuberous sclerosis: Report of three patients and a review of the literature. *Q J Med* 40:115, 1971.

49. Ellis RH. Familial incidence of diffuse interstitial pulmonary fibrosis. *Postgrad Med J* 41:150, 1965.

50. Eriksson S. Pulmonary emphysema and alpha$_1$-antitrypsin deficiency. *Acta Med Scand* 175:197, 1964.

51. Eriksson S. Studies in α_1-antitrypsin deficiency. *Acta Med Scand Suppl* 432:1, 1965.

52. Eriksson S. Alpha$_1$-antitrypsin deficiency: Lessons learned from the bedside to the gene and back again: Historic perspectives. *Chest* 95:181, 1989.

53. Eriksson S, Carlson J, Velez R. Risk of cirrhosis and primary liver cancer in alpha$_1$-antitrypsin deficiency. *N Engl J Med* 314:736, 1986.

54. Eriksson S, Hagerstrand I. Cirrhosis and malig-

nant hepatoma in alpha$_1$-antitrypsin deficiency. *Acta Med Scand* 195:451, 1974.

55. Erkulvrawatr S, et al. Intrathoracic meningoceles and neurofibromatosis. *Arch Neurol* 36:557, 1979.

56. Fagerhol MK, Cox DW. The PI polymorphism: Genetic, biochemical, and clinical aspects of human α$_1$-antitrypsin. *Adv Hum Genet* 11:1, 1981.

57. Fallot RJ, et al. ^{133}Xe ventilation studies in alpha$_1$-antitrypsin deficiency. *J Nucl Med* 14:5, 1972.

58. Ford GT, Abboud RT, Guenter CA. Current status of alpha-1-antitrypsin replacement therapy: Recommendations for the management of patients with severe hereditary disease. *Can Med Assoc J* 146:841, 1992.

59. Frank MD, Simon L, Dawson BH. The lymphangiomyomatosis syndrome. *Cancer* 72:428, 1968.

60. Fryer AE, et al. Evidence that the gene for tuberous sclerosis is on chromosome 9. *Lancet* 1:659, 1987.

61. Fulmer JD, et al. Distribution of HLA antigens in idiopathic pulmonary fibrosis. *Am Rev Respir Dis* 118:141, 1978.

62. Gadek JE, et al. Danazol-induced augmentation of serum α$_1$-antitrypsin levels in individuals with marked deficiency of this antiprotease. *J Clin Invest* 66:82, 1980.

63. Gadek JE, et al. Replacement therapy of alpha$_1$-antitrypsin deficiency. Reversal of protease-antiprotease imbalance within the alveolar structures of PiZ subjects. *J Clin Invest* 68:1158, 1981.

64. Garay SM, et al. Hermansky-Pudlak syndrome. Pulmonary manifestations of a ceroid storage disease. *Am J Med* 66:737, 1979.

65. Garver RI, et al. Alpha$_1$-antitrypsin deficiency and emphysema caused by homozygous inheritance of non-expressing alpha$_1$-antitrypsin genes. *N Engl J Med* 314:762, 1986.

66. Garver RI Jr, et al. Clonal gene therapy: Transplanted mouse fibroblast clones express human α$_1$-antitrypsin gene in vivo. *Science* 237:762, 1987.

67. Geddes DM, Webley M, Brewerton DA. α$_1$-Antitrypsin phenotypes in fibrosing alveolitis and rheumatoid arthritis. *Lancet* 2:1049, 1977.

68. Gibson GJ. Familial pneumothoraces and bullae. *Thorax* 32:88, 1977.

69. Glasgow JFT, et al. α$_1$-Antitrypsin deficiency in association with both cirrhosis and chronic obstructive lung disease in two sibs. *Am J Med* 54:181, 1973.

70. Gomez MR. *Tuberous Sclerosis* (2nd ed). New York: Raven, 1988.

71. Gomez MR. Varieties of expression of tuberous sclerosis. *Neurofibromatosis* 1:330, 1988.

72. Gottlieb AJ, et al. Serologic factors in idiopathic diffuse interstitial pulmonary fibrosis. *Am J Med* 39:405, 1965.

73. Grossman RF, et al, the Toronto Lung Transplant Group. Results of single-lung transplantation for bilateral pulmonary fibrosis. *N Engl J Med* 322:727, 1990.

74. Guenter CA, et al. The pattern of lung disease associated with α$_1$-antitrypsin deficiency. *Arch Intern Med* 122:254, 1968.

75. Haines JL, et al. Localization of one gene for tuberous sclerosis within 9q32-9q34, and further evidence for heterogeneity. *Am J Hum Genet* 49:764, 1991.

76. Harbitz F. Extensive calcification of the lungs as a distinct disease. *Arch Intern Med* 21:139, 1918.

77. Hardcastle SW, Hendricks ML. Neurofibromatosis (von Recklinghausen's disease)—An unusual cause of parenchymal lung disease. A case report. *S Afr Med J* 66:959, 1984.

78. Hauck RW, et al. Tuberous sclerosis with pulmonary involvement. *Respiration* 57:289, 1990.

79. Hilton RC, Pitkeathly DA. Familial association of rheumatoid arthritis and fibrosing alveolitis. *Ann Rheum Dis* 33:191, 1974.

80. Hubbard R, et al. Biochemical efficacy and safety of monthly augmentation therapy for α$_1$-antitrypsin deficiency. *JAMA* 260:1259, 1988.

81. Hubbard RC, et al. Delivery of proteins for therapeutic purposes by aerosolization: Direct augmentation of anti-neutrophil elastase defenses of the lower respiratory tract in alpha$_1$-antitrypsin deficiency with an aerosol of alpha$_1$-antitrypsin. *Ann Intern Med* 111:206, 1989.

82. Hubbard RC, et al. Recombinant DNA-produced alpha$_1$-antitrypsin administered by aerosol augments lower respiratory tract anti-neutrophil elastase defenses in individuals with alpha$_1$-antitrypsin deficiency. *J Clin Invest* 84:1349, 1989.

83. Hughes EW. Familial interstitial pulmonary fibrosis. *Thorax* 19:515, 1964.

84. Hunninghake GW, et al. Mechanisms of neutrophil accumulation in the lungs of patients with idiopathic pulmonary fibrosis. *J Clin Invest* 68:259, 1981.

85. Hutchison DCS, Tobin MJ, Cook PJL. Alpha$_1$-antitrypsin deficiency: Clinical and physiological features in heterozygotes of Pi type SZ. A survey by the British Thoracic Association. *Br J Dis Chest* 77:28, 1983.

86. Janoff A. Mediators of tissue damage and leukocytes lysosomes: Further studies on human granulocyte elastase. *Lab Invest* 22:228, 1970.

87. Janoff A. Elastases and emphysema: Current assessment of the protease-antiprotease hypothesis. *Am Rev Respir Dis* 132:417, 1985.

88. Janus ED, Phillips NT, Carrell RW. Smoking,

lung function, and α_1-antitrypsin deficiency. *Lancet* 1:152, 1985.

89. Javaheri S, et al. Idiopathic pulmonary fibrosis in monozygotic twins. *Chest* 78:591, 1980.

90. Jeppsson J-O, et al. Prenatal diagnosis of alpha$_1$-antitrypsin deficiency by direct analysis of fetal blood obtained at fetoscopy. *Pediatr Res* 15:254, 1981.

91. Jeppsson J-O, Larsson C, Eriksson S. Characterization of α_1-antitrypsin in the inclusion bodies from the liver in α_1-antitrypsin deficiency. *N Engl J Med* 293:576, 1975.

92. Jones DK, Godden D, Cavanagh P. Alpha$_1$-antitrypsin deficiency presenting as bronchiectasis. *Br J Dis Chest* 79:301, 1985.

93. Journel H, et al. Prenatal diagnosis of familial tuberous sclerosis following detection of cardiac rhabdomyoma by ultrasound. *Prenat Diag* 6:283, 1986.

94. Kabiraj MU, et al. Bronchial reactivity, smoking, and alpha$_1$-antitrypsin. A population-based study of middle-aged men. *Am Rev Respir Dis* 126:864, 1982.

95. Karlinsky JB, Snider GL. Animal models of emphysema. *Am Rev Respir Dis* 117:1109, 1978.

96. Kent G, Gilbert ES, Meyer HH. Pulmonary microlithiasis: Microlithiasis alveolaris pulmonum. *Arch Pathol Lab Med* 60:556, 1955.

97. Kidd VJ, et al. Prenatal diagnosis of α_1-antitrypsin deficiency by direct analysis of the mutation site in the gene. *N Engl J Med* 310:639, 1984.

98. Kino T, Kohara Y, Tsuji S. Pulmonary alveolar microlithiasis. A report of two young sisters. *Am Rev Respir Dis* 105:105, 1972.

99. Kleinerman J, et al. The effect of the specific elastase inhibitor, alanyl alanyl prolyl alanine chloromethyl ketone, on elastase induced emphysema. *Am Rev Respir Dis* 121:381, 1980.

100. Koch B. Familial fibrocystic pulmonary dysplasia: Observations in one family. *Can Med Assoc J* 92:801, 1965.

101. Kueppers F, Black LF. α_1-Antitrypsin and its deficiency. *Am Rev Respir Dis* 110:176, 1974.

102. Kueppers F, Fallat R, Larson RK. Obstructive lung disease and α_1-antitrypsin deficiency gene heterozygosity. *Science* 165:899, 1969.

103. Kurachi K, et al. Cloning and sequence of cDNA coding for α_1-antitrypsin. *Proc Natl Acad Sci USA* 78:6826, 1981.

104. Larsson C. Natural history and life expectancy of severe α_1-antitrypsin deficiency, PiZ. *Acta Med Scand* 204:345, 1978.

105. Laurell CB, Eriksson S. The electrophoretic α_1-globulin pattern of serum in alpha$_1$-antitrypsin deficiency. *Scand J Clin Lab Invest* 15:132, 1963.

106. Leites V, Tannenbaum E. Familial spontaneous pneumothorax. *Am Rev Respir Dis* 82:240, 1960.

107. Lenler-Petersen P, et al. Familial spontaneous pneumothorax. *Eur J Respir* 3:342, 1990.

108. Lenoir S, et al. Pulmonary lymphangiomyomatosis and tuberous sclerosis: Comparison of radiographic and thin-section CT findings. *Radiology* 175:329, 1990.

109. Lie JT, Miller RD, Williams DE. Cystic disease of the lungs in tuberous sclerosis. Clinicopathologic correlation, including body plethysmographic lung function studies. *Mayo Clin Proc* 55:547, 1980.

110. Lieberman J. Heterozygous and homozygous α_1-antitrypsin deficiency in patients with pulmonary emphysema. *N Engl J Med* 281:279, 1969.

111. Lieberman J. Alpha$_1$-Antitrypsin Deficiency and Related Disorders. In AEH Emery, DL Rimoin (Eds), *Principles and Practice of Medical Genetics* (2nd ed). Edinburgh: Churchill-Livingstone, 1990. Pp 1179–1205.

112. Lieberman J, Gawad MA. Inhibitors and activators of leukocytic proteases in the purulent sputum: Digestion of human lung and inhibition by α_1-antitrypsin. *J Lab Clin Med* 77:713, 1971.

113. Lieberman J, Winter B, Sastre A. Alpha$_1$-antitrypsin Pi-types in 965 COPD patients. *Chest* 89:370, 1986.

114. Listernick R, Charrow J. Neurofibromatosis type 1 in childhood. *J Pediatr* 116:845, 1990.

115. Lubs M-LE, et al. Lisch nodules in neurofibromatosis type 1. *N Engl J Med* 324:1264, 1991.

116. MacMillan JM. Familial pulmonary fibrosis. *Dis Chest* 20:426, 1951.

117. Mahadeo R, et al. Hermansky-Pudlak syndrome with granulomatous colitis in children. *J Pediatr* 118:904, 1991.

118. Malfait R, Gorus F, Sevens C. Electrophoresis of serum protein to detect α_1-antitrypsin deficiency: Five illustrative cases. *Clin Chem* 31:1397, 1985.

119. Martin GI, et al. Computer assisted cranial tomography in early diagnosis of tuberous sclerosis. *JAMA* 235:2323, 1976.

120. Massaro D, Katz S. Fibrosing alveolitis: Its occurrence, roentgenographic and pathologic features of von Recklinghausen's neurofibromatosis. *Am Rev Respir Dis* 93:934, 1966.

121. McCarty KS, et al. Pulmonary lymphangiomyomatosis responsive to progesterone. *N Engl J Med* 303:1461, 1980.

122. McDonaugh DJ, et al. Assessment of α_1-antitrypsin deficiency heterozygosity as a risk factor in the etiology of emphysema: Physiological comparison of adult normal and heterozygous protease inhibitor phenotype subjects from a random population. *J Clin Invest* 63:299, 1979.

123. Menon AG, et al. Chromosome 17p deletions and p53 gene mutations associated with the formation of malignant neurofibrosarcomas in von

Recklinghausen neurofibromatosis. *Proc Natl Acad Sci USA* 87:5435, 1990.

124. Merchant RN, et al. Computerized tomography in the diagnosis of lymphangioleiomyomatosis. *Am Rev Respir Dis* 131:295, 1985.

125. Mittman C. The PiMZ phenotype: Is it a significant risk factor for the development of chronic obstructive disease (editorial)? *Am Rev Respir Dis* 118:649, 1978.

126. Monteforte WJ, Kohnen PW. Angiomyolipomas in case of lymphangiomyomatosis syndrome: Relationship to tuberous sclerosis. *Cancer* 34:317, 1974.

127. Moroz SP, et al. Liver disease associated with α_1-antitrypsin deficiency in children. *J Pediatr* 88:19, 1976.

128. Morse JPO. α_1-Antitrypsin deficiency (parts I and II). *N Engl J Med* 299:1045, 1099, 1978.

129. Mulvihill JJ, et al. Neurofibromatosis 1 (Recklinghausen disease) and neurofibromatosis 2 (bilateral acoustic neurofibromatosis): An update. *Ann Intern Med* 113:39, 1990.

130. Musk AW, et al. Genetic studies in familial fibrosing alveolitis: Possible linkage with immunoglobulin allotypes (Gm). *Chest* 89:206, 1986.

131. National Institutes of Health Consensus Development Conference. Neurofibromatosis. Conference statement. *Arch Neurol* 45:575, 1988.

132. Nickoladze GD. Surgical management of familial spontaneous pneumothorax. *Respir Med* 84:107, 1990.

133. Okayama H, et al. Rapid, non-radioactive detection of mutations in the human genome by allele specific amplification. *J Lab Clin Med* 114:105, 1989.

134. O'Neill RP, Cohn JE, Pelligrino ED. Pulmonary alveolar microlithiasis—A family study. *Ann Intern Med* 67:957, 1967.

135. Orel SR, Mazodier P. Pathological Findings in Alpha$_1$-antitrypsin Deficiency. In C Mittman (ed), *Pulmonary Emphysema and Proteolysis*. New York: Academic, 1972. P 69.

136. Owen MC, et al. Mutation of antitrypsin to antithrombin: α_1-Antitrypsin Pittsburgh (358Met→Arg), a fatal bleeding disorder. *N Engl J Med* 309:694, 1983.

137. Owen MC, Lorier M, Carrell RW. α_1-Antitrypsin structural relationships of the substitutions of the S and Z variants. *FEBS Lett* 88:234, 1978.

138. Palombini BC, et al. Bronchopulmonary lavage in alveolar microlithiasis. *Chest* 80:242, 1981.

139. Peabody JW Jr, Hayes EW, Hayes EW Jr. Idiopathic pulmonary fibrosis: Its occurrence in identical twin sisters. *Dis Chest* 18:330, 1950.

140. Porterfield JK, Pyeritz RE, Traill TA. Pulmonary hypertension and interstitial fibrosis in von Recklinghausen neurofibromatosis. *Am J Med Genet* 25:531, 1986.

141. Prakash UBS, et al. Pulmonary alveolar microlithiasis. A review including ultrastructural and pulmonary function studies. *Mayo Clin Proc* 58:290, 1983.

142. Psacharopoulos HT, et al. Outcome of liver disease associated with α_1-antitrypsin deficiency (PiZ). *Arch Dis Child* 58:882, 1983.

143. Putnam CW, et al. Liver replacement for alpha$_1$-antitrypsin deficiency. *Surgery* 81:258, 1977.

144. Rees G. Neurofibroma of the recurrent laryngeal nerve. *Chest* 60:414, 1971.

145. Riccardi VM. von Recklinghausen neurofibromatosis. *N Engl J Med* 305:1617, 1981.

146. Riccardi VM, Eicher JE. *Neurofibromatosis: Phenotype, Natural History, and Pathogenesis*. Baltimore: Johns Hopkins University Press, 1986.

147. Sandoz E. Uber zwei falle von totaler bronchiektasie. *Beitr Pathol Anat* 41:495, 1907.

148. Sawicka EH, Morris AJR. A report of two long-term surviving cases of pulmonary lymphangioleimyomatosis and response to progesterone therapy. *Br J Dis Chest* 79:400, 1985.

149. Schallreuter KU, King RA, Witkop CJ. Thioredoxin reductase activity in Hermansky-Pudlak syndrome. A method for identification of putative heterozygotes. *J Invest Dermatol* 90:372, 1988.

150. Schinella RA, et al. Hermansky-Pudlak syndrome with granulomatous colitis. *Ann Intern Med* 92:20, 1980.

151. Schmidt MA, Michels VV, Dewald GW. Cases of neurofibromatosis with rearrangements of chromosome 17 involving band 17q11.2. *Am J Med Genet* 28:771, 1987.

152. Sears MR, Chang AR, Taylor AJ. Pulmonary alveolar microlithiasis. *Thorax* 26:704, 1971.

153. Seizinger BR, et al. Genetic linkage of von Recklinghausen neurofibromatosis to the nerve growth factor receptor. *Cell* 49:589, 1987.

154. Sharp HL, et al. Cirrhosis associated with alpha$_1$-antitrypsin deficiency: A previously unrecognized inherited disorder. *J Lab Clin Med* 73:934, 1969.

155. Shepherd CW, et al. Causes of death in patients with tuberous sclerosis. *Mayo Clin Proc* 66:792, 1991.

156. Silverman EK, et al. Variability of pulmonary function in alpha-1-antitrypsin deficiency: Clinical correlates. *Ann Intern Med* 111:983, 1989.

157. Silverstein EF, et al. Pulmonary lymphangiomyomatosis. *AJR* 120:832, 1974.

158. Slingerland JM, et al. Pulmonary manifestations of tuberous sclerosis in first degree relatives. *Thorax* 44:212, 1989.

159. Snider GL. Pulmonary disease in α_1-antitrypsin deficiency (editorial). *Ann Intern Med* 111:957, 1989.

160. Snodgrass SR. Usefulness of magnetic resonance imaging in tuberous sclerosis. *Arch Neurol* 44:898, 1987.

161. Sosman MC, et al. The familial occurrence of pulmonary alveolar microlithiasis. *AJR* 77:947, 1957.
162. Starzl TE, et al. Evolution of liver transplantation. *Hepatology* 2:614, 1982.
163. Stovin PGI, et al. The lungs in lymphangiomyomatosis and in tuberous sclerosis. *Thorax* 30:497, 1975.
164. Sveger T. Liver disease in alpha₁-antitrypsin deficiency detected by screening of 200,000 infants. *N Engl J Med* 294:1316, 1976.
165. Sveger T. Prospective study of children with α_1-antitrypsin deficiency: Eight-year-old follow-up. *J Pediatr* 104:91, 1984.
166. Talamo RC, Blennerhassett JB, Austen KF. Familial emphysema and α_1-antitrypsin deficiency. *N Engl J Med* 275:1301, 1966.
167. Talamo RC, et al. α_1-Antitrypsin deficiency: A variant with no detectable α_1-antitrypsin. *Science* 181:70, 1973.
168. Tao L-C. Microliths in sputum specimens and their relationship to pulmonary alveolar microlithiasis. *Am J Clin Pathol* 69:482, 1978.
169. Taylor JR, et al. Lymphangioleiomyomatosis: Clinical course in 32 patients. *N Engl J Med* 323:1254, 1990.
170. Thind GS, Bhatia JL. Pulmonary alveolar microlithiasis. *Br J Dis Chest* 72:151, 1978.
171. Tobin MJ, Cook PJL, Hutchison DCS. Alpha₁-antitrypsin deficiency: The clinical and physiological features of pulmonary emphysema in subjects homozygous for Pi type Z. A survey of the British Thoracic Society. *Br J Dis Chest* 77:14, 1983.
172. Tobin MJ, Duncan CS, Hutchison BM. An overview of the pulmonary features of α_1-antitrypsin deficiency. *Arch Intern Med* 142:1342, 1982.
173. Travis J, Salveson GS. Human plasma proteinase inhibitors. *Annu Rev Biochem* 52:655, 1983.
174. Trulock EP, et al, the Washington University Lung Transplantation Group. The Washington University-Barnes Hospital experience with lung transplantation. *JAMA* 266:1943, 1991.
175. Turner-Warwick M, Doniach D. Auto-antibody studies in interstitial pulmonary fibrosis. *Br Med J* 1:886, 1965.
176. Valensi QJ. Pulmonary lymphangiomyoma: A probable forme fruste of tuberous sclerosis. *Am Rev Respir Dis* 108:1411, 1973.
177. Viskochil D, et al. Deletions and a translocation interrupt a cloned gene at the neurofibromatosis type 1 locus. *Cell* 62:187, 1990.
178. Wallace G, et al. Tuberous sclerosis presenting with fetal and neonatal cardiac tumors. *Arch Dis Child* 65:377, 1990.
179. Wallace MR, et al. Type I neurofibromatosis gene: Identification of a large transcript disrupted in three neurofibromatosis 1 patients. *Science* 249:181, 1990.
180. Ward K, et al. Diagnosis of neurofibromatosis I by using tightly linked, flanking DNA markers. *Am J Hum Genet* 46:943, 1990.
181. Webb WR, Goodman PD. Fibrosing alveolitis in patients with neurofibromatosis. *Radiology* 122:289, 1977.
182. Wellen F, et al. Combined heart-lung transplantation for terminal pulmonary lymphangioleiomyomatosis. *J Thorac Cardiovasc Surg* 89:872, 1985.
183. Wewers MD, et al. Replacement therapy for alpha₁-antitrypsin deficiency associated with emphysema. *N Engl J Med* 316:1055, 1987.
184. Wilson WG, Aylsworth AS. Familial spontaneous pneumothorax. *Pediatrics* 64:172, 1979.
185. Winzelberg GG, et al. CT evaluation of pulmonary alveolar microlithiasis. *J Comput Assist Tomogr* 8:1029, 1984.
186. Witkop CJ Jr, et al. Reliability of absent platelet dense bodies as a diagnostic criterion for Hermansky-Pudlak syndrome. *Am J Hematol* 26:305, 1987.
187. Witkop CJ Jr, et al. Albinism. In CR Scriver et al (Eds), *The Metabolic Basis of Inherited Disease* (6th ed). New York: McGraw-Hill, 1989. Pp 2905–2947.
188. Witkop CJ, et al. The Role of Ceroid in Lung and Gastrointestinal Disease in Hermansky-Pudlak Syndrome. In EA Porta (Ed), *Lipofuscin and Ceroid Pigments*. New York: Plenum, 1990. Pp 283–297.
189. Xu G, et al. The neurofibromatosis type 1 gene encodes a protein related to GAP. *Cell* 62:599, 1990.
190. Yoshida A, et al. Molecular abnormality of PiS variant of human alpha₁-antitrypsin. *Am J Hum Genet* 29:233, 1977.
191. Yoshida A, et al. Molecular abnormality of human α_1-antitrypsin variant (PiZZ) associated with plasma activity deficiency. *Proc Natl Acad Sci USA* 73:1324, 1976.
192. Young WA. Familial fibrocystic pulmonary dysplasia: A new case in a known affected family. *Can Med Assoc J* 94:1059, 1966.
193. Yunis EJ, Agostini RM Jr, Glew RH. Fine structural observations of the liver in α_1-antitrypsin deficiency. *Am J Pathol* 82:265, 1976.

71

Vascular and Other Genetic Diseases Affecting the Lungs

Irwin A. Schafer

Pulmonary Arteriovenous Fistulas

Abnormal arteriovenous communications in the lung may occur as single or multiple lesions. Both genetic and sporadic forms are recognized [32]. When pulmonary arteriovenous fistulas are associated with hereditary hemorrhagic telangiectasia (Rendu-Osler-Weber disease), the cause is clearly genetic with dominant inheritance [40]. The patient and other family members may show small, dilated arteriovenous connections on the mucous membranes of the mouth, lips, conjunctiva, and skin. The lesions may occur anywhere, including the gastrointestinal tract, urinary bladder, lungs, and central nervous system [20]. With hereditary hemorrhagic telangiectasia, pulmonary arteriovenous fistulas tend to be multiple, while single pulmonary lesions are most frequently found in the sporadic nonfamilial disease [32,89]. In the individual patient it may be difficult to differentiate the genetic from the sporadic form of pulmonary arteriovenous fistula without extensive examination of other family members for telangiectasia.

The pathogenesis of pulmonary arteriovenous fistula is probably related to the persistence of fetal anastomotic capillaries [144]. These offer low resistance to flow, allowing a shunt of unoxygenated blood to empty directly into the pulmonary vein. The lesion tends to expand slowly, transmitting increasing quantities of blood; therefore, patients may not become symptomatic until the second or third decade of life. Most patients are asymptomatic, and the lesion is first detected on routine chest roentgenogram, which shows single or multiple coinlike nodules, most frequently in the lower lobes [32,140].

Symptoms, when they develop, include dyspnea, hemoptysis, palpitations, and chest pain.

Physical findings may include cyanosis, digital clubbing, a vascular murmur, and erythrocytosis. A murmur present in 50 percent of cases may be heard over the lesion as a continuous hum or only during systole with accentuated deep inspiration [40]. If the shunt is large enough, there is arterial hypoxemia uncorrectable with 100% oxygen breathing. Hypoxemia produces increased red cell mass and eventually high-output heart failure [103]. Cerebrovascular accidents and brain abscess can complicate the course; however, bleeding from rupture of the malformation either into the bronchus or into the pleural cavity is the most frequent cause of death [78].

Diagnosis is established on clinical and roentgenographic findings. The presence of telangiectasia on mucosal surface associated with single or multiple nodules in the lung should suggest the diagnosis of hereditary telangiectasia with pulmonary arteriovenous fistula. In the patient with an isolated pulmonary lesion or with multiple pulmonary lesions without evidence of telangiectasia, the diagnosis can be established by fluoroscopy if the lesion is seen to pulsate or change in size with changes in intrathoracic pressure [145]. Angiography may be necessary and is almost always diagnostic (Figs. 71-1 and 71-2). This procedure should certainly be carried out before surgical excision of the lesion.

Surgical resection is the only definitive treatment. Operative intervention should be considered in patients with large shunts, complications, or the familial form of the disease [32,140]. The prognosis is good following operation, but repeated surgery may be necessary if previously undetected lesions enlarge and produce symptoms. Forty percent of symptomatic patients die from rupture of the fistula, cerebrovascular accidents, or brain abscess if not treated by surgical

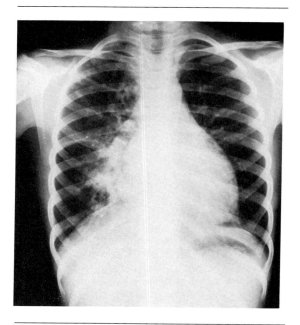

Fig. 71-1. An irregular density in the right lower lobe in a patient with arterial hypoxemia, a continuous murmur, dyspnea, and palpitations.

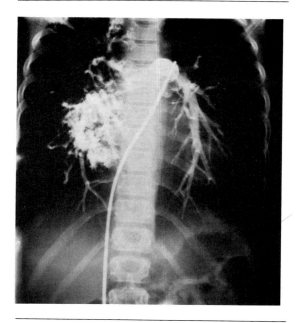

Fig. 71-2. Angiographic demonstration of a single pulmonary arteriovenous fistula in the patient shown in Fig. 71-1.

resection [78]. Embolotherapy, using silicone balloons or coiled springs to occlude the fistula, produces a reduction in flow through the shunt; this alternate to surgical resection is reported to be safe and effective [156]. Pulmonary arteriovenous fistulas are found in 15 percent of patients with hereditary hemorrhagic telangiectasia [65]. This diagnostic possibility also should be considered in every patient with arteriovenous fistulas, especially if they are multiple, even if the patient shows no mucosal telangiectasia, since dominant genes may show variable penetrance. Examination of other family members coupled with pedigree analysis should differentiate most familial from sporadic cases. In most large series, 60 percent or more of all patients with pulmonary arteriovenous fistulas have the lesion in association with hereditary hemorrhagic telangiectasia [20,32,140,144].

Familial Primary Pulmonary Hypertension

The cause of primary pulmonary hypertension remains an enigma. The disorder is characterized by increased pulmonary arterial pressures associated with sclerosis of small vessels within the lungs with no obvious cause, plus hypertrophy of the right side of the heart. Sporadic and familial cases have been described. Most patients are between 20 and 40 years of age, and women outnumber men by 4 or 5 to 1 [154,164]. In familial cases, the disease may appear in childhood.

Genetics

At least 20 reports have been published documenting the familial occurrence of primary pulmonary hypertension in 19 families. In 10 of these families, more than one generation was affected, which suggests autosomal dominant inheritance. In the remaining 9 families, only members of the same generation have been found to have the disease, which suggests autosomal recessive inheritance [79]. The phenotype probably reflects mutations at two or more loci that produce different modes of inheritance in different families. Until the causes of pulmonary hypertension are better defined, genetic counseling will depend on pedigree analysis, which can be uncertain in individual families. The concept of genetic heterogeneity is supported by variation in the age of onset and the sex ratios of familial cases occurring in a single generation and those occurring in families showing a dominant pattern of inheritance. In the recessively inherited forms, symptoms appear at a younger age and the sexes are more equally affected [70].

Pathophysiology

The main abnormality in primary pulmonary hypertension is an increase in pulmonary vascular resistance of 10 to 20 times over normal values, associated with muscular hypertrophy and intimal and medial fibrosis of the pulmonary arteries [139]. These findings may or may not be associated with intravascular thrombosis [153]. The high pulmonary arterial pressure leads to right ventricular hypertrophy and eventually right-sided heart failure. Pulmonary function test values are usually normal.

Pulmonary hypertension secondary to chronic vasoconstriction of the pulmonary vasculature, platelet-induced endothelial damage, and abnormal metabolism of adrenergic analogues have all been invoked as primary etiologic determinants, but none of these hypotheses has been scientifically validated [109]. The disease is difficult to study in humans, since at least a 50 percent reduction in the pulmonary vascular bed occurs before the patient becomes symptomatic [39].

Diagnosis

Symptoms appear when pulmonary hypertension is well established and include dyspnea, ankle swelling, and sometimes syncopal attacks. Some patients complain of retrosternal chest pain. About one third of the cases are associated with Raynaud's disease, scleroderma, and other collagen diseases [154,158]. Hoarseness secondary to compression of the left recurrent laryngeal nerve by an enlarged pulmonary artery and hemoptysis can complicate advanced disease. The more constant physical findings include increased intensity of the pulmonary component of the second heart sound that is often palpable. In patients with severe pulmonary hypertension, a pulmonary diastolic murmur may develop along with the signs of right-sided heart failure. The ECG shows right-axis deviation and right ventricular hypertrophy, while the chest film may show only prominence of the main pulmonary artery segment.

Pulmonary hypertension is a common secondary complication of many diseases of the heart and lungs. The more obvious ones should be apparent by clinical presentation. The diagnosis of pulmonary hypertension secondary to thromboembolism affecting the small vessels of the lung may be difficult [4]. Cardiac catheterization and pulmonary angiography may be required to distinguish primary pulmonary hypertension from some secondary causes [136] (see Chap 51).

Prognosis and Treatment

The clinical course is progressive and usually fatal in 2 to 8 years after the onset of symptoms. A few patients with the familial form of the disease live longer. Except for one patient, a 10-year-old girl, regression of the disease has not been recorded [14].

There is no effective therapy. Anticoagulants are frequently prescribed because thrombotic episodes are likely to complicate the course and recurrent pulmonary emboli are difficult to exclude. Anticoagulants do not appear to alter the natural history of the disease, and their therapeutic value remains uncertain [154].

Treatment is directed at symptomatic relief. In a few patients early in their disease, parenteral administration of isoproterenol, methamphetamine, and tolazoline hydrochloride decreased pulmonary artery pressures [5,88]. Although vasodilator therapy in primary pulmonary hypertension has improved symptoms in individual patients, it has been disappointing as a standard therapy for this disease [115,136].

Drugs have been shown to produce pulmonary hypertension with vascular lesions histologically identical with those of primary pulmonary hypertension. These include adrenergic analogues used clinically as appetite suppressants. Aminorex, used as a dietary aid in Europe in the 1960s, was associated with an epidemic of pulmonary hypertension that disappeared when the drug was removed from the market [92]. Another anorexic drug, fenfluramine, plus chemically related compounds have been associated with pulmonary hypertension [34]. Pulmonary hypertension in a patient with tryptophan-induced eosinophilia-myalgia syndrome cleared after discontinuation of tryptophan [162]. In the evaluation of individual patients, drug-related pulmonary hypertension should be considered.

Pregnancy apparently adversely affects pulmonary hypertension [154]. Oral contraceptives have also been implicated, with exacerbations of the disease in young women with predisposing risk factors [80]. These risk factors include mild pulmonary hypertension secondary to surgical corrections of congenital heart lesions, systemic lupus, or a family history of pulmonary hypertension [111]. It seems clear that oral contraceptives are contraindicated in these women.

Scimitar Syndrome

Over 95 cases of the scimitar syndrome have been described. The basic features of this disorder include hypoplasia of the right lung associated with dextroposition of the heart, systemic arterial supply to the right lung, and anomalous right pulmonary venous drainage to the inferior vena cava [74]. The most constant feature is anomalous venous drainage. The entire right lung is usually drained by a single vein that runs parallel to the right border of the heart to join the inferior vena cava between the right atrium and the hepatic veins. The site of junction is usually below the diaphragm. The arterial supply to the right lung is variable and can arise from the pulmonary, bronchial, and systemic arterial systems. Typically, arteries arise from the aorta, often below the diaphragm [38]. Hypoplasia or absence of the right upper lung segment is frequent [86]. Congenital heart lesions, especially atrial septal defects, are seen in one fourth of patients, and the right leaf of the diaphragm may be abnormal, with eventration or with an accessory posterolateral leaf [83].

The cause of the syndrome is undefined, but it probably arises early in right-lung bud development secondary to the persistence of embryonic connections of the pulmonary plexus with the cardinal veins [59]. The syndrome can show familial clustering. An affected father and daughter have been reported, which suggests autosomal dominant inheritance [105].

The majority of cases appear to be sporadic; however, the fact that affected individuals may be asymptomatic and are discovered accidentally by routine chest roentgenogram complicates ascertainment. A systematic study of first- and second-degree relatives of affected individuals could clarify the genetic component of this syndrome.

Approximately one third of patients are diagnosed in childhood because of clinical symptoms of recurrent pulmonary infections and dyspnea [77,83]. The remaining patients become symptomatic as adults or are discovered accidentally by chest roentgenogram. Both sexes are affected. The peculiar diagnostic characteristic that gives

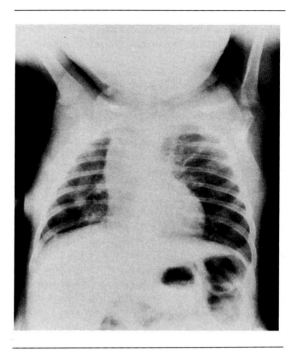

Fig. 71-3. Scimitar syndrome in a child. The pulmonary vein on the right runs parallel to the right atrium to its connection with the inferior vena cava below the diaphragm.

scimitar syndrome its name is seen on the routine chest x-ray film. The anomalous vein that courses downward parallel to the right atrium to its connection with the inferior vena cava produces an arclike shadow that resembles the blade of a Turkish sword or scimitar, with the shaft of the heart to the right due to the hypoplastic right lung (Fig. 71-3). The clinical and roentgenographic overlap of components of this syndrome with those of pulmonary sequestration and pulmonary hypoplasia due to pulmonary artery deficiency should be considered in diagnosis [85]. Prognosis relates to the severity of infection in the hypoplastic right lung. Medical treatment is limited to control of infections with antibiotics and measures to improve the bronchial clearing. In patients with serious recurrent respiratory infections, surgical resection of the affected lobe or pneumonectomy may be required. Improved function may be obtained in selected patients by surgical correction of pulmonary venous blood flow to the left atrium [77].

In patients with symptoms attributable to a shunt and with supradiaphragmatic drainage, surgery carries a low risk and is successful.

Infradiaphragmatic drainage can be confidently predicted by ultrasound studies and favors conservative management, since this anatomy poses special problems [112].

Immunodeficiency States

Major elements that interact to protect the respiratory tract from infection include mucociliary clearance, lymphocytes, macrophages, polymorphonuclear leukocytes, immunoglobulins, and complement. These host defenses act as a complex interacting unit in the face of infection and are under specific genetic control. Many inherited immune defects produce pulmonary disease. The diagnostic possibility of immune deficiency should be considered in patients with recurrent or chronic pulmonary infections who have no underlying structural defect to account for their problem. Useful reviews are available on lung defense mechanisms [66,108] and specific primary immunodeficiency states [25,131–134,150]. The inherited immune defects included in this section were selected because pulmonary disease is prominent in the clinical presentation of affected individuals.

Infantile Sex-Linked Immunodeficiency

This X-linked disorder of B-cell function presents within the first 2 years of life with recurrent pyogenic infections. Males are affected, while most female carriers are asymptomatic. Lymphocytic tissues show germinal centers, plasma cells are absent, and circulating blood lymphocytes have no surface immunoglobulins. Serum immunoglobulin levels are low. The gene has been localized to X q21.3–q22 and genetic linkage with restriction fragment length polymorphism (RFLP) has been established [75,93]. Using these probes, gene tracking in individual families may potentially be used for the detection of carriers and for prenatal diagnoses. Carrier detection of several X-linked primary immunodeficiency diseases including agammaglobulinemia has been accomplished using X-chromosome inactivation analyses [157]. Treatment of acute infections with antibodies plus replacement of immunoglobulin G (IgG) by intramuscular or intravenous injection may control infections [3]. Viral and fungal infections are normally tolerated by most patients, but in some, persistent viral or parasitic infections have been documented [132].

Complement Deficiencies

Inherited deficiencies of most complement components have been described. Affected patients show variable clinical syndromes. Hereditary C3 deficiency results in increased susceptibility to pyogenic infection. The disorder is inherited as an autosomal recessive trait. Affected individuals show concentrations of serum C3 of less than 2.5 $\mu g/ml$ (normal, 1000 to 2000 $\mu g/ml$), while the concentrations of other components of the complement system are normal [2]. Other genetic defects that affect the function of the complement system include C1 inhibitor deficiency in hereditary angioneurotic edema; C2, C4 deficiency associated with increased frequency of connective-tissue disorders; and C5 deficiency that presents shortly after birth with infection, seborrheic dermatitis, persistent diarrhea, and failure to thrive. C1 inhibitor deficiency is inherited as an autosomal dominant trait, C2 and C5 deficiency as autosomal recessive traits. Pulmonary involvement is not the major problem in C1 and C2 deficiency, but it may be in some patients with C5 deficiency [25,100].

Chronic Granulomatous Disease

Both X-linked and autosomal recessively inherited forms of chronic granulomatous disease have been documented. The X-linked disorder of childhood is characterized by widespread granulomas of skin, lymph nodes, bone, and spleen. Pulmonary involvement is manifested by hilar enlargement, bronchopneumonia, empyema, and lung abscesses [160]. Response to appropriate antibiotic therapy is slow, and bacterial pneumonia may persist for weeks. Infectious agents most frequently isolated are catalase-positive bacteria including *Serratia*, *Klebsiella*, *Enterobacter*, *Pseudomonas*, *Escherichia coli*, *Proteus*, *Salmonella*, and fungi. The functional defect resides in neutrophils and monocytes, which can ingest bacteria and fungi but cannot kill the organisms effectively. Prolonged retention of material in leukocytes resulting from this functional deficiency probably leads to granuloma formation [7]. The basic molecular defect is a deficiency of the heme-containing protein cytochrome b558. The defect in oxidative metabolism is the basis of the nitroblue tetrazolium reduction test used in diagnosis and for the detection of carriers [8]. Female carriers show two populations of leukocytes, one with defective reducing capacity and one with normal function. In contrast, affected males have 90 to 95 percent defective cells. The prognosis is poor. The disease is uniformly fatal, with life spans ranging from several months to adulthood. Treatment consists of prompt recognition of infection followed by aggressive and prolonged therapy with antibiotics. Recombinant human gamma interferon apparently is an effective and well-tolerated treatment that reduces the frequency of serious infections [43].

Genetic heterogeneity is extensive in chronic granulomatous disease. Nearly two-thirds of individuals have defects localized to a membrane component of the oxidase in a cell-free activation system. To date, all these individuals have abnormalities in one or the other of the cytochrome b558 subunits that lead to altered function of the cytochrome [142]. The defect in the 91 kilodalton (kD) glycoprotein subunit is inherited as an X-linked recessive trait, while defects in the 22 kD subunit, which is encoded on chromosome 16, is transmitted as an autosomal recessive trait [31]. A defect in the cytosolic components of the oxidase is found in approximately 40 percent of individuals with chronic granulomatous disease. All affected patients examined to date have had normal levels of cytochrome b558 in their neutrophil membranes and histories that are compatible with autosomal recessive inheritance. The bulk of individuals with cytosol-deficient chronic granulomatous disease lack detectable levels of a 47 kD phosphoprotein necessary for normal reduced nicotinamide adenine dinucleotide phosphate (NADPH) oxidase function [23]. A minority of patients with cytosol-deficient chronic granulomatous disease are missing a 67 kD cytosolic protein [23]. The 47 and 67-phox proteins appear to be critical for the translocation of the known cytosolic oxidase components to the membrane. Nitroblue tetrazolium (NBT) dye reduction testing of fetal blood neutrophils is the most commonly used for prenatal diagnosis [107]. Although the gene coding for the gp 91-phox protein subunit has been cloned, few families show detectable deletions [135]. At present, prenatal diagnosis for most families depends on the identification of specific family-based mutations or on RFLP using probes for the gene or closely linked flanking markers [142]. Recent reports indicate that deletion analyses for X-linked chronic granulomatous disease using the cDNA probe may be useful for both prenatal diagnoses and carrier determination [116,157].

Chédiak-Higashi Syndrome

Chédiak-Higashi syndrome is characterized by the presence of giant granules in the leukocytes of the peripheral blood in patients with recurrent infections and depigmentation of skin, hair, and eyes. Phagocytic killing, especially by mononuclear cells, may be defective. The basic defect in this recessively inherited disorder is not defined but may be related to a membrane abnormality or a defect in microtubular function leading to inappropriate granule fusion. Carriers may sometimes be detected by the presence of occasional giant granules in smears of peripheral blood. Prognosis is poor, and most patients die in childhood. Treatment is limited to the aggressive use of antibiotics and such preventive measures as seem warranted. Bone marrow transplant with durable engraftment of all hematopoietic elements in one patient resulted in the reconstitution of normal hematopoietic and immunologic function. The correction of the natural killer cell deficiency characteristic of this disease has led to prolonged disease-free survival in the patient [53]. Lymphoreticular malignancies occur with a high frequency [76,126,130].

Severe Combined Immunodeficiency

This is a genetically heterogeneous group of disorders in which both humoral and cellular responses may be impaired. T and B lymphocytes are usually depleted and do not show a normal lymphoproliferative response to mitogens. Levels of serum immunoglobulins may be low. Patients show no delayed hypersensitivity after skin tests, do not reject allogeneic skin grafts, lack isohemagglutinins, and fail to make antibodies after immunization with typhoid antigens or diphtheria toxoid [63].

Clinically, patients present within the first year of life with bronchitis; pneumonia; infection of the skin and mucosal surfaces, usually with *Candida;* gastroenteritis; diarrhea with malabsorption; and failure to grow in length. Progressive deterioration occurs with no control of infection by standard methods of treatment. The pneumonia is usually interstitial with tachypnea and hyperinflation of the lungs and is due to *Pneumocystis carinii.* Lymphadenopathy is strikingly absent, as are the tonsils and adenoids. X-ray film of the chest shows a small or absent thymus.

Family studies describe recessive, dominant, and X-linked patterns of inheritance. In small outbred sibships, the X-linked and autosomal recessive disease may be clinically and pathologically indistinguishable. At least two forms of recessively inherited severe combined immunodeficiency disease are recognized. In certain families, affected individuals lack the enzyme adenosine deaminase (ADA) in tissues, while patients from other families show normal activity of this enzyme [48]. Parents of ADA-deficient patients show ADA activity that is approximately 50 percent of the normal mean, which indicates that they are carriers of a mutant autosomal recessive gene. Pathologically, the thymus differs in patients with and without ADA deficiency. The thymus in the ADA-deficient patient is small but shows some evidence of differentiation of thymic vessels, suggesting atrophy. The thymus from patients with normal ADA activity usually weighs less than 2 gm, is frequently found in an anatomically abnormal position, and is devoid of lymphocytes, Hassall's corpuscles, and normal vasculature. These findings suggest that early differentiation may occur in the ADA-deficient form followed by atrophy, while in patients with normal ADA activity the thymus never undergoes embryonic transformation to its normal lymphoid morphology [72]. A deficiency of nucleoside phosphorylase, another enzyme of the purine salvage pathway, has been described in nine patients from six families who showed cellular immunodeficiency [113]. Only ADA deficiency has been diagnosed in utero [64].

Adenosine deaminase deficiency can be diagnosed antenatally by measurement of ADA activity in cultured amniotic fluid cells [64], fetal blood [33], and samples of chorionic villus tissue [11]. Gene tracking by direct analyses of DNA, using fragment length polymorphism, can be carried out on cultured cells, lymphocytes from fetal blood, or chorionic villus tissue. The gene for X-linked severe combined immunodeficiency has been mapped to X q11–q13 by linkage analyses. Restriction fragment length polymorphisms used to localize the gene in these studies should provide a useful probe for the antenatal diagnoses [11].

The diagnosis of the specific immune defect is based on the clinical picture coupled with pedigree analysis and appropriate laboratory studies. The prognosis in patients with combined immunodeficiencies diseases is poor. Most patients die within the first 2 years of life, despite aggressive therapy with antibiotics, administration of immunoglobulins, and other supportive measures.

Lethal graft-versus-host reactions can occur after whole blood transfusions if histoincompatible lymphocytes are administered. Bone marrow transplant is the therapy of choice. Fetal liver and thymus implants have been tried to replace the missing lymphoid stem cell, and some successes have been reported [69]. In the absence of a suitable donor, enzyme replacement therapy has been achieved in a few ADA-deficient patients with red cell transfusions, while other patients do not respond to transfusion therapy [120,134]. Intramuscular injection of polyethylene glycol modified adenosine deaminase reverses the biochemical consequences of the enzyme deficiency and may be preferable to red cell transfusions [62].

Recently, transfer of the ADA gene into the hematopoietic cells of a patient with adenosine deaminase was accomplished using a modified retroviral vector. Somatic cell gene therapy may be practical in this disorder. A long-term follow-up study of this patient is anxiously awaited [28].

Variable Immunodeficiency

This is a heterogeneous group of disorders with onset of clinical symptoms in adults [45]. Pulmonary difficulties include virus-like upper-respiratory infections, sinusitis, pneumonia, and chronic progressive bronchiectasis. Many patients also develop gastrointestinal symptoms with malabsorption and a spruelike state often due to *Giardia lamblia* infestation [61]. Progressive loss of immunologic function due to failure of plasma cell production, abnormalities of B- and T-cell response, and deficiency of IgG, IgA, IgD, and IgE have been reported. Because of the variability of the clinical and laboratory findings in affected individuals, interpretation of family data is difficult [161]. At this point, no monogenic mechanisms of gene transmission can be substantiated. The reports of autosomal recessive and autosomal dominant forms of transmission in specific families could be due to common environmental exposures as well as inheritance.

Variable immunodeficiency is the most common form of immunodeficiency observed clinically. Clarification of a genetic component in this group of disorders may provide therapeutic insights that will reduce morbidity in affected individuals and their families. Treatment now consists of specific antibiotic therapy for recurrent infections, supportive therapy, and, in some patients, replacement of immunoglobulins, if markedly deficient. Intravenous gamma globulin replacement has superseded intramuscular injections as the preferred mode of therapy [163].

Chromosome Abnormalities

The 46 chromosomes of the human genome can now be unambiguously identified with newer cytogenetic techniques that permit recognition of subtle rearrangements in chromosome structure in addition to detection of increases or decreases in chromosome number. It is not yet clear why patients affected with certain chromosome abnormalities show an increased frequency of infection and malignancy. Efforts directed at identifying the location of specific genes on specific chromosomes may provide some answers. The chromosome disorders discussed in this section were selected because they have been associated with defects in immunologic function. In none of these disorders is the pulmonary lesion diagnostic. Problems related to the lung reflect systemic defects in host resistance.

Down Syndrome

Trisomy of chromosome 21 was the first chromosomal abnormality described in humans and is the most frequent autosomal anomaly. The clinical phenotype is well known and is usually recognized at birth. Early diagnosis is important because mental retardation is a consistent feature. The dysmorphoses observed include a small, round head with a flat occiput, palpebral fissures that slant upward and outward with the inner angle marked by epicanthal folds, and irises that show a ring of small, round, irregular whitish spots (Brushfield's spots). The ears are usually small. The nape of the neck is short, flat, and broad with redundant skin folds. Infants always show marked muscle hypotonia. The fifth finger is short and incurved, and the hands may show a single palmar crease (simian crease). Associated structural defects are found in the heart in 40 percent of patients. Malformations of the gastrointestinal tract include duodenal stenosis or atresia, annular pancreas, and anal atresia. Infection, leukemia, other cancers, and thyroid disease occur with increased frequency [141]. These clinical observations may be related to the qualitative and quantitative defects in the immune response described in affected individuals. Stimulation of

lymphocytes with mitogens is decreased [127]. Immunoglobulin G levels of affected newborn infants are low [101], while older children and adults have higher levels of IgG but lower IgM levels than do normal persons [147]. The frequencies of hepatitis-associated antigens are increased [36]. These observations have not been integrated to explain the decrease in host resistance to infection but suggest a biologic link among gene dosage, chromosome 21, and the immune system. The lung in Down syndrome may show pulmonary hypoplasia because of a diminished number of alveoli in relation to acini. The resultant decrease in alveolar surface area may account for the severe pulmonary hypertension observed in some Down syndrome patients [26]. Other contributory factors that produce pulmonary hypertension unassociated with, and out of proportion to, congenital heart disease include the obstructive sleep apnea syndrome. Pulmonary hypertension due to this etiology may be reversible by relieving airway obstruction [94].

The clinical diagnosis of Down syndrome should be confirmed by cytogenetic analysis, which is indispensable for genetic counseling. The majority of cases (90 percent) show three chromosomes of the G21 group resulting from nondisjunction at the time of the first or second meiotic division. The patients have 47 chromosomes instead of the normal number of 46. Trisomy 21 can be considered an isolated accident, with the risk of recurrence related to parental age. The frequency of trisomy 21 is about 1 in 1000 births. In women at age 20, its frequency is on the order of 1 in 2000 births, but the frequency increases exponentially to 1 in 50 births after 45 years of age [71]. Approximately 5 percent of Down syndrome patients show a chromosome number of 46, with the extra 21 chromosome attached to another autosome, usually one of the D group. This translocation is a sporadic event in half the cases. In the remaining translocation patients, a balanced translocation is demonstrated in one of the parents who is phenotypically normal. In these families, the risk of recurrence is high, ranging from 5 percent if the father is the carrier to 16 percent if the mother is the carrier. Down syndrome can be diagnosed before birth with amniocentesis by chromosome analysis of fetal cells. This option may be considered by families with the translocation form of Down syndrome or in women over age 35 because of the statistical rise for nondisjunction [102].

Chromosome Instability

Ataxia-telangiectasia and Bloom's syndrome are recessively inherited diseases that have in common chromosome instability of cells cultured in vitro, a high incidence of malignancy and immune dysfunction, and an increased incidence of pulmonary infections. At least two other inherited disorders, xeroderma pigmentosum and Fanconi's syndrome, also show chromosome instability and a high incidence of malignancy. These two diseases are not discussed because the immune deficiencies are not clearly associated with an increased frequency of pulmonary infections. The relationship between immunologic deficiency, chromosome fragility, and a predisposition to malignancies remains an unsolved biologic problem. The increased frequency of pulmonary infections in ataxia-telangiectasia and Bloom's syndrome is presumably a direct consequence of immune dysfunction.

ATAXIA-TELANGIECTASIA

Ataxia-telangiectasia is a recessively inherited disease characterized by ataxia, telangiectasia of the bulbar conjunctiva, and sinopulmonary infections [117]. Cerebellar ataxia becomes evident when the child begins to walk. Oculocutaneous telangiectasia may be delayed until 2 to 6 years. Neurologic dysfunction is progressive, with complete incapacitation by 12 years of age. Death usually occurs in adolescence either from pulmonary infection or lymphoreticular malignancy. Patients who do not develop pulmonary disease or cancer live to the fifth decade [96]. Sinopulmonary infections indicate immunodeficiency. In over 70 percent of patients studied, serum IgA and IgE levels are decreased or not detectable. Cell-mediated immune deficiency evidenced by diminished cutaneous delayed hypersensitivity reactions, delayed skin allograft rejections, and inhibition of in vitro lymphocyte response to mitogens [12]. Pathologically, there is depletion of lymphocytes in lymphoid tissues with a predominance of reticular epithelial cells. The central nervous system shows diffuse atrophy of Purkinje's and granular cells of the cerebellum, degeneration of the olivary and dentate nuclei, and diffuse demyelination and axonal degeneration of the spinocerebellar tracts and posterior columns. Between 10 and 30 percent of patients develop lymphoreticular malignancies or other neoplasms [57,118]. The syndrome appears to be causally related to a basic repair defect in the DNA of ataxia-telangiectasia cells. Cultured cells from patients show increased numbers of breaks, gaps, and rearrangements [57]. The majority of chromosomal breaks are clustered at chromosome 14q12 with translocations to chromosomes 6, 7, and X. Ring formation of chromosome 14 also has been noted [95]. There are no definitive tests to detect carriers of the mutant gene, although family members may show some degree of anergy, delayed hypersensitivity responses, or IgE deficiency. In complementation groups A and C, which comprise 80 to 85 percent of families with ataxia-telangiectasia, linkage analysis has localized the ATA and ATC genes to chromosome 11q22–23. The genes have not yet been cloned [52].

Treatment is supportive and consists of antibiotics to control respiratory infections, aggressive pulmonary toilet, immunization with killed vaccines only, and physical therapy for the neurologic dysfunction. Replacement of immunoglobulins is generally ineffective for IgA deficiency but may be considered if IgG and other specific antibody levels are significantly depressed [12].

BLOOM'S SYNDROME

The major clinical features of Bloom's syndrome are dwarfism with normal body proportions, a narrow face with nasal prominence, dolichocephaly, and sun-sensitive telangiectatic erythema of the face, usually showing a butterfly distribution. Affected children are small at birth. This disorder is inherited as an autosomal recessive trait, predominantly among Ashkenazic Jews. During the first decade of life, infections of the upper and lower respiratory tracts are frequent [46]. The increased incidence of infection is associated with immune dysfunction, which may include a poor lymphoproliferative response to pokeweed mitogen and variable changes in serum immunoglobulin levels [73,149]. The predisposition to cancer shown by these patients may be related to either chromosome instability or an immune defect. The cytogenetic abnormality consists of a marked increase of sister and nonsister homologous chromatid exchange in cultured cells. This finding is consistent and is of diagnostic value. Although the molecular basis of Bloom's syndrome is not defined, several genes have been proposed to cause the hypermutability in Bloom's syndrome cells. Several of these genes have now been cloned, but their roles in producing Bloom's syndrome phenotype remain to be defined [110]. The diagnosis of Bloom's syndrome is suggested in dwarfed children with normal body proportions who show facial dysmorphism and sun-sensitive telangiectatic skin lesions of the face. The prognosis is poor, with death occurring before age 20 from cancer or infection. There are no laboratory tests for carrier detection. Treatment of pulmonary complications is symptomatic [47].

Heritable Disorders of Connective Tissue

Connective-tissue proteins are complex and interdependent in their anatomic arrangement and physical properties. The major proteins of connective tissue are collagen, elastin, and proteoglycans. A large number of enzymes participate in the biosynthesis and degradation of these proteins. Genetic mutations affecting biosynthetic enzymes at the level of transcription or translation may alter the primary structure of the protein. Mutations also could alter the function of enzymes involved in the posttranslational modification of the protein, thereby affecting its secondary or tertiary structure. A change in protein structure could be expected to alter the normal organization and function of connective tissue to produce disease. Genetic mutations affecting enzymes involved in the degradation of connective-tissue proteins are well documented as producing diseases through the accumulation of material in lysosomes.

Several reviews relate the biochemistry of collagen, elastin, and proteoglycans to connective-tissue disease [56,67,121,123,137]. The disorders selected for discussion in this section illustrate the progress made in defining the biochemical basis for certain connective-tissue disorders that affect the lungs. They also point out the need for research in this area. The heritable disorders of connective tissue provide models that define the functions of specific connective-tissue proteins in normal pulmonary function.

Marfan Syndrome

Marfan syndrome in its classic form is characterized by ectopia lentis, aneurysm of the ascending aorta with aortic regurgitation, and limbs that are inappropriately long compared with the trunk. In addition, arachnodactyly, pectus deformity, scoliosis, and joint laxity are common. The disorder

is inherited as an autosomal dominant trait. As with most dominantly inherited conditions, spontaneous mutations occur frequently. This accounts for those individuals who clearly show the phenotype but have normal parents and other family members. In addition, expressivity of the classic Marfan gene varies widely, which leads to clinical heterogeneity and problems in diagnosis [124].

The diagnosis of Marfan syndrome is based on clinical assessment. The salient criteria include a family history, ocular finding, cardiovascular abnormalities, and skeletal features described previously. At least two features should be present to make the diagnosis. In classic cases, three or four are usually evident. Since each of the clinical features of the syndrome occurs with variable frequency in the general population, it is to be expected that several can occur by chance alone in some individuals. Determining whether such individuals are affected with Marfan syndrome will tax the acumen of the best clinician.

The basic genetic defect that produces Marfan syndrome has now been identified. The syndrome is due to a mutant fibrillin gene that has been localized to the long arm of chromosome 15 [30]. The fibrillin monomer is a 350 kD glycoprotein that is associated with microfibrillar fibers. These fibers are integral components of elastic elements and are also present in a variety of other cells and tissues. A decreased content of fibrillin has been documented in the microfibrils of tissues from patients with Marfan syndrome and in cultured Marfan fibroblasts using monoclonal antibodies to fibrillin. In addition, there appears to be a direct relationship between the decreased content of fibrillin and the presence of symptoms [68].

A second fibrillin gene has now been identified in a phenotypically related, but distinct, disorder [87]. The availability of cDNA probes makes possible genetic linkage analyses in families for prenatal diagnoses or presymptomatic diagnoses of affected individuals. They also provide methods for laboratory confirmation of clinical diagnosis.

Approximately 10 percent of Marfan patients have pulmonary lesions, including emphysema associated with cystic change [91]. Spontaneous pneumothorax is the most frequent cause of pulmonary symptoms in affected individuals [35, 151]. Clinical observations indicate that 4.4 percent of patients with Marfan syndrome have a spontaneous pneumothorax. Those who show apical bullous changes once the lung reinflates are at high risk for recurrence. If either bullous lung changes are detected, or if an air leak persists, then resection of the bulla and apical pleurodesis should be performed [55].

Patients with homocystinuria may phenotypically resemble patients with Marfan syndrome. Homocystinuria is inherited as an autosomal recessive trait and is frequently associated with mental retardation. A deficiency in the activity of cystathionine B synthetase, an enzyme required for the methylation of homocysteine to cystathionine, is the most common enzyme defect; however, at least three other enzyme lesions have been described. As a result of the enzyme defect, large amounts of homocysteine accumulate in the extracellular fluid and are excreted in the urine. The cyanide nitroprusside test is a simple urine screening procedure that is useful in the differential diagnoses of homocystinuria and Marfan syndrome. Homocysteine gives a positive deep-red to magenta reaction with the nitroprusside test and is not found in the urine of Marfan patients [104].

Ehlers-Danlos Syndrome

The classic clinical features of the Ehlers-Danlos syndrome include hyperelastic skin, hyperextensible joints, fragile tissues, and a bleeding diathesis; however, the clinical phenotype is variable. At least 11 variants are recognized based on clinical, genetic, and biochemical criteria. Only the more common forms of the syndromes are summarized. The biochemical defect is not known for types I, II, and III, which are inherited as dominant traits. They are classified by the severity of the clinical features described above. Type I patients have gross skin extensibility, severe joint hypermobility, fragile skin, poor wound healing, and a moderate bleeding diathesis. They are frequently born prematurely with rupture of fetal membranes before the mother goes into labor, since these tissues are derived from the fetus and share the same connective-tissue defect [9]. Musculoskeletal deformities are common. Patients with the type II variants are less severely affected, while type III patients may show only hypermobile joints.

The ecchymotic form or type IV variant is characterized by a bleeding diathesis, arterial rupture, and intestinal perforation. Both dominant and recessively inherited kindreds have been described. In all patients studied, a unifying biochemical abnormality is a defect in the synthesis, structure, or secretion of type III collagen [122,125,148]. Biochemical studies on several patients indicate a deficiency of mature type III collagen. The gene for type III collagen has been localized to the long arm of chromosome 2q31–32 [19]. Analyses of lung tissue from a patient with type IV Ehlers-Danlos who developed recurrent pneumothoraces and whose apical bullae were resected showed that the relative proportion of type III collagen in the lungs was markedly decreased. These data suggested that the structural abnormalities in the lung that led to pneumothorax were due to a deficiency of type III collagen [22].

Type V is inherited as an X-linked trait. Clinically, it is characterized by joint hypermobility limited to the fingers and hyperextensible skin. Fragile skin, poor wound healing, and easy bruising may occur but are relatively mild. Deficiency in activity of the enzyme lysyl oxidase, which catalyzes the initial step in the cross-linking of collagen, has been demonstrated in cultured skin fibroblasts [29]. These data have not been confirmed.

Patients with the type VI variant show the same clinical features as do those with type I, but the disorder is inherited as a recessive trait. A deficiency of the enzyme lysyl hydroxylase has been demonstrated in cultured fibroblasts. This enzyme is required for the posttranslational modification of lysine to hydroxylysine in the biosynthesis of collagen [82,119].

Type VII patients have minimal tissue fragility but show other clinical features of the syndrome. They are short in stature and frequently present with dislocation of the hips. This variant is inherited as a recessive trait. In cultured fibroblasts, a deficiency of the enzyme procollagen peptidase has been described that normally modifies procollagen after its secretion from the cell [90]. Recently, fibroblasts from these patients have been reexamined. The results do not indicate a deficiency of procollagen peptidase but rather a structural mutation in the pro-alpha-2 collagen chain that prevents normal enzymatic removal of the aminopropeptide from the collagen chain [146]. Another variant with a different structural defect in the alpha-2 (I) chain of type I collagen has been defined due to addition of approximately 15 to 20 amino acid residues [37]. Other variants undoubtedly will be identified. The gene coding for the alpha-1 (I) (COL_1A_1) chain has been localized to chromosome 17q21–22, while the gene coding for the alpha-2 (I) chain (COL_1A_2) is located on chromosome 7q21–22 [18,19]. The biochemical abnormalities found in the X-linked and recessively inherited variants of the syndrome clearly indicate that the clinical phenotype for the Ehlers-Danlos syndrome can result when collagen is defective.

Pulmonary pathology results from kyphoscoliosis, rupture of the lung, mediastinal emphysema, and pneumothorax [114]. In patients who died from rupture of an artery, large emphysematous subplural bullae have been described [97]. Pulmonary function has not been extensively studied in affected individuals, but thus far no consistent spirometric or lung volume abnormalities have been detected [6].

Cutis Laxa

Cutis laxa is a heterogeneous group of disorders for which generalized cutaneous laxity and changes in elastic fibers have been proposed as minimal diagnostic criteria. The relatively benign autosomal dominant form of the syndrome shows as its main clinical characteristic loose folds of skin over all parts of the body, but especially on the face and around the eyes. Sagging jowls give the patient a bloodhound appearance. The changes in facial skin also give the appearance of premature aging (Fig. 71-4). Pendulous skin over the abdomen may cover the genitalia. In contrast to the Ehlers-Danlos syndrome, a bleeding diathesis, poor wound healing, and joint hypermobility are not seen in cutis laxa [58].

Systemic manifestations are primarily pulmonary. Emphysema occurs in severe cases [99]. In the autosomal recessive form, it may begin in infancy and lead to death before age 2 from cor pulmonale [54,152]. Tissue examination by light microscopy shows a sparsity, fragmentation, and granular disruption of elastic fibers in the skin, lungs, and large arteries [51]. With electron microscopy, the microfibrillar component of elastic tissue appears normal, but elastin is diminished and unevenly distributed [58]. The syndrome can be inherited as an autosomal dominant or recessive or an X-linked trait [17]. The biochemical basis of the connective-tissue defect is not completely defined. A deficiency of lysyl oxidase has been detected in the cultured fibroblasts of one patient with the X-linked form. This enzyme is capable of affecting both elastin and collagen cross-linking; therefore, both proteins may be abnormal in this condition. Supporting this concept is the distinctive profile of chemically modified collagen peptides described in the skin of another patient with the recessively inherited form. Recent studies indicate that a structurally distinct colla-

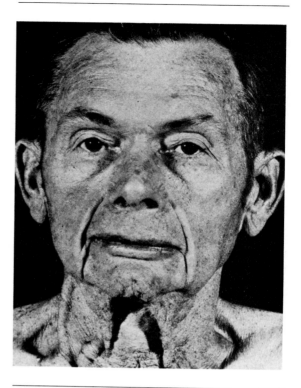

Fig. 71-4. Connective-tissue manifestations in a patient with cutis laxa. (Reproduced from K Hashimoto, T Kanzaki. Cutis laxa: Ultrastructural and biochemical studies. *Arch Dermatol* 111:861, 1975, by permission. Copyright 1975, American Medical Association.)

gen (type VI) with a molecular weight of 140,000 accumulates in the medium of cultured fibroblasts in some patients [27]. It is likely that a heterozygous group of metabolic derangements is involved in producing the laxity of the skin and the pulmonary changes in this disorder. The X-linked form of cutis laxa is now classified by some as Ehlers-Danlos syndrome, type IX [123].

The Lung in Lysosomal Storage Disease

Lysosomes are pleomorphic cellular organelles that contain a variety of hydrolytic enzymes with an acid pH optimum. These acid hydrolases are synthesized in the endoplasmic reticulum, transported through the Golgi apparatus, and finally packaged in lysosomes, where they degrade biologic macromolecules. The sequence by which macromolecules are degraded is complex, involving several enzymes acting in a coordinated sequential fashion. The deficiency of a single degradative enzyme leads to the accumulation of the macromolecule or its partially degraded metabolite within the lysosome; such accumulation produces disease. The best-characterized groups of lysosomal storage disorders are the mucopolysaccharidoses and the glycosphingolipidoses [106].

In the mucopolysaccharidoses, glycosaminoglycans are stored in lysosomes. Hurler's syndrome is the prototype to which at least 13 variants are compared. This disorder is inherited as a recessive trait. The biochemical basis for the disease is a deficiency of the enzyme alpha-L-iduronidase. As a result of the enzyme deficiency, dermatan sulfate and heparin sulfate are stored in cells throughout the body, which produces multiple organ dysfunction. Pulmonary problems develop secondary to kyphoscoliosis and deformities of the ribs, which reflect storage of mucopolysaccharides in bone. By the second decade of life, upper-airway obstruction is frequent due to storage of polysaccharides in lymphoid tissue and deformity of tracheal cartilage. As a result, respiratory acidosis develops. Intercurrent infections produce respiratory decompensation with anoxia. Bronchopneumonia is a frequent cause of death [137].

The pulmonary problems in the mucopolysaccharidoses are but one component of a systemic metabolic disorder. The clinical appearance of the patient with Hurler's syndrome suggests the diagnosis, which can be confirmed by appropriate biochemical studies. The other variants may show similar pulmonary problems to those described for Hurler's syndrome, especially as the patients enter the second decade of life. All variants are inherited as autosomal recessive traits except for type II (Hunter's syndrome), which shows X-linked inheritance. The clinical phenotype, biochemical defects, and genetics of the other established disorders of mucopolysaccharide metabolism are detailed in a review [98].

By contrast, two disorders of glycosphingolipid metabolism may present with pulmonary symptoms. The chronic nonneuropathic form of Gaucher's disease may produce respiratory difficulties because of diffuse pulmonary involvement (Fig. 71-5). In some patients this process is severe enough to produce cor pulmonale. Lung infiltrates may predispose to pneumonia, which is a major cause of death in younger patients [129]. Gaucher's disease is inherited as a recessive trait. The biochemical basis for the storage of glucosyl

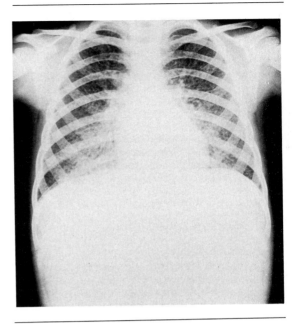

Fig. 71-5. Chronic nonneuropathic Gaucher's disease in a child showing diffuse pulmonary infiltrates.

ceramide in lysosomes is a deficiency of the enzyme glucocerebrosidase, which is required for the hydrolysis of glucocerebroside to ceramide and glucose [15].

The second group of lysosomal storage diseases involving glycosphingolipids that may present with pulmonary symptoms comprises the nonneuropathic forms of Niemann-Pick disease. The lungs on X-ray film show diffuse reticular infiltrates. Histologic examination at autopsy frequently shows foam cells in the alveoli, lymphatic vessels, and branches of the pulmonary artery [42]. This disorder is also inherited as an autosomal recessive trait. The biochemical basis for the lysosomal storage of sphingomyelin is a deficiency of the enzyme sphingomyelinase, which is required for the hydrolysis of sphingomyelin to ceramide and phosphocholine [16]. The gene has been localized to chromosome 11p15 [106].

In both Gaucher's and Niemann-Pick disease, patients usually show hepatosplenomegaly in addition to pulmonary infiltrates, which should suggest these diagnostic possibilities. Although aspiration and pneumonia may cause death in the other glycosphingolipidoses, the pulmonary problems in these patients are secondary to involvement of the central nervous system with attendant difficulties in handling secretions and swallowing.

The gene for Gaucher's disease has been localized to chromosome 1q21. Several allelic mutations have been identified, but whether a specific mutation predisposes to pulmonary involvement is not clear. Enzyme replacement therapy with macrophage-targeted glucocerebrosidase appears to produce improvement in the hematologic and visceral responses of patients with type I Gaucher's disease [10]. It will be of interest to determine whether this type of replacement therapy will improve pulmonary function.

Pulmonary Amyloidosis

Amyloid is a fibrillar protein that is deposited in tissues as rigid, fine, nonbranching fibrils having a width of approximately 100 Å [24]. The polypeptide chains are arranged perpendicularly to the axis of the fibril, forming a beta-pleated sheet conformation [13]. The term *amyloidosis* is applied to a family of systemic diseases that has as its common denominator the extracellular deposition of amyloid protein. Histologic staining of tissues with alkaline Congo red shows homogeneous eosinophilic deposits exhibiting dichroic birefringence under polarized light. This pathologic picture may be systemic in its distribution or localized to the heart and lungs. Systemic forms of amyloidosis have been classified as primary when the disease occurs without known predisposing factors and secondary when found in association with chronic infections, rheumatoid arthritis, multiple myeloma, tumors, and other chronic diseases [49,84].

Several heredofamilial forms of amyloidosis are now recognized, but the only entity that shows prominent pulmonary involvement is familial Mediterranean fever. This disorder is inherited as an autosomal recessive trait in which pulmonary deposits of amyloid may be found early in the course of the disease [60]. Familial aggregation has been reported in primary systemic amyloidosis without predisposing cause, but whether this represents a distinct genetic entity is not known [49,143].

Other forms of genetic amyloidosis present as sensorimotor polyneuropathies in which some patients may show systemic accumulations of amyloid with pulmonary involvement. The neuropathic amyloidoses appear to be inherited as autosomal dominant traits [49]. An interesting variant that is probably genetic is amyloid cardio-myopathy. Only two families have been reported. Amyloid deposits in the myocardial interstitial tissue produce symptoms of congestive heart failure appearing in the third decade of life [1,41].

The biochemical basis for the deposition of amyloid in tissue remains undefined. In familial Mediterranean fever, the origin of the protein is not known. In the systemic amyloidoses associated with plasma cell myeloma, primary macroglobulinemia, and other lymphoid system neoplasms, the amyloid is derived from immunoglobulins [50]. Sorting out the varying forms of systemic amyloidosis is in progress.

Pulmonary involvement with diffuse deposition of amyloid in alveolar septa, pulmonary vessels, and capillary membranes occurs in 40 to 50 percent of patients with primary systemic amyloidosis. Nodular pulmonary deposits of amyloid have been described as incidental findings at autopsy and produce no symptoms during life [21,143].

There are no clinical or laboratory findings diagnostic of amyloidosis. For practical purposes, the diagnosis depends on the demonstration of green birefringent material under polarized light in Congo red–stained tissue sections. The selection of biopsy sites depends on the site of involvement, the patient's clinical status, and the clinician's judgment. Diagnosis of pulmonary amyloidosis by transbronchial biopsy has been reported using flexible fiberoptic bronchoscopy [81].

Hereditary Mucoepithelial Dysplasia

Hereditary mucoepithelial dysplasia is inherited as an autosomal dominant trait. Patients present clinically with micropapillary lesions of the oral mucosa; keratoconjunctivitis; cataracts; coarse, scanty hair; and follicular keratosis. Bladder infections are common, as are abnormal cervical epithelial cells in affected females. Of 10 affected individuals in one family, 8 showed evidence of significant pulmonary disease characterized by recurrent pneumonia leading to pulmonary fibrosis and cor pulmonale at an early age. This syndrome is of particular interest because of unique cytologic features found in epithelial cells. Paranuclear vacuolation is observed with strand-shaped cytoplasmic inclusions. The inclusions resemble gap junction and desmosomal structures. It is probable that the molecular defect represents the first recognized example of a disease involving gap junction and desmosomal organization of epithelial cells [138,159].

References

1. Allensworth DC, Rice GJ, Lowe GW. Persistent atrial standstill in a family with myocardial disease. *Am J Med* 47:775, 1969.
2. Alper CA, Rosen F. Increased Susceptibility to Infection in Patients with Defects Affecting C₃. In D Berfisma (Ed), *Immunodeficiencies in Man and Animals* (National Foundation of Birth Defects Original Article Series, Vol 11, No. 1). Sunderland, MA: Sinauer, 1975. Pp 301–395.
3. Ammann AJ, et al. Use of intravenous alpha-globulin in antibody immunodeficiency states. *Clin Immunol Immunopathol* 22:60, 1982.
4. Anderson EG, Simon G, Reid L. Primary and thromboembolic pulmonary hypertension: A quantitative pathological study. *J Pathol* 110: 273, 1973.
5. Aviado DM, Jr, Schmidt FM. Effect of sympathomimetic drugs on pulmonary circulation with special reference to a new pulmonary vasodilator. *J Pharmacol Exp Ther* 120:512, 1974.
6. Ayres JG, et al. Abnormalities of the lungs and thoracic cage in the Ehlers-Danlos syndrome. *Thorax* 40:300, 1985.
7. Baehner RL. The Growth and Development of Our Understanding of Chronic Granulomatous Disease. In JA Bellanti, DH Day (Eds), *The Phagocytic Cell in Host Resistance.* New York: Raven Press, 1975. P 173.
8. Baehner RL, Nathan DG. Quantitative nitroblue tetrazolium test in chronic granulomatous disease. *N Engl J Med* 278:971, 1968.
9. Barabas AP. Ehlers-Danlos syndrome: Associated with prematurity and premature rupture of fetal membranes; possible increase in incidence. *Br Med J* 2:682, 1966.
10. Barton NW, et al. Replacement therapy for inherited enzyme deficiency—macrophage targeted glucocerebrosidase for Gaucher's disease. *N Engl J Med* 324:1464, 1991.
11. Basile G de Saint, et al. Close linkage of the locus for X chromosome–linked severe combined immunodeficiency to polymorphic DNA markers in X q11–q13. *Proc Natl Acad Sci USA* 84:7576, 1987.
12. Biggar WD, Good RA. Immunodeficiency in Ataxia-telangiectasia. In D Bergsma (Ed), *Immunodeficiency in Man and Animals* (National Foundation of Birth Defects Original Article Series, Vol 11, No. 1). Sunderland, MA: Sinauer, 1975. P 271.
13. Bonar L, Cohen AS, Skinner MM. Characterization of the amyloid fibrils as a cross-B protein. *Proc Soc Exp Biol Med* 131:1373, 1969.
14. Bourdillon PDV, Oakley CM. Regression of primary pulmonary hypertension. *Br Heart J* 38:264, 1976.
15. Brady RO, et al. Demonstration of a deficiency of glucocerebroside-clearing enzyme in Gaucher's disease. *J Clin Invest* 45:112, 1966.
16. Brady RO, et al. The metabolism of sphingomyelin II: Evidence of an enzymatic deficiency in Niemann-Pick disease. *Proc Natl Acad Sci USA* 55:366, 1966.
17. Breighton P. The dominant and recessive forms of cutis laxa. *J Med Genet* 9:216, 1972.
18. Byers PH. Disorders of Collagen Biosynthesis and Structure. In CR Scriver et al. (Eds), *The Metabolic Basis of Inherited Disease* (6th ed). New York: McGraw-Hill, 1989. Pp 2802–2845.
19. Byers PH, Holbrook K. Molecular basis of clinical heterogeneity in the Ehlers-Danlos syndrome. *Ann NY Acad Sci* 460:298, 1985.
20. Chandler D. Pulmonary and cerebral fistula with Osler's disease. *Arch Intern Med* 116:277, 1965.
21. Chen KTK. Amyloidosis presenting in the respiratory tract. *Pathol Annu* 24:253, 1989.
22. Clark JG, Kuhn C, III, Uitto J. Lung collagen in type IV Ehlers-Danlos syndrome: Ultrastructural and biochemical studies. *Am Rev Respir Dis* 122:971, 1980.
23. Clark RA, et al. Genetic variants of chronic granulomatous disease: Prevalence of deficiencies of two cytosolic components of the NADH oxidase system. *N Engl J Med* 321:647, 1989.
24. Cohen AS, Calkins E. Electron microscopic observation on a fibrous component of amyloid in diverse organs. *Nature* 183:1202, 1959.
25. Colton HR, Alper CA, Rosen FS. Genetics and biosynthesis of complement proteins. *N Engl J Med* 304:653, 1981.
26. Conney TP, Thurlbeck WM. Pulmonary hypoplasia in Down's syndrome. *N Engl J Med* 307:1170, 1982.
27. Crawford SW, et al. Characterization of a type VI collagen-related Mᵣ 140,000 protein from cutis-laxa fibroblasts in culture. *Biochem J* 227:494, 1985.
28. Culver W, et al. Lymphocyte Gene Therapy for Adenosine Deaminase Deficiency (abstract). *Pediatr Res* Annual Meeting 1992 Society Pediatric Research. 31:149a, 1992.
29. DeFerrante N, et al. Lysal oxidase deficiency in Ehlers-Danlos syndrome type V. *Connect Tissue Res* 3:49, 1975.
30. Dietz HC, et al. Marfan syndrome caused by a recurrent de novo missense mutation in the fibrillin gene. *Nature* 352:337, 1991.
31. Dinauer MD, et al. Human neutrophil cytochrome-β light chain (p 22-phox): Gene structure, chromosome location and mutations in cytochrome-negative autosomal recessive chronic granulomatous disease. *J Clin Invest* 86:1729, 1990.

32. Dines DE, et al. Pulmonary arteriovenous fistulas. *Mayo Clin Proc* 49:460, 1974.

33. Dooley TA, et al. First trimester diagnoses of adenosine deaminase deficiency. *Prenat Diagn* 7:561, 1987.

34. Douglas JG, et al. Pulmonary hypertension and fenfluramine. *Br Heart J* 283:881, 1983.

35. Dwyer EM, Jr, Troncale F. Spontaneous pneumothorax and pulmonary disease in the Marfan syndrome: Report of two cases and review of the literature. *Ann Intern Med* 62:1285, 1965.

36. Esber HJ, et al. Hepatis associated antigens and immunoglobulin composition in patients with Down's anomaly. *Am J Clin Pathol* 59:872, 1973.

37. Eyre DR, Shapiro FD, Aldrige JF. A heterozygous collagen defect in a variant of the Ehlers-Danlos syndrome type VII. *J Biol Chem* 2608: 11322, 1985.

38. Farnsworth AE, Ankeney JL. The spectrum of the scimitar syndrome. *J Thorac Cardiovasc Surg* 68:37, 1974.

39. Fishman AP. Pulmonary Circulation. In AP Fishman, AB Fisher, SD Geiger (Eds), *The Respiratory System*. Philadelphia: American Physiological Society, 1985. Pp. 93–165.

40. Foley RE, Boyd DP. Pulmonary arteriovenous aneurysms. *Surg Clin North Am* 41:801, 1961.

41. Frederiksen T, et al. Primary familial amyloidosis with severe amyloid heart disease. *Am J Med* 33:328, 1962.

42. Fredrickson DS, Sloan HR. Sphingomyelin Lipidosis: Niemann-Pick Disease. In JB Stanbury, JB Wyngaarden, DS Fredrickson (Eds), *The Metabolic Basis of Inherited Disease*, (3d ed). New York: McGraw-Hill, 1973. P 783.

43. Gallin JI, and the International Chronic Granulomatosis Disease Cooperative Study Group. A controlled trial of interferon gamma to prevent infection in chronic granulomatosis disease. *N Engl J Med* 324:509, 1991.

44. Garland HG, Anning ST. Hereditary hemorrhagic telangiectasia: Genetic and bibliographic study. *Br J Dermatol* 62:289, 1950.

45. Geha RG, et al. Heterogeneity of "acquired " or common variable agammaglobulinemia. *N Engl J Med* 291:1, 1974.

46. German J. Bloom's syndrome: Genetic and clinical observations in the first twenty-seven patients. *Am J Hum Genet* 21:196, 1969.

47. German J. Bloom's Syndrome II: The Prototype of Human Genetic Disorders Predisposing to Chromosome Instability and Cancer. In J German (Ed), *Chromosomes and Cancer*. New York: Wiley, 1974. P 601.

48. Giblett ER, Polmar SH. Inherited Immunodeficiency: Relationship to Lymphocyte Metabolic Dysfunction. In A Steinberg, et al. (Eds), *Progress in Medical Genetics*, Vol 3. Philadelphia: Saunders, 1979. P 185.

49. Glenner GG, Agnaczak TF, Page DL. The Inherited Systemic Amyloidoses and Localized Amyloid Deposits. In JB Stanbury, JB Wyngaarden, DS Fredrickson (Eds), *The Metabolic Basis of Inherited Disease*. New York: McGraw-Hill, 1973. P 1308.

50. Glenner GG, et al. Amyloid fibril proteins: Proof of homology with immunoglobulin light chains by sequence analysis. *Science* 172:1150, 1971.

51. Glotz RW, et al. Cutis laxa: A manifestation of generalized elastolysis. *Arch Dermatol* 92:373, 1965.

52. Gotti RA, et al. Ataxia telangiectasia: An interdisciplinary approach to pathogenesis. *Medicine* 70:99, 1991.

53. Griscelli C, Virelizier JL. Bone Marrow Transplant in a Patient with the Chediak-Higashi Syndrome. In RJ Wedgewood, FS Rosen, FS Paul (Eds), *Primary Immunodeficiency Diseases*. New York, Alan R. Liss, 1983. Pp 333–334.

54. Hajjar BA, Joyner EN, III. Congenital cutis laxa with advanced cardio-pulmonary disease. *J Pediatr* 73:116, 1968.

55. Hall JR, et al. Pneumothorax in the Marfan syndrome: Prevalence and therapy. *Ann Thorac Surg* 37:500, 1984.

56. Hance AJ, Crystal RG. The connective tissue of the lung. *Am Rev Respir Dis* 112:657, 1975.

57. Harnden DG. Ataxia Telangiectasia Syndrome: Cytogenetic and Cancer Aspects. In JG German (Ed), *Chromosomes and Cancer*. New York: Wiley, 1974. Pp 619–636.

58. Hashimoto K, Kanzaki T. Cutis laxa: Ultrastructural and biochemical studies. *Arch Dermatol* 103:661, 1971.

59. Healey JE. An anatomic survey of anomalous pulmonary veins. Their clinical significance. *J Thorac Surg* 23:433, 1952.

60. Heller H, et al. Amyloidoses in familial Mediterranean fever. *Arch Intern Med* 107:539, 1961.

61. Hermans PE, Diaz-Buxo JA, Stobo JD. Idiopathic late-onset immunoglobulin deficiency, clinical observations in 50 patients. *Am J Med* 61:221, 1976.

62. Hershfield MS, et al. Treatment of adenosine deaminase deficiency with polyethylene glycol–modified adenosine deaminase. *N Engl J Med* 316:589, 1987.

63. Hirschhorn R. Defects of purine metabolism: Immunodeficiency diseases. *Prog Clin Immunol* 3:67, 1977.

64. Hirschhorn R, Beratis NG. Prenatal diagnoses of adenosine deaminase deficiency. *Lancet* 2:1270, 1976.

65. Hodgson CH, et al. Hereditary hemorrhagic telangiectasia and pulmonary arteriovenous fistula. *N Engl J Med* 261:625, 1959.

66. Holian A, Scheule RK. Alveolar macrophage biology. *Hosp Pract* 25:53, 1990.

67. Hollister DW, Byers PH, Holbrook KA. Genetic disorders of collagen metabolism. *Adv Hum Genet* 12:1, 1982.

68. Hollsster DW, et al. Immunohistologic abnormalities of the micro fibrillin-fiber system in the Marfan syndrome. *N Engl J Med* 323:152, 1990.

69. Hong R, et al. Reconstitution of B and T cell lymphocyte function in severe combined immunodeficiency disease after transplantation with thymic epithelium. *Lancet* 2:1270, 1976.

70. Hood WB, Jr, et al. Primary pulmonary hypertension: Familial occurrence. *Br Heart J* 30:336, 1968.

71. Hook EB. Risk of Down's syndrome in relation to maternal age. *Lancet* 2;465, 1976.

72. Huber J, Kersey J. Pathological Findings in Combined Immunodeficiency Diseases and Adenosine Deaminase Deficiency. In HJ Meuwissen, et al. (Eds), *Combined Immunodeficiency Diseases and Adenosine Deaminase Deficiency: A Molecular Defect.* New York: Academic Press, 1975. P 279.

73. Hutteroth TH, Litwin SD, German J. Abnormal immune responses in Bloom's syndrome lymphocytes in vitro. *J Clin Invest* 56:1, 1965.

74. Jue KL, et al. Anomalies of the great vessels associated with lung hypoplasia. The scimitar syndrome. *Am J Dis Child* 111:35, 1966.

75. Karin SP, et al. Mapping the X-linked agammaglobulinemia locus by the use of restriction fragment-length polymorphism. *J Clin Invest* 77:649, 1986.

76. Katz P, et al. Mechanism of human cell-mediated cytotoxicity: II. Correction of the selective defect in natural killing in the Chédiak-Hagashi syndrome with inducers of intracellular cyclic GMP. *J Immunol* 129:297, 1982.

77. Kiely B, et al. Syndrome of anomalous venous drainage of the right lung to the inferior vena cava. *Am J Cardiol* 20:1, 1967.

78. King TKC, Norum RA. Unusual Inherited Pulmonary Disorders which Provide for Pulmonary Physiology and Function. In SD Litwin (Ed), *Lung Biology in Health and Disease*, Vol 11: *Genetic Determinants of Pulmonary Disease.* New York: Marcel Dekker, 1978. Pp 167–171.

79. King TKC, Norum RA. Unusual Inherited Pulmonary Disorders which Provide for Pulmonary Physiology and Function. In SD Litwin (Ed), *Lung Biology in Health and Disease*, Vol 11: *Genetic Determinants of Pulmonary Disease.* New York: Marcel Dekker, 1978. Pp 171–173.

80. Kleiger RE, et al. Pulmonary hypertension in patients using oral contraceptives: A report of six cases. *Chest* 69:143, 1976.

81. Kline LR, et al. Diagnosis of pulmonary amyloidosis by transbronchial biopsy. *Am Rev Respir Dis* 132:191, 1985.

82. Krane SM, Pinnell SR, Erbe RW. Lysyl-protocollagen hydroxylase deficiency in fibroblasts from siblings with hydroxylysine-deficient collagen. *Proc Natl Acad Sci USA* 69:2899, 1972.

83. Kuiper-Oosterwal CH, Moulaert A. The scimitar syndrome in infancy and childhood. *Eur J Cardiol* 1:55, 1973.

84. Kyle R, Bayrd ED. Amyloidoses—Review of 236 cases. *Medicine* 54:271, 1975.

85. Landing BH. Congenital malformations and genetic disorders of the respiratory tract (larynx, trachea, bronchi, and lungs). *Am Rev Respir Dis* 120:151,1979.

86. Landing BH, Wells TR. Tracheobronchial anomalies in children. *Perspect Pediatr Pathol* 1:1, 1973.

87. Lee B, et al. Linkage of Marfan syndrome and a phenotypically related disorder to two different fibrillin genes. *Nature* 352:334, 1991.

88. Lee TD, Jr, Roveti GC, Ross RS. The hemodynamic effects of isoproterenol on pulmonary hypertension in man. *Am Heart J* 65:361, 1963.

89. LeRoux BT. Pulmonary hamartoma. *Thorax* 19:236, 1964.

90. Lichtenstein JR, et al. Procollagen peptidase deficiency in a form of the Ehlers-Danlos syndrome. *Trans Assoc Am Physicians* 86:333, 1973.

91. Lipton RA, Greenwald RA, Seriff NS. Pneumothorax and bilateral honeycomb lung in Marfan syndrome: Report of a case and review of the pulmonary abnormalities in this disorder. *Am Rev Respir Dis* 104:924, 1971.

92. Lockart A, Reeves JT. Pleurogenic pulmonary hypertension: What's new? *Clin Sci* 67:1, 1984.

93. Malcolm S, et al. Close linkage of random DNA fragments from X q21.3–22 to X-linked agammaglobulinemia (XLA). *Hum Genet* 77:172, 1987.

94. Marcus CL, et al. Obstructive sleep apnea in children with Down syndrome. *Pediatrics* 88:132, 1991.

95. McCaw BK, et al. Somatic rearrangement of chromosome 14 in human lymphocytes. *Proc Natl Acad Sci USA* 72:2071, 1975.

96. McFarlin DE, Straber W, Waldman TA. Ataxia telangiectasia. *Medicine* 51:281, 1972.

97. McKusick VA. *Heritable Disorders of Connective Tissue* (4th ed). St. Louis: Mosby, 1972. P 329.

98. McKusick VA, Neufeld EF. The Mucopolysaccharide Storage Diseases. In JB Stanbury, (Eds), *The Metabolic Basis of Inherited Disease* (5th ed). New York: McGraw-Hill, 1983. P 751.

99. Merten DF, Rooney R. Progressive pulmonary emphysema associated with congenital gener-

alized elastolyses (cutis laxa). *Radiology* 113: 691, 1974.

100. Miller ME, Nilsson UR. A familial deficiency of the phagocytosis enhancing activity of serum related to a dysfunction of the fifth component of complement (C5). *N Engl J Med* 282:354, 1970.

101. Miller ME, et al. Depressed immunoglobulin G in newborn infants with Down's syndrome. *Pediatrics* 371:715, 1966.

102. Milunsky A. Prenatal diagnosis of genetic disorders. *N Engl J Med* 245:377,1976.

103. Moyer JH, Glantz HG, Brest AN. Pulmonary arteriovenous fistulas: Physiologic and clinical consideration. *Am J Med* 32:417, 1962.

104. Mudd SH, Levy HL. Disorders of Transulfuration. In JB Stanbury, et al. (Eds), *The Metabolic Basis of Inherited Disease.* New York: McGraw-Hill, 1983. P 522.

105. Neill CA, et al. The familial occurrence of hypoplastic right lung with systemic arterial supply and venous drainage: "Scimitar syndrome." *Bull Johns Hopkins Hosp* 107:1, 1960.

106. Neufeld EF. Lysosomal storage diseases. *Annu Rev Biochem* 60:257, 1991.

107. Newburger PE, et al. Prenatal diagnosis of chronic granulomatous disease. *N Engl J Med* 300:178, 1979.

108. Newhouse M, Sanchis J, Bienenstock J. Lung defense mechanisms. *N Engl J Med* 295:990, 1976.

109. Newman JH, Loyd JE. Genetic basis for pulmonary hypertension. *Semin Respir Med* 7:343, 1986.

110. Nicotera TM. Molecular and biochemical aspects of Bloom's syndrome. *Cancer Genet Cytogenet* 53:1, 1991.

111. Oakley C, Somerville J. Oral contraceptives and progressive pulmonary vascular disease. *Lancet* 1:890, 1968.

112. Oakley D, et al. Scimitar vein syndrome: Report of nine new cases. *Am Heart J* 107:596, 1984.

113. Osborne WRA, Scott CR. Genetic Heterogeneity in Purine Nucleoside Phosphorylase Deficiency. In *Inborn Errors of Specific Immunity* (Birth Defects Institute Symposium IX). Albany, NY, 1978. P 279.

114. Packer BD, Blades JF. Dermatorrhexis: A case report; the so-called Ehlers-Danlos syndrome. *Va Med Monthly* 81:21, 1954.

115. Packer M. Vasodilator therapy for primary pulmonary hypertension. *Ann Intern Med* 103:255, 1985.

116. Pelham A, et al. RFLP and deletion analysis for X-linked chronic granulomatous disease using the cDNA probe: Potential for improved prenatal diagnosis and carrier determination. *Blood* 76:820, 1990.

117. Perry WH. Clinical spectrum of hereditary hemorrhagic telangiectasia (Osler-Weber-Rendu Disease). *Am J Med* 82:989, 1987.

118. Peterson RDA, Kelly WD, Good RA. Ataxia telangiectasia, its association with a defective thymus, immunological deficiency disease and malignancy. *Lancet* 1:1189, 1964.

119. Pinnell SR, et al. A heritable disorder of connective tissue: Hydroxylysine-deficient collagen disease. *N Engl J Med* 286:1013, 1972.

120. Polmar SH, et al. Enzyme replacement therapy for adenosine deaminase deficiency and severe combined immunodeficiency. *N Engl J Med* 295:1337, 1976.

121. Poole AR. Proteoglycans in health and disease: Structures and functions. *Biochem J* 236:1, 1986.

122. Pope FM, et al. Patients with Ehlers-Danlos syndrome type IV lack type III collagen. *Proc Natl Acad Sci USA* 72:1314, 1975.

123. Prockop DJ, Kivirikko KI. Heritable diseases of collagen. *N Engl J Med* 311:376, 1984.

124. Pyeritz RE, McKusick VA. The Marfan syndrome: Diagnosis and management. *N Engl J Med* 300:772, 1979.

125. Pyeritz RE, et al. Ehlers-Danlos syndrome due to a novel defect in type III procollagen. *Am J Med Genet* 19:607, 1984.

126. Rausch PG, Pryzwansky BS, Spitznagel JK. Immunocytochemical identification of azurophilic and specific granule markers in the giant granules of Chediak-Higashi neutrophils. *N Engl J Med* 298:693, 1978.

127. Regas DA, Elsasser AP, Hecht F. Impaired in vitro response of circulating lymphocytes to phytohemagglutinin in Down's syndrome. *Int Arch Allergy Appl Immunol* 39:587, 1970.

128. Rich S, Levy PS. Characteristics of surviving and nonsurviving patients with primary pulmonary hypertension. *Am J Med* 76:573, 1984.

129. Roberts WC, Fredrickson DS. Gaucher's disease of the lung causing severe pulmonary hypertension with associated acute recurrent pericarditis. *Circ Res* 35:783, 1967.

130. Root RK, Rosenthal AS, Balestra DJ. Abnormal bactericidal metabolic and lysosomal function of Chediak-Higashi syndrome leukocytes. *J Clin Invest* 51:649, 1972.

131. Rosen FS. Immunodeficiency. In B Benacerraf (Ed), *Immunogenetics and Immunodeficiency.* Baltimore: University Park Press, 1975. P 229.

132. Rosen FS, Cooper MD, Wedgwood RJP. The primary immunodeficiencies (first of two parts). *N Engl J Med* 311:235, 1984.

133. Rosen FS, Cooper MD, Wedgwood RJ. The primary immunodeficiencies (second of two parts). *N Engl J Med* 311:300, 1984.

134. Rosen FS, et al. Primary immunodeficiency diseases: Report prepared for the WHO by a sci-

entific group on immunodeficiency. *Clin Immunol Immunopathol* 28:450, 1983.

135. Royer-Pokora B, et al. Cloning the gene for an inherited disorder—chronic granulomatous disease—on the basis of its chromosomal location. *Nature* 322:32, 1986.

136. Rubin LJ. Approach to the diagnoses and treatment of pulmonary hypertension. *Chest* 96:659, 1989.

137. Schafer IA. The Genetic Mucopolysaccharidoses: Clinical and Chemical Correlates in Diagnosis. In DS Young, JM Hicks (Eds), *The Neonate*. New York: Wiley, 1976. P 171.

138. Scheman AJ, et al. Hereditary mucoepithelial displasia. Case report and review of the literature. *J Am Acad Dermatol* 21:351, 1989.

139. Shepherd JT, Edwards JE, Burchell HB, Swan HJC, Wood EHH. Clinical, physiological and pathological considerations in patients with idiopathic pulmonary hypertension. *Br Heart J* 19:70, 1957.

140. Sluiter-Eringa H, Orie NGM, Sluiter HJ. Pulmonary arteriovenous fistula: Diagnosis and prognosis in non-compliant patients. *Am Rev Respir Dis* 100:177, 1969.

141. Smith DW, Wilson AC. *The Child with Down's Syndrome*. Philadelphia: Saunders, 1973.

142. Smith RM, Curnutte JT. Molecular Basis of Chronic Granulomatous Disease. *Blood* 77:673, 1991.

143. Smith RRL, et al. Type and distribution of pulmonary parenchymal and vascular amyloid. *Am J Med* 66:96, 1979.

144. Spencer H. *Pathology of the Lung* (2d ed). Oxford: Pergamon, 1968.

145. Standefer JE, Tabakin BS, Hanson JS. Pulmonary arteriovenous fistula: Case report with cine-angiographic studies. *Am Rev Respir Dis* 89:95, 1966.

146. Steinmann B, et al. Evidence for a structural mutation of procollagen in a patient with Ehlers-Danlos syndrome type VII. *Eur J Pediatr* 130:203, 1979.

147. Stiehm ER, Fudenberg HH. Serum levels of immune globulin in health and disease: A survey. *Pediatrics* 75:996, 1969.

148. Stolle CA, et al. Synthesis of an altered type III procollagen in a patient with type IV Ehlers-Danlos syndrome. *J Biol Chem* 260:1937, 1985.

149. Tanisuchi N, et al. Impaired B-cell differentiation and T-cell regulation in four patients with Bloom's syndrome. *Clin Immunol Immunopathol* 22:242, 1982.

150. Trappeiner G. Disease states in genetic complement deficiencies. *Int J Dermatol* 21:175, 1982.

151. Turner JAM, Stanley NN. Fragile lung in the Marfan syndrome. *Thorax* 31:771, 1976.

152. Van Maldergem L, et al. Severe congenital cutis laxa with pulmonary emphysema: A family with three affected sibs. *Am J Med Genet* 31:455, 1988.

153. Wagenvoort CA, Wagenvoort N. Primary pulmonary hypertension: A pathological study of the lung vessels in 156 clinically diagnosed cases. *Circulation* 42:1163, 1970.

154. Walcott GH, Burchell HB, Brown AL, Jr. Primary pulmonary hypertension. *Am J Med* 49:76, 1970.

155. Weening RS, et al. Cytochrome b deficiency in an autosomal form of chronic granulomatous disease. *J Clin Invest* 75:915, 1985.

156. White RI, Jr, et al. Pulmonary arteriovenous malformation: Techniques and long-term outcome of embolotherapy. *Radiology* 169:663, 1988.

157. Winkelstein JA, Fearon E. Carrier detection of the X-linked primary immunodeficiency diseases using X-chromosome inactivation analyses. *J Allergy Clin Immunol* 85:1090, 1990.

158. Winters WL, Joseph RR, Learner N. Primary pulmonary hypertension and Raynaud's phenomenon. *Arch Intern Med* 114:821, 1964.

159. Witkop CJ, Jr, White JG, Waring GO. Hereditary mucoepithelial dysplasia: A disease of gap junction and desmosome formation. *Birth Defects* 18:493, 1982.

160. Wolfson JJ, et al. Roentgenologic manifestations in children with a genetic defect of polymorphonuclear leukocyte function: Chronic granulomatous disease of children. *Radiology* 91:37, 1968.

161. Wollheim FA. Primary Acquired Hypogammaglobulinemia: Genetic Defect or Acquired Disease? In D Bergsma, RA Good (Eds), *Immunologic Deficiency Diseases in Man* (Original Article Series IV, No. 1). White Plains, NY: The National Foundation March of Dimes, 1968. P 311.

162. Yakovlevitch M, et al. Pulmonary hypertension in a patient with tryptophan-induced eosinophilia-myalgia syndrome. *Am J Med* 90:272, 1991.

163. Yocum MW, Kelso JM. Common variable immunodeficiency: The disorder and treatment. *Mayo Clin Proc* 66:83, 1991.

164. Yu PN. Primary pulmonary hypertension: Report of 6 cases and review of literature. *Ann Intern Med* 49:1138, 1958.

XI

Pleural Diseases

Pleural Anatomy, Pleural Fluid Dynamics, and the Diagnosis of Pleural Disease

Alfred F. Connors, Jr.   *Murray D. Altose*

Pleural Anatomy and Histology

The pleura is a thin serous membrane that covers the lungs, mediastinum, diaphragm, and inner surface of the chest wall. It is made up of visceral and parietal layers. The visceral pleura covers all surfaces of the lung, including the interlobar fissures. The parietal pleura lines all the inside surfaces of the thoracic cavity, including the surface of the chest wall, the mediastinum, and the diaphragm. The visceral and parietal pleurae meet at each hilum and in a fold of the pleura, the pulmonary ligament, which extends posteriorly and downward from the hilum.

The pleural space is a potential space with only a very small amount of fluid between the visceral and parietal surfaces. The fluid acts as a lubricant to allow free motion of the lung in the pleural space in response to changes in lung volume with respiration. The right and left pleural spaces are separated by the mediastinum and do not communicate.

The pleura is lined by a single layer of mesothelial cells. These cells are 20 to 40 μm wide, from 0.1 to 0.4 μm thick, and have microvilli on their surface [46,47]. The microvilli are distributed over the entire pleura but are most prominent on the caudal as compared to the cephalad portions and on the visceral as compared to the parietal pleura [46,47]. They increase the surface area of the pleura and thus enhance membrane transport and other membrane-dependent metabolic functions [23]. They also may be important in reducing friction between the lung and the chest wall.

Mesothelial cells reproduce slowly and are easily damaged by exposure to the air [47]. Defects in the pleura are repaired by a combination of migration of cells and mitosis. Mesothelial cells that are dislodged from the pleura can be transformed into macrophages and, possibly, fibroblasts. Activated mesothelial cells are active in prostacyclin synthesis and fibrinolysis.

Blood to the parietal pleura is supplied by systemic capillaries [4]. The chest-wall pleura is perfused by small branches of the intercostal and internal mammary arteries, whereas the mediastinal pleura is supplied by the pericardiophrenic and internal mammary arteries. The musculophrenic and superior phrenic arteries supply blood to the diaphragmatic pleura. The visceral pleura receives its blood supply from both the pulmonary and the systemic circulations. The mediastinal and interlobular surfaces are supplied predominantly by the bronchial circulation. The costal and most of the diaphragmatic surfaces of the visceral pleura are supplied by branches of both the bronchial and pulmonary arteries.

The various arteries supplying the visceral pleura terminate in a loose capillary network, notable for the unusual size of the individual capillaries. The capillaries have a diameter of 30 μm and are three or four times as large as alveolar capillaries [18]. These "giant capillaries" empty into the pulmonary veins. Because of the very large capacitance of the capillary bed, the pressures tend to be low, approximating that in the pulmonary circulation.

The costal pleural lymph vessels drain into the dorsal internal intercostal lymph nodes or into sternal lymph nodes located along the internal thoracic artery [4]. The diaphragmatic and mediastinal pleura drain into middle, anterior, and posterior diaphragmatic lymph nodes. The visceral pleural lymphatics consist of a superficial plexus located in the subpleural connective-tissue layer of the visceral pleura. The density of this plexus is greatest in the lung bases. The lymph is removed from this plexus either via subpleural collecting vessels, which course along the surface of the lung and drain into mediastinal lymphatics through the root of the lung, or via small lymphatic vessels located in the interlobular septa, which pass directly into the lung and anastomose with terminal intrapulmonary lymphatics at the level of the terminal bronchioles [4]. These intrapulmonary lymphatics drain to the hilum via the perivenous or peribronchial lymphatics.

The parietal pleural lymphatics are in direct communication with the pleural space via multiple stomata, which range from 2 to 6 nm in diameter [23]. These stomata are found mostly in the mediastinal pleural and low on the costal surface. They are connected to lacunae, dilated submesothelial lymphatic vessels, which drain into the costal and mediastinal vessels [45,46]. The stomata and their associated lacunae are important in removing red blood cells and particulate matter from the pleural space.

Pleural Fluid Dynamics

The volume of fluid in the pleural space is normally only about 0.1 to 0.2 ml/kg body weight [42]. The small pleural fluid volume is maintained because of equilibrium between the rate of fluid formation and resorption (Table 72-1). This equilibrium is based on (1) Starling forces, which govern the movement of fluid into and out of pleural capillaries; (2) the efficiency of the pleural lymphatic system in removing fluid and protein from the pleural space; and (3) the surface area of the pleura.

The Starling relationship is summarized in the following equation:

$$F = K\,[(P_{cap} - P_{pl}) - \sigma(\pi_{cap} - \pi_{pl})]$$

where F is the net fluid movement of fluid into or out of the pleural space, K is the filtration coefficient of the pleural membrane, P_{cap} is the capillary hydrostatic pressure, P_{pl} is the pleural hydrostatic pressure, σ is the reflection coefficient (i.e., the effectiveness of the membrane in

Table 72-1. **The forces governing pleural fluid production and removal from the pleural space**

Starling forces	Parietal pleura		Pleural space		Visceral pleura
Hydrostatic (gradient)	+30	(+35) →	−5	(+17) ←	+12
Oncotic (gradient)	+34	(+30) ←	+4	(+30) →	+34
Net gradient		+5 →		−13 →	

Note: The balance between the hydrostatic forces, which tend to move fluid into the pleural space, and the oncotic forces, which tend to remove fluid from the pleural space, is shown. The net result is a pressure gradient from the parietal pleura into the pleural space and from the pleural space to the visceral pleura.

preventing the flow of solute compared with the flow of water), π_{cap} is the capillary plasma oncotic pressure, and π_{pl} is pleural fluid oncotic pressure. The hydrostatic pressure gradient $(P_{cap} - P_{pl})$ tends to move fluid from the capillaries into the pleural space, while the oncotic pressure gradient $(\pi_{cap} - \pi_{pl})$ tends to move fluid from the pleural space into the capillaries. The reflection coefficient is between 0.9 and 1.0.

It is generally considered that the capillary hydrostatic pressure in the parietal pleural capillaries is that of the systemic vascular system, while the capillary hydrostatic pressure in the visceral pleura is that of the pulmonary vascular system [17,28]. This results in a balance of pressures as shown in Table 72-1. The parietal pleural hydrostatic forces exceed the oncotic forces and result in a net movement of fluid into the pleural space. The visceral pleural hydrostatic forces, on the other hand, are less than the oncotic forces and favor absorption of fluid from the pleural space. The net gradient for fluid absorption through the visceral pleura is greater than that for fluid formation through the parietal pleura, so that the volume of residual pleural fluid is very small. Fluid resorption is also enhanced by the greater surface area of the visceral pleura made up by the interlobar fissures and by the microvilli on the visceral pleural mesothelial cells.

Since the visceral pleura is supplied over most of its surface by the bronchial circulation either alone or together with the pulmonary arterial circulation, the capillary hydrostatic forces in the visceral pleura in humans may be closer to those of the systemic capillaries [42]. If this were the case, fluid would move into the pleural space from both the visceral and parietal surfaces. Removal of fluid from the pleural space would then depend entirely on lymphatic drainage.

Pleural fluid, proteins, cells, and particulate matter are removed from the pleural space via the pleural stomata, which open into lacunae. The lymphatics remove considerable amounts of fluid from the pleural space, from 400 to 700 ml fluid per day [19,43].

Clinical Manifestations of Pleural Disease

Symptoms

The main symptoms of pleural disease are pain, cough, and dyspnea. The pain of pleural disease is caused by irritation of the parietal pleura. In contrast, the visceral pleura has no sensory nerve endings. The intercostal nerves supply the parietal pleura and the periphery of the diaphragm. Inflammation in these areas is appreciated in the overlying chest wall. The central diaphragmatic tendon is innervated by the phrenic nerve. Consequently, inflammation of this portion of the pleura results in pain that is referred to the ipsilateral shoulder.

Pain from the pleura is generally severe and well localized, and usually has an abrupt onset. The pain is commonly sharp, although it can be dull or aching in quality. It is made worse by coughing or by taking a deep breath and can be relieved by splinting the affected side. Irritation of the anterior or lateral costal pleura can result in upper-quadrant abdominal pain. Pain in both the upper abdomen and ipsilateral shoulder is diagnostic of inflammation of the diaphragmatic pleura.

Patients with pleural effusion frequently complain of a nonproductive cough. The cause of the cough is not clear, but it may be directly related to the pleural inflammation or result from compression of lung parenchyma causing the activation of airway irritant receptors.

Dyspnea commonly accompanies a pneumothorax, pleural effusion, or pleural fibrosis. The shortness of breath may be severe, even with a relatively small pleural effusion or pneumothorax. The mechanism of dyspnea with pleural effusions is unclear. Mechanical distortion of the lung and chest wall may stimulate vagal mechanoreceptors, which influence central respiratory neuronal activity. Alternatively, changes in respiratory impedance may increase the strain on the respiratory muscles. Hypoxemia can contribute to the sensation of dyspnea, but the hypoxemia associated with pleural effusion and pneumothorax is usually mild unless substantial underlying parenchymal lung disease is also present.

The vital capacity is often reduced in the presence of large pleural effusions. Since pleural effusions tend to displace rather than compress underlying lung, changes in lung volume are small [3]. Removal of even large volumes of pleural fluid results in only relatively small increases in vital capacity.

Physical Signs

The heart rate and breathing frequency of patients with pleural effusion are normal or slightly elevated. Prominent tachycardia in a patient with pneumothorax, especially in the presence of hypotension, suggests a tension pneumothorax, and this requires prompt intervention.

With pleural effusion and pneumothorax, the resting volume of the involved hemithorax is usually increased slightly. When the pleural pressure exceeds atmospheric pressure, as with a tension pneumothorax, the involved hemithorax may be enlarged with a loss of the concave shape of the intercostal spaces. On the other hand, if the underlying lung is collapsed because of a large airway obstruction, the hemithorax may be smaller and the intercostal spaces retracted even in the presence of a pleural effusion. The position of the trachea provides information about displacement of the mediastinum. The trachea shifts away from a hemithorax with a large pleural effusion or a pneumothorax. A midline trachea in a patient with a large pleural effusion suggests an obstructed mainstem bronchus, a trapped lung, or fixation of the mediastinum with an inflammatory or malignant process.

The presence of fluid, air, or fibrous tissue between the lung and chest wall impedes the transmission of sound vibrations from the vocal apparatus to the chest wall and results in reduction in auditory and tactile fremitus. The boundary between normal and reduced fremitus is useful in localizing the upper border of a pleural effusion.

The percussion note is flat over a pleural effusion but hyperresonant over a pneumothorax.

Changes in the tone of the percussion note along the chest wall are also useful in assessing the extent of a pleural effusion. In the upright position, dullness to percussion is most prominent at the lung base. Changes in the location of percussion dullness with changes in posture indicate free pleural fluid.

Breath sounds are diminished in intensity or totally absent over a pleural effusion, pneumothorax, or fibrothorax. Often breath sounds have a distinct bronchial quality just above the upper boundary of a pleural effusion because of enhanced sound transmission through compressed lung parenchyma.

Diagnostic Approaches

The recognition and diagnostic evaluation of pleural abnormalities require a careful history and physical examination along with a chest roentgenogram. Ultrasonography of the thorax is also useful in assessing the location and extent of a pleural effusion. The most important and direct diagnostic procedure is thoracentesis, which will allow the classification and diagnosis of most pleural effusions. Other invasive diagnostic procedures such as pleural biopsy, either closed or open, and thoracoscopy may be needed in certain patients. Occasionally, bronchoscopy is required to determine the cause of an exudative pleural effusion.

Chest Roentgenography

PLEURAL EFFUSION

The normal or "typical" distribution of fluid in the pleural space is determined by two physical phenomena: gravity and the tendency of the lung to maintain its shape as it changes volume. This latter characteristic is termed *form elasticity* [11]. Because of gravity and the elastic properties of the lung, fluid first accumulates at the base of the hemithorax under the lung; the lung, in essence, "floats" above the effusion. Pleural effusions of up to 300 to 500 ml can maintain an infrapulmonary location without spilling into the costophrenic angles [12] (Fig. 72-1).

There are several roentgenographic signs that suggest an infrapulmonary accumulation of fluid [31]: (1) The peak of the pseudodiaphragm on the posteroanterior view is lateral to the position of the expected peak of the true hemidiaphragm, (2) the space between the top of the left pseudodiaphragm and the top of the gastric bubble is increased, (3) the posterior costophrenic sulcus on the lateral view may be blunted even though the lateral costophrenic sulcus is sharp on the posteroanterior view, and (4) fluid on the left side may accumulate along the lower mediastinum, producing a wedge-shaped opacity.

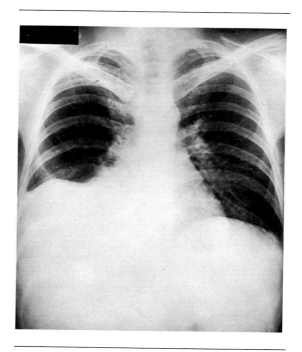

Fig. 72-1. A characteristic right infrapulmonary effusion.

When the volume of pleural fluid exceeds a certain amount, it spills first into the posterior costophrenic sulcus. This causes obliteration of the sharp costophrenic angle, replacing it with a tissue-density shadow that has a meniscus-shaped upper border. The meniscus is due to capillary action, which draws fluid upward on the chest wall surrounding the lung because of the surface tension of the fluid itself. As fluid continues to accumulate, first the lateral and then the anterior costophrenic sulci become obliterated. The typical configuration of moderate to large pleural effusion consists of a homogeneous tissue-density shadow with an upper meniscus extending from the anterior to the posterior wall on the lateral view and from the mediastinum to the lateral chest wall on the posteroanterior view [12]. Fluid also may accumulate within interlobar fissures.

Lateral decubitus roentgenographic views of

the chest effectively confirm the presence of free-flowing fluid in the pleural space. It is preferable to obtain both right and left decubitus views regardless of the side of apparent pleural fluid accumulation. Bilateral decubitus views often identify a contralateral effusion that may not be apparent on an upright view. Also, in the decubitus position with the diseased hemithorax elevated, fluid gravitates toward the mediastinum so that parenchymal infiltrates, masses, or atelectasis may come into view. Free pleural fluid appears as a homogeneous density between the chest wall and the lung with a rather sharp border between the fluid and the aerated lung. Decubitus views are particularly useful in identifying very small pleural effusions.

It may be difficult to recognize even large pleural effusions on chest roentgenograms taken with patients in the supine position. Large pleural effusions appear as a homogeneous hazy density over the entire lung field, since fluid is as likely to collect at the apex or laterally as it is to collect at the lung base. Several signs distinguish parenchymal infiltrates from the diffusely increased density of a pleural effusion [23]. With a pleural effusion, the density is homogeneous and not patchy, as is commonly seen with parenchymal infiltrates. Air bronchograms are seen with diffuse infiltrates but not with pleural effusions. Finally, the vascular structures of the lung are visible through the increased density of a pleural effusion but are obscured by a parenchymal infiltrate.

Atypical patterns of pleural fluid accumulation suggest underlying parenchymal disease or pleural fibrosis [11]. Parenchymal diseases produce patchy changes in lung elasticity, and pleural fluid tends to accumulate over regions with the greatest elastic recoil. Fibrous adhesions between the visceral and parietal pleural surfaces or within interlobar fissures result in loculated effusions. Loculations between the lung and chest wall are smooth, sharply demarcated, homogeneous densities that compress the underlying lung parenchyma [12]. They are often D-shaped, with the base of the D against the chest wall and the convexity projecting into the lung parenchyma. With large loculations or loculations at the base of the lung, the lower border of the fluid collection is often not clearly discernible.

Fluid that is loculated in interlobar fissures is best seen on lateral views, where it appears as a sharply defined shadow in the shape of a biconvex lens along the course of the major or minor fissures [49]. On the posteroanterior radiograph, loculated interlobar fluid may be mistaken for a mass lesion. These are referred to as *pseudotumors*. Interlobar fluid collections, particularly in the minor fissure, are commonly seen in congestive heart failure.

PNEUMOTHORAX

Since air is less dense than lung tissue, a pneumothorax tends to collect in the least dependent portions of the chest. The diagnosis of a pneumothorax requires the identification of a visceral pleural line displaced from the chest wall. The visceral pleura appears as a thin, sharply defined line that separates the lung parenchyma with its visible lung markings from the clear pleural space, which contains air and is devoid of lung markings. The hemithorax may be enlarged because of the loss of apposition of the lung to the chest wall. The diaphragm may be slightly depressed, and the mediastinum may be shifted contralaterally.

A small pneumothorax may not be readily apparent on a standard chest roentgenogram. It may be more easily seen, however, in views taken in full exhalation, which reduces the volume of the lung relative to the volume of the pneumothorax. Also, lateral decubitus views with the side with the suspected pneumothorax up may allow identification of air between the lung and the lateral chest wall when small collections of air at the apex cannot be discerned because of confounding rib shadows.

A tension pneumothorax results when the intrapleural pressure exceeds atmospheric pressure. This is usually caused by a ball-valve mechanism that allows air to enter the pleural space during inspiration but does not permit air to leave the pleural space during expiration. A tension pneumothorax is more likely to occur during positive-pressure mechanical ventilation. Because of the large volume of air under pressure in the pleural space, the diaphragm is depressed, the mediastinum is shifted to the contralateral side, and the lung is severely compressed. Venous return may be impeded, leading to shock. When circulatory changes or signs of respiratory distress are noted in a patient with a pneumothorax, the pleural space must be evacuated of air immediately.

PLEURAL FIBROSIS AND PLEURAL PLAQUES

Pleural thickening is a common finding on chest roentgenographs and usually represents fibrosis of the visceral pleura caused by a previous pleuropulmonary inflammatory condition. The extent and thickness of the pleural line depends on the type and severity of the inflammatory disorder. Thick pleural plaques and calcifications result from hemothorax, pyothorax, or healed tuberculous pleuritis. These are generally unilateral and may be seen in continuous sheets of calcification or in discrete plaques [12]. Extensive fibrosis of the parietal pleura with pleural plaques may follow the inhalation of asbestos fibers. Bilateral calcifications of the diaphragmatic pleura are pathognomonic of asbestos-related pleural disease.

Pleural thickening may be confined to the apical regions of the lung alone. Apical capping is a common finding, particularly in those over the age of 45 years [35]. It is caused by a variety of previous inflammatory conditions and is not necessarily a reflection of old tuberculosis. Markedly asymmetrical apical thickening, particularly if changes in the radiographic appearance are seen over several months, suggests a neoplastic process such as a superior sulcus tumor.

Computed Tomography

Computed tomography (CT) has only limited applicability in the evaluation of patients with pleural disease. It is rarely required to establish the presence of free pleural fluid, and the localization of both free and loculated pleural fluid is better accomplished by ultrasonography. Computed tomography is useful for locating the parenchymal lung disease that caused the pleural effusion, evaluating mediastinal lymphadenopathy, and evaluating the condition of the lung parenchyma hidden behind a pleural effusion. It is helpful in distinguishing between malignant and benign disease in patients with diffuse pleural disease [20]. Computed tomography may also be useful in establishing parietal pleural fibrosis in cases of suspected asbestos-related disease and in distinguishing pleural plaques from peripheral pulmonary nodules.

Ultrasonography

Ultrasonography of the thorax is useful in the evaluation of pleural effusions. Pleural fluid is recognized sonographically as an echo-free space between the proximal echoes from the skin and chest-wall structures and the distal echoes from the lung parenchyma. Volumes of pleural fluid as small as 10 ml can be identified [1]. The width of the echo-free space correlates well with the actual amount of pleural fluid.

If the presence of free fluid cannot be confirmed in decubitus views of the chest, ultrasonography can localize loculated pleural fluid collections. Ultrasonography also locates the optimal point for thoracentesis. This is particularly important when the pleural effusion is very small. Thoracentesis should be performed immediately after ultrasonography, with the patient in the same position as that during the ultrasound examination. Ultrasound also increases the yield of pleural biopsy by identifying focal pleural abnormalities for biopsy [6].

Thoracentesis and Pleural Fluid Analysis

THORACENTESIS

Thoracentesis is almost invariably required to establish the cause of a pleural effusion. A successful thoracentesis depends on selection of a proper site. A common mistake is to insert the needle too low. When the effusion is large, the thoracentesis site can be determined by physical examination. Small or loculated effusions may require ultrasonography for localization.

Thoracenteses are preferentially performed from behind, with the patient sitting upright on the side of a bed, arms crossed, and elbows supported on a raised bedside stand. Only rarely is it necessary to perform a thoracentesis with the patient in a supine or lateral decubitus position.

Premedication is usually not necessary, although some physicians administer atropine to prevent vasovagal reactions. Particularly anxious patients can be given a small dose of a benzodiazepine before the procedure.

The skin is cleansed, and the area is draped. A local anesthetic such as 2% lidocaine is injected first intradermally at the inferior margin of the intercostal space using a 25-gauge needle. The needle is gradually advanced in small increments. After each advance, the plunger of the syringe is pulled back to ensure that a blood vessel has not been entered, and small amounts of anesthetic are injected. When the anesthetizing needle enters the pleural space, a small amount of fluid is aspirated; then the anesthetizing needle is removed. A 22-gauge needle attached to a 20- to 50-ml syringe with a three-way stopcock interposed is used for the thoracentesis. When the pleural space is entered, a Kelly clamp is attached to the needle at the skin surface to hold the needle in place and to prevent inadvertent deeper penetration of the needle into the chest. Some prefer to use a plastic catheter threaded through a needle, which is then withdrawn, to prevent puncture or laceration of the lung during therapeutic thoracentesis.

As little as 5 to 10 ml of pleural fluid may be adequate for diagnostic purposes, but in general, volumes of 50 to 100 ml are needed to perform a full battery of diagnostic tests.

Thoracentesis is generally safe, but complications can occur. The lung can be punctured by the needle, resulting in a pneumothorax. Contamination of the pleural space at the time of thoracentesis may cause an empyema. Laceration of an intercostal artery may produce a hemothorax. Finally, the removal of large amounts of pleural fluid during a therapeutic thoracentesis can result in hypovolemia or reexpansion pulmonary edema caused by very high negative pleural pressures.

TRANSUDATIVE AND EXUDATIVE PLEURAL EFFUSIONS

For diagnostic purposes, pleural effusions are categorized as transudative or exudative (Table 72-2). Transudative pleural effusions result from an imbalance of the Starling forces that govern the movement of fluid into and out of the pleural space. Congestive heart failure, cirrhosis, renal disease, or hypoproteinemia is responsible for the vast majority of transudative effusions. In contrast, exudative effusions result from increases in vascular permeability to protein and fluid or from abnormalities of protein clearance from the pleural space by the lymphatics. Exudative effusions are most commonly caused by pleural space infection, malignancy, immune inflammatory diseases, or pulmonary emboli. As a generalization, transudative pleural effusions are a manifestation of systemic disorders, whereas exudative effusions are an indication of a pathologic process within the respiratory system. A list of diagnostic tests to analyze pleural fluid is shown in Table 72-3.

Transudative and exudative effusions can be distinguished by pleural fluid concentrations and/or pleural fluid to serum ratios of protein and lactic dehydrogenase [23,27]. The criteria for an exudative effusion include (1) pleural fluid lactic dehydrogenase (LDH) greater than 200 IU or greater than two thirds of the laboratory's upper-normal limit for serum LDH, (2) pleural fluid–serum lactic dehydrogenase ratio greater than 0.6, and (3) pleural fluid–serum protein ratio greater than 0.5. If all three criteria are met, the effusion can be classified as an exudate with a sensitivity of 99 percent and a specificity of 98 percent [14].

Other analyses of pleural fluid provide little additional information in distinguishing transudates from exudates. Pleural fluid specific gravity is an index of protein concentration but is clearly less accurate than direct measurements of protein concentration. Cell counts are of some value. Only 15 percent of transudative effusions contain greater than 15,000 red blood cells/mm^3, and only 20 percent of transudates have a white blood cell count greater than 1000 cells/mm^3 [25]. Pleural fluid glucose and amylase levels and pH do not help in distinguishing between transudates and exudates.

A two-stage approach to pleural fluid analysis may be more cost effective [30]. The first stage involves only the measurement of protein and lactate dehydrogenase concentrations. Only those fluids that are clearly exudative are analyzed further for cell counts and chemical constituents. This approach would substantially reduce the cost of pleural fluid analysis by eliminating unnecessary testing of transudative effusions.

PLEURAL FLUID APPEARANCE

A thorough examination of pleural fluid obtained at thoracentesis is critical in establishing the cause of an exudative pleural effusion. It is important to note the color, turbidity, viscosity, and odor of the pleural fluid. Red- or brown-tinged fluid suggests the presence of blood. Turbid fluid is due to large numbers of cells or a high lipid concentration. These can be distinguished by centrifuging the fluid: The supernatant is clear if the turbidity is due to cells but remains cloudy if lipid concentrations are high. Pleural fluid is viscous in the case of mesothelioma because of elevated levels of hyaluronic acid and in longstanding empyemas, probably because of the high content of cellular debris. Empyemas caused by anerobic infections have a strong putrid odor.

GLUCOSE

The pleural fluid glucose concentration should approximately equal that in the serum. A low pleural fluid glucose (<60 mg/dl) or pleural fluid–serum glucose ratio less than 0.5 limits the differential diagnosis of exudative pleural effusions (Table 72-4) to empyema (or complicated parapneumonic effusion), malignancy, rheumatoid disease, systemic lupus erythematosus,

Table 72-2. **Differential diagnosis of pleural effusion**

Transudative pleural effusions	Thromboembolic disease
Cardiovascular disease	Pulmonary embolus*
Congestive heart failure	Pulmonary infarction
Fluid overload	Immune-mediated diseases
Constrictive pericarditis	Rheumatoid disease
Superior vena caval obstruction	Systemic lupus erythematosus
Liver disease	Drug-induced lupus
Cirrhosis	Wegener's granulomatosis
Renal disease	Sarcoidosis*
Nephrotic syndrome	Postcardiac injury syndrome
Peritoneal dialysis	Angioimmunoblastic lymphadenopathy
Acute glomerulonephritis	Sjögren's syndrome
Urinary tract obstruction	Progressive systemic sclerosis
Other causes	Intraabdominal disorders
Myxedema*	Pancreatitis
Pulmonary emboli*	Esophageal perforation
Meigs' syndrome*	Subphrenic abscess
Sarcoidosis*	Intrahepatic abscess
Iatrogenic	Splenic abscess
Exudative pleural effusions	Esophageal variceal sclerotherapy
Infections	After abdominal surgery
Bacterial	Postpartum
Empyema	Drug-induced pleural disease
Parapneumonic effusions	Nitrofurantoin
Tuberculous	Methysergide
Viral	Dantrolene
Fungal	Bromocriptine
Parasitic	Procarbazine
Mycoplasmal	Practolol
Rickettsial	Methotrexate
Neoplasms	Inhalation of inorganic dusts
Direct pleural involvement	Asbestosis
Metastases	Other causes
Direct invasion from surrounding structures	Meigs' syndrome*
Primary pleural malignancy	Yellow nail syndrome
Indirect causes	Uremic pleuritis
Lymphoma	Radiation pleuritis
Ovarian neoplasm (Meigs' syndrome)	Myxedema*
	Spontaneous pneumothorax
	Familial Mediterranean fever
	Trapped lung

*Pleural effusions due to pulmonary emboli, sarcoidosis, myxedema, and Meigs' syndrome can be either transudates or exudates.

esophageal rupture, or tuberculosis [38]. The low glucose concentrations of empyema fluid are thought to be due to increased glucose metabolism by bacteria and leukocytes that exceeds the rate of glucose transport into the pleural space. A pleural fluid glucose level of less than 40 mg/dl has been proposed as an indication for chest tube drainage of parapneumonic effusions [32,33].

A low pleural fluid glucose concentration is not very common in malignant effusions, but when it is present, it has important prognostic implications [36]. The pleural fluid glucose concentration is thought to be reduced by the metabolism of malignant cells. Low-glucose malignant effusions are likely to contain cancer cells, and tumor is commonly identified in biopsy samples of pleura. There is a poor response to pleurodesis, and the overall survival time in these patients is short [36].

In rheumatoid disease involving the pleura, there is a selective block of glucose transfer from the blood to the pleural fluid, and pleural fluid glucose concentrations are characteristically low [9].

Table 72-3. **Diagnostic tests of pleural fluid**

Essential tests
  Total protein
  Lactic dehydrogenase
Tests commonly obtained for initial fluid analysis
  Glucose
  Amylase
  pH
  White blood cell count and differential
  Red blood cell count
  Gram stain
  Cultures (aerobic and anaerobic bacteria, myco-
    bacteria, and fungi)
Tests obtained when clinically indicated
  Cytology
  Countercurrent immunoelectrophoresis
  Complement levels (C3, C4, CH50)
  Antinuclear antibody, lupus erythematosus cells
  Rheumatoid factor
  Lipid studies: cholesterol, triglycerides, lipopro-
    tein, electrophoresis

Table 72-4. **Differential diagnosis of a low pleural fluid glucose level**

Differential diagnosis	Estimated incidence (%)
Empyema or complicated parapneumonic effusion	80–90
Malignant effusion	30–40
Rheumatoid pleuritis	85–90
Lupus pleuritis	20–30
Esophageal rupture	50
Tuberculous pleuritis	20–30

Note: Low pleural fluid glucose level is defined as glucose less than 60 mg/dl or pleural fluid–serum glucose ratio of less than 0.5.
Source: Modified from SA Sahn. Pathogenesis and Clinical Features of Diseases Associated with a Low Pleural Fluid Glucose. In J Chretien, J Bignon, A Hirsch (Eds), *The Pleura in Health and Disease*, Vol 30: *Lung Biology in Health and Disease.* New York: Marcel Dekker, 1985. Pp 267–285.

AMYLASE

Pleural fluid amylase concentrations exceed the normal serum levels in only three diseases: pancreatic disease (pancreatitis or pseudocyst), malignancy, and esophageal rupture [24]. Pleural effusions develop in about 15 percent of patients with pancreatitis, and in most instances, amylase levels are elevated. The pleural fluid amylase level is also elevated in about 10 percent of ma-

lignant pleural effusions not associated with pancreatic disease. High levels of amylase, probably of salivary origin, are found in the pleural fluid soon after esophageal rupture. In essentially all other pleural effusions the amylase level is normal.

CELL COUNTS

Blood-tinged pleural fluid (red blood cell counts between 5000 and 100,000 cells/mm³) is seen in 40 percent of all exudative pleural effusions [25]. Red blood cell counts in this range are of no diagnostic significance. A grossly bloody pleural fluid with greater than 100,000 cells/mm³ or a hematocrit of over 2 percent suggests malignancy, pulmonary embolus, or trauma. A pleural fluid hematocrit greater than half the serum hematocrit indicates a frank hemothorax, and drainage by tube thoracostomy is usually necessary.

A pleural fluid white blood cell count greater than 1000 cells/mm³ is found in up to 20 percent of transudative effusions [27]. A white blood cell count greater than 10,000 cells/mm³ in the pleural fluid can be seen in a variety of exudative effusions. Empyema is suggested by pleural fluid white cell counts of 20,000 to 50,000 cells/mm³ or higher, but other pleural inflammatory processes also can give rise to cell counts in this range in the absence of infection.

The differential white blood cell count is very helpful in establishing the cause of an exudative effusion. A predominant polymorphonuclear leukocytosis in the pleural fluid is indicative of an acute inflammatory process. Greater than 50 percent lymphocytes in the pleural fluid suggests a diagnosis of tuberculosis or malignancy. Pleural fluid eosinophilia (greater than 10 percent) is most commonly caused by air or blood in the pleural space, drug reactions, parasitic infections, or fungal disease [23]. Mesothelial cells are characteristically scant or absent from the pleural fluid of tuberculous effusions, as well as in complicated parapneumonic effusions and other types of fibrinous pleuritis [16]. Activated mesothelial cells may be confused with malignant cells.

pH

The normal pleural fluid pH is usually higher than the blood pH because of active transport of bicarbonate into the pleural space [37]. Transudative pleural effusions always have a pH greater than 7.30 to 7.40. On the other hand, approximately 30 percent of exudative effusions have a pH of less than 7.30. The several causes of pleural

Table 72-5. **Differential diagnosis of a low pleural fluid pH**

Differential diagnosis	Estimated incidence (%)
Empyema (complicated parapneumonic effusion)	100
Malignant effusion	30–40
Rheumatoid pleuritis	100
Esophageal rupture	100
Lupus pleuritis	25–35
Tuberculous pleuritis	10–20
Hemothorax	20
Systemic acidosis	?

Note: Low pH is defined as a pH of less than 7.30.
Sources: Modified from SA Sahn. Pleural Fluid pH in the Normal State and in Diseases Affecting the Pleural Space. In J Chretien, J Bignon, A Hirsch (Eds), *The Pleura in Health and Disease.* New York: Marcel Dekker, 1985. Pp 253–266; and RW Light et al. Diagnostic significance of pleural fluid pH and PCO_2. *Chest* 64:591, 1973.

effusions with pH less than 7.30 [26,37] are listed in Table 72-5. Pleural fluid acidosis in these disorders results from the accumulation of lactic acid produced by anaerobic glycolysis [39]. This leads to increased pleural fluid CO_2 tensions. The diffusion of carbon dioxide out of the pleural space is impaired by pleural inflammation, while in malignant effusions the diffusion of hydrogen ions out of pleural fluid is also slowed. The lowest values of pleural fluid pH (less than 6.0) are seen with esophageal rupture, which permits the extravasation of gastric acid into the pleural space.

The pH of parapneumonic effusions is commonly used as a guideline for chest tube drainage. A pH below 7.0 is indicative of an actual or impending empyema that is likely to require tube drainage. On the other hand, a parapneumonic effusion with a pH of greater than 7.20 is considered unlikely to develop into an empyema. The management of simple parapneumonic effusions with pH values between 7.00 and 7.20 is less clear. In the absence of signs of loculation of empyema, conservative management with monitoring of pleural fluid pH is generally indicated.

CYTOLOGY

The diagnosis of malignancy can be made by cytologic examination of pleural fluid. False-positive results are rare, but atypical mesothelial cells can be confused with cancer cells. The proper handling of specimens is critical. The pleural fluid should be anticoagulated. If analysis is delayed, the fluid should be refrigerated to prevent deterioration of cellular structures. Pleural fluid from an initial thoracentesis is positive for cancer cells in about 50 percent of malignant pleural effusions [25,40]. With two or three repeat thoracenteses, a positive diagnosis can be made by cytologic examination in 70 to 80 percent of malignant effusions [25,40].

Several new techniques may enhance the cytologic evaluation of pleural fluid. Monoclonal antibodies are useful in distinguishing among adenocarcinoma, mesothelioma, and benign mesothelial cells [7,48]. Flow cytometry is helpful in identifying malignant cells by the presence of abnormal numbers of chromosomes [8]. Finally, chromosomal analysis may be useful in establishing the presence of malignancy.

STAINS AND CULTURES

Since the pleural space is normally sterile, the presence of bacteria, mycobacteria, or fungi in pleural fluid is diagnostic of infection. A Gram stain, a Ziehl-Neelsen stain, and cultures for aerobic and anaerobic bacteria, mycobacteria, and fungi should be performed routinely on exudative pleural fluid obtained at diagnostic thoracentesis. Tests for specific antigens (counterimmunoelectrophoresis or latex particle agglutination) may be helpful in providing evidence of certain types of pleural infection when the stains and cultures are negative. Although the results are promptly available, only few bacterial agents may be detected by commercially produced reagents. These include *Streptococcus pneumoniae*, group B streptococci, *Haemophilus influenzae* type B, and *Neisseria meningitidis*.

LIPID ANALYSIS

Several conditions yield a milky or opalescent pleural fluid. A turbid supernatant after centrifugation suggests a chylothorax or pseudochylothorax. Chylous effusions contain high levels of triglycerides. The pleural fluid triglyceride levels are usually greater than 110 mg/dl and more than twice that in the serum [41]. Cholesterol levels in chylothorax vary from less than 50 to more than 200 mg/dl. The presence of chylomicrons on lipoprotein electrophoresis is diagnostic of chylothorax or chylous effusion [41]. Pseudochylous effusions are characterized by low triglyceride levels and the absence of chylomicrons in the pleural fluid. The cholesterol concentration is elevated, and cholesterol crystals are found in the pleural fluid sediment.

IMMUNOLOGIC STUDIES

Collagen-vascular diseases, most commonly systemic lupus erythematosus and rheumatoid arthritis, may be associated with pleuritis and pleural effusions in which pleural fluid complement levels are reduced. This includes total hemolytic complement (CH_{50}), C3, and C4 [2,13,15]. A CH_{50} below 10 units/ml and a C3 to total protein ratio below 0.005 are rarely seen in disorders other than systemic lupus erythematosus and rheumatoid arthritis [2,15]. Elevated levels of immune complexes in the pleural fluid are somewhat less specific for collagen-vascular disease because these are also found in other types of exudative effusions [2,13]. A high rheumatoid factor titer in the pleural fluid is not diagnostically specific; this can be found in parapneumonic as well as malignant effusions [22]. However, in the appropriate clinical context, a pleural fluid rheumatoid factor titer of greater than 1 : 360 strongly supports a diagnosis of rheumatoid pleuritis, whereas a negative rheumatoid factor measurement essentially excludes this diagnosis [23]. Antinuclear antibodies (ANA) are only found in the fluid of lupus pleuritis. Increased ANA titers in pleural fluid may simply reflect the high level in the serum, so that the determination of pleural ANA may not be necessary if serum values are high [2].

Transthoracic Needle Biopsy

A sample of parietal pleura can be obtained by transthoracic needle biopsy to establish the cause of exudative effusions, particularly when tumor or granulomatous disease is suspected. Pleural biopsy is not helpful when the effusion is clearly secondary to pneumonia, pulmonary emboli, pancreatitis, or collagen-vascular disease. An empyema is a contraindication to pleural biopsy because of the risk of abscess formation along the needle track.

For the diagnosis of a suspected malignant effusion, the information obtained from a pleural biopsy complements that from pleural fluid cytology examination, and both tests should be performed. Although pleural biopsies are positive in only 40 to 60 percent of malignant pleural effusions, biopsies may show evidence of malignant disease even when pleural fluid cytology is normal or equivocal [34,40]. The combination of a pleural biopsy and cytologic examination of three separate samples of pleural fluid will yield a positive diagnosis in 85 to 90 percent of malignant effusions [40].

Tuberculosis causing a pleural effusion also can be diagnosed by pleural biopsy. Acid-fast bacilli are rarely seen in the pleural fluid of tuberculous effusions, and even pleural fluid cultures are positive in fewer than 50 percent of patients [12]. On the other hand, a positive diagnosis from cultures of pleural biopsy material and from the histologic demonstration of noncaseating granulomas is made in 60 to 80 percent of cases of pleural tuberculosis [10,44]. A second pleural biopsy will sometimes establish the diagnosis if the first biopsy is negative [10]. Granulomas in a pleural biopsy in conjunction with a positive tuberculin skin test and a pleural fluid lymphocytosis are virtually diagnostic of a tuberculous effusion.

Pleural biopsy is most safely performed in the presence of significant quantities of pleural fluid. It is, however, also possible to biopsy the pleura with a cutting needle even in the absence of pleural fluid. In these circumstances, the risk of lung injury and pneumothorax is increased and the procedure is best avoided.

Thoracoscopy (Pleuroscopy)

Thoracoscopy or pleuroscopy is an alternative to open pleural biopsy in suspected neoplastic disease when a diagnosis cannot be made even after repeated thoracenteses and pleural biopsies [5,29]. This procedure can be carried out under local anesthesia, but general anesthesia is preferable. A small chest incision is made, and a pneumothorax is induced. A rigid scope introduced into the pleural space enables direct visualization and multiple biopsies.

Bronchoscopy

Bronchoscopy with endobronchial or transbronchial lung biopsy is sometimes helpful in establishing the cause of exudative pleural effusions when lung parenchymal abnormalities are evident on the chest roentgenogram. The demonstration of lung masses or infiltrates often requires the removal of most of the pleural fluid by thoracentesis or decubitus views of the chest to displace the fluid. In the absence of roentgenographic parenchymal changes, routine bronchoscopy seldom aids in making a specific diagnosis in the case of pleural effusions [10].

References

1. Adams FV, Galati V. M-mode ultrasonic localization of pleural effusions. *JAMA* 239:1761, 1978.
2. Andrews BS, et al. The role of immune complexes in the pathogenesis of pleural effusions. *Am Rev Respir Dis* 124:115, 1981.
3. Anthonisen NR, Martin RR. Regional lung function in pleural effusion. *Am Rev Respir Dis* 116:201, 1977.
4. Bernaudin JF, Fleury J. Anatomy of the Blood and Lymphatic Circulation of the Pleural Serosa. In J Chretien, J Bignon, A Hirsch (Eds), *The Pleura in Health and Disease*, Vol 30: *Lung Biology in Health and Disease*. New York: Marcel Dekker, 1985. Pp 101–124.
5. Boutin C, et al. Thoracoscopy in malignant pleural effusions. *Am Rev Respir Dis* 124:588, 1981.
6. Chang DB, et al. Ultrasound-guided pleural biopsy with Tru-Cut needle. *Chest* 100:1328, 1991.
7. Croonen AM, et al. Cytology, immunopathology and flow cytometry in the diagnosis of pleural and peritoneal effusion. *Lab Invest* 50:725, 1988.
8. Dewald G, et al. Usefulness of chromosome examination in the diagnosis of malignant effusions. *N Engl J Med* 295:1494, 1976.
9. Dodson WH, Hollingsworth JW. Pleural effusion in rheumatoid arthritis: Impaired transport of glucose. *N Engl J Med* 275:1337, 1966.
10. Feinsilver SH, Barrows AA, Braman SS. Fiberoptic bronchoscopy and pleural effusion of unknown origin. *Chest* 90:516, 1986.
11. Fleischner FG. Atypical arrangement of free pleural effusion. *Radiol Clin North Am* 1:347, 1963.
12. Fraser RG, Paré JAP. *Diagnosis of Diseases of the Chest* (2d ed). Philadelphia: Saunders, 1977.
13. Halla JT, Schrohenloher RE, Volanakis JE. Immune complexes and other laboratory features of pleural effusion. *Ann Intern Med* 92:748, 1980.
14. Health and Policy Committee, American College of Physicians. Diagnostic thoracentesis and pleural biopsy in pleural effusions. *Ann Intern Med* 103:799, 1985.
15. Hunder GG, McDuffie FC, Hepper NGG. Pleural fluid complement in systemic lupus erythematosus and rheumatoid arthritis. *Ann Intern Med* 76:357, 1972.
16. Hurwitz S, Leiman G, Shapiro C. Mesothelial cells in pleural fluid: TB or not TB? *S Afr Med J* 57:937, 1980.
17. Kinasewitz GT, Fishman AP. Influence of alterations in Starling forces on visceral pleural fluid movement. *J Appl Physiol* 51:671, 1981.
18. Krahl VE. Anatomy of the Mammalian Lung. In WO Fenn, H Rahn (Eds), *Handbook of Physiology*, Section 3: *Respiration*, Vol 1. Washington, DC: American Physiologic Society, 1964. Pp 213–284.
19. Leckie WJH, Tothill P. Albumin turnover in pleural effusions. *Clin Sci* 29:339, 1965.
20. Leung AN, Müller NL, Miller RR. CT in differential diagnosis of diffuse pleural disease. *AJR* 154:487, 1990.
21. Levine H, et al. Diagnosis of tuberculous pleurisy by culture of pleural biopsy specimen. *Arch Intern Med* 126:269, 1970.
22. Levine H, et al. Rheumatoid factor in nonrheumatoid pleural effusions. *Ann Intern Med* 69:487, 1968.
23. Light RW. *Pleural Diseases*. Philadelphia: Lea & Febiger, 1983.
24. Light RW, Ball WC. Glucose and amylase in pleural effusions. *JAMA* 225:257, 1973.
25. Light RW, Erozan YS, Ball WC, Jr. Cells in the pleural fluid: Their value in differential diagnosis. *Arch Intern Med* 132:854, 1973.
26. Light RW, et al. Diagnostic significance of pleural fluid pH and PCO_2. *Chest* 64:591, 1973.
27. Light RW, et al. Pleural effusions: The diagnostic separation of transudates and exudates. *Ann Intern Med* 77:507, 1972.
28. Mellins RB, Levine OR, Fishman AP. Effect of systemic and pulmonary venous hypertension on pleural and pericardial fluid accumulation. *J Appl Physiol* 29:564, 1970.
29. Oldenburg FA, Newhouse MT. Thoracoscopy: A safe, accurate diagnostic procedure using the rigid thoracoscope and local anesthesia. *Chest* 75:45, 1979.
30. Peterman TA, Speicher CE. Evaluating pleural effusions: A two-stage laboratory approach. *JAMA* 252:1051, 1984.
31. Petersen JA. Recognition of infrapulmonary pleural effusion. *Radiology* 74:34, 1960.
32. Potts DE, Levin DC, Sahn SA. Pleural fluid pH in parapneumonic effusions. *Chest* 70:328, 1976.
33. Potts DE, Taryle DA, Sahn SA. The glucose-pH relationship in parapneumonic effusions. *Arch Intern Med* 138:1378, 1978.
34. Prakash UBS. Comparison of needle biopsy with cytologic analysis for the evaluation of pleural effusion: Analysis of 414 cases. *Mayo Clin Proc* 60:158, 1985.
35. Renner RR, et al. The apical cap. *Radiology* 110:569, 1974.
36. Sahn SA. Malignant pleural effusions. *Clin Chest Med* 6:113, 1985.
37. Sahn SA. Pleural Fluid pH in the Normal State and in Diseases Affecting the Pleural Space. In J Chretien, J Bignon, A Hirsch (Eds), *The Pleura in Health and Disease*, Vol 30: *Lung Biology in Health and Disease*. New York: Marcel Dekker, 1985. Pp 253–266.
38. Sahn SA. Pathogenesis and Clinical Features of Diseases Associated with a Low Pleural Fluid Glucose. In J Chretien, J Bignon, A Hirsch (Eds), *The Pleura in Health and Disease*, Vol 30: *Lung Biology in Health and Disease*. New York: Marcel Dekker, 1985. Pp 267–285.

39. Sahn SA, Taryle DA, Good JT. Experimental empyema: Time course and pathogenesis of pleural fluid acidosis and low pleural fluid glucose. *Am Rev Respir Dis* 120:355, 1979.

40. Salyer WR, Eggleston JC, Erozan YS. Efficacy of pleural needle biopsy and pleural fluid cytopathology in the diagnosis of malignant neoplasm involving the pleura. *Chest* 67:536, 1975.

41. Staats BA, et al. The lipoprotein profile of chylous and nonchylous pleural effusions. *Mayo Clin Proc* 55:700, 1980.

42. Staub NC, Wiener-Kronish JP, Albertine KH. Transport Through the Pleura: Physiology of Normal Liquid and Solute Exchange in the Pleural Space. In J Chretien, J Bignon, A Hirsch (Eds), *The Pleura in Health and Disease*, Vol 30: *Lung Biology in Health and Disease.* New York: Marcel Dekker, 1985. Pp 169–193.

43. Stewart PB. The rate of formation and lymphatic removal of fluid in pleural effusions. *J Clin Invest* 42:158, 1963.

44. Von Hoff DD, LiVolsi V. Diagnostic reliability of needle biopsy of the parietal pleura. *Am J Clin Pathol* 64:200, 1975.

45. Wang NS. The preformed stomas connecting the pleural cavity and the lymphatics in the parietal pleura. *Am Rev Respir Dis* 111:12, 1975.

46. Wang NS. Anatomy and physiology of the pleural space. *Clin Chest Med* 6:1, 1985.

47. Wang NS. Mesothelial Cells in Situ. In J Chretien, J Bignon, A Hirsch (Eds), *The Pleura in Health and Disease*, Vol 30: *Lung Biology in Health and Disease.* New York: Marcel Dekker, 1985. Pp 23–42.

48. Warnok ML, Stoloff A, Thor A. Differentiation of adenocarcinoma of the lung from mesothelioma: Periodic acid–Schiff, monoclonal antibodies, B72.3, and Leu M1. *Am J Pathol* 133:30, 1988.

49. Weiss W, Boucet KR, Getter WI. Localized interlobar effusion in congestive heart failure. *Ann Intern Med* 38:1177, 1953.

73

Pleural Inflammation and Pleural Effusion

Alfred F. Connors, Jr.   *Murray D. Altose*

Transudative Pleural Effusions

Transudative pleural effusions accumulate as a result of imbalances in the normal relationships between capillary hydrostatic pressure and colloid osmotic pressure. Three basic mechanisms lead to the formation of transudative pleural effusions: (1) systemic venous hypertension, (2) pulmonary venous hypertension, and (3) reduced plasma oncotic pressure. Because the pleural surfaces are not affected, the protein concentration and lactic dehydrogenase levels in the fluid are low. Also, white and red blood cell counts are low, and pleural fluid glucose and amylase levels are close to those in the plasma. Transudates can also result from the direct leakage of fluid from the interstitial space of the lungs [12].

Congestive Heart Failure

Congestive heart failure is one of the most common causes of pleural effusion. Elevations of systemic and pulmonary venous pressure increase the production of pleural fluid by the parietal pleura and reduce reabsorption of fluid by the visceral pleura [57,78]. In addition, high systemic venous pressure impedes lymphatic drainage from the pleural space. The rate of pleural fluid production for a given elevation of systemic venous pressure is about twice that for the same elevation of pulmonary venous pressure [78]. Right ventricular failure from cor pulmonale causes substantial systemic venous hypertension and peripheral edema, but pleural effusions are uncommon. Pleural effusions are also uncommon when left atrial pressure alone is elevated, as in mitral stenosis [17]. On the other hand, pleural effusions regularly develop with biventricular heart failure in the presence of both systemic and

pulmonary venous hypertension [34]. In the presence of hydrostatic pulmonary edema, pleural transudates may arise directly from the interstitial space of the lungs.

Sixty to 70 percent of patients with symptomatic congestive heart failure have pleural effusions [83,84]. Symptoms include dyspnea on exertion, orthopnea, and paroxysmal nocturnal dyspnea. Physical examination reveals jugular venous distension, pulmonary congestion, ventricular gallops, and dependent edema. The chest roentgenogram shows cardiomegaly and, in most cases, bilateral pleural effusions [83,84]. When the pleural effusion of congestive heart failure is unilateral, it is more commonly on the right. Unilateral effusion on the left side of the chest and bilateral effusions of unequal size and without cardiomegaly suggest a diagnosis other than congestive heart failure.

Cirrhosis

Pleural effusions are seen in only about 5 percent of patients with cirrhosis and ascites [63]. Fluid accumulates primarily because of the direct passage of ascitic fluid across the diaphragm either through defects in the diaphragm [63] or via transdiaphragmatic lymphatic channels [53]. Hypoproteinemia in cirrhosis also may contribute to pleural fluid accumulation, but this is not an important factor.

Pleural effusions rarely, if ever, develop from cirrhosis in the absence of ascites. Usually, the pleural effusions of cirrhosis are found on the right side only, but in about a third of cases the fluid accumulates only on the left or bilaterally [53,63]. The effusions can be large with high intrapleural pressures. Pleural effusions in association with ascites also can be caused by pancreatitis, neoplastic disease, and peritonitis. These effusions, however, are exudative rather than transudative.

Although there is no specific treatment for pleural effusion due to cirrhosis, the volume of fluid can be reduced by salt restriction and by diuresis. Surgical procedures to shunt peritoneal fluid to the systemic venous system also may be helpful. Removal of pleural fluid by repeated thoracentesis or by tube drainage is not recommended because this may cause dangerous reductions in intravascular fluid volume and serum protein levels. Furthermore, pleural fluid tends to reaccumulate rapidly.

In a few reported cases, chemical pleurodesis has been effective in controlling pleural effusions due to cirrhosis when large effusions cause respiratory embarrassment [30]. Extreme care must be taken in monitoring hemodynamic status during the chest tube drainage preliminary to pleurodesis.

Nephrotic Syndrome

Pleural effusions develop in about 20 percent of patients with nephrotic syndrome [16]. This results from reductions in intravascular oncotic pressure that allow an increased movement of fluid out of pleural capillaries and into the pleural space. The pleural effusions are usually bilateral and are commonly infrapulmonary in location [34]. The effusions usually resolve when the underlying disorder is corrected. Treatment is aimed at increasing plasma protein concentration and minimizing the renal loss of protein. Therapeutic thoracentesis is ineffective in controlling the effusions and will worsen the hypoproteinemia. Large effusions that cause disabling shortness of breath can be controlled by chemical pleurodesis.

In nephrotic syndrome secondary to renal vein thrombosis, pulmonary embolism is responsible for about 20 percent of pleural effusions [72]. Therefore, ventilation-perfusion lung scanning should be performed in all patients with pleural effusions complicating nephrotic syndrome. When lung scanning does not provide a definitive diagnosis, the appropriate tests should be carried out to exclude deep venous thrombosis.

Other Renal Diseases

PERITONEAL DIALYSIS
Pleural effusions are regularly found in patients undergoing peritoneal dialysis. The mechanisms are similar to those responsible for pleural effusions in association with cirrhosis and ascites [88]. Within several hours of starting dialysis, symptoms of dyspnea develop. The pleural fluid, which has the same composition as the dialysis fluid, tends to resolve when dialysis is stopped, but at times prolonged drainage via the peritoneal catheter is required [88]. No additional therapy is usually necessary. Severe respiratory distress can be alleviated with pleural fluid removal by thoracentesis.

ACUTE GLOMERULONEPHRITIS
Acute glomerulonephritis in children is associated with pleural effusions in about half the cases [59]. The effusions are usually transudative, and they result from fluid overload and increased systemic venous pressure.

URINARY TRACT OBSTRUCTION
Urinary tract obstruction is a rare cause of pleural effusions. A *urinothorax* can result from hydronephrosis when urine extravasates into the retroperitoneal space and then dissects into the pleural space [98].

Other Causes of Transudative Effusions

MYXEDEMA
The pleural effusions of myxedema are transudative and generally occur in association with pericardial effusions [96]. The effusions resolve after thyroid hormone replacement therapy.

PULMONARY EMBOLISM
Pleural effusions due to pulmonary embolism are transudative about 25 percent of the time [13]. Transudative effusions seem to result from the systemic venous hypertension of right ventricular failure. When no obvious cause of a transudative effusion is apparent, pulmonary embolism should be considered.

IATROGENIC TRANSUDATIVE PLEURAL EFFUSIONS
Misplacement of a central venous catheter into the pleural space or mediastinum can result in the infusion of intravenous fluids into the pleural space. The effusions are usually unilateral but may be bilateral when fluid is mistakenly infused into the mediastinum. This occurrence is suggested by the rapid accumulation of pleural fluid following placement of a central venous line and is confirmed by demonstrating pleural fluid glu-

cose and protein concentrations equal to those of the infused fluid.

OTHERS

Meigs' syndrome [24,77] and pleural disease due to sarcoidosis are usually associated with an exudative effusion and are discussed in detail below. Both can rarely present as transudative effusions.

The superior vena cava syndrome is another rare cause of a transudative right pleural effusion. Superior vena cava obstruction, usually caused by malignancy, raises systemic venous pressure and increases filtration from parietal pleural capillaries [39].

Exudative Pleural Effusions

Exudative pleural effusions occur as the result of (1) increased permeability of the pleural capillaries to protein, (2) reduced reabsorption of fluid by the visceral pleura, (3) impaired removal of protein and fluid by the pleural lymphatics, and (4) abnormally subatmospheric pleural pressures due to local or generalized reduction of lung compliance. Exudative effusions are most commonly associated with inflammatory processes, infections, and neoplastic involvement.

Parapneumonic Effusions

BACTERIAL INFECTIONS

About half of all bacterial pneumonias are associated with parapneumonic pleural effusions, which cause greater morbidity and mortality than pneumonia alone. Exudative parapneumonic effusions usually contain no bacteria and resolve promptly with treatment of the underlying pulmonary infection. Some so-called complicated parapneumonic effusions persist, become loculated, and undergo organization and fibrosis. An empyema may result when the pleural fluid becomes infected and large numbers of polymorphonuclear leukocytes accumulate.

Pathogenesis. There are three stages in the development of a parapneumonic pleural effusion [2]. The initial exudative stage is a result of inflammation of the pleura over an area of parenchymal infection. The inflamed pleura leaks fluid and protein, and inflammatory cells are attracted to the pleural space. Most commonly, the process is arrested at this point. If appropriate antibiotic treatment is not given, or if host defenses are impaired, a subsequent fibropurulent stage may develop. Bacteria invade the pleural space, and large numbers of white blood cells accumulate. Fibrin is deposited over the visceral and parietal pleural surfaces, and fluid loculation can result. The pH and glucose levels fall, and lactic dehydrogenase increases. Finally, in the stage of organization, a thick, fibrous peel encases the visceral pleura of the lung, restricting lung expansion.

Bacteriology. The incidence of parapneumonic effusions and the frequency of bacterial contamination of pleural fluid depend on the specific bacterial type of pneumonia. The causes of bacterial empyema have changed over the past several decades. Thirty to 40 years ago, empyema most commonly followed streptococcal pneumonia [32]. Later, staphylococcal pneumonia was most likely to produce complicated parapneumonic effusions [97,105]. In recent years, empyemas are more likely to occur with gram-negative or anaerobic pulmonary infections [7,102]. The bacteria most commonly responsible for parapneumonic effusions and empyemas are listed in Table 73-1.

Clinical Features. Aerobic bacterial pneumonia generally presents as an acute illness with fever, chest pain, sputum production, and leukocytosis. There are no specific symptoms that signal the

Table 73-1. **Incidence of pleural effusions and empyema associated with bacterial pneumonia in adults**

Bacteria causing pneumonia	Percent effusions	Percent positive cultures
Anaerobic bacteria	35	90
Aerobic bacteria		
Gram positive		
Streptococcus pneumoniae	40–60	5
Staphylococcus aureus	40	20
Streptococcus pyogenes	75	35
Gram negative		
Escherichia coli	40	80
Pseudomonas species	50	40
Klebsiella pneumoniae	20	20
Haemophilus influenzae	45	20
Proteus species	20	50

Sources: Modified from RW Light. *Pleural Diseases.* Philadelphia: Lea & Febiger, 1983; and RW Light. Parapneumonic effusions and empyema. *Clin Chest Med* 6:55, 1985.

presence of pleural effusion in these patients. However, the persistence of fever for more than 48 hours after starting antibiotic therapy does suggest the presence of a complicated parapneumonic effusion. Persistent fever is not always a reliable sign and fever may be altogether absent with acute aerobic pneumonia and empyema in severely debilitated or immunocompromised patients.

Anaerobic parapneumonic effusions usually produce a subacute illness [7]. Fever, weight loss, and anemia are common. Most patients are predisposed to aspiration as a result of alcoholism, seizure disorder, or a loss of consciousness. Significant periodontal disease is often observed.

Empyemas due to aerobic bacteria may follow thoracic surgical procedures, particularly pneumonectomy. They tend to develop within 1 to 4 weeks of surgery and often present as an unexplained febrile illness. Other findings that suggest an empyema include purulent drainage from the surgical incision site and a new air-fluid level in a previously airless pleural space.

Diagnosis. Parapneumonic pleural effusions are readily detected by physical examination and on chest roentgenogram. Decubitus views are sometimes required to verify the presence of free pleural fluid and to allow better visualization of the lung parenchyma. Preexisting pleural adhesions can cause the loculation of parapneumonic effusions, which can be localized by ultrasonography.

Small parapneumonic effusions, measuring less than 10 mm in thickness on a lateral decubitus radiograph of the chest, are not clinically significant and resolve with antibiotic therapy alone. Larger effusions should be sampled by thoracentesis and the fluid carefully analyzed. In the event of multiple loculations, it is important that fluid be sampled from each loculation, since only one may contain pus and bacteria [7].

The pleural fluid may be clear and straw colored or grossly purulent. A putrid odor is a definite sign of an anaerobic infection but only 60 percent of anaerobic empyemas are malodorous [5]. Gross pus and/or bacteria in the pleural space demonstrated by culture or Gram stain, or both, are indicative of a frank empyema. The finding of a pleural fluid pH of less than 7.0 and a glucose concentration of less than 40 mg/dl strongly suggests a complicated parapneumonic effusion in a fibropurulent stage [70,82,90].

Management. The first step in the management of a parapneumonic effusion is the appropriate antibiotic therapy of the underlying pneumonia. However, antibiotic dosage does not usually need to be adjusted when a parapneumonic effusion is present.

The decision as to whether a parapneumonic pleural effusion requires tube drainage is based on the result of pleural fluid analysis. In general, tube thoracostomy for drainage is instituted in cases of complicated parapneumonic effusions and frank empyemas. The indications for tube thoracostomy are summarized in Table 73-2, and an algorithm for the management of parapneumonic effusions is shown in Figure 73-1.

Proper drainage of complicated parapneumonic effusions and empyemas must be instituted without delay. This can usually be achieved by closed-tube drainage. A large-bore chest tube is inserted at the most dependent point of the effusion and connected to an underwater seal to which negative pressure is applied. Drainage of large, nonpurulent loculated parapneumonic effusions may be aided by the intrapleural instillation of streptokinase. This could reduce the need for multiple chest tubes or surgical drainage [44].

Since, particularly with anaerobic pleural infections and multiple loculated pleural effusions, closed chest tube drainage may not be sufficient, open drainage is required. Segments of one or more ribs overlying the dependent portion of an

Table 73-2. **Indications for tube thoracostomy in parapneumonic effusions**

Complicated parapneumonic effusion (tube thoracostomy should be performed)
  Gross pus in the pleural space
  Organisms present on Gram stain or pleural fluid culture
  Pleural fluid pH less than 7.0
  Pleural fluid glucose less than 40 mg/dl

Possible complicated parapneumonic effusion (tube thoracostomy may be indicated; careful observation with repeat thoracentesis in 8 to 12 hours is indicated)
  Pleural fluid pH between 7.0 and 7.2
  Pleural fluid lactic dehydrogenase over 1000 IU/liter

Complicated parapneumonic effusion unlikely (observe; effusion will resolve with therapy of the pneumonia)
  Pleural fluid pH greater than 7.2
  Pleural fluid glucose greater than 40

Sources: Modified from Light [65], Potts et al. [82], and Sahn [90].

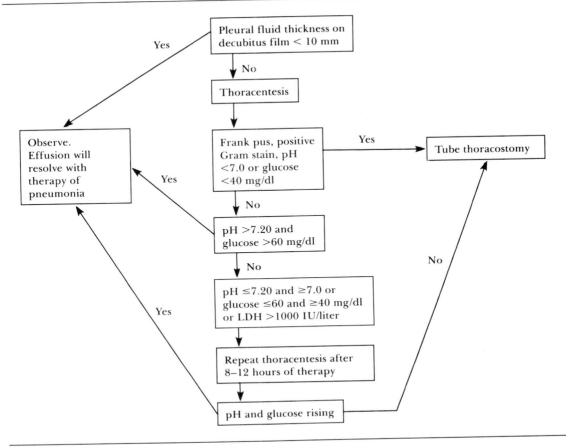

Fig. 73-1. An algorithm demonstrating the approach to a patient with pneumonia and pleural effusion. LDH = lactic dehydrogenase.

empyema are resected. Then, either large-bore tubes are inserted into the pleural space or, alternatively, an open (Eloesser) flap is constructed whereby muscle and skin are sewn in to line the tract between the chest surface and the pleural space. In both instances, the pleural space is open directly to the atmosphere, but extensive pleural adhesion bordering the empyema prevents the lung from collapsing.

Another approach to the treatment of chronic loculated empyemas is decortication. Through a full thoracotomy incision, all fibrin and pus are evacuated and fibrous tissue is removed from the pleural space. This is a major thoracic surgical procedure and should not be considered in severely ill and debilitated patients. On the other hand, decortication avoids long-term drainage through an open chest wound.

TUBERCULOUS INFECTIONS

Pleural effusion in tuberculosis usually occurs during the primary infection. It results from the rupture of a small subpleural caseous focus and release of bacilli into the pleural space [10]. Tuberculoprotein in the pleural space initiates a delayed hypersensitivity reaction, as evidenced by the presence of activated T lymphocytes in the pleural fluid [28]. Increased pleural capillary permeability to protein and decreased clearance of protein through pleural lymphatic pores cause the accumulation of pleural fluid, which usually contains relatively few tubercle bacilli. The occasional finding of a negative tuberculin skin test may be associated with compartmentalization of sensitized lymphocytes in the pleural fluid or with high levels of suppressor T cells in the blood [28]. The skin test will usually convert to positive within 6 to 8 weeks.

Tuberculous pleuritis is an acute or subacute

disease that presents with symptoms of nonproductive cough, fever, and pleuritic chest pain of 1 to 4 weeks' duration [10]. Some patients present with more chronic symptoms of low-grade fever, cough, and weight loss. Tuberculous effusions are usually unilateral and of small to moderate size [10]. In up to one half of cases, tuberculous pleural effusions are accompanied by parenchymal infiltrates. The roentgenographic appearances may include lower-lobe infiltrates and intrathoracic lymphadenopathy. Cavitary infiltrates in the upper lobes or superior segments of the lower lobes, typical of reactivation tuberculosis, may also be found [95]. In the majority of cases, the diagnosis of a tuberculous effusion largely depends on identifying tubercle bacilli in the pleural fluid or pleural biopsy, or on demonstrating pleural noncaseating granulomas in conjunction with a positive tuberculin skin test. The combination of culture and histologic examination of the pleura is generally the most sensitive diagnostic test for pleural tuberculosis. When the pleural effusion is accompanied by parenchymal infiltrates, sputum specimens are likely to be culture positive.

There are several important characteristics of the pleural fluid in tuberculous pleuritis. In the earliest phases, the white blood cells in the pleural fluid are predominantly polymorphonuclear leukocytes [62]. With time, however, lymphocytes in the pleural fluid predominate. Tuberculous effusions rarely contain mesothelial cells [50]. Greater than 5 percent mesothelial cells in pleural fluid is suggestive evidence against the diagnosis of tuberculosis. Similarly, greater than 10 percent eosinophils is rarely seen in untreated and uncomplicated tuberculous effusions [65]. A low glucose concentration is suggestive of tuberculosis but is not specific or diagnostic, since the glucose concentration of pleural fluid in a tuberculous effusion is commonly no lower than in a malignant effusion. Adenosine deaminase levels in pleural fluid are elevated in tuberculosis pleural effusions and may be a useful diagnostic marker [5]. Tubercle bacilli in pleural fluid are usually not seen on Ziehl-Neelsen stains, and pleural fluid cultures for mycobacteria are positive in only 25 percent of patients with tuberculous effusions [10].

Cultures for mycobacteria and histologic examination for granulomas of tissue obtained at pleural biopsy are most useful in making the diagnosis of tuberculous pleuritis. Often, two or three attempts at pleural biopsy are required to establish the diagnosis [93].

When untreated, tuberculous effusions generally resolve within a month or two, but more than half the patients will develop active tuberculosis within a decade [86]. This can be prevented and the symptoms relieved by appropriate drug therapy. Corticosteroid therapy speeds the resolution of the fever and pleural effusion and may reduce the amount of residual pleural thickening [100]. Even so, approximately one half of patients with pleural tuberculosis will be left with residual pleural thickening after antituberculosis drug treatment is completed [6].

Tuberculous effusions also may accompany disseminated or miliary disease or present as an empyema due to rupture of a caseous lesion or lung cavity. In the past, pleural effusion and empyema occurred as a complication of therapeutic pneumothorax.

VIRAL INFECTIONS

Viral infections are a common cause of exudative pleural effusions. Pleural effusions accompany infections by adenovirus, respiratory syncytial virus, influenza, measles, cytomegalovirus, and herpes simplex [65]. Five percent of patients with infectious mononucleosis [60] and as many as 70 percent of patients with infectious hepatitis [54] have pleural effusions. Pleural effusions due to viral disease are usually small. On occasion, there may be little evidence of an underlying pneumonia because the extent of consolidation is small or the parenchymal infiltration is obscured by the pleural effusion. The effusions are exudative, with predominantly mononuclear cells. A definite diagnosis is made by culturing the organism from sputum or pleural fluid or by demonstrating a significant rise in specific antibody titers in the blood. Pleural effusions secondary to viral infections are usually self-limited.

FUNGAL INFECTIONS

A variety of fungal diseases may cause pleural effusions. Pleural aspergillosis, for example, can be a very late complication of extensive tuberculosis treated with artificial pneumothorax [47]. It may occur following thoracic surgery for lung resection, when it is almost always associated with a bronchopleural fistula [45]. Rarely, immunosuppressed patients with disseminated systemic aspergillosis will develop pleural involvement [45]. The diagnosis is best made by identifying the organism in the pleural fluid. Precipitin tests for antibodies against *Aspergillus* are nonspecific. Optimal therapy includes the systemic administration of amphotericin B followed by surgical excision of the involved pleura and resection of the underlying diseased lung [45,47]. In debilitated patients who cannot undergo extensive chest surgery, open or closed drainage procedures should be performed with irrigation of the pleural space with amphotericin B.

Neither histoplasmosis [20,94] nor blastomycosis [58] commonly produces pleural effusion; lung parenchymal involvement predominates. Pleural effusions, when present, are exudative, with high lymphocyte counts, and they may contain significant numbers of eosinophils. Diagnosis may be made by identifying organisms on pleural fluid stains and cultures and by finding granulomas in tissue obtained by pleural biopsy [58]. Serologic tests are helpful in the diagnosis of histoplasmosis but presently are not available for the diagnosis of blastomycosis. Pleural effusions secondary to histoplasmosis generally do not require specific antimicrobial therapy [94].

Extension of a subpleural nodule into the pleural space is responsible for pleural cryptococcosis [106]. Usually, the pleural involvement is unilateral and there is clear radiographic evidence of underlying parenchymal abnormalities. The exudative pleural fluid is predominantly lymphocytic and may contain up to 15 percent eosinophils. Pleural fluid cultures are regularly positive for *Cryptococcus*, but histologic examination of lung tissue or pleura may be required for diagnosis. The detection of cryptococcal antigens in blood or cerebrospinal fluid is important in diagnosis and in shaping treatment. Antimicrobial therapy is necessary in debilitated and immunocompromised patients.

Primary coccidioidomycosis commonly causes pleuritic chest pain, but unilateral pleural effusions, often without radiographic evidence of parenchymal infiltrates, are seen in only 10 percent of symptomatic patients [27]. The effusions are sometimes large, filling over half of the hemithorax [73]. The exudative effusion is predominantly lymphocytic. Whereas blood eosinophilia is common, there are generally few eosinophils in the pleural fluid. The diagnosis is made on the basis of pleural fluid cultures, cultures and histologic examination of pleural biopsy specimens, skin tests, and serologic studies [73]. Treatment is not required unless there is evidence of dissemination. The rupture of a coccidioidal cavity into the pleural space produces a bronchopleural fistula and a hydropneumothorax [27]. Immediate chest tube drainage and systemic treatment with amphotericin B are required.

ACTINOMYCOSIS AND NOCARDIOSIS

The pleural disease produced by these bacteria resembles that associated with mycobacterial or fungal infections. Pleural effusions and pleural thickening are present in most cases of pulmonary actinomycosis [33]. Symptoms include chronic cough, weight loss, fever, and hemoptysis [37]. The typical chest radiographic findings are a localized pulmonary lesion with chest-wall involvement, pleural thickening, and pleural effusion. The lung lesion has the appearance of a lung mass with surrounding infiltrate. Cavitation is often present. Chest-wall abscesses and sinus tracts, although uncommon, are characteristic of the disease [33]. The diagnosis is made by anaerobic culture of pleural fluid, sinus drainage, or sputum and by biopsy of draining sinus walls. Gram staining of these fluids reveals "sulfur granules," 1- to 2-mm masses of filamentous organisms. Pleural fluid can range from a serous exudate to a grossly purulent empyema. Penicillin is the drug of choice. Prolonged therapy at high doses is necessary for cure. Serous effusions usually resolve with therapy, but if the pleural fluid is purulent, chest tube drainage is required.

Infections with *Nocardia asteroides* most commonly occur in immunocompromised patients [35] or in patients with chronic pulmonary diseases such as alveolar proteinosis, bronchiectasis, or sarcoidosis [80]. Pleural effusions are seen in 25 percent of patients with pulmonary nocardiosis and can range from a serous exudate to frank pus. The organism is easily seen in Gram stain or modified acid-fast stain of the pleural fluid, sputum, or lung biopsy. The treatment consists of prolonged sulfonamide therapy and chest tube drainage of empyemas.

PARASITIC INFECTIONS

Pleural effusions are seen in approximately a third of patients with liver disease due to *Entamoeba histolytica* [51]. They are generally right sided and often very large. Serous effusions result primarily from subphrenic inflammation. Pleural fluid with the appearance of "anchovy paste" is caused by the rupture of a hepatic cyst into the pleural space [85]. Patients often present with rapidly progressive respiratory distress, sepsis, and shock. Occasionally, the clinical course is subacute. The diagnosis of transdiaphragmatic rupture of an amebic abscess suggested by the characteristic appearance of the pleural fluid may be confirmed by serologic tests for amebiasis. Patients respond well to chest drainage and specific antiamebic therapy.

Pleural involvement occurs rarely with infections due to *Echinococcus granulosus, Pneumocystis carinii,* and *Paragonimus westermani.*

MYCOPLASMA AND RICKETTSIAL INFECTIONS

Pneumonitis due to *Mycoplasma pneumoniae* is associated with pleural effusion in 20 percent of cases [31]. Pleural effusions are generally small in size. The diagnosis is made serologically by the presence of cold agglutinins and a fourfold increase in specific antibody titers.

Q fever due to *Coxiella burnetii* is a rickettsial disease that causes small pleural effusions in about a third of cases [52]. It is seen in farmers and stockyard workers exposed to infected livestock. The diagnosis is usually made by observing a fourfold rise in specific antibody titers. Tetracycline or chloramphenicol is the treatment of choice.

Malignant Effusions

The spread of cancer to the pleura or to mediastinal lymph nodes is the most common cause of exudative pleural effusions. Three quarters of all malignant pleural effusions are caused by bronchogenic carcinoma, breast cancer, and lymphoma.

Pleural metastases increase the permeability of pleural surfaces to allow a greater influx of protein. However, the primary mechanism for fluid accumulation is probably impaired lymphatic drainage of the pleural space. Abnormal lymphatic drainage is the result of either direct involvement of the visceral and parietal pleural lymphatics with tumor or mediastinal lymph node involvement.

Malignant pleural effusions commonly accompany carcinoma of the lung and are seen in over half the patients with disseminated lung cancer. Nearly half the patients with disseminated breast carcinoma also develop pleural effusions, usually in association with lymphangitic spread of the tumor. Another common cause of malignant pleural effusions is lymphoma, Hodgkin's disease, or leukemia with involvement of hilar and mediastinal lymph nodes. The spread of many other tumors, including ovarian carcinoma, stomach cancer, and some sarcomas, also results in pleural effusions. In about 5 percent of malignant pleural effusions, a primary site is not identified.

The prognosis in patients with malignant pleural effusion is very poor. The mean survival is only about 1 year, but it is considerably shorter when the pleural fluid glucose level and pH are low.

Not all pleural effusions in patients with malignant disease represent involvement of the pleura or mediastinal lymph nodes. With lobar atelectasis consequent to bronchial obstruction from a bronchogenic carcinoma, the pleural pressure becomes more negative. The resulting alteration in the Starling balance promotes the accumulation of pleural fluid. Hypoproteinemia due to malnutrition or liver dysfunction from metastases and pulmonary embolism are some of the other factors that may be responsible for pleural effusion associated with cancer. Finally, pleural effusions can result from the effects of cancer treatment. Radiation therapy may lead to pleural effusions consequent to impaired mediastinal lymphatic drainage. Also, chemotherapeutic agents such as methotrexate and cyclophosphamide can cause pleuritis and effusions.

CLINICAL FEATURES

Common symptoms of malignant pleural effusions are dyspnea and dull, aching chest pain [18]. The effusions are generally large in size. Massive effusions occupying the entire hemithorax strongly suggest malignancy [74]. Evidence of underlying lung cancer is often seen in chest roentgenogram, but it may be obscured by the pleural effusion. There also may be enlargement of hilar or mediastinal lymph nodes in lymphoma or leukemia. However, the lung parenchyma and mediastinum are often normal in metastatic pleural disease from extrathoracic tumors.

Malignant effusions are exudates. All have elevated lactic dehydrogenase levels, but only 80 percent of malignant effusions have pleural fluid–serum protein ratios of greater than 0.5 [71]. The pleural fluid may be bloody or blood tinged. Malignancy is the most common cause of a pleural fluid red cell count greater than 100,000 cells/mm^3 [69]. The white blood cell count ranges from 1000 to 10,000 cells/mm^3, usually with a predominance of lymphocytes. Fifteen percent of malignant effusions have a glucose concentration less than 60 mg/dl and/or a pH less than 7.2 [38,89]. These findings suggest extensive pleural involvement, and pleural fluid cytology and pleural biopsies are usually positive for malignancy.

DIAGNOSIS

The diagnosis of a malignant pleural effusion requires fluid sampling by thoracentesis and often a pleural biopsy. Three separate pleural fluid specimens will yield a positive diagnosis by cytologic examination in 70 to 80 percent of patients [69,92]. The addition of a transthoracic pleural needle biopsy will increase the diagnostic yield to 85 to 90 percent [92]. Thereafter, thoracoscopy is useful in establishing the diagnosis in patients in whom pleural malignancy is strongly suspected, and when repeated thoracenteses and pleural biopsies do not provide a definite diagnosis. Thoracoscopy allows inspection of approximately 75 percent of the visceral pleural surface as well as the parietal pleural surface. The diagnostic accuracy of thoracoscopy is over 90 percent and major complications, such as hemothorax, empyema, and arrhythmia, are less than 3 percent [81].

TREATMENT

The presence of a pleural effusion in a patient with bronchogenic carcinoma does not completely exclude the possibility of a curative resection of the tumor, since pleural effusions need not be the result of malignant involvement of the pleura or mediastinum [23]. When there is no cytologic or histologic evidence of pleural involvement with tumors and no other signs of metastases, a mediastinoscopy followed by an exploratory thoracotomy should be considered. Occasionally, these patients can be cured by surgical resection [23].

Systemic chemotherapy is helpful in the palliation of pleural effusions caused by the spread of carcinoma of the lung, breast carcinoma, and lymphoma. When systemic chemotherapy is not effective, mediastinal radiation can be of benefit in managing chylothorax caused by tumor infiltration of the thoracic duct.

When malignant pleural effusions become sufficiently large, disabling impairment in ventilatory function can result. Patients may suffer from severe dyspnea and may be unable to carry out even simple tasks of daily living. When other specific therapies have failed, these adverse effects can be ameliorated in some instances by chemical pleurodesis. Before undertaking pleurodesis, it is important to ascertain that removal of pleural fluid does indeed relieve symptoms and improve ventilatory function and gas exchange. Also, pleurodesis may not be necessary if pleural fluid reaccumulates very slowly after removal. Such patients are best managed by repeated thoracentesis. An important prerequisite for successful pleurodesis is the ability of the lung to reexpand after removal of pleural fluid so that symphysis between visceral and parietal surfaces can take place. Lung expansion will not occur if

there is extensive atelectasis beyond a major bronchus obstructed with tumor or if the lung is trapped because of visceral pleural or marked parenchymal involvement with tumor. An algorithm for the management of malignant effusions is presented in Figure 73-2.

The first step in pleurodesis is a tube thoracotomy to drain all pleural fluid. Once the lung is fully expanded and the pleural surfaces are in contact, a sclerosing agent is instilled through the chest tube. Chemical pleuritis leading to pleurodesis can be achieved by a variety of agents, including nitrogen mustard, radioisotopes, quinacrine, talc, and bleomycin. Tetracycline is preferred by many. It is effective, easy to administer, and produces few side effects [8]. However, injectable tetracycline hydrochloride for pleurodesis is no longer being manufactured. In its place some are using doxycycline [76]. Following instillation of the sclerosing agent, the chest tube is clamped and the patient is systematically repositioned to allow contact of the agent with all pleural surfaces. Thereafter, chest tube drainage with suction is reinstated for at least 24 hours or until the volume of tube drainage falls below 150 ml per day.

Pulmonary Embolism

Pulmonary embolism is a commonly overlooked cause of pleural effusions. Pleural effusions associated with pulmonary embolism are produced in two different ways. Pulmonary hypertension resulting from multiple pulmonary emboli may lead to right-sided heart failure and elevated systemic venous pressure. This in turn causes increased formation of fluid, resulting in a transudative effusion [78]. About 25 percent of pleural effusions due to pulmonary embolism are transudative [13]. A more common mechanism is visceral pleural ischemia consequent to occlusion of the pulmonary artery. The increased permeability of the capillaries in the ischemic pleura leads to the accumulation of fluid and protein in the pleural space.

About half the patients with pulmonary embolism have pleural effusions. These effusions produce no distinguishing symptoms. When chest pain is present, it is on the side of the effusion, which is usually small and unilateral [14].

The findings in the pleural fluid of patients with pulmonary embolism are variable and nonspecific. The fluid may be either exudative or transudative. The fluid is often blood tinged, but the red blood cell count can be less than 10,000

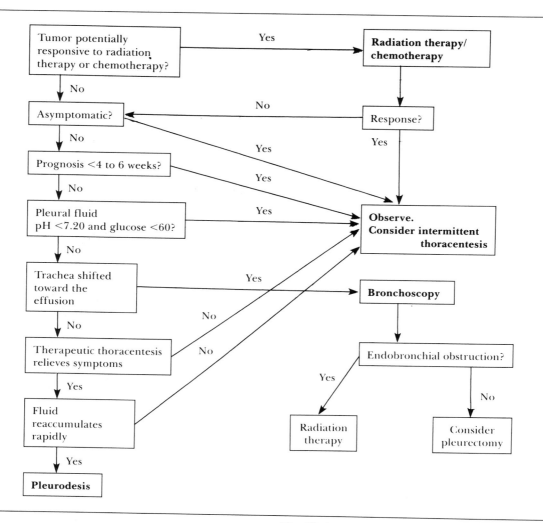

Fig. 73-2. An algorithm demonstrating the evaluation and therapy of a patient with malignant pleural effusion.

cells/mm³ in up to a third of patients [13]. The white blood cell count varies from 100 to as high as 50,000 cells/mm³. There is usually a predominance of polymorphonuclear lymphocytes, and there may be increased numbers of eosinophils.

Pulmonary embolism should be considered in all cases of pleural effusion. When the cause of an effusion is not apparent after a careful clinical evaluation, including radiographic examination and diagnostic thoracentesis, then a search for deep vein thrombosis or pulmonary embolism employing impedance plethysmography, venography, or ventilation-perfusion scanning should be initiated.

A bloody pleural effusion is not a contraindication to anticoagulant therapy. However, if the effusion increases in size after anticoagulant therapy and the hematocrit of the pleural fluid rises, anticoagulation should be discontinued.

Collagen-Vascular Diseases

Rheumatoid arthritis and systemic lupus erythematosus (SLE) are the two collagen-vascular diseases most likely to cause pleuritis and pleural effusions. Pleuritic chest pain is a symptom in one quarter of patients with rheumatoid disease, but frank pleural effusions are found in only about 5 percent [103]. Pleural involvement is most commonly seen in middle-aged men with a long history of moderate to severe arthritis, subcutaneous nodules, and high rheumatoid factor titers [103,104]. Most commonly, pleural disease develops after the onset of joint symptoms. Rarely, pleurisy is the first sign of rheumatoid disease. On occasion, pleural effusions are found on physical examination or chest roentgenogram in the absence of symptoms of pleuritis. The pleural effusions are unilateral and are slightly more common on the right side [104]. They are small to moderate in size. There is coexisting rheumatoid lung disease in a third of patients.

Rheumatoid pleural effusions vary from clear straw colored to turbid. The white blood cell count can be as high as 20,000 cells/mm³ [91]. In acute, active pleuritis, polymorphonuclear leukocytes predominate, but in chronic effusions, the majority of cells are lymphocytes. Typically, the glucose levels and pH are low, and the lactic dehydrogenase level is high. Pleural fluid CH50, C3, and C4 levels are low, and pleural fluid rheumatoid factor is usually greater than 1 : 320 [41]. A low pleural fluid glucose concentration is characteristic of rheumatoid pleuritis. The pleural fluid glucose level is less than 50 mg/dl in 80 percent of patients with rheumatoid pleuritis and below 30 mg/dl in about two thirds. This is due to a block of glucose transport from the blood into the pleural space [25] and to increased glucose metabolism consequent to pleural inflammation [4,91]. Glucose metabolism increases the production of carbon dioxide and lactic acid so that the low pleural fluid glucose concentration is associated with low pleural fluid pH levels. Some rheumatoid pleural effusions contain cholesterol crystals or high levels of cholesterol. Pleural biopsies generally show only chronic inflammation or fibrosis. Rheumatoid nodules are rarely found on pleural biopsies.

Rheumatoid pleural effusions often resolve slowly over weeks to months. The first line of treatment is nonsteroidal anti-inflammatory drugs such as aspirin or ibuprofen. This results in symptomatic relief and control of pleural fluid volume in the majority of patients. If, however, the pleural effusion persists, a trial of corticosteroid therapy is recommended. Occasionally, severe pleural fibrosis develops that necessitates decortication.

Pleuritis is a feature of SLE in about three quarters of patients and is occasionally the presenting manifestation [43]. Pleural involvement is heralded by pleuritic chest pain. More than half the patients complain of dyspnea or cough [40]. Fever and a pleural friction rub are regular findings. Pleural effusions are also common in drug-induced SLE with antinuclear antibodies [40]. The most important offending drugs are hydralazine, procainamide, isoniazid, phenytoin, and chlorpromazine [42]. A number of other drugs can produce a lupus-like syndrome without antinuclear antibodies. Drug-induced lupus is clinically indistinguishable from idiopathic SLE except for the lower likelihood of renal involvement.

The pleural fluid in lupus pleuritis ranges from clear and yellow in color to turbid or blood tinged. The leukocyte count is generally around 5000 cells/mm³, but can be as high as 20,000 cells/mm³ [40]. In the acute inflammatory phase, the cells are predominantly polymorphonuclear leukocytes, but lymphocytes predominate in chronic effusions. The pleural fluid glucose, pH, and lactic dehydrogenase (LDH) levels are helpful in distinguishing SLE from rheumatoid pleuritis. In SLE, the pH is greater than 7.35, the glucose concentration is above 80 mg/dl, and the LDH level is less than 500 IU/liter [41]. The presence of pleural fluid antinuclear antibodies, low complement levels, and LE cells is important in establishing the diagnosis of lupus pleuritis [1,15,61]. Immunofluorescence studies of pleural biopsy material demonstrate the characteristic diffuse and speckled staining pattern of the cell nuclei considered to be diagnostic of SLE.

The pleuritis of SLE responds well to corticosteroid therapy. Usually no specific treatment is required for drug-induced lupus pleuritis, since signs and symptoms resolve promptly after the responsible drug is withdrawn.

Other collagen-vascular diseases that occasionally cause pleuritis and pleural effusions include Wegener's granulomatosis, Sjögren's syndrome, and familial Mediterranean fever.

Other Immunologic Disorders

SARCOIDOSIS
Sarcoidosis is a granulomatous disorder of unknown etiology. An imbalance of helper to suppressor T lymphocytes seems to play a role in mediating granuloma formation in this disease. Pleural disease, which is uncommon in this disorder, is in the form of a noncaseating granu-

lomatous pleuritis and pleural effusion [9,19]. There is usually extensive parenchymal lung disease. Chest pain and dyspnea are common symptoms. The effusions are small and more often unilateral than bilateral. The fluid is exudative, with a predominance of lymphocytes. Rarely, a transudative pleural effusion is found. The pleural effusions of sarcoidosis must be distinguished from tuberculous pleuritis by skin tests and cultures of pleural fluid and biopsy material. Sarcoid pleuritis is best managed with systemic corticosteroid therapy.

POSTCARDIAC INJURY SYNDROME

The postcardiac injury syndrome is characterized by the development of pleuritis, pneumonitis, and pericarditis several weeks after myocardial infarction, cardiac surgery, or other thoracic trauma [26,64,101]. The incidence of the syndrome is related to the extent of myocardial and pericardial injury, and may be as high as 15 percent in patients with large transmural myocardial infarctions [101]. High titers of antimyocardial antibodies may be detected [64], suggesting an immunologic basis for the disorder. Symptoms include fever and chest pain. Pericardial friction rubs are commonly heard. There is peripheral leukocytosis and an elevated erythrocyte sedimentation rate. The chest roentgenogram shows cardiac enlargement and pleural effusions, which are bilateral in a third of patients. Over half the patients have evidence of pericardial effusions. The pleural fluid is serosanguinous or frankly bloody [99]. The white blood cell count is elevated, and there is a predominance of polymorphonuclear leukocytes. The fluid is exudative with normal pH and glucose levels. The diagnosis of postcardiac injury syndrome is established after ruling out congestive heart failure, bacterial pneumonia, and pulmonary embolism. This syndrome usually responds well to treatment with aspirin or indomethacin. In severe cases, systemic corticosteroid therapy may be required.

ANGIOIMMUNOBLASTIC LYMPHADENOPATHY

This is a rare disorder caused by the proliferation of B lymphocytes and hypergammaglobulinemia [49]. There is generalized lymphadenopathy, hepatosplenomegaly, and anemia. Pleural effusions are seen on chest radiographs in about 12 percent of patients [22]. The fluid is an exudate with a predominance of lymphocytes. The diagnosis is based on the microscopic finding of material from lymph node biopsy.

Intraabdominal Disorders

PANCREATITIS

Pleural effusions develop in approximately 15 percent of patients with acute pancreatitis [55]. This is due to the transdiaphragmatic passage of exudative fluid from the abdomen through diaphragmatic lymphatic channels, sinus tracts, and anatomic defects in the diaphragm. This fluid is rich in pancreatic enzymes. It causes pleural inflammation and increased capillary permeability and results in further accumulation of pleural fluid.

Pleural effusions in patients with acute pancreatitis often cause dyspnea and chest pain. The effusions are generally small to moderate in size. Approximately 60 percent are left sided, 30 percent are right sided, and 10 percent are bilateral [55]. Other radiographic signs such as an elevated hemidiaphragm and basilar parenchymal infiltrates are commonly seen. In chronic pancreatitis, pleural effusions are more likely to be massive because of pancreaticopleural fistulas. These effusions reaccumulate rapidly after removal by thoracentesis.

Pleural fluid amylase levels are invariably elevated, usually to levels higher than those in the serum. This alone, however, is not diagnostic of pancreatitis, since pleural amylase levels are also high in some cases of malignant pleural effusion and after esophageal rupture. Other than the amylase concentration, there are no specific characteristics of the fluid. It is an exudate and can be serosanguinous or frankly bloody in appearance. The white blood cell count is usually between 1000 and 15,000 cells/mm^3, and the cells are predominantly polymorphonuclear leukocytes [67]. Generally, the pleural effusions clear within a couple of weeks as the pancreatitis resolves. Persistent effusions suggest the presence of a pancreatic abscess or a pancreatic pseudocyst. Pleural thickening and fibrosis can complicate a chronic pancreatic effusion.

ESOPHAGEAL DISORDERS

Esophageal perforation is a rare complication of endoscopy and intubation [56,79]. Rupture of the esophagus also may follow esophageal carcinoma or occur spontaneously after severe vomiting. The major symptom is excruciating chest pain, often with hematemesis. Pleural effusions, usually on the left side, are associated with pneumothorax and subcutaneous and mediastinal emphysema. The pleural fluid has a high amylase level and a very low pH, and may contain food particles or squamous epithelial cells. A pleural fluid pH of less than 6.0 should raise suspicion of esophageal perforation. The diagnosis is then confirmed by contrast studies of the esophagus.

Sclerotherapy of esophageal varices to control or prevent bleeding is associated with pleural effusions in approximately half the patients [3]. The effusions are due to inflammation induced by the sclerosant. Symptoms include fever and epigastric chest pain. The effusions occur on the right and left sides with equal frequency and can be bilateral. They are usually small to moderate in size. The lactic dehydrogenase level is always elevated in the pleural fluid, but the pleural fluid–serum protein ratio is often less than 0.5. Cell counts are typically elevated, with 1000 to 5000 white blood cells and 5000 to 40,000 red blood cells/mm^3.

SUBPHRENIC, INTRAHEPATIC, AND SPLENIC ABSCESSES

Ipsilateral pleural effusions are seen in about 70 percent of subphrenic abscesses as a result of inflammation of the diaphragm and increased permeability of the capillaries in the diaphragmatic pleura [21]. Typically, about 1 to 3 weeks after an abdominal surgical procedure, abdominal pain, fever, and leukocytosis develop, often in association with pleuritic chest pain and dyspnea. Basilar parenchymal infiltrates, atelectasis, and elevation of the diaphragm are often noted on chest roentgenograms along with the pleural effusion.

Intrahepatic abscesses are associated with pleural effusion in 20 percent of cases, and pleural effusions are seen in about a third of patients with splenic abscess [87]. The fluid is almost always exudative, with a predominance of polymorphonuclear leukocytes. Abdominal computed tomographic (CT) scanning is the procedure of choice in diagnosing intraabdominal abscesses. Ultrasonography is also useful in diagnosis and in monitoring the responses to therapy.

EFFUSIONS AFTER ABDOMINAL SURGERY AND POSTPARTUM PLEURAL EFFUSIONS

Small pleural effusions are seen in about half the patients within a few days of abdominal surgery [68]. The fluid is usually exudative, but it resolves spontaneously without therapy. Similarly, small pleural effusions are common in the postpartum period following uncomplicated deliveries [48]. These may be due to the increased blood volume and decreased colloid osmotic pressure of late pregnancy. The effusions are of no consequence and resolve spontaneously.

Miscellaneous Causes of Exudative Pleural Effusions

UREMIA

Pleuritis develops in about 3 percent of patients with uremia [11]. Symptoms of fever, chest pain, cough, and dyspnea occur in half the patients with uremic pleuritis. A pleural friction rub may be the only finding, or a large pleural effusion may be present. Involvement tends to be unilateral. The pleural fluid is exudative and is usually serosanguinous or frankly bloody. In general, the pleuritis and pleural effusions resolve with dialysis. Rarely, pleural fibrosis may develop.

MEIGS' SYNDROME

Meigs' syndrome is characterized by benign solid ovarian tumors in association with ascites and pleural effusion [77]. Ascites occurs in about 40 percent of ovarian tumors, and about 3 percent of these are associated with pleural effusions [24]. Ascites results from the generalized secretion of fluid from the tumor, and the pleural effusion follows from the passage of fluid through pores in the diaphragm. The effusions are usually right sided and can be quite large. The pleural effusions of Meigs' syndrome usually have high protein levels and are generally not transudative. After surgical removal of the tumor, the pleural effusions resolve.

DRUG REACTIONS

In addition to those drugs that produce lupus-like reactions, several others, including nitrofurantoin, some serotonin antagonists, dantrolene, radium, bromocriptine, practolol, procarbazine, and methotrexate, have been reported to cause pleuritis [65].

BENIGN ASBESTOS PLEURAL EFFUSION

Benign inflammatory exudative pleural effusions occasionally occur in workers exposed to asbestos. These tend to develop from 5 to 20 years after the initial asbestos exposure [29]. The development of the effusion is chronic with few or no symptoms, but some patients complain of chest heaviness, pleuritic chest pain, or dyspnea [29,36]. The effusions are usually unilateral. They often resolve spontaneously, only to recur on the same or the contralateral side. There also may be radiographic signs of pleural thickening or parenchymal fibrosis. The pleural fluid is exudative and serous or serosanguinous in appearance, with a white blood cell count as high as 20,000 to 30,000/mm³ [36]. There may be a predominance of either polymorphonuclear leukocytes or lymphocytes. Differential cell counts of pleural fluid sometimes reveal eosinophils in excess of 40 percent. In about 20 percent of patients, benign asbestos pleural effusions lead to extensive pleural fibrosis, but malignant mesotheliomas only rarely develop.

YELLOW NAIL SYNDROME

The yellow nail syndrome is characterized by lymphedema of the extremities, pleural effusions, and a yellowing dystrophy of the nails [46,75]. The condition is due to a generalized hypoplasia of lymphatic vessels. The condition is rare but is more often seen in women. The onset may occur at any age.

The pleural effusions are either unilateral or bilateral, and range in size from small to massive. They persist and tend to recur rapidly after removal by thoracentesis. The fluid is a serous exudate. There is no specific treatment, but pleurodesis may help when effusions are large and symptomatic.

References

1. Andrews BS, et al. The role of immune complexes in the pathogenesis of pleural effusions. *Am Rev Respir Dis* 124:115, 1981.
2. Andrews NC, et al. Management of nontuberculous empyema. *Am Rev Respir Dis* 85:935, 1962.
3. Bacon BR, Bailey-Newton RS, Connors AF. Pleural effusions after endoscopic variceal sclerotherapy. *Gastroenterology* 88:1910, 1985.
4. Ball GV, Whitfield CL. Studies on rheumatoid disease pleural fluid. *Arthritis Rheum* 9:846, 1966.
5. Banales JL, et al. Adenosine deaminase in the diagnosis of tuberculous pleural effusions: A report of 218 patients and review of the literature. *Chest* 99:355, 1991.
6. Barbas CSV, et al. The relationship between pleural fluid findings and the development of pleural thickening in patients with pleural tuberculosis. *Chest* 100:1264, 1991.
7. Bartlett JG, Finegold SM. Anaerobic infections of the lung and pleural space. *Am Rev Respir Dis* 110:56, 1974.
8. Bayly TC, et al. Tetracycline and quinacrine in the control of malignant pleural effusions. *Cancer* 41:1188, 1978.
9. Beekman JF, et al. Spectrum of pleural involvement in sarcoidosis. *Arch Intern Med* 136:323, 1976.
10. Berger HW, Mejia E. Tuberculous pleurisy. *Chest* 63:88, 1973.
11. Berger HW, et al. Uremic pleural effusion: A study in 14 patients on chronic dialysis. *Ann Intern Med* 82:362, 1975.
12. Broaddus VC, Wiener-Kronish JP, Staub NC. Clearance of lung edema into the pleural space of volume-loaded anesthetized sheep. *J Appl Physiol* 68:2623, 1990.
13. Bynum LJ, Wilson JE. Characteristics of pleural effusion associated with pulmonary embolism. *Arch Intern Med* 136:159, 1976.
14. Bynum LJ, Wilson JE, III. Radiographic features of pleural effusions in pulmonary embolism. *Am Rev Respir Dis* 117:829, 1978.
15. Carel RS, et al. Lupus erythematosus cells in pleural effusion. *Chest* 72:670, 1977.
16. Cavina C, Vichi G. Radiological aspects of pleural effusions in medical nephropathy in children. *Ann Radiol Diagn* 31:163, 1958.
17. Chen JT, et al. Correlation of roentgen findings with hemodynamic data in pure mitral stenosis. *AJR* 102:280, 1968.
18. Chernow B, Sahn SA. Carcinomatous involvement of the pleura. *Am J Med* 63:695, 1977.
19. Chusid EL, Siltzbach LE. Sarcoidosis of the pleura. *Ann Intern Med* 81:190, 1974.
20. Connell JV, Jr, Muhm JR. Radiographic manifestations of pulmonary histoplasmosis: A ten-year review. *Radiology* 121:281, 1976.
21. Connell TR, et al. Upper abdominal abscess: A continuing and deadly problem. *AJR* 134:759, 1980.
22. Cullen MH, et al. Angioimmunoblastic lymphadenopathy: Report of ten cases and review of the literature. *Q J Med* 189:151, 1979.
23. Decker DA, et al. The significance of a cytologically negative pleural effusion in bronchogenic carcinoma. *Chest* 74:640, 1978.
24. Dockerty MB. Ovarian neoplasms: A collective review of the recent literature. *Int Obstr Surg* 81:179, 1945.
25. Dodson WH, Hollingsworth JR. Pleural effusion in rheumatoid arthritis: Impaired transport of glucose. *N Engl J Med* 275:1337, 1966.
26. Dressler W. The post-myocardial infarction syndrome. *Arch Intern Med* 103:28, 1959.
27. Drutz DJ, Catanzaro A. Coccidioidomycosis. *Am Rev Respir Dis* 117:727, 1978.
28. Ellner JJ. Pleural fluid and peripheral blood lymphocyte function in tuberculosis. *Ann Intern Med* 89:932, 1978.
29. Epler GR, McLoud TC, Gaensler EA. Prevalence and incidence of benign asbestos pleural effusion in a working population. *JAMA* 247:617, 1982.
30. Falchuk KR, et al. Tetracycline-induced pleural

symphysis for recurrent hydrothorax complicating cirrhosis. *Gastroenterology* 72:319, 1977.

31. Fine NL, Smith LR, Sheedy PF. Frequency of pleural effusions in mycoplasma and viral pneumonias. *N Engl J Med* 283:790, 1970.

32. Finland M, Barnes MW. Changing ecology of acute bacterial empyema: Occurrence and mortality at Boston City Hospital during 12 selected years from 1935 to 1972. *J Infect Dis* 137:274, 1978.

33. Flynn MW, Felson B. The roentgen manifestations of thoracic actinomycosis. *AJR* 110:707, 1970.

34. Fraser RG, Paré JAP. *Diagnosis of Diseases of the Chest* (2d ed). Philadelphia: Saunders, 1977.

35. Frazier AR, Rosenow EC, III, Robert GD. Nocardiosis: A review of 25 cases occurring during 24 months. *Mayo Clin Proc* 50:657, 1975.

36. Gaensler EA, Kaplan AI. Asbestos pleural effusion. *Ann Intern Med* 74:178, 1971.

37. George RB, Penn RL, Kinasewitz GT. Myobacterial, fungal, actinomycotic, and nocardial infections of the pleura. *Clin Chest Med* 6:63, 1985.

38. Good JT, Taryle DA, Sahn SA. The diagnostic value of pleural fluid pH. *Chest* 78:55, 1980.

39. Good JT, Jr, et al. Superior vena cava syndrome as a cause of pleural effusion. *Am Rev Respir Dis* 125:246, 1982.

40. Good JT, Jr, et al. Lupus pleuritis: Clinical features and pleural fluid characteristics with special reference to pleural fluid antinuclear antibodies. *Chest* 84:714, 1983.

41. Halla JT, Schrohenloher RE, Volanakis JE. Immune complexes and other laboratory features of pleural effusion. *Ann Intern Med* 92:748, 1980.

42. Harpey JP. Lupus-like syndromes induced by drugs. *Ann Allergy* 33:256, 1974.

43. Harvey AM, et al. Systemic lupus erythematosus: Review of the literature and clinical analysis of 138 cases. *Medicine* 33:291, 1954.

44. Henke CA, Leatherman JW. Intrapleurally administered streptokinase in the treatment of acute loculated non-purulent parapneumonic effusions. *Am Rev Respir Dis* 145:680, 1992.

45. Herring M, Pecora D. Pleural aspergillosis: A case report. *Am Surg* 42:300, 1976.

46. Hiller E, Rosenow EC, III, Olsen AM. Pulmonary manifestations of the yellow nail syndrome. *Chest* 61:452, 1972.

47. Hillerdal G. Pulmonary *Aspergillus* infections invading the pleura. *Thorax* 36:745, 1981.

48. Hughson WG, et al. Postpartum pleural effusion: A common radiologic finding. *Ann Intern Med* 97:856, 1982.

49. Hunninghake GW, Fauci AS. Pulmonary involvement in the collagen-vascular diseases. *Am Rev Respir Dis* 119:471, 1979.

50. Hurwitz S, Leiman G, Shapiro C. Mesothelial cells in pleural fluid: TB or not TB? *S Afr Med J* 57:937, 1980.

51. Ibarra-Perez C. Thoracic complications of amebic abscess of the liver: Report of 501 cases. *Chest* 79:672, 1981.

52. Jacobson G, Denlinger RB, Carter RA. Roentgen manifestations of Q fever. *Radiology* 53:739, 1949.

53. Johnston RF, Loo RV. Hepatic hydrothorax: Studies to determine the source of the fluid and report of thirteen cases. *Ann Intern Med* 61:385, 1964.

54. Katsilabros L, et al. Pleural effusions and hepatitis. *Gastroenterology* 63:718, 1972.

55. Kaye MD. Pleuropulmonary complications of pancreatitis. *Thorax* 23:297, 1968.

56. Keszler P, Buzna E. Surgical and conservative management of esophageal perforation. *Chest* 80:158, 1981.

57. Kinasewitz GT, Fishman AP. Influence of alterations in Starling forces on visceral pleural fluid movement. *J Appl Physiol* 51:671, 1981.

58. Kinasewitz GT, Penn RL, George RB. The spectrum and significance of pleural disease in blastomycosis. *Chest* 86:580, 1984.

59. Kirkpatrick JA, Jr, Fleischer DS. The roentgen appearance of the chest in acute glomerulonephritis in children. *J Pediatr* 64:492, 1964.

60. Lander P, Palayew MJ. Infectious mononucleosis: A review of chest roentgenographic manifestations. *J Can Assoc Radiol* 25:303, 1974.

61. Leechawengwong M, Berger HW, Sukumaran M. Diagnostic significance of antinuclear antibodies in pleural effusion. *Mt Sinai J Med* 46:137, 1979.

62. Levine H, Szanto PB, Cugell DW. Tuberculous pleurisy: An acute illness. *Arch Intern Med* 122:329, 1968.

63. Lieberman FL, et al. Pathogenesis and treatment of hydrothorax complicating cirrhosis with ascites. *Ann Intern Med* 64:341, 1966.

64. Liem KL, et al. Incidence and significance of heart muscle antibodies in patients with acute myocardial infarction and unstable angina. *Acta Med Scand* 206:473, 1979.

65. Light RW. *Pleural Diseases*. Philadelphia: Lea & Febiger, 1983.

66. Light RW. Parapneumonic effusions and empyema. *Clin Chest Med* 6:55, 1985.

67. Light RW, Ball WC. Glucose and amylase in pleural effusions *JAMA* 225:257, 1973.

68. Light RW, George RB. Incidence and significance of pleural effusion after abdominal surgery. *Chest* 69:621, 1976.

69. Light RW, Erozan YS, Ball WC, Jr. Cells in pleural fluid: Their value in differential diagnosis. *Ann Intern Med* 132:854, 1973.

70. Light RW, et al. Parapneumonic effusions. *Am J Med* 69:507, 1980.
71. Light RW, et al. Pleural effusions: The diagnostic separation of transudates and exudates. *Ann Intern Med* 77:507, 1972.
72. Llach F, Arieff AI, Massry SG. Renal vein thrombosis and nephrotic syndrome: A prospective study of 36 adult patients. *Ann Intern Med* 83:8, 1974.
73. Lonky SA, et al. Acute coccidioidal pleural effusion. *Am Rev Respir Dis* 114:681, 1976.
74. Maher GG, Berger HW. Massive pleural effusion: Malignant and nonmalignant causes in 46 patients. *Am Rev Respir Dis* 105:458, 1972.
75. Mambretti-Zumwalt J, Seidman JM, Higano N. Yellow nail syndrome: Complete triad with pleural protein turnover studies. *South Med J* 73:995, 1980.
76. Masson T. Treatment of malignant pleural effusion with doxycycline. *Scand J Infect Dis* 53:29, 1988.
77. Meigs JV, Cass JW. Fibroma of the ovary with ascites and fibrothorax: With a report of seven cases. *Am J Obstet Gynecol* 33:249, 1937.
78. Mellins RB, Levine OR, Fishman AP. Effect of systemic and pulmonary venous hypertension on pleural and pericardial fluid accumulation. *J Appl Physiol* 29:564, 1970.
79. Michel L, Grillo HC, Malt RA. Operative and nonoperative management of esophageal perforations. *Ann Surg* 194:57, 1981.
80. Murray JF, et al. The changing spectrum of nocardiosis. *Am Rev Respir Dis* 83:315, 1961.
81. Page RD, Jeffrey RR, Donnelly RJ. Thoracoscopy: A review of 121 consecutive surgical procedures. *Ann Thorac Surg* 48:66, 1989.
82. Potts DE, Taryle DA, Sahn SA. The glucose-pH relationship in parapneumonic effusions. *Arch Intern Med* 138:1378, 1978.
83. Rabin CB, Blackman NS. Bilateral pleural effusion: Its significance in association with a heart of normal size. *J Mt Sinai Hosp* 24:45, 1957.
84. Race GA, Scheifley CH, Edwards JE. Hydrothorax in congestive heart failure. *Am J Med* 22:83, 1957.
85. Rasaretnam R, Paul ATS, Yoganathan M. Pleural empyema due to ruptured amebic liver abscess. *Br J Surg* 61:713, 1974.
86. Roper WH, Waring JJ. Primary serofibrinous pleural effusion in military personnel. *Am Rev Respir Dis* 71:616, 1955.
87. Rubin RH, Swartz MN, Malt R. Hepatic abscess: Changes in clinical, bacteriologic, and therapeutic aspects. *Am J Med* 57:601, 1974.
88. Rudnick MR, et al. Acute massive hydrothorax complicating peritoneal dialysis: Report of two cases and a review of the literature. *Clin Nephrol* 12:38, 1979.
89. Sahn SA. Malignant pleural effusions. *Clin Chest Med* 6:113, 1985.
90. Sahn SA. Pleural Fluid pH in the Normal State and in Diseases Affecting the Pleural Space. In J Chretien, J Bignon, A Hirsch (Eds), *The Pleura in Health and Disease*, Vol 30: *Lung Biology in Health and Disease*. New York: Marcel Dekker, 1985. Pp 253–266.
91. Sahn SA, et al. Rheumatoid pleurisy: Observations on the development of low pleural fluid pH and glucose level. *Arch Intern Med* 140:1237, 1980.
92. Salyer WR, Eggleston JC, Erozan YS. Efficacy of pleural needle biopsy and pleural fluid cytopathology in the diagnosis of malignant neoplasm involving the pleura. *Chest* 67:536, 1975.
93. Scharer L, McClement JH. Isolation of tubercle bacilli from needle biopsy specimens of parietal pleura. *Am Rev Respir Dis* 97:466, 1968.
94. Schub HM, Spivey CG, Baird GD. Pleural involvement in histoplasmosis. *Am Rev Respir Dis* 94:225, 1966.
95. Seibert AF, et al. Tuberculous pleural effusion: Twenty year experience. *Chest* 99:883, 1991.
96. Smolar EN, et al. Cardiac tamponade in primary myxedema and review of the literature. *Am J Med Sci* 272:345, 1976.
97. Snider GL, Saleh SS. Empyema of the thorax in adults: Review of 105 cases. *Chest* 54:12, 1968.
98. Stark DD, et al. Biochemical features of urinothorax. *Arch Intern Med* 142:1509, 1982.
99. Stelzer TJ, et al. The pleuropulmonary manifestations of the postcardiac injury syndrome. *Chest* 84:383, 1983.
100. Tani P, Poppius H, Makipaja J. Cortisone therapy for exudative tuberculous pleurisy in the light of the follow-up study. *Acta Tuberc Scand* 44:303, 1964.
101. Toole JC, Silverman ME. Pericarditis of acute myocardial infarction. *Chest* 67:647, 1975.
102. Varkey B, et al. Empyema thoracis during a ten-year period: Analysis of 72 cases and comparison to a previous study (1952 to 1967). *Arch Intern Med* 141:1771, 1981.
103. Walker WC, Wright V. Rheumatoid pleuritis. *Ann Rheum Dis* 26:467, 1967.
104. Walker WC, Wright V. Pulmonary lesions and rheumatoid arthritis. *Medicine* 47:501, 1968.
105. Yeh TJ, Hall DP, Ellison RG. Empyema thoracis: A review of 110 cases. *Am Rev Respir Dis* 88:785, 1963.
106. Young EJ, et al. Pleural effusions due to *Cryptococcus neoformans*: A review of the literature and a report of two cases with cryptococcal antigen determinations. *Am Rev Respir Dis* 121:743, 1980.

74

Hemothorax, Chylothorax, Pneumothorax, and Other Pleural Disorders

Alfred F. Connors, Jr.   *Murray D. Altose*

Hemothorax

The diagnosis of *hemothorax*, or blood in the pleural space, is confirmed when the pleural fluid hematocrit is greater than half that of peripheral blood. Trauma is the most common cause of hemothorax, but significant amounts of blood in the pleural space also can be caused by the spread of cancer to the pleura, anticoagulant therapy, and complications of percutaneous insertion of central venous catheters, thoracentesis, and pleural biopsy. Hemothorax should always be considered following blunt or penetrating chest trauma. The diagnosis is usually suspected when pleural effusion is noted on the chest radiograph of a patient with thoracic trauma. An upright chest roentgenogram should be taken, since the hemothorax may not be apparent on a supine view [11]. Chest films should also be repeated 24 hours after chest trauma since 24 percent of hemothoraces are not present on the admission radiograph [11]. There is a close association between hemothorax and pneumothorax following both blunt and penetrating chest trauma [11,14].

Immediate chest tube drainage is required in the case of hemothorax. Chest tube drainage allows quantitation of the extent of bleeding, will help stop bleeding from pleural lacerations, and will reduce the risk of empyema and the likelihood of fibrothorax [3,30]. When vascular injury, cardiac tamponade, or bronchial rupture is suspected, an emergency thoracotomy is required. Thoracotomy is also indicated for pleural bleeding that continues despite chest tube drainage. Empyemas develop in about 1 to 4 percent of

cases of hemothorax [3,14]. The risk of empyema is highest in patients with contamination of the pleural space at the time of the initial injury and in those patients with shock, abdominal injuries, or prolonged pleural space drainage. Some patients retain clotted blood in the pleural space despite chest tube drainage. The presence of blood clots does not increase the risk of empyema, and recovery is usually complete without any specific therapy [32].

After chest tubes are removed from patients recovering from chest trauma and hemothorax, about one quarter go on to develop pleural effusions [32]. These tend to resolve spontaneously, but about 25 percent are associated with empyema. Thus, early diagnostic thoracentesis is recommended to rule out pleural infection. Fibrothorax is a rare complication and occurs in only about 1 percent of patients with hemothorax. It is most likely to result when the hemothorax is complicated by pneumothorax or empyema. Several months of observation are required before decortication should be considered, since, in most cases, the pleural thickening tends to resolve.

A number of disorders other than trauma can cause hemothorax. These are summarized in Table 74-1. Metastatic malignancy is the most common cause of nontraumatic hemothorax. Rarely, a significant hemothorax will occur with spontaneous pneumothorax. Hemothorax also can complicate anticoagulant therapy for pulmonary embolism. The bleeding is usually on the same side as the pulmonary embolus. The treatment consists of reversing anticoagulation and prompt tube thoracostomy.

Table 74-1. **Causes of hemothorax**

Trauma
    Penetrating or nonpenetrating trauma
    Iatrogenic
Malignancy
    Metastatic
    Primary
Anticoagulant therapy
Spontaneous
    Secondary to bleeding disorder
    Spontaneous pneumothorax
    Rupture of intrathoracic vessels or aneurysms
    Ruptured pancreatic pseudocyst
    Thoracic endometriosis
    Intrathoracic extramedullary hematopoiesis
    Idiopathic

Chylothorax

Chylothorax is caused by chyle leaking from the thoracic duct or collaterals into the pleural space. The thoracic duct originates in the retroperitoneal space. It ascends in the posterior mediastinum between the aorta, the esophagus, and the azygos vein to the right of the midline. It crosses the midline near the level of the fifth thoracic vertebra and enters the left subclavian vein near its junction with the internal jugular vein. Disruption of the duct below the fifth thoracic vertebra produces a right chylothorax, whereas perforation above this level leads to a left-sided effusion. The milky, opalescent chyle contains chylomicrons, triglycerides, and cholesterol. Between 1500 and 2000 ml chyle is produced per day, but the flow of chyle can increase severalfold with a high dietary fat intake [6,31]. The most common cause of chylothorax is thoracic neoplasm, particularly lymphoma. Chylothorax also can occur after cardiovascular surgery in which the left subclavian artery is mobilized, after cervical lymph node dissection, and as a complication of subclavian vein thrombosis [6,25,29,31]. Penetrating trauma to the chest or neck can sever the thoracic duct causing chylothorax. Chylothorax also can follow closed thoracic trauma associated with hyperextension of the thoracic spine or fracture of thoracic vertebral bodies. About 15 percent of cases are idiopathic and are probably due to minor trauma associated with coughing, vomiting, or hiccupping [29]. Chylothorax is the most common form of pleural effusion in neonates and seems to be caused by thoracic duct trauma during delivery. Other uncommon causes of chylothorax include pulmonary lymphangiomyomatosis, lymphadenopathy, cirrhosis, heart failure, filariasis, thoracic aortic aneurysms, and various lymphatic disorders [29]. Chest pain and fever are rare with nontraumatic chylothorax, since chyle causes little pleural irritation. Patients with large volumes of pleural fluid complain of dyspnea.

The diagnosis of chylothorax is made by thoracentesis, which yields white, milky fluid. Empyema can be excluded by centrifuging the fluid and examining the supernatant. The supernatant is clear in empyema, since the turbidity is due to cellular material and debris. The fluid remains opaque with chylothorax or pseudochylothorax because of the high lipid content of the fluid. In chylothorax, the pleural fluid triglyceride level is greater than 50 mg/dl [28]. A triglyceride level greater than 110 mg/dl is highly suggestive of chylothorax [28]. Lipoprotein analysis that reveals the presence of chylomicrons is diagnostic. Although cholesterol levels may range from 20 to 250 mg/dl, cholesterol crystals are not seen on examination of the pleural fluid sediment.

The management of chylothorax can be difficult, since the removal of fat, lymphocytes, and electrolytes by chest tube drainage or repeated thoracenteses can cause malnutrition and immunocompromise. While in many cases chylothorax resolves spontaneously, delaying definitive therapy too long can result in cachexia and increased morbidity and mortality.

The management of traumatic chylothorax is aimed at relief of dyspnea by evacuation of the pleural space, reduction of chyle formation, and prevention of malnutrition. Little recommends the pleuroperitoneal shunt as the best means of removing chyle from the pleural space [20]. Since immunocompromise and malnutrition are avoided because the chyle is not removed from the body, more time is allowed for spontaneous closure of the defect in the thoracic duct.

Tube thoracostomy can also be performed to remove chyle from the pleural space and relieve symptoms of dyspnea. Tube drainage ensures expansion of the lung and also may result in pleurodesis. Malnutrition due to the removal of large volumes of chyle must be avoided. With both tube drainage and pleuroperitoneal shunt, chyle formation should be kept to a minimum by discontinuing oral feedings and by employing constant nasogastric suction [29]. Nutritional support is best provided by total parenteral hyperalimentation. Bed rest is necessary, since lymph flow increases with activity. Reducing the formation of chyle also seems to facilitate spontaneous healing of thoracic duct defects. The flow of chyle following traumatic chylothorax generally decreases substantially within a week of the injury. Exploratory thoracotomy and ligation of the thoracic duct may be required if the chylothorax cannot be controlled. This definitive therapy should not be delayed when the patient's nutritional status is deteriorating, since debilitation may lead to death.

The effective treatment of nontraumatic chylothorax requires that the cause be established first. In the case of lymphoma (the most common nontraumatic cause of chylothorax) or malignant neoplastic disease, mediastinal radiation or systemic chemotherapy usually stops the flow of chyle [25,29]. If the chylothorax persists, chemical pleurodesis with tetracycline may be effective. For patients without evidence of lymphoma or metastatic carcinoma, the therapy is the same as that for traumatic chylothorax. With chest tube drainage and discontinuation of oral feedings, the chylothorax will usually resolve within a week. If the chylothorax persists, exploratory thoracotomy with examination of the mediastinum and ligation of the thoracic duct should be considered.

Pseudochylothorax is a pleural effusion that has a high lipid content but is not due to disruption of the thoracic duct [7]. It is usually found in patients with chronic pleural effusions of several years' duration and with thickened and calcified pleura. It is commonly seen in chronic rheumatoid and tuberculous pleuritis [7,13]. The predominant material in the pleural fluid is cholesterol, which appears to originate from degenerating red and white blood cells. Frequently, cholesterol crystals are seen on smears of pleural fluid sediment. Pleural fluid triglyceride levels are generally low in pseudochylothorax, but may, on occasion, exceed 250 mg/dl [28]. Pseudochylothorax is distinguished from chylothorax by the absence of chylomicrons [28]. Table 74-2 demonstrates how the clinical presentation and the results of pleural fluid analysis are used to distinguish chylothorax from pseudochylothorax.

Pneumothorax

Spontaneous Pneumothorax

Spontaneous pneumothorax develops in the absence of any trauma to the chest. When no obvious diseases of the lung are present, a spontaneous pneumothorax is considered to be primary. In contrast, secondary spontaneous pneumothoraces develop as a complication of a wide variety of diseases of the airways and lungs.

Primary spontaneous pneumothorax is predominantly a disease of young males and is six times more common in men than in women [22]. It results from the rupture of small apical subpleural emphysematous blebs that either are congenital or are caused by bronchiolar inflammation and obstruction. Primary spontaneous pneumothorax is more likely to occur in tall, thin individuals [33]. It has been suggested that in tall men with longer lungs, the pleural pressure is more subatmospheric at the apex and as a result apical alveoli are more greatly distended. This may play a role in bleb formation in those who are congenitally predisposed. Cigarette smoking also increases the likelihood of primary spontaneous pneumothorax [16]. The relative risk of spontaneous pneumothorax was 102 times greater in heavy smokers (>22 cigarettes per day) in a recent study [5].

Primary spontaneous pneumothorax is not precipitated by exertion. It usually occurs when the patient is at rest and only infrequently develops during exercise. Chest pain and dyspnea are the most common symptoms, and only rarely are both these symptoms absent [26]. The chest pain is sudden in onset and pleuritic in nature; shoulder pain reflects irritation of the diaphragmatic

Table 74-2. Distinguishing between chylothorax and pseudochylothorax: History and pleural fluid analysis

	Chylothorax	Pseudochylothorax
History	Acute onset, no inflammation	Chronic effusion, pleural thickening
Pleural fluid analysis		
Triglycerides	>110 mg/dl	<50 mg/dl diagnostic
Cholesterol	20–250 mg/dl	20–300 mg/dl
Chylomicrons	Present	None
Cholesterol crystals	None	Present

pleura. Compression and collapse of the lung under a pneumothorax causes cough in over half the patients.

The characteristic findings on physical examination include impaired expansion of the involved hemithorax, a hyperresonant percussion note, and diminished or absent fremitus and breath sounds. Marked respiratory distress with cyanosis, tachycardia, and hypotension signals a tension pneumothorax.

The diagnosis is made by identifying a visceral pleural line on the chest radiograph. A small pneumothorax is often best visualized on radiographs taken in full expiration. In about 20 percent of cases, there is an associated small pleural effusion. This appears as an air-fluid level.

The treatment of primary spontaneous pneumothorax is determined by the size of the pneumothorax and history of prior pneumothoraces. Patients with a small, stable pneumothorax can be treated without tube thoracostomy because the air in the pleural space will spontaneously resorb. The rate of resorption, however, is very slow and amounts to less than 1.5 percent of the volume of the pneumothorax per day [17]. Resorption can be speeded by having patients breathe high concentrations of oxygen, which increases the nitrogen gradient between the pleural air space and the blood.

Patients with pneumothoraces larger than 15 percent are best managed with tube thoracostomy using small chest tubes (7–13 F) connected to water seal or a Heimlich valve [19]. This causes the lungs to rapidly reexpand and tends to minimize the likelihood of a persistent air leak. In fewer than 5 percent of patients with primary spontaneous pneumothorax, an open thoracotomy is required for persistent air leakage or failure of the lung to reexpand [26]. Open thoracotomy permits oversewing of apical pleural blebs and pleurodesis to prevent recurrences.

Recurrences of primary spontaneous pneumothorax are common when thoracotomy is not performed. In about half of all patients, a subsequent spontaneous pneumothorax will develop within 2 to 3 years of the initial episode [26]. After a second pneumothorax, the likelihood of recurrence increases yet further. After a second spontaneous pneumothorax, steps should be taken to prevent recurrence. This is most readily accomplished by pleurodesis. In the event of recurrences after attempted pleurodesis, thoracotomy may be required to oversew subpleural blebs and for pleural scarification.

Spontaneous pneumothorax is also a common complication in patients with underlying lung diseases, most commonly chronic obstructive pulmonary disease. Other lung diseases associated with secondary spontaneous pneumothorax are listed in Table 74-3.

Patients with underlying lung disease in whom a secondary spontaneous pneumothorax develops tend to have severe symptoms and gas-exchange abnormalities [10]. Most complain of shortness of breath and chest pain, but the shortness of breath is often out of proportion to the size of the pneumothorax [27]. Severe hypoxemia, cyanosis, and hypotension can occur. The mortality may be as high as 15 percent [10,15,27]. The clinical diagnosis is often difficult in the patient with severe chronic obstructive pulmonary

***Table 74-3.* Causes of pneumothorax**

Primary spontaneous pneumothorax
Secondary spontaneous pneumothorax
  Obstructive pulmonary disease
    Chronic airways obstruction
    Asthma
  Malignancy
    Primary lung cancer
    Pleural metastatic disease
  Infectious disease
    Lung abscess
    Tuberculosis
    Pneumocystis carinii pneumonia
  Pulmonary infarction
  Diffuse lung disease
    Idiopathic pulmonary fibrosis
    Eosinophilic granuloma
    Scleroderma
    Rheumatoid disease
    Tuberous sclerosis
    Sarcoidosis
    Lymphangiomyomatosis
    Idiopathic pulmonary hemosiderosis
    Alveolar proteinosis
  Pneumoconiosis
    Silicosis
    Berylliosis
  Congenital disease
    Cystic fibrosis
    Marfan syndrome
  Catamenial pneumothorax
  Neonatal pneumothorax
Traumatic pneumothorax
  Penetrating thoracic trauma
  Sudden chest compression
  Iatrogenic

disease who may have overinflated lungs, decreased breath sounds, and hyperresonance to percussion. A chest radiograph is required to establish the diagnosis. This can sometimes be difficult in the presence of marked emphysema or bullous disease. Under these circumstances, the diagnosis of pneumothorax should be made only if a visceral pleural line can be demonstrated.

Tube thoracostomy is usually necessary in secondary spontaneous pneumothorax, particularly if the patient is undergoing mechanical ventilation. As many as a third of patients will require a second chest tube for complete reexpansion of the lung, and 20 percent will have a persistent air leak after 7 days [27]. Because of the danger of recurrence, pleurodesis should be performed after the lung is reexpanded and the air leak has stopped. The persistence of an air leak for greater than 7 to 10 days in patients with underlying lung disease poses a difficult problem, since the mortality may be as high as 10 percent [10]. In patients with mild lung disease and good general condition, open thoracotomy seems to be the treatment of choice. For patients with severe underlying lung disease, prolonged chest tube drainage will often result in reexpansion of the lung and cessation of the air leak. In patients with pneumothorax secondary to tuberculosis, the air leak may not close until after 6 weeks of tube drainage and antituberculous therapy. Because of the risks of open thoracotomy in patients with tuberculosis, this procedure should only be undertaken after several weeks of tube thoracostomy drainage.

On occasion, a pneumothorax will develop in patients with extensive atelectasis secondary to bronchial obstruction from bronchogenic carcinoma. In these patients, it may be inadvisable to institute closed-tube drainage, since the lung cannot expand to fill the hemithorax. A chest tube in a persistent large pleural airspace may eventually lead to the development of an empyema.

Traumatic Pneumothorax

Traumatic pneumothorax is most often due to penetrating chest trauma, but it also can occur with closed chest trauma consequent to alveolar rupture from thoracic compression, fracture of a bronchus, esophageal rupture, or rib fractures that lacerate the pleura [15]. Tube thoracostomy is required to evacuate air and blood from the pleural space. The air leak will stop within 3 days in most patients. Hemoptysis and persistent air leakage in patients with substantial trauma to the upper anterior chest suggest the possibility of a tracheal or bronchial fracture [15]. The prompt diagnosis by bronchoscopy of fracture of the trachea or major bronchus is required to ensure timely surgical correction.

Iatrogenic Pneumothorax

Pneumothorax is also a common complication of central venous line insertion, thoracentesis, pleural biopsy, percutaneous needle aspiration of the lung, and transbronchial lung biopsy. The management of an iatrogenic pneumothorax depends on its size and the degree of respiratory embarrassment. Small pneumothoraces of less than 10 or 15 percent that show no signs of enlarging can be managed expectantly. The administration of supplemental oxygen will speed resorption of the pneumothorax. Larger pneumothoraces and those that appear to be increasing in size are best evacuated through a small chest tube.

Barotrauma from high airway and alveolar pressure leads to pneumothorax in about 5 percent of patients undergoing mechanical ventilation [9,34]. The likelihood of barotrauma and pneumothorax increases with the level of the peak positive airway pressure during mechanical ventilation. When peak pressures consistently exceed 55 to 60 cmH$_2$O, the prophylactic placement of chest tubes should be considered.

Tension Pneumothorax

When the pressure in a pneumothorax exceeds atmospheric pressure, a tension pneumothorax is said to exist. It most commonly occurs during mechanical ventilation or cardiopulmonary resuscitation, but it may complicate any type of spontaneous or traumatic pneumothorax [9,21, 34]. A tension pneumothorax develops when a ball-valve mechanism allows air to move from the lung to pleural space but prevents air movement in the opposite direction. This generally causes severe respiratory distress, diaphoresis, tachycardia, and hypotension. Hypoxemia is marked, and cyanosis may be apparent.

Characteristic findings on chest radiogram include a shift of the mediastinum away from the pneumothorax and ipsilateral depression of the diaphragm. Since tension pneumothorax is a medical emergency, the diagnosis must be made clinically. Treatment cannot be delayed until a chest radiograph is obtained. When a tension pneumothorax is suspected, the patient should be given a high inspired oxygen concentration and a large-bore needle should be inserted into the pleural space through the second anterior intercostal space about 2 to 3 cm from the edge of the sternum. A tension pneumothorax is confirmed by a rush of air through the needle and an alleviation of respiratory distress. Once the presence of a tension pneumothorax is confirmed, a chest tube should be inserted immediately.

Other Pleural Disorders

Fibrothorax

Fibrous pleural adhesions are common findings on chest roentgenograms and at autopsy. They are often the result of previous tuberculous or pyogenic infections. The pleural peel surrounding the lung may become exceedingly thick and calcified along its inner aspect, to produce a restrictive ventilatory impairment. Usually no treatment is necessary. Provided no underlying parenchymal disease is present, decortication may produce functional improvement when the ventilatory defect is marked and symptoms are severe. Since decortication is a major surgical procedure, it should not be performed in severely ill or debilitated patients.

Asymptomatic fibrous thickening of the pleura is also caused by the inhalation of asbestos [8]. The parietal pleura, including that over the diaphragm, is preferentially affected with cell-poor collagenous connective tissue that may eventually calcify [4,24]. Asbestos bodies are not seen on conventional microscopy, but uncoated fibers can be identified by electron microscopy or in ashed tissue using polarized microscopy [4]. Pleural plaques cause little or no impairment in ventilatory function in the absence of parenchymal fibrosis from asbestosis.

Mesothelioma and Other Asbestos-Related Pleural Disorders

There are both benign and malignant mesotheliomas. Benign fibrous mesothelioma is an uncommon condition that is not related to asbestos exposure [23]. These tumors usually arise from the parietal surface and are thought to originate from the mesothelial cell or from subpleural fibroblasts [12,23]. The tumors are discrete and localized but may invade the adjacent lung and chest wall. Pleural effusions are evident in 10 per-

cent of cases. Patients are often asymptomatic or complain of cough, chest pain, or dyspnea. Hypertrophic pulmonary osteoarthropathy is common, particularly with tumors greater than 7 cm in diameter [23]. Another paraneoplastic syndrome that is seen with benign fibrous mesothelioma is hypoglycemia. Treatment is by surgical resection.

Malignant mesothelioma is largely a disease of people who have been exposed to asbestos [2,18]. There is, however, no relationship between the degree or extent of asbestos exposure and development of the tumor, which may take place 20 to 40 years after the first exposure [1]. The tumor grows rapidly, encases the lung, and spreads to involve the pericardium, heart, and other mediastinal structures. Tumors may penetrate the diaphragm to involve the peritoneum. The extent of disease is best evaluated by chest computed tomographic scans. Distant metastases are found in about 50 percent of patients. There are three main histologic types: epithelial, mesenchymal, and mixed. It is often difficult to distinguish the epithelial type from metastatic adenocarcinoma, and special stains and electron microscopy may be necessary. The pleural effusions of malignant mesotheliomas may be very large. The fluid is a serous or serosanguineous exudate, often with low glucose and pH levels. The fluid may be highly viscid due to large amounts of hyaluronic acid. Although malignant mesothelial cells are regularly found in the pleural fluid, a definite diagnosis requires an open-lung biopsy.

References

1. Aisner J, Weirnik PH. Malignant mesothelioma: Current status and future prospects. *Chest* 74: 438, 1978.
2. Antman KH. Clinical presentation and natural history of benign and malignant mesothelioma. *Semin Oncol* 8:313, 1981.
3. Beall AC, Jr, Crawford HW, DeBakey ME. Considerations in the management of acute traumatic hemothorax. *J Thorac Cardiovasc Surg* 52:351, 1966.
4. Becklake MR. Asbestos-related disease of the lung and other organs: Their epidemiology and implications for clinical practice. *Am Rev Respir Dis* 114:187, 1976.
5. Bense L, Ecklund G, Wiman LG. Smoking and the increased risk of contracting spontaneous pneumothorax. *Chest* 92:1009, 1987.
6. Bower GC. Chylothorax: Observations in 20 cases. *Dis Chest* 46:464, 1964.

7. Coe JE, Aikawa JK. Cholesterol pleural effusion. *Arch Intern Med* 108:163, 1961.
8. Craighead JE, Mossman BT. The pathogenesis of asbestos-related diseases. *N Engl J Med* 306:1446, 1982.
9. De Latorre FJ, et al. Incidence of pneumothorax and pneumomediastinum in patients with aspiration pneumonia requiring ventilatory support. *Chest* 72:141, 1977.
10. Dines DE, Clagett OT, Payne WS. Spontaneous pneumothorax in emphysema. *Mayo Clin Proc* 45:481, 1970.
11. Drummond DS, Craig RH. Traumatic hemothorax: Complications and management. *Am Surg* 33:403, 1967.
12. Ellis K, Wolff M. Mesotheliomas and secondary tumors of the pleura. *Semin Roentgenol* 12:303, 1977.
13. Ferguson GC. Cholesterol pleural effusion in rheumatoid lung disease. *Thorax* 21:577, 1966.
14. Graham JM, Mattox KL, Beall AC, Jr. Penetrating trauma of the lung. *J Trauma* 19:665, 1979.
15. Guest JL, Anderson JN. Major airway injury in closed chest trauma. *Chest* 72:63, 1977.
16. Jansveld CAF, Dijkman JH. Primary spontaneous pneumothorax and smoking. *Br Med J* 4:559, 1975.
17. Kircher LT, Jr, Swartzel RL. Spontaneous pneumothorax and its treatment. *JAMA* 155:24, 1954.
18. Legha SS, Muggia FM. Pleural mesothelioma: Clinical features and therapeutic implications. *Ann Intern Med* 87:613, 1977.
19. Light RW. *Pleural Diseases* (2nd ed). Philadelphia: Lea & Febiger, 1990. Pp 237–249.
20. Little AG, et al. Pleuroperitoneal shunting: Alternative therapy for pleural effusions. *Ann Surg* 208:443, 1988.
21. Ludwig J, Kienzle GD. Pneumothorax in a large autopsy population. *Am J Clin Pathol* 70:24, 1978.
22. Melton LJ, Hepper NGG, Offord KP. Incidence of spontaneous pneumothorax in Olmsted County, Minnesota: 1950 to 1974. *Am Rev Respir Dis* 120:1379, 1979.
23. Okike N, Bernatz PE, Woolner LB. Localized mesothelioma of the pleura: Benign and malignant variants. *J Thorac Cardiovasc Surg* 75:363, 1978.
24. Roberts GH. The pathology of parietal pleural plaques. *J Clin Pathol* 24:348, 1971.
25. Roy PH, Carr DT, Payne WS. The problem of chylothorax. *Mayo Clin Proc* 42:457, 1967.
26. Serremetis MG. The management of spontaneous pneumothorax. *Chest* 57:65, 1970.
27. Shields TW, Oilschlager GA. Spontaneous pneumothorax in patients 40 years of age and older. *Ann Thorac Surg* 2:377, 1966.
28. Staats BA, et al. The lipoprotein profile of chylous and nonchylous pleural effusions. *Mayo Clin Proc* 55:700, 1980.
29. Strausser JL, Flye MW. Management of non-traumatic chylothorax. *Ann Thorac Surg* 31:520, 1981.
30. Weil PH, Margolis IB. Systematic approach to traumatic hemothorax. *Am J Surg* 142:692, 1981.
31. Williams KR, Burford TH. The management of chylothorax. *Ann Surg* 160:131, 1964.
32. Wilson JM, et al. Traumatic hemothorax: Is decortication necessary? *J Thorac Cardiovasc Surg* 77:489, 1979.
33. Withers JN, et al. Spontaneous pneumothorax. *Am J Surg* 108:772, 1964.
34. Zwillich CW, et al. Complications of assisted ventilation: A prospective study of 354 consecutive episodes. *Am J Med* 57:161, 1974.

Index